T0200000

THE WASHINGTON MANUAL
OF SURGICAL PATHOLOGY

Third Edition

John D. Pfeifer, MD, PhD
Professor of Pathology and Immunology
Professor of Obstetrics and Gynecology
Department of Pathology and Immunology
Washington University School of Medicine
St. Louis, Missouri

Peter A. Humphrey, MD, PhD
Professor of Pathology
Director, Genitourinary Pathology
Yale School of Medicine
New Haven, Connecticut

Jon H. Ritter, MD
Ladenson Professor of Surgical Pathology
Department of Pathology and Immunology
Washington University School of Medicine
St. Louis, Missouri

Louis P. Dehner, MD
Professor of Pathology and Immunology
Professor of Pathology in Pediatrics
Department of Pathology and Immunology
Washington University School of Medicine
St. Louis, Missouri

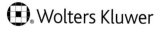

. Wolters Kluwer

Philadelphia · Baltimore · New York · London
Buenos Aires · Hong Kong · Sydney · Tokyo

Acquisitions Editor: Ryan Shaw
Development Editor: Ariel S. Winter
Editorial Coordinator: Tim Rinehart
Marketing Manager: Julie Sikora
Production Project Manager: Linda Van Pelt
Design Coordinator: Stephen Druding
Manufacturing Coordinator: Beth Welsh
Prepress Vendor: Aptara, Inc.

3rd edition

9 8 7 6 5 4 3 2

Printed in China

Library of Congress Cataloging-in-Publication Data

Names: Pfeifer, John D., editor. | Dehner, Louis P., 1940- editor. |
  Humphrey, Peter A., editor.
Title: Washington manual of surgical pathology / John D. Pfeifer, Louis P.
  Dehner, Peter A. Humphrey.
Other titles: Surgical pathology
Description: 3rd edition. | Philadelphia : Wolters Kluwer, [2020] | Includes
  bibliographical references and index.
Identifiers: LCCN 2019002092 | ISBN 9781496367785 (pbk.)
Subjects: | MESH: Pathology, Surgical | Handbook
Classification: LCC RD57 | NLM WO 39 | DDC 617/.07–dc23
LC record available at https://lccn.loc.gov/2019002092

RRS1912

JDP: For Lee, David, and Jennifer, who make it all worthwhile

PAH: For Kay, Tom, and Jennifer

JHR: For Hannah and the kids, and all of the residents and fellows who continue to inspire us to do what we do

LPD: For Becky, Helen, and our six children and grandchildren

Contributors

Brooj Abro, MD
Resident Physician
Department of Pathology and Immunology
Washington University School of Medicine
St. Louis, Missouri

Cory Bernadt, MD, PhD
Assistant Professor
Department of Pathology and Immunology
Washington University School of Medicine
St. Louis, Missouri

Elizabeth M. Brunt, MD
Professor Emeritus of Pathology
Department of Pathology and Immunology
Washington University School of Medicine
St. Louis, Missouri

Dengfeng Cao, MD, PhD
Professor
Department of Pathology and Immunology
Washington University School of Medicine
St. Louis, Missouri

Deyali Chatterjee, MD
Assistant Professor
Department of Pathology and Immunology
Washington University School of Medicine
St. Louis, Missouri

Tiffany Y. Chen, MD
Resident Physician
Department of Pathology and Immunology
Washington University School of Medicine
St. Louis, Missouri

Rebecca D. Chernock, MD
Associate Professor
Department of Pathology and Immunology
Washington University School of Medicine
St. Louis, Missouri

John S.A. Chrisinger, MD
Assistant Professor
Department of Pathology and Immunology
Washington University School of Medicine
St. Louis, Missouri

Leigh Compton, MD, PhD
Assistant Professor of Pathology and
  Immunology
Assistant Professor of Medicine (Dermatology)
Department of Pathology and Immunology
Washington University School of Medicine
St. Louis, Missouri

Sonika M. Dahiya, MBBS, MD
Associate Professor
Department of Pathology and Immunology
Washington University School of Medicine
St. Louis, Missouri

Louis P. Dehner, MD
Professor of Pathology and Immunology
Professor of Pathology in Pediatrics
Department of Pathology and Immunology
Washington University School of Medicine
St. Louis, Missouri

Samir K. El-Mofty, DMD, PhD
Professor Emeritus of Pathology
Department of Pathology and Immunology
Washington University School of Medicine
St. Louis, Missouri

John L. Frater, MD
Associate Professor
Department of Pathology and Immunology
Washington University School of Medicine
St. Louis, Missouri

Joseph Gaut, MD, PhD
Assistant Professor of Pathology and
  Immunology
Assistant Professor of Medicine
Associate Chief, Division of Anatomic and
  Molecular Pathology
Department of Pathology and Immunology
Washington University School of Medicine
St. Louis, Missouri

Brian Goetz, BS
Senior Biorepository Manager
Siteman Cancer Center
Washington University School of Medicine
St. Louis, Missouri

Dikson Dibe Gondim, MD
Head and Neck Pathology Fellow
Department of Pathology and Immunology
Washington University School of Medicine
St. Louis, Missouri

Iván González, MD
Resident Physician
Department of Pathology and Immunology
Washington University School of Medicine
St. Louis, Missouri

Ian S. Hagemann, MD, PhD
Assistant Professor of Pathology and
Immunology
Assistant Professor of Obstetrics and
Gynecology
Department of Pathology and Immunology
Washington University School of Medicine
St. Louis, Missouri

George J. Harocopos, MD
Associate Professor of Ophthalmology and
Visual Sciences
Associate Professor of Pathology and
Immunology
Department of Ophthalmology and Visual
Sciences
Washington University School of Medicine
St. Louis, Missouri

Anjum Hassan, MD
Associate Professor
Department of Pathology and Immunology
Washington University School of Medicine
St. Louis, Missouri

Mai He, MD, PhD
Associate Professor
Department of Pathology and Immunology
Washington University School of Medicine
St. Louis, Missouri

Matthew Hedberg, MD, PhD
Resident Physician
Department of Pathology and Immunology
Washington University School of Medicine
St. Louis, Missouri

Kirk Hill, MD
Resident Physician
Department of Pathology and Immunology
Washington University School of Medicine
St. Louis, Missouri

Peter A. Humphrey, MD, PhD
Professor of Pathology
Director of Genitourinary Pathology
Yale School of Medicine
New Haven, Connecticut

H. Michael Isaacs, BS
Director of Informatics
Department of Pathology and Immunology
Washington University School of Medicine
St. Louis, Missouri

Farhan A. Khan, MD
Surgical Pathology Fellow
Department of Pathology and Immunology
Washington University School of Medicine
St. Louis, Missouri

Friederike Kreisel, MD
Associate Professor
Department of Pathology and Immunology
Washington University School of Medicine
St. Louis, Missouri

Hannah R. Krigman, MD
Associate Professor
Department of Pathology and Immunology
Washington University School of Medicine
St. Louis Missouri

Satoru Kudose, MD
Renal Pathology Fellow
Vagelos College of Physicians and Surgeons
Columbia University
New York City, New York

Yi-Shan Lee, MD, PhD
Assistant Professor
Department of Pathology and Immunology
Washington University School of Medicine
St. Louis, Missouri

Ta-Chiang Liu, MD, PhD
Assistant Professor
Department of Pathology and Immunology
Washington University School of Medicine
St. Louis, Missouri

Horacio M. Maluf, MD
Professor
Department of Pathology and Immunology
Washington University School of Medicine
St. Louis, Missouri

Patrick Mann, MD
Molecular Genetic Pathology Fellow
Department of Pathology and Immunology
Washington University School of Medicine
St. Louis, Missouri

Mena Mansour, MD
Assistant Professor
Department of Pathology and Immunology
Washington University School of Medicine
St. Louis, Missouri

Aidas J. Mattis, MD, PhD
Resident Physician
Department of Pathology and Immunology
Washington University School of Medicine
St. Louis, Missouri

Heidi Miers, BS
Lab Supervisor/QA Manager
Tissue Procurement Core
Siteman Cancer Center
Washington University School of Medicine
St. Louis, Missouri

Julie Neidich, MD
Associate Professor
Department of Pathology and Immunology
Washington University School of Medicine
St. Louis, Missouri

Richard J. Perrin, MD, PhD
Assistant Professor
Department of Pathology and Immunology
Washington University School of Medicine
St. Louis, Missouri

Jessica Petrone, MD
Cytopathology Fellow
Department of Pathology and Immunology
Washington University School of Medicine
St. Louis, Missouri

John D. Pfeifer, MD, PhD
Professor of Pathology and Immunology
Professor of Obstetrics and Gynecology
Vice Chairman For Clinical Affairs
Chief (Interim), Division of Anatomic and
  Molecular Pathology
Department of Pathology and Immunology
Washington University School of Medicine
St. Louis, Missouri

Margareth Pierre-Louis, MD, MBA
Medical Director
Twin Cities Dermatology Center
Minneapolis, Minnesota

Neda Rezaei, MD
Resident Physician
Department of Pathology and Immunology
Washington University School of Medicine
St. Louis, Missouri

Jon H. Ritter, MD
Ladenson Professor of Surgical Pathology
Department of Pathology and Immunology
Washington University School of Medicine
St. Louis, Missouri

Ilana S. Rosman, MD
Assistant Professor of Medicine (Dermatology)
Assistant Professor of Pathology and
  Immunology
Department of Medicine
Washington University School of Medicine
St. Louis, Missouri

Marianna Ruzinova, MD
Assistant Professor
Department of Pathology and Immunology
Washington University School of Medicine
St. Louis, Missouri

Behzad Salari, MD
Resident Physician
Department of Pathology and Immunology
Washington University School of Medicine
St. Louis, Missouri

Souzan Sanati, MD
Assistant Professor
Department of Pathology and Immunology
Washington University School of Medicine
St. Louis, Missouri

Robert E. Schmidt, MD, PhD
Professor
Chief, Division of Neuropathology
Department of Pathology and Immunology
Washington University School of Medicine
St. Louis, Missouri

Jennifer K. Sehn, MD
Assistant Professor
Department of Pathology and Immunology
Washington University School of Medicine
St. Louis, Missouri

Kevin D. Selle, MBA, MT(ASCP), HTL
Program Manager
Department of Surgical Pathology
Barnes-Jewish Hospital
St. Louis, Missouri

Morton E. Smith, MD
Professor Emeritus of Ophthalmology and Visual Sciences
Department of Ophthalmology and Visual Sciences
Washington University School of Medicine
St. Louis, Missouri

Lulu Sun, MD, PhD
Molecular Genetic Pathology Fellow
Department of Pathology and Immunology
Washington University School of Medicine
St. Louis, Missouri

Deborah Veis, MD, PhD
Professor of Medicine
Professor of Pathology and Immunology
Department of Medicine
Washington University School of Medicine
St. Louis, Missouri

Mark A. Watson, MD, PhD
Associate Professor
Department of Pathology and Immunology
Washington University School of Medicine
St. Louis, Missouri

Cody Weimholt, DO
Instructor
Department of Pathology and Immunology
Washington University School of Medicine
St. Louis, Missouri

Frances V. White, MD
Associate Professor
Department of Pathology and Immunology
Washington University School of Medicine
St. Louis, Missouri

Chen Yang, MD
Resident Physician
Department of Pathology and Immunology
Washington University School of Medicine
St. Louis, Missouri

Lily Zhang, MD
Resident Physician
Department of Pathology and Immunology
Washington University School of Medicine
St. Louis, Missouri

Lingxin Zhang, MD
Resident Physician
Department of Pathology and Immunology
Washington University School of Medicine
St. Louis, Missouri

Preface

Welcome to the third edition of *The Washington Manual of Surgical Pathology*. As with the first and second editions, this edition draws on the rich traditions that are the heritage of surgical pathology at Barnes Hospital, now Barnes-Jewish Hospital, which began with Lauren V. Ackerman, MD. When Dr. Ackerman first came to this institution in 1948 as the Director of Surgical Pathology, he was the first trained and board-certified pathologist to occupy a position previously held by surgeons. Dr. Ackerman initiated the paradigm of diagnostic excellence with the central focus on the patient, and advanced the vital role of the surgical pathologist as a consultant to clinicians. He was also keenly aware of the surgical pathologist as an educator and an investigator of diseases from the observational perspective, and of the central role of the pathologist in correlating those findings with the clinical behavior of disease processes. Today the basics remain in place, but the complexity has expanded with the need to incorporate pertinent molecular aspects for therapeutic and prognostic purposes.

Although multivolume textbooks, as well as subspecialty texts, continue to have a central role in education and in everyday clinical practice, this manual is focused on meeting the immediate needs of an ever-accelerating world. Specifically, this manual aims to meet the needs of pathology residents and fellows who never seem to have enough time to "get it all done," pathologists in practice who never seem to be able to sign out cases quickly enough to satisfy their clinical colleagues, and their clinical colleagues themselves who need a ready and available reference in surgical pathology when the pathologist is not immediately available. As with the first and second editions, it is our goal that this latest edition, continuing in the fast-access *Washington Manual* outline format, will fill this niche in our hectic world. A companion website offers the fully searchable text and an online image bank of over 2,800 full-color images (see the inside front cover for website access information).

This edition of *The Washington Manual of Surgical Pathology* includes significant revisions of all chapters, with special emphasis on the ancillary information obtained from specialized methods (e.g., flow cytometry, immunohistochemistry, molecular genetic testing) that is an integral part of surgical pathology diagnosis and vitally important for directing appropriate therapy.

As with the first and second editions, most of the individuals who have contributed to this work are in their surgical pathology training in the Lauren V. Ackerman Laboratory of Surgical Pathology at Barnes-Jewish Hospital, or are members of the faculty in the Department of Pathology and Immunology. As is the tradition of all *Washington Manual* series, residents and fellows have contributed to many of the chapters.

Finally, we dedicate this edition of the *Washington Manual of Surgical Pathology* to Dr. John Kissane, a member of the faculty for over 50 years, and a model physician, colleague, mentor, and friend. He is especially missed by one of us (LPD), who came to know him as a second-year medical student in 1963, and for whom he and Dr. Ackerman had a determinative influence on the professional direction of my life. Although another one of us (JDP) did not come to know him until 1988, Dr. Kissane likewise had a profound influence on the direction of my career.

John D. Pfeifer, MD, PhD
Peter A. Humphrey, MD, PhD
Jon H. Ritter, MD
Louis P. Dehner, MD

Acknowledgments

The third edition of *The Washington Manual of Surgical Pathology* would not have been possible without the participation of our colleagues who so willingly and generously provided their time and expertise to the project. All authors are, or were, faculty or house staff in the Department of Pathology at the Washington University School of Medicine, which emphasizes that academic surgical pathology at Washington University has always been a collaborative venture between faculty and trainees.

We extend special thanks to our administrative assistants, Elease Barnes and Linda Hankins, who handled most of the logistical and secretarial work required to make the third edition a reality. We also acknowledge Jared Amann-Stewart, who expertly edited all the electronic figures found at the associated website. We are lucky to continue to have had the opportunity to work with the wonderful people at Lippincott Williams & Wilkins/Wolters Kluwer including Jonathan W. Pine, Jr., Senior Executive Editor and Ryan Shaw, Senior Acquisitions Editor, both of whom enthusiastically suggested that we produce a third edition of the manual. And especially Tim Rinehart, Editorial Coordinator, who provided the necessary structure and deadlines, but always with patience and good humor.

And we thank our families. Their love and support have again made the book possible.

John D. Pfeifer
Peter A. Humphrey
Jon H. Ritter
Louis P. Dehner

Contents

Head and Neck

<table>
<tr><td>1</td><td>

Oral Cavity and Oropharynx

Rebecca D. Chernock and Dikson Dibe Gondim
</td></tr>
</table>

I. NORMAL ANATOMY

A. Oral Cavity. The anterior aspect of the oral cavity extends from the mucocutaneous junction (vermillion border) of the lips to include the buccal mucosa (inside of cheek), maxillary and mandibular arches (teeth), retromolar trigone, anterior two-thirds of the tongue (oral tongue), floor of mouth, and hard palate. Posteriorly, the oral cavity freely communicates with the oropharynx; the border between the two is marked by the junction of the hard and soft palates superiorly and the line of circumvallate papillae on the dorsal tongue (junction between the anterior two-thirds and posterior one-third of the tongue) inferiorly.

The oral tongue is freely mobile and composed mainly of skeletal muscle. It has a dorsal (exposed) surface, ventral surface, and tip. The dorsal surface contains numerous papillae that have specialized taste receptors. The floor of the mouth lies beneath the tongue and is divided into sides by the midline frenulum (mucosal fold) of the tongue. It contains ostia of the submandibular and sublingual salivary glands, whereas the main duct of the parotid gland (Stensen duct) enters the oral cavity through the buccal mucosa. The hard palate forms the roof of the oral cavity and consists of portions of the maxillary and palatine bones.

The oral cavity is lined by stratified squamous mucosa with prominent mucoserous glands in the submucosa. Most of the mucosa is nonkeratinizing with the exception of the hard palate, gingiva, and dorsal tongue, which become keratinized due to the friction of mastication.

B. Oropharynx. The oropharynx is the space posterior to the oral cavity that communicates with the nasopharynx superiorly and the larynx and hypopharynx inferiorly. The soft palate marks the superior aspect of the oropharynx and is suspended from the posterior aspect of the hard palate. In contrast to the hard palate, the soft palate is fibromuscular without a bony skeleton. Whereas the oral aspect is covered with nonkeratinizing stratified squamous epithelium, the nasal surface is covered by pseudostratified ciliated columnar (respiratory-type) epithelium. Numerous mucoserous glands lie in its submucosa. The uvula extends down from the posterior aspect of the soft palate and has an identical histology. The posterior one-third of the tongue (base of tongue) is rich in lymphoid tissue (known as the lingual tonsil); the palatine and lingual tonsils, together with the pharyngeal tonsil in the nasopharynx, are collectively known as Waldeyer ring.

II. GROSS EXAMINATION, TISSUE SAMPLING, AND HISTOLOGIC SLIDE PREPARATION

A. Open and Endoscopic Biopsies.
The majority of specimens from the oral cavity and oropharynx consist of open biopsies of lesions that can be visualized by the naked eye. The small biopsy pieces should be placed immediately into 10% buffered formalin or other appropriate fixative. Processing of the biopsies should include gross description of the tissue fragments with documentation of the number of pieces; the biopsies should be entirely submitted, with three levels cut from each paraffin block for hematoxylin and eosin (H&E) examination.

B. Resections

1. Open procedure specimens are widely variable depending on the location of the tumor. Because many lesions encroach on or invade the bone of the mandible or maxilla, composite resections with bone and soft tissue are common. As a generalization, all specimens need to be oriented appropriately, the soft tissue margins inked, and the mucosal and soft tissue margins evaluated followed by sectioning of the tumor relative to bone and soft tissue margins. Margins should be evaluated by either shave or radial sections, depending on the nature of the specimen. If the tumor is relatively distant from a margin, 1- to 2-mm shave sections are preferred. If the tumor is close to a margin, radial sections should be taken.

2. Partial resections with a CO_2 laser under an operating microscope are becoming more common. Because the inherent approach of this procedure is to excise the tumor piece by piece, the surgeon inks the individual pieces as s/he alone knows what constitutes the true margin. In the gross room all that is therefore required is to measure the pieces provided, describe them, and submit them entirely sectioned perpendicular to the ink.

C. Frozen Sections
are a critical element of surgical therapy for tumors of the head and neck region. Although practices vary, at most institutions shave margins are taken by the surgeon from the periphery of the surgical defect after the tumor has been removed, and separately submitted. In other cases, the surgeon may sample the tumor or suspicious sites to confirm and/or map the lesion, with additional samples from areas where the tumor is felt to be closest to the surgical margin.

For frozen sections, the tissue is submitted in saline to the pathology lab and then frozen in its entirety. The tissue pieces should be evaluated grossly for mucosa (typically the shiny and pink-tan surface of the tissue) and, if mucosa is present, the specimen should be oriented in the frozen section block to demonstrate this surface on edge. If the surgeon has inked the true margin, the tissue should be submitted radial to the ink as well. It is critical to cut deeply into the block to obtain sections that represent the entire tissue submitted so that small foci of tumor are not missed by inadequate sampling; cutting three rather than two H&E frozen section slides reduces sampling errors.

In some instances, the surgeon may send an oriented mucosal ellipse with intact margins for frozen section evaluation. In these cases, the margins should first be inked to maintain orientation. Close margins should be submitted radially and remote margins can be shaved.

The tissue that remains after frozen section is submitted for evaluation by permanent sections, which helps assure adequate sampling. Permanent sections can help resolve a number of issues from the frozen sections themselves including freezing and cautery artifact, volume of tumor, and orientation (note that the margins of the main resection specimen should also be evaluated throughout their entirety because separate frozen section specimens almost never cover the entire margins of a resection specimen).

III. DIAGNOSTIC FEATURES OF COMMON BENIGN DISEASES

A. Inflammation.
Lichen planus, pemphigus vulgaris, and cicatricial pemphigoid are autoimmune disorders that predominately affect middle-aged adults and occur more frequently in women than men. They are diseases that affect mucosal sites as well as skin, so the oral cavity is sometimes involved as well.

1. Lichen planus. This disorder commonly affects the oral mucosa. Whereas skin involvement is usually self-limited, oral lichen planus follows a more protracted waxing and waning course. The oral lesions are multifocal and typically asymptomatic unless ulceration occurs.

Any oral mucosal surface can be involved, and several patterns can be seen. The classic pattern is reticular with intersecting white keratotic streaks (Wickham striae); the lesions are ill-defined and the background may be erythematous due to mucosal atrophy. Some lesions may be mostly erythematous with minimal keratotic streaks, whereas others may show extensive keratinization and/or ulceration or form bullae. Microscopically, a dense submucosal band of lymphocytes is present, which may be less distinct in ulcerated lesions (e-Fig. 1.1). The rete ridges may be hyperplastic (saw-toothed) or flattened. There is loosening of the basal layer of the epithelium, with degeneration of individual keratinocytes that may form eosinophilic colloid (cytoid or Civatte) bodies (e-Fig. 1.2). The surface may show hyper- or parakeratosis. Although the histologic findings of lichen planus have been well defined, they are nonetheless not specific; for example, some oral lesions with a similar histologic picture may be due to a contact hypersensitivity reaction. In addition, a lichenoid infiltrate may accompany dysplastic lesions.

Asymptomatic patients require no treatment, but steroids (particularly topical) are often used for erosive or erythematous lesions. Some data suggest that there is an increased risk of malignant transformation in the erythematous, ulcerative, and bullous forms of oral lichen planus. Although this proposed risk of malignancy is controversial, these lesions at least require closer clinical follow-up.

2. Pemphigus vulgaris. This is an uncommon disorder that causes superficial ulceration of the skin and mucous membranes. Involvement of the oral mucosa may precede the development of skin lesions. The disease is caused by auto-antibodies to desmogleins 1 and 3 (cellular transmembrane proteins involved in the assembly of desmosomes). Cell-to-cell adhesion is impaired in the suprabasal epithelium, leading to clefting and ulceration. Flaccid bullae that easily rupture to form painful erosions can be seen on any oral mucosal surface. The lesions heal without scarring. Microscopically, intraepithelial separation with edema and acantholysis, which imparts a "tombstone" appearance to the remaining attached basal cell layer (e-Fig. 1.3), is seen at the edge of the ulcer. Acute and chronic inflammation are frequently present in the submucosa. Direct immunofluorescence is positive for immunoglobulin G (IgG) along cell membranes throughout the epidermis.

Paraneoplastic pemphigus, which is associated with an underlying malignancy, may be distinguished from pemphigus vulgaris by the identification of a different pattern of antibody staining by direct immunofluorescence.

3. Cicatricial or mucous membrane pemphigoid. This is a rare disease caused by various antibodies that target the basement membrane of mucous membranes and occasionally the skin. The oral mucosa is almost always involved, most commonly the gingiva. In contrast to pemphigus vulgaris, the variably sized bullae are not flaccid, and ruptured bullae heal with scarring. Microscopically, there is clefting between the epithelium and basement membrane, and the space may be filled with serous fluid containing sparse inflammatory cells. Direct immunofluorescence shows a linear band of IgG and C3 on the basement membrane. Treatment is with immunosuppression, but the disease is often progressive despite therapy.

B. Infections. Only a few of the most common of the numerous infections that may involve the oral cavity are discussed here.

1. Fungal. *Candida* species cause most of the fungal infections of the oral cavity. Other fungal infections that occur less frequently in the oral cavity include histoplasmosis, blastomycosis, and coccidioidomycosis. *Candida* species are a part of the normal oral flora; candidiasis occurs due to overgrowth, usually in the setting of a predisposing factor, and *Candida albicans* is the most frequently isolated species. Local and systemic factors that favor overgrowth include immunosuppression, use of steroids or antibiotics, radiation therapy, xerostomia, use of dentures, and anemia. The extremes of ages are more often affected as well, and infection may be acute or chronic.

Symptoms include a burning sensation or foul odor, although the infection may be asymptomatic.

Several clinical patterns of oral candidiasis are seen. White plaques that are easily scraped off underlying erythematous mucosa are called pseudomembranous candidiasis (oral thrush); this is the most common type of oral candidiasis. Erythematous candidiasis appears as a red patch due to atrophy of the mucosa. Median rhomboid glossitis is a type of erythematous candidiasis that occurs in a specific location, namely a rhomboid-shaped area on the midline dorsal tongue, which over time may develop a nodular appearance. Angular cheilitis causes red fissuring and scaling at the labial commissures; predisposing factors include drooling and ill-fitting dentures. Chronic hyperplastic candidiasis presents as asymptomatic white patches (due to the thickened hyperplastic mucosa) that cannot be removed by scraping. This pattern is more common in immunocompetent individuals and may predispose to the development of carcinoma, although a causal relationship between the two has not been clearly demonstrated.

Microscopically, an intraepithelial infiltrate of neutrophils is seen in all types of candidal infection. The epithelium may be ulcerated, although in chronic hyperplastic candidiasis it is thickened and hyperkeratotic (e-**Fig. 1.4**). Fungal pseudohyphae may be difficult to identify on routine H&E-stained slides. However, methenamine silver or periodic acid–Schiff (PAS) stains will highlight the fungal elements within the keratin and in the superficial squamous epithelium (e-**Fig. 1.4, inset A**).

2. Viral. Oral viral infections are highly prevalent, although frequently asymptomatic.

    a. Human papillomavirus (HPV) does not cause specific clinically symptomatic infection but is associated with several benign and malignant neoplasms in the oral cavity and oropharynx including squamous papillomas and squamous cell carcinoma (SCC) (see below).

    b. Herpes simplex virus (HSV) causes a common oral viral infection with seroprevalence rates of up to 80% of the population. There are two common serotypes (HSV-1 and HSV-2), and HSV-1 is primarily associated with oral lesions. Gingivostomatitis occurs in 10% of initial infections, predominately in children, and is characterized by fever and a vesicular rash. The virus then latently infects sensory ganglia and may be reactivated periodically throughout life. Recurrent disease is manifested by clusters of vesicles that may cause a burning sensation at the mucocutaneous junction of the lip or nose. Intraoral lesions can also occur.

    Microscopically, the lesional mucosa is often ulcerated and acantholytic, with marked acute and chronic inflammation. There are typically individual necrotic squamous cells. Identification of the classic intranuclear eosinophilic inclusions within squamous epithelial cells is diagnostic of herpes virus infection; the inclusion-harboring cells are often single, detached, and multinucleated (e-**Fig. 1.5**). Immunohistochemical stains may be useful to confirm the diagnosis.

    c. Epstein–Barr virus (EBV). Acute EBV infection, although frequently asymptomatic, may cause pharyngitis and tonsillitis. The virus enters the host through oral epithelial cells, where it then gains access to and infects B lymphocytes. Acute EBV infection may produce reactive changes in the tonsils and lymph nodes that can mimic a hematopoietic malignancy.

    Latent EBV infection is virtually universal in adults and is usually asymptomatic. However, an EBV-driven proliferation of tongue epithelial cells, known as **oral hairy leukoplakia,** occurs in immunosuppressed patients, approximately 80% of whom are HIV positive. The lesions are asymptomatic unless superinfection with Candida occurs. Grossly, hairy leukoplakia appears as a flat, white, shaggy plaque on the lateral tongue. Microscopically, the epithelium is acanthotic with hyper- and parakeratosis. Perinuclear clearing forming "balloon cells" is characteristic (e-**Fig. 1.6**), and viral replication may cause "nuclear beading" (e-**Fig. 1.7**). Inflammation is typically sparse. Definitive diagnosis relies on detection of EBV within the lesion by in situ hybridization (e-**Fig. 1.8**). Oral hairy leukoplakia is self-limited with no propensity for malignant transformation.

Latent EBV infection has been implicated in the development of a variety of hematopoietic and nonhematopoietic malignancies as well as (see Chapters 3 and 41).

3. Bacterial. Cervicofacial actinomycosis ("lumpy jaw"). *Actinomyces* are gram-positive, saprophytic anaerobes that are part of the normal oral flora. The organisms are often incidentally found in sections of the tonsillar crypts. Occasionally, they are introduced into the soft tissues through trauma, particularly from dental manipulations, where an acute or chronic infection may ensue. *Actinomyces israelii* is the most common pathogenic species.

Acute infections are suppurative, creating a nontender fluctuant mass. In the chronic phase, infections may form a more extensive firm fibrous mass mimicking a neoplasm. Sinus tracts may exit either the skin or mucosa (e-**Fig. 1.9**) and often discharge yellow clusters of tightly adherent *Actinomyces* bacteria that have the appearance of sulfur granules. Osteomyelitis may develop in adjacent bone. Microscopically, collections of radiating, filamentous organisms are seen in a background of neutrophils with surrounding granulation tissue and/or fibrosis. Cultures are often negative due to overgrowth of other organisms. Prolonged treatment with antibiotics is usually successful, although incision and drainage may be necessary.

C. Other Nonneoplastic Lesions

1. Fibrous lesions. A number of different types of fibrous lesions occur in and around the oral cavity.

a. Irritation fibroma. These are the most common oral mucosal mass lesions. They are painless reactive proliferations of fibrous tissue that develop in response to trauma from teeth or dentures. The lateral tongue and buccal mucosa along the bite line are the most common sites. Multiple fibromas may be seen in inherited syndromes including Cowden syndrome and tuberous sclerosis. Linear, grooved fibromas occurring in the mucosa opposing the teeth or sulcus of the alveolar ridge are called epulis fissuratum and are denture-related.

Grossly, irritation fibroma is usually pink to white, dome-shaped, and only a few millimeters in maximal diameter. Microscopically, there is a nodular deposition of dense collagen with associated chronic inflammation and overlying thinned mucosa (e-**Fig. 1.10**). Trauma-related changes such as hyperkeratosis and ulceration may be seen. The fibroblasts are spindled and indistinct; if larger, stellate fibroblasts are present, the lesion is called a **giant cell fibroma,** which in contrast to irritation fibromas, is not associated with trauma and occurs at a younger age (e-**Fig. 1.11**). Whereas typical irritation fibromas do not recur after simple resection, giant cell fibromas may recur.

b. Gingival fibromatosis. This is generalized, but not necessarily symmetrical, enlargement of the gingiva which may be hereditary, drug-induced, related to poor oral hygiene, or idiopathic. When it is drug-induced, it is called fibrous gingival hyperplasia and frequently regresses with cessation of the inciting drug.

Grossly, the gums are enlarged, smooth-surfaced, and firm. Microscopically, the submucosa shows dense eosinophilic to slightly basophilic fibrous tissue with associated mild chronic inflammation (e-**Fig. 1.12**). The surface squamous epithelium may have chronic inflammation or extreme elongation of the rete, but is otherwise unremarkable.

2. Inflammatory papillary hyperplasia is a denture-associated lesion and is typically located beneath a denture base in the hard palate and alveolar ridges. It is occasionally seen in patients without dentures and may be associated with poor oral hygiene.

Clinically, the mucosa looks "pebbly" with numerous small, papular projections. Microscopically, the mucosa may be atrophic or demonstrate pseudoepitheliomatous hyperplasia. The underlying submucosa may vary from edematous to fibrotic, with mild chronic inflammation. Individual nodules may resemble an irritation fibroma or pyogenic granuloma. The condition is not premalignant, may subside with less denture wear, or may require surgical excision.

3. **Torus palatinus, torus mandibularis, and buccal exostosis** are common developmental anomalies that continue to grow throughout life and typically present in
adulthood. They are site-specific. Torus palatinus occurs in the midline of the hard
palate, torus mandibularis occurs on the lingual surface of the mandible near the
bicuspid teeth, and buccal exostosis is found on the facial surface of the alveolar bone.
Any identical appearing bony proliferations at other oral sites are generically termed
"bony exostosis" or "osteoma" and are not developmental, but rather trauma-related
or true neoplasms that can be associated with Gardner syndrome.

Grossly, these lesions are broad-based, single, or lobulated masses with smooth
surfaces (e-**Fig. 1.13**). Microscopically, they are composed of dense lamellar bone
with scattered osteocytes and variable amounts of marrow. Ischemic changes with
marrow fibrosis and loss of osteocytes from lacunae may be seen. Resection is not
necessary except for cosmetic reasons or if the lesions become large. There is little risk
of recurrence, and the lesions have no malignant potential.

4. **Fordyce granules.** Sebaceous glands are normally found in the skin associated
with hair follicles. When they are ectopically present in the oral mucosa they are
called Fordyce granules. They are common (present in up to 80% of adults) and
can occur on any oral mucosal surface, although the buccal mucosa is most common. Most appear as scattered, 1 to 3 mm in diameter, white to yellow papules.
Microscopically, normal sebaceous glands are present in the submucosa without
associated hair follicles; occasionally, Fordyce granules coalesce to form the larger
cauliflower-like lesion termed sebaceous hyperplasia. No treatment is necessary
unless for cosmetic reasons (biopsies are rarely performed as the diagnosis is usually clinically apparent).

5. **Cysts.** Included here are several of the more common soft tissue true cysts that have
an epithelial lining. Odontogenic cysts, bone cysts, and salivary gland–derived cysts,
including pseudocysts (lacking a true epithelial lining) are discussed in Chapter 4.

   a. **Epidermoid cyst.** Intraoral epidermoid cysts are much less common than their
   counterparts in the skin and are thought to represent inclusions of surface epithelium or cystic change in odontogenic rests. They often present in teenagers
   and young adults. The most common site is the gingiva. Clinically, they are small
   (<1 cm) superficial nodules. When they occur in the midline floor of mouth,
   however, they can become much larger (>5 cm) and interfere with swallowing.
   Microscopically, they are lined by thin stratified squamous epithelium, with or
   without a granular cell layer, and are often filled with keratinous debris. Rupture
   with spillage of keratinous debris may elicit a granulomatous inflammatory reaction. Treatment is by simple surgical excision.

   b. **Dermoid cysts.** These are similar to epidermoid cysts but contain adnexal structures, such as sebaceous glands or hair follicles, in the cyst wall. If other tissue
   types are present, the lesion is termed a teratoid cyst.

   c. **Nasolabial cysts.** These rare cysts occur at the base of the nostril or at the superior aspect of the upper lip. They are thought to be derived from remnants of the
   embryonic nasolacrimal duct. Seventy-five percent of cases occur in women. More
   than 10% are bilateral. They present as slow growing masses, usually <1.5 cm, and
   they may have irregular contours. Soft tissue swelling with loss of the nasolabial
   fold or elevation of the nasal ala or floor may occasionally cause nasal obstruction.
   Pressure erosion of underlying bone is possible.

   Microscopically, the cysts may be lined by respiratory type, cuboidal, and/
   or stratified squamous epithelium with scattered mucus-filled goblet cells, with
   surrounding chronic inflammation. A fibrous or epithelial connection to the nasal
   mucosa is almost always present. Simple surgical excision is curative.

   d. **Lymphoepithelial cyst.** These cysts are thought to develop from invaginations
   of crypt epithelium within accessory tonsillar tissue. Clinically, they are painless
   submucosal nodules that are almost always <6 mm in diameter and typically occur
   in teenagers or young adults. Half of cases occur in the floor of the mouth; the

lateral and ventral tongue, as well as the soft palate, are also common sites. They do not occur in the alveolar soft tissue.

Microscopically, the cyst lining is an attenuated squamous epithelium with a poorly formed granular layer. The cyst is filled with orthokeratin and surrounded tightly by lymphoid aggregates with variable numbers of germinal centers. The cysts may become dissociated from the epithelium or remain connected, often with keratin plugging. Microscopically, the prominent lymphoid aggregates distinguish this cyst from an epidermoid cyst. Similar appearing cysts can be seen within the tonsils themselves from blockage of the crypt connection with the surface.

6. Pseudoepitheliomatous hyperplasia is a generic term for benign, downward proliferation of the epithelium that is important to distinguish from invasive well-differentiated SCC. Pseudoepitheliomatous hyperplasia is characteristically seen in association with specific lesions including inflammatory papillary hyperplasia, submucosal granular cell tumors, and fungal infections. It can also be seen adjacent to ulcers or in association with myriad other lesions. Microscopically, irregular and pseudoinfiltrative nests of keratinizing squamous epithelium are sometimes seen beneath a thickened surface epithelium; the papillae of the squamous epithelium may be markedly elongated and extend deeply into the submucosa (**e-Fig. 1.14**). However, in contrast to squamous dysplasia and carcinoma, cytologic atypia is absent.

7. Amalgam tattoo. Amalgam is a material used for dental fillings that is composed of a combination of metals. It can be inadvertently implanted into oral mucosa during a dental procedure, creating a tattoo that may be mistaken clinically for melanoma. The lesions present as painless, blue-gray pigmented macules that are variable in size and location. Microscopically, pigmented particles are seen scattered in the submucosa around vessels and along reticulin fibers (**e-Figs. 1.15** and **1.16**). There is typically no tissue reaction.

IV. NEOPLASTIC LESIONS. The 2017 World Health Organization (WHO) classification of tumors of the oral cavity and oropharynx is listed in Tables 1.1 and 1.2, respectively.

TABLE 1.1	**WHO Histologic Classification of Tumors of the Oral Cavity and Mobile Tongue**
Malignant surface epithelial tumors	**Soft tissue and neural tumors**
Squamous cell carcinoma	Granular cell tumor
Oral potentially malignant disorders and oral epithelial dysplasia	Rhabdomyoma
	Lymphangioma
Oral potentially malignant disorders	Hemangioma
Oral epithelial dysplasia	Schwannoma and neurofibroma
Proliferative verrucous leukoplakia	Kaposi sarcoma
Papillomas	Myofibroblastic sarcoma
Squamous cell papilloma	**Oral mucosal melanoma**
Condyloma acuminatum	**Salivary type tumors**
Verruca vulgaris	Mucoepidermoid carcinoma
Multifocal epithelial hyperplasia	Pleomorphic adenoma
Tumors of uncertain histogenesis	**Hematolymphoid tumors**
Congenital granular cell epulis	CD30-positive T-cell lymphoproliferative disorder
Ectomesenchymal chondromyxoid tumor	Plasmablastic lymphoma
	Langerhans cell histiocytosis
	Extramedullary myeloid sarcoma

From El-Naggar AK, Chan JKC, Grandis JR, Takata T, Slootweg PJ, eds. *WHO Classification of Head and Neck Tumours.* Lyon, France: IARC Press; 2017. Used with permission.

| **TABLE 1.2** | **WHO Histologic Classification of Tumors of the Oropharynx** |

Squamous cell carcinoma	**Hematolymphoid tumors**
Squamous cell carcinoma, HPV-positive	Hodgkin lymphoma
Squamous cell carcinoma, HPV-negative	Burkitt lymphoma
Salivary gland tumors	Follicular lymphoma
Pleomorphic adenoma	Mantle cell lymphoma
Adenoid cystic carcinoma	T-lymphoblastic leukemia/lymphoma
Polymorphous adenocarcinoma	Follicular dendritic cell sarcoma

From El-Naggar AK, Chan JKC, Grandis JR, Takata T, Slootweg PJ, eds. *WHO Classification of Head and Neck Tumours.* Lyon, France: IARC Press; 2017. Used with permission.

A. Epithelial
1. Benign
  a. **Squamous papilloma.** Squamous papillomas are benign squamous proliferations caused by HPV. They are most common in the larynx but also occur as solitary lesions in the oral cavity and oropharynx.

   Squamous papillomas are strongly associated with the nononcogenic HPV types 6 and 11, but have a very low infectivity so do not appear contagious. In the oral cavity and oropharynx, they occur in adults between 30 and 50 years of age, most commonly on the hard and soft palate and uvula.

   Squamous papillomas have a characteristic morphology. Grossly, they are soft, exophytic, granular, and pink-red or tan. Microscopically, they consist of arborizing, papillary fronds of thickened but maturing squamous epithelium with nuclei that are slightly enlarged and irregular but not overtly dysplastic. Mitotic activity is usually present but is modest. Sometimes there is slight hyperplasia of the basal layer. Cells in the mid-layer often have cytoplasmic clearing but frank koilocytosis is not regularly observed. Although typically absent, surface keratinization may be seen (**e-Fig. 1.17**).

   Squamous papillomas are cured by simple excision. They have limited growth potential, rarely recur, and have essentially no risk of malignant transformation.
  b. **Condyloma acuminatum and verruca vulgaris.** Both of these lesions, although much more common on the skin, can also occur in the oral cavity. Condylomas are considered a sexually transmitted disease and usually occur in young adults on the lips and soft palate as clusters of pink nodules that coalesce into more exophytic masses. They have more blunted, papillary fronds and more hyperkeratosis than squamous papillomas.

   Verrucae also can occur intraorally, particularly in children, commonly on the lips and anterior tongue. They have a morphology identical to that of verruca of the skin with a broad base, marked papillomatosis, and hyperkeratosis with parakeratosis.
  c. **Verruciform xanthoma.** This is a peculiar lesion of the oral cavity which has no relation to HPV and may be reactive in nature. It occurs in middle-aged to older adults and is most common on the alveolar ridges. Clinically it is a well-demarcated, painless, and soft, slightly elevated mass. It may have a yellow or white color with a roughened surface. Microscopically, it consists of broad papillae with intervening cleft-like spaces covered by a slightly thickened, nondysplastic squamous epithelium with hyperkeratosis and parakeratosis. The diagnostic cells, which lie in the superficial submucosa, are foamy macrophages with abundant pale, flocculent cytoplasm and round to oval, bland nuclei (**e-Fig. 1.18**); these cells are filled with lipid and should be distinguished from the eosinophilic granular cells of granular cell tumor (see below).

Verruciform xanthoma is treated by conservative excision and has no risk of malignant transformation. Recurrences are rare.

2. **Precursor (premalignant) squamous lesions.** Precursor lesions are defined as altered squamous epithelium with an increased risk of progression to SCC, and are strongly associated with smoking and alcohol use. They may present as leukoplakia (white, thickened epithelium; see **e-Fig. 1.19**), erythroplakia (thin, erythematous, and red epithelium), or speckled erythroplakia (a mixture of both erythroplakia and leukoplakia).

The terms dysplasia or intraepithelial neoplasia should be used for these lesions. The likelihood of malignant change relates to the severity of dysplasia, although carcinoma can develop from any grade of dysplasia (as well as from normal epithelium). Atypia, on the other hand, is not considered synonymous with dysplasia and is used in a more general sense because the term may also describe changes seen in reactive epithelium. There are a number of changes that occur in dysplasia including nuclear abnormalities, architectural/organizational abnormalities, and abnormal keratinization. Unfortunately, there is poor agreement among pathologists about the minimum histopathologic changes that constitute dysplasia, and about the grading of dysplasia. Oral dysplasia is generally classified as mild, moderate, or severe. Some experts advocate a binary system (low-grade dysplasia versus high-grade dysplasia) but clinical validation of the binary scheme is still needed.

3. **Malignant.** SCC is overwhelmingly the most common malignant tumor of the oral cavity and oropharynx. SCC has a high male to female ratio (3:1) and a strong relationship to tobacco smoking and alcohol consumption, with a multiplicative rather than additive relative risk. Although not as extreme, the risk of SCC is also increased with the use of snuff and chewing tobacco. Betel quid, commonly used in some parts of the world, is another major risk factor. Finally, HPV, particularly type 16, has a major causative role in oropharyngeal SCC, leading to carcinomas that have less aggressive behavior and usually, but not always, show a distinct nonkeratinizing morphology. Since HPV status is prognostic and may alter treatment strategies, HPV testing should be performed on all oropharyngeal SCCs. p16 immunohistochemistry as a surrogate marker for HPV-positivity is the preferred initial test (see below; see also the College of American Pathologists Guidelines for HPV testing in head and neck carcinomas available at: http://www.cap.org/ShowProperty?nodePath =/UCMCon/Contribution%20Folders/WebContent/pdf/hpv-testing-in-head-and-neck-carcinomas-summary.pdf). HPV-positive tumors are not graded, as they often have a poorly differentiated nonkeratinizing or basaloid appearance that does not reflect the favorable biologic behavior of HPV-positive SCC.

a. **Conventional or keratinizing SCC.** The gross appearance of keratinizing-type SCC is quite variable, ranging from fungating, exophytic tumors to endophytic, ulcerated tumors with raised edges. Most tumors elicit stromal fibrosis and thus have firm and tan-white cut surfaces. Microscopically, these tumors consist of nests and sheets of cells with squamous differentiation. The cells are typically polygonal in shape and have distinct cell borders, eosinophilic cytoplasm, and round to oval nuclei, often with prominent nucleoli. Well-differentiated tumors retain abundant pink or clear cytoplasm, often show intercellular-bridges representing desmosomes, and sometimes show keratin "pearl" formation (**e-Fig. 1.20**). Moderately differentiated tumors (the majority of cases) have cells with more pleomorphism and a higher nucleus to cytoplasm ratio while still retaining a moderate amount of eosinophilic cytoplasm (**e-Fig. 1.21**). Poorly differentiated tumors often have single cells or small nests of cells with more mitotic activity and less cytoplasm (**e-Fig. 1.22**). Grading should be performed, unless the tumor is HPV-positive and oropharyngeal, but has not been shown to predict clinical behavior. Perineural, lymphatic, and vascular space invasion are commonly seen.

Treatment for oral cavity and oropharyngeal SCC typically consists of surgery followed by postoperative radiotherapy, the latter depending somewhat on the stage of disease. Small primary lesions without neck lymph node metastases, or with a small lymph node metastasis without extracapsular extension, may be treated by surgery alone. Radiotherapy, sometimes with chemotherapy and/or epidermal growth factor receptor (EGFR)-targeted drugs, is sometimes used, particularly for large tumors that are not surgically resectable. The overall survival for conventional keratinizing SCC of the oral cavity is approximately 50% to 55% at 5 years but varies greatly by tumor stage. A minority of oropharyngeal keratinizing SCCs (about 20%) are HPV-positive and these tumors have the more favorable prognosis of HPV-related SCC. HPV is rare in oral cavity SCC.

b. **Nonkeratinizing (HPV-positive) SCC.** Nonkeratinizing SCC is almost exclusively seen in the palatine tonsils and base of tongue, and is virtually always p16-positive and HPV-associated (HPV16 can be demonstrated in more than 90% of cases). Patients with nonkeratinizing SCC are, on average, 5 years younger than those with conventional SCC. A significant minority are nonsmoker, and those that do smoke are less likely to be heavy smokers. Nonkeratinizing SCC arises in the invaginated crypts of the tonsillar tissue (palatine tonsils and base of tongue or lingual tonsil), so the tumors tend to be subsurface and thus clinically subtle. This feature, combined with the tumor's strong propensity for early metastasis to cervical lymph nodes, explains why the most common presentation is as a painless neck mass often without a clinically obvious primary tumor. For this reason, HPV testing of unknown primary SCC in the neck (specifically upper and mid jugular lymph nodes) is recommended, as a positive result strongly favors tonsillar or base of tongue origin.

Grossly, nonkeratinizing SCC is endophytic, firm, and tan in most cases. However, because the tumors are often small and do not elicit much desmoplasia in the surrounding stroma, they can be quite difficult to identify grossly. Microscopically, they consist of ribbons of tumor cells lining the crypt epithelium and of nests and sheets of cells with smooth borders in the submucosa. The overlying surface epithelium is typically intact without dysplasia (e-**Fig. 1.23**). The cells are basal in appearance, with round to oval to spindled nuclei, relatively homogeneous chromatin without nucleoli, minimal cytoplasm, and very brisk mitotic activity with abundant apoptosis (e-**Fig. 1.24**). Central (comedo) necrosis is common in the tumor cell nests.

In situ hybridization and/or polymerase chain reaction (PCR) are positive for HPV16 or other high-risk HPV types in almost all cases; more recently, assays specific for high-risk HPV RNA transcripts have been applied. Immunohistochemistry is positive for p16 (a tumor suppressor protein that is aberrantly overexpressed in cells infected by HPV) (e-**Fig. 1.25**). Strong and diffuse p16 immunoreactivity has become increasingly recognized as a clinically useful surrogate marker for HPV-driven SCCs of the oropharynx and is the preferred initial HPV testing method.

Treatment is most often by surgical resection with neck dissection followed by postoperative radiation therapy. Numerous studies have shown that the prognosis for HPV-positive SCC of the oropharynx, which is usually nonkeratinizing, is better than for HPV-negative SCC, despite the fact that tumors commonly present with lymph node metastases. Therefore, as mentioned above, HPV testing is indicated for all oropharyngeal SCCs.

c. **Verrucous carcinoma** (VC) is a specific, well-differentiated and nonmetastasizing variant of SCC. It occurs in the larynx and oral cavity and grossly appears as a well-circumscribed, warty and exophytic, broad-based, white or tan mass (e-**Fig. 1.26**). It can become very large and dramatically invade soft tissues and bone. Microscopically, VC consists of very thick surface squamous epithelium with club-shaped papillae that have a broad pushing base. There is usually prominent surface hyperkeratosis, and the sheets of tumor are composed of bland cells with abundant eosinophilic or clear cytoplasm, sometimes described as glassy in appearance. There is no cytologic atypia. The stroma directly beneath the tumor typically demonstrates prominent chronic inflammation, often with abundant plasma cells (e-**Fig. 1.27**).

Pure VC is a tumor type in which the cells have not invaded through the basement membrane, and as such has an excellent prognosis. Although the tumor can be large and locally destructive, complete surgical resection is often curative. Radiation is also an acceptable treatment, particularly in poor surgical candidates. Conventional invasive SCC sometimes arises from VC; when this occurs, the prognosis and behavior is the same as for conventional SCC. Thus, the lesion must be thoroughly sampled histologically before a diagnosis of pure VC is made.

d. **Spindle cell carcinoma** (SpCC) is the head and neck mucosal form of sarcomatoid carcinoma, a variant of SCC consisting of spindled or pleomorphic tumor cells that simulate a true sarcoma. It is clear from ultrastructural, immunohistochemical, and molecular studies that the sarcomatoid cells represent a clone of poorly differentiated, or divergently differentiated, carcinoma cells. SpCC has demographics similar to those of conventional SCC, occurring in the fifth to sixth decade, showing a strong association with smoking and alcohol use, and having a very high male to female ratio. It occurs most commonly in the larynx (particularly the glottis) followed by the oral cavity, hypopharynx, and nasal cavity. Up to 20% of patients have a history of previous radiation to the originating site, which is higher than that for conventional SCC.

Grossly, the vast majority of laryngeal and hypopharyngeal SpCC, and approximately 50% of oral SpCC, have a polypoid growth pattern resulting in an exophytic mass with a smooth and extensively ulcerated surface. Up to 75% of SpCC are biphasic tumors with areas of conventional SCC admixed with areas of spindled and/or pleomorphic tumor cells (e-**Fig. 1.28**); the spindled component usually predominates. The conventional squamous component may take the form of squamous dysplasia, carcinoma in situ, or invasive carcinoma; because the tumors are usually exophytic with extensive surface ulceration, the noninvasive component may be only a focal finding or may be effaced altogether. SpCC has a wide variety of architectural patterns including fascicular (e-**Fig. 1.29**), storiform, lace-like, or myxoid. On occasion, the tumor cells may be widely spaced in an edematous stroma mimicking granulation tissue with cytologic atypia, a diagnostic pitfall. Approximately 5% of tumors will have definable heterologous sarcomatous differentiation, usually either osteo- or chondrosarcomatous. Immunohistochemistry in the spindle cell component is positive for cytokeratins and/or epithelial membrane antigen in approximately two-thirds of cases, and positive for p63 in a similar percentage; vimentin is always positive, and a significant minority of tumors will be positive for smooth muscle actin.

Although any malignant spindle cell lesion of the mucosa of the upper aerodigestive tract should be considered an SpCC until proven otherwise, the differential diagnosis includes a true sarcoma, spindle cell melanoma, nodular fasciitis, and ulcers and granulation tissue with reactive atypia (particularly after radiation). When a conventional squamous carcinoma component is present intermingled with the spindle cells, the diagnosis of SpCC is confirmed without the need for additional studies.

Because SpCC is inherently a carcinoma, current treatment recommendations are essentially identical to those for conventional SCC, and taking all patients together, the prognosis does not appear different from conventional SCC. However, the prognosis is worse for oral cavity SpCC, and patients with endophytic tumors do worse than those with exophytic tumors.

e. **Papillary SCC** is a rare variant of SCC that is defined as more than 50% of the tumor having an exophytic, papillary growth pattern (e-**Figs. 1.30** and **1.31**). It is more common in the larynx than in the oral cavity and oropharynx, and has a good prognosis.

f. **Adenosquamous carcinoma** is another rare variant consisting of a mixture of SCC and adenocarcinoma with true gland formation, often with mucin production (e-**Fig. 1.32**). The oral cavity and oropharynx are less common sites than the larynx. These tumors are typically more aggressive than conventional SCC.

g. **Basaloid squamous cell carcinoma (BSCC)** is a variant that is rare in the oral cavity but is slightly more common in the oropharynx, larynx, and hypopharynx. It is characterized by molded nests forming a "jigsaw" pattern. The tumor cells are basaloid with hyperchromatic, round to oval nuclei, and scant cytoplasm (e-**Fig. 1.33**). Extracellular mucoid or hyaline material may be present. Abrupt squamous differentiation or overlying squamous dysplasia is seen (e-**Fig. 1.34**). While generally considered an aggressive variant, BSCC in the oropharynx is frequently HPV-positive, and the subset of HPV-positive tumors has a favorable prognosis as is typical of an HPV-positive oropharyngeal SCC.

B. **Melanocytic.** Melanoma is not uncommon in the oral cavity. It occurs in adults with an average age of approximately 60 years, with a very even incidence from age 20 to 80 years. Unlike cutaneous melanoma, in which sun damage underlies the development of most cases, no major etiology has been identified for oral lesions. There is a slight male preponderance and, also unlike cutaneous melanoma, oral lesions occur relatively equally among several races. Oral melanomas present as incidental pigmented lesions identified by a dentist or physician, as masses arising in a pre-existing pigmented lesion, or simply as a new mass growing over a few months. The most common oral site is the hard palate (~40%), followed by the maxillary gingiva (~25%) (e-**Fig. 1.35**), the buccal mucosa, mandibular gingiva, and lip. Melanomas of the oropharynx are rare.

Grossly, most tumors are heavily pigmented and heterogeneous, with a brown, gray, or black color. There are sometimes satellite lesions without intervening pigmentation. Microscopically, most melanomas are deeply invasive, but two-thirds retain a surface in situ component as well. Architecturally, the tumors consist of single cells and ill-defined sheets and nests of either epithelioid cells, spindle cells, or both. The large epithelioid cells have abundant cytoplasm (which can be eosinophilic to gray) and round to oval nuclei with a characteristic single, large, cherry red nucleolus (e-**Fig. 1.36**). Melanin pigment is commonly present. Spindle cells are less common and have cigar-shaped nuclei and moderate clear to eosinophilic cytoplasm. Plasmacytoid and rhabdoid cells can also be seen. Intranuclear cytoplasmic inclusions that are typical of melanomas at other sites are uncommon in oral melanomas. By immunohistochemistry, oral melanomas express the same proteins as other melanomas, namely Melan A, MART-1, HMB-45, S-100, and tyrosinase.

Treatment consists of radical resection with radiation, with or without chemotherapy. Neck dissection is performed only for clinically detected disease. The prognosis is poor; numerous studies have demonstrated a collective 5-year survival between 15% and 25%. Breslow thickness, unlike cutaneous lesions, is of very limited prognostic utility. Approximately 40% of patients will develop cervical lymph node metastases, and common distant metastatic sites include the lung, liver, and brain.

C. **Neuroendocrine Carcinomas** are uncommon tumors in the head and neck region in general, and are very uncommon in the oral cavity and oropharynx. They are essentially all high grade with a small cell morphology, composed of cells with scant cytoplasm, crush artifact, granular chromatin without nucleoli, and extensive necrosis with brisk mitotic activity (i.e., morphologically identical to small cell carcinomas of the lung and other organs) (e-**Figs. 1.37** and **1.38**). Large cell neuroendocrine carcinoma is rare. Some are mixed with a component of SCC. Low-grade neuroendocrine carcinomas ("carcinoid tumors") almost never occur in the oral cavity and oropharynx.

The prognosis for high-grade neuroendocrine carcinoma is very poor, with rapid progression of disease including the development of cervical lymph node metastases and distant metastatic disease. Although high-grade neuroendocrine carcinomas in the oropharynx are often HPV-positive, they do not share the favorable prognosis of HPV-related oropharyngeal SCC. It should also be noted that p16 immunohistochemistry is not a good surrogate marker for HPV in neuroendocrine carcinomas, which frequently overexpress p16 even when HPV-negative.

D. Vascular

1. **Pyogenic granulomas** (or lobular capillary hemangiomas) are benign lesions of the oral cavity that are usually solitary, and are most common on the lips, tongue, gingival and buccal mucosa. They occur in patients of all ages but have a particular predilection for the gingiva of pregnant women and, thus, are often referred to as a "pregnancy tumor" in this setting. They usually present as small (a few centimeters or less) exophytic masses that bleed easily. They may grow rapidly and cause false clinical concern for a malignant neoplasm.

   Grossly, they are polypoid or pedunculated, pink to red, and have a smooth surface. Microscopically, they consist of lobules of small capillaries with plump endothelial cells that have round to oval nuclei and occasional mitoses (e-Fig. 1.39), with larger central "feeder" vessels. Extensive surface ulceration with associated fibrin is usually present. The cells are positive for endothelial immunohistochemical markers such as CD34, CD31, and factor VIII–related antigen.

   Pyogenic granulomas are benign neoplasms that are cured by simple excision. A small percentage may recur. Pregnancy-related lesions often regress postpartum and thus may be hormonally driven.

2. **Hemangioma and lymphangioma** are benign tumors composed of abundant blood or lymphatic vessels, respectively. Hemangiomas of the oral cavity usually occur in adults. They occur most commonly on the lip, buccal mucosa, and lateral tongue borders and present as painless, nodular or well-circumscribed, red or blue masses (e-Fig. 1.40) measuring less than 2 cm in maximal dimension. Microscopically, they consist of blood vessels ranging from small capillaries to large cavernous spaces. The endothelial lining cells can be plump and may have mitotic activity, a feature more common in children. There are a number of named histologic variants, most of which have no clinical significance.

   Lymphangiomas (or cystic hygromas) are composed of dilated lymphatic channels. About 75% occur in the head and neck and, when presenting in the oral cavity, they are almost always found in children younger than 3 years. Histologically, they typically consist of very dilated lymphatic channels lined by bland inconspicuous endothelial cells, with associated intraluminal eosinophilic material, lymphocytes, and occasional red blood cells. There often are interstitial aggregates of lymphocytes.

   Both hemangioma and lymphangioma are benign lesions cured by conservative excision. Hemangiomas can be sclerosed as well. Large lymphangiomas are often debulked, often via serial resections to avoid major morbidity.

3. **Kaposi sarcoma (KS)** is a locally aggressive tumor uniformly associated with human herpesvirus 8 (HHV-8) that predominantly involves the skin but can also involve mucosal sites. When KS involves the oral cavity, usually as a complication of AIDS, it is most commonly found in the palate, followed by the gingiva and dorsal tongue. Clinically, KS appears as purple, red-blue, or brown macules or plaques. Later in the disease course the lesions become nodular and may ulcerate.

   The three histologic stages of KS (patch, plaque, and nodular; all discussed in more detail in Chapter 38) can all be associated with oral KS (e-Fig. 1.41). There are frequently associated collections of extravasated red blood cells and hemosiderin-laden macrophages. A characteristic feature that is sometimes seen is the pale, eosinophilic hyaline globule, which probably represents degenerating red blood cells. Immunohistochemistry is positive for the common endothelial markers CD34 and CD31.

   The behavior of oral KS is variable. It is generally indolent in nonimmunocompromised patients but is more aggressive in patients with AIDS. However, the mortality related to KS is highly dependent on other comorbidities such as opportunistic infections and systemic symptoms.

E. Neural/Neuroectodermal.

Granular cell tumors are benign, slow growing tumors of neural origin that occur at many anatomic sites. Approximately 50% occur in the head and neck region, and half of these occur in the tongue. They also occur in the buccal mucosa, floor of mouth, and palate; are twice as common in women as men; and approximately 10% to 20% are multiple. Grossly, they are smooth, sessile, and firm with a pink or tan-white color. Microscopically, they consist of infiltrative nonencapsulated sheets and cords of bland cells with abundant eosinophilic granular cytoplasm and indistinct cell borders (e-**Fig. 1.42**). There is usually no significant stromal reaction. The nuclei are small, oval, and hyperchromatic with minimal atypia and no mitotic activity. A common feature is pseudoepitheliomatous hyperplasia of the overlying squamous epithelium, which can closely mimic SCC. Conservative excision is the treatment of choice, with a risk of recurrence of <10%. Malignant granular cell tumors (see Chapter 44) are very rare but do occur.

F. Mesenchymal

1. **Peripheral ossifying fibroma** is a reactive proliferation of fibrous tissue on the gingiva which shows focal bone formation. It occurs over a broad age range, but young adults are most commonly affected. The lesions range from a few millimeters up to 2 cm in maximal dimension. They are essentially exclusive to the gingiva, particularly along the incisors, and present as sessile pink nodules, usually with surface ulceration. Microscopically, they consist of randomly distributed plump (but not atypical) fibroblasts with foci of mineralization ranging from dystrophic calcification, to cementum-like material, to a well-formed bone (e-**Fig. 1.43**). Rare giant cells can be seen. Even when excised down to the periosteum the lesion will recur in 15% to 20% of cases.

2. **Peripheral giant cell granuloma** is another reactive proliferation of the gingiva, particularly along the incisors, caused by chronic irritation. It presents over a wide age range, particularly in middle-aged to older adults, as a solitary broad-based nodule that is reddish or blue and <2 cm in diameter. Microscopically, it consists of a mixture of multinucleated osteoclast-like giant cells and plump spindled to oval mononuclear cells (e-**Fig. 1.44**). Hemosiderin, chronic inflammation, and foci of metaplastic bone are frequent. The differential diagnosis includes brown tumor of hyperparathyroidism, cherubism, and central (intraosseous) giant cell granuloma. The lesion is treated by local excision down to the bone; recurrence occurs in approximately 10% of cases.

3. **Congenital granular cell epulis** is a rare benign mesenchymal tumor that classically arises from the anterior alveolar ridge of a newborn. Girls are more frequently affected than boys by a ratio of 9:1. The tumor presents as a smooth, nonulcerated mass about 1 cm in size arising from the gingiva over the lateral incisor/canine area of the maxilla, or less commonly, the mandible. Grossly, it is polypoid and has a homogeneous firm pink or tan cut surface. Microscopically, it consists of a sheet of large cells that have abundant, granular, eosinophilic cytoplasm and round to oval, bland nuclei. The surface squamous epithelium is intact and shows no hyperplasia. By immunohistochemistry, the cells are positive only for vimentin, and specifically are negative for S-100.

Congenital granular cell epulis is not the newborn equivalent of a granular cell tumor and shows no neural differentiation. The tumor stops growing at birth and regresses over time, but most cases still require surgical resection. There is no recurrence, even after incomplete removal.

V. PATHOLOGIC REPORTING OF ORAL CAVITY AND OROPHARYNGEAL MALIGNANCIES

A. Staging.
The American Joint Committee on Cancer (AJCC) now has separate staging systems for oral cavity and oropharyngeal carcinoma (Amin MB et al., eds. *AJCC Cancer Staging Manual.* 8th ed. New York: Springer, 2017). Oropharyngeal carcinoma staging is further separated based on p16/HPV status to reflect the unique biology of HPV-positive as compared with HPV-negative oropharyngeal SCCs. These staging guidelines are applicable to all forms of carcinoma; any nonepithelial tumor type is excluded. Staging is extremely important for clinical management and establishing prognosis. A specific and very important point in staging involves bone involvement by tumor. To qualify as a T4 lesion, the tumor must erode through the bone cortex; superficial bone erosion is not sufficient for classification as T4.

It is important to note that mucosal melanomas of the head and neck, including the oral cavity, have their own staging system.

B. Additional Pertinent Pathologic Features. As with carcinomas at all upper aerodigestive tract sites, margin status, tumor differentiation, and the presence or absence of perineural or lymphovascular space invasion should be reported. Perineural invasion is particularly common in oral cavity carcinomas and is correlated with a poorer prognosis. The pattern of infiltration as well as the presence or absence of a host inflammatory response may also be reported, because both features have been correlated in many studies with a higher rate of local recurrence, a poorer prognosis, or both. Reporting should follow recommended guidelines (e.g., Protocol for the Examination of Specimens from Patients with Cancers of the Lip and Oral Cavity, Protocol for the Examination of Specimens From Patients With Cancers of the Pharynx; available at http://www.cap.org).

ACKNOWLEDGMENT

The authors thank James S. Lewis Jr., an author of the previous editions of this chapter.

SUGGESTED READINGS

Amin MB, Edge S, Greene F, et al. *Head and Neck Section. American Joint Committee on Cancer.* 8th ed. Springer international publishing; 2017.

Bouquot JE, Muller, S, Nikai H. Lesions of the oral cavity. In: Gnepp DR, ed. *Diagnostic Surgical Pathology of the Head and Neck.* 2nd ed. Philadelphia, PA: W.B. Saunders Publishers; 2009.

El-Naggar AK, Chan JKC, Grandis JR, Takata T, Slootweg PJ, eds. *World Health Organization Classification of Head and Neck Tumours.* Lyon: IARC Press; 2017.

Lewis JS Jr, Beadle B, Bishop JA, et al. Human papillomavirus testing in head and neck carcinomas: guideline from the College of American Pathologists. *Arch Pathol Lab Med* 2018;142(5):559–597. doi: 10.5858/arpa.2017-0286-CP

Lewis JS. Malignant neoplasms of the oropharynx. Chapter 10. In: Thompson LDR, Bishop JA, eds. *Head and Neck Pathology, A Volume in the Series Foundations in Diagnostic Pathology.* 3rd ed. Philadelphia, PA: Elsevier; 2019.

Muller S. Malignant neoplasms of the oral cavity. Chapter 9. In: Thompson LDR, Bishop JA, eds. *Head and Neck Pathology, A Volume in the Series Foundations in Diagnostic Pathology.* 3rd ed. Philadelphia, PA: Elsevier; 2019.

2 Larynx

Mena Mansour and Rebecca D. Chernock

I. NORMAL ANATOMY

A. Macroscopic/gross. The larynx is a unique organ designed to produce phonation by modulation of the respiratory airstream. It includes several cartilaginous structures: the thyroid, cricoid, and arytenoid cartilages and the epiglottis. The hyoid bone sits at the superior aspect and is connected to the larynx by the thyrohyoid membrane (Fig. 2.1). The thyroid (and lesser so, cricoid) cartilages ossify in adults. In functional terms, the larynx is divided into three subsites: the supraglottis, glottis, and subglottis. The subsites are particularly useful for tumor management and staging purposes. The supraglottis includes the epiglottis, aryepiglottic folds, arytenoid cartilages, false cords and ventricle, the deeper recess of which is referred to as the saccule. The glottis includes the true vocal cords and extends approximately 1 cm below the level of the free edge of the cords. The true cords, with a hypocellular stroma called Reinke space, are designed to vibrate for phonation, and the ventricle amplifies this further. The cords are manipulated by muscles that attach to and move the arytenoid cartilages, which sit at the posterior aspect of the vocal cords. The subglottis refers to the area approximately 1 cm below the free edge of the true vocal cord to the inferior border of the cricoid cartilage.

B. Microscopic. The larynx is covered by a mixture of squamous and pseudostratified ciliated columnar (respiratory-type) epithelium. The true cords themselves are always **covered** by squamous epithelium. The supra- and subglottis are typically lined by respiratory-type epithelium. In smokers, however, much of the endolarynx undergoes squamous metaplasia. The true cords contain a lamina propria area called Reinke space, which lies between the epithelium and the vocal ligament, deep to which lies the vocalis muscle. Reinke space consists of loose connective tissue with few capillaries and no lymphatics (**e-Fig. 2.1**). The submucosa of the false cords is rich in seromucinous glands.

II. GROSS EXAMINATION, TISSUE SAMPLING, AND HISTOLOGIC SLIDE PREPARATION

A. Endoscopic Biopsies. The majority of specimens from this region consist of endoscopic forceps biopsies. The tissue samples should be placed immediately into 10% **buffered** formalin or other appropriate fixative. These should undergo gross examination and description documenting the exact number of pieces present, and then be entirely submitted with three levels cut from each paraffin block for hematoxylin and eosin (H&E) examination.

B. Resections

1. Partial. These are widely variable specimens depending on the location of the tumor. Standard procedures include vertical hemilaryngectomy and supraglottic or supracricoid laryngectomy. As a generalization, these specimens need to be oriented, the soft tissue margins inked, and margins demonstrated by shave or radial section followed by sectioning of the tumor relative to cartilage/bone and soft tissue margins. The use of either shave or radial sections depends on the nature of the specimen. If the tumor is relatively distant from a margin, 1- to 2-mm shave sections are preferred. If the tumor approximates a margin to less than 1 to 2 mm, radial sections are taken.

Partial resections with a CO_2 laser under an operating microscope are becoming more common because of their low morbidity. Since an inherent part of this procedure is to cut into the tumor or to remove tumor in more than one piece, surgeons ink the individual pieces themselves as they alone know what constitutes the true margin. In the pathology lab, the pieces are measured, described, and submitted entirely in sections perpendicular to the ink.

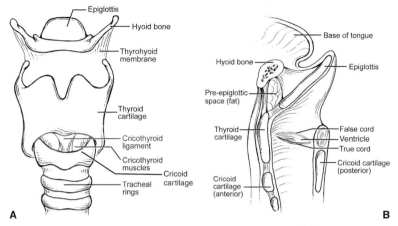

Figure 2.1 Larynx anatomy: (**A**) anterior view, (**B**) sagittal cross-section.

2. Total. For years, total laryngectomy has been the standard operation for malignancy. However, partial resections with preservation of function are increasingly common. Total laryngectomy is currently used most often for large tumors or as salvage therapy for recurrences after partial surgery or definitive radiation and chemotherapy (e-**Fig. 2.2**).

The usual approach to grossing a total laryngectomy is to initially ink the peripheral nonmucosal soft tissue margins and then open the larynx by a posterior vertical midline cut with scissors, propping it wide open with a small stick. After overnight formalin fixation, the specimen is ready for prosection. After orientation and measurement in three dimensions, the tumor is measured and described, specifically noting what structures are involved. The specimen typically includes the entire larynx including cartilages and hyoid bone, as well as small portions of hypopharyngeal mucosa bilaterally adjacent to the aryepiglottic folds. Standard sections (Fig. 2.2) are taken as follows: (i) Margins: shaved inferior tracheal ring; shaved right and left hypopharyngeal mucosa; shaved postcricoid soft tissue; radial sections demonstrating anterior, anterolateral, and base of tongue inked soft tissue margins. (ii) Soft tissue/mucosa: bilateral vertical glottis (including both true and false cords); vertical anterior commissure; vertical midline epiglottis showing pre-epiglottic soft tissue space; bilateral aryepiglottic folds; four sections of tumor if not included in the previous sections. (iii) Cartilage/bone: vertical sections showing tumor and thyroid as well as cricoid cartilages (at closest or at sites of gross invasion); sections of right and left wings of the hyoid bone (where closest to or involved by tumor). Typically, all soft tissue and margin sections are taken first, and the entire specimen is bisected in the midline vertically and decalcified *in toto* overnight followed by cartilage and/or bone section acquisition.

C. Frozen Sections. Frozen sections are a critical element of surgical therapy for tumors of the head and neck region. Although practices vary, most institutions have margins taken as separate pieces by the surgeon from the periphery of the surgical defect after the tumor has been removed. Because laryngeal resections are quite variable, the sites where frozen sections are taken are not standard; with total laryngectomies, sometimes no frozen sections are clinically necessary. The surgeon may sample the tumor or suspicious sites to confirm and/or map the tumor, and then take margins from the area of closest approach. The tissue pieces are submitted individually to pathology in saline and frozen in their entirety, with two to three H&E slides generated at representative levels. It is

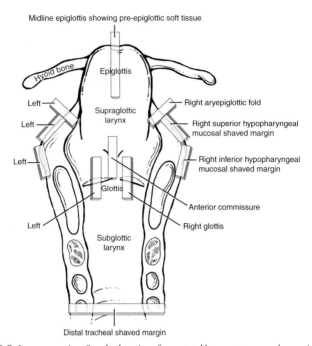

Midline epiglottis showing pre-epiglottic soft tissue

Hyoid bone

Epiglottis

Left — Right aryepiglottic fold

Supraglottic
larynx

Left — Right superior hypopharyngeal
mucosal shaved margin

Left — Right inferior hypopharyngeal
mucosal shaved margin

Glottis

Anterior commissure

Left — Right glottis

Subglottic
larynx

Distal tracheal shaved margin

Figure 2.2 Larynx grossing. Standard sections from a total laryngectomy are shown. Additional sections include sections of tumor (4 to 5 total), right and left postcricoid soft tissue shaved margins, and anterior soft tissue margins (either shaved or radial). After decalcification, additional sections should include cartilage deep to the tumor showing involvement or nearest approach, any surrounding lymph nodes in neck soft tissue, and the hyoid bone (when closest to tumor or grossly involved by it). If necessary, sections of tracheostomy skin, thyroid lobe(s), and neck skin should also be submitted.

critical to obtain sections that represent the entire tissue submitted so that small foci of tumor are not missed by sampling error (i.e., missing significant but focal findings in the tissue at the time of frozen section by not sampling the tissue adequately). This is best done by making sure the second and third sections are taken from deep into the tissue. The pieces should be evaluated grossly for mucosa—typically shiny and pink tan on one surface of the tissue; if present, the specimen should be oriented to demonstrate this surface on edge with the submucosa below. If the surgeon has inked the true margin, the tissue should be submitted radially to the ink. Additional sections should be cut if needed to assure that quality sections are obtained.

In some instances, the surgeon may send an oriented mucosal ellipse with intact margins for frozen section evaluation. In these cases, the margins should first be inked to maintain orientation. Close margins should be submitted radially and remote margins can be shaved.

The tissue that remains after frozen section is submitted for evaluation by permanent sections. This process can help resolve a number of issues from frozen section including freezing and cautery artifact, amount of tumor represented, and orientation or embedding issues. The margins of the main resection specimen are also evaluated via permanent sections throughout their entirety because the separate frozen section specimens are small and almost never cover the entire margin of a resection.

III. DIAGNOSTIC FEATURES OF COMMON DISEASES

A. **Inflammation and Infection.** Inflammation of the larynx (laryngitis) is quite common clinically, and can be divided into acute and chronic forms, which are variable by age. Laryngitis rarely necessitates tissue biopsy for pathologic evaluation. Infections can be caused by a myriad of agents including viruses, bacteria, fungi, and parasites. The pathologist must be alert to the possibility of infection, and helpful information includes the immune status of the patient as many of these patients will be immunocompromised.

Inflammation is essentially never present in the normal larynx, so the presence of inflammatory cells is a diagnostic clue. Depending on the organism, the inflammation can take a number of different forms, almost all of which are typical for the type of organism when it presents in other locations. Examples of some of the major infections include cytomegalovirus, herpes simplex virus, tuberculosis, rhinoscleroma (*Klebsiella rhinoscleromatis*), candidiasis, histoplasmosis, blastomycosis, cryptococcosis, coccidioidomycosis, or rhinosporidiosis (*Rhinosporidium seeberi*). The resulting inflammation may cause mucosal ulceration, acute and chronic inflammation, necrosis, or granulomas. Viral cytopathic effect may be noted in viral infections. Special stains (such as Gomori methenamine silver [GMS], acid-fast bacillus [AFB], or periodic acid–Schiff [PAS]) should be utilized to look for organisms.

B. **Nonneoplastic Lesions**

1. **Traumatic**

   a. **Vocal cord nodules and polyps.** These are nonneoplastic degenerative stromal lesions of Reinke space that are usually related to trauma due to misuse or vocal excess. As such, they have been referred to as singer's or screamer's nodules. They are more common in women and are commonly bilateral, characteristically occurring at the junction of the anterior and middle one-third of the vocal cord as this is the point of maximal vibration during phonation. Macroscopically, they appear as gray or white broad-based nodules or polyps (e-**Fig. 2.3**). Microscopically, they consist of squamous mucosa with or without hyperkeratosis, are only rarely ulcerated, and overlie an altered sparsely cellular myxoid, edematous, fibrous, fibrinous, and/or vascular stroma. The myxoid appearance is most common and it may demonstrate small cystic spaces (e-**Figs. 2.4** and **2.5**). So-called vocal cord polyps are histologically identical but clinically present unilaterally, and in men and smokers with more regularity.

   b. **Contact ulcer.** Also referred to clinically as *contact granulomas* or just *granulomas*, these occur on the vocal process of the arytenoids classically as a result of forceful vocalization in individuals who must affect a low, deep, forceful voice. However, they also may result after endotracheal intubation or as a result of gastroesophageal reflux disease. They are more common in men, can be unilateral or bilateral, and present as polypoid lesions. Microscopically, they are essentially granulation tissue polyps with an ulcerated mucosa covered by fibrin, with a stroma containing abundant small vessels in a zonal configuration with plump endothelial cells (e-**Fig. 2.6**). The stroma may be rich in lymphocytes, plasma cells, neutrophils, or histiocytes (sometimes including giant cells).

2. **Cysts.** Laryngeal cysts can be divided into three main categories: (i) ductal cysts, (ii) laryngoceles, and (iii) saccular cysts. All are cured by simple excision.

   a. **Ductal cysts.** These are the most common and result from obstruction of a minor salivary gland duct. Ductal cysts are typically small "bumps" on endoscopy and have a predilection for the cords, ventricle, aryepiglottic folds, and epiglottis. The lining may be ductal, squamous, or oncocytic.

   b. **Laryngocele.** A laryngocele is an asymptomatic dilatation of the saccule (the deep aspect of the ventricle). It may remain internal and manifest as a supraglottic mucosal bulge, or may herniate above the thyroid cartilage to project externally into the neck soft tissue and present as a neck mass. Microscopically, it is lined by respiratory-type mucosa (e-**Fig. 2.7**).

c. Saccular cyst. This represents a mucin-filled dilatation of the saccule, either developmental or acquired due to obstruction. It is also typically lined by respiratory-type mucosa, but the lining can be squamous or oncocytic on occasion.

3. Metabolic

a. Amyloidosis. The larynx is a well-established, though infrequent, site of localized amyloidosis. It most commonly involves the false cord, followed by the true cord and ventricle. A subset of patients has multifocal disease, with approximately one-third having tracheal disease as well. Most patients have only localized disease, but systemic disease also occurs in a subset of patients. All patients should have a workup to rule out systemic amyloidosis with or without an associated plasma cell dyscrasia. The amyloid in localized laryngotracheal amyloidosis is of the AL (or immunoglobulin) type.

Laryngeal amyloidosis usually macroscopically presents as a polypoid nodule covered by intact mucosa. Microscopically, it consists of sheets and nodular masses of amorphous, hypocellular eosinophilic material in the stroma (**e-Fig. 2.8**) and in blood vessel walls, encasing and compressing mucoserous glands. The diagnosis is confirmed by Congo red special staining demonstrating "apple-green" birefringence by polarized light microscopy. Thioflavin T staining with examination under fluorescence microscopy is also sometimes used. Amyloid typing can be performed by mass spectrometry.

C. Neoplastic Lesions. The 2017 World Health Organization (WHO) classification of tumors of the larynx, hypopharynx, and trachea is listed in Table 2.1.

1. Benign

a. Squamous papillomas are squamous proliferations caused by human papillomavirus (HPV) and are the most common benign tumors of the larynx. They are most common in the larynx, but also occur in the trachea and bronchi. They also occur occasionally in the oral cavity and pharynx. There are two separate clinical settings: juvenile or juvenile-onset laryngeal papillomatosis (JOLP) and adult (or adult-onset) laryngeal papillomatosis (AOLP). Juvenile papillomas most often begin before age 5 years and are much more likely than adult papillomas to be multifocal and to have an associated clinical impact. In a significant minority of patients, carpeting of the larynx occurs, requiring repeated laser excisions and occasionally tracheostomy or even laryngectomy for control and airway management. Papillomas tend to recur rapidly, but the disease severity usually regresses in early adulthood. In adult papillomas, the peak age is between 20 and 40 years, disease is usually unifocal or limited, and even when multifocal it is less aggressive. Only occasionally does it present as multifocal disease that recurs after excision.

Squamous papillomas are strongly associated with HPV types 6 and 11, which are thought to be transmitted from the mother to the upper aerodigestive tract (UADT) of the neonate during vaginal delivery, thus explaining the occurrence in childhood. There is minimal risk of transformation to invasive carcinoma.

Regardless of the clinical context, squamous papillomas have a typical morphology. Grossly, they appear as exophytic, granular, and friable pink, red, or tan lesions. Microscopically, they consist of arborizing papillary fronds of thickened but maturing squamous epithelium with slight hyperplasia of the basal layer (**e-Fig. 2.9**). Cells in the midlayer often have cytoplasmic clearing, but frank koilocytosis is not regularly observed. The nuclei are slightly enlarged and irregular but not overtly dysplastic appearing, and mitotic activity is usually present but modest. Characteristically, there is minimal surface keratinization (**e-Fig. 2.10**). Frank dysplasia can be seen in some lesions and should be reported, and graded as in nonpapillary squamous mucosa (see section III.C.2). However, there is no consistent correlation of overt dysplasia with the development of subsequent invasive carcinoma.

b. Granular cell tumors are benign, slowly growing tumors of neural origin that occur in a multitude of anatomic locations. They are particularly common in the head and neck region with a minority occurring in the larynx. They are slightly more common in African Americans and typically present with hoarseness. Grossly,

TABLE 2.1	2017 WHO Histologic Classification of Tumors of the Hypopharynx, Larynx, and Trachea

Malignant surface epithelial tumors
Conventional squamous cell carcinoma
Verrucous squamous cell carcinoma
Basaloid squamous cell carcinoma
Papillary squamous cell carcinoma
Spindle cell squamous cell carcinoma
Adenosquamous carcinoma
Lymphoepithelial carcinoma

Precursor lesions
Dysplasia
Squamous cell papilloma and squamous cell papillomatosis

Neuroendocrine tumors
Well-differentiated neuroendocrine carcinoma
Moderately differentiated neuroendocrine carcinoma
Poorly differentiated neuroendocrine carcinoma

Salivary gland tumors
Adenoid cystic carcinoma
Pleomorphic adenoma
Oncocytic papillary cystadenoma

Soft tissue tumors
Granular cell tumor
Liposarcoma
Inflammatory myofibroblastic tumor

Cartilage tumors
Chondroma
Chondrosarcoma

Hematolymphoid tumors

From El-Naggar AK, Chan JKC, Grandis JR, Takata T, Slootweg PJ, eds. *WHO Classification of Head and Neck Tumours*. 4th ed. Lyon, France: IARC Press; 2017. Used with permission.

they are smooth, white polypoid tumors involving the posterior true cords, anterior commissure, false cords, or subglottis. Microscopically, they consist of infiltrative, nonencapsulated sheets and cords of bland cells with abundant eosinophilic granular cytoplasm and indistinct cell borders. There is usually no significant stromal reaction. The nuclei are small, oval, and eccentric with minimal atypia and no mitotic activity. A common feature is pseudoepitheliomatous hyperplasia of the overlying squamous epithelium, which can be quite alarming; when pseudoepitheliomatous hyperplasia is present it should always prompt a search of the submucosa for a granular cell tumor (e-**Fig. 2.11**). Conservative endoscopic excision is the treatment of choice with a less than 10% risk of recurrence.

c. **Paragangliomas** are tumors recapitulating the paraganglia, specialized organs of the autonomic nervous system derived from the neural crest. They occur in numerous locations throughout the body, and their behavior is largely dependent on site. Laryngeal paragangliomas are benign and are divided into two groups: superior and inferior. Superior paragangliomas are much more common and occur in the supraglottic larynx, from the false cord up into the aryepiglottic fold.

They are polyploid submucosal lesions. Inferior paragangliomas occur along the cricoid cartilage in the subglottic region and often present as dumbbell-shaped lesions with both intra- and extralaryngeal components.

Microscopically, these tumors are identical to those arising elsewhere. They consist of sheets and nests of polygonal to spindled cells with abundant eosinophilic to slightly basophilic cytoplasm, and round to oval nuclei with a slightly granular chromatin. They are very vascular with stellate large vessels throughout (e-**Fig. 2.12**). Nuclear pleomorphism may be striking, but there is minimal mitotic activity. The cells are arranged in nests (classically termed *zellballen*) (e-**Fig. 2.13**). By immunohistochemistry, the cells are strongly positive for synaptophysin and chromogranin A, virtually always negative for epithelial markers such as epithelial membrane antigen (EMA) and cytokeratin, and show the typical sustentacular (or supporting) cell staining for S-100 around the periphery of the nests while the tumor cells themselves are negative.

2. Precursor (premalignant) squamous lesions are defined as altered squamous epithelium with an increased risk of progression to squamous cell carcinoma. The term dysplasia or intraepithelial neoplasia should be used for these lesions. Atypia, in contrast, is not considered synonymous with dysplasia or risk of squamous carcinoma and is used in a more general sense, and may describe changes seen in reactive epithelium as well.

Unfortunately, there is poor agreement about the histopathologic changes that constitute dysplasia and about its grading. Also, there is poor correlation between the varying grades of dysplasia and subsequent risk of carcinoma. Several grading systems have been proposed (Table 2.2). Precursor lesions are strongly associated with smoking and alcohol use. Most precursor lesions present along the true cords, and are often bilateral. This presentation is likely due to early dysfunctional symptoms of the cords from the dysplasia; at other sites in the larynx, symptoms do not usually develop until there is established invasive malignancy.

There are a number of changes that occur in dysplasia including nuclear abnormalities, architectural abnormalities, and abnormal keratinization. Hyperplasia manifests as thickening of the epithelium without any cytologic atypia. The changes of dysplasia, particularly mild dysplasia, are difficult to distinguish from hyperplasia or reactive change, and similarly, the varying degrees of dysplasia are difficult to distinguish from each other. In broad terms, mild dysplasia shows nuclear enlargement; hyperchromasia; and increased nucleus to cytoplasm ratios limited to the lower third of the epithelium (e-**Fig. 2.14**), moderate dysplasia into the middle third (e-**Fig. 2.15**), and severe dysplasia into the upper third or full thickness (e-**Fig. 2.16**). However, severe dysplasia in particular may manifest as an expanded basal cell layer with maturation in the upper layers, particularly with bulbous or down-streaming

TABLE 2.2	Precursor Lesion Classification Schemes		
Ljubljana Classification Squamous Intraepithelial Lesions (SIL)	**Squamous Intraepithelial Neoplasia (SIN)**	**2005 World Health Organization Classification**	**2017 World Health Organization Classification**
Squamous cell (simple) hyperplasia	N/A	Squamous cell hyperplasia	Low-grade dysplasia
Basal/parabasal cell hyperplasia	SIN 1	Mild dysplasia	
Atypical hyperplasia	SIN 2	Moderate dysplasia	
Atypical hyperplasia	SIN 3	Severe dysplasia	High-grade dysplasia
Carcinoma in situ	SIN 3	Carcinoma in situ	

N/A, not applicable.

tongues of basal epithelium toward the submucosa (e-**Fig. 2.17**). The epithelium is usually thickened but sometimes thinned, and hyperkeratosis may or may not be present.

3. Malignant

a. Conventional squamous cell carcinoma

is the overwhelmingly most common malignant tumor of the larynx. It occurs with a peak in the sixth and seventh decades and, just as with other UADT squamous cancers, has a high male-to-female ratio (5:1) and a strong relationship to tobacco use and alcohol consumption, with a multiplicative rather than additive relative risk when both are used. HPV is found in a small minority of tumors (<10%), but the etiologic role of the virus and clinical impact are not clear. Most tumors involve the glottis or supraglottic region. Glottic tumors present earliest and at the smallest size because of functional compromise and symptomology.

The gross appearance of squamous cell carcinoma is quite variable, ranging from fungating, exophytic tumors to endophytic, ulcerated tumors with raised edges. Microscopically, the term "squamous cell carcinoma, keratinizing type" is used to describe the common version of the cancer and to distinguish it clearly from the numerous variant squamous carcinoma types that exist. Keratinizing-type squamous cell carcinoma consists of nests and sheets of cells with abundant eosinophilic cytoplasm and round to oval nuclei, often with prominent nucleoli. Well-differentiated tumors retain abundant pink or clear cytoplasm and often show keratin "pearl" formation (e-**Fig. 2.18**). Moderately differentiated tumors have more pleomorphism and a higher nucleus to cytoplasm ratio in many of the cells while still retaining moderate eosinophilic cytoplasm (e-**Fig. 2.19**). Poorly differentiated tumors often have single cells or small nests of cells with more mitotic activity and less cytoplasm (e-**Fig. 2.20**). Grading should be performed, although it has not been shown to consistently predict the clinical behavior of individual tumors; the majority of UADT squamous cell carcinomas are moderately differentiated. Although frank keratin formation is commonly seen in well- and moderately differentiated carcinomas, its presence or absence does not have any clinical significance for laryngeal carcinoma.

i. Verrucous carcinoma

(VC) is a specific, well-differentiated, and nonmetastasizing variant of squamous cell carcinoma also known as "Ackerman's tumor." It occurs in the larynx and oral cavity and grossly appears as a well-circumscribed, warty and exophytic, broad-based, white, granular, and friable mass. Microscopically, VC consists of very thick, club-shaped papillae with a broad pushing base. There is usually prominent surface hyperkeratosis, and the sheets of tumor have bland cells with abundant eosinophilic to clear cytoplasm, sometimes described as "glassy" in appearance. There is no cytologic atypia, mitotic activity is very low and basal, and there is a smooth interface with the stroma. The stroma directly beneath the tumor typically demonstrates prominent plasma cell–rich chronic inflammation (e-**Figs. 2.21** to **2.23**).

The prognosis for pure VC is excellent. Although it can be large and locally destructive, complete surgical resection is often curative. Radiation is also an acceptable treatment, particularly in poor surgical candidates. However, routine invasive squamous cell carcinoma often arises from VC. When this occurs, the prognosis and behavior are the same as for typical squamous cell carcinoma.

ii. Spindle cell carcinoma

(SpCC) is the term for a poorly differentiated carcinoma that adopts a sarcomatoid, spindled, or mesenchymal-appearing morphology but which is, nevertheless, of epithelial origin. It is frequently biphasic with a spindled component and intermingled with either in situ or invasive squamous cell carcinoma. The tumor has the same demographics as routine squamous cell carcinoma.

Grossly, SpCC is characteristically polypoid with an ulcerated surface. The glottis is the most common laryngeal site. Microscopically, these tumors can be quite variable; among the patterns encountered are sheets of spindle cells mimicking a fibrosarcoma (e-**Fig. 2.24**), and broad regions of pleomorphic hyperchromatic cells widely separated in an edematous stroma mimicking a pleomorphic undifferentiated sarcoma (e-**Fig. 2.25**). There is usually brisk mitotic activity and necrosis. Foci of recognizable sarcomatous differentiation such as chondrosarcoma, osteosarcoma, or rhabdomyosarcoma sometimes occur. As noted above, most cases are "biphasic," showing some component of in situ or invasive squamous cell carcinoma (e-**Fig. 2.26**), but it may take extensive sectioning to demonstrate the routine squamous component.

If the tumor consists of spindle or pleomorphic cells only, immunohisto-chemistry for epithelial markers such as pancytokeratin, EMA, and *p63* or *p40* is usually very helpful; these immunostains are positive in one-fourth to one-third of cases. With markedly extended panels utilizing antibodies to more than 10 different individual keratins, approximately three-quarters of tumors will demonstrate staining; however, in everyday practice, utilization of pancytokeratin (AE1/AE3) as well as 34βE12 or cytokeratin 5/6 will suffice to demonstrate keratin expression. SpCC stains for some mesenchymal markers as well, such as vimentin (every case), smooth muscle actin, and muscle-specific actin. Nevertheless, a malignant spindle cell neoplasm involving/arising along the mucosa of the UADT should be considered an SpCC until proven other-wise, because sarcomas are distinctly uncommon at these sites. The differential diagnosis includes a granulation tissue polyp, true sarcoma, or inflammatory myofibroblastic tumor. The positive epithelial marker immunohistochemistry will usually distinguish SpCC from these other entities.

iii. **Basaloid squamous cell carcinoma** (BSCC) is a variant of squamous carcinoma composed almost entirely of basaloid cells giving it a "blue cell" appearance. It has the same demographics as routine squamous cell carcinoma but has a predilection for the supraglottic larynx, the oropharynx, and the hypopharynx, particularly the pyriform sinus. While oropharyngeal BSCCs are usually HPV positive, laryngeal and hypopharyngeal tumors are almost always HPV negative. HPV-negative BSCC typically presents at high stage and is more aggressive than typical squamous cell carcinoma stage for stage, with high rates of distant metastasis.

Grossly, BSCC presents as a centrally ulcerated mass with thickening at the edges, and commonly with extensive submucosal induration and spread at the periphery. Microscopically, there are two components. The first is pre-dominant and consists of nests of basaloid cells with hyperchromatic round nuclei, inconspicuous nucleoli, and scant cytoplasm. A "jigsaw puzzle" pattern in which the tumor nests mold to one another is characteristic. Comedo-type central necrosis is common. The second component is typical keratiniz-ing-type squamous cell carcinoma, either in situ or invasive, which is always focal (e-**Fig. 2.27**). The basaloid component of many tumors shows a charac-teristic hyalinized, eosinophilic basement membrane–like stroma around the tumor cells, and as small round nodules within tumor nests akin to that seen in cylindromas of the skin (e-**Fig. 2.28**).

The differential diagnosis includes neuroendocrine carcinoma or the solid variant of adenoid cystic carcinoma. The former expresses neuroendocrine markers in most cases and is negative for high–molecular-weight cytokeratins such as 34βE12 and 5/6. Solid adenoid cystic carcinoma shows some evidence of myoepithelial differentiation on staining for *p63* manifested as scattered staining at the periphery of tumor nests; in contrast, BSCC stains diffusely throughout the tumor (as with squamous epithelium and squamous carci-noma, which also show strong staining).

iv. **Papillary squamous cell carcinoma** (PSCC) is an uncommon variant of squamous cell carcinoma which has the same demographics as typical squamous carcinoma. The larynx is among the most common sites of involvement, the supraglottis and glottis in particular; only very rarely does the tumor arise in the subglottis. Grossly it is a soft, polypoid, and friable tumor. Microscopically it is defined by having a predominantly (>50%) papillary growth pattern with fibrovascular cores lined by full-thickness, markedly dysplastic squamous cells which are most often very immature and basaloid appearing. There is usually minimal keratinization. Stromal invasion may or may not be present, but when it is, it has the appearance of typical squamous cell carcinoma. However, PSCC is considered by definition invasive even in the absence of clear-cut histologic stromal invasion.

The differential diagnosis includes squamous papilloma, VC, and typical squamous cell carcinoma with a partially exophytic growth pattern. The prognosis of PSCC is better than for typical squamous carcinoma. PSCC frequently recurs locally, but metastases are infrequent.

v. **Adenosquamous carcinoma.** The larynx is the most common site for adenosquamous carcinoma, followed by the oral cavity and sinonasal region. Adenosquamous carcinoma has the same demographics and clinical presentation as typical squamous cell carcinoma. It does not have a unique gross appearance, and is either exophytic or ulcerated with indurated edges. Microscopically, it consists of both true squamous carcinoma and adenocarcinoma. The two components are usually close to each other but still have a tendency to segregate. The squamous component, which is usually of the keratinizing type, can be either invasive or in situ carcinoma and has the same appearance as typical squamous carcinoma. It usually predominates in the superficial aspects of the tumor, whereas the adenocarcinoma component, which may either be isolated glands or glandular structures within larger sheets of tumor, tends to occupy the deeper aspects and therefore may be missed in a superficial biopsy (e-**Fig. 2.29**). The glands are often "punched out" with round, smooth edges. Mucin production is not required for the diagnosis but is very frequently present (e-**Fig. 2.30**); mucicarmine or other mucin stains can be quite helpful to highlight its presence. Adenosquamous carcinomas are more aggressive than typical squamous cell carcinoma, and the literature shows that the prognosis for adenosquamous carcinoma is worse than conventional squamous cell carcinoma.

The differential diagnosis includes mucoepidermoid carcinoma, acantholytic or adenoid squamous cell carcinoma, and squamous cell carcinoma invading seromucinous minor salivary gland tissue. Mucoepidermoid carcinoma is the most important consideration (Table 2.3).

b. **Neuroendocrine carcinomas** of the larynx are relatively uncommon and are divided into three major categories: well-differentiated neuroendocrine carcinoma ("carcinoid tumor"), moderately differentiated neuroendocrine carcinoma

TABLE 2.3	Adenosquamous Carcinoma vs. Mucoepidermoid Carcinoma: Histologic Features	
Adenosquamous Carcinoma	**Mucoepidermoid Carcinoma**
Squamous carcinoma in situ	No squamous carcinoma in situ
Origin from squamous epithelium	Origin from seromucinous glands
Keratin pearls	Limited keratin pearls
Glands at lower invasive parts	Glands widely intermingled
No lobular arrangement	Lobular arrangement
No intermediate cells	Intermediate cells

("atypical carcinoid tumor"), and poorly differentiated neuroendocrine carcinoma. The latter category is further divided into two subtypes: small cell and large cell. There is a clear spectrum of behavior among the subtypes ranging from very indolent to highly aggressive.

Most neuroendocrine carcinomas of the larynx occur in the sixth to the eighth decade, and there is a strong male predominance. They are almost exclusively supraglottic, and smoking is associated with moderately and poorly differentiated neuroendocrine carcinomas only.

The histology of these tumors directly parallels those within the lung. Well-differentiated neuroendocrine carcinoma is characterized by nests, trabeculae, and sheets of round, regular tumor cells with moderate eosinophilic to partially clear cytoplasm. The tumor nuclei are round, regular, and show the typical "salt and pepper" or stippled chromatin. Mitotic activity is less than 2 per 10 high-power fields. Moderately differentiated tumors have a similar appearance but are less organized and show more cellular pleomorphism, focal necrosis, and more prominent mitotic activity (2 to 10 per 10 high-power fields). Small cell neuroendocrine carcinoma consists of sheets of blue cells with nuclear molding, crush artifact, and delicate chromatin with indistinct nucleoli (**e-Fig. 2.31**). Large cell neuroendocrine carcinoma is also high grade, akin to small cell carcinoma, but has larger cells with more generous eosinophilic cytoplasm, prominent nucleoli, and frequently a more organized growth pattern with peripheral palisading. There is brisk mitotic activity and prominent necrosis in both forms of high-grade neuroendocrine carcinoma.

All of these neuroendocrine neoplasms stain with neuroendocrine markers by immunohistochemistry (synaptophysin, chromogranin A, CD56/NCAM), but there tends to be less staining with the high-grade tumors. In particular, in small cell neuroendocrine carcinoma the staining can become quite focal and sometimes is only present for one of the several neuroendocrine markers.

Well-differentiated tumors have an excellent prognosis despite frequent local recurrence, and metastases are uncommon. Moderately differentiated neuroendocrine carcinoma is an aggressive tumor with frequent cervical lymph node and distant metastases. Both well- and moderately differentiated tumors are treated surgically. Poorly differentiated neuroendocrine carcinomas, whether small cell or large cell, have a dismal prognosis with frequent neck nodal and distant metastases; patients with high-grade neuroendocrine carcinomas are typically treated with radiation and chemotherapy rather than surgery.

c. Mesenchymal tumors. A great variety of mesenchymal tumors occasionally occur in the larynx, the most common of which are the cartilaginous tumors chondrosarcoma and chondroma. Chondrosarcomas are the most common sarcoma of the larynx, occur in older adults, and are decidedly more common in men. They originate from the cricoid or thyroid lamina (3:1, cricoid to thyroid) and tend to present differently by site of origin with slowly progressive dyspnea for cricoid tumors, or an anterior neck mass for thyroid cartilage tumors. Symptoms are usually present for a long period of time (often several years). Grossly, the neoplasms consist of well-circumscribed, shiny white, or gray lobulated masses with gritty areas of calcification and a glistening cut surface (**e-Fig. 2.32**). Microscopically, they consist of lobules of cartilage which, relative to normal, show increased cellularity and nuclear atypia with variability in size, more than one nucleus in individual lacunae, and binucleated cells (**e-Fig. 2.33**). The periphery of the tumor is typically pushing and not infiltrative but shows destructive growth into soft tissue and/or surrounding bone.

The grading system is identical to that for chondrosarcomas elsewhere in the body. As the grade increases, the cells show increased atypia with enlarged nuclei and nucleoli, but mitotic activity is only seen in high-grade tumors. It can be remarkably challenging to differentiate low-grade chondrosarcomas from chondromas, particularly on biopsy specimens. Chondrosarcomas display cytologic atypia with increased cellularity and nucleoli in chondrocytes, and show at least some areas of destructive growth at the periphery.

The vast majority of laryngeal chondrosarcomas are low grade (grade 1). However, grade does not seem to affect prognosis. Surgery is directed at larynx-sparing complete excision, with total laryngectomy reserved for recurrence or uncontrolled local disease. Survival is about 85% at 10 years.

IV. PATHOLOGIC REPORTING OF LARYNGEAL CARCINOMA

A. Staging. Staging of laryngeal carcinomas is extremely important for clinical **management** and prognosis. The most recent staging system is that of the 2017 Tumor, Node, Metastasis (TNM) American Joint Committee on Cancer staging classification (Amin MB, Edge SB, Greene FL, et al., eds. *AJCC Cancer Staging Manual*. 8th ed. New York: Springer; 2017). For T-staging purposes, the larynx is divided into the supraglottis, glottis, and subglottis. Although squamous cell carcinoma is the overwhelmingly most common type of malignancy, staging guidelines are applicable to all forms of carcinoma. Any nonepithelial tumor type is excluded. The staging guidelines often require both clinical and pathologic input (e.g., vocal cord fixation or not) for proper classification.

B. Additional Pertinent Pathologic Features. As with carcinomas at all UADT sites, margin status, tumor differentiation, and the presence or absence of perineural or **lymphovascular** space invasion should be reported. Reporting should follow recommended guidelines (e.g., College of American Pathologists Protocol for the Examination of Specimens From Patients With Cancers of the Larynx, available at http://www.cap.org).

ACKNOWLEDGMENT

The authors thank James S. Lewis Jr., author of the previous editions of this chapter.

SUGGESTED READINGS

Bishop JA. Chapter 5: Benign neoplasms of the larynx, hypopharynx, and trachea. In: Thompson LDR, Bishop JA, eds. *Head and Neck Pathology, A Volume in the Series Foundations in Diagnostic Pathology*. 3rd ed. Philadelphia, PA: Elsevier; 2019.

Brandwein-Gensler MS, Mahadevia P, Gnepp DR. Nonsquamous pathologic diseases of the hypopharynx, larynx, and trachea. In: Gnepp DR, ed. *Diagnostic Surgical Pathology of the Head and Neck*. Philadelphia, PA: W.B. Saunders Publishers; 2009.

El-Naggar AK, Chan JKC, Grandis JR, Takata T, Slootweg PJ, eds. Chapter 3: Tumours of the hypopharynx, larynx, trachea and parapharyngeal space. In: *WHO Classification of Head and Neck Tumors*. Lyon, France: IARC Press; 2017.

Slootweg PJ, Richardson M. Squamous cell carcinoma of the upper aerodigestive system. In: Gnepp DR, ed. *Diagnostic Surgical Pathology of the Head and Neck*. Philadelphia, PA: W.B. Saunders Publishers; 2009.

Thompson LDR. Chapter 4: Non-neoplastic lesions of the larynx, hypopharynx, and trachea. In: Thompson LDR, Bishop JA, eds. *Head and Neck Pathology, A Volume in the Series Foundations in Diagnostic Pathology*. 3rd ed. Philadelphia, PA: Elsevier; 2019.

Thompson LDR. Chapter 6: Malignant neoplasms of the larynx, hypopharynx, and trachea. In: Thompson LDR, Bishop JA, eds. *Head and Neck Pathology, A Volume in the Series Foundations in Diagnostic Pathology*. 3rd ed. Philadelphia, PA: Elsevier; 2019.

3

Nasal Cavity, Paranasal Sinuses, and Nasopharynx

Samir K. El-Mofty, Mena Mansour, and Dikson Dibe Gondim

I. NORMAL ANATOMY

A. **Nasal Cavity.** The normal sinonasal region consists of the central nasal cavity, paired bilateral paranasal sinuses, and the nasopharynx. The nasal cavity consists anteriorly of the nasal vestibule, the small hair-bearing region just inside the nasal ostia, with the remainder representing the nasal antrum; the nasal cavity has four walls, a central dividing septum, and paired upper, middle, and lower turbinates. The nasal vestibule lining is an extension of the surrounding facial skin and as such has a stratified, keratinizing squamous epithelium with associated skin-type appendages and hair; it extends for 1 to 2 cm into the nasal cavity. The nasal antrum is lined by pseudostratified ciliated columnar (respiratory-type) epithelium of ectodermal origin referred to as the Schneiderian membrane (e-**Fig. 3.1**). The lamina propria beneath consists of minor-salivary gland-type mucoserous glands embedded in fibrovascular connective tissue with small ducts that convey their secretions to the surface. The turbinates have a more richly vascular stroma. The roof of the nasal cavity contains the cribriform plate with olfactory mucosa, a modified respiratory-type epithelium with olfactory nerve cells and supporting cells.

B. **Paranasal Sinuses.** The paranasal sinuses consist of the maxillary (largest), frontal, sphenoid, and ethmoid sinuses. They drain into the nasal cavity and are air-filled, intraosseous, and open. The ethmoid sinuses are small and complex (referred to as the ethmoid labyrinth or air cells). All paranasal sinuses are in continuity with the nasal cavity so they have a similar, although thinner, mucosa. The lamina propria is also thinner, looser, and less vascular than in the nasal cavity, although it does contain prominent seromucinous glands.

C. **Nasopharynx.** The nasopharynx is the most cephalad portion of the pharynx and is a cuboidal structure. Its roof is formed by the pharyngeal tonsil. The lateral walls are the most pathologically important because they contain the opening of the Eustachian tubes, and a depression posterior to the torus tubarius called the fossa of Rosenmüller. The fossa of Rosenmüller is the most common site of origin for nasopharyngeal carcinoma (NPC). Because the nasopharynx is surrounded by bone and vital structures, it is poorly accessible for surgery. The epithelial lining consists of a mixture of stratified squamous, intermediate (or transitional), and respiratory-type epithelium.

II. GROSS EXAMINATION, TISSUE SAMPLING, AND HISTOLOGIC SLIDE PREPARATION

A. **Endoscopic Biopsies.** The majority of specimens from this region consist of endoscopic forceps biopsies. The small tissue pieces should be placed immediately into 10% buffered formalin or other appropriate fixative. If there is a suspicion of lymphoma, a minimum of three biopsy passes should be submitted in saline or RPMI medium and sent directly for an appropriate hematopathology workup. Standard formalin-fixed specimens should undergo gross examination and description documenting the exact number of pieces present, and then should be entirely submitted for histologic examination (three hematoxylin and eosin [H&E] levels cut per block). For very small specimens, or where few pieces are obtained from clinical masses, it is strongly recommended that additional unstained slides be cut from the block on initial submission for potential use for immunohistochemistry or special stains.

B. **Functional Endoscopic Sinus Surgery (FESS; "sinus contents").** The tissue consists of fragments of ethmoid and maxillary ostium sinus bone and mucosa, resected inflammatory polyps, and nasal cavity and sinus tissue obtained by suction devices. These samples should be described, measured, and submitted for histologic examination. If firm or dense tissue fragments are identified, they should be entirely submitted as they may represent an unsuspected neoplasm. Otherwise, pieces of intact tissue should be collected from the blood and fluid from the suction device, inspected grossly, and measured in aggregate. Only one cassette of these fragments need to be submitted for histologic examination with decalcification in EDTA or formic acid if gross pieces of bone are identified.

C. Resections. Surgical resections for sinonasal tumors are complex and varied, and are guided by tumor location, extent, and type. They always consist of soft tissue, mucosa, and bone. Margins are in large part guided by frozen section. The main specimen should be oriented, the tumor identified, and mucosal, soft tissue, and bone margins identified. The main specimen should be described and measured; the soft tissue margins are inked and then mucosal and soft tissue margin sections sampled. If the tumor is relatively distant from a margin, 1- to 2-mm thick shave sections are preferred; if the tumor approximates a margin (within 1 to 2 mm), radial sections are preferred. After this, the tumor is sectioned and sampled. Four to five sections should be taken from the tumor, or if small, lesion should be entirely submitted for histologic examination. Often sectioning requires a saw to cut through bone to demonstrate the relationship of the lesion to the adjacent structures; the bone should be decalcified, and shave sections from the bone margins as well as sections demonstrating tumor involving bone should be taken.

D. Frozen Sections are a critical element of surgical therapy for head and neck tumors. Although practices vary, most institutions have margins taken as small pieces by the surgeon from the periphery of the surgical defect after the tumor has been removed. The pieces should be evaluated grossly for mucosa (which is typically shiny and pink-tan on one surface of the tissue); if present, the tissue should be oriented to demonstrate this mucosal surface on one edge of the section. Two to three high quality sections should be obtained with the second and third levels taken deep into the tissue to ensure adequate sampling.

The tissue that remains after a frozen section should be submitted for evaluation on permanent sections. This is done to further assure adequate sampling of the tissue and to help resolve possible questions from the time of frozen section including freezing and cautery artifacts, amount of tumor represented, and orientation/embedding issues. The final margin status is therefore a conglomerate of the frozen section slides, permanent slides of the frozen tissue, and the margins of the resection specimen itself.

III. DIAGNOSTIC FEATURES OF COMMON DISEASES

A. Inflammation and Infection. These processes are extremely common necessitating a large amount of medical care and surgery.

1. **Acute rhinosinusitis.** Acute sinusitis is rarely seen by the pathologist because it is treated medically. However, typical histologic findings include neutrophils migrating through, and present in, the respiratory-type mucosa with luminal contents showing necrotic material, apoptotic neutrophil nuclear debris, and mucin with abundant neutrophils.

2. **Chronic rhinosinusitis.** Chronic inflammation of the nasal cavity can result from allergy, upper respiratory tract infections, or cystic fibrosis. Sinusitis is thought to occur secondary to obstruction of the outflow of the paranasal sinuses by myriad etiologies such as edema and inflammation, or anatomic abnormalities (particularly in children). Some of the most common obstructing agents are inflammatory polyps, a deviated septum, or concha bullosa (air pocket in the middle turbinate). Finally, rare genetic conditions such as immotile cilia syndrome (Kartagener syndrome) cause chronic sinusitis. Complications include secondary bacterial infection and, in chronic allergic sinusitis, the development of inflammatory polyps.

Specimens from FESS in chronic sinusitis typically show edema of the submucosa with a mixture of lymphocytes, plasma cells, and eosinophils, the latter sometimes being quite prominent. The abundance and distribution of eosinophils histologically do not have a clinical correlate other than suggesting allergy as an underlying etiology for the sinusitis.

3. **Wegener granulomatosis** is an autoimmune disorder characterized by a necrotizing vasculitis that affects the nasal cavity and paranasal sinuses, pulmonary, and/or renal systems. Manifestations of nasal cavity/paranasal sinus involvement include rhinorrhea, sinusitis, headache, nasal obstruction, anosmia, and sometimes middle ear and mastoid symptoms if inflammation obstructs the Eustachian tube.

Histologically, in biopsies of the sinonasal region, the diagnosis can be quite difficult. Features include mucosal ulceration, acute and chronic inflammation, necrosis, and granulomas. Wegener granulomatosis causes a vasculitis which is often obscured by the inflammation, so elastic stains such as Verhoeff Van Gieson may be helpful to demonstrate the elastic fibers of inflamed vessels. The vasculitis involves arterioles, small arteries, and veins with changes ranging from fibrinoid necrosis with neutrophils and associated extravasated red blood cells and fibrin thrombi, to granulomatous inflammation with multinucleated giant cells and histiocytes (e-**Fig. 3.2**). It is very important to correlate the histologic findings with clinical information and laboratory investigation, the latter of which reveals cytoplasmic antineutrophil antibodies (cANCA) in approximately 90% of patients.

4. **Inflammatory polyps.** Sinonasal inflammatory polyps are nonneoplastic mucosal and submucosal projections that arise in longstanding chronic rhinitis, usually associated with allergy or asthma. They are seen most commonly in adults but can be seen in children as well, particularly in those with cystic fibrosis. Symptoms include headache, nasal obstruction, and rhinorrhea. They are multiple, often bilateral, and most commonly arise from the lateral nasal wall. Although nonneoplastic, they are capable of dramatic behavior including deviation of the septum, destruction of bone, extension into the nasopharynx, and rarely extension into the orbit or cranial cavities.

Grossly, inflammatory polyps can measure up to several centimeters and are boggy, gelatinous, and partially translucent with broad bases. Microscopically, there is a highly edematous or myxoid stroma with a mixed inflammatory infiltrate of lymphocytes, plasma cells, and a variable number of eosinophils. There are few small vessels and minimal bland spindled stromal cells. Inflammatory polyps are typically devoid of seromucinous glands, a feature that is particularly helpful in identifying them when they are in fragmented pieces (e-**Fig. 3.3**). The surface is typically intact and lined by respiratory epithelium with a variably thickened basement membrane; squamous metaplasia is occasionally present.

5. **Fungal infections** are relatively frequent and can involve any of the paranasal sinuses. They can be broadly classified as "invasive" and "noninvasive" (Table 3.1).

   a. **Noninvasive.** Immunocompetent patients usually develop noninvasive fungal disease, either allergic fungal sinusitis or mycetoma ("fungus ball"). Clinically, they have similar presentations with symptoms of chronic sinusitis including headache, nasal discharge, stuffiness, and facial pressure.

   Allergic fungal sinusitis patients have asthma (present in >90% of cases), eosinophilia, atopy, and elevated total fungus-specific immunoglobulin E (IgE) concentrations. Endoscopy reveals thick, sticky, greenish or black to brown mucus, often described as the consistency of peanut butter. Microscopically, abundant brightly eosinophilic hypocellular mucin is present, distinct from slightly basophilic normal mucin. The mucin contains sheets of eosinophils that are degenerating and degranulating. These granules may coalesce to form the classic Charcot–Leyden crystals (e-**Fig. 3.4**). The most common causative organisms are dematiaceous fungi such as *Bipolaris, Curvularia, Alternaria,* and also *Aspergillus.* Fungal hyphae are fragmented and widely scattered in the mucin so they are rarely visible by H&E; special stains such as Grocott's Methenamine Silver (GMS) are usually necessary to demonstrate the presence of hyphae. If the typical histologic picture is present without identifying organisms, the term *allergic mucin* is used. If hyphae are identified, the term *allergic fungal sinusitis* is used.

TABLE 3.1	Fungal Sinusitis		
Entity	Clinical	Histology	Organism
Noninvasive: Allergic fungal sinusitis	Chronic sinusitis; inflammatory polyps; allergic symptoms; pan-sinusitis	Eosinophilic mucus; sheets of degenerating eosinophils; Charcot–Leyden crystals; sometimes fragmented hyphae in mucus	*Aspergillus;* dematiaceous fungi: *Bipolaris, Alternaria, Curvularia, Cladosporium*
Noninvasive: Mycetoma ("Fungus ball")	Chronic sinusitis, mass lesion on imaging—usually one sinus cavity; usually nonallergic type presentation	Large intraluminal collections of fungal hyphae; minimal mucus; minimal inflammation	*Aspergillus;* dematiaceous fungi: *Bipolaris, Alternaria, Curvularia, Cladosporium*
Invasive: Acute invasive fungal sinusitis	Severe acute sinusitis; fever; nasal discharge; ocular or neurologic deficits	Necrosis; thrombosis; hemorrhage; angioinvasive fungal hyphae in viable tissue; minimal inflammation	Common: Mucorales order—*Mucor, Rhizopus, Absidia, Cunninghamella* Uncommon: *Aspergillus, Curvularia, Alternaria*
Invasive: Chronic invasive fungal sinusitis	Slow, progressive onset; neurologic or orbital deficits; mass on imaging	Necrosis; angioinvasive fungal hyphae; granulomas	*Aspergillus*

Patients with mycetoma have chronic sinusitis but less often allergic symptoms. On endoscopy, the single affected sinus has mucopurulent, cheesy, or claylike material that microscopically consists of sheets of fungal hyphae with minimal mucin and inflammatory cells (e-**Fig. 3.5**).

b. Invasive. Patients with invasive fungal disease are usually immunocompromised, usually due to diabetes mellitus, bone marrow or solid organ transplantation, or occasionally human immunodeficiency virus (HIV) infection, and are at great risk of morbidity and mortality.

Patients are often severely ill with fever, cough, nasal discharge, headache, and mental status changes. They sometimes have ophthalmologic symptoms or neurologic deficits due to orbital or cranial involvement. On endoscopy, there are dark ulcers on the mucosa and associated black, greasy necrotic tissue. The fungi are angioinvasive so they cause extensive hemorrhage and necrosis. In the viable tissue, the microscopic findings include minimal inflammation and blood vessels filled with refractile fungal hyphae (e-**Fig. 3.6**). The order *Mucorales* is the most common (e.g., *Mucor, Rhizopus, Absidia*), but other fungi including *Aspergillus* species may be causative. The morphology of *Mucor* species includes bizarre, angulated hyphal fragments and elongated hyphae that are wide, irregular, and thick walled. Typically there is 90-degree angle branching without septation. Diabetics may also develop a chronic pattern of invasive fungal disease, often presenting as a slowly progressive orbital mass; microscopically, angioinvasive hyphae or granulomas are often present in these patients.

B. Nonneoplastic Lesions. A number of lesions, developmental or mechanical, can occur in the sinonasal region and can be mass-like and simulate true neoplasms.

1. Mucous impaction is an uncommon lesion that occurs mostly in children and young adults with a long history of chronic sinusitis. It represents impaction of a large amount of mucus within the maxillary antrum. Grossly, it consists of translucent gray to pink material. Microscopically, it simply consists of slightly basophilic to eosinophilic extracellular mucin with a mixture of plasma cells, lymphocytes, and neutrophils with desquamated respiratory-type epithelium.

2. **Paranasal sinus mucoceles** are chronic, nonneoplastic cysts that form from obstruction of the sinus outlet by any of a number of processes. They occur most commonly in the ethmoid and frontal sinuses. Grossly, they consist of a cyst filled with mucoid or gelatinous material. Microscopically, they consist of extracellular mucin with a flattened respiratory-type epithelial lining that may have secondary squamous metaplasia.

3. **Respiratory epithelial adenomatoid hamartoma** (REAH) is a rare, benign lesion characterized by an adenomatoid proliferation of respiratory-type epithelium that occurs primarily on the posterior nasal septum. Microscopically, it consists of a polypoid proliferation of variably sized, round to oval glands lined by respiratory-type epithelium with a markedly thickened basement membrane and no cytologic atypia or significant mitotic activity (e-**Fig. 3.7**). The gland-like structures are often in direct continuity with the surface epithelium (e-**Fig. 3.8**). The stroma is edematous and resembles that of an inflammatory polyp.

C. **Neoplastic Lesions.** A wide array of neoplasms occur in the sinonasal region, paranasal sinuses, and nasopharynx (Tables 3.2 and 3.3, respectively).

1. **Benign**

a. **Schneiderian papillomas.** The ectodermally derived Schneiderian membrane gives rise to three different types of benign papillomas: exophytic, inverted, and oncocytic (Table 3.4). The distinction of these papillomas is important because of their differences in behavior and risk of carcinoma development. For this reason, it is critical to submit all papilloma tissue for microscopic examination.

i. **Exophytic papilloma** (fungiform papilloma). The vast majority of these occur on the nasal septum, particularly anteriorly, in adults 20 to 50 years old. They are more common in men. Human papillomavirus (HPV; specifically the low risk types HPV 6 and 11) has been detected in a significant number of cases, so the virus may be important for pathogenesis. Exophytic papillomas are usually solitary and discrete, and patients present with epistaxis, unilateral nasal obstruction, or an asymptomatic mass.

Clinically and grossly they are warty, gray-pink, nontranslucent growths with a broad base. Microscopically, they consist of exophytic papillary fronds lined by a variably thickened epithelium that varies from squamous to respiratory-type to a transitional form with features of both (e-**Fig. 3.9**). Scattered mucin-containing cells are usually present, and the lining characteristically has abundant intraepithelial neutrophils, some in small collections simulating microabscesses. Surface keratinization is absent except in rare cases in which the lesion has been traumatized. There is minimal mitotic activity and no cytologic atypia.

After complete removal, exophytic papillomas recur locally in less than 25% of cases. However, there is no significant risk for developing carcinoma.

ii. **Inverted papilloma.** This is the most common type of Schneiderian papilloma and occurs primarily in adults between 40 and 70 years old. It characteristically arises from the lateral nasal wall in the region of the middle turbinate and ethmoid recesses, frequently extending into the sinuses. Only 8% of inverted papillomas arise from the nasal septum. They are only rarely bilateral. HPV, of numerous different serotypes, can be detected in up to 50% of cases.

Grossly, the lesion is fleshy, pink-tan, and papillary or polypoid. Microscopically, inverted papillomas are composed of numerous basement membrane–enclosed, rounded ribbons of thickened epithelium identical to that seen in exophytic papillomas, ranging from squamous to transitional to respiratory-type (e-**Figs. 3.10** and **3.11**). There is minimal mitotic activity, no significant cytologic atypia, and the epithelium characteristically has abundant intraepithelial neutrophils, singly and in clusters, as well as numerous

TABLE 3.2	WHO Histologic Classification of Tumors of the Nasal Cavity, Paranasal Sinuses, and Skull Base

Carcinomas

Keratinizing squamous cell carcinoma

Nonkeratinizing squamous cell carcinoma

Spindle cell squamous cell carcinoma

Lymphoepithelial carcinoma

Sinonasal undifferentiated carcinoma

NUT carcinoma

Neuroendocrine carcinoma
    Small cell neuroendocrine carcinoma
    Large cell neuroendocrine carcinoma

Adenocarcinoma
    Intestinal-type adenocarcinoma
    Nonintestinal-type adenocarcinoma

Teratocarcinosarcoma

Sinonasal papillomas

Sinonasal papilloma, inverted type

Sinonasal papilloma, oncocytic type

Sinonasal papilloma, exophytic type

Respiratory epithelial lesions

Respiratory epithelial adenomatoid hamartoma

Seromucinous hamartoma

Salivary gland tumors

Pleomorphic adenoma

Malignant soft tissue tutors

Fibrosarcoma

Undifferentiated pleomorphic sarcoma

Leiomyosarcoma

Rhabdomyosarcoma, NOS

Embryonal rhabdomyosarcoma

Alveolar rhabdomyosarcoma

Pleomorphic rhabdomyosarcoma, adult type

Spindle cell rhabdomyosarcoma

Angiosarcoma

Malignant peripheral nerve sheath tumor

Biphenotypic sinonasal sarcoma

Borderline/low-grade malignant soft tissue tutors

Desmoid-type fibromatosis

Sinonasal glomangiopericytoma

Solitary fibrous tumor

Epithelioid hemangioendothelioma

Benign soft tissue tutors

Leiomyoma

Hemangioma

Schwannoma

Neurofibroma

Other tumors

Meningioma

Sinonasal ameloblastoma

Chondromesenchymal hamartoma

Hematolymphoid tumors

Extranodal NK/T-cell lymphoma

Extraosseous plasmacytoma

Neuroectodermal/melanocytic tumors

Ewing sarcoma/primitive neuroectodermal tumor

Olfactory neuroblastoma

Mucosal melanoma

From El-Naggar AK, Chan JKC, Grandis JR, Takata T, Slootweg PJ, eds. *WHO Classification of Head and Neck Tumours.* Lyon, France: IARC Press; 2017. Used with permission.

mucin-filled microcysts. Some inverted papillomas can have a prominent exophytic-appearing component. However, any Schneiderian papilloma with a significant inverted and/or downward pushing component (more than just rare nests) should be diagnosed as an inverted papilloma.

Uncommonly, there is surface keratinization, and 5% to 20% of these lesions show varying degrees of dysplasia. Interestingly, dysplasia by itself does not signify malignancy or a different clinical course for the patient, but it does make it important to thoroughly evaluate the lesion for coexisting carcinoma. Approximately 10% to 15% of inverted papillomas are complicated by carcinoma, mostly squamous cell carcinoma. A significant number of inverted papillomas will recur, particularly after conservative removal.

iii. **Oncocytic papillomas** are the least common Schneiderian papillomas and have a variety of alternate names including cylindrical cell and columnar cell

TABLE 3.3 WHO Histologic Classification of Tumors of the Nasopharynx

Carcinomas	**Soft tissue tumors**
Nasopharyngeal carcinoma	Nasopharyngeal angiofibroma
Nonkeratinizing squamous cell carcinoma	**Hematolymphoid tumors**
Keratinizing squamous cell carcinoma	Diffuse large B-cell lymphoma
Basaloid squamous cell carcinoma	Extraosseous plasmacytoma
Nasopharyngeal papillary adenocarcinoma	Extramedullary myeloid sarcoma
Salivary gland tumors	**Notochordal tumors**
Adenoid cystic carcinoma	Chordoma
Salivary gland anlage tumor	
Benign borderline lesions	
Hairy polyp	
Ectopic pituitary adenoma	
Craniopharyngioma	

From El-Naggar AK, Chan JKC, Grandis JR, Takata T, Slootweg PJ, eds. *WHO Classification of Head and Neck Tumours.* Lyon, France: IARC Press; 2017. Used with permission.

papilloma. They occur in the same sites as inverted papillomas, namely, the lateral nasal wall and paranasal sinuses. Unlike other Schneiderian papillomas, they have an equal male to female ratio, and studies have not identified an association with HPV.

Microscopically, they typically have a mixture of exophytic and endophytic components and are lined by a unique two- to eight-cell layer of tall columnar oncocytic cells that have abundant granular eosinophilic cytoplasm. The nuclei are slightly more atypical than in other Schneiderian papillomas with a wrinkled, dark to slightly vesicular appearance with small nucleoli. The epithelium contains numerous mucin-filled microcysts and intraepithelial neutrophils (e-**Fig. 3.12**).

Oncocytic papillomas have a risk of local recurrence and carcinoma similar to that of inverted papillomas.

TABLE 3.4 Schneiderian Papillomas

Type	Common Location	Pathology	Behavior
Exophytic	Nasal septum	Exophytic fronds of bland epithelium—squamous, transitional, or respiratory-type; intraepithelial neutrophils and microcysts; thin basement membranes	Local recurrence; essentially no risk of invasive carcinoma
Inverted	Lateral nasal wall; paranasal sinuses	Pushing, endophytic nests of bland epithelium—squamous, transitional, or respiratory-type; lesser exophytic component at times; intraepithelial neutrophils and microcysts; thin basement membranes	Local recurrence; ~10% risk of invasive carcinoma
Oncocytic	Lateral nasal wall; paranasal sinuses	Exophytic and endophytic pushing nests of columnar, oncocytic cells with abundant, granular eosinophilic cytoplasm; intraepithelial neutrophils and microcysts	Local recurrence; ~5–15% risk of invasive carcinoma

b. **Verruca vulgaris (nasal vestibule).** As the nasal vestibule is essentially an extension of the surrounding nasal skin, verrucae occur in this location and have the same morphology as elsewhere (see Chapter 38).

2. **Malignant**

a. **Sinonasal undifferentiated carcinoma (SNUC).** This tumor is a clinicopathologically distinct, aggressive form of sinonasal carcinoma. Patients are most commonly in their sixth decade and present with symptoms of short duration including nasal obstruction and epistaxis, and often have orbital or cranial nerve deficits. The tumor most often arises in the nasal cavity, particularly anteriorly, or in the maxillary or ethmoid sinuses. It is usually bulky, often involving contiguous sites.

There are no unique gross features. Tumors are usually greater than 4 cm, poorly defined, and invade bone. Microscopically, different growth patterns can be seen including nested, trabecular, or lobular, although the nests are not usually well defined. The tumor cells are small to moderate in size, have a small to moderate amount of cytoplasm with distinct cell borders, and have nuclei that range from hyperchromatic to vesicular, often with prominent nucleoli. Despite being overtly malignant, the individual tumor cells are remarkably regular in size. There is abundant apoptosis, brisk mitotic activity, and often prominent necrosis (e-**Fig. 3.13**). By definition, there is a lack of definable differentiation.

Immunohistochemistry is positive for pan-cytokeratin and epithelial membrane antigen. More specifically, simple keratins such as 7, 8, and 19 are present, whereas complex keratins such as 5/6 are absent. Neuron-specific enolase (NSE) is positive in up to 50% of cases, but more specific neuroendocrine markers such as chromogranin A and synaptophysin are negative or show very minimal staining.

SNUC is very aggressive with a mean survival of 4 to 18 months despite aggressive surgery and radiation therapy.

b. **Nasopharyngeal carcinoma (NPC).** Although still relatively uncommon in the United States, NPC is important because of its relationship to Epstein–Barr Virus (EBV) and because of specific geographic predilections (it is particularly common in the so-called "endemic" areas of Asia and North Africa). The World Health Organization (WHO) classification (2017) recognizes three major types: keratinizing squamous cell carcinoma, nonkeratinizing squamous cell carcinoma, and basaloid squamous cell carcinoma (Table 3.3). NPC occurs in all age groups, with a peak incidence between 30 and 50 years of age. It is not uncommon in adolescents. Patients present with symptoms of a sinonasal mass, including nasal obstruction and epistaxis but may also have serous otitis media from Eustachian tube obstruction or, not infrequently, an asymptomatic neck mass from metastasis. The clinical and macroscopic appearance is nondescript.

Microscopically, the keratinizing type has a morphology identical to that of keratinizing squamous cell carcinoma elsewhere in the head and neck and is graded similarly, from well to poorly differentiated (e-**Fig. 3.14**).

The nonkeratinizing type is often subclassified morphologically into undifferentiated and differentiated subtypes which have no clinical or prognostic importance. Histologically, the differentiated subtype can have surface disease with stratified cells that have an appearance similar to that of urothelial carcinoma of the urinary bladder. The cells are moderately atypical with well-defined cell borders and a sharp interface of tumor with the surrounding stroma (e-**Fig. 3.15**). The undifferentiated subtype is more common, most distinctive, and most challenging. It consists of syncytial aggregates/sheets of tumor cells with moderate eosinophilic cytoplasm; large, vesicular nuclei with prominent nucleoli; and a brisk mixed chronic inflammatory infiltrate (e-**Fig. 3.16**). Occasionally, the cells are dispersed in small clusters or as single cells making the diagnosis of carcinoma difficult. Apoptosis and brisk mitotic activity are invariably present.

Basaloid squamous cell carcinoma, the least common type, has a morphology identical to that seen in the same tumor in other regions of the head and neck (e-**Figs. 3.17** and **3.18**).

NPC has a number of interesting clinicopathologic features. First, given the location and anatomy of the nasopharynx, radiation therapy is the first-line treatment modality. Surgery is uncommon and usually reserved for salvage therapy. Second, although EBV is strongly related to the tumorigenesis of nonkeratinizing NPC, in keratinizing NPC this relationship is tenuous at best. Third, nonkeratinizing NPC tends to metastasize to lymph nodes early (60% to 85% overall), often to the posterior triangle (level V), and these tumors have a different staging system that reflects this unique behavior (see AJCC staging below). Finally, despite advanced disease, nonkeratinizing NPC responds well to systemic therapy (5-year survival of approximately 65% in the United States). Keratinizing NPC, although it more often presents with localized disease, does not respond well to therapy (5-year survival of approximately 20% to 40% in the United States).

c. **Squamous cell carcinoma/cylindrical cell carcinoma.** Squamous cell carcinoma is the most common carcinoma in most head and neck anatomic subsites, and constitutes approximately 65% of carcinomas in the nasal cavity and paranasal sinuses. When it occurs in the nasopharynx, it is designated *keratinizing squamous cell carcinoma*. Keratinizing, or typical, squamous cell carcinoma of the nasal cavity and paranasal sinuses has the same morphology as that occurring elsewhere in the upper aerodigestive tract. Squamous cell carcinoma of this subsite, unlike other head and neck subsites, has only a modest association with smoking. However, tumors have been related to other exposures including nickel, chlorophenols, and textile dust.

A distinct variant of nonkeratinizing squamous cell carcinoma occurs in this region, the so-called cylindrical cell (Schneiderian or transitional) carcinoma. The recent WHO classification simply terms it *nonkeratinizing carcinoma*. It has a papillary configuration with ribbons of invaginating tumor composed of pleomorphic cells without keratinization. These ribbons have a smooth border without clear stromal infiltration, which makes identification of invasion difficult (e-**Fig. 3.19**). This tumor type has been associated with HPV and is also reported to have a better prognosis, although the latter contention is still controversial.

d. **HPV-related carcinoma with adenoid cystic-like features** is a provisional entity in the 2017 edition of the WHO classification, only mentioned as a differential diagnosis of nonkeratinizing squamous cell carcinoma. It is not yet considered a distinct pathologic entity due to the small number of cases reported, variable histology, and uncertain prognostic significance. The tumor occurs over a wide age range (40 to 73 years), with a mean of 55 years, and arises in the nasal cavity and paranasal sinuses. Like other tumors of the sinonasal tract, the presenting symptoms are nonspecific, including nasal obstruction and epistaxis.

There are no unique gross features. Histologically, HPV-related carcinoma with adenoid cystic-like features shows morphologic characteristics that resemble true adenoid cystic carcinoma. It consists of a cellular proliferation of basaloid cells growing as solid nests and trabeculae, with the majority of cases showing focal cribriform architecture with microcystic spaces. The basaloid cells have hyperchromatic, angulated nuclei, a high nucleus-to-cytoplasmic ratio, and can have some cell spindling or clearing. In addition, the tumor can harbor inconspicuous ducts with eosinophilic cuboidal cells. Mitotic figures are evident and necrosis is often present. Another distinct feature found in most cases is the presence of squamous dysplasia of the surface epithelium. In contrast to true adenoid cystic carcinomas, perineural invasion is uncommon.

HPV-related carcinoma with adenoid cystic-like features shows similar immunophenotypic features of true adenoid cystic carcinoma, with two cell populations. The basaloid cells stain with myoepithelial markers such as S100, calponin, p63, and actin. The tumor ductal cells are positive for c-kit and CK7. The tumor is positive for high-risk HPV types (positive for p16 by RNA in situ hybridization), with most cases harboring the uncommon HPV type 33. Contrary to classical adenoid cystic carcinoma, the tumor does not contain an *MYB* gene fusion.

Prognostic data are limited due to the small number of cases reported and absence of long-term follow-up. However, the available data (median follow-up of 15 months) show that most patients are alive without evidence of disease, or with local recurrence.

e. **NUT carcinoma** was recently included in the 2017 edition of the WHO classification. It is a poorly differentiated carcinoma (often with evidence of squamous differentiation) defined by rearrangement of the *NUT* gene. This rare tumor can affect patients of any age (0.1 to 82 years), though it is more common in young patients (median 22 years). Most cases from the head and neck occur in the nasal cavity and paranasal sinuses, but the tumor can affect virtually any site. The tumor is generally, but not always, located in the midline (hence also known as NUT midline carcinoma). Patients with NUT carcinoma present with nonspecific symptoms of a rapidly growing mass, including nasal obstruction, epistaxis, pain, and orbital symptoms. Imaging frequently shows extensive local invasion into neighboring structures such as the orbit and cranial cavity. Approximately half of cases present with lymph node involvement or distant metastases.

There are no unique macroscopic features. The histology is that of an undifferentiated/poorly differentiated carcinoma, with tumor cells growing in sheets (e-**Figs. 3.20** and **3.21**). The nuclei are round to oval, with moderate nuclear enlargement. The chromatin is vesicular with distinct nucleoli. The cytoplasm varies from scant to moderate, and can be clear. Mitotic figures are conspicuous and necrosis is often present. Intratumoral acute inflammation may be present. The two histologic hallmarks of NUT carcinoma are monotonous tumor cells and the presence of abrupt keratinization; glandular and mesenchymal differentiation, although described, is infrequent.

The diagnosis of NUT carcinoma is established by demonstration of *NUT* rearrangement by immunohistochemistry (nuclear staining in >50% of tumor cells), which has 87% sensitivity and 100% specificity. Other methods of demonstrating *NUT* rearrangement include FISH, RT-PCR, conventional cytogenetics, and targeted next-generation sequencing. Other than NUT, the tumor cells are commonly immunopositive for p63, p40, and cytokeratins; CD34 is positive in 55% of cases. Occasional positivity for neuroendocrine markers, P16, and TTF-1 has been described.

The differential diagnosis of NUT carcinoma is broad and includes olfactory neuroblastoma, primitive neuroectodermal tumor, melanoma, squamous cell carcinoma, and SNUC. The tumor has a poor prognosis (medial overall survival of 9.8 months) despite treatment.

f. **SMARCB1-deficient carcinoma** is part of a family of malignant tumors that have in common the loss of the tumor suppressor gene *SMARCB1* (*INI-1*). This neoplasm is considered an emerging entity but was not recognized as a distinct tumor type in the 2017 WHO classification. It is rare, presenting in patients over a wide age range (19 to 89 years, median 52 years), with a slight male predominance. The nasoethmoidal region is the most frequently affected site. Patients develop nonspecific symptoms caused by a rapidly growing mass such as nasal obstruction, facial pain, and epistaxis. Most patients (80%) present with high stage tumors (pT4).

Macroscopically, SMARCB1 carcinoma is a large destructive lesion associated with degeneration and necrosis. Histologically, the tumor has an undifferentiated/basaloid morphology and can resemble SNUC or nonkeratinizing carcinoma (e-**Figs. 3.22** and **3.23**). The distinct morphologic feature is the presence of rhabdoid to plasmacytoid cells that are arranged in clusters or as isolated, scattered cells. By immunohistochemistry, the tumor cells are negative for INI-1, react with several cytokeratins and p40, and show variable reactivity for p63, CK5/6, and

CK7. The tumor cells can also show focal staining for the neuroendocrine markers synaptophysin, chromogranin, and CD56, but usually not all three.

Treatment consists of radical surgery with combined chemoradiation but, in spite of treatment, there is rapid clinical progression and consequently high mortality (56% of patients die of disease with a median survival of 15 months).

g. Salivary gland–type tumors constitute a small percentage of sinonasal neoplasms. They arise from submucosal seromucinous glands. The most common are adenoid cystic carcinoma and pleomorphic adenoma, although almost all other types have been described (e-Figs. 3.24 to 3.26). They are morphologically identical to their counterparts elsewhere.

h. Adenocarcinoma. Primary nonsalivary gland type adenocarcinomas of the sinonasal region are uncommon. The WHO classifies them as intestinal and nonintestinal types, the latter of which are subdivided into high and low grade tumors.

i. Intestinal type. Primary intestinal-type adenocarcinomas (ITACs) of the sinonasal region typically arise from the ethmoid sinuses or high in the nasal cavity. They have a strong association with long-term occupational exposures, specifically wood dust (in carpenters), leather dust, nickel, or chromium compounds. The latency period is several decades. Microscopically, these tumors recapitulate gastrointestinal adenocarcinomas, including very well-differentiated tumors resembling colonic adenomas, typical "colonic-appearing" tumors with columnar glands with or without mucinous differentiation (e-Fig. 3.27), and high-grade tumors with a signet-ring cell morphology.

By immunohistochemistry, they are positive for cytokeratin 20, CDX-2, MUC2, and villin, similar to gastrointestinal adenocarcinoma. Cytokeratin 7 is variably positive and carcinoembryonic antigen (CEA) is usually positive. As such, they stain essentially identical to gastrointestinal adenocarcinomas, so it can be very difficult to separate them from the rare metastasis to this region from a primary gastrointestinal adenocarcinoma.

ITACs should be graded from poorly to well-differentiated, and the type (colonic, mucinous, papillary, signet ring cell, or solid) specified, as both have prognostic significance. The mortality rate is approximately 50% overall.

ii. Nonintestinal type. These are uncommon tumors, most of which are low grade and have a predilection for the ethmoid sinus. Low-grade tumors have a glandular or papillary growth pattern with numerous uniform, small glands arranged back-to-back and lined by a single layer of cuboidal to columnar cells with a moderate amount of eosinophilic to clear cytoplasm and round nuclei. There is only mild nuclear pleomorphism, modest mitotic activity without atypical forms, and no necrosis. High-grade tumors typically occur in the maxillary sinus and have similar histologic features, but also have solid areas and show moderate to severe nuclear pleomorphism with brisk mitotic activity and necrosis.

By immunohistochemistry, nonintestinal-type adenocarcinomas are positive for cytokeratin 7 and negative for cytokeratin 20, CDX-2, and MUC2. Smooth muscle actin and p63 are negative. The prognosis for low-grade tumors is excellent, but for high-grade tumors is quite poor.

i. Neuroendocrine carcinomas occasionally arise in the sinonasal region and are morphologically identical to those arising in the lung.

i. Low-grade neuroendocrine carcinoma (i.e., carcinoid tumor) is extremely rare in this region.

ii. High-grade neuroendocrine carcinoma (small cell carcinoma) is a rapidly proliferating, aggressive neoplasm that presents with epistaxis, nasal obstruction, and exophthalmos. It usually presents at an advanced stage with extensive local disease and lymph node or distant metastases. Microscopically, it consists of nests and sheets of small- to intermediate-sized blue cells with minimal cytoplasm, speckled chromatin, frequent nuclear molding, and crush artifact (e-**Fig. 3.28**). Apoptosis is abundant, and there is brisk mitotic activity and necrosis. By immunohistochemistry, it is positive for pancytokeratin with a "dotlike" paranuclear staining pattern (e-**Fig. 3.29A**). It is variably positive for the neuroendocrine markers CD56, synaptophysin, and chromogranin A, but in most cases at least one of these markers is positive on careful inspection (e-**Fig. 3.29B**). The tumor is negative for S-100, CD99 (O13), and cytokeratin 20.

j. Melanoma. Primary malignant melanoma of the sinonasal tract constitutes approximately 1% of all melanomas. It is more common in the nasal cavity than in the paranasal sinuses, and most patients are over 50 years old. The tumor most often occurs on the middle or inferior turbinates, or anterior septum. Although variable, the typical macroscopic appearance is a sessile or polypoid lesion with mucosal ulceration. Most lesions are heavily pigmented with a brown or black color. Microscopically, melanoma has a wide range of appearances, although usually it is composed of high grade epithelioid cells. Some tumors have a mixture of epithelioid and spindle cells. A junctional component with pagetoid spread of melanocytes in the intact mucosa is also sometimes present.

Immunohistochemistry results are the same as for melanomas at other sites, with virtually all tumors expressing S-100, HMB-45, and melan-A. Cytokeratin reactivity, if present, is only focal.

Metastasis of melanoma to the sinonasal region from another primary site is not particularly uncommon and should always be considered. Although metastases can recapitulate a primary lesion, a junctional component in the surface mucosa essentially rules out metastasis.

The prognosis for sinonasal melanoma is very poor, with frequent local recurrence. Sinonasal melanomas have their own AJCC staging system, and unlike cutaneous melanomas, tumor (Breslow) thickness has not been shown to predict behavior.

k. Olfactory neuroblastoma. This unique tumor arises almost exclusively in the upper nasal cavity from olfactory mucosa on the cribriform plate, upper lateral nasal wall, and superior turbinate. The presumed cell of origin is the reserve cell that gives rise to neuronal and sustentacular cells of the olfactory mucosa. The tumor occurs at any age but most commonly in the third and fourth decades, with symptoms of nasal obstruction, epistaxis, and anosmia.

The neoplasm is usually a unilateral, polypoid mass, microscopically composed of small, round cells that are slightly larger than lymphocytes. The nuclei are round, with uniform to delicately stippled chromatin without nucleoli. Many tumors have areas with fibrillary eosinophilic material reminiscent of neuropil (e-**Fig. 3.30**). Some tumors have a very lobulated and nested growth pattern, whereas others have a diffuse pattern. Homer–Wright rosettes (that have no central lumen) are relatively common. Mitotic activity is low. Necrosis and dystrophic calcification are uncommon. Some tumors have been reported to show significant nuclear pleomorphism and high mitotic activity; however, this is very uncommon and merits consideration of another neoplasm, particularly, high-grade neuroendocrine carcinoma. Rare findings include ganglion cells, melanin-containing cells, and divergent differentiation including glandular, squamous, and teratomatous features.

By immunohistochemistry, olfactory neuroblastoma shows strong cytoplasmic staining for synaptophysin, chromogranin A, and NSE (e-**Fig. 3.31**). S-100 often highlights sustentacular cells at the periphery of tumor nests, but is negative in tumor cells themselves. Although unusual, cytokeratin reactivity has been reported in up to 35% of cases, specifically CAM 5.2 and less often AE1/AE3. The staining is typically weaker and more focal than would be expected in a carcinoma.

Grading systems have been proposed, but their correlation with prognosis has not been consistently demonstrated.

I. Soft tissue tumors

i. Angiofibroma (nasopharyngeal angiofibroma).

This unique tumor is thought to arise from a fibrovascular nidus in the posterolateral nasal wall adjacent to the sphenopalatine foramen. It occurs virtually exclusively in boys aged 10 to 20 years. The tumor often presents as a nasopharyngeal mass due to its pushing, well-circumscribed border, which bulges posteriorly into the nasopharynx as it enlarges, causing nasal obstruction and epistaxis.

Grossly, the tumor is gray-white to tan, smooth, and lobulated, with a homogeneous cut surface. Microscopically, it consists of abundant vessels ranging from capillaries to large vessels, the latter often assuming a "staghorn" appearance (e-**Fig. 3.32**). The vessels are lined by a single layer of endothelial cells that can be flat to slightly plump without cytologic atypia. The vessel wall is typically devoid of smooth muscle and blends imperceptibly with the stromal component of the tumor, which has regularly distributed, plump, stellate spindle cells embedded in a dense collagenous stroma. The stromal cells have vesicular chromatin, sometimes with small nucleoli, but no atypia is present and there is minimal mitotic activity. By immunohistochemistry, the stromal cells are positive for vimentin and negative for smooth muscle actin. The endothelial cells are positive for CD34. Otherwise, the tumors are negative for S-100, desmin, and cytokeratin.

Although the tumor is benign, pressure erosion of the adjacent bone is not uncommon. The virtually exclusive occurrence in adolescent boys, with growth around puberty, is consistent with the fact that androgen receptors can be demonstrated in most cases.

ii. Glomangiopericytoma (sinonasal-type hemangiopericytoma or hemangiopericytoma-like tumor).

This is a somewhat uncommon tumor of perivascular myoid-type cells. All ages can be affected, but patients in their seventh decade predominate. Unilateral nasal cavity involvement is most common, and the tumor is grossly polypoid, beefy-red to gray-pink, and soft. Microscopically, the tumor consists of numerous variably sized vascular channels that classically have a staghorn appearance. The intervascular stroma consists of a proliferation of closely packed cells with round to ovoid nuclei and small amounts of eosinophilic cytoplasm. The tumor cells grow in short fascicles, sometimes with a storiform pattern. There is minimal nuclear pleomorphism, little mitotic activity, and no necrosis (e-**Fig. 3.33**). By immunohistochemistry, the cells are strongly and diffusely positive for smooth muscle and muscle-specific actins, and for vimentin and factor XIIIa. The tumor cells lack strong, diffuse CD34 staining. The prognosis is excellent, with >90% survival at 5 years after surgery, with only a modest recurrence rate.

iii. Alveolar rhabdomyosarcoma.

Rhabdomyosarcoma is a malignant tumor with skeletal muscle differentiation and is the most common sarcoma in childhood. In children, up to 50% of rhabdomyosarcomas occur in the head and neck involving the parameninges, orbit, oral cavity, nasopharynx, sinuses, ear, and neck. Alveolar rhabdomyosarcoma occurs predominantly in children with a median age of 7 to 9 years, but may also arise in adolescents and young adults. In the head and neck region, the alveolar subtype most commonly involves the nose and paranasal sinuses, and presents as a polypoid mass causing dyspnea, epistaxis, facial swelling, and visual disturbances.

Grossly, the lesion has a fleshy to firm tan-gray appearance. Microscopically, the tumor is composed of small to medium-sized cells with hyperchromatic nuclei and scant eosinophilic cytoplasm growing as loosely cohesive sheets separated by fibrous septa (e-**Fig. 3.34**). Multinucleated giant cells with peripheral nuclei are often readily identified (e-**Fig. 3.35**). Cytodifferentiation may be seen, particularly after treatment, manifesting as cells with more abundant eosinophilic fibrillary cytoplasm. By immunohistochemistry, the cells are positive for desmin, muscle specific actin, myoglobin, myoD1, and myogenin (e-**Fig. 3.36**), but negative for cytokeratins. Although the cells may be, confusingly, positive for synaptophysin and chromogranin-A, such staining is not indicative of a neuroendocrine neoplasm.

Alveolar rhabdomyosarcoma is nearly always characterized by one of two characteristic translocations, namely t(1;13), resulting in a *PAX7-FOXO1* fusion transcript (approximately 20% of cases) and t(2;13) resulting in a *PAX3-FOXO1* fusion transcript (approximately 80% of cases). The former is thought to be associated with a better prognosis, but only in the setting of metastatic disease.

iv. **Biphenotypic Sinonasal Sarcoma (BSNS)** was included in the 2017 edition of the WHO classification. It is a low grade spindle cell neoplasm with associated respiratory epithelium, shows reactivity for neural and myogenic markers, and has a distinct *PAX3-MAML3* gene fusion. BSNS tends to occur in females, with a female-to-male ratio of 2:1. The reported age range is 24 to 85 years (mean of 52 years). BSNS typically involves multiple sites in the sinonasal tract, specially the superior aspect of the nasal cavity and ethmoid sinus. Patients with BSNS present with nonspecific symptoms caused by mass effect, such as nasal obstruction and facial pressure.

The typical specimen received in the pathology lab consists of multiple polypoid fragments of red-pink to tan-grey tissue which can be as large as 4 cm in greatest aggregate dimension. Microscopically, the tumor is characterized by an infiltrative spindle cell proliferation arranged in fascicles or in a herringbone pattern (e-**Figs. 3.37** and **3.38**). Hemangiopericytoma-like vessels are common. Tumor nuclei are slender and relatively uniform; mitotic figures and necrosis are inconspicuous. A particular feature of this tumor is its tendency to entrap benign downward invaginations of the sinonasal epithelium which become intimately admixed with the neoplastic spindle cells; this entrapped epithelium can become hyperplastic and undergo squamous or oncocytic metaplasia, mimicking sinonasal papillomas. Rhabdomyoblastic differentiation can be seen in approximately 10% of cases.

By immunohistochemistry, BSNS is immunopositive for S100, SMA, and/or MSA, although these markers show varying degrees of staining from focal to patchy, to diffuse. Focal and/or weak reactivity for CD34, desmin, MYOD1, myogenin, EMA, and cytokeratins has been described in several cases.

As noted above, BSNS characteristically harbors rearrangements of *PAX3*, with the most common partner being *MAML3*. Interestingly, tumors that show rhabdomyoblastic differentiation can have *PAX3-NCOA1* or *PAX3-FOXO1* fusions characteristic of alveolar rhabdomyosarcoma. BSNS normally shows slow, progressive growth. Although nearly half of patients experience local recurrence (as long as 9 years after initial treatment), there are no reports of metastases or death from disease.

IV. PATHOLOGIC REPORTING OF SINONASAL MALIGNANCIES

A. **Staging.** Clinical staging of sinonasal cancers is important for prognosis and treatment, and differs by site. The most recent staging system is that of the American Joint Committee on Cancer (AJCC 8th edition), which includes classification schemes for epithelial malignancies of the nasopharynx, as well as for the nasal cavity and paranasal sinuses. A separate staging scheme is used for mucosal melanomas of the head and neck.

B. **Additional pertinent pathologic features.** A number of pathologic features not reflected in the AJCC staging have been proven important for head and neck squamous cell carcinomas, as well as for numerous tumor types, including perineural invasion, lymphovascular space invasion, and positive margin status. All of these latter features have been demonstrated in numerous studies to correlate with a higher risk of local recurrence, a poorer prognosis, or both. Reporting should follow recommended guidelines (e.g., College of American Pathologists Protocol for the Examination of Specimens From Patients With Cancers of the Nasal Cavity and Paranasal Sinuses; available at http://www.cap.org).

ACKNOWLEDGMENT

The authors thank Heather N. Wright and James S. Lewis Jr., authors of the previous editions of this chapter.

SUGGESTED READINGS

Amin MB, Edge S, Greene F, et al., eds. *AJCC Cancer Staging Manual*. 8th ed. New York: Springer; 2017.

El-Naggar AK, Chan JKC, Grandis JR, Takata T, Slootweg PJ, eds. *World Health Organization Classification of Head and Neck Tumours*. Lyon: IARC Press; 2017.

Prasad ML, Perez-Ordonez B. Nonsquamous lesions of the nasal cavity, paranasal sinuses, and nasopharynx. In: Gnepp DR, ed. *Diagnostic Surgical Pathology of the Head and Neck*. Philadelphia, PA: W.B. Saunders Publishers; 2009.

Thompson LDR, Bishop JA, eds. *Head and Neck Pathology, A Volume* in *the Series Foundations in Diagnostic Pathology*, 3rd ed, Philadelphia, PA: Elsevier; 2019.

Tumors and Cysts of the Jaws

Mena Mansour and Samir K. El-Mofty

I. NORMAL ANATOMY. Of all the bones of the skeleton, the jaws are uniquely distinguished by harboring the odontogenic apparatus of the deciduous and permanent dentitions. The teeth germs are composed of three main components: the enamel organ, the dental papilla, and the tooth follicle. The enamel organ is composed of ectodermally derived epithelial cells, the ameloblasts, and is responsible for enamel formation. The dental papilla is of ectomesenchymal origin and produces the dentine. The tooth follicle is also ectomesenchymal; it surrounds the developing tooth and provides the supporting structures of the formed teeth, the periodontium. The odontogenic tissues may also be a source of a bewildering array of odontogenic cysts and tumors. Nonodontogenic cysts and tumors of the jaws will also be discussed in this chapter.

II. ODONTOGENIC AND NONODONTOGENIC CYSTS. Odontogenic cysts of the mandible and maxilla are relatively common and can present over a large age range. Accurate diagnosis is simplified by location, radiographic correlation, and microscopic examination (e-**Fig. 4.1**). Odontogenic tumors by contrast are uncommon. They may be epithelial, mesenchymal, or mixed; may be noncalcifying; or they may contain hard structures that mimic enamel, dentine, cementum, or bone. Although malignant odontogenic tumors are extremely rare, odontogenic carcinoma, sarcoma, and carcinosarcoma do occur.

A. Odontogenic Cysts. With the exception of a few cysts that may develop along embryonic lines of fusion (known as nonodontogenic cysts), most jaw cysts are lined with epithelium that is derived from the odontogenic epithelium. Odontogenic cysts are classified as either developmental or inflammatory. Various types of odontogenic cysts are listed in Table 4.1.

1. Developmental Odontogenic Cysts

    a. *Dentigerous cyst (follicular cyst)* is a unilocular cyst that forms in association with the crown of an impacted tooth, and is usually associated with a molar or canine. Patients usually present with an asymptomatic, well-defined, expansive, radiolucent lesion. Microscopic examination shows a thin layer of cuboidal to slightly flattened epithelial cells. Focal keratinization, mucous cells, inflammation, and dystrophic calcification are possible. Enucleation and excision of the associated tooth are the treatment of choice. *Eruption cyst* is a subclass of dentigerous cysts associated with the erupting primary or permanent tooth.

    b. *Odontogenic keratocyst (keratocystic odontogenic tumor)* usually presents as an asymptomatic unilocular cyst in the mandible or maxilla. While more frequent in the second to fourth decades, it can be seen at any age. Its incidence is higher in Caucasians and men, and roughly 5% of patients with odontogenic keratocysts have nevoid basal cell carcinoma (Gorlin) syndrome. Gross examination typically yields a cyst containing keratinous debris. Microscopic examination shows palisading basal cells covered by a few layers of squamous cells under a corrugated parakeratotic surface (e-**Fig. 4.2**). A key diagnostic feature is the lack of rete pegs. Satellite cysts and intramural epithelial cell proliferation are more commonly found in the syndrome-associated cases. Exceptionally, dysplasia and carcinoma develop in the cyst. Treatment is surgical excision, and recurrence is common.

    c. *Lateral periodontal cyst* generally presents as a well-demarcated radiolucent lesion in asymptomatic patients in their fifth to seventh decades. The typical locations are the lateral surface of the roots of the mandibular premolar teeth,

TABLE 4.1	Odontogenic Cysts

Developmental
Dentigerous cyst and eruption cyst
Keratocystic odontogenic tumor (odontogenic keratocyst)
Lateral periodontal cyst
Gingival cyst of the adult
Calcifying cystic odontogenic tumor (calcifying odontogenic cyst, Gorlin cyst)
Glandular odontogenic cyst

Inflammatory
Periapical (radicular) cyst
Residual periapical (radicular) cyst

although rare presentations in the maxilla may be encountered. Microscopic examination shows a thin layer of nonkeratinized epithelium with focal thickening and possible clear cells (e-**Fig. 4.3**). The adjacent soft tissue is not inflamed. A rare polycystic variant (botryoid odontogenic cyst) is characterized by rapid growth and an elevated probability of recurrence. Simple excision is typically curative.

d. *Gingival cyst of the adult* is an infrequent lesion appearing on the buccal gingival of the mandible near the premolars and canines. It represents the soft tissue counterpart of the lateral periodontal cyst. Patients are typically in the fifth to sixth decades, and present with a <1-cm gingival cyst that has a normal to bluish overlying mucosal surface. While usually unicystic, rare multicystic gingival cysts (gingival botryoid odontogenic cyst) may be seen. Microscopic examination shows a cyst lined by a thin layer of epithelium with rare focal thickening; the adjacent soft tissue is fibrotic and does not show inflammation. Treatment is simple excision.

e. *Calcifying cystic odontogenic tumor* (calcifying odontogenic cyst, Gorlin cyst) presents as a radiolucent asymptomatic lesion of the maxilla or mandible. The tumor can be unicystic, multicystic, and occasionally solid. Focal radiopaque areas may be identified. The incidence peaks in the second and third decades, although cases occur in all age groups. Microscopic examination shows a proliferating layer of columnar palisaded basal cells similar to ameloblasts. The superficial layers frequently have larger ghost cells characterized by eosinophilic cytoplasm without nuclei (e-**Fig. 4.4**). Calcification of the tumor and adjacent soft tissue can be identified in some cases. Treatment is surgical excision and recurrence is uncommon.

f. *Glandular odontogenic cyst* is a recently defined lesion that has also been referred to as sialo-odontogenic cyst. The majority occur as a radiolucent cyst in the anterior mandible or anterior maxilla. Patients typically present with pain and swelling, but some cases are asymptomatic. Microscopic examination demonstrates a unilocular/multilocular cyst with nonkeratinized epithelium, mucos producing cells, and focal solid areas (e-**Fig. 4.5A,B**). The major histologic criteria include: (1) variable thickness of the lining epithelium, (2) hobnail cells, (3) intraepithelial microcysts, (4) apocrine metaplasia, (5) clear cells, (6) papillary projections, (7) mucus cells, (8) epithelial spheres, (9) cilia, and (10) cystic compartments. The presence of seven or more features is highly suggestive of glandular odontogenic cyst. Care should be taken to differentiate between a glandular odontogenic cyst and a central mucoepidermoid carcinoma. Glandular odontogenic cyst is negative for *MAML2* rearrangement. Surgical excision is the treatment of choice.

2. **Inflammatory Odontogenic Cysts.** *Radicular (periapical) cysts* are associated with a nonviable carious teeth. The usual location is the apical third of the tooth root, with occasional cases involving the lateral root surface. The cyst is more common in the mandible. The typical age of patients is the third to sixth decades. The most common presentation is pain and swelling, but presentation as an incidental finding on routine radiographic examination is not unusual. Microscopic examination reveals

an inflamed, nonkeratinizing, stratified epithelium. Cholesterol crystals, foamy macrophages, dystrophic calcifications, and intraepithelial hyaline bodies (Rushton bodies) may be identified (e-**Fig. 4.6A,B**). The *residual cyst* is a variant of radicular cyst that is seen at the site of an extracted tooth.

B. **Nonodontogenic Cysts.** This class of lesions includes a group of epithelium-lined cysts, as well as nonepithelium-lined bone cysts. The epithelial-lined cysts are believed to arise from epithelial remnants entrapped along embryonic lines of fusion and are referred to as fissural cysts (e-**Fig. 4.7**).

1. **Epithelial-lined nonodontogenic cysts (fissural cysts)**

   a. *Nasopalatine duct cyst (incisive canal cyst)* is the most common of the fissural cysts. It is believed to arise from remnants of the nasopalatine duct. The cyst can develop almost at any age, but is most common in the fourth to sixth decades of life. Most studies show a slight male predilection. The most common presenting symptoms include swelling of the anterior palate, drainage, and pain.

      Radiographs usually demonstrate a well-circumscribed radiolucency, in or near the midline of the anterior maxilla, between and apical to the central incisor teeth. The lesion most often is round oval or pear-shaped. Microscopically, the epithelial lining of the cyst may be stratified squamous, pseudostratified columnar, simple columnar, or cuboidal. Commonly more than one epithelial type is present. Because the cyst arises within the incisive canal, moderate-sized nerves and small muscular arteries and veins are usually found in the cyst wall (e-**Fig. 4.8**). Surgical enucleation is the treatment of choice.

   b. *Globulomaxillary cyst* is believed to develop from epithelium entrapped during fusion of the globular portion of the medial nasal process with the maxillary process, although its origin continues to be a subject of debate.

      The cyst classically develops between the lateral incisor and cuspid teeth, although occasional it has been reported between the central and lateral incisors. Radiographically, the cyst presents as is well-circumscribed unilocular radiolucency between and apical to the teeth. The radiolucency is often pear-shaped. As the cyst expands, tilting of the adjacent teeth may occur. Microscopically, many of the cysts are lined with stratified squamous epithelium. Occasionally, however, the lining epithelium is of pseudostratified columnar ciliated type. Enucleation is the treatment of choice.

   c. *Median palatal cysts (median palatine cysts)* are rare fissural cysts. They are believed to develop from epithelium entrapped along the embryonic line of fusion of the lateral palatal shelves of the maxilla. The cyst may be difficult to distinguish from the nasopalatine duct cysts, and some cases may actually represent a posteriorly placed nasopalatine duct cyst.

      Clinically, the cyst presents as a firm or fluctuant swelling in the midline of the hard palate, posterior to the incisive papilla. It is more frequent in young adults and is often asymptomatic. The average size is 2×2 cm, but these cysts may become quite large. Radiographs demonstrate a well-circumscribed lucency in the midline of the hard palate. Microscopically, the cyst is commonly lined by stratified squamous epithelium, but areas of pseudostratified columnar epithelium may be seen. Surgical removal is the treatment of choice.

2. **Nonepithelial-lined nonodontogenic bone cysts of the jaws**

   a. *Simple bone cysts* are known by multiple names including unicameral bone cyst, solitary bone cyst, progressive bony cavity, hemorrhagic cyst, and traumatic bone cyst. The typical patient is under 20 years old and has a well-demarcated osteolytic solitary lesion in the posterior mandible. Unusual cases have been seen in the maxilla. The cyst cavity is lined by fibrovascular tissue with hemosiderin laden macrophages. Reactive bone and osteoclasts may be identified.

   b. *Aneurysmal bone cyst* is a rapidly enlarging blood filled cystic lesion usually identified in the first three decades of life. The majority are well demarcated, unilateral pseudocysts located in the mandible (60%) and maxilla (40%). Aneurysmal bone cyst may be identified alone, or in conjunction with another lesion (e.g., chondroblastoma, osteoblastoma). CT and MRI studies show characteristic layering of blood cells and serum. Microscopic examination shows a fibrotic stroma with giant cells, macrophages, and hemosiderin granules (e-Fig. 4.9A,B). Areas of ossification may be present. A t(16;17) translocation producing a *CDH11–USP6* gene fusion is seen in about 70% of primary aneurysmal bone cysts. Treatment is curettage and enucleation, and about 25% of the lesions recur.

III. ODONTOGENIC TUMORS. Odontogenic tumors are classified according to their composition into epithelial, mesenchymal, or mixed. Epithelial odontogenic tumors are composed only of odontogenic epithelium, while mesenchymal odontogenic tumors are composed principally of ectomesenchymal elements. Mixed odontogenic tumors contain epithelial and ectomesenchymal tissues. Inductive interactive action between the epithelial and ectomesenchymal elements may mimic normal odontogenesis and thus dental hard tissues may, on occasions, be found in these tumors. As stated above, malignant odontogenic tumors are rare, but carcinomas, sarcomas, and carcinosarcomas do occur.

Odontogenic tumors are listed in Table 4.2.

A. Epithelial Odontogenic Tumors

1. *Ameloblastoma* is the most common clinically significant odontogenic tumor. Its relative frequency equals the combined frequency of all other odontogenic tumors, excluding odontoma. Ameloblastoma is slow-growing, locally invasive neoplasm. The tumor is encountered over a wide age range; it is rare in children and is most prevalent in the third to the seventh decades of life. There is no gender predilection.

About 85% of ameloblastomas occur in the mandible, most often in the molar-ascending ramus area. About 15% of ameloblastoma occur in the maxilla, usually in the posterior region. Painless swelling or expansion of the jaw is the usual clinical presentation. If untreated, the lesion may grow slowly to massive or grotesque proportions. Pain and paresthesia are uncommon, even in large tumors. Radiographically, the most typical feature is that of a multilocular radiolucent lesion. Cortical expansion is frequently present. Microscopically, the lesion may present several patterns; these microscopic patterns have no bearing on the behavior of the tumor, and large tumors often show a combination of patterns.

The follicular pattern is the most common and recognizable. It is composed of nests of epithelium that resemble the enamel organ of the developing teeth, dispersed in a mature fibrous connective tissue stroma. The core of the nests is composed of loosely arranged angular cells that resemble the stellate reticulum of the enamel organ. A single layer of tall columnar ameloblast-like cells surround the central core. The nuclei of these cells are placed away from the basement membrane (so-called reversed polarity) (e-Fig. 4.10). Cyst formation is common and may vary from microcysts forming within the follicles, to large macroscopic cysts that may be several centimeters in diameter.

The plexiform type of ameloblastoma consists of long anastomosing cords or large sheets of odontogenic epithelium bound by ameloblastic cells as seen in the follicular pattern, with similar stellate reticulum-like cores. Cyst formation is rare (e-Fig. 4.11).

The desmoplastic type consists of cuboidal peripheral cells with central spindle cells surrounded by a dense fibrous stroma.

Genetically, 90% of ameloblastomas have mutations in genes of the MAPK pathway, the majority being BRAF V600E mutations. *KRAS, NRAS, HRAS,* and *FGFR2* mutations have also been identified.

Unless removed in its entirety, ameloblastoma has a high recurrence rate. The tumor cells tend to infiltrate the surrounding marrow spaces, and the actual margin of the tumor often extends beyond its apparent radiographic or clinical margin. Marginal resection is therefore the most widely used treatment, but it is still associated with recurrence rates of up to 15%, and thus many surgeons advocate that the margin of resection should be at least 1 cm past the radiographic limit of the tumor. BRAF-targeted therapy has been used alongside surgical management in experimental studies.

TABLE 4.2 WHO Histologic Classification of Odontogenic Tumors

Benign epithelial odontogenic tumors
Ameloblastoma
  Ameloblastoma, unicystic type
  Ameloblastoma, extraosseous/peripheral type
  Metastasizing ameloblastoma
Squamous odontogenic tumor
Calcifying epithelial odontogenic tumor
Adenomatoid odontogenic tumor

Benign mixed epithelial and mesenchymal odontogenic tumors
Ameloblastic fibroma
Primordial odontogenic tumor
Odontoma
  Odontoma, compound type
  Odontoma, complex type
Dentinogenic ghost cell tumor

Benign mesenchymal odontogenic tumors
Odontogenic fibroma
Odontogenic myxoma/myxofibroma
Cementoblastoma
Cemento-ossifying fibroma

Odontogenic cysts of inflammatory origin
Radicular cyst
Inflammatory collateral cysts

Odontogenic and non-odontogenic developmental cysts
Dentigerous cyst
Odontogenic keratocyst
Lateral periodontal cysts and botryoid odontogenic cyst
Gingival cyst
Glandular odontogenic cyst
Calcifying odontogenic cyst
Orthokeratinized odontogenic cyst
Nasopalatine duct cyst

Fibro-osseous and osteochondromatous lesions
Ossifying fibroma
Familial gigantiform cementoma
Fibrous dysplasia
Cemento-osseus dysplasia
Osteochondroma

Giant cell lesions and bone cysts
Central giant cell granuloma
Peripheral giant cell granuloma
Cherubism
Aneurysmal bone cyst
Simple bone cyst

Odontogenic carcinomas
Ameloblastic carcinoma
Primary intraosseous squamous cell carcinoma, NOS
Sclerosing odontogenic carcinoma
Clear cell odontogenic carcinoma
Ghost cell odontogenic carcinoma

Odontogenic carcinosarcoma

Odontogenic sarcomas

Hematolymphoid tumors
Solitary plasmacytoma of bone

Modified from El-Naggar AK, Chan JKC, Grandis JR, Takata T, Slootweg PJ, eds. *WHO Classification of Head and Neck Tumors.* Lyon, France: IARC Press; 2017. Used with permission.

2. *Calcifying epithelial odontogenic tumor (Pindborg tumor)* is a rare tumor that presents as a slowly growing painless expansive lesion that favors the posterior mandible. The peak age of incidence is the third to seventh decades, and the male/female ratio is equal. The radiographic appearance of the tumor changes over time. Early on, the tumor appears as a radiolucent lesion that can be mistaken for a cyst. As the lesion ages it develops a poorly demarcated border and multiple radiopaque foci. The lesion may be multilocular.

   On microscopic examination, the tumor is characterized by clusters of pleomorphic polyhedral epithelial cells with a well-defined cell border and dense nuclear staining. The cells show mild to moderate nuclear pleomorphism, rare mitotic figures, and may contain multiple nuclei. Layered calcifications and amyloid-like globules are usually present (e-**Fig. 4.12**). Calcifying epithelial odontogenic tumors are generally treated surgically. Because they tend to be infiltrating tumors, treatment should include removal with a border of clinically and radiographically normal bone.

3. *Adenomatoid odontogenic tumor (adenoameloblastoma)* typically presents as a slowly growing asymptomatic mass in the anterior portion of the maxilla or mandible in patients younger than 30 years. Women are affected twice as often as men. Radiographic examination demonstrates a radiolucent, well-defined lesion involving the crown of an unerupted/impacted tooth. Adjacent teeth may show root divergence without root resorption. Gross examination reveals a well-defined encapsulated mass of soft tissue with focal cystic and granular areas. Microscopic examination shows a well-defined fibrotic capsule surrounding a multinodular mass of eosinophilic spindle and polyhedral cells. Scattered among these cells are amphophilic globules with variable levels of calcification and lamination; these globules are Periodic acid-Schiff (PAS) positive and diastase resistant. In addition to the globules, small cystic spaces lined by a single layer of cuboidal to columnar cells with foamy cytoplasm and basally orient nuclei are present (e-**Fig. 4.13**). Treatment is enucleation, and recurrence is extremely rare.

4. *Squamous odontogenic tumors* are benign lesions that occur in patients over a wide age distribution. Patients generally present with tooth loosening in the absence of periodontal disease. Radiology demonstrates a radiolucent mass in the anterior maxilla or posterior mandible with tooth root involvement. Microscopic examination shows a lesion is characterized by nodules of bland squamous cells with peripheral flattening of the basal cells, separated by a fibrous stroma (e-**Fig. 4.14**). Treatment is surgical excision with associated tooth removal.

5. *Malignant ameloblastoma and ameloblastic carcinoma.* Very rarely ameloblastoma exhibits frank malignant behavior with development of metastasis. The frequency of such an event is difficult to determine but probably occurs in far less than 1% of all ameloblastomas.

   By definition, malignant ameloblastoma is a tumor that shows histomorphologic features of a benign ameloblastoma, yet metastasizes. Metastasis is most often to the lungs, which has been regarded as aspiration or implant metastasis. In such cases the first evidence of metastasis is often discovered 1 to 30 years after surgical treatment of the primary lesion.

   The term ameloblastic carcinoma should be reserved for an ameloblastoma that has the cytologic features of malignancy in the primary tumor, in a recurrence, or in any metastatic deposit (e-**Fig. 4.15**). Ameloblastic carcinoma has similar *BRAF* mutations as in its benign counterpart. The lesion typically follows a markedly aggressive local course but metastasis does not always occur.

B. Mesenchymal Odontogenic Tumors

1. *Odontogenic myxoma* is a benign tumor that has the potential for local infiltration with extensive bone destruction, and a relatively high recurrence rate. It is thought to be derived from the ectomesenchyme. Microscopically, it resembles the dental papilla of a developing tooth. Myxomas are most common in the second and third decades of life; although they occur in patients from 5 to 72 years old, they are uncommon

in patients younger than 10 years or older than 50 years. Some studies show a female predilection. They have been associated with tuberous sclerosis and nevoid basal cell carcinoma. The lesion may be found at any location in the jaws, although some studies show a predominance of maxillary tumors.

Myxomas vary in their radiographic appearance, from small and unilocular, to large and multilocular with a "soap bubble" appearance. Tooth displacement and cortical expansion are common in larger lesions. Maxillary tumors often extend into the maxillary sinus. Microscopic examination reveals a bland, monotonous, hypocellular proliferation of loose mesenchymal fibrous tissue. The cells are spindled or stellate, with long cytoplasmic processes. The nuclei are small and may be hyperchromatic. Mitoses are scarce. Small nests of odontogenic epithelium may be present but are not necessary for the diagnosis (e-Fig. 4.16A,B).

Because of their lack of encapsulation and infiltrative growth, myxomas tend to extend beyond their clinically anticipated boundaries. Recurrence rates are as high as 25%, and thus close follow-up is recommended (recurrences are usually due to incomplete excision). Some recurrences occur years after excision.

2. **Benign cementoblastoma (true cementoma)** is a distinctive mesenchymal odontogenic tumor which is intimately associated with the roots of teeth. It is characterized by the formation of calcified cementum-like tissue deposited on the tooth root, most commonly mandibular molars. Although the tumor is detected in patients over a wide age range, it most commonly affects teenagers and young adults. Pain is a frequent symptom. The radiographic appearance of cementoblastoma is characteristic and is almost pathognomonic, namely, a radiopaque mass that obliterates the radiographic details of the root of the affected tooth.

On microscopic examination, the peripheral part of the tumor resembles osteoblastoma. Centrally, thick trabeculae of cementum, which are strongly basophilic, are deposited on the intact or partially resorbed tooth root. Peripherally, bone-like trabeculae are rimmed with plump cementoblasts. The intervening fibrovascular tissue shows dilated vessels and occasional clusters of multinucleated osteoclast-like giant cells (e-Fig. 4.17).

Cementoblastoma is a slowly growing benign neoplasm, but it may attain a large size if not treated. The recommended treatment is surgical excision with extraction of the affected tooth. Recurrence is usually a result of incomplete removal.

3. **Cemento-ossifying fibroma** (COF) of the jaws is synonymous with ossifying fibroma and cementifying fibroma. It is a benign odontogenic neoplasm that is limited to the tooth bearing areas of the jaws. COF is more often seen in the mandible (90%) and in women (83%). Most patients are in their third to fourth decades, and present with a small asymptomatic expanding bone mass that does not erode the adjacent cortical bone. Larger lesions present with facial deformation and pain. Radiographic examination demonstrates a well circumscribed radiolucent lesion with patchy focal radiopaque areas that does not encase the teeth roots. Tooth displacement, resorption, and root divergence may be seen.

Microscopic examination shows a lesion characterized by a fibrous stroma with bone trabecula and associated variable mineralized material that resembles dental cementum; either component may dominate in an individual lesion. The stroma is usually hypercellular; the bone trabeculae are usually woven but lamellar bone may also be seen. Osteoblastic rimming may vary in extent (e-Fig. 4.18).

Most COFs are small tumors that can be shelled out or curetted out of the jaw bone with relative ease. Recurrence after adequate removal is rare. Incompletely excised tumors continue to grow slowly, but may attain a large size.

C. Mixed Odontogenic Tumors

1. **Odontomas** represent the most highly differentiated of the mixed odontogenic tumors. They are considered by some pathologists to be hamartomas. Two types of odontomas are recognized: **compound** and **complex**. Compound odontoma is composed of many, sometimes even dozens, of small miniature teeth that are surrounded

by a dental follicle, the same tissue that surrounds a normal developing tooth. This form of odontoma shows the highest degree of histodifferentiation and morphodifferentiation (e-**Fig. 4.19**). In contrast, the complex odontoma is composed of a mass of intermixed enamel and dentine with no resemblance to normal or miniaturized teeth (e-**Fig. 4.20**).

Compound odontoma occurs most often in the anterior segment of the jaws, particularly the canine area in association with an impacted canine tooth. It is the most common odontogenic tumor. It is found most often in the second decade of life, and is more common in males than in females by a 3:2 ratio.

Complex odontomas occur most often in the posterior segment of the jaws, primarily in association with an impacted third molar tooth. They are the second most common odontogenic tumor and are usually discovered in the early third decade of life. Like compound odontomas, there is a male gender predilection of 2:1.

Odontomas are typically discovered when radiographic examination is performed because of a delay in eruption of a tooth. They may be mostly radiolucent with areas of opacity, and may be associated with an odontogenic cyst (particularly dentigerous cyst) or with calcifying odontogenic cyst. They are treated by surgical excision.

2. **Ameloblastic fibroma** is a true neoplasm composed of both epithelial and mesenchymal types of tissues, but with without calcified structures. The tumor is typically seen in adolescent patients. The average age is 14 years and there is an equal male/female distribution. About 80% of patients present with a well-defined unilocular or multilocular lesion in the mandible. Association with an unerupted tooth is common. Gross examination demonstrates a smooth well-defined lesion with a tan white cut surface. Microscopic examination demonstrates a lesion characterized by a background of immature connective tissue that resembles dental papilla with cords, strands, and nests of cuboidal to columnar epithelial cells. The epithelial nests are indistinguishable from those seen in follicular ameloblastoma, with a central stellate reticulum-like component and peripheral palisaded columnar cells showing reversed nuclear polarity. A prominent basement membrane separates the epithelial cells from the stroma (e-**Fig. 4.21**). Treatment is by enucleation and thorough curettage, and if necessary, extraction of the involved tooth. Recurrence is uncommon. Malignant transformation is extremely rare but has been documented.

3. **Ameloblastic fibrosarcoma and odontogenic carcinosarcoma.** Sarcomatous transformation of the mesenchymal component of ameloblastic fibroma, in association with benign epithelial elements, is designated **ameloblastic fibrosarcoma.**

Tumors with both a sarcomatous and carcinomatous component are termed **odontogenic carcinosarcoma.**

Ameloblastic fibrosarcoma typically presents as an expansive mandibular mass measuring 4 to 6 cm in maximum dimension in an adolescent or young adult. The tumor has high propensity for recurrence if conservatively treated, and can occasionally metastasize. Death more frequently results from aggressive local growth.

Microscopically, the architecture of ameloblastic fibrosarcoma resembles ameloblastic fibroma, albeit with a malignant connective tissue component. The epithelial cords and nests are widely separated by a hypercellular stroma. The fibroblast cells are round or fusiform and pleomorphic, with hyperchromatic nuclei and a high mitotic rate (e-**Fig. 4.22**). Ameloblastic fibrosarcoma can arise in an existing or recurrent ameloblastic fibroma. Multiple recurrences are usually associated with increasingly malignant cytologic features.

Odontogenic carcinosarcoma is extremely rare. One case developed in a preexisting ameloblastic fibroma in a 19-year-old pregnant woman, exhibited sudden growth, and was painful to palpation. The lesion was radiolucent and extended from the left body of the mandible into the ramus, reaching the condyle. Microscopically, areas of benign ameloblastic fibroma were associated with malignant epithelial and mesenchymal components. Interestingly, Ki67 labeling scores differed significantly between the two components of the tumor: the carcinosarcoma's score was much higher than that of the ameloblastic fibroma. The tumor was resected en block with no evidence of recurrence after 2 years of follow-up.

IV. **NONODONTOGENIC TUMORS.** The jaws, like other bones in the skeleton, can be a site of a wide variety of benign and malignant bone tumors; these entities are discussed in Chapter 46. This chapter will mainly address tumors and tumor-like lesions that occur predominantly or exclusively in the jaws (Table 4.3).

A. *Benign Fibro-osseous Lesions* are a group of lesions that share similar histomorphologic features although they have differing clinical and radiographic presentations and behavior. Microscopically, fibro-osseous lesions are composed of fibrous connective tissue stroma containing mineralized structures which may be bone or cementum. Proper diagnosis requires correlation of history, clinical, and radiographic findings. The more important types of fibro-osseous lesions of the jaws are discussed here.

1. *Fibrous dysplasia* is a skeletal anomaly in which normal bone is replaced by poorly organized and inadequately mineralized immature woven bone and fibrous connective tissue. Fibrous dysplasia is separated into two forms; the polyostotic form involves multiple bones while the monostotic form is limited to a single site. Polyostotic fibrous dysplasia is less common, and a few of these cases may be associated with skin pigmentation and endocrine anomalies, a condition known as the McCune-Albright syndrome. The craniofacial skeleton is involved in 20% to 25% of cases of monostotic fibrous dysplasia, particularly the mandible and maxilla.

Craniofacial fibrous dysplasia is not strictly monostotic but may extend by continuity to adjoining bones across suture lines. The maxilla is involved more often than the mandible. Most patients present in their second to third decades with a painless expanding bone mass. The mass does not involve the overlying bone cortex and growth halts when the patient reaches skeletal maturity. The radiographic appearance can be variable, but the majority of patients present with a poorly defined lesion that is radio-lucent when small, but becomes radiopaque as it enlarges, often described as having a ground glass appearance. The lesion blends imperceptibly with the surrounding bone.

Microscopic examination demonstrates a bland fibrovascular stroma with numerous irregular trabeculae of woven bone merging to form complex shapes described as resembling Chinese letters. The bone trabeculae are not rimmed with osteoblasts and lamellar bone is rarely identified (e-**Fig. 4.23**). Genetically, *GNAS* mutations are present in monostotic and polyostotic fibrous dysplasias. Repair of the deformity is usually attempted after the cessation of growth with skeletal maturity. Radiation is contraindicated due to the elevated risk of radiation induced sarcomas.

TABLE 4.3	Nonodontogenic Tumors

Benign fibro-osseous lesions

Fibrous dysplasia

Juvenile ossifying fibroma
   Trabecular
   Psammomatoid

Cemento-osseous dysplasia
   Periapical
   Florid

Giant cell lesions

Central (intro-osseous) giant cell granuloma

Brown tumor of hyperparathyroidism

Cherubism

Aneurysmal bone cyst

2. **Juvenile ossifying fibroma** (JOF), also known as juvenile active and juvenile aggressive ossifying fibroma, is used in the literature to describe two distinct clinicopathologic entities: *trabecular JOF (TrJOF)* and *psammomatoid (PsJOF).*

a. **Trabecular juvenile ossifying fibroma (TrJOF).** The great majority of the patients are children and adolescents, with an equal gender distribution. Clinically, the lesions are characterized by progressive and sometimes rapid expansion. The maxilla is more commonly affected than the mandible. Radiographically, the tumor is expansive and may be fairly well demarcated, with cortical thinning and perforation. Depending on the amount of calcification the lesion may show varying degrees of radiodensity.

Microscopically, TrJOF is composed of a cell-rich fibrous stroma containing bundles of cellular osteoid and bone trabeculae, without osteoblastic rimming. Aggregates of multinucleated giant cells are invariably present in the stroma (**e-Fig. 4.24**). Cystic degeneration and aneurysmal bone cyst formation may occur. The clinical course of TrJOF following conservative treatment is characterized by recurrence; eventual complete cure can be achieved by re-excision without resorting to radical surgery. Malignant transformation has not been reported.

b. **Psammomatoid juvenile ossifying fibroma (PsJOF).** Unlike TrJOF, PsJOF is a lesion that affects predominantly the extragnathic skull bones, particularly the periorbital bones. Occasional cases are encountered in the jaws, particularly the mandible. Affected patients tend to be older than those who have TrJOF. There is no sex predilection.

On radiographic examination the tumor appears expansive with well-defined borders that may be corticated. Sclerotic changes within the lesion may impart a ground glass appearance. The tumors vary in size from 2 to 8 cm. Cystic changes are not uncommon and present as areas of low density in the CT scans.

Microscopically, the tumor is noteworthy for multiple, round, uniform, small ossicles that are basophilic and resemble psammoma bodies. The psammomatoid structures are embedded in relatively cellular stroma composed of stellate and spindle-shaped cells (**e-Fig. 4.25**). Aneurysmal bone cyst formation is not uncommon. Surgical excision is the treatment of choice; multiple recurrences are not unusual. No malignant changes are observed.

3. **Cemento-osseous dysplasia** of the jaws is a nonneoplastic, presumably dysplastic, fibro-osseous lesion of the tooth bearing areas of the jaws. Two types are recognized: *periapical cemento-osseous dysplasia (PCOD)* and *florid cemento-osseous dysplasia*

a. **Periapical cemento-osseous dysplasia (PCOD),** also known as periapical cementoma, is a relatively common condition, particularly in middle aged black female patients. The anterior mandibular teeth are typically the site of this lesion. The condition is non-expansive, asymptomatic, and is typically identified in routine dental radiographs as periapical radiolucencies which become progressively mineralized in older lesions. Microscopic examination shows a poorly demarcated lesion consisting of fibrovascular stroma with trabeculae of bone and smooth globular masses of cementum-like material (**e-Fig. 4.26**). The bone and cementum may merge with adjacent bone, but will not involve adjacent teeth. No treatment is required. It is of importance to distinguish PCOD from periapical inflammatory disease.

b. **Florid cemento-osseous dysplasia (FCOD)** is uncommon. It usually presents in middle aged or older black women, is usually asymptomatic, and may be incidentally discovered on routine radiographic examination. Pain is rarely manifested. Radiographically, FCOD is characterized by extensive sclerotic areas often involving the posterior quadrants of the mandible and maxilla bilaterally in the tooth bearing areas, usually symmetrically (**e-Fig. 4.27**). Microscopically, FCOD and PCOD are analogous. However, large sclerotic masses that are hypocellular, extremely dense, and have small marrow spaces and more likely to form in FCOD. It is of importance to recognize the clinical radiographic features of

FCOD so that the patient is not subject to surgical intervention. In fact, surgery is contraindicated because it may result in local infection, pain, and a complicated clinical course.

B. *Giant Cell Lesions of the Jaws.* Giant cell lesions of the jaws are heterogeneous clinical entities that share similar microscopic features.

1. *Central giant cell granuloma (CGCG),* or intra-osseous granuloma of the jaws, is also known as giant cell reparative granuloma. It is a localized osteolytic lesion of the mandible (66% of cases) and maxilla (33% of cases). The majority of patients are under 30 years old, and women outnumber men by a ratio of 2:1.

Giant cell granulomas are typically nonaggressive and present on routine dental radiographs as a small radio-lucent expansive masses that do not erode into the cortex. The majority of CGCG occur in the anterior mandible, commonly crossing the midline. Microscopically, the lesions are unencapsulated and are composed of focal or evenly dispersed aggregates of multinucleated osteoclast-like giant cells in a richly vascular stroma with little collagen deposition (e-Fig. 4.28). Two types of mononuclear stromal cells are identified: spindle shaped fibroblastic cells and polygonal macrophage-like cells. Areas of ossification and hemosiderin granules may be present.

A rare aggressive variant characterized by pain, rapid growth, and cortical perforation with a marked tendency for recurrence may be an example of "true" giant cell tumor of bone. The lesion may show increased mitotic activity and evenly distributed larger giant cells that have an increased number of nuclei.

CGCG of the jaws is usually treated by curettage. Recurrent lesions often respond to further conservative surgery. A number of alternative nonsurgical approaches have been used in recent years, including intralesional corticosteroids injections, subcutaneous calcitonin injections, and interferon alpha therapy.

2. **Brown tumor of hyperparathyroidism** is an osseous lesion that develops in bones affected by primary or secondary hyperparathyroidism. It is currently less frequently encountered since the diagnosis of hyperparathyroidism is now often made on the basis of elevated serum calcium levels in asymptomatic adults.

The lesions may be solitary or multifocal, and the mandible is a common site of involvement. Radiographically, brown tumors are well-defined lytic lesions that are microscopically identical to CGCG. Treatment is aimed at correction of the hyperparathyroid state; complete resolution usually occurs within 6 months after removal of a parathyroid adenoma.

3. *Cherubism* is a rare dominant genetic disease with complete male penetrance and 50% to 70% penetrance in women. It typically presents as painless bilateral symmetric jaw expansion in children 1 to 5 years old which slowly increases in size until puberty; at puberty the lesion undergoes variable regression. The lesions may be unilocular or multilocular with a 'soap bubble' appearance on radiographic examination.

Microscopically, the lesions are essentially similar to CGCG. However, the giant cells in cherubism tend to be less numerous, and placed in a less cellular stroma. The pathologic process in cherubism is self-limited and treatment is dictated by cosmetic and functional needs. Curettage and contouring of bone are the treatments of choice.

ACKNOWLEDGMENT

The authors thank David E. Spence, an author of the previous edition of this chapter.

SUGGESTED READINGS

Delair D, Bejarano P, Peleg M, El-Mofty SK. Ameloblastic carcinosarcoma arising in ameloblastic fibroma: a case report and review of literature. *Oral Surg Oral Med Oral Pathol Oral Radiol Endod* 2007;103(4):516–520.

El-Mofty SK. Cemento-ossifying fibroma and benign cementoblastoma. *Semin Diagn Pathol* 1999;16(4):302–307.

El-Mofty SK. Psammomatoid and trabecular juvenile ossifying fibroma of the craniofacial skeleton: Two distinct clinicopathologic entities. *Oral Surg Oral Med Oral Pathol Oral Radiol Endod* 2002;93(3):269–304.

El-Mofty SK. Bone lesions. In: Gnepp DR, ed. *Diagnostic Surgical Pathology of the Head and Neck.* 2nd ed. Philadelphia, PA: WB Saunders Co; 2009:729–784.

El-Mofty SK, Kyriakos M. Soft tissue and bone lesions. In: Gnepp DR, ed. *Diagnostic Surgical Pathology of the Head and Neck.* Philadelphia, PA: WB Saunders Co; 2001:505–604.

Nevill BW, Damm DD, Allen CM, Bouquot JE, eds. Odontogenic cysts and tumors. *Oral, and Maxillofacial Pathology.* 4th ed. St. Louis, MO: Elsevier, 2015:632–689.

El-Naggar AK, Chan JKC, Grandis JR, Takata T, Slootweg PJ, eds. Odontogenic and maxillofacial bone tumors. *WHO Classification of Head and Neck Tumors.* Lyon, France: IARC Press; 2017.

El-Mofty SK, Nelson B, Toyosawa S. Ossifying fibroma In: El-Naggar AK, Chan JKC, Grandis JR, Takata T, Slootweg PJ, eds. *WHO Classification of Head and Neck Tumors.* Lyon, France: IARC Press; 2017.

The Eye

George J. Harocopos and Morton E. Smith

I. DISEASES OF THE CONJUNCTIVA

A. **Degenerative.** Two benign degenerative lesions on the conjunctiva are the **pinguecula** and the **pterygium**, which are manifestations of chronic actinic damage to the inter-palpebral bulbar conjunctiva. The pinguecula is confined to the conjunctiva, appearing clinically as a yellowish nodule, whereas the pterygium extends onto the peripheral cornea, appearing clinically as a vascular, wing-shaped lesion. Histologically, a pinguecula shows elastotic (actinic) degeneration and may show variable degrees of chronic inflammation (e-**Fig. 5.1**). The pterygium may show these same findings, but the most prominent feature is congested vessels (e-**Fig. 5.2**).

B. **Inflammatory.** A variety of infectious and noninfectious conditions may cause conjunctivitis.

1. **Sarcoidosis** often affects the conjunctiva, manifesting clinically as small, tan nodules in the inferior forniceal conjunctiva, often in noninjected, asymptomatic eyes. Sarcoidosis may also cause symptomatic inflammation in all parts of the eye, including conjunctivitis, uveitis, retinal phlebitis, optic neuritis, and so on. Conjunctival biopsy may provide the most expedient way of diagnosing this systemic disease, even in cases where there are no visible nodules clinically, though the diagnostic yield is highest when an obvious nodule is present. Histology shows noncaseating granulomatous tubercles in the stroma, with a variable (but usually minimal) cuff of lymphocytes and plasma cells (e-**Fig. 5.3**).

2. **Ocular cicatricial pemphigoid (OCP)** is a form of cicatrizing conjunctivitis that typically also involves other mucous membranes and sometimes involves the skin. When conjunctival biopsy is performed to establish the diagnosis, half the specimen should be submitted in formalin for routine histology, and half in Michel's medium or saline for immunofluorescence studies. Histology shows epithelial bullae (or blebs) and a subepithelial band of chronic inflammation composed predominantly of plasma cells (e-**Fig. 5.4**). Immunofluorescence demonstrates IgG, IgA, and/or IgM immunoglobulins, and/or complement (C3) positivity in the epithelial basement membrane zone. The sensitivity of immunofluorescence may be as low as 50%, and accordingly, a negative result does not rule out OCP.

C. **Neoplasms** of the conjunctiva fall mostly into one of three categories: squamous (surface epithelium), melanocytic, or lymphoid.

1. Neoplasms arising from the surface epithelium range from benign **papillomas** (e-**Fig. 5.5**) to **ocular surface squamous neoplasia (OSSN)** which is further subdivided into **conjunctival intraepithelial neoplasia (CIN)** (e-**Fig. 5.6**) versus invasive **squamous cell carcinoma** (e-**Fig. 5.7**). Histologic sections of a papilloma show finger-like projections of hyperplastic epithelium draped over fibrovascular cores. The epithelium may exhibit loss of goblet cells and surface keratinization if the lesion was exposed (i.e., not covered adequately by the tear film due to its size).

OSSN histologically exhibits epithelial hyperplasia with loss of goblet cells, nuclear hyperchromasia, and cellular pleomorphism, and often shows surface keratinization, dyskeratosis, and increased mitotic figures. In the most severe cases, squamous eddies or keratin whorls/pearls may be seen. There is frequently a subepithelial chronic inflammatory response. The most important distinction histologically in terms of prognosis is whether the lesion is confined by the epithelial basement membrane, (i.e., CIN) versus whether the lesion has broken through the basement membrane and invaded the stroma (i.e., invasive squamous carcinoma). The most recent staging scheme for conjunctival squamous carcinoma can be found in the 2017 Tumor, Node, Metastasis (TNM) American Joint Committee on Cancer (AJCC) staging classification (Amin MB, Edge S, Greene F, et al., eds. *AJCC Cancer Staging Manual*. 8th ed. New York: Springer; 2017). Treatment options for OSSN include excision with 3- to 4-mm margins and cryotherapy to the edges of excision versus topical chemotherapy with agents such as interferon (IFN) α-2b, 5-fluorouracil (5-FU), or mitomycin C (MMC). Topical chemotherapy may also be used as pre- or postoperative adjuvant treatment.

2. Melanocytic lesions of the conjunctiva range from benign to malignant.

   a. Conjunctival **melanocytic nevi** (e-Fig. 5.8) are benign lesions that bear similarities to cutaneous melanocytic nevi. Clinically, they may be pigmented or amelanotic. On histology, as with melanocytic nevi of the skin, the melanocytes are typically arranged in nests which may be junctional, intrastromal, or compound. Another important feature generally seen in conjunctival nevi is microepithelial inclusion cysts in association with the melanocytes.

   b. Intraepithelial melanocytic lesions of the conjunctiva include **benign acquired melanosis** (BAM) (also known as racial melanosis) (e-Fig. 5.9), which appears clinically as bilateral, flat, patchy brown pigmentation in dark-skinned individuals, and **primary acquired melanosis (PAM)** which has a similar clinical appearance except that it is generally unilateral in Caucasians. Histologically, BAM appears as a lentiginous proliferation of normal-appearing melanocytes confined to the basal layer of the epithelium, similar to lentigo simplex of the skin.

   PAM is subdivided into PAM without atypia, which appears histologically identical to BAM (and accordingly has no to minimal risk of future malignant transformation) versus PAM with atypia (e-Fig. 5.10). In PAM with atypia (similar to melanoma in situ of the skin), the melanocytic proliferation extends into the more superficial epithelial layers to varying degrees, and the melanocytes exhibit discohesiveness and may have epithelioid morphology; however, the lesion is still confined by the epithelial basement membrane. A subepithelial chronic inflammatory response may be present. In the ophthalmic nomenclature on conjunctival neoplasms, the term *melanoma* in situ is generally reserved for PAM with severe atypia involving at least 75% of the epithelial thickness. PAM with atypia carries a significant risk of future malignant transformation, with the risk being proportional to the degree of atypia. It is therefore generally treated via complete excision with 4-mm wide margins and cryotherapy to the edges of excision, similar to squamous neoplasms. Topical chemotherapy may also be a treatment option for very extensive lesions deemed too large for excision, though the success rate with this treatment is not as high as with squamous lesions.

   c. **Melanoma** of the conjunctiva (e-Fig. 5.10) generally arises from PAM with atypia, may arise de novo, or, less commonly, may arise from a nevus. When melanoma arises from PAM with atypia, histology demonstrates an area where the melanocytic proliferation violates the epithelial basement membrane and invades the stroma. Particularly when the focus of invasion is relatively small, immunostains such as melanA-red may be helpful in distinguishing the focus of invasion from the surrounding chronic inflammatory response, and in delineating the deep margin of invasion. The most recent staging scheme for melanomas of the conjunctiva can be found in the 2017 TNM AJCC staging classification (Amin MB, Edge S, Greene F, et al., eds. *AJCC Cancer Staging Manual*. 8th ed. New York: Springer; 2017). Conjunctival melanoma is generally treated via complete excision with at least 4-mm margins and cryotherapy to the edges of excision.

3. Lymphocytic lesions of the conjunctiva include **lymphoid hyperplasia** and **lymphoma**, either of which may be unilateral or bilateral. Lymphomas can range from primary localized lesions (even if bilateral), to lesions associated with systemic disease. Most conjunctival/orbital lymphomas are low-grade B-cell lymphomas, with the single most common type being extranodal marginal zone lymphoma (e-**Fig. 5.11**) that are generally localized to the conjunctiva. Histologically, marginal zone lymphoma shows a sheet of lymphocytes infiltrating the subepithelial region of the substantia propria (stroma) without well-defined follicles; scattered lymphocytes may extend into the epithelium. Immunohistochemistry for B- and T-cell markers (e-**Fig. 5.12A** and e-**Fig. 5.12B**) as well as in situ hybridization for kappa and lambda light chains (e-**Fig. 5.13A** and e-**Fig. 5.13B**) are very helpful diagnostically. Other techniques for establishing clonality such as IgH gene rearrangement testing by PCR and flow cytometry are also useful, particularly in cases where in situ hybridization proves insufficient. Fluorescence in situ hybridization (FISH) may also be used if needed to test for specific genetic translocations.

Follicular lymphomas are also seen in the conjunctiva. Less commonly, diffuse large B-cell, mantle cell, Burkitt, Hodgkin, plasmacytoma, or T-cell lymphoma may also occur. Lower-grade lymphomas are more often localized to the conjunctiva, whereas higher-grade lymphomas are more likely to be associated with systemic disease. If lymphoma is localized to the conjunctiva, the treatment is generally orbital radiation. Another treatment option is subconjunctival injections of IFN or intravenous rituximab. In contrast, if systemic lymphoma is present, then it is treated accordingly with chemotherapy; if systemic remission is achieved, the conjunctival lesion(s) will likewise resolve. The most recent staging scheme for conjunctival/orbital lymphoma can be found in the 2017 TNM AJCC staging classification (Amin MB, Edge S, Greene F, et al., eds. *AJCC Cancer Staging Manual*. 8th ed. New York: Springer; 2017).

  4. Other neoplasms. **Oncocytoma**, also known as **apocrine cystadenoma** or **oxophylic cystadenoma** (e-**Fig. 5.14**), is a benign lesion that arises most commonly in the caruncle of elderly females. Histologically, it is an adenoma composed of apocrine or accessory lacrimal gland epithelial cells which exhibit distinctive eosinophilic cytoplasm and surround gland-like spaces.

  Any neoplasm seen in the orbit may also occasionally arise in the conjunctiva, including neural, vascular, fibrous, and muscular tumors. Additionally, metastatic lesions to the conjunctiva rarely occur.

II. DISEASES OF THE CORNEA. The host tissue from a corneal transplant procedure is traditionally referred to as a corneal "button"; the surgical procedure itself is a keratoplasty (KP). Most often, full-thickness cornea is removed, (i.e., penetrating keratoplasty or PKP). More recently, however, surgical techniques have been developed such that, for certain disorders, only the diseased layer(s) of the cornea need be transplanted, for example, deep anterior lamellar keratoplasty (DALK), in which only the epithelium and stroma are removed, versus Descemet's stripping endothelial keratoplasty (DSEK), in which only Descemet's membrane and endothelium are removed. In the gross room, corneal buttons are bisected, and each half is embedded with the cut side down. The most common reasons for keratoplasty to be performed are Fuchs endothelial dystrophy, pseudophakic/aphakic bullous keratopathy, keratoconus, infectious keratitis (especially herpetic), and graft failure.

A. Fuchs Endothelial Dystrophy (e-**Fig. 5.15**) exhibits an autosomal dominant inheritance pattern or may be sporadic, generally becoming symptomatic in middle-aged to older individuals. The corneal endothelial cells diminish in number significantly faster than is normal for aging, ultimately leading to chronic edema of the cornea. If conservative therapy is unsuccessful, then keratoplasty (either PKP or DSEK) is necessary. Histologically, Fuchs dystrophy demonstrates loss of the endothelial cells and the presence of anvil-shaped excrescences, known as guttae, along a thickened Descemet's membrane. Often secondary epithelial bullae are seen (i.e., bullous keratopathy).

B. Pseudophakic Bullous Keratopathy (e-**Fig. 5.16**) is the term used when endothelial cell decompensation follows (usually months or years later) cataract extraction with intraocular lens implantation. Endothelial decompensation following cataract surgery without lens implantation is referred to as **aphakic bullous keratopathy**. Generally, around 5%

of endothelial cells are lost during an anterior segment procedure, but occasionally 50% or more of the endothelial cells may be lost if the surgery is highly complex/traumatic. The endothelium may then decompensate, either immediately if the residual endothelial cells are too few, or sometime later, after the endothelial cell population declines further with age. Keratoplasty (either PKP or DSEK) may ultimately be required. Although cataract surgery is the most common intraocular procedure performed, bullous keratopathy may similarly occur following other intraocular procedures, for example, multiple glaucoma surgeries or retinal surgeries. Histologically, endothelial cell loss is seen, but without guttae of Descemet's membrane; epithelial bullae are present.

C. **Keratoconus** is a condition generally presenting in teenagers and young adults in which the cornea is more ectatic (i.e., cone-shaped) than normal, causing myopia and astigmatism. Both genetic and environmental/acquired factors may be involved, since keratoconus is associated with both hereditary connective tissue disorders such as Marfan syndrome, as well as with excessive eye rubbing such as in chronic atopic conjunctivitis or chronic blepharitis associated with Down syndrome. In the early phases of the disease, the patient may be managed with spectacle or contact lens correction, but if the condition progresses to the extent that a corneal stromal scar forms at the apex of the cone (by which time the patient is often middle-aged), then keratoplasty (either PKP or DALK) is required for visual rehabilitation. The corneal button shows central thinning, breaks in Bowman's layer, and often loss of Bowman's layer with anterior stromal fibrosis at the apex of the cone correlating with the apical scar seen clinically (e-**Fig. 5.17**).

D. Corneal buttons with **ulcerative keratitis** may or may not reveal the offending microorganism when special stains are performed (e.g., Gram for bacteria; Gomori's Methenamine Silver [GMS] and periodic acid–Schiff [PAS] for fungi; GMS and PAS for *Acanthamoeba*). Lack of microorganisms on histology despite a history of positive cultures is generally attributable to antecedent antimicrobial therapy, as an attempt is generally made to sterilize the ulcer prior to keratoplasty. This scenario is frequently encountered with bacterial corneal ulcers, whereas fungi (e-**Fig. 5.18**) and amoebal cysts (e-**Fig. 5.19**) are often more difficult to eradicate with medical treatment and are therefore generally still present on histology. Herpes simplex keratitis has a characteristic histopathologic appearance including patchy loss of Bowman's layer, stromal fibrosis and vascularization, interstitial keratitis (consisting of plasma cells and lymphocytes in the corneal stroma), and often granulomatous inflammation near Descemet's membrane (e-**Fig. 5.20**).

E. When a PKP fails (for example, due to immunologic rejection, infectious ulcerative keratitis, or most commonly, simply gradual loss of endothelial cells over time), a re-graft may be necessary. On histology, the button may be identified as a re-graft by peripheral discontinuities in Bowman's layer and peripheral stromal scars (e-**Fig. 5.21**) that represent the entry sites of sutures and sometimes the graft–host interface (i.e., if the surgeon chose to make the re-graft of a slightly larger diameter than the prior graft). Residual suture material may be present, or may be absent if all the sutures were removed at some point after the initial procedure. Chronic inflammatory cells are often present along the suture tracks. The most essential histologic feature of graft failure is generally endothelial cell loss. In many cases there is also a fibrous retrocorneal membrane.

F. Other rare entities for which a PKP is performed include hereditary stromal dystrophic diseases, for example, macular dystrophy (due to acid mucopolysaccharide accumulation); granular dystrophy (due to hyaline deposition); lattice dystrophy (due to amyloid); and combined granular-lattice (Avellino) dystrophy in which both hyaline and amyloid deposits are seen (e-**Fig. 5.22A** and e-**Fig. 5.22B**).

III. **VASCULAR AND INFECTIOUS DISEASES AND TRAUMA.** Eyes are often removed when they become "blind and painful." The reasons for an eye becoming blind and painful are numerous, but often the final common pathway involves the development of secondary angle-closure glaucoma and/or chronic retinal detachment, and optic atrophy. The antecedent event can range from previous accidental trauma or previous surgical trauma, to specific disease entities such as retinal vascular disease (including diabetes, or central retinal artery or vein occlusion), intraocular infection (endophthalmitis), chronic inflammatory disease, or primary retinal detachment. Surgical methods of removing an eye include enucleation, in which the entire eye is removed intact, or evisceration, in which only the intraocular contents (lens, retina, uvea) and possibly cornea are removed with retention of the sclera in the eye socket to house the orbital implant. Exenteration, in which the eye along with surrounding orbital soft tissues are removed, is sometimes required to achieve complete excision of an eyelid/orbital tumor (see below).

A. **Secondary Glaucoma.** The key histopathologic finding in most cases of secondary glaucoma is an anterior chamber angle closed by peripheral anterior synechiae. The term "closed angle" means that the anatomical angle normally formed by the cornea and iris, and occupied by the trabecular meshwork (the main outflow channel for aqueous humor), is occluded by the peripheral iris. If this occlusion is chronic, then permanent adhesions form between the peripheral iris and trabecular meshwork, that is, peripheral anterior synechiae (e-**Fig. 5.23**). These adhesions may be induced by chronic inflammation, such as in various forms of chronic uveitis, or by the abnormal proliferation of capillaries (neovascular glaucoma) as seen in proliferative diabetic retinopathy or retinal vascular occlusion (see below). Occasionally, in contrast to the closed-angle appearance, post-contusion angle recession may be seen in cases of blunt trauma. The retina in glaucoma exhibits atrophy of the nerve fiber layer and loss of ganglion cells; the optic nerve shows cupping (e-**Fig. 5.24**) and atrophy.

B. **Chronic Retinal Detachment.** Retinal detachment may be idiopathic, trauma-induced, related to inflammation or infection, or secondary to proliferative retinopathy of various etiologies (diabetic, post-vascular occlusion, and so on). Often an attempt is made to repair the detachment surgically, but severe cases in which surgery fails or the detachment repeatedly recurs may ultimately be treated by enucleation (e-**Fig. 5.25**).

C. **Retinal Vascular Diseases.** Eyes with severe retinal vascular disease (most commonly diabetic retinopathy, or central retinal arterial or venous occlusion) often exhibit both secondary angle closure due to neovascularization of the iris (e-**Fig. 5.26**) and angle (neovascular glaucoma), as well as chronic tractional retinal detachment due to proliferative retinopathy. In cases of diabetic retinopathy, microscopic examination of the retina reveals the key features of diabetes: lipoproteinaceous exudates, intraretinal hemorrhages, and neovascularization of the inner surface of the retina (proliferative diabetic retinopathy) (e-**Fig. 5.27**), often with tractional retinal detachment and hemorrhage into the vitreous. In cases of old central retinal vein or artery occlusion, the retina exhibits atrophy and cystoid degeneration of the inner two-thirds of the retina, lipoproteinaceous exudates, and in the case of venous occlusion, often a persistence of hemorrhage. There may also be a neovascular epiretinal membrane with tractional retinal detachment and vitreous hemorrhage. As with neovascular glaucoma of any etiology, eyes with severe diabetic retinopathy or central retinal vascular occlusion also exhibit atrophy and possibly cupping of the optic nerve.

D. **Intraocular Inflammation and Infection.** Endophthalmitis most commonly occurs via an exogenous source (e.g., following a surgical procedure, trauma, or perforated corneal ulcer), or may arise from an endogenous source (e.g., secondary to bacteremia or fungemia). Endophthalmitis is generally treated with intravitreal antibiotics and/or antifungals, and possibly vitrectomy surgery to clear the abscess. However, in severe cases treatment may not be successful, and evisceration or enucleation may ultimately be performed. On histology (e-**Fig. 5.28**), such cases demonstrate intraocular abscess formation and retinal detachment/destruction; depending on the degree of chronicity, optic nerve atrophy may also be seen.

Other severe inflammatory or infectious diseases that can lead to a blind and painful eye include diffuse uveitis of unknown etiology; juvenile rheumatoid arthritis-associated uveitis or uveitis associated with other collagen vascular/autoimmune diseases; diffuse granulomatous uveitis secondary to sympathetic ophthalmia (e-**Fig. 5.29**), sarcoidosis, or toxoplasmosis; and necrotizing retinitis (as seen in cytomegalovirus [CMV] retinitis or herpetic retinitis).

E. Trauma. Many eyes are enucleated because of severe trauma. If there is no attempt at repair by the ophthalmologist because the rupture is too extensive, the pathology specimen usually consists of a ruptured globe with massive intraocular hemorrhage and total retinal detachment (e-**Fig. 5.30**). Often there is loss of intraocular contents such as the lens and a portion of the uvea, and possibly also the retina. If an attempt has been made by the surgeon to salvage the ruptured globe, but the eye later has to be enucleated because it has become blind and painful, the histopathologic findings vary depending on the degree of chronicity; in cases of recent rupture, the findings may be the same as described above (i.e., massive intraocular hemorrhage, total retinal detachment, and loss of intraocular contents) or may also include additional findings such as endophthalmitis. In cases with a more distant history of rupture, there may be total retinal detachment with gliosis and loss of intraocular contents, intraocular granulation tissue or fibro-connective tissue emanating from the rupture site, and often osseous metaplasia of the retinal pigment epithelium (see below). Angle closure or post-contusion angle recession may also be present depending on the location of the rupture and the nature of the traumatic forces. Optic nerve atrophy is generally also seen.

F. Phthisis Bulbi. When an eye has undergone a previous insult such as severe trauma, complications of surgery, proliferative retinopathy, or chronic inflammation, and has a chronic total retinal detachment, a gradual degenerative process eventually ensues in which the eye undergoes shrinkage, that is, phthisis (from the Greek verb "to wither"). Clinically, the eye has hypotony (very low intraocular pressure) and is visibly shrunken. Histologically, the retina is totally detached, with marked diffuse atrophy and archi-tectural distortion of all layers of the eye including such severe retinal gliosis as to render the retina barely recognizable. Often the retinal pigment epithelium undergoes osseous metaplasia, and bone may occupy a significant portion of the intraocular cavity (e-**Fig. 5.31**). Choroidal effusion may be seen. The optic nerve is atrophic.

IV. INTRAOCULAR NEOPLASMS

A. Gross room processing of enucleated globes follows a standard protocol to generate the pupil–optic nerve (p.o.) section, as shown in Figure 5.1. Larger cassettes are required for processing. The figure shows the standard transverse plane that is often used for cutting the section, but the globe may be opened along any plane that best captures the particular area of interest. For eyes enucleated due to intraocular tumors, especially primary uveal melanoma, the tumor may be localized by transillumination prior to cutting the eye. Transillumination is achieved by shining onto the cornea a very bright light source that is about 1 cm or less in diameter. The normal uvea will not block the transmission of light, and hence the sclera will glow. However, a uveal tumor will block light transmission, thereby casting a shadow over the corresponding portion of sclera.

B. The most common primary intraocular neoplasm is **melanoma of the uvea** (choroid, ciliary body, or less commonly, iris). Melanomas usually occur in adults of light com-plexion. Melanomas of the iris have a better prognosis than do melanomas of the ciliary body and/or choroid. Although some intraocular melanomas can be treated by excision or brachytherapy, some patients do not seek medical attention until the melanoma has become so large that the only course of management is enucleation of the globe. If the diagnosis is in doubt, fine-needle aspiration biopsy (FNAB) may be performed to con-firm the diagnosis (e-**Fig. 5.32**). In cases of smaller-to-medium-sized melanomas treated with radioactive plaque brachytherapy, some ocular oncologists routinely perform FNAB at the time of plaque placement so as to obtain a sample for gene expression profiling (GEP), as this provides useful prognostic information.

Large uveal melanomas are generally treated with enucleation. Primary uveal mel-anoma usually arises from the ciliary body or choroid as an ellipse or almond-shaped mass (e-**Figs. 5.33** and **5.34**) which eventually breaks through Bruch's membrane and becomes mushroom-shaped (e-**Fig. 5.35**). Microscopically, intraocular melanomas are composed of cells ranging from spindle to epithelioid, with the latter having a worse prognosis (e-**Figs. 5.36** and **5.37**). Other histopathologic features that predict prognosis are size (e-**Fig. 5.38**); extrascleral extension (e-**Fig. 5.38**); and location (those arising

Left Eye   Right Eye
Posterior View

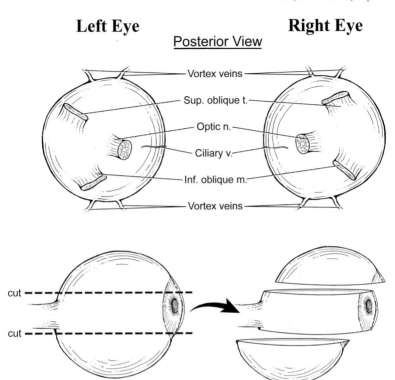

Figure 5.1 The globe is identified as to right eye or left eye using anatomic landmarks (*upper panel*). Two cuts (traditionally referred to as the pupil–optic nerve [p.o.] sections) are then made in a transverse plane, passing in relation to the pupil and optic nerve as shown (*lower panel*). The superior cap (also known as calotte) and inferior cap are usually not processed unless abnormalities are seen or the eye has an intraocular tumor.

from the iris have a better prognosis, whereas those involving the ciliary body [e-**Fig. 5.39**] or peripapillary region have a poorer prognosis). Other factors associated with a worse prognosis include necrosis and mitotic figures. When uveal melanoma metastasizes, it most commonly spreads first to the liver, via hematogenous dissemination. The staging scheme for melanoma of the uvea is described in the 2017 TNM AJCC staging classification (Amin MB, Edge S, Greene F, et al., eds. *AJCC Cancer Staging Manual.* 8th ed. New York: Springer; 2017) and diagrammed in Figure 5.2.

As alluded to above, GEP of uveal melanoma provides useful prognostic information. GEP classifies uveal melanomas via a 12-gene expression profile as either Class 1A tumors, which are associated with 95% survival at about 7.5 years, or as Class 2 tumors, which are associated with only about 30% survival at 7.5 years; Class 1B tumors are associated with an intermediate prognosis. Uveal melanomas in general often exhibit early in tumorigenesis (i.e., too early to be predictive of prognosis) mutations in the *GNAQ* or *GNA11* genes. Unlike cutaneous and conjunctival melanomas, uveal melanomas do not exhibit *BRAF* or *NRAS* mutations. Later in tumorigenesis, Class 2 tumors are characterized by downregulation of genes on chromosome 3 and upregulation of genes on chromosome 8q, correlating with the earlier cytogenetic discovery that loss of

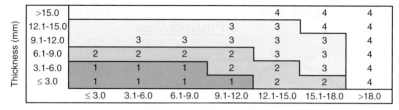

Thickness (mm)	≤ 3.0	3.1-6.0	6.1-9.0	9.1-12.0	12.1-15.0	15.1-18.0	>18.0
>15.0					4	4	4
12.1-15.0				3	3	4	4
9.1-12.0		3	3	3	3	3	4
6.1-9.0	2	2	2	2	3	3	4
3.1-6.0	1	1	1	2	2	3	4
≤ 3.0	1	1	1	1	2	2	4

Largest basal diameter (mm)

Figure 5.2 Size categories for ciliary body and choroidal melanoma based on thickness and diameter.

heterozygosity of chromosome 3 is associated with a relatively higher risk of metastatic disease, while adjunctive gains in chromosome 8q increase the risk of metastatic disease yet further. In particular, Class 2 tumors are frequently characterized by mutation in the *BAP1* tumor suppressor gene on chromosome 3. Some patients with Class 2 uveal melanomas have been found to harbor a germline (rather than somatic) mutation in the *BAP1* gene; these patients may exhibit one or more additional primary neoplasms elsewhere in the body, for example, mesothelioma, less commonly cutaneous melanoma, basal cell carcinoma, ovarian carcinoma, renal clear-cell carcinoma, or occasionally breast or lung adenocarcinoma. Conversely, in the gene expression profile of Class 1 tumors, a mutation in the *EIF1AX* gene predicts a low risk for metastatic disease; furthermore, Class 1A tumors typically have low *CDH1/RAB31* expression, whereas Class 1B tumors have high *CDH1/RAB31* expression. Most recently, GEP has demonstrated that metastatic disease in Class 1 tumors (though much less common than metastatic disease in Class 2 tumors) is strongly associated with *PRAME* expression (which has also been found to be a useful biomarker for distinguishing melanomas of the skin from benign nevi). Mutations in *SF3B1* are also associated with metastasis of Class 1 tumors, though not as strongly as *PRAME* expression. Due to the strong association between metastasis of Class 1 tumors and *PRAME* expression, the genetic differentiation of Class 1 uveal melanomas into Class1[PRAME-] and Class1[PRAME+] categories may ultimately supplant the Class 1A and Class 1B designations in the stratification of patients into low–metastatic-risk and intermediate-metastatic-risk categories, respectively.

Genetic classifications aside, the importance of tumor size with regard to prognosis cannot be understated. Recent research on prognosis of uveal melanoma has demonstrated retrospectively that early treatment (i.e., when the maximal basal tumor diameter is still <12 mm) is associated with a high 5-year progression-free survival rate (≥ 90%), regardless of GEP class.

C. Retinoblastoma is the most common ocular neoplasm in children. The usual age for clinical presentation in nonfamilial cases is 1 year, whereas familial cases are generally screened within the first few weeks of life and therefore present earlier. The usual clinical appearance is leukocoria (white pupil). In nonfamilial cases, the tumor is generally large and unilateral, and accordingly treated with enucleation. In familial cases, tumors are generally seen bilaterally. The tumor may be much larger in one eye than the other, in which case the eye with the large tumor is often enucleated, whereas the eye with smaller tumor(s) may be salvaged via laser or cryotherapy applied to the tumor foci, possibly with antecedent adjuvant systemic chemotherapy. Some centers utilize intra-arterial chemotherapy (delivered to the ophthalmic artery) to treat unilateral or bilateral tumors, thereby potentially salvaging eyes that would otherwise need to be enucleated. Intravitreal chemotherapy may be used for vitreous tumor seeding. Some centers utilize periocular injection of chemotherapy.

With regard to the genetics of tumorigenesis, retinoblastoma arises when there is a mutation in both alleles of the *RB1* tumor suppressor gene (which was the first tumor suppressor gene to be discovered), located at chromosome 13q14.2. In familial cases, there is a germline mutation in one of the *RB1* alleles, and a somatic mutation occurs within the tumor in the second *RB1* allele. The second, intratumoral somatic mutation occurs in multiple retinal foci such that familial cases exhibit multifocal/bilateral involvement. In contrast, unilateral/unifocal cases most often harbor somatic mutations in both *RB1* alleles (but the tumor tends to occupy much of the posterior segment in these cases, as such cases are typically not diagnosed clinically until leukocoria is noted). However, it is also possible (though less common) for a unilateral/unifocal case, even with no family history of retinoblastoma, to be associated with a germline *RB1* mutation, and therefore blood testing to screen for a germline RB1 mutation is recommended in all unilateral/unifocal cases since the discovery of a germline mutation would obviously have significant implications in terms of genetic counseling, with each offspring of the germline-mutation index case having a 50% chance of inheriting the germline mutation, with retinoblastoma (assuming the germline mutation is passed on) having >95% penetrance.

Histopathologically, retinoblastoma arises from the retina (e-**Fig. 5.40**) and is composed of basophilic cells intermingled with anastomosing pools of pink necrosis giving rise to the traditional description of "islands of blue tumor in a sea of pink necrosis" (e-**Fig. 5.41**). Scattered flecks of purple calcium are often seen. Cytologically, the tumor is composed of cells with hyperchromatic, oval-shaped nuclei with scant cytoplasm; the nuclei are densely packed together and thus show nuclear molding. There are many apoptotic bodies and numerous mitotic figures. More differentiated retinoblastomas often exhibit Flexner–Wintersteiner rosettes (e-**Fig. 5.42**). Extension into the optic nerve, and especially presence of tumor at the surgical margin of the nerve, predicts a poor prognosis (e-**Fig. 5.43**). The other factor predictive of poor prognosis is massive invasion of the choroid. If optic nerve invasion past the lamina cribrosa or massive choroidal invasion is seen on histology, then the patient is treated with adjuvant systemic chemotherapy. (Some practitioners have a lower threshold for adjuvant chemotherapy than others; the optimal algorithm for post-enucleation chemotherapy has not been definitively established.) The most recent staging scheme for retinoblastoma can be found in the 2017 TNM AJCC staging classification (Amin MB, Edge S, Greene F, et al., eds. *AJCC Cancer Staging Manual*. 8th ed. New York: Springer; 2017).

V. DISEASES OF THE LACRIMAL GLAND AND LACRIMAL SAC

A. Lacrimal gland lesions are similar to lesions of the parotid gland (see Chapter 6). Infiltrative lesions include dacryoadenitis, sarcoidosis, lymphoid hyperplasia, and lymphoma. Intrinsic lesions of the lacrimal gland include pleomorphic adenoma, adenoid cystic carcinoma, and mucoepidermoid carcinoma. The most recent staging scheme for lacrimal gland carcinoma can be found in the 2017 TNM AJCC staging classification (Amin MB, Edge S, Greene F, et al., eds. *AJCC Cancer Staging Manual*. 8th ed. New York: Springer; 2017).

B. Generally occurring in middle aged to elderly individuals, a stone (dacryolith) may form in the lacrimal sac, causing obstruction of the nasolacrimal drainage system which generally presents as chronic severe watering of the eye (epiphora). Lacrimal sac dacryolithiasis often contains *Actinomyces* organisms (e-**Fig. 5.44A** and e-**Fig. 5.44B**). Alternatively, Streptococcal or fungal organisms may be seen. Tumors of the lacrimal sac include papillomas, nonkeratinizing squamous cell carcinoma, and other rare entities such as plasmacytoma or lymphoma.

VI. DISEASES OF THE ORBIT.
Lesions of the orbit include all the aforementioned lesions of the lacrimal gland; lesions elsewhere in the orbit include lymphoma, cavernous hemangioma in young to middle-aged adults, capillary hemangioma in children, idiopathic orbital inflammation (also known as inflammatory pseudotumor), schwannoma, neurofibroma, infectious abscess, dermoid cyst, and lymphangioma. Less common lesions include rhabdomyosarcoma, granular cell tumor, Rosai–Dorfman disease, optic nerve glioma, meningioma of the optic nerve sheath or sphenoid wing, alveolar soft part sarcoma, fibrous histiocytoma, melanoma, plasmacytoma, and metastatic carcinoma.

The morphologic features of all these lesions are the same as when they occur in other soft tissue sites. The recent staging scheme for sarcomas of the orbit can be found in the

2017 TNM AJCC staging classification (Amin MB, Edge S, Greene F, et al., eds. *AJCC Cancer Staging Manual*. 8th ed. New York: Springer; 2017).

VII. DISEASES OF THE EYELID. The common benign and malignant lesions of the eyelid are identical to those that occur at other cutaneous sites. The most recent staging scheme for carcinoma of the eyelid can be found in the 2017 TNM AJCC staging classification (Amin MB, Edge S, Greene F, et al., eds. *AJCC Cancer Staging Manual*. 8th ed. New York: Springer; 2017). Sometimes basal cell, squamous cell, or sebaceous gland carcinomas of the eyelid become so extensive as to invade the orbit and ocular surface, in which case exenteration may be required to achieve complete excision. Exenteration is sometimes also required for tumors arising in the orbit/sinuses. In processing an exenteration specimen, the eye should be dissected out of the surrounding soft tissue; the soft tissue should then be processed in the usual fashion for soft tissue tumors, and the eye should be placed separately in fixative for at least 24 hours. The eye may then be processed as described previously under gross room processing of enucleated globes. In such cases, there may be varying degrees of optic atrophy due to optic nerve compression by the tumor, but the intraocular contents are often normal on histology.

SUGGESTED READINGS

Eagle RC. *Eye Pathology, An Atlas and Text*. 2nd ed. Philadelphia, PA: Lippincott Williams & Wilkins; 2011.

Field MG, Decatur CL, Kurtenbach S, et al. PRAME as an independent biomarker for metastasis in uveal melanoma. *Clin Cancer Res* 2016;22(5):1234–1242.

Font RL, Croxatto JO, Rao NA. Volume 5. In: *AFIP Atlas of Tumor Pathology, Series 4*. Washington, DC: ARP Press; 2006.

Goldstein AM. Germline BAP1 mutations and tumor susceptibility. *Nat Genet* 2011;43: 925–926.

Harbour JW, Onken MD, Roberson EDO, et al. Frequent mutation of BAP1 in metastasizing uveal melanomas. *Science* 2010;330(6009):1410–1413.

Onken MD, Worley LA, Ehlers JP, Harbour JW. Gene expression profiling in uveal melanoma reveals two molecular classes and predicts metastatic death. *Cancer Research* 2004; 64(20):7205–7209.

Smith ME, Kincaid MC, West CE. In: Krachmer JH, ed. *The Requisites in Ophthalmology*. St. Louis, MO: Mosby; 2002; chapters 3–9;23.

Van Raamsdonk CD, Bezrookove V, Green G, et al. Frequent somatic mutations of GNAQ in uveal melanoma and blue naevi. *Nature* 2009;457:599–602.

Van Raamsdonk CD, Griewank KG, Crosby MB, et al. Mutations in GNA11 in uveal melanoma. *N Engl J Med* 2010;363:2191–2199.

Walter SD, Chao DL, Feuer W, Schiffman J, Char DH, Harbour JW. Prognostic implications of tumor diameter in association with gene expression profile for uveal melanoma. *JAMA Ophthalmol* 2016;134(7):734–740.

Yanoff M, Sassani JW. *Ocular Pathology*, 7th ed. New York, Philadelphia, PA, St. Louis, MO: Elsevier/Saunders; 2015.

Salivary Glands

Mena Mansour and Samir K. El-Mofty

I. NORMAL ANATOMY

A. Macroscopic/Gross. Salivary glands are exocrine organs that secrete components of saliva that both break down carbohydrates and lubricate the passage of food. There are three major paired salivary glands: the parotid, the submandibular, and the sublingual. There are also numerous minor salivary glands located in the submucosa of the entire upper aerodigestive tract (UADT), from the lips and nasal cavity to the major bronchi.

The parotid glands are the largest major salivary glands and are located between the ramus of the mandible and the mastoid process. Each gland is composed of a superficial lobe and a smaller deep lobe, and the facial nerve is intimately associated with both lobes. Each gland normally contains approximately 20 intraglandular lymph nodes. The secretions of the parotid gland empty via Stensen duct into the buccal mucosa of the oral cavity near the second maxillary molar.

The submandibular glands (also referred to as the submaxillary glands) are located just medial to the body of the mandible, and are smaller than the parotid glands. Their secretions drain through Wharton duct into the floor of the mouth.

The sublingual glands are the smallest of the major salivary glands and are located in the floor of the mouth between the genioglossus muscle and mandible. Their secretions drain into the floor of the mouth directly via small ducts or through the larger (Bartholin) duct which drains into Wharton duct.

B. Microscopic. The major salivary glands are enclosed by a connective tissue capsule and divided into lobules composed of ducts and acini, whereas the minor salivary glands are unencapsulated. The acini are composed of mucinous and/or serous epithelial cells surrounded by a layer of myoepithelial cells which contract to aid in the movement of glandular secretions. Myoepithelial cells are inconspicuous in normal salivary gland sections.

A single acinus may be composed of a mixture of serous and mucous cells. Serous cells are pyramidal in shape and contain basophilic zymogen granules within their cytoplasm that are periodic acid–Schiff (PAS)-positive. Mucous cells are more rounded, have basally oriented nuclei, and contain abundant clear mucin. The parotid gland is almost exclusively serous, the sublingual gland almost exclusively mucinous, and the submandibular gland is mixed serous and mucinous (e-**Figs. 6.1** to **6.3**). The acini secrete fluid into the intercalated ducts, which are lined by a low simple cuboidal epithelium. Intercalated ducts are also the source of reserve cells that can repopulate the acinar system. The intercalated ducts join to form striated ducts, which merge to form interlobular ducts, which ultimately empty into the large named ducts.

II. GROSS EXAMINATION, TISSUE SAMPLING, AND HISTOLOGIC SLIDE PREPARATION

A. Biopsies of many salivary gland lesions are taken prior to surgery to characterize the lesion and direct management.

   1. Fine needle aspiration (FNA) is the procedure of choice for initial characterization of salivary gland lesions for many reasons (see Cytopathology of the Salivary Glands section below).

   2. Core needle and incisional biopsies of the parotid gland can damage the facial nerve branches, so are rarely performed.

B. Resections. Some salivary gland masses are removed in their entirety without a previous tissue diagnosis. Superficial parotidectomy remains the initial procedure of choice for benign parotid gland tumors. Submandibular gland resections are usually performed without taking any significant periglandular soft tissue, although more tissue may be included with the specimen for submandibular or parotid tumors that are known or suspected to be malignant. The rare sublingual gland tumor necessitates a resection of the floor of mouth that is qualitatively similar to those performed for mucosal-based squamous carcinomas of the same area.

In general, salivary gland specimens are small enough to prosect the day of receipt. The gland should be described, and its dimensions recorded. The deep (covered by muscle and fascia) and superficial (covered by subcutaneous fat) surfaces of the parotid gland can sometimes be deciphered, and should be differentially inked. The specimen should be serially sectioned, and any tumor (or other mass) should be described including dimensions, color, texture, and distance to the margins. Four to five sections of the tumor, including representative areas of the closest inked margins, should be taken. At least one section of the normal surrounding gland should also be taken. For the parotid gland, the surrounding gland should be thoroughly searched for intraparenchymal lymph nodes, which should be separately submitted.

III. DIAGNOSTIC FEATURES OF COMMON DISEASES

A. Inflammation and Infection. Sialadenitis, or inflammation of the salivary glands, can be divided into infectious causes (bacterial and viral) and autoimmune disease.

1. Bacterial sialadenitis is rare and is generally a result of obstruction by stones (sialolithiasis). The causative organism is usually *Staphylococcus aureus*, followed by *Streptococcus viridans* and gram-negative rods. Surgical specimens from bacterial sialadenitis are almost never seen. However, sialadenitis may lead to an abscess that requires drainage. Gross specimens may show a purulent exudate or a relatively intact gland. Microscopic sections can show an abscess, cystic degeneration, and/or bacterial colonies.

2. Viral sialadenitis is most commonly caused by mumps (paramyxovirus), but can also be associated with Epstein–Barr, coxsackie, influenza A, and parainfluenza viruses. Surgical specimens are rarely encountered. Grossly infected glands are boggy and edematous, and chronic inflammation may be seen microscopically.

3. Autoimmune sialadenitis is relatively common, and usually presents as Sjögren syndrome characterized by facial swelling, dry mouth, and dry eyes (termed Sicca syndrome) with inflammatory arthritis and elevated autoantibodies. On physical examination, bilateral symmetric enlargement of the salivary and lacrimal glands is seen. Diagnosis may be facilitated by a minor salivary gland biopsy, typically taken from the inner lip.

Grossly, the major glands usually have a discrete, tan nodularity. Microscopically, in early disease, there is a lymphoplasmacytic septal inflammatory infiltrate with little to no abnormality of the parenchyma. The so-called focus score, a nodular collection of >50 lymphocytes, is considered diagnostic of autoimmune sialadenitis in the appropriate clinical context. In larger glands or in more severe disease, there is typically an extensive lymphoid infiltrate with germinal centers (e-**Fig. 6.4**). The acini are often atrophic, and interstitial fibrosis may be seen. In late disease, acini may be completely absent leaving only isolated residual ducts, termed "epimyoepithelial islands," with an associated dense intraepithelial lymphocytosis. In Sjögren syndrome, the lymphocytic infiltrate is polyclonal, which can be used to exclude a mucosa-associated lymphoid tissue (MALT) lymphoma.

4. Chronic sialadenitis (or chronic sclerosing sialadenitis) is usually unilateral and clinically can mimic a true salivary gland neoplasm. When it occurs in the submandibular gland, it is known as Kuttner tumor. Chronic sialadenitis most commonly results from sialolithiasis with obstruction, although some cases may be due to radiation therapy or duct strictures. It can have no structural or obvious etiology, and recently most of these cases have been shown to be an autoimmune-related IgG4-related sclerosing disease. Grossly, it is characterized by a very hard, fibrotic gland with lobulation and septation (e-**Fig. 6.5**). Histologic examination of the gland early in the disease process shows dilated ducts filled with secretions with an associated lymphocyte and plasma cell rich infiltrate, occasionally with germinal center formation. As the disease progresses, fibrosis surrounds the ducts and results in lobulation of the gland (e-**Fig. 6.6**) with acinar atrophy and broad fibrous bands. Immunohistochemistry for IgG4 and IgG to establish a ratio of IgG4 to IgG positive plasma cells should be used if IgG4-related disease is suspected. Surgical excision may be required.

5. **Necrotizing sialometaplasia** is a rare inflammatory/destructive lesion that simulates malignancy and is thought to be secondary to an ischemic injury. Although it can occur anywhere along the UADT, the vast majority of cases occur in the hard palate. Men are slightly more commonly affected, and the average patient age is 46 years. Clinically, the lesion consists of a sharply defined and deep ulcer that develops rapidly (over a few days) and can persist for months. Grossly, the lesion consists of loose tissue with a surface ulcer and no distinguishing mass lesion. Microscopically, the most typical feature is coagulative necrosis of the minor salivary gland lobules with a prominent associated inflammatory response. There is extensive squamous metaplasia of the ducts (which can be an alarming microscopic feature), but the lesion retains its overall lobular architecture (e-**Fig. 6.7**). The surface squamous mucosa may show pseudoepitheliomatous hyperplasia. Given the clinical and microscopic presentation, the lesion may be mistaken for a malignant neoplasm, however, the lack of peripheral infiltration and the retained lobular architecture are keys to its benign nature. No specific therapy is indicated because the lesion is self-healing.

B. Cystic Lesions

1. **Human immunodeficiency virus salivary gland disease** (HIV-SGD, AIDS-related parotid cysts) manifests as benign lymphoepithelial cysts. Patients present with unilateral or bilateral, painless, slowly enlarging parotid masses that may be the initial presentation of HIV infection. They sometimes have associated cervical lymphadenopathy and/or nasopharyngeal swelling. Grossly, these lesions have multiple cystic spaces usually containing serous fluid. Microscopically, HIV-SGD consists of cysts that most often have a squamous epithelial lining, although the lining is sometimes cuboidal or columnar with goblet cells. Below the epithelium, the cyst wall has dense lymphoid tissue with germinal centers. Occasionally, lesions within the gland can lack cystic change and appear similar to epimyoepithelial islands.

Unlike autoimmune sialadenitis, the vast majority of HIV patients with HIV-SGD have no autoimmune symptoms, no sicca syndrome from glandular dysfunction, and no serum autoantibodies. The etiology of HIV-SGD is thus unclear. Patients usually have bilateral disease by radiologic examination, even if there are no symptoms and no clinical mass in the contralateral gland. If the diagnosis is established by radiologic imaging and cytology, surgery is not necessary for other than cosmetic reasons.

2. **Benign lymphoepithelial cysts** are unifocal lesions that occur in patients in their fifth and sixth decades. They most commonly involve the parotid gland, but are occasionally seen in the oral cavity. There is no association with systemic disease. Grossly, they consist of well-circumscribed unilocular cysts with contents ranging from serous to mucoid to caseous; keratinous debris may be present. Microscopically, they consist of a cyst lined by benign mature squamous epithelium without papillary projections. In rare cases, the lining is cuboidal or columnar with goblet cells. Below the epithelium, the cyst wall has dense lymphoid tissue with germinal centers (e-**Fig. 6.8**). Excision is curative, and the lesion does not recur.

3. **Mucoceles** are the most common non neoplastic lesion of salivary gland tissue and are defined as pooling of mucin in a cystic cavity. Two types of mucoceles are recognized. In the retention type, the mucin is within a dilated duct. In the extravasation type, the mucin accumulates in the soft tissue. The lower lip is the most common site of mucoceles, followed by the tongue, the floor of the mouth (where the lesion is termed a ranula), and the buccal mucosa. The peak incidence of mucoceles is in the third decade. Grossly, a mucocele presents as a cystic cavity in the connective tissue that is filled with glistening fluid. Microscopically, the cyst wall may or may not have an epithelial lining, depending on the type. Those of the retention type have a lining and usually no surrounding inflammation, whereas those of the extravasation type consist of mucin with surrounding inflammatory cells without a lining. Some late lesions consist only of

a collection of foamy histiocytes containing mucin (**e-Fig. 6.9**), which can be confirmed by PAS or mucicarmine stains. Surgical excision is generally curative.

IV. **NEOPLASMS.** Neoplasms of the salivary gland can be roughly classified based on the cell type of the normal salivary gland toward which they differentiate: acinar, myoepithelial, or ductal. However, most neoplasms have dual differentiation because almost all show some myoepithelial differentiation. Most benign neoplasms have a malignant counterpart. The World Health Organization (WHO) classification of tumors of the salivary gland is listed in Table 6.1.

A. **Benign Neoplasms**

1. **Pleomorphic adenoma** (PA) is the most common neoplasm of the salivary glands. Ninety percent of PAs occur in the parotid gland, and PAs represent 60% of parotid gland neoplasms; the majority of the remaining cases occur in the hard palate or submandibular gland. The tumor occurs in a wide age range of patients, but the peak incidence is in the fourth and fifth decades. The tumor presents as a slowly growing painless mass that usually is between 2 and 5 cm in diameter. On gross examination, these tumors appear well-circumscribed and are not usually encapsulated (they are never encapsulated when occurring in minor salivary glands). Sectioning reveals a rubbery, myxoid, tan-white mass (**e-Fig. 6.10**). The microscopic appearance, as

---

TABLE 6.1 WHO Histologic Classification of Tumors of the Salivary Glands

Malignant tumors	Benign tumors
Mucoepidermoid carcinoma	Pleomorphic adenoma
Adenoid cystic carcinoma	Myoepithelioma
Acinic cell carcinoma	Basal cell adenoma
Polymorphous adenocarcinoma	Warthin tumor
Clear cell carcinoma	Oncocytoma
Basal cell adenocarcinoma	Lymphadenoma
Intraductal carcinoma	Cystadenoma
Adenocarcinoma, NOS	Sialadenoma papilliferum
Salivary duct carcinoma	Sebaceous adenoma
Myoepithelial carcinoma	Canalicular adenoma and other ductal adenomas
Epithelial–myoepithelial carcinoma	**Nonneoplastic epithelial lesions**
Carcinoma ex pleomorphic adenoma	Sclerosing polycystic adenosis
Secretory carcinoma	Nodular oncocytic hyperplasia
Sebaceous adenocarcinoma	Lymphoepithelial sialadenitis
Carcinosarcoma	Intercalated duct hyperplasia
Poorly differentiated carcinoma	**Hematolymphoid tumors**
Undifferentiated carcinoma	Extranodal marginal zone lymphoma of mucosa-associated lymphoid tissue (MALT lymphoma)
Large-cell neuroendocrine carcinoma	
Small-cell neuroendocrine carcinoma	
Lymphoepithelial carcinoma	
Squamous cell carcinoma	
Oncocytic carcinoma	
Uncertain malignant potential	
Sialoblastoma	

TABLE 6.2	Key Molecular Alteration in Salivary Gland Tumors	
Tumor	Chromosomal Alteration	Genes
Pleomorphic adenoma	8q12 and 12q13-15 rearrangements	PLAG1-HMGA2
Mucoepidermoid carcinoma	t(11;19)(q21;p13)	CRTC1-MAML2 (80%)
	t(11;15)(q21;q26)	CRTC3-MAML2
Adenoid cystic carcinoma	t(6;9)(q22-23;p23-24)	MYB-NFIB
Secretory carcinoma	t(12;15)(p13;q25)	ETV6-NRTK3 (100%)
Clear cell carcinoma	t(12;22)(q21;q12)	EWSR1-ATF1 (≈100%)
Salivary duct carcinoma	17q21.1 amplification	ERBB2 (HER2/neu)

the name suggests, is highly variable, but always shows an intimate admixture of epithelial and mesenchymal elements. The epithelial component consists of ductal structures with an associated myoepithelial layer but also may contain collections of myoepithelial cells that may be spindled, clear, plasmacytoid, or basaloid. The mesenchymal, or stromal, component is typically myxoid, hyaline, or chondroid (e-Fig. 6.11). Although defined subcategories have no clinical significance, PAs have been divided into a myxoid type (>80% mesenchymal-type tissue), cellular type (>80% epithelial-type tissue), and mixed or classic type (generally an equal mix of components). Genetically, PLAG1-HMGA2 fusion genes are frequently present (Table 6.2).

Treatment requires complete excision because PAs are likely to recur if tumor is left behind or transected. Multinodular growth is uncommon in primary tumors but is frequent in recurrent disease, yielding a so-called buckshot pattern (e-Fig. 6.12). Therapy for recurrence is consequently more difficult.

2. **Warthin tumor** (papillary cystadenoma lymphomatosum) is the second most common benign salivary gland tumor and is found exclusively in the parotid gland. It is the most common bilateral or multifocal salivary gland tumor, usually presents in the sixth or seventh decade, and is associated with smoking. Grossly, it presents as a soft, brown or yellow mass that is composed of cysts that are classically filled with viscous brown fluid. Microscopically, the lesion has a classic and highly reproducible morphology with papillary projections into cystic spaces which have an epithelial lining composed of two layers of cells with oncocytic features (e-Fig. 6.13). The epithelium overlies a dense polyclonal lymphoid component that forms germinal centers. Warthin tumors may show a giant cell reaction, fibrosis, or squamous metaplasia from trauma and/or cyst rupture. Surgical excision is almost always curative as recurrence is rare. Associated malignancy is also very rare and takes the form of either squamous cell carcinoma or lymphoma.

3. **Basal cell adenomas** are benign tumors that are composed of small basaloid cells. They generally occur in adults, and 75% occur in the parotid gland. They usually present as an asymptomatic, slowly growing mass. The membranous subtype (dermal anlage tumor) may be multicentric, and the occurrence of numerous basal cell adenomas, dermal cell cylindromas, and trichoepitheliomas is called Brooke–Spiegler syndrome.

On gross examination, these tumors are usually solid, well-circumscribed, and pink to brown. Some may be cystic. Microscopically, four patterns are recognized: tubular, solid, trabecular, and membranous (Table 6.3). In all patterns, the tumor is

TABLE 6.3	Four Major Patterns of Basal Cell Adenoma
Tubular	
Solid	
Trabecular	
Membranous ("dermal anlage tumor")	

composed of two cell types. Small cells with little cytoplasm typically lie at the neoplasm's edge, frequently show peripheral palisading, and give the tumor its basaloid appearance. Polygonal basaloid cells with slightly more cytoplasm and round to oval nuclei with more open chromatin usually lie in the center of the nests. The trabecular and membranous patterns have a "jigsaw puzzle" appearance with rounded nests of tumor cells shaped like puzzle pieces (e-**Fig. 6.14**). The membranous pattern additionally shows hyalinized, eosinophilic, linear, or nodular basement membrane–like material around the nests (e-**Fig. 6.15**). The tubular pattern consists of tubular, gland-like structures (e-**Fig. 6.16**), and the solid pattern consists of solid cell nests. The tumor cells express myoepithelial markers including pan-cytokeratin, S-100, smooth muscle actin, and p63.

The differential diagnosis for basal cell adenoma includes basal cell adenocarcinoma and adenoid cystic carcinoma, both of which, unlike basal cell adenoma, show infiltrative growth and/or perineural invasion. Simple excision of basal cell adenoma is usually curative and recurrence is rare, except in the membranous type where the recurrence rate approaches 25%.

4. Canalicular adenomas are benign salivary tumors thought to arise from the excretory ducts of the minor salivary glands, particularly of the upper lip. They are frequently multifocal (e-**Fig. 6.17**). Women and African Americans are more commonly affected, and the peak incidence is in the seventh decade. Canalicular adenomas present clinically as an asymptomatic, fluctuant, or firm 1- to 2-cm submucosal nodule that grows slowly.

On gross examination, they are well-circumscribed but unencapsulated, and have a tan to pink, cystic or solid cut surface. Histologically, canalicular adenomas are composed of long strands or tubules of columnar epithelial cells with a loose collagenous stroma (e-**Fig. 6.18**). There are typically two rows of columnar cells situated opposite each other; the rows may take on a beaded appearance, with tubules coming together and then separating. The epithelial cells lining the tubules have eosinophilic cytoplasm and range from cuboidal to columnar. There is no significant pleomorphism, and mitotic counts are low. The epithelial cells express cytokeratin and S-100, but are negative for calponin.

The differential diagnosis for canalicular adenoma includes PA and basal cell adenoma. However, the pattern of growth of canalicular adenoma is virtually always distinctive enough to make the diagnosis. Simple local excision is performed with an attempt to obtain clear margins. Recurrence is rare.

5. Myoepitheliomas are benign tumors composed almost exclusively of myoepithelial cells, though ductal cells may occasionally be present. In this regard, myoepitheliomas are sometimes considered to lie at one end of a biologic spectrum, with PA in the middle, and basal cell adenoma at the opposite end. Myoepitheliomas occur with approximately equal frequency in the parotid gland and minor salivary glands, particularly the hard and soft palate, and present as slowly growing, painless masses in adults. Men and women are affected equally.

Grossly, these neoplasms are well-circumscribed and encapsulated with a tan to white cut surface. Histologically, they consist of sheets and cords of tumor cells that can be classified into four major subtypes: spindle cell, hyaline, plasmacytoid, and clear cell. All subtypes generally have a collagenous or myxoid stroma. The spindle cell type can show an interlacing, fascicular pattern of growth (e-**Fig. 6.19**). Loosely cohesive myoepithelial cells with eosinophilic cytoplasm and eccentric round nuclei are present in the plasmacytoid variant (e-**Fig. 6.20**). The clear cell type is composed of sheets and aggregates of clear cells (e-**Fig. 6.21**). The tumor cells express typical myoepithelial markers such as S-100, pan-cytokeratin, smooth muscle actin, and p63.

Simple excision is generally the treatment of choice unless malignant features, such as infiltrative growth or perineural invasion, are encountered, in which the diagnosis is myoepithelial carcinoma. Myoepitheliomas have a slightly lower recurrence rate than PAs.

B. Malignant Neoplasms

1. **Mucoepidermoid carcinoma** is a malignant glandular tumor composed of mucous, intermediate, and epidermoid (or squamoid) cells and is the most common salivary gland malignancy. The major salivary glands account for more than half of all cases, with most arising in the parotid gland. The tumor also arises from minor salivary glands in the oral cavity, particularly in the hard palate, buccal mucosa, lip, and retromolar trigone. It may also develop intraosseously in the mandible and maxilla, but such tumors are considered odontogenic in origin and have a different clinical behavior. Mucoepidermoid carcinomas are slightly more common in women, and the mean age of affected patients is approximately 45 years. The tumor also occurs in children and is the most common pediatric salivary gland carcinoma. Patients usually present with a painless, slowly growing mass, but may also present with a blue-red superficial nodule along the oral mucosa mimicking a mucocele or vascular lesion.

   Grossly, both solid and cystic components may be present, often with mucinous material within the cysts. Microscopically, the hallmark of these tumors is the presence of the three different cell types. The three cell types are present in variable proportions in individual tumors and form sheets, nests, duct-like structures, and/or cysts. Intermediate cells frequently predominate, and range from small basal cells with minimal basophilic cytoplasm to larger oval cells with pale eosinophilic cytoplasm. The mucous cells occur singly or in clusters and have pale, foamy cytoplasm, distinct cell membranes, and eccentric small nuclei (e-**Fig. 6.22**); they frequently line cystic spaces and are positive with mucicarmine and PAS stains. Squamoid cells have abundant eosinophilic cytoplasm and vesicular nuclei with open chromatin; they are not truly squamous as they lack intercellular bridges, and only very rarely is there true keratinization. A population of glycogen rich clear cells is often scattered throughout the tumor.

   The differential diagnosis includes necrotizing sialometaplasia, which is discerned by its residual normal lobules of minor salivary gland tissue, presence of necrosis, associated dense inflammatory infiltrate, and lack of cytologic atypia. Adenosquamous carcinoma and squamous cell carcinoma are also in the differential, but both have true squamous differentiation with intercellular bridges or keratinization, and are frequently associated with surface squamous dysplasia or carcinoma in situ. Most mucoepidermoid carcinomas possess a t(11;19)(q21;p13) forming a *CRTC1-MAML2* gene fusion (Table 6.2). Tumors that carry the rearrangement are usually of low or intermediate grade, although recent studies have found the translocation in high-grade tumors as well. The clinical utility of testing for the translocation has yet to be established.

   Prognosis is highly dependent on the grade of the tumor, and the grade is in turn dependent on the relative amounts of the various cell types. Low-grade lesions are markedly cystic and have abundant well-differentiated mucous cells. High-grade lesions are more solid with squamous and intermediate cells predominating. Different grading systems have been proposed with inconsistent results, although the Brandwein-Gensler grading system (Table 6.4) has gained acceptance for its reproducibility and ability to stratify for outcomes.

   Wide local excision is recommended. Radiation therapy has not been shown to be beneficial except for palliation of unresectable or recurrent disease. The prognosis for low-grade tumors is excellent (>90% survival at 5 years) but drops greatly for high-grade tumors (about 50% survival at 5 years).

2. **Polymorphous adenocarcinoma** (PAC) is the second most common intraoral salivary gland tumor and accounts for 25% of all minor salivary gland tumors. The tumor's most common site is the palate, particularly at the junction of the hard and soft palate. Less common sites include the upper lip, buccal mucosa, retromolar region, base of tongue, major salivary and lacrimal glands, nasopharynx, and nasal cavity. PAC arises more commonly in women and tends to present in the fourth

TABLE 6.4	Brandwein-Gensler Grading System for Mucoepidermoid Carcinoma
Parameter	**Point Value**
Cystic component <25%	+2
Tumor front invades in small nests and islands	+2
Pronounced nuclear atypia	+2
Lymphatic and/or vascular invasion	+3
Neural invasion	+3
Necrosis	+3
4+ mitoses/10 HPF	+3
Bony invasion	+3
Grade	**Point Score**
Low (I)	0
Intermediate (II)	2–3
High (III)	4 or more

Adapted from Brandwein MS, Ivanov K, Wallace DI, et al. Mucoepidermoid carcinoma: a clinicopathologic study of 80 patients with special reference to histological grading. *Am J Surg Pathol* 2001;25(7):835–845.

to sixth decades, often as a very slowly growing mass that may be present for years before coming to clinical attention.

On gross examination, PAC is a circumscribed, nonencapsulated, and pale yellow or tan mass that generally ranges from 1 to 3 cm in greatest dimension. Microscopically, the architectural features are quite variable, as the name suggests, showing solid nests, lobules, cribriform gland-like structures, duct-like arrangements, and/or a characteristic concentric whirling of the cellular nests in a single file arrangement that has been termed "the eye of the storm." Stromal hyalinization with a grayish hue is characteristic. The periphery of the tumor shows markedly infiltrative growth, and perineural invasion is common (e-**Fig. 6.23**). Cytologically, in contrast to the architecture, the tumor cells are very uniform with moderate eosinophilic cytoplasm and characteristic round to oval nuclei with open chromatin (e-**Fig. 6.24**). There is minimal mitotic activity and no necrosis. The differential diagnosis includes PA, which usually exhibits myxochondroid areas that are not seen in PAC, and adenoid cystic carcinoma, which consists of basaloid cells with more hyperchromatic nuclei than those of PAC.

Conservative resection is the treatment of choice. Local recurrence occurs in 10% to 33% of patients. Neck dissection is only recommended for significant clinical adenopathy or proven metastasis because lymph node metastases are distinctly uncommon. Distant metastases are even less common. Patients have an excellent long-term prognosis even in the presence of recurrent/metastatic disease, and deaths due to PAC are extremely uncommon.

3. **Acinic cell carcinoma** accounts for only 6.5% of salivary gland tumors. It occurs evenly through the second to seventh decades and can be seen in childhood (in fact, it is the second most common childhood salivary gland malignancy). About 80% of cases arise in the parotid gland, usually presenting as a slowly growing mass which is occasionally painful.

Grossly, acinic cell carcinoma presents as a single, usually circumscribed solid mass that can undergo cystic degeneration. Histologically, the architecture can be solid/lobular, microcystic, papillary-cystic, or follicular. Mixed architectural patterns are common as is a background inflammatory infiltrate with germinal center formation (e-**Fig. 6.25**). Small tumors can be easily missed because the acinar cells may be very well differentiated. The acinic cell is characteristic and has the appearance of a salivary acinar cell with abundant granular, basophilic cytoplasm and a small, round, eccentrically placed nucleus (e-**Fig. 6.25**). PAS stains highlight the cytoplasmic zymogen granules, which are resistant to diastase digestion. An immunostain for DOG-1 is positive in all tumors, and strong staining may be used to support the diagnosis. A number of other cell types can also be present including eosinophilic, clear, and vacuolated cells. The periphery of the tumor may not be infiltrative, but this finding should not be interpreted as evidence of benignancy. A common finding is a tumor-associated lymphoid proliferation which may be extensive and should not be confused with lymph node involvement.

The differential diagnosis differs depending on the architecture and predominant cell type, and includes normal parotid gland, oncocytoma/oncocytic carcinoma, secretory carcinoma, and clear cell lesions. The papillary variant of acinic cell carcinoma must be differentiated from cystadenoma/adenocarcinoma.

Recurrence after excision occurs in approximately one third of cases. Although classically regarded as a low-grade malignancy, 10% to 15% of these tumors will metastasize to regional lymph nodes or distantly, particularly to the lungs and bones. Survival is approximately 80% at 5 years and 70% at 10 years. Tumor grade does not correlate well with behavior (the majority of tumors are well-differentiated) although high-grade transformation (also known as dedifferentiation) (e-Fig. 6.26) has consistently been associated with a poor outcome.

4. **Adenoid cystic carcinoma** is one of the most recognizable salivary gland tumors. It comprises 10% of all salivary gland malignancies, and is the most common malignancy of the minor salivary glands. Although the tumor occurs in patients over a wide age range, the peak incidence is in patients between 40 and 60 years of age. The tumor is slowly growing, but nonetheless relentlessly progressive. Perineural invasion is extremely common, so cranial nerve involvement, including facial nerve palsy, may be the presenting symptom, with or without associated pain.

Grossly, the tumor is solid, light tan, firm, and well circumscribed. Histologically, several architectural patterns are found including cribriform, tubular, solid, and mixed. Tumors are graded based on the predominant pattern (Table 6.5). The tubular pattern consists of double cell-lined ducts with inner epithelial and outer myoepithelial layers (e-Fig. 6.27). The most common and recognizable pattern is cribriform (e-Fig. 6.28) which consists of nests of cells arranged around gland-like spaces filled with reduplicated basement membrane material (which appears as pink and hyaline) or glycosaminoglycans (which appear as basophilic mucoid material). The solid pattern consists of rounded nests of basaloid tumor cells with no, or virtually no, tubule formation (e-Fig. 6.29). The cells in adenoid cystic carcinoma are basaloid with little cytoplasm, and have round to oval nuclei that are dark and hyperchromatic without nucleoli. The cells are usually regular with little mitotic activity, except in the solid type, in which mitotic activity may be prominent. Perineural invasion is seen in the majority of cases, particularly at the tumor's periphery. The tumors are predominantly composed of epithelial cells, which express pancytokeratin and EMA, and much less prominent myoepithelial cells, which express S-100, SMA, calponin, and p63, particularly as scattered cells at the periphery of the nests (e-Fig. 6.30). The myxoid stromal material in and around the nests stains for collagen type IV and laminin. Genetically, the majority of adenoid cystic carcinomas have a t(6;9) resulting in *MYB-NFIB* gene fusion (Table 6.2).

The differential diagnosis for low-grade (tubular) adenoid cystic carcinomas most importantly includes polymorphous adenocarcinoma, epithelial–myoepithelial

TABLE 6.5	Grading of Adenoid Cystic Carcinoma
Predominant Pattern	**Grade**
Tubular	I
Cribriform	II
Solid	III

carcinoma, and basal cell adenocarcinoma, but none of these tumors shows the basaloid and hyperchromatic nuclei characteristic of adenoid cystic carcinoma. High-grade neuroendocrine carcinomas and basaloid squamous cell carcinoma enter the differential diagnosis of solid-type adenoid cystic carcinoma, but adenoid cystic carcinoma lacks neuroendocrine staining and squamous differentiation. Solid adenoid cystic carcinoma will have a patchy p63 staining pattern with positive cells at the periphery of the nests, while in basaloid squamous cell carcinoma, the staining is diffuse.

Despite its somewhat bland appearing morphology, adenoid cystic carcinoma causes progressive disease. Five- and ten-year survival rates are only 62% and 40%. Local recurrence is extremely common, particularly in the first 5 years after surgery, although late recurrences also occur. Involvement of bone, submandibular gland origin, and solid histologic type (grade III) all adversely affect prognosis. Identification of perineural invasion may adversely affect prognosis as well.

5. **Secretory carcinoma (mammary analogue secretory carcinoma)** is a recently described low-grade neoplasm that morphologically resembles mammary secretory carcinoma and is characterized by the presence of the *ETV6-NTRK3* gene fusion. Historically, these tumors were diagnosed as zymogen-poor acinic cell carcinomas but are now a distinct entity with a specific histological, immunohistochemical, and molecular profile. Secretory carcinomas are more common in males and occur over a wide age range of 21 to 75 years, the mean being 46 years. The majority arise as a painless slowly growing mass in the parotid gland, but the tumor may occur in other major and minor salivary glands.

Grossly, the tumor is circumscribed but unencapsulated with a lobulated architecture that may occasionally form cystic structures. Microscopically, the tumor border is often infiltrative, but may be pushing. The mass is lobulated with fibrous septae and shows micro/macrocystic, solid, tubular, papillary, or follicular growth patterns. On low power, the tumor cells characteristically have an eosinophilic, vacuolated (bubbly) cytoplasm with round nuclei and minimal atypia (e-**Fig. 6.31**). Abundant bluish to deep pink intraluminal secretions are usually present. There are rare reports of high-grade transformation that is characterized by anaplastic cells, necrosis, marked nuclear pleomorphism, and perineural invasion. Immunohistochemically, lesional cells are strongly reactive to S100 and mammaglobin (e-**Fig. 6.32**). Detection of t(12;15) (p13;q25) chromosomal translocation resulting in *ETV6-NTRK3* gene fusion using FISH or RT-PCR can be used as a confirmatory test (Table 6.2). To date, secretory carcinoma is the only salivary gland tumor with this gene fusion.

Secretory carcinoma is an indolent malignancy with occasional lymph node metastasis but very rare distant metastasis. Complete surgical resection is the treatment of choice.

6. **Clear cell carcinoma (CCC)** is an uncommon low-grade salivary gland carcinoma that most commonly arises from the palate and base of tongue, but may also be seen in major salivary glands. Typically, these tumors present in the fifth to eighth decade of life as an asymptomatic mass, however, it may be painful in the presence of ulceration and bone invasion.

Grossly, the lesion appears as a gray-white poorly circumscribed mass with a scar-like appearance if extensive hyalinization is present. As the name implies, CCCs are composed of malignant cells with clear cytoplasm with or without surrounding hyalinization. The lesion is poorly circumscribed and the cells are arranged in solid sheets, nests, cords, trabeculae, and/or single cells. Prominent hyalinized stroma surrounding cell nests are present in most cases (e-**Fig. 6.33**). Overt squamous and mucinous differentiation may be present.

To make a diagnosis of CCC, the tumor must have a squamoid phenotype and lack features of other salivary gland carcinomas that contain clear cells. By immunohistochemistry, the tumor should be positive for p63 expression but negative for S100 expression. Clear cell variants of oncocytoma, myoepithelioma, mucoepidermoid, and squamous cell carcinomas must be ruled out.

Genetically, CCC shows an *EWSR1-ATF1* gene fusion (e-**Fig. 6.34**). Demonstration of the fusion is helpful in cases with prominent squamous and mucinous differentiation. CCC is treated surgically and has a good prognosis.

7. **Malignant mixed tumor** is a broad term that is used to encompass true malignant mixed tumors, carcinoma ex pleomorphic adenoma, and metastasizing mixed tumor.

   a. **Carcinosarcoma** is a malignant neoplasm that is composed of both carcinomatous and sarcomatous components, and is exceedingly rare with less than 100 reported cases. The mean age of affected individuals is in the sixth to seventh decade, and one third of patients have evidence of a pre-existing PA. Approximately two-thirds of cases arise in the parotid gland, 15% in the submandibular gland, and 15% in the minor salivary glands of the palate.

   Grossly, there is typically a firm, tan-white mass with hemorrhage, necrosis, and, on occasion, grittiness or calcification. Microscopically, there is an intimate admixture of the two components. The carcinomatous component typically takes the form of adenocarcinoma, NOS (e-**Fig. 6.35**). The sarcomatous component is usually chondrosarcoma or osteosarcoma, but fibrosarcoma, leiomyosarcoma, and even liposarcoma occur. Treatment consists of wide local excision combined with radiotherapy. The tumors are very aggressive, with up to two-thirds of patients dying of disease, usually within 30 months.

   b. **Carcinoma ex pleomorphic adenoma** is defined as a mixed tumor in which carcinoma is present. This tumor accounts for more than 95% of malignant mixed tumors, and is most common in the parotid gland, followed by the minor salivary glands, submandibular gland, and sublingual gland. Most patients are in their sixth or seventh decade, which is approximately one decade older than the age of most patients who have PAs. The classic history is that of a patient with a longstanding mass that undergoes rapid growth over a period of several months.

   Grossly, these tumors can reach up to 25 cm in diameter, and the average size is more than twice that of PAs. The carcinomatous component is usually an infiltrative, hard, white to tan-gray mass with hemorrhage and necrosis. Microscopically, the proportions of the carcinoma and PA are quite variable, and the PA component may be replaced by scarring or overgrown by the malignant component. The malignant component most often is a high-grade adenocarcinoma, typically a salivary duct carcinoma or adenocarcinoma not otherwise specified (e-**Figs. 6.36** and **6.37**). Low-grade carcinomas such as myoepithelial carcinoma occur in 35% of cases.

   Prognosis and management are highly dependent on the type of carcinoma and extent of invasion. The malignant component should be classified as noninvasive (intracapsular), minimally invasive (<4 to 6 mm in greatest extent), or invasive. Extent of invasion shows superior prognostic significance compared with pT classification. As with PAs, *PLAG1-HMGA2* rearrangements are detected and may be helpful in cases where a clear PA component cannot be readily identified. Wide resection is the treatment of choice, with lymph node dissection and radiation therapy reserved for widely invasive tumors or tumors with obvious cervical lymph node metastases.

   c. **Metastasizing pleomorphic adenoma** is the least common form of malignant mixed tumor. These tumors are histologically identical to PA, but metastasize either to local lymph nodes or distantly, usually to bone and lung. Often there is a protracted clinical course with many recurrences at the primary site. Overall mortality due to the tumor is 40%.

8. **Salivary duct carcinoma** is one of the most aggressive primary salivary gland tumors. It histologically resembles high-grade ductal carcinoma of the breast, and accounts for <10% of salivary gland tumors. Men are more commonly affected in a ratio of 4:1. Patients generally present in the sixth decade with a rapidly growing parotid mass with facial nerve involvement.

   Grossly, the tumors are solid and white with hemorrhage, necrosis, and cystic areas. Infiltration of the surrounding tissue is usually apparent. Microscopically, ductal carcinoma in situ with a cribriform pattern is present in a pattern similar to that of breast ductal carcinomas, often with comedo-type necrosis (e-**Fig. 6.38**). The tumor's invasive component consists of large cells with abundant eosinophilic cytoplasm and large, round nuclei with vesicular chromatin and prominent nucleoli (e-**Fig. 6.39**). The neoplasm shows marked tissue infiltration with stromal desmoplasia and brisk mitotic activity, and vascular and perineural invasion are common. Salivary duct carcinomas express low- and high-molecular weight cytokeratins, carcinoembryogenic antigen (CEA), androgen receptors, and human epidermal growth factor receptor 2 (HER2)/neu. The differential diagnosis includes metastatic breast carcinoma, poorly differentiated squamous cell carcinoma, and mucoepidermoid carcinoma. The presence of intraductal carcinoma is an important finding that argues strongly for a diagnosis of a primary salivary duct carcinoma rather than a metastasis.

Salivary duct carcinoma is the most aggressive salivary gland tumor. Approximately one third of patients develop local recurrence, half develop distant metastases, and 65% of patients die of their disease, most within 4 years of diagnosis. Wide local excision with neck dissection and postoperative radiotherapy is the treatment of choice.

9. **Epithelial–myoepithelial carcinoma** is a low-grade carcinoma that accounts for only 0.5% to 1% of salivary gland neoplasms. It arises in the parotid gland, and occasionally from the minor salivary glands of the larynx or paranasal sinuses.

Grossly, the tumor is firm and well-demarcated, averaging 2 to 3 cm in diameter. Microscopically, the tumor is usually partially encapsulated, with invasion by tumor into the adjacent parenchyma. The classic morphology is of ductal structures lined by an inner layer of eosinophilic epithelial cells and an outer layer of clear myoepithelial cells (e-**Fig. 6.40**), which lie in an eosinophilic hyaline stroma. In rare cases, the myoepithelial cell component may be present as large sheets or nests of cells with only focal ductal differentiation. The individual tumor cells are bland with minimal mitotic activity. The epithelial cells express low–molecular-weight cytokeratins, and the myoepithelial cells express calponin, smooth muscle actin, and p63. The differential diagnosis includes PA, myoepithelioma/myoepithelial carcinoma, and the tubular variant of adenoid cystic carcinoma.

Epithelial–myoepithelial carcinoma is a moderately aggressive tumor with a recurrence rate of 40%. Metastases to lymph nodes, lung, or liver occur in 15% of patients, and overall survival at 5 years is about 80%. Treatment is wide local excision with or without radiotherapy.

10. **Squamous cell carcinoma** is only rarely primary to the salivary glands. Metastases to the intraparotid lymph nodes from primary skin cancers of the head and neck (particularly of the scalp, ear, and face) are much more common. Most patients are in their sixth to eighth decade. About 80% of tumors arise in the parotid gland and 20% in the submandibular gland. The tumors typically are high stage at the time of diagnosis. By definition, the diagnosis of primary squamous cell carcinoma is restricted to the large salivary glands, because tumors arising in the minor salivary glands cannot be reliably distinguished from primary squamous carcinoma of the surrounding mucosa.

Grossly, the neoplasm is a firm, white, infiltrative, and nonencapsulated mass. Microscopically, it is identical to typical squamous cell carcinomas of the UADT, although cases arising in a salivary gland tend to be well-differentiated. Prominent desmoplasia is common, and perineural invasion and extension of the tumor into periglandular soft tissue are frequently present.

The differential diagnosis most importantly includes metastatic squamous cell carcinoma. High-grade mucoepidermoid carcinoma can have a largely squamoid appearance but lacks keratinization, has a more heterogeneous cell population, and almost always demonstrates mucous cells.

Primary squamous carcinomas are aggressive tumors, and the 5-year survival of patients is approximately 25%. Treatment involves radical surgery, neck dissection, and radiotherapy.

11. **Malignant counterparts to benign salivary gland tumors** are relatively uncommon and microscopically resemble benign salivary gland tumors in differentiation and cellular components but show aggressive features such as an invasive growth, perineural invasion, lymphovascular invasion, cellular anaplasia, necrosis, and/or metastasis). The more common types are basal cell adenocarcinoma (e-**Fig. 6.41**) and myoepithelial carcinoma (e-**Fig. 6.42**), although the majority of benign salivary gland tumors have a reported malignant counterpart.

12. **Metastasis to the salivary glands** or, more commonly, to intra- or periglandular lymph nodes, is a frequent occurrence.

    The parotid contains an average of 20 lymph nodes which drain the scalp, face, ear skin, external auditory canal, and tympanic membrane. Skin tumors such as squamous cell carcinoma and melanoma, therefore, account for approximately 80% of metastases to the gland. The remaining metastases are from non–head and neck primary tumors, most commonly lung, kidney, and breast carcinomas.

    The opposite distribution of metastases is seen for the submandibular gland, which does not contain lymph nodes. More than 85% of metastases arise from infraclavicular primary tumors, most commonly breast, kidney, and lung carcinomas, particularly pulmonary small-cell carcinoma.

13. **Pediatric tumors** are uncommon. Hemangioma is the most frequent, but most salivary gland neoplasms that occur in adults can also occur in children. There are two congenital tumors worth specific mention.

    a. **Sialoblastoma** is an extremely rare, potentially aggressive neoplasm that recapitulates the embryonic stage of salivary gland development and is thought to develop from retained blastematous cells. Clinically, it is seen in the perinatal to neonatal period; it usually involves the parotid gland but may also involve the submandibular gland. The tumor may grow quickly and cause skin ulceration or airway compromise.

       Grossly, the mass is lobulated and partially circumscribed. Microscopically, it is composed of nests or nodules of basaloid cells with accompanying ductal structures. The basaloid cells have scanty cytoplasm, round to oval nuclei, and fine chromatin with small nucleoli. Ducts are small and lined by cuboidal to low columnar cells. Complete surgical excision with a rim of normal tissue is the treatment of choice. Although local recurrence is relatively common, occurring in up to 30% of cases, metastasis is extremely uncommon.

    b. **Salivary anlage tumor,** also referred to as a congenital PA, occurs in male neonates in the first 2 weeks of life and is associated with respiratory obstruction or difficulty feeding. Sometimes, the mass is spontaneously passed or inadvertently removed by airway suctioning. On examination, a mass attached by a thin stalk to the posterior nasal mucosa or nasopharynx is sometimes present.

       Grossly, salivary anlage tumors are firm and tan-yellow with a smooth surface. Microscopically, the tumor's surface shows nonkeratinizing squamous epithelium, with a deeper stroma composed of bland spindled cells and intervening squamous islands. The overall histology suggests a hamartoma rather than a true neoplasm. The treatment is simple excision of the mass, and the lesion does not recur or spread.

V. PATHOLOGIC REPORTING OF MALIGNANT SALIVARY GLAND TUMORS

A. **Staging:** Clinical staging of salivary gland cancers is important for prognosis and treatment decisions. The most recent AJCC staging manual (Amin MB, Edge SB, Greene FL, et al., eds. *AJCC Cancer Staging Manual.* 8th ed. New York: Springer; 2017.) has a staging system for malignancies arising in the major salivary glands. Minor salivary gland tumors are staged according to the primary site in which they arise (e.g., oral cavity, sinus, larynx).

B. **Additional Pertinent Pathologic Features.** Pathologic features such as tumor grade, positive resection margins, and skin or bone invasion have been demonstrated in numerous studies to correlate with a higher risk of local recurrence, a poorer prognosis, or both, and so should always be reported. Perineural and lymphovascular space invasion should also always be reported when observed, because they have been correlated with distant metastases in some studies, even though they are not predictive of recurrence or poorer prognosis. Reporting should follow suggested guidelines (e.g., see the College of American Pathologists Protocol for the Examination of Specimens from Patients with Carcinomas of the Major Salivary Glands, at http://www.cap.org).

ACKNOWLEDGMENT

The authors thank Joshua I. Warrick, Elease L. Krejci, and James S. Lewis Jr., authors of the previous edition of this chapter.

Cytopathology of the Salivary Glands

Cory Bernadt

The parotid and minor salivary glands are superficially located and palpable, and so salivary gland lesions are readily amenable to percutaneous fine-needle aspiration (FNA). A pattern approach is typically utilized for the evaluation of FNA specimens for diagnosis, classification, and clinical management of patients.

I. NONNEOPLASTIC CONDITIONS

A. **Chronic Sialadenitis.** Chronic inflammation can cause diffuse or focal enlargement which by palpation can be indistinguishable from a neoplasm. However, chronic sialadenitis is very tender on FNA, which can be a helpful clue to diagnosis. Aspiration smears are hypocellular with benign ductal epithelial groups which have a minimal degree of nuclear atypia. Acinar elements can be scant or absent due to the underlying destructive nature of the process. A variable mixture of large and small lymphocytes is present. Acinic cell carcinoma is an important differential diagnostic consideration when presented with bland acinar type cells and lymphocytes on aspirate smears.

B. **Lymph Nodes.** The parotid is a common site of intraparenchymal lymph nodes which can be clinically difficult to distinguish from a neoplasm. Aspirate smears will show a mixture of lymphocytes in the pattern typically seen with reactive lymphoid hyperplasia.

II. BENIGN NEOPLASMS

A. **Warthin Tumor.** This tumor commonly arises in the parotid gland and by aspiration shows a mixture of lymphocytes and cohesive groups of oncocytic-type epithelial fragments (e-**Figs. 6.43** and **6.44**). The lymphoid elements are intimately admixed with the oncocytic cells, and the background usually shows cystic change with macrophages and granular debris.

B. **Pleomorphic Adenoma.** Aspiration smears can show a wide variety of patterns and cellular elements. Commonly, there is a mixture of bland epithelial, spindled, and myoepithelial-like cells which occur as single cells and are intimately admixed with a variable amount of fibromyxoid stroma (e-**Figs. 6.45** and **6.46**). The relative proportions of these elements can vary significantly between cases. Diff-Quik staining of smears helps to highlight the metachromatic fibromyxoid stroma. When present in the customary pattern, a definitive diagnosis can be rendered.

C. **Basal Cell Adenoma.** Aspiration smears are cellular and contain small uniform basaloid cells with scant cytoplasm and round to oval nuclei with indistinct nucleoli. The dense extracellular material present, usually less than that seen in pleomorphic adenoma, tends to be arranged in globules and trabecular-tubular configurations (e-**Fig. 6.47**). This pattern typically is classified as a basaloid neoplasm and the differential diagnosis includes adenoid cystic carcinoma, since the cytomorphologic pattern on aspiration does not permit definitive classification.

III. MALIGNANT NEOPLASMS

A. Adenoid Cystic Carcinoma. Aspiration shows small basaloid cells with globules of dense matrix material. The cells are monomorphic with round to oval nuclei, even chromatin, indistinct nucleoli, and scant cytoplasm. Aspirates are usually cellular with cell groups arranged in syncytial and three-dimensional fragments. The extracellular matrix consists of dense amorphous material with tubular and/or globular shapes (e-**Figs. 6.48** to **6.50**). Classically, the cells appear to surround the round globules. Because of the cytomorphologic overlap with other basaloid tumors, definitive classification is not possible.

B. Mucoepidermoid Carcinoma. These neoplasms vary in their cellular composition, and this difference is reflected in the patterns and cellular elements encountered by FNA. For low-grade neoplasms, aspiration smears are hypocellular and contain thick mucoid-like material with granular debris. The three cell types that characterize the tumor (squamoid or epidermoid, mucous, and intermediate) are all present, and they can be arranged separately or be admixed. The nuclear features of all three cell types are bland (e-**Figs. 6.51** and **6.52**). For high-grade neoplasms, aspirate smears are cellular with groups and sheets of cells with a squamoid appearance. Nuclei are large with coarse chromatin and prominent nucleoli; the cytoplasm is dense, and moderate in amount with well-defined cell borders. Mucin cells with intracytoplasmic vacuoles are usually few and can be difficult to identify (e-**Figs. 6.53** and **6.54**).

C. Acinic Cell Carcinoma. Aspirate smears are cellular with a mixture of single cells, small groups of cells, and three-dimensional clusters. The large polygonal cells have round nuclei with nucleoli, and the cytoplasm demonstrates features of acinar differentiation with delicate vacuoles and granules (e-**Figs. 6.55** and **6.56**). While usually clean, the background can show stripped (naked) tumor cell nuclei and lymphoid elements. As these are richly vascular neoplasms, delicate blood vessels surrounded by neoplastic cells may be present.

ACKNOWLEDGMENT

The author thanks Brian Collins, author of the previous edition of this section.

SUGGESTED READINGS

Chiosea SI, Thompson LDR. Malignant neoplasms of the salivary glands. In: Thompson LDR, Bishop, JA, eds. *Head and Neck Pathology*. Philadelphia, PA: Elsevier; 2019:284–362.

El-Naggar AK, Chan JKC, Grandis JR, Takata T, Slootweg PJ, eds. Tumours of salivary glands, Chapter 7 (159-201). *WHO Classification of Head and Neck Tumors*. Lyon, France: IARC Press; 2017.

Faquin WC, Powers CN. *Salivary Gland Cytopathology: Essentials in Cytopathology*. New York: Springer; 2008.

Gnepp DR, Henley JD, Simpson RHW, Eveson J. Salivary and lacrimal glands. In: Gnepp DR, ed. *Diagnostic Surgical Pathology of the Head and Neck*. Philadelphia, PA: W.B. Saunders Publishers; 2009;413–562.

Layfield L. *Cytopathology of the Head and Neck*. Chicago, IL: ASCP Press; 1997.

Powers CN, Frable WJ. *Fine Needle Aspiration Biopsy of the Head and Neck*. Boston, MA: Butterworth Heinemann; 1996.

Richardson MS. Non-neoplastic lesions of the salivary glands. In: Thompson LDR, ed. *Head and Neck Pathology*. Philadelphia, PA: Elsevier; 2019:241–260.

Richardson MS. Benign neoplasms of the salivary glands. In: Thompson LDR, ed. *Head and Neck Pathology*. Philadelphia, PA: Elsevier; 2019:261–283.

Wenig BM. Major and minor salivary glands. In: Wenig BM, ed. *Atlas of Head and Neck Pathology*. Saunders Elsevier: Philadelphia, PA; 2016:805–1072.

7 The Ear

Peter A. Humphrey and Rebecca D. Chernock

I. **NORMAL ANATOMY.** The ear is composed of the external ear, the middle ear, and the inner ear. The external ear is made up of the auricle, which leads to the external auditory canal. The auricle has a supporting plate of elastic cartilage, which also helps form the outer two-thirds of the external auditory canal. Skin covers both the auricle and the canal; the main distinctive histologic features of this skin are that the squamous lining of the inner half of the canal is thinned, and that modified apocrine glands called ceruminal glands are present in the outer third of the canal. The clustered ceruminal glands are lined by cuboidal epithelial cells that have an eosinophilic cytoplasm that often harbors a granular golden-yellow pigment (**e-Fig. 7.1**).

The middle ear, or tympanic cavity, lies within the temporal bone. It is separated from the external auditory canal by the tympanic membrane, a thin fibrous sheet that has an external keratinizing squamous epithelial lining and an inner cuboidal cell lining. The middle ear contains the three auditory ossicles (malleus, incus, and stapes), ossicle ligaments, tendons of the ossicular muscles, the auditory tube, the tympanic cavity itself, and the epitympanic recess, mastoid cavity, and chorda tympani of the facial nerve (cranial nerve VII). The auditory or Eustachian tube connects the tympanic cavity with the nasopharynx. The tympanic cavity is lined by a single layer of flattened to cuboidal respiratory epithelium, whereas most of the auditory tube is lined by a low ciliated epithelium.

The inner ear is located within the petrous portion of the temporal bone and is composed of a membranous labyrinth surrounded by an osseous labyrinth. The membranous labyrinth houses the cochlea and the vestibular apparatus, both of which are supplied by cranial nerve VIII. There are several parts to the cochlea: the cochlear duct with the organ of Corti (the end organ of hearing), and the scala vestibuli and scala tympani which hold perilymph. The organ of Corti has thousands of neurotransmitting hair cells. The vestibular apparatus, which functions in motion and position sensing, consists of three semicircular canals and the utricle and saccule. The ampullae of the canals have a sensory end organ, the crista ampullaris, with neurosensory hair cells. The utricle and saccule also possess a sensory end organ, the macula, which has neurosensory hair cells and otoliths. There is also a blind sac in the membranous labyrinth known as the endolymphatic sac, which is lined by tall columnar epithelium arranged on papillae.

II. **GROSS EXAMINATION AND TISSUE SAMPLING**

A. **External Ear.** Biopsy and excision specimens should be handled as skin specimens from other anatomic sites (see Chapter 38).

B. **Middle and Inner Ear.** Samples from the middle ear are often obtained in cases of suspected cholesteatoma. For these cases, it should be noted whether bone fragments are present. Standard hematoxylin and eosin (H&E) slide preparation is sufficient. Ossicles from the middle ear can be processed by gross examination only unless microscopic examination is requested by the surgeon. For middle ear and inner ear neoplasms, which are uncommon, use of ink to mark the peripheral margins is not usually possible because these specimens are typically received as small fragments. In those rare cases in which the patient has a history of lymphoma or lymphoma is suspected clinically, fresh tissue should be processed according to the standard lymphoma work-up protocol. For all other middle ear samples, all tissue should be submitted for histologic examination.

III. COMMON DISEASES OF THE EXTERNAL EAR

A. **Nonneoplastic Diseases.** The common diseases of skin that involve the pinna and external ear canal are covered in the chapter on skin (Chapter 38). Some diseases have a particular predilection for the skin of the ear, including gout, keloids (often secondary to ear piercing), relapsing polychondritis, angiolymphoid hyperplasia with eosinophilia (epithelioid or histiocytoid hemangioma), and chondrodermatitis nodularis (the latter is discussed below).

1. **Congenital anomalies of the ear** that may be seen by the surgical pathologist include accessory tragi, branchial cleft abnormalities, congenital aural sinuses, and salivary gland ectopia.

   a. **Accessory tragi** are found at birth and clinically and macroscopically are most often solitary, sessile, or pedunculated polyps in the preauricular area. Microscopically, skin, hair follicles, and a central fibrofatty core with or without cartilage are observed (e-**Fig. 7.2**). They should not be misdiagnosed as a papilloma, fibroma, or chondroma.

   b. **Anomalies of the first branchial cleft** present near the ear as cysts, sinuses, and fistulas. The epithelial lining can be squamous or respiratory; Type I or pure squamous cell–lined cysts can be confused with keratinous cysts histologically. Lymphoid tissue in the wall (e-**Fig. 7.3**) is less frequently found in first branchial cleft cysts than in the much more common second branchial cleft cysts which arise in the lateral neck. Type II defects can harbor skin including adnexal structures or cartilage (e-**Fig. 7.4**); associated salivary gland tissue may also be present when the process extends into or near the parotid gland.

   c. **Congenital aural sinuses** are distinguished from branchial cleft anomalies by location: Branchial cleft abnormalities are found in infra- or postauricular sites, whereas congenital aural sinuses are present in a preauricular location.

2. **Chondrodermatitis nodularis helicis** is a condition of uncertain etiology that occurs on the skin of the external ear, usually on the upper part of the helix. Clinically, middle-aged or older, typically male, patients present with a small (<1 cm) painful nodule that can be ulcerated and can exhibit a crust. This appearance can clinically simulate actinic keratosis or squamous cell carcinoma. Microscopically, there is a somewhat funnel-shaped ulcer with associated dermal collagen edema and degeneration. There may be surrounding pseudoepitheliomatous squamous cell hyperplasia (e-**Fig. 7.5**), granulation tissue and fibrosis, and a predominantly lymphocytic inflammatory cell infiltrate, although the infiltrate can be mixed. A perichondritis with destruction of cartilage can be seen but is uncommon. Superficial or shave biopsies may show only a few of the above findings. Curettage and cautery are used for treatment, with recurrence in a minority of patients.

3. **Otitis externa** is inflammation of the external auditory canal and/or pinna and is very common. Biopsy is generally not indicated.

4. **Necrotizing (malignant) otitis externa** is usually caused by *Pseudomonas aeruginosa* infecting diabetic patients, but fungi can also be the causative agent. Microscopically, the response is one of necrotizing inflammation.

B. **Neoplasms of the External Ear.** The 2017 World Health Organization histologic classification of tumors of the ear is given in Table 7.1. The most common neoplasms of the external ear are **basal cell carcinoma** and **squamous cell carcinoma** of the skin of the ear (discussed in Chapter 38). Of the tumors of the external ear, only the rare ceruminous gland tumors are specific for this site and are discussed below.

1. **Benign ceruminous gland tumors** include ceruminous adenoma, chondroid syringoma, and syringocystadenoma papilliferum. The latter two entities have the same histopathologic features as when they occur at other sites. Ceruminous adenomas are rare, and are seen in adult patients who present with a painless mass of the outer half of the external auditory canal. Grossly, they are 0.4- to 4-cm polypoid growths. Microscopically, there are regular oxyphilic glands and small cysts lined by an inner ceruminous cell layer and an outer spindled to cuboidal myoepithelial cell layer

Tumors of the external auditory canal
Squamous cell carcinoma
Ceruminous adenocarcinoma
Ceruminous adenoma

Tumors of the middle and inner ear
Squamous cell carcinoma
Aggressive papillary tumor
Endolymphatic sac tumor
Otosclerosis
Cholesteatoma
Vestibular schwannoma
Meningioma
Middle ear adenoma

From: El-Naggar AK, Chan JKC, Grandis JR, Takata T, Slootweg PJ, eds. Tumours of the ear. Chapter 9. *WHO Classification of Head and Neck Tumors.* Lyon, France: IARC Press; 2017. Used with permission.

(**e-Fig. 7.6**). Cerumen pigment, cytokeratin 7 (CK7) expression in ceruminal cells, and *p63* and CK5/6 expression in the myoepithelial cells can be helpful in the distinction from adenocarcinoma and middle ear adenoma. There is about a 10% recurrence rate, which is associated with incomplete excision.

2. **Malignant tumors of ceruminous glands** include adenocarcinoma, adenoid cystic carcinoma, and mucoepidermoid carcinoma. The latter two are histologically identical to the same entities arising in salivary glands. Ceruminous adenocarcinomas show infiltrative growth and range from cytologically bland to markedly atypical with an increase in mitotic activity. Perineural invasion is uncommon, but can be a useful diagnostic clue favoring adenocarcinoma, especially in small biopsy samples. Ceruminous adenocarcinomas are locally aggressive.

3. **Other unusual neoplasms and tumorlike conditions of the external ear** include malignant melanoma, benign fibro-osseous lesion, osteoma and exostosis, and idiopathic pseudocystic chondromalacia (which is a nonneoplastic swelling of the pinna due to fluid accumulation within the cartilage of the ear).

IV. **COMMON DISEASES OF THE MIDDLE EAR**
   A. **Nonneoplastic Middle Ear Diseases.** The common disorders include choristoma, inflammation, infection, cholesterol granuloma, cholesteatoma, and otosclerosis.
   1. **Choristomas** (heterotopic tissues) in the middle ear are composed of benign salivary gland, glial, or sebaceous gland tissue. Glial heterotopia is histologically identical to the more commonly occurring encephalocele; the two must be distinguished clinically (**e-Fig. 7.7A,B**).
   2. **Otitis media** is one of the most common diseases of childhood. Most acute purulent cases are due to bacterial infection by *Streptococcus pneumoniae* or *Haemophilus influenzae*. Tissue samples are not usually procured, but in chronic cases tissue may be removed. Microscopically, granulation tissue, scar tissue, chronic inflammation, calcific debris, and sclerotic or reactive bone can be seen. Occasionally, neutrophils and foreign body–type giant cells are present. There may be associated polypoid granulation tissue, cholesterol granulomas, cholesteatoma, or tympanosclerosis. Entrapped metaplastic glands should not be mistaken for neoplastic glands.
   3. **Cholesterol granulomas** are found in a number of chronic ear diseases. Cholesterol clefts, a foreign body–type giant cell reaction, and hemosiderin deposition are characteristic (**e-Fig. 7.8**).
   4. **Cholesteatoma** may be congenital or acquired. The congenital form is found in infants and young children, is defined as occurring in the presence of an intact tympanic membrane, and may result from an epidermoid cell rest (epidermoid

formation). In the more common acquired form, seen mainly in older children and adults, there is an association with severe otitis media and a perforated tympanic membrane. Histologically, there are three major elements: keratin (e-**Figs.** 7.9 and 7.10), stratified squamous epithelium, and fibrous and/or granulation tissue. Since squamous epithelium is not normally found in the middle ear, the diagnosis is usually straightforward. Downgrowth of the epithelium into underlying subepidermal connective tissue may be appreciated. Marked vascular congestion and abscess formation may also be found. Cholesteatoma is not a neoplasm, but can be locally destructive; ossicle(s) and the bony wall of the middle ear can be eroded. There is an increased cell proliferation index in the squamous epithelium of cholesteatoma and overexpression of cathepsin enzymes, abnormalities that may be related to the local growth but are not required for diagnosis.

5. **Otosclerosis** is a disease of unknown etiology that leads to progressive fixation of the stapes footplate and, as a result, conductive hearing loss. The onset is typically in adulthood and women are more often affected than men. The initial histologic changes include resorption of bone and replacement by cellular fibrovascular tissue. Over time, this is replaced by dense sclerotic bone (e-**Fig.** 7.11). Patients are treated with stapedectomy.

B. **Neoplasms of the Middle Ear** include paraganglioma, adenoma of the middle ear, papillary tumors, meningioma, and squamous cell carcinoma (Table 7.1).

1. **Paraganglioma** (also known as glomus tumor, glomus tympanicum, or chemodectoma) is the most common tumor of the middle ear (but is nonetheless still rare). It usually presents clinically with hearing loss or tinnitus in patients in the fifth and sixth decade of life. The neoplasm can be solitary or part of a familial paraganglioma–pheochromocytoma syndrome caused by germline mutations in *SDHB, SDHC,* or *SDHD* genes; the head and neck paragangliomas in the familial syndrome are often bilateral/multicentric. Clinically, the tumor is bulging, red, pink, or bluish (and not white like a cholesteatoma). Biopsy may result in brisk bleeding.

   Microscopically, sections usually demonstrate the classical "zellballen" appearance with nests of small uniform epithelioid cells that have a peripheral layer of flattened cells (e-**Figs.** 7.12 and 7.13). Sclerosis and vascularity can be pronounced in some tumors; in the former circumstance, the nested pattern may not be apparent (e-**Fig.** 7.14). Immunohistochemical stains can be confirmatory and particularly contributory in small biopsy samples (which may display significant crush artifact). Chromogranin A and synaptophysin immunostains are positive, whereas carcinoembryonic antigen and keratin immunostains are negative. Only a few S-100 positive peripheral sustentacular cells may be present.

   These tumors grow slowly and can recur after surgery and/or radiation treatment. Intracranial extension develops in a small minority of patients, and about 1% to 2% of patients suffer from metastatic spread. It is not possible to predict aggressive behavior based on histopathologic features.

2. **Middle ear adenoma** is a benign glandular neoplasm with variable neuroendocrine and mucin-secreting differentiation. The typical clinical presentation is in an adult (mean age in the 40s) with muffled hearing, tinnitus, and/or a sensation of pressure and/or fullness. The neoplasms are variably colored and only uncommonly penetrate through the tympanic membrane. Microscopic architectural patterns are variable and include closely packed small glands with solid, glandular, and/or trabecular arrangements (e-**Fig.** 7.15). The glands lack a myoepithelial layer. Cytologically, the cuboidal to columnar glandular cells are bland, with uniform small nuclei and rare nucleoli (e-**Fig.** 7.16). Mitoses should not be present. The immunoprofile includes positivity for cytokeratin and neuroendocrine markers such as chromogranin and synaptophysin. In the past, this immunophenotype was viewed as being indicative of a carcinoid tumor of the middle ear, but it is now recognized that expression of neuroendocrine markers is a characterized feature of most middle ear adenomas. Recurrence has been reported in a minority of cases, usually after incomplete surgical excision.

3. **Papillary tumors of the middle ear** include aggressive papillary tumor and inverted papilloma, although only a few cases of the latter have been described. Aggressive papillary tumors are more common, and are also known as low-grade papillary adenocarcinomas and endolymphatic sac tumors (Heffner tumor). Typically, patients in their fourth decade present with hearing difficulty and vertigo; 15% of patients have a family history of von Hippel–Lindau syndrome. Microscopically, there are complex interdigitating papillae with fibrous cores covered by cuboidal to columnar cells that have bland nuclear cytology and eosinophilic cytoplasm. Mitoses are absent. The papillae may overly granulation tissue causing diagnostic confusion with reactive processes. Cystic spaces with a colloid-like material simulating thyroid follicles can also be present. Immunostains show positivity for keratin, with variable S-100, glial fibrillary acidic protein, and synaptophysin immunoreactivity; thyroglobulin and PAX8 immunostaining is negative. Despite the bland histologic appearance, the tumor is a slowly growing, locally aggressive, but nonmetastasizing neoplasm. Temporal bone invasion is common, and the tumor may extend into the cerebellum. Outcome is related to size of the tumor and adequacy of excision; radical surgical excision affords the best chance for cure. Recurrence is seen in about 20% of cases, with tumor-specific death in about 13% of patients.

4. **Meningioma** in the middle ear is a rare neoplasm that is more likely to represent secondary extension from an intracranial meningioma than from a primary middle ear meningioma. Patients with primary middle ear meningiomas present at a mean age of 50 years with hearing changes and sometimes otitis and pain. The histopathologic features are similar to intracranial meningiomas, with meningothelial meningioma predominating (e-**Fig. 7.17**). Vimentin, progesterone receptor, and epithelial membrane antigen immunostains are positive; cytokeratin immunostains are negative. Meningiomas are slowly growing neoplasms and can recur following incomplete surgical excision. The 5-year survival is 83%.

5. **Squamous cell carcinoma** in the middle ear is uncommon and is typically advanced at presentation. Its development is not clearly related to chronic otitis media and is not related to cholesteatoma. Microscopically, the carcinoma is keratinizing and displays a variable degree of differentiation. Outcome is related to tumor extent and margin status at surgery, but not histologic grade. The 5-year survival is roughly 50%.

6. **Other rare neoplasms of the middle ear** include embryonal rhabdomyosarcoma (e-**Fig. 7.18**), lipoma, hemangioma, osteoma, ossifying fibroma, and teratoma.

7. **Metastasis** to the ear is uncommon, accounting for only 2% to 6% of all neoplasms of the ear. Most patients have known, widely disseminated cancer. The middle ear is the most common site for metastatic spread. Breast, lung, and prostate are, in order, the common primary sites of origin for the metastatic deposits.

V. NEOPLASMS OF THE INNER EAR. Vestibular schwannoma, lipoma, and hemangioma are the most common neoplasms of the inner ear. Endolymphatic sac tumors also arise in the inner ear (the aforementioned aggressive papillary tumor of the middle ear is thought to represent an endolymphatic sac tumor with extension into the middle ear).

A. **Vestibular Schwannoma (Acoustic Neuroma)** is relatively common. Unilateral vestibular schwannoma accounts for 5% to 10% of all intracranial tumors, and has been found in about 1% of autopsies. Bilateral vestibular schwannoma, found in 5% of all vestibular schwannoma cases, is characteristic of neurofibromatosis type 2 (an autosomal dominant disease due to mutations in the *NF2* gene on 22q12). Patients, usually in their 40s or 50s, present with progressive hearing loss and tinnitus. Grossly, the size range of the tumor is a few millimeters up to 6 cm in maximal dimension. The smaller tumors are round to oval, whereas large tumors can assume a mushroom shape. The cut surfaces are yellow and can exhibit hemorrhage and cystic change. Microscopically, the attributes are the same as in soft tissue schwannomas (e-**Fig. 7.19**), with Antoni A regions with Verocay bodies, and Antoni B areas. Mitotic figures should be rare. Degenerative nuclear atypia should not be taken as a sign of malignancy. S-100 immunoreactivity is strong.

B. Lipomas of the Internal Auditory Canal resemble lipomas at other anatomic sites, except that cranial nerves VII or VIII or their branches may be present in the lipoma.

SUGGESTED READINGS

El-Naggar AK, Chan JKC, Grandis JR, Takata T, Slootweg PJ, eds. Tumours of the ear. Chapter 9. *WHO Classification of Head and Neck Tumors*. Lyon, France: IARC Press; 2017.

Mills SE, Stelow EB, Hunt JL. Tumors of the ear. Chapter 16. *Tumors of the Upper Aerodigestive Tract and Ear*. Silverspring, Maryland: ARP Press; 2012.

Thompson LDR. Benign neoplasms of the ear and temporal bone. Chapter 18. *Head and Neck Pathology, A Volume in the Series Foundations in Diagnostic Pathology*. 3rd ed. Philadelphia, PA: Elsevier; 2019.

Thompson LDR. Malignant neoplasms of the ear and temporal bone. Chapter 19. *Head and Neck Pathology, A Volume in the Series Foundations in Diagnostic Pathology*. 3rd ed. Philadelphia, PA: Elsevier; 2019.

Thompson LDR. Non-neoplastic lesions of the ear and temporal bone. Chapter 17. *Head and Neck Pathology, A Volume in the Series Foundations in Diagnostic Pathology*. 3rd ed. Philadelphia, PA: Elsevier; 2019.

SECTION II

Thorax

Lung
Jon H. Ritter and Hannah R. Krigman

I. **NORMAL ANATOMY.** The lung is defined by airway branching, first into right and left lobes, then segments, and finally, the functional unit of the lung, the lobule. Arteries follow the airways, while veins and lymphatics flow toward the lobular septa and finally to the hilum and main pulmonary veins. Bronchi are lined by a pseudostratified respiratory epithelium that includes goblet cells, which is separated by a basement membrane from a delicate submucosa. Larger airways have a smooth muscle wall that contains minor salivary glands and a cartilaginous skeleton; bronchioles have lost the latter components. Each lobule has a central bronchovascular bundle; the interstitial space between the pulmonary artery branches and the bronchioles is eventually continuous with the alveolar interstitium. Lymph nodes occur within the lung, and also are discontinuous along the bronchi.

Progressive branching of the airways leads to the alveolar ducts, from which alveoli spring. Normal alveolar walls are very delicate and have a fine elastic tissue matrix. The barrier between the blood in capillaries and the air in the alveolar space consists of the endothelial cell, the basement membrane, the wispy alveolar interstitium, epithelial cell basement membrane, and the flattened type 1 pneumocyte. Type 2 pneumocytes can proliferate to replace injured type 1 cells.

The visceral pleura consists of an inner vascular layer that abuts the alveolar tissue, a connective tissue layer, and an outer layer of mesothelium. The visceral pleura is reflected back at the hilum and becomes continuous with the parietal pleural layer that lines the chest cavity.

II. **SPECIMEN HANDLING AND REPORTING**

A. **Samples.** Biopsies of lung tissue for diagnosis are obtained endoscopically (transbronchial or endobronchial biopsy), via radiologically guided procedures (usually needle core biopsies), or for peripheral disease, via wedge biopsies. Resections can involve a single lobe (lobectomy), two lobes (bilobectomy), or an entire lung (pneumonectomy.)

B. **Gross Examination and Sampling**

1. **Endoscopic biopsies** are usually submitted in a single cassette. The fragments are small; the use of a nylon mesh bag or a filter paper wrap is preferable to submission on biopsy sponges since tissue can be compressed or lost in the pores of sponges. The number of fragments, range of size, and color should be recorded. Three hematoxylin and eosin (H&E)-stained levels should be examined. For smaller biopsies, additional unstained levels may be cut at the time of initial sectioning in case special stains are needed, and this also provides slides that can be used for subsequent molecular studies in the case of neoplasms.

Core biopsies of nodules presumed to represent neoplasms are obtained under CT guidance, or in the setting of endobronchial ultrasound guidance. They should be processed as for endoscopic biopsies.

2. Wedge resections are performed for either nonneoplastic or neoplastic processes. The specimen should be measured in three dimensions and weighed. Assessment of alveolar architecture may be improved by gently inflating the specimen by injection of formalin at multiple sites. If the specimen is inflated, the gross description should include this fact. Wedge biopsies generally have multiple staple lines, which should be cut off as close to the staples as possible; ideally, sections are taken perpendicular to the staple line. The entire specimen should be submitted in nonneoplastic cases; levels are usually not necessary. If the specimen is obtained for diagnosis of a neoplasm, the presence and dimensions of any masses should be described, as well as the distance to the staple line(s) and pleura.

3. Lung resections should be described as a segmentectomy, lobectomy, bilobectomy, or right or left pneumonectomy. The specimen should be measured in three dimensions and weighed. Any additional designation by the surgeon (e.g., sutures) should be described. If a portion of chest wall is attached to the specimen, its size in three dimensions and the number of ribs or other attached structures should be noted. For lobectomy and pneumonectomy specimens, insufflation by injection of formalin into the bronchial orifices improves fixation and visualization of changes. Occasionally, obstruction of bronchi by tumor makes this technique ineffective, in which case the lung can be expanded by injection of formalin at multiple sites. The pleural surface should be described; areas of puckering, dullness, or adhesions should be noted, as should adhesions of lobes together in multilobe resections. Areas of pleural distortion over a mass should be marked with ink. The hilar area should be examined and the number and size of bronchial stumps noted. The lung can be sectioned in either parasagittal or in coronal planes; it is important to choose planes to highlight the extent of tumor, pleural invasion, invasion of adjacent structures, proximity to the hilum, and relationship to major airways and vessels. At least four sections of tumor should be taken, including one or two with the closest pleural surface (which may be at the hilum). If tumor is invading structures such as a rib, chest wall, or mediastinal soft tissue, a section that shows tumor in the lung in continuity with the involved structure should be taken. Other sections should include normal-appearing lung, areas distal to the tumor that show obstructive pneumonia, and any additional nodules or lesions. Vascular and bronchial margins, hilar lymph nodes, and peribronchial lymph nodes should be submitted as well.

C. Adjunct Information. For both nonneoplastic and neoplastic samples, the radiographic findings are an important adjunct to diagnosis. Either review the radiograph directly, or review its interpretation; old films may provide information on the pace of disease. The distribution of abnormalities, the presence of lymphadenopathy, and the extent of disease all contribute to the final diagnosis. For nonneoplastic cases, a review of the clinical history, including the presence of systemic illnesses, medications, and exposures; laboratory data including cultures and serologic studies; and pulmonary function tests all may assist in interpretation of the findings.

D. Microscopic Description

1. A description of small biopsies includes the number of pieces and their constituent elements: alveolar tissue, bronchial wall, and superficial detached fragments of epithelium. The number of fragments is not insignificant; six fragments are considered to be representative of lung. The low-power impression of normal or abnormal alveolar architecture should be included. Expansion of the alveolar septa may be by inflammatory tissue, cellular tissue, or acellular fibrosis. Alveolar spaces may be empty, or filled with blood, histiocytes, or exudates. The vasculature may be unremarkable, thickened, show inflammation or vasculitis, or contain tumor or thromboemboli. The bronchial epithelium can be columnar, squamous, or dysplastic. The absence or presence and type of granulomas should be described. Inflammatory cells should be noted and characterized as to the type and distribution, whether alveolar, septal, peribronchial, perivascular, or diffuse. The results of special stains for organisms or fibrosis should be reported.

Biopsies for a neoplasm should include the same quantitation of the biopsy fragments as for nonneoplastic samples, as well as a description of the neoplasm. An in situ or dysplastic component should be described, if present. Detectable vascular space invasion should be noted.

2. The pathology report of wedge resections for nonneoplastic processes should contain the same information as for smaller biopsies, but should also include additional assessment of larger airways and vessels, and distribution of any nonneoplastic processes. Fibrosis, for example, can be diffuse, peripheral, or sparing the periphery. Similarly, inflammation or granulomas can be perivascular, peribronchial, or distributed along the septa.

3. Definitive resections of neoplasms, from wedge resections to pneumonectomies, should provide as much information as possible. Prior sampling (endoscopic biopsy, mediastinoscopy, or previous wedge resections) and prior treatment (chemotherapy or irradiation) should be included in the pathology report. Margins should be evaluated, and the nonneoplastic lung should be described.

III. NONNEOPLASTIC DISEASE

A. Acute Lung Injury Patterns. When evaluating lung biopsies taken for medical diseases, identification of patterns of acute lung injury should be a major point of emphasis. These patterns represent the response of the lung to an acute injury, and immediately switch the diagnostic considerations away from the chronic fibrosing interstitial lung diseases. The commonly recognized patterns of acute lung injury include diffuse alveolar damage (DAD), bronchiolitis obliterans/organizing pneumonia, and acute interstitial pneumonia (AIP). All three processes share key findings: they all feature fibrosis characterized by loose, fibroblast-rich, new fibrous tissue; they are temporally uniform; and they may be potentially reversible, at least before significant collagen fibrosis develops.

1. Diffuse alveolar damage (DAD) is the prototypical pattern of acute lung injury (**e-Fig. 8.1**). It is the pattern of histologic changes underlying the clinical syndrome of acute respiratory distress syndrome (ARDS), the clinical triad of diffuse lung infiltrates, hypoxemia, and decreased pulmonary compliance. DAD has myriad causes, as detailed in Table 8.1. DAD is caused by cellular injury to pulmonary epithelial and endothelial cells. The initial insult causes edema from leaky capillaries, and the sloughed cellular material and fibrinous exudate form hyaline membranes; there is often surprisingly little inflammation in this early phase, known as the exudative stage. By 6 to 7 days after the initializing injury, the edema and hyaline membranes begin to disappear, and hyperplastic and regenerative type 2 pneumocytes are prominent. By 7 days, the process of organization is well underway, with interstitial and airspace fibroblastic proliferations; this stage is known as the proliferative or organizing phase. During organization, the alveolar exudates may be incorporated into the alveolar wall if proliferating type 2 pneumocytes grow on top of the exudate rather than along the original alveolar basement membrane. Likewise, alveolar collapse may lead to further remodeling of prior airspaces. This process of organization and fibrosis may resolve at some point, or can continue along the path of fibrosis leading to the appearance of honeycomb lung within 3 to 4 weeks.

The hallmark of biopsies with DAD is spatial and temporal uniformity; that is, the process is similar across all areas of the tissue because the inciting injury is diffuse. By the time most patients are sick enough to come to biopsy, this process has been present for at least several days, and hence is in the organizing phase. A search for such etiologic clues as viral inclusions or fungus by silver stains is important, but the identification of the etiology for DAD is generally a clinicopathologic correlation exercise. When patients recover, they may be essentially normal, or may be left with some degree of lung impairment. Trichrome or similar stains may be helpful when reviewing these biopsies. Cases that show cellular fibrosis but in which trichrome

TABLE 8.1 Etiology of Diffuse Alveolar Damage

Category	Selected Agents
Infectious	Viruses
	Mycoplasma
	Other infections in immunocompromised patients
Inhaled toxins	Oxygen
	Smoke
Drugs	Chemotherapeutic agents
	Amiodarone
	Nitrofurantoin
Shock	Traumatic
	Cardiogenic
	Other
Sepsis	Any organism
Miscellaneous	Radiation
	Burns
	Cardiopulmonary bypass
	Pancreatitis
	Lupus

stains do not show significant collagen deposition are thought to be reversible; however, once significant collagen is present in the areas of fibrosis, the process is not likely to resolve.

2. **Acute interstitial pneumonia** (AIP). AIP is histologically similar to DAD, but has no definable cause and could thus also be considered as idiopathic DAD. The patients, often young adults, present with rapid onset of respiratory failure. There is often a history of a flu-like illness, and some studies have suggested that a herpes-like virus may be present in some cases. By the time patients come to biopsy, the lung almost always shows a picture identical to that of organizing phase DAD. Most patients die of the disease within 2 months. This rapid form of interstitial lung disease was classically described as the Hamman–Rich syndrome.

3. **Bronchiolitis obliterans–organizing pneumonia** (BOOP) is another manifestation of acute lung injury (e-**Fig. 8.2**). Some authors now advocate substitution of the term cryptogenic organizing pneumonia (COP). The causes are detailed in Table 8.2. Idiopathic cases tend to present in older adults with fever, cough, and some dyspnea; there may be an antecedent respiratory infection. Radiographs show patchy, peripheral air-space–filling opacities that may appear in different areas of the lung over

TABLE 8.2 Process Associated With Bronchiolitis Obliterans–Organizing Pneumonia Response

- Idiopathic BOOP
- Collagen vascular diseases
- Toxins
- Organizing infection
- Proximity to a variety of space-occupying lesions including neoplasms, granulomas, infarcts, and abscesses
- Distal to bronchiectasis
- Acute infection
- Immune-mediated pneumonitis

time. Histologic sections show a very distinctive pattern of immature fibroblastic tissue within terminal bronchioles and alveolar ducts, which often has an elongated or hook-like configuration; these are often referred to as Masson bodies and can also be seen in peribronchiolar alveolar spaces. Because of the luminal filling of terminal bronchioles, there is often an associated localized obstructive pneumonia in the form of accumulation of lipid-filled macrophages. Since BOOP is centered on terminal airways, low-power views of wedge biopsies show a somewhat nodular configuration in contrast to the diffuse nature of injury in DAD. Thus, BOOP shares the temporal uniformity of DAD, but not the homogeneous spatial appearance; nonetheless, the basic lesion of epithelial and endothelial cell injury is identical to that seen in DAD. It is important to emphasize that many, if not most, cases of BOOP are secondary to some other process. Consequently, the finding of a pattern of BOOP on a biopsy should lead to a careful search of the tissue for lesions that can be associated with BOOP, such as granulomas, vasculitis, or viral inclusions indicative of viral infection.

While the distinction between nodular versus diffuse involvement (and consequently, distinction between BOOP and DAD/AIP) may be obvious in wedge biopsies, transbronchial biopsies may show features such as organizing airspace fibrosis and type 2 pneumocyte hyperplasia without a clear indication of the spatial distribution of the process. In such cases, a more generic diagnosis of "organizing acute lung injury" may be used. This conveys the essential information for patient care—that is, the diagnosis defines the patient as having an acute injury with attendant lung response, as opposed to a chronic idiopathic interstitial lung disease.

B. Idiopathic Interstitial Pneumonitis

1. Usual interstitial pneumonitis (UIP) is the prototypical chronic interstitial pneumonitis. It is so named because it represents the underlying pathology in at least 80% of cases that fall under the clinical term of idiopathic pulmonary fibrosis. UIP is most often a disease of older adults, but has been reported in all age groups, including children. By the time of diagnosis, patients have often had several years of slowly developing shortness of breath. Pulmonary function tests show restrictive disease corresponding to the small lungs seen by chest x-ray examination. CT scans demonstrate honeycombing, most commonly at the lung bases and lung periphery, as well as traction bronchiectasis (**e-Fig. 8.3**). Gross examination shows coarse sponge-like lung corresponding to the honeycombing seen on radiographs. Microscopically, the disease is characterized by spatial and temporal heterogeneity. Temporal heterogeneity refers to the coexistence of old honeycomb scars (defined as cystic spaces lined by bronchiolar-type epithelium) with areas of ongoing fibrosis (fibroblastic foci). The fibroblastic foci represent small areas of developing fibrosis, consistent with the insidious progression of this disease. Acute inflammation is often restricted to the honeycomb areas, which may contain mucoid debris. Spatial heterogeneity refers to the finding that the most severe fibrosis is in the subpleural areas and along the lobular septa; more central parts of the pulmonary lobule typically show less severe disease. Chronic inflammation is mild and patchy within areas of fibrosis; autoimmune or connective tissue disorders (CTDs) should be considered in cases with more extensive chronic inflammation. Related changes in the lung include secondary pulmonary hypertension and type 2 pneumocyte hyperplasia. The clinical course both before and after diagnosis is variable; most patients die within 5 years of diagnosis, although some patients have a more protracted course. In the process known as acute exacerbation of UIP, histologic sections show DAD superimposed on a background of UIP; the precise etiology for acute exacerbation of UIP is not known (which parallels the fact that the etiology of UIP itself is generally unknown).

2. Nonspecific interstitial pneumonitis (NSIP) is the second most common form of idiopathic interstitial pneumonitis. As with UIP, patients tend to be middle aged or older adults. Many patients have underlying CTDs such as rheumatoid arthritis or lupus. Pulmonary function tests show a restrictive pattern. CT scans disclose significant differences from those in UIP; honeycombing is rarely a prominent feature in

NSIP, but ground-glass opacities, linear opacities, and small nodular infiltrates are frequently present (e-**Fig. 8.4**).

Microscopically, the process has a more homogeneous appearance than UIP. Biopsies usually lack subpleural accentuation, but instead show more uniform involvement of both central and peripheral parts of the lobule. The process is generally more cellular than UIP with a mixed interstitial acute and chronic inflammatory infiltrate. Cases may show features of organizing pneumonia or BOOP, and small nondescript granulomas may be seen in some cases. Honeycombing, if seen on microscopic sections, is usually more focal and should not be a dominant pattern. The forgoing findings are characteristic of the cellular and the mixed patterns of NSIP; since they bear significant resemblance to processes such as chronic hypersensitivity pneumonia or unresolved or slowly resolving organizing pneumonia, it is not clear that cases labeled as NSIP do not represent some unusual variants of the latter groups. Many cases of NSIP are also related to connective tissue disease or autoimmune diseases involving the lung. A third pattern of NSIP, namely the sclerotic variant, consists of hyaline-like interstitial fibrosis. Although the full characterization of NSIP is still evolving, the one unifying feature of NSIP is that the patients survive longer, and with less disability than those patients whose biopsies show UIP. Many cases of NSIP may also benefit from immune-modulating drugs, unlike UIP, so separation of NSIP and UIP may also drive therapy.

3. **Desquamative interstitial pneumonia and related lesions** (DIP) is a rare form of interstitial pneumonia characterized by abundant macrophage exudates that fill the alveolar spaces. In most patients, this process is related to cigarette smoking, although rare examples have been reported in nonsmokers; most patients are middle aged to older adults. Radiographic studies are dominated by ground-glass opacities reflective of the filling of alveolar spaces, and microscopic sections feature dramatic filling of the alveolar spaces by macrophages which tend to be light brown due to the smoking-related pigment (e-**Fig. 8.5**). DIP is spatially homogeneous in that virtually any microscopic field from the involved lung will show identical features. The alveolar walls may be thin and delicate, or may show some mild inactive hyaline fibrosis. Honeycomb changes are rare. DIP has an excellent prognosis; in cases related to cigarette use, the primary therapy is smoking cessation.

Less dramatic findings along the same spectrum of smoking-related changes include **respiratory bronchiolitis** (RB) and **respiratory bronchiolitis–associated interstitial lung disease** (RB-ILD). RB shows similar macrophages as in DIP, but limited to the lumen of terminal airways; it is often most prominent in the upper lobes and is thought to be the precursor of centriacinar emphysema (e-**Fig. 8.6**). RB-ILD is similar with the addition of mild interstitial fibrosis surrounding the terminal bronchioles.

4. **Lymphoid interstitial pneumonitis** (LIP) is another rare idiopathic form of interstitial pneumonitis. LIP can occur in patients of any age. When LIP occurs in children, it is often a harbinger of HIV infection; similarly, LIP has been described in immunocompromised patients as a manifestation of EBV infection. Some cases of LIP are related to the Sjögren syndrome. Chest radiographs demonstrate infiltrates of a variety of patterns. Microscopically, there is diffuse expansion of the pulmonary interstitium by a mixed inflammatory cell infiltrate that includes small lymphocytes, plasma cells, germinal centers, and histiocytes. There may be some associated interstitial fibrosis. Many cases previously described as LIP likely represent examples of pulmonary MALToma or related neoplasms. Immunostains should show a mixed pattern of CD3-positive T-cells and CD20-positive B-cells. In cases of suspected LIP, flow cytometry or molecular studies to assess clonality are very useful to exclude lymphoma.

5. **Giant cell interstitial pneumonitis** is very rare. Most cases are now known to represent a reaction to various heavy metals. Consequently, optimum diagnosis is made by the combination of accurate history and spectrophotometric analysis of the lung tissue.

6. Smoking-related interstitial fibrosis (SRIF) is a recent addition to the list of smoking-related lung diseases (*Hum Pathol* 2010;41:316). SRIF is often found in lobectomy specimens of resected lung carcinomas in patients with no preoperative clinical symptoms or imaging diagnosis of interstitial lung disease. The fibrosis typically has a hyaline or sclerotic appearance that somewhat resembles the sclerotic form of NSIP. Also, the fibrosis is almost always superimposed on significant emphysema.

C. Other Noninfectious, Nonneoplastic Pulmonary Processes

1. Connective tissue/autoimmune disorders. Lung involvement in CTDs is extremely common and variable. Prominent patterns of involvement for selected disorders are summarized in Table 8.3. There is significant overlap among these entities and assignment to a specific entity should not be made on the basis of pulmonary findings. Also, many of the lung findings in CTDs overlap with the idiopathic interstitial lung diseases. The role of autoimmune disorders in interstitial lung disease has become much more widely recognized, and many examples of NSIP are currently thought to be manifestations of autoimmune disease in the lung. In addition, some cases with a UIP-like pattern can also be seen in the setting of autoimmunity. Thus, it is critical when evaluating cases of interstitial disease that appropriate serologic studies for autoimmunity have been performed. Many other cases will show interstitial chronic inflammation and patterns of fibrosis that do not fit neatly into the prototypical categories of NSIP or UIP. When appropriate clinical and serologic findings of autoimmune disease are present, such cases maybe be labeled as interstitial pneumonia with autoimmune features (IPAF). Examples of autoimmune-related lung disease are also often treated with and will respond to immunosuppressing drugs (*J Eur Respir* 2015;46:976–987).

2. Pleuropulmonary fibroelastosis. Pleuropulmonary fibroelastosis (PPFE) is a relatively new entity in the lexicon of interstitial lung disease. The disease usually occurs in older adults, where PPFE may be idiopathic, although a subset of cases have been described in patients with altered immune status, including lung transplant recipients.

TABLE 8.3 Pulmonary Manifestations of Connective Tissue Disorders

Disease	Pleural Changes	Pulmonary Changes
Rheumatoid arthritis	Nonspecific pleuritis Necrobiotic nodules	Interstitial pneumonia and fibrosis Bronchiolitis Necrobiotic nodules Vasculitis Pulmonary hypertension Systemic amyloidosis
Systemic lupus erythematosus	Fibrinous pleuritis Effusions Pleural fibrosis	Chronic interstitial pneumonia Diffuse alveolar damage Intra-alveolar hemorrhage Vasculitis, both large vessel and capillaritis Pulmonary hypertension
Scleroderma		Interstitial fibrosis with UIP-like pattern Interstitial fibrosis with NSIP-like pattern Pulmonary hypertension
Polymyositis and dermatomyositis		Interstitial fibrosis Bronchiolitis obliterans–organizing pneumonia
Sjögren syndrome		Lymphocytic inflammation of tracheobronchial glands, atrophy of glands Peribronchiolar lymphocytic inflammation Lymphoid hyperplasia/lymphoid interstitial pneumonitis Lymphomas including MALToma

TABLE 8.4	Pulmonary Manifestations of Drug Reactions

- Chronic interstitial pneumonia
- Diffuse alveolar damage
- Bronchiolitis obliterans–organizing pneumonia
- Obliterative bronchiolitis
- Eosinophilic pneumonia
- Pulmonary hemorrhage
- Pulmonary edema
- Pulmonary veno-occlusive disease
- Large- and small-vessel vasculitis

PPFE (e-**Fig. 8.3e, f**) is characterized by elastotic tissue that forms a rind-like thickening around the subpleural lung. This elastosis can extend irregularly into the lung along the septae, and there can be fibroblast-like foci at the interface of the elastotic tissue and normal lung. FPPE does not feature the prominent honeycombing that characterizes UIP. The disease is slowly progressive and there is no particularly effective medical therapy at this point (*Chest* 2004;126:2007–2013).

3. **Drug-induced pulmonary changes.** Prominent pathologic findings associated with drug reactions are listed in Table 8.4. It is clear from this list that drug reactions can mimic virtually any nonneoplastic condition, which emphasizes the need for accurate history and correlation with the clinical setting.

   a. **Amiodarone.** Perhaps 5% to 10% of patients treated with amiodarone experience a pulmonary complication. The drug inhibits phospholipase, so the hallmark of exposure is accumulation of phospholipids, which in the lung manifests as accumulations of foamy macrophages (e-**Fig. 8.7**); note that accumulation of foamy macrophages is seen in almost all patients on the drug to varying degrees, and does not by itself indicate toxicity. Toxicity occurs as early as 1 month after initiation of therapy, with an average of 10 to 12 months, and is associated with higher doses. Patients present with a variety of symptoms, such as cough, dyspnea, chest pain, fever, and myalgias. Radiographs can show a mixture of airspace infiltrates, interstitial disease, or even isolated collections. Microscopically, toxicity has several manifestations, including a cellular chronic interstitial pneumonitis characterized by chronic inflammation in the interstitium, pneumocyte hyperplasia, and fibrosis; foamy alveolar macrophages are also present, as is lipid within pneumocytes and within cells in the interstitium. Rarer cases show a dose-independent reaction that resembles hypersensitivity pneumonia (HP). Still other cases show a pattern of DAD and/or BOOP-like injury.

   b. **Methotrexate** therapy is also commonly complicated by pulmonary toxicity in perhaps 5% to 10% of patients, which does not seem to be related to the total dose. Radiographically, patients have diffuse infiltrates. Microscopically, there are multiple patterns of injury including: (1) cellular interstitial pneumonitis with nodular collections of lymphocytes, plasma cells, histiocytes, eosinophils, and poorly formed granulomas; (2) HP (many of these patients are on low-dose therapy); and (3) BOOP (with poorly formed granulomas), DAD, and severe pulmonary edema.

4. **Hypersensitivity pneumonitis** (HP), also known as extrinsic allergic alveolitis (EAA), is a disease caused by exposure to organic antigens. Classically the exposure is to thermophilic *Actinomyces*, but a variety of organic agents have been implicated (Table 8.5). Acute HP occurs with exposure to a large amount of antigen; within 4 to 6 hours of dyspnea, cough, fever, and diffuse infiltrates develop. Pulmonary function tests show moderate to severe restriction and decreased DLCO; severe hypoxemia is also present. Radiology studies show airspace disease, ground-glass opacities, and some small nodular opacities. Symptoms improve in 12 to 18 hours, and within 2 to 3 days the

TABLE 8.5 **Agents Implicated in Hypersensitivity Pneumonitis**

- Thermophilic actinomyces
- Molds
- Animal proteins
- Rarely, exposure to drugs (i.e., methotrexate, amiodarone)

radiographic findings resolve. Microscopically, acute inflammation, edema, and exudates may be seen, but because of the rapid course of the disease, it is rarely biopsied.

Chronic HP is due to repeated or prolonged exposure to small amounts of antigen; it is typically due to episodic exposure to some organic antigen, but the offending antigen is eventually identified in only 1/3 to 1/2 of cases. Chronic HP has several histopathologic characteristic (e-**Fig. 8.8**) including chronic interstitial inflammation with many CD8+ T-cells, vague granulomas or giant cells in the interstitium, and chronic bronchiolitis, sometimes with BOOP. Eosinophils are not part of the disease, despite the hypersensitivity label. Most patients respond to therapy or have a stable disease, with a minority progressing to fibrosis and end-stage lung disease. There is overlap between chronic HP and some cases labeled as NSIP, and the two diseases may actually be the same process.

5. Sarcoidosis is a systemic disease of uncertain etiology. While some molecular genetic studies suggest that the sarcoid represents a hypersensitivity-like reaction to mycobacterial infection, standard stains and cultures do not show organisms. There is frequent lung involvement, although it is usually mild and as many as 2/3 of patients are asymptomatic. Most cases involve the hilar and mediastinal nodes as well as the lung, but isolated involvement of either site can occur. In symptomatic patients, pulmonary function tests show mixed restriction and obstruction and decreased DLCO; lung volumes tend to be preserved.

The basic histologic lesion of the sarcoid is a noncaseating granuloma with enveloping fibrosis (e-**Fig. 8.9**). The individual granulomas can coalesce to form larger nodules. The granulomas follow the lymphatic routes and so are present along airways; for this reason, transbronchial lung biopsies produce a diagnosis in up to 80% of cases. The giant cells in the granulomas may contain various structures, including Schaumann bodies, asteroid bodies, and oxalate crystals (the latter are produced endogenously by the giant cells, and thus polarizable material in the giant cells should not be taken as evidence of foreign body exposure). The sarcoid also includes varying degrees of interstitial lymphoid infiltrates. Stains for fungi and mycobacteria should be performed in all cases. Some cases otherwise typical for sarcoid show minimal central fibrinoid material in the granulomas; however, true caseation should raise concern that the diagnosis is not sarcoidosis.

Unusual clinicopathologic features of the sarcoid include massive pleural effusions associated with chest pain suggesting mesothelioma or pleural tumors, or one large nodule or multiple nodules with cavitation mimicking primary or metastatic tumor within the lung. Rare cases of sarcoidosis produce peripheral infiltrates that simulate eosinophilic pneumonia, or granulomatous vascular impingement that can simulate veno-occlusive disease. End-stage cases often are dominated by the presence of apical bullous disease; the granulomas at this stage may be largely "burnt out" and replaced by hyalinized fibrous tissue that tracks along the lymphatic routes.

The differential diagnosis of the sarcoid is always granulomatous infection, and it is important to note that up to 10% to 15% of biopsies with granulomas and negative special stains are culture positive. Infection should always be suspected if the granulomas are necrotizing. The differential diagnosis also includes a drug reaction, berylliosis, and aluminum exposure.

6. Pulmonary eosinophilic granuloma (EG) (also called Langerhans cell histiocytosis, or histiocytosis X) is a disease of adults, with most cases presenting in the third and fourth decades of life. There is a history of cigarette smoking in almost 90% of cases, indicating that this disease should be considered as another facet of smoking-induced lung disease. Patients with pulmonary EG have disease limited to the lung; although some are asymptomatic, most complain of cough, dyspnea, fever, or weight loss. Pneumothorax is another documented presentation of EG. Radiologic studies show an upper-lobe predominance; cysts and small stellate nodules can be seen by high-resolution CT scans. Because of the smoking history, there is often coexistent emphysema, desquamative interstitial pneumonitis, RB, or RB-ILD.

The characteristic histologic picture of EG (e-**Fig. 8.10**) is a stellate interstitial collection, often near small airways, of eosinophils and Langerhans cells. Langerhans cells feature a unique convoluted nucleus and a moderate amount of cytoplasm; some binucleated forms may also be present. An admixture of pigmented alveolar macrophages (the so-called smoker's macrophages) is also often present. Langerhans cells can be easily demonstrated by immunostains for S-100 and CD1a; alveolar macrophages stain for CD68 but not S-100 or CD1a. In contrast to the cellular lesions just described, resolved or "burnt out" lesions in chronic disease may consist only of hyalinized stellate scars in the upper lung zones; immunostains may highlight a few Langerhans cells in these scars, or may be completely negative. About 10% to 20% of cases progress to fibrosis, but most patients improve with cessation of smoking; rare patients develop severe pulmonary hypertension. Eosinophilic pneumonia is one important differential consideration in small biopsies, but can be easily dismissed by correlation with radiographic and clinical features; in addition, the macrophages in eosinophilic pneumonia will be negative for S-100 and CD1a. Eosinophilic pleuritis may develop after pneumothorax, and may raise concern for EG in the lung, but reactive mesothelial cells are negative for S-100 and CD1a.

7. **Lymphangioleiomyomatosis** (LAM) is a disease that essentially occurs only in women of reproductive age. Although classified as an interstitial disease, it features preserved lung volumes, unlike most fibrosing diseases. CT scans show diffuse involvement of the lung by cysts of rather uniform size that feature some mural thickening around the cystic spaces, a finding that serves to distinguish LAM from processes such as emphysema. In fact, high-resolution CT images are so characteristic that the first pathologic specimen seen in many patients is explanted lungs. Patients present with obstructive lung symptoms or spontaneous pneumothorax, and also may demonstrate large chylous pleural effusions. Microscopic sections of LAM (e-**Fig. 8.11**) show a proliferation of abnormal smooth muscle–like cells in the lung. In many cases these cells seem to swirl away from the native smooth muscle of airways and vessels. Vascular compromise is linked to microhemorrhages, and so many cases show abundant hemosiderin within the lung. While LAM is centered in the lung, it also involves lymph nodes in the pulmonary hilum, mediastinum, and abdomen in most cases. The smooth muscle–like cells stain with vimentin, desmin, and smooth muscle actin, and also may express estrogen and progesterone receptor. LAM also shows cross-lineage staining with melanoma markers including HMB-45 and melan-A. In this regard, the cells of LAM share the staining attributes of the neoplasms of the PEComa family (including the sugar tumor of the lung), renal angiomyolipomas, and some soft tissue tumors (see Chapter 44). LAM also shows overlap with tuberous sclerosis (TS) in that some TS patients develop an identical cystic lung disease, and both LAM and TS share an association with angiomyolipomas in the kidney and elsewhere. The course of the disease is unpredictable; transplantation has been the only long-term option for those with severe disease.

8. **Alveolar proteinosis** refers to a peculiar accumulation of intra-alveolar eosinophilic, granular PAS-positive protein and phospholipid. It was initially reported as an idiopathic process, but a relation to immune deficiency, hematologic malignancies, infections, and various exposures is now recognized. Classic exposure-related cases are associated with massive acute silica exposure, which is believed to poison the alveolar macrophages and thus inhibit their ability to clear alveolar debris.

Clinically, patients present with slowly progressive alveolar infiltrates and complain of dyspnea, cough, or sputum production with fever; CT scans show the so-called crazy paving with alveolar infiltrates and septal-line thickening. The diagnosis is often apparent from the milky appearance of lavage fluid; biopsies show complete filling of the alveolar spaces by granular eosinophilic debris that is PAS-positive and diastase-resistant (e-Fig. 8.12). Findings often include cholesterol clefts (acicular clefts), globular eosinophilic debris, and macrophages. In most cases the underlying alveolar structure appears normal, although some chronic cases may eventually show fibrosis. Secondary infection of the fluid by *Nocardia*, mycobacteria, and fungi has been reported. *Pneumocystis* infection can microscopically mimic alveolar proteinosis, although the material in alveolar proteinosis lacks the frothy appearance characteristic of *Pneumocystis* infection.

D. "Allergic" Diseases

1. **Eosinophilic pneumonia** can be divided into acute and chronic forms. The acute forms include the simple form also known as the Löffler syndrome; this is an acute, self-limited process with fleeting infiltrates and peripheral blood eosinophilia and is rarely biopsied. The tropical form is usually linked to *Filaria* infection, and also presents as an acute illness. The chronic form is more likely to require biopsy for diagnosis.

   Chronic eosinophilic pneumonia (CEP) has a variable presentation from acute illness with fever, dyspnea, and weight loss, to vague respiratory complaints. Many patients have a history of asthma, and laboratory tests reveal elevated blood IgE and peripheral blood eosinophilia. Chest radiographs show patchy nonsegmental infiltrates, often peripheral, that may cross fissures, a pattern that is sometimes described as the photographic negative of pulmonary edema. There are myriad underlying causes; major categories include drugs (antibiotics such as nitrofurantoin, sulfonamides, penicillins, anti-inflammatory agents, and chemotherapeutics), fungus (*Aspergillus* and *Candida*), parasites, nickel vapor, and idiopathic cases. Histologic sections of CEP (e-Fig. 8.13) show an alveolar-filling process consisting of a mixture of eosinophils and macrophages. Necrosis of eosinophils may be present, forming an eosinophilic abscess. Charcot–Leyden crystals will also be present, as well as interstitial and perivascular eosinophils, lymphocytes, plasma cells, and areas of BOOP.

2. **Mucoid impaction of bronchi** (MIB) is the filling of bronchi by viscous mucus, usually caused by another underlying disease such as asthma, cystic fibrosis, or chronic bronchitis. Patients present with evidence of lobar collapse or an irregular branching mass–like density. Histologic sections of the impacted material in most cases show the so-called allergic mucin that consists of laminated collections of eosinophils, eosinophil debris, and mucinous exudates. Fungal hyphae, most often *Aspergillus* (e-Fig. 8.14), may also be present in a pattern that overlaps with allergic bronchopulmonary aspergillosis (ABPA). A related process is plastic bronchitis which is impaction of airways by neutrophilic debris.

3. **Allergic bronchopulmonary aspergillosis (ABPA)** is a related form of hypersensitivity to fungal organisms, most often *Aspergillus*. The disease almost always occurs in asthmatic patients, and is usually diagnosed by a combination of clinical features that include pulmonary infiltrates and proximal bronchiectasis, skin testing that shows reaction to fungal antigens, precipitating antibodies to fungal antigen, elevated IgE levels, and peripheral blood eosinophilia. Tissue sections show a combination of eosinophilic pneumonia, MIB, and bronchocentric granulomatosis (granulomatous destruction of bronchioles).

4. **Pulmonary amyloidosis** occurs in several forms.

   a. Tracheobronchial amyloidosis is rare, and features focal or diffuse amyloid deposition in the airway submucosa and around bronchial glands. The amyloid may show calcification or ossification. The patients may have symptoms of wheezing, lobar collapse, or recurrent infections, and the airways are prone to bleeding. This form does not feature systemic involvement.

TABLE 8.6 Pulmonary Hemorrhage Syndromes

Syndrome	Capillaritis	Immunofluorescence
Goodpasture	+/–	+, linear staining
Idiopathic hemosiderosis	–	–
Wegener	+	–
Microscopic polyarteritis	+	–
Collagen vascular disease (SLE)	+	–
Idiopathic rapidly progressive GN	+	+, granular staining
Toxins	–	–

b. Nodular pulmonary amyloid is also typically confined to the lung, with no systemic disease. Patients are usually asymptomatic but have a well-circumscribed peripheral nodule or nodules evident on radiographic studies. Grossly, the mass is often described as waxy or lardaceous. Microscopic sections show nodules of amyloid with an associated foreign body reaction, lymphoplasmacytic infiltrate, and foci of calcification and metaplastic bone formation (e-**Fig. 8.15**).

c. In contrast to the previous types of pulmonary amyloid, the diffuse septal form is most often seen with disseminated primary amyloidosis. Patients present with dyspnea, hypoxemia, and an increased A/a gradient. Chest radiographs show diffuse fine reticulonodular infiltrates. Microscopic sections show deposits in the alveolar interstitium, around vessels, and sometime in the airways and pleura (e-**Fig. 8.16**).

E. Vasculitis and Related Diseases. Vasculitis and related diseases constitute an important collection of lung diseases, many of which have been historically included together in the category of "angiitis and granulomatosis." Patients with vasculitis and related lesions often present alveolar hemorrhage, the causes of which can be categorized (Table 8.6) based on the histologic finding of capillaritis (see below) and immunofluorescent findings. Large pulmonary vessels may also be involved by vasculitis (e-**Fig. 8.17**); common etiologies of large-vessel pulmonary artery vasculitis are presented in Table 8.7.

1. Granulomatosis with polyangiitis (Wegener granulomatosis) is the prototypical lung vasculitis. It most often presents in the middle age with pulmonary symptoms including cough, hemoptysis, and fever. Other patients present with upper respiratory complaints or renal failure, depending on the dominant sites of the disease. Chest radiographs may show alveolar filling due to hemorrhage, multiple nodules with cavitation, or even a single massive nodule. Microscopic features in the lung reflect a classic triad of findings (e-**Fig. 8.17**): (1) Vasculitis which involves arteries, veins, and capillaries (capillaritis). Acute vascular lesions show fibrinoid necrosis; chronic lesions may show only vascular scarring or perivascular chronic inflammation. Capillaritis consists of neutrophils, nuclear dust, and fibrin microthrombi in lung capillaries, analogous to leukocytoclastic vasculitis in the skin. (2) Necrosis that is often described as geographic necrosis, and classically

TABLE 8.7 Differential Diagnosis of Pulmonary Large-Vessel Vasculitis

Involvement by systemic vasculitides	Polyarteritis nodosa, Behçet, Takayasu, giant cell arteritis
Classic causes	Wegener, necrotizing sarcoid granulomatosis, Churg–Strauss syndrome
Other primary entities with large-vessel vasculitis	Collagen vascular disease, malignancy, toxins, and drugs
Secondary	Infection, pulmonary hypertension, others

has an abscess-like appearance with a hematoxyphilic hue, surrounded by palisaded histiocytes. (3) Granulomatous inflammation comprised of palisades of histiocytes, scattered giant cells, and poorly formed granulomas.

Other microscopic features can include acute or chronic alveolar hemorrhage; airway bronchocentric granulomatosis–like lesions, BOOP, chronic bronchitis, and bronchiolitis; interstitial lesions including fibrosis and nonspecific chronic inflammation; DAD; and pleural lesions such as fibrinous pleuritis, granulomas, or chronic inflammation. Serology studies in most cases reveal c-ANCA positivity; the antineutrophil antibodies will show a cytoplasmic pattern of staining, and PR3 is usually the antigen. Rarely, p-ANCA will be positive.

2. **Microscopic polyarteritis** is the lung equivalent of leukocytoclastic vasculitis. It is often associated with p-ANCA and has many other associations including drug-related cases, infection (e.g., hepatitis B, bacteria), Henoch–Schönlein purpura, collagen vascular disease, cryoglobulinemia, and idiopathic. The basic lesion is capillaritis, which has two main features: neutrophils in the alveolar septae and capillary walls with neutrophilic nuclear dust, and microscopic fibrin thrombi in capillaries (e-**Fig. 8.18**). Arteriolitis or venulitis is also often present. Since the differential diagnosis includes acute lung injury or acute pneumonia, microscopic polyarteritis is a diagnosis of exclusion.

3. **Churg–Strauss syndrome** (allergic angiitis and granulomatosis) is another ANCA-related vasculitis. Nearly all patients have a history of asthma. Many patients also have skin lesions, neuropathy, CNS disease, or heart failure; most cases are diagnosed by biopsy of sites other than the lung. The histopathologic findings are a combination of two features: (1) Vasculitis that can affect both arteries and veins, with giant cell infiltration of vessel walls. There may also be transmural eosinophilia with fibrinoid necrosis and small palisaded granulomas. (2) Eosinophilic infiltrates that resemble eosinophilic pneumonia consisting of a combination of histiocytes and eosinophils that fill alveoli.

F. **Bronchiolitis**

1. **Obliterative bronchiolitis** (constrictive bronchiolitis, bronchiolitis obliterans), though it has a name that is similar to BOOP, is a completely different disease that is characterized by the progressive narrowing and luminal compromise of small airways by subepithelial fibrosis. Conditions associated with this process are listed in Table 8.8, many of which have some immunologic basis. Patients present with insidious onset of shortness of breath and obstructive pulmonary functions with air trapping. Wedge biopsies are often required for diagnosis, and it is common to see a spectrum of small airway changes in such biopsies ranging from virtually normal, to partial scarring, to total luminal obliteration by fibrous tissue (e-**Fig. 8.19**). Inflammation is variable, and there will be mucus trapped distal to areas of severe luminal compromise. Although the disease may stabilize for some time, the changes are generally irreversible.

2. **Cellular bronchiolitis** is a descriptive name given to forms of bronchiolitis that feature marked acute and chronic bronchiolar inflammation. Conditions associated with this lesion are listed in Table 8.9.

IV. **INFECTIOUS PROCESSES**

A. **Viral Infections.** Typically, viral infections of the lung are self-limited and do not require biopsy for diagnosis. However, in the setting of immunocompromise or severe pulmonary dysfunction from infection, an attempt to identify the etiology of pneumonia by

TABLE 8.8 Causes of Obliterative Bronchiolitis

• Idiopathic	• Rheumatoid arthritis
• Chronic lung allograft rejection	• Postinfection (viruses)
• Graft versus host disease	• "Pop-corn lung"
• Immunodeficiency states	• Inhaled toxins
• Drugs (penicillamine)	

TABLE 8.9 Conditions Associated With Cellular Bronchiolitis

- Infections: bacteria, viral, mycoplasma
- Toxin/fume exposures
- Asthma
- Bronchiectasis
- Central obstruction

- Collagen vascular diseases (i.e., Sjögren)
- Wegener granulomatosis
- Transplant rejection/graft vs. host disease
- Diffuse pan-bronchiolitis (Homa disease)

tissue biopsy is often made. Viral cultures may require 1 to 4 weeks for growth, and so in some instances a biopsy can provide a specific diagnosis in far less time. In addition to the findings in H&E-stained slides, immunostains, electron microscopy, and serology can be used to increase diagnostic sensitivity.

1. **Cytomegalovirus** (CMV) typically affects immunocompromised patients; since most people are exposed to CMV in childhood, many cases represent activation of latent infection. Patients may develop fever, cough, or shortness of breath. Chest x-rays show diffuse infiltrates, and biopsies show interstitial pneumonitis as well as DAD or nodular inflammation. Enlarged cells with nuclear and/or cytoplasmic inclusions are pathognomonic for CMV infection. In H&E-stained sections, nuclear inclusions have an eosinophilic core (6 μ) with a surrounding cleared zone, while the cytoplasmic deposit is basophilic (e-**Fig. 8.20**). Epithelial cells, vascular cells, and even stromal cells can exhibit inclusions. Immunohistochemistry for CMV will decorate the enlarged cells; electron microscopy demonstrates virions in the inclusions, while a PAS stain with diastase highlights the cytoplasmic deposits.

2. **Herpesvirus** (HSV). Both HSV types 1 and 2 can induce pneumonitis, and immunocompromised hosts are more prone to herpes viral pneumonia. Clinically, HSV pneumonia may result from extension of upper airway disease with primarily bronchiolar inflammation, or from systemic infection which presents as multiple small perivascular inflammatory nodules. Three findings are characteristic of HSV: necrosis, individual cells with inclusions (e-**Fig. 8.21**) (featuring eosinophilic nuclear inclusions with perinuclear clearing; amphophilic nucleoplasm in single cells may represent early inclusions or giant cell formation), and herpes viral giant cells (which contain two or more nuclei with ground-glass central nuclear clearing and coarsely granular, sharply defined nuclear borders; the nuclei are often molded against one another). Immunohistochemistry using antibodies to HSV decorates the giant cells and the individual cells with inclusions.

3. **Varicella zoster virus** (VZV) is the causative agent for chicken pox and shingles. Primary infection in healthy adults and immunocompromised children can result in pneumonia. The underlying lung injury pattern can be either DAD with hyaline membranes and proteinaceous exudates, or nodular inflammation with central necrosis that calcifies and persists on chest radiographs. Biopsies of VZV infections show giant cells similar to those of HSV.

4. **Adenovirus** infection generally presents with symptoms typical of an upper respiratory infection; pneumonia develops in a small percentage of healthy and immunocompromised children and adults. Two patterns of infection evolve. Some patients develop necrotizing bronchiolitis and pneumonia, while others respond with DAD with hyaline membranes and exudates. In adenoviral infections, both alveolar lining cells and bronchial epithelial cells may exhibit blurred and hyperchromatic nuclear chromatin (the so-called smudge cells) (e-**Fig. 8.22**). The bronchial damage of adenovirus may result in fibrosis or constricting bronchiolitis.

5. **Respiratory syncytial virus** (RSV) affects primarily small children and infants; premature infants and immunocompromised children are particularly prone to infection. RSV infection exhibits some seasonality, and is more common in fall and winter. RSV can induce bronchiolitis with symptoms of cough, wheezing, and respiratory distress. Biopsies show necrotizing bronchiolitis and/or interstitial pneumonia.

6. Measles virus. With the advent of vaccination, infection by measles virus is rare, and evolution to pneumonia even rarer. Most patients are immunocompromised, and the characteristic skin rash is present. The underlying pathology is DAD, with associated individual and giant cells with viral inclusions; the alveolar spaces may contain exudates, and necrosis may be present. Both eosinophilic intranuclear and cytoplasmic inclusions develop in both alveolar and vascular lining cells. Measles pneumonia features a distinctive multinucleate giant cell thought to derive from coalescence of type 2 pneumocytes, the Warthin–Finkeldey giant cell, which contains up to 60 nuclei.

7. Parainfluenza and influenza generate nonspecific patterns consisting of varying degrees of DAD, bronchial necrosis, and peribronchial inflammation.

B. Bacterial Infections

1. Mycoplasma induces acute and chronic bronchiolitis, with necrosis and denudement of bronchial epithelium. The bronchial lumina may contain acute inflammatory cells admixed with denuded epithelium. Acute and chronic inflammatory cells often traverse the bronchial wall. Alveolar spaces may exhibit bronchopneumonia, with BOOP or DAD.

2. Mycobacterial infections are typically grouped into tuberculosis (TB) and other (atypical) mycobacterial infections. The most common stain used to demonstrate organisms in tissue sections is the Ziehl–Neelsen stain; immunofluorescent (auramine–rhodamine) and immunohistochemical stains can also be used to identify mycobacteria. PCR-based genetic methods can also be used to detect (and speciate) the organism in tissue sections.

  a. Tuberculosis (TB). Multidrug resistance has emerged in this organism and consequently the pathologic spectrum of tubercular infection is expanding. The causative organism is *Mycobacterium tuberculosis*, which is transmitted via inhalation of organisms. Histologically, the tubercular granuloma is a classic palisaded necrotizing granuloma. Granulomas may caseate and coalesce, creating nodules with central necrosis, or even cavitary masses. Organisms may be found in multinucleate giant cells or at the periphery of necrosis (e-**Fig. 8.23**). Lymph nodal involvement may be present. Miliary TB is unlikely to be sampled in biopsy or resection specimens.

  b. Atypical mycobacterial infection. *Mycobacterium avium-intracellulare* (MAI) is the most common of the atypical mycobacterial infections, and is more common among immunocompromised patients where it presents with nonspecific fever and malaise. Radiographs show diffuse or patchy infiltrates. Histologic findings vary from more typical nonnecrotizing punctuate granulomas, to necrotizing granulomatous pneumonia, to diffuse pneumonitis (in which abundant pneumocytes or interstitial cells contain abundant organisms by acid-fast stains).

C. Fungal Infections

1. *Candida* infection arises in several contexts. Mucocutaneous candidiasis can arise in immunocompetent adults, but arises more frequently in immunocompromised patients; the trachea or bronchial tree can have plaques of fungus admixed with desquamated cells and neutrophils. Impaired host defenses potentiate invasive disease; in the lungs, vascular invasion results in hemorrhagic necrosis. Direct inoculation into the bloodstream from iatrogenic sources (catheters, surgery) or other inoculation (drug abuse) results in disseminated disease. Transplant patients can develop infection at the sites of anastomosis. *Candida albicans* is the most prevalent species; other species more often infect compromised hosts. All species exhibit the same basic morphology: nonbranching, aseptate pseudohyphae forming "boxcar"-like chains of cells; yeast forms bud from pseudohyphae (e-**Fig. 8.24**). Yeast forms are visible in sections stained with H&E, PAS, or silver stains.

2. Mucormycosis. Several members of *Phycomycetes* result in clinically and morphologically identical disease, including *Mucor*, *Absidia*, and *Rhizopus*, among others. Almost all cases occur in the setting of diabetic ketoacidosis (sinonasal or rhinocerebral disease) or immunosuppression from hematologic malignancies. Lung involvement may be the primary focus, or develop secondary to head and neck disease. Lung lesions are typified by hemorrhagic pneumonia; fungal thrombi with distal infarction are often present. The dual circulation of the lung (bronchial and pulmonary arterial systems) results in perfusion of infarcted areas with resulting hemorrhagic necrosis, associated with varying amounts of inflammation. A key to recognition of the infection is identification of wide, ribbon-like nonseptate hyphae with irregular wide-angle branching. The pseudohyphae are often described as empty, and stain poorly with most special stains.

3. **Aspergillus** species cause a wide spectrum of disease, dependent on both host immune status and site of growth. Colonization with *Aspergillus* can induce an allergic response, including ABPA, sinusitis, and HP. *Aspergillus* can also colonize mucus or grow in a preexisting cavity, and sinus or cavitary lung lesions both can harbor fungus balls. Transplant anastomoses are also prone to colonization by *Aspergillus* species (e-**Fig. 8.25**). The characteristic lung lesion is the target lesion with a sharply delineated hemorrhagic border, which reflects the fact that the fungus is frequently vasoinvasive and produces hemorrhagic infarcts. In well-preserved areas, organisms have relatively uniform septa which are thinner than those of *Mucor*. The hyphae branch at ~45 degrees; the reproductive form (fruiting body) is only rarely seen in tissues. Degenerate hyphae can be mistaken for *Mucor*, with empty or dilated forms; acute-angle branching, occasional septa, and more intact forms indicate the correct diagnosis.

4. **Cryptococcus.** The most common pathogen of this genus is *Cryptococcus neoformans*, which is usually an opportunistic infection but rarely also infects normal hosts after massive exposure. The common portal of entry is the lungs; patients remain virtually asymptomatic while the fungus spreads to other sites. The organism is present in the lung as the so-called naked masses of organisms, to intracellular forms resembling those of histoplasmosis, to granulomas with surrounding fibrosis (the so-called cryptococcomas) (e-**Fig. 8.26**). The organisms are much larger than *Candida* or *Histoplasma* with an average diameter of 4 to 10 μ; only yeast forms are found in tissue. The diameter of cryptococcal forms varies in large part with capsule thickness, a function of host immune status, and mucicarmine stains the capsule strongly (generally considered a diagnostic feature). Capsule-deficient forms are common in cancer or AIDS patients, and may be much more difficult to diagnose definitively.

5. **Blastomycosis** is generally seen in the middle of the United States. Infection usually involves lungs and skin; spore inhalation is the mode of transmission for virtually all cases. Pulmonary blastomycosis takes several forms; the most common is a solitary focus of infection with variable-associated lymph nodal disease, which usually heals and leaves a fibrous scar. Progressive disease is less common, in which infection spreads throughout the lung as miliary foci which range from neutrophil-rich abscesses to tubercle-like granulomas. The causative agent maintains a variably sized yeast form in tissue ranging from 5 to 25 μ, and has a thick, refractile, double-contoured wall; unlike *Cryptococcus*, this wall is negative or very weakly mucin positive (e-**Fig. 8.27**).

6. **Histoplasmosis.** In the United States, infection is usually caused by *Histoplasma capsulatum* from bird or bat droppings. In tissue, the fungus reverts to a primitive yeast, 2 to 5 μ in diameter with occasional unequal budding. Primary histoplasmosis produces a mild, self-limited febrile illness in most cases, with hyalinized granulomas as the result (e-**Fig. 8.28**); however, it can also result in a progressive, disseminated, fatal disease. Cases with active disease can also produce a granulation tissue–like pattern, with vague granulomas. The organism can also induce secondary scarring forms of inflammation, such as sclerosing mediastinitis with calcified granulomas in which organisms are often not identified.

7. **Coccidioidomycosis** is caused by *Coccidioides immitis*, a soil-borne saprophyte typically found in the southwestern United States. Patients typically have travel histories to that region, and present with an acute febrile illness (some infections are asymptomatic). Infection develops in both immunocompetent and immunocompromised individuals. The inhaled organisms transform into spherules, thick-walled sacs 60 to 80 μ in

diameter containing multiple endospores (**e-Fig. 8.29**); reproduction in tissue results from rupture of the spherule with release of endospores. Microscopically, the organisms create a nodule, typically with noncaseating granuloma formation; cavitation may occur. Lymph nodal involvement may be present and disseminated infection may result. The organisms can be demonstrated with GMS or PAS stains.

8. ***Pneumocystis carinii* pneumonia** (PCP). *P. carinii* was formerly considered a protozoan, but genetic analysis suggests that it is best classified as a fungus. Infection is generally seen among immunocompromised patients. The chest radiograph classically shows diffuse infiltrates which correspond to the diffuse alveolar infiltrates that are almost diagnostic microscopically (**e-Fig. 8.30**). Cytologically, the infiltrate exfoliates in lavage specimens as alveolar casts. PCP can induce interstitial pneumonitis or granulomatous inflammation; these variant forms are often seen in chronic disease or with partially treated disease, may progress to cavitating or cystic disease in the upper lobes, and are associated with extrapulmonary disseminated disease. The cysts stain well with GMS in most cases; in degenerate cases, immunostains may be of some help. The organism has a helmet or cup shape, often referred to as a "dented ping-pong ball."

D. Parasite Infections

1. **Dirofilariasis**. *Dirofilaria* are nematodes, the most common pathogen of which is *Dirofilaria immitis*, the common dog heartworm. While this parasite does not have a life cycle in the human host, occasional infection can develop with adult nematodes via transmission by a mosquito bite. Infection can result in noncaseating granulomas presenting as a nodule in the lung (or other organ). Cross sections of the organism's refractile cuticle (10 to 14 μ in greatest diameter) may be seen in histologic sections. Endovascular thrombi with organisms have been reported as well.

V. SELECTED PNEUMOCONIOSES

A. Asbestosis. Asbestosis is an interstitial lung disease caused by asbestos. It usually occurs in workers heavily exposed, for a prolonged period of time. There is often a long latency period, usually at least 15 years, between exposure and the disease. Mild disease shows no symptoms; with increasing severity, patients complain of dyspnea, dry cough, weight loss, and chest pain. Radiographic findings are characterized by small irregular opacities, most prominent in the bases of the lung. The American Thoracic Society has defined six clinical criteria a clinical diagnosis of asbestosis, including exposure, a latency period, rales, decreased lung volumes and DLCO by PFTs, and chest radiograph infiltrates. Thankfully, pathologic criteria include just two required findings: the presence of peribronchiolar fibrosis (known as fibroelastosis) and associated asbestos bodies (**e-Fig. 8.31**). Grading of asbestosis can be performed: grade 1, fibrosis confined to respiratory bronchioles; grade 2, fibrosis involves alveolar ducts, or two tiers of alveoli; grade 3, fibrosis involves all alveoli between two bronchioles; grade 4, honeycombing. The lungs show a high fiber burden: 98% to 99% of cases have at least 2,000 asbestos bodies per gram of wet lung tissue; most have 10,000 to 100,000 or more asbestos bodies per gram of wet lung tissue which correlates with at least several asbestos bodies per tissue slide in the majority of cases (iron stains often help to demonstrate asbestos bodies). If pathologic examination of biopsy or lung resections suggests asbestosis, or if there is clinical suspicion for asbestosis, it is prudent to set tissue aside for fiber analysis (fiber studies on either fresh lung tissue or formalin fixed and embedded tissue), although it is not required for diagnosis in most cases. Classically, asbestosis is required to attribute pulmonary carcinomas to asbestos exposure; asbestosis plus smoking increases the risk for lung carcinomas by a multiplicative factor, to perhaps 50× nonsmoking, nonasbestotic controls. Pleural plaques and mesothelioma, which are also asbestos-related pleuropulmonary lesions, are discussed in the chapter on serosal membranes (Chapter 11).

B. Silicosis. Silicosis is produced by silica deposition in the lung. Occupations at risk include sandblasting, grinding, mining, plastering, and masonry, among many others. Silicosis typically produces infiltrates in the mid-lung zones, in contrast to other types of pulmonary fibrosis. Lymph nodes in the chest will also show the characteristic so-called egg-shell calcifications on x-ray. The characteristic lung lesion is the silica nodule; nodules have a lymphangitic distribution, so are seen along the bronchovascular tree and in the pleura (e-**Fig. 8.32**). Early nodules are cellular and composed of a swirling collection of fibrohistiocytic cells; birefringent particles can be seen in these nodules with polarized microscopy. Older lesions become progressively hyalinized; they may coalesce to form irregular masses that can mimic pulmonary neoplasms. The relationship of silicosis to the development of pulmonary neoplasms is debated, but appears to be a small risk, if present at all. Nodules may also include other material such as iron or carbon, in which case a diagnosis of mixed dust fibrosis is appropriate.

VI. PULMONARY TRANSPLANTATION

A. Gross Processing of Transplant Specimens.
Pulmonary transplantation is now a well-established therapy for various end-stage lung diseases including emphysema/chronic obstructive pulmonary disease, cystic fibrosis, LAM, pulmonary hypertension, and pulmonary fibrosis of various causes. Examination of the explanted, native lungs should include thorough documentation of the underlying disease process. A minimum of one section per lobe should be submitted for diffuse processes, as well as sections of the hilar lymph nodes; cases of pulmonary hypertension may require additional sections to document plexiform lesions. Any mass or focal abnormality should be sampled thoroughly. Examination should be comprehensive enough to exclude foci of malignancy, or infections which may recur due to the immunocompromise of transplant recipients.

The allograft is surveyed by transbronchial biopsy, and occasional wedge biopsies, both at scheduled protocol intervals, as well as in response to changes in clinical condition. A minimum of five pieces of alveolar tissue is considered adequate for assessment in this setting. In general, three levels of H&E-stained sections are obtained; some institutions employ protocols with adjunct special stains for infectious organisms on all biopsies.

B. Microscopic Features of Transplant Biopsies

1. Preservation injury is the first change seen in posttransplant biopsies. This change reflects ischemic damage that develops in the lung in the interval between removal from the donor and reimplantation. Preservation injury produces a picture of classic lung injury that may exhibit features of DAD or BOOP (e-**Fig. 8.33**). The appearance sometimes suggests viral infection, but for biopsies taken in the first 1 to 2 weeks after transplant, it is generally too early for opportunistic infections to become manifest. One important differential diagnosis for early acute graft injury is humoral or hyperacute rejection (discussed below).

2. Opportunistic infections. Biopsies after the first week or two must be surveyed for opportunistic infections, the most frequent of which is CMV, the features which are detailed above (e-**Fig. 8.20**). Important clues of CMV infection include interstitial neutrophils and alveolar fibrin exudates, findings which warrant immunostains for CMV since transplant patients may not always develop classic inclusions. CMV may produce perivascular inflammation, a finding that mimics acute rejection (see below). Other viral infections often seen include herpesvirus (e-**Fig. 8.21**) and adenovirus (e-**Fig. 8.22**), and a variety of nonspecific pneumonitis patterns may actually represent responses to other viral pathogens. The results of culture, serologic, and molecular tests for infectious organisms must be integrated with biopsy data by the transplant clinician.

Since most transplant patients currently receive prophylactic therapy against *Pneumocystis* infection, PCP is a rare complication. Fungal infections seen more commonly are due to *Aspergillus* or *Candida* colonization of the bronchial tissue in the region of the airway anastomosis, likely related to tissue ischemia (e-**Fig. 8.25**); invasive growth within the lung is much less common. The presence of foamy macrophages in a transbronchial biopsy may be an indicator of fungal infection and should be followed with silver stains to exclude intrahistiocytic organisms such as *Histoplasma*.

3. Acute rejection is a primary concern in all follow-up biopsies. The 2007 revised lung allograft rejection scheme is provided in Table 8.10. The basic lesion of acute

TABLE 8.10	Revised Scheme for Lung Allograft Rejection[a]

A: Acute rejection
  A0: None
  A1: Minimal
  A2: Mild
  A3: Moderate
  A4: Severe

B: Small airway inflammation/lymphocytic bronchiolitis
  B0: None
  B1R: Low grade (previous B1, B2)
  B2R: High grade (previous B3, B4)
  BX: Ungradeable

C: Chronic airway rejection—bronchiolitis obliterans
  C0: Absent
  C1: Present

D: Chronic vascular rejection

[a]After Stewart S, Fishbein MC, Snell GI, et al. Revision of the 1996 Working Formulation for the Standardization of nomenclature in the diagnosis of lung rejection. *J Heart Lung Trans* 2007;26:122.

rejection is lymphocytic infiltration surrounding blood vessels and airways. The perivascular inflammation is reflected in the "A" scores (e-**Fig. 8.34**). T-cells are the main cell type present in acute rejection; more severe rejections feature larger, more activated cells, and will also show eosinophils and neutrophils. Table 8.11 presents more details of the histologic patterns of rejection.

Airways are the other target of rejection and are reflected in the "B" scores (e-**Fig. 8.35**; Table 8.11). Airway inflammation is less specific for rejection, and can be seen with chronic airway infections, obstruction, and preservation injury among

TABLE 8.11	Key Characteristics/Features in the Grading of Allograft Cellular Rejection

"A" Lesions

Grade	Circumferential Perivascular Infiltrates	Cytologic Features of Infiltrate	Endothelialitis	Airway Infiltrate
A0	None	N/A	N/A	Usually absent
A1	Rare, hard to see at scanning power 1–2 cell thick cuffs	Small, "resting" lymphocytes	Usually absent	Often modest
A2	More vessels with infiltrate, easily seen at scanning power, 2–5 cell thick cuffs	More "activated" lymphocytes, also eosinophils	Sometimes	Common
A3	Often many vessels, infiltrates into the adjacent septa, "stellate"	More activated, many eosinophils, can be neutrophils	Almost always	Usually present
A4	May be confluent, associated lung injury	Similar to A3	Almost always, vasculitis like	Usually present, severe

"B" Lesions

Grade	Severity	Epithelial Damage
B0	None	N/A
B1R	Mild	No
B2R	Moderate to severe	Yes, individual cell apoptosis, to ulcers, total denudation of epithelium

other causes. In general, A and B grades tend to follow each other, although they can be discordant, particularly if small biopsies are obtained.

4. **Humoral rejection** is a form of acute rejection that has been recognized more recently. It often occurs in cases that show donor–recipient crossmatch positivity in which the recipient has antidonor antibodies. The most dramatic example of antibody-mediated rejection is **hyperacute rejection**, where there may be immediate graft dysfunction, noted even in the operating room, as a result of extensive vascular thrombosis and acute inflammation. Histologic features of hyperacute rejection include neutrophil infiltrates in the interstitium and fibrinoid vasculitis that leads to necrosis and hemorrhage. In contrast, cases of humoral rejection seen outside of the immediate postoperative period are characterized by more subtle disease; although lesions may include features similar to hyperacute rejection with capillaritis and necrosis, in many cases the only lesion detected in biopsies will be acute interstitial inflammation or a lung injury pattern such as DAD or BOOP. In analogy to renal or cardiac transplantation, it has been suggested that immunostains for C4d may be helpful to identify cases of humoral rejection. The postulated pattern of positivity is diffuse capillary staining; however, the role of C4d immunostaining in the lung remains to be clarified.

5. **Chronic airway rejection** is a major problem in lung transplantation. Bronchiolitis obliterans syndrome (BOS) is the clinical feature of chronic airway rejection, defined by a drop of FEV below 80% of the posttransplant maximum value. Chronic airway rejection is reflected in the "C" score. The pathologic lesion is subepithelial fibrosis of airways that leads to a picture of obliterative bronchiolitis (e-**Fig. 8.36**). This subepithelial fibrosis pushes the mucosa toward the center of the lumen, with progressive luminal compromise; the findings in individual airways range from partial eccentric thickening, to complete obliteration of the airway resulting in a small fibrous scar next to an accompanying artery. Features of localized obstructive pneumonitis may also be seen due to bronchiolar dysfunction. The development of chronic rejection is correlated with increasing episodes of acute rejection, and also with the severity of the lymphocytic infiltrate around airways, although the mechanisms of chronic rejection are still poorly understood.

6. **Posttransplant lymphoproliferative disorder** (PTLD) is another serious posttransplant process. Changes in immunosuppressive regimens have resulted in a decreased incidence of the disease. In lung transplant patients there is a propensity for PTLD to develop in the transplanted lung, although lymph nodes, the gastrointestinal tract, and tonsils appear to be other preferred sites. The vast majority of cases, in particular those that occur early in the transplant course, are EBV positive with a B-cell phenotype. There should be a high index of suspicion for PTLD in any lung allograft biopsy that shows an intense infiltrate with cytologic atypia or necrosis, or where the clinical history suggests nodules or a mass. Cases usually fall into three general categories: plasma cell hyperplasia, consisting of cases that show low-grade findings; polymorphous PTLD, which is comprised of a mixed population of atypical lymphoid cells; and monomorphous PTLD, consisting of cases that consist of a monotonous population of high-grade, malignant-appearing cells (e-**Fig. 8.37**). Monomorphous cases are much less likely to regress following diminution of immunosuppression as compared with the lower-grade lesions; thus, higher-grade cases are likely to require cytotoxic therapy. In allograft biopsies, if there is a question of PTLD versus a rejection-related infiltrate, a simple panel of CD3, CD20/CD79a, and EBV immunostains will provide dichotomous results: the infiltrate in severe rejection or infections is almost always a CD3-predominant infiltrate, while the infiltrate in PTLD is positive for CD20 and CD79a, as well as EBV, in the great majority of cases. Adjunctive studies to indicate clonality may also be of value in terms of diagnosis, classification, and prognosis. It is important to note that rare examples of PTLD may have the morphology of Hodgkin disease, and that late cases of EBV-negative lymphoid neoplasms (4 or 5 years after transplant) which resemble non-Hodgkin lymphomas can also develop.

7. Recurrent disease. With the exception of a few cases of the sarcoid, recurrence of the native lung disease in allografts is not a significant problem. There are reports of occasional cases of carcinoma arising in transplanted lungs, as well as in the native lung in the setting of unilateral transplant; these patients fare poorly.

VII. NEOPLASMS. A modified WHO classification of lung neoplasms is presented in Table 8.12. Malignancies of the lung are the most common cause of cancer-related mortality in the United States. Despite decades of warnings, cigarette smoking remains the predominant risk factor for the development of pulmonary carcinoma. There has been speculation that a shift in the location and cell type for pulmonary carcinomas is related to changes in cigarette usage. Some data suggest that filtered cigarettes, which remove larger tar particles, have allowed carcinogens to penetrate to more distal parts of the lung and produce peripheral adenocarcinomas instead of central squamous carcinomas or small cell carcinomas caused by larger particles. Changes in tobacco formulation over the years may also have played some role in these changes. Other risk factors for lung carcinoma, either proven or speculative, include asbestos exposure, radiation, various chemicals, heavy metals, viral infection, fibrosing lung diseases, immunosuppression, and genetic syndromes. Outside of these causes, there remain some cases of lung carcinomas for which there is no clear etiologic factor.

Up to 10% of patients with head and neck carcinomas may harbor a concurrent lung primary carcinoma; therefore, the finding of a lung nodule in a head and neck cancer patient should not automatically be assumed to represent metastatic disease. Similarly, 2% to 5% of lung carcinoma patients present with apparent synchronous lung primary tumors (which may be due to the greatly improved resolution of CT techniques which can now detect additional small nodules in patients with dominant lung masses). Histologic sampling of these lesions often shows alveolar proliferations with varying degrees of atypia which may represent precursor lesions in the peripheral lung similar to squamous dysplasia in the more central airways.

A. Pathologic Reporting. The important data to be included in a diagnostic report of a primary pulmonary neoplasm are summarized in Table 8.13; templates are available with suggested guidelines for reporting (e.g., see the College of American Pathologists Protocol for the Examination of Specimens From Patients With Primary Non-Small Cell Carcinoma, Small Cell Carcinoma, or Carcinoid Tumor of the Lung, available at http://www.cap.org). The most recent AJCC staging scheme (*Arch Pathol Lab Med* 2018;142:645) emphasizes that the tumor size has become an important factor with all the stages now dependent on the tumor size. T2 and T3 lesions now have a defined size range (3 to 5 cm and 5 to 7 cm, respectively). Tumors under 3 cm are designated as T1 lesions; tumors larger than 7 cm up are now in the T4 category, which was previously limited largely to tumors that had extended outside of the lung in some manner. In the past, the tumor size was assessed by gross examination, and this measurement usually suffices unless there is confounding fibrosis or peritumoral pneumonia. An exception to the use of gross tumor size is in the setting of nonmucinous adenocarcinomas with a lepidic component, where only the invasive component is included for tumor size and staging (see nonmucinous AIS below). In addition, in cases with multiple nodules of lepidic-predominant adenocarcinoma, these can now be staged as independent primaries if all of the invasive foci have their own associated foci of adenocarcinoma in situ (AIS); in the past these cases would have been considered to be stage 3 tumors based on multiple tumor nodules. The extension of tumor through the pleura covering the lung (visceral pleura) or into the pleura lining the chest wall (parietal pleura) should be noted; an elastin stain can delineate these layers in some cases. Lymphatic, arterial, and venous invasion should be noted separately. The status of the margins of resection should be listed, and any abnormalities in the adjacent lung should be described.

In the past, therapy of non–small cell lung carcinomas was largely independent of histology. However, recent developments in the therapy make histologic classification important. Therapy with pemetrexed has been demonstrated to be efficacious in pulmonary adenocarcinomas, and bevacizumab is contraindicated in squamous carcinomas due to bleeding complications. Furthermore, mutation testing is indicated in

TABLE 8.12	Modified WHO Histologic Classification of Tumors of the Lung

Malignant epithelial tumors

Squamous cell carcinoma
  Papillary
  Clear cell
  Small cell
  Basaloid
Small cell carcinoma
  Combined small cell carcinoma
Adenocarcinoma
  Adenocarcinoma in situ
    Nonmucinous
    Mucinous
  Minimally invasive adenocarcinoma
  Adenocarcinoma, mixed subtype
  Acinar adenocarcinoma
  Lepidic predominant
  Papillary
  Micropapillary
  Papillary adenocarcinoma
  Enteric adenocarcinoma
  Solid adenocarcinoma with mucin production
  Fetal adenocarcinoma
  Mucinous ("colloid") carcinoma
  Mucinous cystadenocarcinoma
  Signet-ring adenocarcinoma
  Clear cell adenocarcinoma
Large cell carcinoma
  Large cell neuroendocrine carcinoma
    Combined large cell neuroendocrine carcinoma
  Basaloid carcinoma
  Lymphoepithelioma-like carcinoma
  Clear cell carcinoma
  Large cell carcinoma with rhabdoid phenotype
Adenosquamous carcinoma
Sarcomatoid carcinoma
  Pleomorphic carcinoma
  Spindle cell carcinoma
  Giant cell carcinoma
  Carcinosarcoma
  Pulmonary blastoma
Carcinoid tumor
  Typical carcinoid
  Atypical carcinoid
Salivary gland tumors
  Mucoepidermoid carcinoma
  Adenoid cystic carcinoma
  Epithelial–myoepithelial carcinoma
Preinvasive/dysplastic lesions
  Squamous carcinoma in situ
  Atypical adenomatous hyperplasia
  Diffuse idiopathic pulmonary neuroendocrine cell hyperplasia

(continued)

TABLE 8.12	Modified WHO Histologic Classification of Tumors of the Lung (*Continued*)

Mesenchymal tumors
   Epithelioid hemangioendothelioma
   Angiosarcoma
   Pleuropulmonary blastoma
   Chondroma
   Congenial peribronchial myofibroblastic tumor
   Diffuse pulmonary lymphangiomatosis
   Inflammatory myofibroblastic tumor
   Lymphangioleiomyomatosis
   Synovial sarcoma
      Monophasic
      Biphasic
   Pulmonary artery sarcoma
   Pulmonary vein sarcoma
   Primary pulmonary myxoid sarcoma with EWSR translocation

Benign epithelial tumors
Papillomas
   Squamous cell papilloma
      Exophytic
      Inverted
   Glandular papilloma
   Mixed squamous cell and glandular papilloma
Adenomas
   Alveolar adenoma
   Papillary adenoma
   Adenomas of the salivary gland type
      Mucous gland adenoma
      Pleomorphic adenoma
      Others
   Mucinous cystadenoma

Lymphoproliferative tumors
   Marginal-zone B-cell lymphoma of the MALT type
   Diffuse large B-cell lymphoma
   Lymphomatoid granulomatosis
   Langerhans cell histiocytosis

Miscellaneous tumors
   Hamartoma
   Sclerosing hemangioma
   Clear cell tumor
   Germ cell tumors
      Teratoma, mature
      Immature
      Other germ cell tumors
   Intrapulmonary thymoma
   Melanoma

Metastatic tumors

From Travis WD, Brambilla E, Burke AP, Marx A, Nicholson AG. *WHO Classification of Tumours of the Lung, Pleura, Thymus and Heart.* Lyon, France: IARC Press; 2017.

TABLE 8.13	Diagnostic Features to be Reported With Lung Carcinoma Resections

- Tumor type
- Grade
- Tumor size
- Pleural involvement
- Lymphatic, arterial, and venous invasion
- Spread through airspaces

- Margins
- Associated conditions in nonneoplastic lung
- T-stage
- N-stage
- M-data

adenocarcinomas. Thus, it is now vital that cases with such features as glandular formation, mucin production, or keratinization should be classified as adenocarcinoma or squamous carcinoma. Cases which have less defined features may be classified by immunostaining; napsin and thyroid transcription factor-1 (TTF-1) are largely restricted to adenocarcinoma, while p63 or cytokeratin 5/6 are largely seen in squamous tumors; however, immunohistochemical classification is still an evolving area, as different experts have recommended various panels in this context (*Am J Surg Pathol* 2011;35:15; *Mod Pathol* 2011;24:1348; *Pathol* 2011;43:103). Also, it remains to be seen whether classification only by immunostaining carries the same therapeutic implications as for cases that can be classified on histology alone, which was the method of classification in the chemotherapy trials discussed above.

B. Non–Small Cell Carcinomas

1. Adenocarcinoma is now the most common subtype of lung carcinoma, accounting for 40% or more of all primary lung carcinomas. This subtype is relatively more common in women. More than two-thirds of cases arise in the periphery of the lung, often in a subpleural location, often with an associated scar (**e-Fig. 8.38**). Pulmonary acinar adenocarcinoma, sometimes designated as adenocarcinoma of no special type, represents the most common form of pulmonary adenocarcinoma. This variant of adenocarcinoma features a glandular, tubular, or solid growth pattern. The cytologic features range from very bland and well differentiated to highly anaplastic. Subtypes of adenocarcinoma include papillary, invasive micropapillary, mucinous, enteric-like, clear cell, glassy cell, and bronchioloalveolar carcinoma (BAC) (see below). Because of the peripheral location of most adenocarcinomas, they have a higher rate of resectability than many other non–small cell carcinomas, and also tend to involve the visceral pleura. Finally, since lymphatic and vascular invasion with consequent lymph node metastases are quite common, relatively small peripheral adenocarcinomas may have mediastinal lymph node involvement.

Electron microscopic and immunostaining studies show that pulmonary adenocarcinomas can resemble the many different respiratory cell types, including bronchial cells, goblet cells, Clara cells, and alveolar pneumocytes. Immunostains show consistent positivity for epithelial membrane antigen (EMA), various cytokeratins including cytokeratin 7, various surfactants and related proteins, and the nuclear marker TTF-1 (**e-Fig. 8.39**). TTF-1 has been shown to be quite useful in differentiating primary pulmonary adenocarcinomas from lung metastases of adenocarcinomas from a variety of other origins, and can also identify metastatic pulmonary adenocarcinomas in distant sites. Since very poorly differentiated adenocarcinomas, as well as some mucinous pulmonary carcinomas, do not express TTF-1, TTF-1 negativity does not provide definitive evidence that a tumor is not of pulmonary origin; such a determination must be based on all available clinical, radiographic, and pathologic information. In addition, TTF-1 is not specific for pulmonary adenocarcinoma and may be expressed by thyroid carcinomas and neuroendocrine carcinomas (NECs) arising at a variety of other anatomic sites. As mentioned below, napsin-A is a marker typically present in lung adenocarcinomas. As expected in many adenocarcinomas, pulmonary adenocarcinoma also expresses many generic carcinoma markers including carcinoma embryonic antigen (CEA), the B72.3-related antigen, CD15, and MOC31.

The recommendations for molecular analysis of lung carcinomas continue to evolve (*Arch Pathol Lab Med* 2018;142:321). Testing is now recommended for adenocarcinoma to include wide spectrum mutation testing for *EGFR*. It has now been convincingly shown that adenocarcinomas with EGFR-activating mutations will respond, sometimes very impressively, to EGFR inhibitors. In multiple trials, such therapy is superior to cytotoxic chemotherapy, with markedly decreased side effects. Thus, EGFR-inhibitor therapy is now the recommended first-line therapy for high-stage adenocarcinomas with *EGFR* mutations. While studies suggest that *EGFR*-mutated adenocarcinomas tend to occur more often in Asian populations, never- or light-smokers, and women, the emergence of *EGFR*-inhibitor therapy and the presence of mutated cases outside of the female/Asian/never/light-smoking population has made testing of all high-stage adenocarcinomas for *EGFR* mutations standard of care. The validity of this approach is emphasized by the fact that approximately 15% of lung adenocarcinomas harbor *EGFR* mutations. Activating mutations in exon 19 and a few other similar activating mutations account for most clinically important *EGFR* mutations; however, testing should include analysis for all clinically significant activating mutations, and in most patients it is also useful to test for resistance mutations, including the most common T790M resistance mutation, which often develops after tyrosine kinase inhibitor treatment. Of note, immunohistochemical testing for specific *EGFR* mutations, which was included as an alternative to molecular studies in prior guidelines, is now not recommended.

Crizotinib and other tyrosine kinase inhibitors target lung adenocarcinomas harboring the *EML4-ALK* translocation. This translocation tends to occur in tumors with mucinous or signet-ring histology, but can occur more rarely in other histiotypes. Overall, 4% to 5% of lung adenocarcinomas harbor this translocation. Tumors harboring a rearrangement in *ROS1* also respond to various tyrosine kinase inhibitors. Thus, analysis for *ALK* and *ROS* rearrangements is now clinically indicated, and may be assessed by FISH analysis. Guidelines also allow for immunohistochemical analysis.

KRAS mutations are also found in a large subset of adenocarcinomas. It has been shown that *KRAS*, *EGFR*, *ALK,* and other mutations are essentially mutually exclusive, and thus some experts advocate that genetic analysis should include testing for *KRAS* mutations, which can be easily and rapidly accomplished. If a *KRAS* mutation is found, testing is essentially complete; if *KRAS* is wild type, additional testing can be performed. While logical, the delays created by this sort of sequential testing and the ability to perform multiplex testing for many mutations at once has for the most part made this approach obsolete.

Beyond these essentially mandatory determinations, current guidelines suggest that there may be some value for additional multiplex testing to assess for mutations in *KRAS*, *BRAF*, *MET*, *HER-2*, *RET*, and others. Given the pace of drug development, it is likely that many of these mutations will become linked to specific drugs in the near future, and thus testing will become clinically mandated. The necessity of testing for such a large number of mutations, and the limited amount of tissue often present in lung carcinoma biopsies, suggest that the use of multiplex NGS sequencing panels is likely to become the testing method of choice.

The last several years have also brought about strides forward in the realm of immunotherapy, mainly in the setting of the so-called checkpoint inhibitors, involving the PD-L1/PD-1 axis (*Immunotargets Ther* 2018;7:63). The drug pembrolizumab has been approved for first-line therapy in the setting of advanced non–small cell lung carcinoma; several other drugs have also been approved for second- and third-line therapy, and there are numerous trials in progress utilizing these checkpoint inhibitor drugs. Thus, immunostain assessment of PD-L1 expression is now a part of the standard assessment of lung carcinomas, in addition to molecular studies as discussed above. Other biomarker studies such as tumor mutation burden, or direct sequencing of the entire exome to detect tumor neoantigens, have been proposed as other ways assess for potential checkpoint inhibitor efficacy, but these are still largely investigative. PD-L1 testing is not limited to adenocarcinoma, and in fact is one of the only targeted therapies that may be utilized for squamous carcinomas or other histologic subtypes. Thus, testing for PD-L1 expression should be part of the ancillary testing for most newly diagnosed lung carcinomas, regardless of histology.

a. Adenocarcinoma in situ (AIS) is a specialized form of pulmonary adenocarcinoma, formerly known as BAC. With the relative and absolute increase of peripheral lung carcinomas, as discussed above, an increasing number of primary lung cancers present as ground-glass opacities on chest imaging. Clinicians and radiologists often characterize these as AIS, but the morphologic diagnosis of AIS is somewhat rare. AIS must grow exclusively with a noninvasive lepidic pattern; cases with any component of destructive invasion, as indicated by desmoplasia, or secondary structures such as papillary growth, should be classified as invasive adenocarcinomas. Pure AIS therefore is rare; it develops relatively more often in women and in nonsmokers. It is much more common as a peripheral component of an invasive adenocarcinoma in which case it should be reported as lepidic-predominant adenocarcinoma.

AIS may present as a solitary peripheral nodule, multiple nodules, with lobar consolidation that mimics pneumonia, or rarely with diffuse involvement of the entire lung. In the pure form, the radiographic description is often that of ground-glass opacity. AIS is generally a well-differentiated neoplasm. The tumor cell nuclei are often only modestly atypical, but are abnormal by their monotonous nature, and may be differentiated from reactive alveolar processes in part by this cellular uniformity. The so-called sclerosing AIS may have some expansion of the alveolar interstitium by fibrosis without invasion, but many postulated examples of this tumor are actually invasive adenocarcinoma. Because AIS grows slowly, there may be a central elastotic scar that is degenerative or involutional and which should not therefore be labeled as invasive growth; these scars may feature calcification or even metaplastic bone. Some examples of AIS can have extensive lymphocytic infiltrates, often with a nodular pattern. AIS can be divided into mucinous and nonmucinous types (formerly known as type 1 and type 2 BAC).

i. Mucinous AIS may resemble pulmonary goblet cells, gastric mucous cells, or intestinal epithelium, both morphologically and in terms of mucin types (**e-Fig. 8.40**). Mucinous AIS is often multifocal and may present with bronchorrhea. The cells grow along alveoli, often with a discontinuous appearance, and mucin and muciphages may fill the involved alveolar spaces. Invasive mucinous carcinomas, including signet-ring lesions, are often found in continuity with mucinous AIS. Also, by definition, mucinous AIS must be limited to tumors 3 cm or less; any apparently in situ lesion larger than 3 cm is considered to be an invasive adenocarcinoma. Another type of adenocarcinoma closely related to mucinous AIS is the so-called enteric-type adenocarcinoma, which closely resembles colonic or other gut carcinomas. Finally, the so-called mucinous cystadenoma may be associated with mucinous AIS; this rare low-grade mucinous lung lesion resembles mucinous cystadenomas in other sites, and so is best considered as a lesion of low malignant potential. Metastatic adenocarcinoma of gastric, pancreatic, or intestinal origin is the most important differential consideration for mucinous AIS.

Mucinous AIS and related invasive adenocarcinomas of the lung often show immunohistochemical coexpression of cytokeratins 7 and 20 (**e-Fig. 8.41**), but may be negative for TTF-1 and Napsin-A. CDX2 staining may also be confusing, since many pulmonary mucinous neoplasms can react with this immunostain. Adequate clinical history and correlation with the appearance and stage of the primary tumor is of great importance in this differential diagnosis.

ii. Nonmucinous AIS cells can resemble several bronchial- and alveolar-type cell types including type 2 pneumocytes and Clara cells (**e-Fig. 8.42**). Nonmucinous tumors, as compared with mucinous tumors, are more likely to present as solitary mass, although multiple nonmucinous tumors do occur. Tumors with type 2 pneumocyte differentiation commonly have intranuclear pseudoinclusions, while Clara cell lesions may show PAS-positive apical granules.

In the setting of adenocarcinoma of the nonmucinous type, with a lepidic component, the tumor size is now determined only by the size of the invasive component. This seems to make some intuitive sense, although the microscopic determination of invasion versus collapse and entrapped noninvasive glands is not always straightforward. Also, some cases may have a large lepidic tumor with separate microscopic foci of invasion, which are not clearly connected. In that setting, guidelines state that the largest contiguous focus of invasion should be reported as the invasive tumor size, and the size should not be based on the distance between separate areas of invasion, or summation of multiple areas of invasion. These rules suggest that tumors with nonmucinous features and a prominent lepidic growth pattern must be sampled extensively enough to appropriately document the extent of invasion.

b. Atypical alveolar hyperplasia (AAH) is a lesion closely related to AIS. In fact, molecular genetic studies show virtually identical abnormalities in cases of AAH and AIS. Key features in the separation of these lesions are presented in Table 8.14. AAH and AIS are best considered as the peripheral lung equivalents of dysplasia and carcinoma in situ, with a postulated role as precursors of invasive peripheral adenocarcinoma.

2. Squamous cell carcinoma (SCC) is most frequently a central lesion arising in larger airways although peripheral lesions do occur; primarily endobronchial tumors are unusual. Postobstructive pneumonia has been reported in up to one-half of SCC. SCC is prone to central necrosis, and cavitation is a common radiologic finding. Squamous dysplasia and carcinoma in situ not infrequently accompany SCC and may be the only material retrieved by endoscopic biopsy. The histology of SCC does not differ significantly from SCC that occurs at other body sites; both keratinizing and nonkeratinizing variants occur, as well as basaloid and clear cell forms (e-**Fig. 8.43**).

Poorly differentiated SCC should not be confused with small cell carcinoma; SCC lacks the individual cell necrosis, crush artifact, and nuclear molding seen in small cell carcinoma. The distinction between small cell carcinoma and SCC can be facilitated by immunostains for p63; SCC generally reacts with antibodies to p63 while small cell carcinoma does not. SCC also seems to be somewhat less prone to nodal metastasis.

3. Large cell carcinoma is an undifferentiated epithelial neoplasm. Neither squamous differentiation (keratin, cytoplasmic bridges) nor glandular features (mucin, acinar formation) are seen by light microscopy, although ultrastructural studies show both squamous and glandular elements. Exhaustive and expensive attempts to subclassify undifferentiated large cell carcinoma into a specific diagnostic category offers no clinical utility; the finding of a tumor so poorly differentiated that standard sampling and diagnostic techniques cannot demonstrate clear cut squamous or glandular

TABLE 8.14	Atypical Alveolar Hyperplasia Versus Bronchioloalveolar Carcinoma	
	Atypical Alveolar Hyperplasia	Bronchioloalveolar Carcinoma
Size	Small, usually less than 5 mm	Greater than 5 mm
Clinical presentation	Often unsuspected, may be found in sections of grossly "normal" lung or in sections of margins	Radiographic and gross lesion is present
Cytologic features	Mildly atypical, but polymorphous	Mildly atypical, monomorphous

differentiation provides prognostic information in itself. These tumors are generally aggressive. Large randomized clinical trials have shown that demonstration of neuroendocrine markers in non-small neoplasms in general, and large cell neoplasms in particular (outside of the defined neuroendocrine tumor types delineated below), does not denote responsiveness to small cell carcinoma–specific chemotherapeutic regimens.

4. **Giant cell carcinoma** is a unique variant of large cell carcinoma. The tumor grows as a large bulky peripheral mass, and often invades the pleura and chest wall. Giant cell carcinoma is composed of large epithelioid cells, many of which are multinucleated (e-**Fig. 8.44**). The cells grow in large sheets and are loosely cohesive. An intense acute and chronic inflammatory cell infiltrate almost always permeates giant cell carcinoma. A spindle cell component often mixes with the giant cell pattern, producing what has sometimes been designated as pleomorphic carcinoma. Unique aspects of giant cell carcinoma include a propensity to metastasize to abdominal sites including the small bowel, and an association with leukemoid reaction. Immunoreactivity for epithelial markers including cytokeratin and epithelial membrane antigen are generally maintained; documentation of these markers in a giant cell carcinoma distinguishes this tumor from such possible mimics as malignant fibrous histiocytoma, anaplastic large cell lymphoma, and choriocarcinoma.

5. **Clear cell carcinoma** does not represent a distinct primary form of pulmonary carcinoma; rather, lung carcinomas with cytoplasmic clearing represent variants of other forms of non–small cell carcinoma. Clearing has been reported in 25% or more of all pulmonary adenocarcinomas, squamous carcinomas, and even large cell carcinomas (e-**Fig. 8.45**). Of course, a pulmonary clear cell neoplasm should raise concern for a metastatic clear cell carcinoma, typically of renal origin, as well as the rare pulmonary clear cell tumor (see below).

6. **Adenosquamous carcinoma** is an uncommon variant of pulmonary carcinoma. These tumors are generally associated with a smoking history. The diagnosis should be reserved for tumors in which there is clearly recognizable differentiation into squamous (intercellular bridges and possibly keratinization) and glandular elements (acini). Solid adenocarcinomas with minimal squamoid differentiation or foci of cytoplasmic eosinophilia should not be interpreted as adenosquamous carcinoma; similarly, SCCs that contain rare droplets of intracytoplasmic mucin are better classified as SCCs. Also, high-grade mucoepidermoid carcinomas in the lung are probably best classified as adenosquamous carcinomas

7. **Other rare types** of lung carcinoma include lymphoepithelial-like carcinoma (e-**Fig. 8.46**), non–small cell carcinoma with rhabdoid features, and invasive micropapillary carcinoma.

C. **Neuroendocrine Neoplasms.** Neuroendocrine neoplasms (see Table 8.15) constitute a spectrum of neoplasms, from lesions of little clinical significance to highly malignant tumors. The exact origin of these neoplasms remains speculative. Although the airways contain neuroendocrine cells known as Kulchitsky cells, the idea that all neuroendocrine tumors arise from preexisting neuroendocrine cells is probably not true; neuroendocrine differentiation may simply be a reflection of the totipotential nature of malignant neoplasms. In general, better differentiated tumors show greater variety in secretory products and have greater number of neuroendocrine granules on ultrastructural examination.

1. **Neuroendocrine cell hyperplasia** is the simplest neuroendocrine lesion seen in the lungs. As its name implies, this process consists of an increased number of neuroendocrine cells in the bronchial and bronchiolar epithelium. This lesion is often not apparent by standard histology and only visualized through the use of immunostains for neuroendocrine markers. The lesion likely represents a reactive process and may be associated with conditions that cause airway inflammation or injury, and is of little or no clinical significance. It is the one lung neuroendocrine lesion that can be safely thought of as benign in essentially all cases.

TABLE 8.15 Features of Pulmonary Neuroendocrine Neoplasms

WHO Terminology	Alternative Terminology	Cell Size	Nuclear Atypia	Mitoses	Necrosis	Malignant Potential
Carcinoid	Grade 1 NEC	Medium to large	None	<2/hpf	None	Low
Atypical carcinoid	Grade 2 NEC	Medium to large	Mild	2–10/hpf	Focal	Intermediate
Large cell neuroendocrine carcinoma	Grade 3 NEC, large cell type	Large	Marked	>10/hpf	Extensive	High
Small cell neuroendocrine carcinoma	Grade 3 NEC, small cell type	Small	Marked	High	Extensive	High

2. **Carcinoid tumors** should be considered grade 1 neuroendocrine carcinomas. Carcinoids can be divided into central lesions which have an association with cartilaginous airways (often designated as typical carcinoids), and peripheral types which lack such an association. Carcinoid tumors tend to occur on average as much as one to two decades earlier than other types of lung carcinomas. In addition, they do not show any convincing relationship to cigarette smoking (in contrast to higher-grade neuroendocrine tumors). The clinical presentation of patients with carcinoid tumors varies based on the tumor's location. Central tumors, which are slowly growing, often present with airway-related symptoms such as wheezing, recurrent pneumonias, and cough (e-**Fig. 8.47**). In contrast, peripheral carcinoids are often asymptomatic and are discovered incidentally as a pulmonary "coin lesion." Unlike small bowel carcinoids, they essentially will never be associated with the carcinoid syndrome, although cases of Cushing syndrome have been reported due to ACTH release.

Grossly, central carcinoid tumors usually present as yellow-tan polypoid intraluminal masses covered by normal respiratory tract mucosa; they almost always measure less than 5 cm. Microscopic sections show a variety of architectural patterns including trabecula, rosettes, papillary formations, and areas of solid growth (e-**Fig. 8.48**). The tumors have vascular stroma which can also feature elements including the amyloid and bone. The individual cells tend to have moderate to abundant cytoplasm, which is often granular and eosinophilic. The tumor cells have nuclei that are regular, and round to oval; the chromatin is granular, and often referred to as having a salt-and-pepper character. Mitotic activity should be essentially absent; the most recent WHO standard is ≤2 mitosis per 10 high-power fields. Necrosis should be absent. Peripheral carcinoid tumors are morphologically identical to central tumors, although peripheral carcinoid tumors often exhibit a spindled morphology. Tumors with a peripheral location and spindled pattern should not be designated automatically as atypical carcinoid tumors (see below).

Carcinoid tumors (which can also be referred to as well-differentiated neuroendocrine carcinomas) contain abundant neurosecretory granules, and show strong expression of chromogranin and synaptophysin; they are also immunopositive for epithelial markers such as cytokeratin. Carcinoid tumors have a low malignant potential. Only about 5% of patients present with lymph node metastases; less than 5% of cases develop distant metastatic disease with spread to the liver, brain, bones, and skin. Long-term survival is in excess of 95%.

a. **Carcinoid tumorlets** are microscopic proliferations (4 mm or less in size) that are otherwise histologically and immunophenotypically identical to carcinoid tumors (e-**Fig. 8.49**); distinction is based solely on the size. Tumorlets tend to occur in distal airways, and may be single lesions incidentally discovered in resection specimens. Rare patients may have hundreds of these lesions in their distal airways. Multiple carcinoid tumorlets have some association with chronic airway diseases. Tumorlets have little or no clinical significance. Rare patients can present with multifocal carcinoids, tumorlets, and airway neuroendocrine cell hyperplasia, which is known as diffuse pulmonary neuroendocrine cell hyperplasia (DIPNECH); this process is associated with small airway obstructive lung disease due to impingement of these proliferating neuroendocrine cells on the bronchiolar lumens.

  b. Paraganglioma features nested cells, a fine fibrovascular stroma, cells with eosinophilic to granular cytoplasm and some spindling, and regular nuclei, and so it can be difficult to distinguish paraganglioma from carcinoid tumor. Although paraganglioma shows immunopositivity for chromogranin and synaptophysin, it is not reactive with antibodies to cytokeratin. In addition, paragangliomas contain S-100–positive sustentacular cells that are not present in carcinoid tumors.

  c. Chemodectomas. Multiple pulmonary chemodectomas were once considered a variant of paraganglioma, but now are known to have no relationship to paraganglioma. Chemodectomas consist of 1- to 2-mm stellate proliferations that fill the pulmonary interstitium and feature bland epithelioid cells in a whirling pattern. These tumors share immunoreactivity for epithelial membrane antigen and vimentin, and have been labeled as minute meningothelial-like nodules. They are of no clinical significance.

3. Atypical carcinoid tumor, better designated as grade 2 neuroendocrine carcinoma, is rarer than carcinoid tumor, and more evenly divided between central and peripheral locations (e-**Fig. 8.50**). Because more tumors are peripheral, airway-related symptoms are less common. In addition, there is a closer relationship to cigarette smoking. These tumors tend to be slightly larger than grade 1 lesions at the time of diagnosis, but it is microscopic features that distinguish grade 2 neuroendocrine carcinoma (atypical carcinoid) from grade 1 neuroendocrine carcinoma (carcinoid). The tumor cells tend to be slightly smaller than those of classic carcinoid tumors, and some modest nuclear pleomorphism is also usually present. Spindling of the cells is also more common with grade 1 cases, and mitotic activity is more frequent; up to 10 mitoses in 10 high-power fields is the accepted criterion. Necrosis may be present, but is usually limited. Because the cells are moderately differentiated, neuroendocrine immunostains tend to be positive.

Atypical carcinoids show significantly greater malignant potential than classic carcinoids. About 25% of patients with atypical carcinoid tumor have lymph nodal metastases at presentation, and approximately 25% of patients are dead of disease at 5 years after diagnosis.

4. Large cell neuroendocrine carcinoma (LCNEC) can also be designated as grade 3 neuroendocrine carcinoma. It is an extremely lethal form of lung carcinoma, and is the most recent variant of neuroendocrine carcinoma to be described. The demographics of LCNEC are similar to those of other lung carcinomas; almost all cases have been reported in cigarette smokers. The vast majority of the tumors are found in the periphery of the lung, and thus they tend to present with the same sort of nonspecific symptoms as do other lung carcinomas. The gross of appearance of LCNEC is similar to that of other non-small cell lung carcinomas, and may include necrosis or cavitation (e-**Fig. 8.51**).

The microscopic features of LCNEC are quite distinctive. The tumor has an organoid appearance in which large solid nests of tumor are separated by scant fibrovascular stroma. In some cases, the tumor seems to fill up the preexisting alveolar spaces. Tumors may show palisading of tumor cells at the periphery of the nests, and spindling or rosettes may also be present. The dominant feature in most cases is extensive necrosis, which may make up the bulk of the tumor mass. The tumor cells themselves are generally polygonal and have a significant amount of cytoplasm. LCNEC can be distinguished from small cell neuroendocrine carcinoma based on several factors: at lower-power microscopy, the nuclei of the tumor do not touch (as do the nuclei in small cell carcinomas, see below); the nuclear–cytoplasmic ratio is significantly lower than that of small cell carcinoma; the nuclear chromatin may be vesicular and nucleoli are often prominent; and finally, crush artifact and nuclear molding are not usually seen.

Mitotic activity is one of the key features of this tumor; the tumor should feature at least 10 mitoses per 10 high-power fields, although the actual rate is generally far higher. Combined with the extensive necrosis described above, it is generally relatively straightforward to separate LCNEC from lower-grade tumors such as atypical carcinoid. In fact, LCNEC probably has greater overlap with non–small cell carcinomas such as poorly differentiated squamous carcinomas. Thus, immunostains can be quite helpful in the diagnosis. LCNEC shows reliable staining with pan-cytokeratin antibodies (because of the increased amount of cytoplasm in the tumor, cytokeratin stains do not show the dot-like pattern that is typical of small cell carcinoma, but rather show strong diffuse cytoplasmic staining). The majority of cases of LCNEC also show positive staining for chromogranin, synaptophysin, CD56, and CD57, although the more poorly differentiated nature of LCNEC is reflected in more focal reactivity for these neuroendocrine markers. LCNEC often also shows positive staining for p53.

The prognosis for LCNEC is quite poor. Although the great majority of patients present with node-negative lesions at diagnosis, most patients rapidly develop recurrent or metastatic disease. The overall survival at 5 and 10 years is poor, approximately 20% and 10%, respectively.

5. Small cell lung carcinoma (SCLC) is classically described as high-grade neuroendocrine carcinoma. The incidence of SCLC is decreasing, but SCLC still accounts for at least 10% of all primary lung carcinomas. This tumor type has a very strong association with cigarette smoking. At least 95% of patients present with a central mass comprised of hilar and/or mediastinal adenopathy; the adenopathy often is larger than any radiographically definable intrapulmonary mass (**e-Fig. 8.52**). The bulky tumor in the mediastinum leads to a variety of clinical presentations, including cough, hemoptysis, lobar collapse, shortness of breath from pleural effusions, chest pain, hoarseness from recurrent laryngeal nerve invasion, or superior vena cava syndrome. A significant number of patients also present with signs or symptoms referable to distant spread, such as neurologic symptoms (brain metastases), bone lesions, or symptoms due to abdominal organ involvement. Paraneoplastic syndromes are common, including the Eaton–Lambert syndrome (inappropriate secretion of the antidiuretic hormone) and the Cushing syndrome (related to ACTH production).

Since small cell carcinomas are rarely resected, the gross features of the tumor are seldom seen in the surgical pathology laboratory. These features include a large central mass that tends to spread along the bronchial tree, with involvement of hilar lymph nodes often in a contiguous fashion with the primary tumor. Some cases show an endobronchial lesion; less than 5% of cases present as a peripheral pulmonary nodule.

The microscopic appearance of small cell carcinoma varies with the method of sampling (**e-Fig. 8.53**). Endobronchial biopsies commonly have the so-called oat cell appearance characterized by small cells (about twice the diameter of a resting lymphocyte) with dark hyperchromatic nuclei. There is scant to barely visible cytoplasm, and crush artifact and nuclear molding are prominent; nucleoli are not usually prominent. Individual apoptotic cells are often seen, and more extensive confluent necrosis may be present. Mitotic figures are frequent. The cells tend to stream through the tissue in irregular sheets, although some cases may show rosettes, palisades, or trabecular growth patterns. Small cell carcinoma often has a slightly different appearance in larger tissue samples, such as resected primary tumors or lymph node biopsies. The cells are oftentimes slightly larger (up to four times the diameter of a resting lymphocyte), but still feature dark hyperchromatic nuclei, often with nucleoli. Crush artifact and nuclear molding may be less prominent. Necrosis is often widespread; one well-known feature of small cell carcinoma with excessive necrosis is the so-called Azzopardi effect, which is the coating of blood vessel walls by nucleic acid to produce dark blue ring-like structures in the midst of otherwise eosinophilic necrotic areas.

Immunostains can be helpful in the diagnosis of small cell carcinoma. Cytokeratin immunostains often produce a dot-like perinuclear pattern of positivity due to the small amount of cytoplasm and the condensation of cytoskeletal elements in the tumor cells. Stains for CD45 can exclude lymphoma. In cases with classic morphology, this simple panel (cytokeratin and CD45) is sufficient for the diagnosis of small cell carcinoma. If additional immunostains are requested to confirm neuroendocrine differentiation, it should be noted that small cell carcinomas have very few neurosecretory granules, and hence chromogranin stains are relatively insensitive. Similarly, synaptophysin and CD57 stains are positive in only approximately 50% to 60% of cases. Stains for NCAM (CD56) are more sensitive, and stains TTF-1 are also positive in the majority of cases of pulmonary small cell carcinoma. The cells of small cell carcinoma may also express CD99, bcl2, p53, and CEA, although these stains generally are not obtained in a diagnostic context.

Since small cell carcinoma has spread extensively at the time of diagnosis in most cases, treatment is generally nonsurgical. Survival remains poor. Modern chemotherapy and radiation regimens produce significant disease remissions in the majority of patients, but relapse within a few months is common. The overall 5-year survival is in the range of 5% to 10%.

Neuroendocrine carcinoma may also be mixed with non–small cell carcinoma. This combination is rarely if ever seen with low-grade lesions, but is seen in a small minority of cases of LCNEC or small cell carcinoma. Admixed non–small cell components are rarely seen in bronchial biopsy specimens, but are detected in up to 10% of resected small cell cancer cases; this discrepancy is probably related to the sampling volume. When recurrences occur after treatment of small cell carcinoma, a dominant non–small cell component may be present; it is likely that this shift in the phenotype represents selective survival of a previously minor admixed non–small cell component not targeted by treatment directed against small cell carcinoma.

D. Sarcomatoid Carcinoma and Related Neoplasms. A subset of primary pulmonary carcinomas has sarcoma-like features. These tumors have been given a variety of names, including carcinosarcoma and spindle cell carcinoma; sarcomatoid carcinoma is the currently preferred designation for all carcinomas with sarcoma-like features. Patients with sarcomatoid carcinoma have a similar age and smoking history as those with other forms of pulmonary carcinoma. Sarcomatoid carcinoma, however, presents in two distinct patterns. Some cases present as a polypoid intraluminal mass within a large central airway; these tumors tend to be small, most likely because patients present with airway-related symptoms early in the course of the tumor's growth. In contrast, other patients present with a bulky peripheral mass, often with pleural and chest wall invasion. Microscopic sections show malignant spindled tumor cells (e-Fig. 8.54) which may transition from areas of non–small cell carcinoma. Various heterologous elements such as malignant cartilage or osteoid may also be seen.

The major differential is with true pulmonary sarcomas and sarcomatoid mesotheliomas. In order to diagnose sarcomatoid carcinoma, the sarcoma-like tumor must be proven to show some evidence of an epithelial lineage. This can be accomplished by immunostaining; reactivity for cytokeratins, epithelial membrane antigen, p63, or other generic carcinoma markers such as carcinoembryonic antigen will be present in the majority of (although not all) examples of sarcomatoid carcinoma. Electron microscopy, with identification of epithelial features such as cell junctions, may be quite useful in this context. In many cases, extensive sampling is enough to demonstrate an epithelial component by showing transition from sarcoma-like areas to classis areas of squamous carcinoma or adenocarcinoma; the finding of such a transition provides definitive evidence as to the nature of the neoplasm. Differentiation from mesothelioma may be difficult in that immunophenotypes may overlap; WT1 and calretinin expression would favor mesothelioma. Clinical presentation as a single intrapulmonary mass may be a critical feature that favors sarcomatoid carcinoma, since mesothelioma tends to present as a diffuse pleural neoplasm.

The behavior of sarcomatoid carcinomas varies with the clinical presentation. Cases presenting as a small intraluminal polypoid airway lesion have a fair prognosis. In contrast, those cases occurring as large bulky peripheral tumors have a poor outcome since high-stage disease at presentation is common.

E. Fetal Adenocarcinoma is also known as monophasic pulmonary blastoma. It is a tumor of adults, although it occurs on average several decades earlier than other non–small cell carcinomas. Most patients are smokers. The tumors generally are found in the periphery of the lung, average 4 to 5 cm, and are usually well circumscribed. Microscopically, the tumor is composed of closely packed glands and tubules with scant intervening stroma (e-**Fig. 8.55**). Cribriform and vaguely papillary patterns can also be seen. The tumor is composed of cytologically bland columnar cells with cytoplasmic clearing that resemble secretory endometrium. The glandular lumina are often filled with solid morules; the cells of these morules have nuclear clearing. Ultrastructural and immunohistochemical studies of fetal adenocarcinomas show pneumocyte-like differentiation, including expression of surfactants and Clara cell antigens. In addition, the glandular and morular cells contain neurosecretory granules with immunoexpression of neuroendocrine markers. The prognosis for this tumor is excellent; more than 80% of patients are cured by surgical resection, an outcome that contrasts markedly with the poor prognosis of biphasic pulmonary blastoma.

F. Biphasic Pulmonary Blastoma. Like sarcomatoid carcinoma, biphasic pulmonary blastoma features both a malignant glandular and malignant stromal component. Biphasic pulmonary blastoma must be distinguished from pleuropulmonary blastoma (PPB; see Table 8.16 and below). Despite the designation as a blastoma, biphasic pulmonary blastoma occurs almost exclusively in adults, albeit at a younger age (third or fourth decade of life) than most non–small cell lung carcinomas. Most patients are smokers and present with a large peripheral mass often accompanied by a pleural effusion and/or adenopathy. On gross examination the tumors are fleshy, and may show necrosis, cystic change, or hemorrhage. Microscopic examination shows a characteristic biphasic pattern with endometrioid-type glands similar to those of monophasic blastoma, although the epithelial component may also be more poorly differentiated and consist of ill-defined cords and sheets of cells without obvious differentiation (e-**Fig. 8.56**). The malignant stromal component may resemble the blastemal component of Wilms tumor, or can include ill-defined spindle cells as well as malignant elements such as chondrosarcoma, osteosarcoma, or a myogenic sarcoma. In contrast to monophasic blastoma, the outcome is poor, with most patients dying within 2 years of presentation.

| | Age at | Smoking | | Malignant | Malignant | |
Tumor Type	Diagnosis	History	Size	Glands	Stroma	Prognosis
Monophasic pulmonary blastoma	3rd–4th decade	Yes	Small	Yes	No	Excellent
Biphasic pulmonary blastoma	3rd–4th decade	Yes	Large, fleshy	Yes	Yes	Poor
Pleuropulmonary blastoma	Children (rare adults)	No	Large, solid and/or cystic	No	Yes	Variable, dependent on type

TABLE 8.16 Blastoma-like Lung Neoplasms

G. Pleuropulmonary Blastoma (PPB) arises almost exclusively in children, although very rare cases have been described in young adults. There is a familial component to many cases of PPB, and many patients have relatives with a variety of other childhood and adult neoplasms. The tumors present in the lung, most often in the subpleural area. PPB is subclassified based on gross features: predominantly cystic (type 1), solid and cystic (type 2), or solid (type 3) (e-**Fig. 8.57**). When cystic, the lesion is often confused with a variety of benign cystic conditions including cystic adenomatoid malformation; the misdiagnosis is often discovered when the lesion recurs. Microscopic sections of the cystic cases show that the cysts are lined by benign epithelium with an underlying stroma that can have a variety of appearances, ranging from mature fibroblastic cells to overtly malignant cells with a sarcomatous appearance. The more solid cases similarly show sarcoma-like malignant cells; rhabdomyoblasts and malignant cartilage may be included. Unlike monophasic and biphasic pulmonary blastoma, PPB does not include a malignant epithelial component. The majority of patients with completely excised cystic lesions that are confined to the lung demonstrate long-term survival; the prognosis is much more guarded for predominantly solid lesions.

H. Salivary Gland Tumors. Minor salivary glands are present all along the tracheobronchial tree. Consequently, the airway can be the site of any of the neoplasms that can occur in the salivary glands. Although rare examples of pleomorphic adenoma (e-**Fig. 8.58**), acinic cell tumor (Fechner tumor), and oncocytoma have been reported, two salivary gland–type neoplasms occur with a high enough frequency to warrant further discussion.

1. Mucoepidermoid carcinoma. Low-grade forms of this tumor tend to present as a polypoid intraluminal mass, and cases have been described in both adults and children. Histologic sections show a mixture of mucus-producing cells, clear cells, and squamous cells (e-**Fig. 8.58**). There is minimal mitotic activity and necrosis is lacking. Many cases have abundant mucus-filled cystic areas. The tumor is generally indolent; local invasion and local recurrence are the primary concerns, and local resection is often curative. The major differential diagnostic considerations include mucus gland adenoma (which lacks the locally invasive character of mucoepidermoid carcinoma) and squamous carcinoma (which tends to show more extensive keratinization and less mucus production). High-grade forms of mucoepidermoid carcinoma similar to those described in the salivary glands also occur in the lung; since such high-grade tumors have a prognosis similar to other forms of non–small cell carcinoma, by convention they are generally considered to represent adenosquamous carcinomas.

2. Adenoid cystic carcinoma (ACC) also occurs in the tracheobronchial tree. It is more common in the trachea, but also arises in the larger bronchi. Most tumors are found in middle-aged to older adults, and many patients present with a long history of airway symptoms such as wheezing; the long history reflects the indolent nature of these tumors. ACC is usually 2 to 5 cm in maximal dimension at the time of diagnosis. The tumor may grossly appear well circumscribed, but microscopically most cases extend beyond the area of gross disease. The histology of the tumor in the lung is identical to the analogous tumor of the salivary glands, with uniform, modestly atypical polygonal cells arranged in nests, cribriform patterns, and solid sheets (e-**Fig. 8.59**). Many of the tumor nests contain characteristic eosinophilic matrix material. As in the salivary glands, perineural invasion is common. Immunostains are consistent with the proposed myoepithelial origin of this tumor, demonstrating immunopositivity for cytokeratin, vimentin, actin, and S-100. Many cases are CD117 positive (it is not clear whether this finding has any therapeutic implications). Positive resection margins are common because of the infiltrative growth pattern; postoperative radiation therapy may help control incompletely resected tumors for extended periods of time. Intrapulmonary metastasis eventually occurs in many cases as a late complication; even these metastases tend to be slow growing and many patients survive with metastatic disease for an extended period of time.

I. **Sarcomas.** Primary sarcomas of the lung are distinctly uncommon. Before concluding that a tumor is a primary pulmonary sarcoma, primary pulmonary sarcomatoid carcinoma and a sarcoma metastatic to the lung must be excluded. It is therefore important to know details of the clinical history and radiographic findings before labeling a lung tumor as a primary lung sarcoma. Fibrohistiocytic, fibroblastic, smooth muscle, and vascular sarcomas have been reported as primary lung sarcomas, as have primary neurogenic, osteogenic, and cartilaginous sarcomas. Small blue cell tumors of the lung include members of the Ewing sarcoma/primitive neuroectodermal tumor (EWS/PNET) family and rhabdomyosarcoma. Lung sarcomas are essentially identical in appearance to their soft tissue counterparts.

1. **Synovial sarcoma** is a tumor that has recently been recognized to occur in both the lung and pleural spaces. It occurs in relatively younger adults than do primary lung carcinomas. The tumor may show calcifications on radiographs, but otherwise has few defining clinical or radiographic features (**e-Fig. 8.60**). Histologic sections show features identical to synovial sarcomas of the soft tissue (see Chapter 44). Immunostains are tremendously helpful for averting a misdiagnosis; synovial sarcomas of the lung demonstrate expression of cytokeratin and epithelial membrane antigen staining in both the glandular and spindle cell areas, and the tumor cells may also be positive for CD34 and CD99. The differential diagnosis includes other biphasic pulmonary tumors such as sarcomatoid carcinoma and biphasic mesothelioma. Molecular demonstration of a t(X;18) translocation can be a helpful aid in diagnosis. As with synovial sarcoma arising in other locations, recurrence or metastasis may take many years to develop, but the ultimate prognosis is poor, with the majority of patients eventually dying of the disease.

2. **Epithelioid hemangioendothelioma** (EH) was originally termed intravascular bronchioloalveolar tumor. EH presents most commonly in women of young to middle age. Patients may be asymptomatic, or present with cough or shortness of breath. Radiology images typically show multiple small pulmonary nodules. Histologic sections show nodules containing pale-staining, hyaline to myxoid stroma in which the preexisting alveolar structure is often still apparent. The neoplastic cells are present within this stoma; they are small and epithelioid and often contain an intracytoplasmic lumen which represents a primitive attempt at vessel formation (**e-Fig. 8.61**). Ultrastructural studies show endothelial cell features such as Weibel–Palade bodies; the cells also react with antibodies for vascular markers, including CD31 and CD34. Although the tumor grows slowly, most patients eventually develop progressive disease with respiratory failure.

3. **Kaposi sarcoma** (KS) is another vascular tumor that may involve the lung. Pulmonary involvement occurs almost exclusively in the setting of immunocompromise, predominantly HIV/AIDS, and rarely in solid organ transplant recipients. Pulmonary KS most often coexists with cutaneous disease. Radiographic studies show nodular infiltrates and a pleural effusion may be present; symptoms include cough, fever, and hemoptysis. KS spreads via lymphovascular routes and thus is seen along the bronchial tree, along pulmonary vessels, and along the pleural and lobular septa. Histology shows typical lesions of KS, with spindled cells arranged to form slit-like vascular spaces, extravasated erythrocytes, and hemosiderin (**e-Fig. 8.62**). Patients who have pulmonary KS have a poor prognosis, determined not only by the response of KS to chemotherapy but also by the course of the underlying HIV infection.

4. **Pulmonary artery sarcoma** is another rare but deadly lung sarcoma. Patients tend to be middle aged or older, and typically present with shortness of breath or signs of right-sided heart failure. Imaging studies often show intravascular filling of the pulmonary artery trunk which may be interpreted as thromboembolic disease. The tumor may be situated in the main pulmonary artery trunk or in one or both of the main right and left artery branches; the sarcoma may extend distally into progressively smaller branches within the lung. The histologic features of pulmonary artery sarcoma are variable, including smooth muscle, fibrohistiocytic, endothelial,

and even chondroid or osteoid differentiation. The prognosis of pulmonary artery sarcoma is poor; even in cases with complete resection, distal recurrences within the ipsilateral lung are the rule. To date, radiation and chemotherapy have not been particularly effective in treating this sarcoma.

5. **Thoracopulmonary small cell tumor,** also known as Askin tumor, is now known to be a member of the EWS/PNET family of neoplasms. This highly malignant tumor most often occurs in children and young adults and is typically very large at presentation; it may literally fill an entire hemithorax (e-Fig. 8.63). The exact site of origin is often unclear, although most tumors probably originate from the chest wall with secondary invasion into the lung. The tumor consists of a classic small blue cell proliferation, growing in sheets or rosettes. Necrosis may be prominent. The tumor shows membrane staining for CD99 as well as various neuroendocrine markers. Most cases demonstrate the t(11;22) translocation characteristic of EWS/PNET (see Chapter 44).

J. Miscellaneous Neoplasms

1. **Pulmonary hamartoma** (chondroid hamartoma) is a benign proliferation usually seen in adults. The tumor usually occurs as a solitary peripheral mass with a radiographic appearance of a so-called coin lesion. A minority of cases involve the more central airways, or even the trachea. Chondroid hamartomas may be part of a heritable syndrome in some cases; the Carney triad consists of pulmonary hamartomas, gastric stromal tumors, and extra-adrenal pheochromocytomas. Grossly, the tumor is a well-circumscribed, nodular lesion (e-Fig. 8.64). Histologic sections disclose a mixture of benign mesenchymal components, including cartilage, mature adipose tissue, and smooth muscle. Bronchial-type epithelium is usually present within the lesion, although this is thought to represent entrapped tissue rather than a true component of the proliferation. Radiographic diagnosis of this lesion can be confidently made based on the presence of adipose tissue and calcifications within the cartilaginous component; for this reason, hamartomas are often not resected.

2. **Pulmonary clear cell tumor,** or sugar tumor, is a unique pulmonary tumor composed of cells with clear cytoplasm. The tumor generally arises in adults and presents as a well-circumscribed, nodular mass; most are found incidentally in asymptomatic patients. The tumor usually measures less than 5 mm in greatest dimension. Histologic sections show epithelioid cells with bland nuclei and abundant clear cytoplasm (e-Fig. 8.65). The cells grow either in nests separated by fine fibrovascular stroma or in a more sheet-like pattern. PAS stains are positive due to abundant intracellular glycogen, as confirmed by ultrastructural studies which may also show premelanosomes within the tumor cells. Immunostains show a unique pattern of vimentin positivity, as well as positivity with melanocyte markers such as HMB-45 and melan-A, with expression of actin and CD117.

The histogenesis of this tumor has long been debated. Most recently it has been suggested that the tumor is a member of the family of tumors known as perivascular epithelioid cell tumors, or PEComas. The most important neoplasm in the differential diagnosis is metastatic renal cell carcinoma; in this regard, it is important to emphasize that pulmonary clear cell tumors uniformly lack expression of epithelial markers such as cytokeratin and epithelial membrane antigen. The behavior of pulmonary clear cell tumor has generally been considered to be benign, although rare tumors show malignant behavior.

3. **Inflammatory myofibroblastic tumor** (IMT) has traditionally been given a variety of names, including inflammatory pseudotumor and plasma cell granuloma. IMT is the most common benign lung tumor in children, but occurs in adults as well. The most common presentation is as a relatively small solitary peripheral nodule; IMT also occurs as an endobronchial lesion. Patients may be asymptomatic, or may present with a variety of systemic signs and symptoms, including fever, anemia, and polyclonal hypergammaglobulinemia; systemic manifestations usually resolve with removal of the tumor. In most cases, the tumor is confined to the lung, although

occasional cases may exhibit more aggressive local behavior, including invasion of mediastinal structures.

Microscopic sections show a proliferation of spindled myofibroblastic cells with a haphazard pattern of vague fascicles (see Chapter 44) (e-**Fig. 8.66**). The spindle cells are characteristically bland and mitotic figures are rare, without abnormal mitotic figures; necrosis is unusual. There is often a marked inflammatory cell infiltrate in the lesion that may include plasma cells, lymphocytes with lymphoid follicles, neutrophils, and eosinophils. The stroma varies from myxoid to densely collagenized and keloid like. Immunohistochemical stains show that the spindle cells are positive for vimentin and smooth muscle actin, and are negative for cytokeratin, CD34, and desmin. ALK-1 is variably expressed in IMTs of the lung, corresponding to those cases that harbor a rearranged *ALK* gene (see Chapter 44). The plasma cells are polyclonal by light chain studies. The immunophenotype of IMT can be used to rule out several tumors in the differential diagnosis such as spindle cell carcinoma, solitary fibrous tumor, and fibrohistiocytic neoplasms.

IMT of the lung is usually cured by surgery. Recurrence is rare, but more common if the lesion has invaded adjacent structures at the time of resection. Extremely unusual cases of malignant transformation to a high-grade fibroblastic or round cell neoplasm have been reported.

It must be emphasized that nonneoplastic inflammatory processes occur in the lung which are also capable of producing a mass-like lesion, such as organizing pneumonia, infarcts, scars, and confluent granulomas. These processes must always be included in the differential diagnosis of IMT.

K. Hematolymphoid Lesions. Hematolymphoid neoplasms and pseudoneoplasms can involve the lung, both primarily and as part of systemic disease. Fresh tissue should be set aside for flow cytometry whenever possible. In cases for which only fixed tissue is available, a variety of molecular studies including gene rearrangement analysis can also be used to evaluate clonality. By definition, primary pulmonary lymphomas should not have evidence of disease outside of the lung or hilar lymph nodes.

1. MALToma. Lymphomas of mucosal associated lymphoid tissue, the so-called MALTomas, commonly arise in the lung and constitute the most common form of primary pulmonary lymphoma. MALTomas for the most part correspond to marginal-zone lymphoma, and many harbor a t(8;11) translocation which may be relatively specific for lung MALTomas. Most cases occur in adults; there is no specific relationship to infection or autoimmune disorders. Pulmonary MALToma may have a nodular or diffuse appearance, with an infiltrate comprised of small lymphocytes, monocytoid cells, and plasmacytoid cells (e-**Fig. 8.67**) that may replace or disrupt the appearance of preexisting germinal centers. The cells also infiltrate the bronchial mucosa with production of lymphoepithelial lesions as are seen with MALToma in other sites. The infiltrating cells are immunopositive for CD19, CD20, and bcl-2, but immunonegative for CD5, CD10, CD23, and cyclin D1.

2. Large cell lymphoma. Pulmonary large cell lymphoma generally presents as a solitary mass lesion involving a single lobe of the lung. These masses may develop central necrosis. Pulmonary large cell lymphomas are usually either of diffuse large cell type or immunoblast, and are of B-cell lineage (e-**Fig. 8.68**).

3. Lymphomatoid granulomatosis (LYG) is the name for a lung lesion now recognized to be a malignant lymphoma, now also known as angiocentric immunoproliferative lesion (AIL). It is an Epstein–Barr virus (EBV)-related B-cell proliferation analogous to PTLD or AIDS-related lymphoma. In fact, patients with LYG often have some underlying immunodeficiency. LYG usually is seen in middle-aged and older adults, and shows multiple nodules that may suggest metastatic disease; concomitant skin and CNS involvement is quite common. Patients have respiratory symptoms such as cough or dyspnea, or may have constitutional symptoms. Microscopically, vasculocentric and angiodestructive lymphoid infiltrates that involve all layers of the vessel are the hallmark of LYG (e-**Fig. 8.69**); this vascular infiltration is hypothesized to result in infarct-like necrosis of the lung seen in the higher-grade cases. Grade 1 lesions have infiltrates composed mainly of small T-cells, plasma cells, and histiocytes; CD20 and EBV stains show only rare atypical B-cells (less than 5 per hpf). Grade 2 cases show a greater number of atypical B-cells (5 to 20 per hpf). Grade 3 cases have abundant large, atypical B-cells.

4. Leukemic infiltrates. The lung may be the site of acute leukemic infiltrates in cases of acute myelogenous leukemia (AML), representing a granulocytic sarcoma or extra-medullary myeloid tumor. Infiltration of airways, interstitial infiltrates, or nodular parenchymal masses are possible manifestations. Histologic clues to a diagnosis of AML include blast-like cells and the presence of immature eosinophilic precursors. Many cases are initially thought to represent a large cell lymphoma; one of the first clues to the correct diagnosis is the absence of expression of both B- or T-cell markers in the presumed lymphomatous cells.

The lung may also show extensive involvement by chronic lymphocytic leukemia/small lymphocytic lymphoma. In this setting, the infiltrate presents as nodular expansions along lymphatic routes in the lung.

5. Other hematolymphoid diseases. The lung has been the reported primary site of a variety of hematolymphoid lesions, including Hodgkin disease, intravascular lymphomatosis, plasmacytomas (e-Fig. 8.70), and Castleman disease. However, it should be reiterated that secondary involvement of the lung in patients with advanced hematolymphoid disease is very common, can occur with essentially all entities, and so must always be excluded.

6. Pseudolymphoma. Small nodular lymphoid deposits in the lung have traditionally been called pseudolymphoma. However, with the advent of more specific diagnostic techniques, many of these lesions have been shown to be lymphomas, such as MALTomas. For lesions that can be demonstrated to be polyclonal, the term lymphoid hyperplasia is more appropriate.

L. Metastatic Tumors. It is prudent to include metastatic disease in the differential diagnosis of every lung tumor. Metastases should be suspected when a tumor type is encountered that would be unusual as a lung primary tumor. Also, presentation as multiple nodules, finding a tumor that is predominantly within lymphatics or vessels, and a tumor that appears very well circumscribed without a host stromal and inflammatory reaction should also raise suspicion for a secondary lung tumor. Clinical history, liberal use of special stains, and radiologic consultation are all important tools to help distinguish metastatic neoplasms in the lung from primary tumors.

Cytopathology of the Lung

Hannah R. Krigman

I. SAMPLE TYPE. Cytology is an appropriate diagnostic modality for both neoplastic and nonneoplastic conditions of the lung. Exfoliative techniques include preparations of sputum, fluid from bronchial washing or lavage, and bronchial brushing. Fine needle aspiration of pulmonary processes can be via a transthoracic, transbronchial, or transesophageal approach. The sensitivity of cytopathologic evaluation depends on the type of procurement technique used. Sputum specimens yield the lowest quantity of exfoliated cells. FNA specimens yield the highest; endobronchial and transthoracic FNA for central and peripheral lung masses, respectively, both yield similarly cellular specimens.

II. SPECIMEN ADEQUACY AND PREPARATION

A. Exfoliated Endoluminal Samples (Sputum, Bronchial Washing, Bronchioloalveolar Lavage, and Bronchial Brushing). Bronchial washing, brushing, and lavage specimens are adequate if sufficient alveolar macrophages are present, or if diagnostic findings are present. Sputum must contain pigmented macrophages to be adequate; if sputum does not contain macrophages, then the cells are likely of oropharyngeal origin. For bronchial brushing specimens, bronchial epithelial cells are also required (**e-Fig. 8.71**). Samples can be submitted fresh or in liquid fixative for liquid-based cytology (LBC). Mucus in the sputum can be dispersed by mechanical disruption or by lytic agents. Air-dried cytospins are stained by the Romanowsky technique; alcohol-fixed samples are best stained by the Papanicolaou technique. Brushing samples can be smeared directly on a slide, but care must be taken to fix smears immediately or air-dry artifact will render the slides uninterpretable. Brushes may be directly fixed in fluid. Dislodged material is processed for either LBC cytospins, or for a formalin-fixed paraffin-embedded cell block.

B. Fine Needle Aspirates of lung masses, whether obtained via endoscopic or transthoracic approaches, are most frequently Wright–Giemsa-stained (Diff-Quik, for air-dried smears) and Papanicolaou stained (after alcohol fixation).

1. Pulmonary. The issue of adequacy for pulmonary lesions is more complex. There are no universally accepted criteria for adequacy in these lesions. Although aspiration of pulmonary elements will result from sampling the lung, and assessment of adequacy requires identification of elements which may explain a mass lesion. In addition to neoplastic groups, aspirates may contain necrosis, inflammation, or granuloma. The Papanicolaou Society suggests the terms "adequate" and "nondiagnostic." Cell block material may be pelleted, formalin-fixed, paraffin-embedded, and stained with H&E.

2. Lymph nodes. Endobronchial ultrasound-guided fine needle aspiration (EBUS-FNA) frequently includes sampling of paratracheal and hilar lymph nodes, in addition to primary lung masses. Sampling may be done for the purposes of staging malignancy, or to assess the etiology of lymphadenopathy. Multiple series have examined the adequacy of EBUS lymph node biopsies. Relatively dense lymphocytes in a background of blood (**e-Fig. 8.72**) in the absence of benign bronchial cells (70 lymphocytes per high-power fields); the presence of tingible body macrophages and blood vessels; and identification of germinal centers have all been proposed as criteria for adequacy.

3. Rapid on-site evaluation (ROSE). ROSE for adequacy is controversial. Some authors assert that ROSE does not improve diagnostic accuracy while others state that the immediate feedback provided by this technique improves triage and maximizes the yield of these specimens. The utility of this technique reflects both the skill of the operator and the confidence of the pathologist. Real-time assessment of the specimen quality provides valuable guidance on needle placement, specimen quality, and appropriate submission of natural for flow cytometry or cultures.

C. Pleural Effusions are generally submitted fresh, from which a well-mixed portion (generally 2 to 300 mL) is used to prepare both Pap- and Diff-Quik-stained cytospins or LBC, and FFPE cell blocks. Benign mesothelial cells are generally found in these specimens (**e-Fig. 8.73**), with or without inflammation. Recent work suggests that at least 75 mL of fluid is required to make an adequate cell block for characterization of malignancies (*Cancer Cytopathol* 2014;122:657).

III. DIAGNOSTIC CATEGORIES. Standardized terminology and nomenclature has recently been proposed for use with respiratory cytology specimens (Table 8.17).

A. Nondiagnostic. The nondiagnostic category includes not only acellular specimens, but also those with obscuring blood, mucus, or inflammation, as well as samples that are limited by poor staining, preparative technique, or fixation. Also included in the nondiagnostic category are those samples for which the findings do not explain a demonstrated mass.

B. Negative for Malignancy/benign. This diagnosis is rendered benign neoplastic, infectious, and inflammatory conditions are identified, correlating to a mass lesion. Granulomatous inflammation, both nonnecrotizing (typically sarcoid) and necrotizing (infectious) is included in this category, as are diagnoses of viral cytopathy, fungal infection, or abscess.

TABLE 8.17 Standardized Terminology and Nomenclature for Respiratory Cytology

Classification	Definitions
Nondiagnostic	Acellular, blood only, specimen limited by preparatory artifact, or benign pulmonary elements not diagnostic for a mass lesion
Benign (specific entities)	Benign neoplasms, inflammatory process, evidence of infection
Atypical	Epithelial, stromal, or lymphoid elements present, with mild atypia, most likely related to benign process, best characterized in a clinicopathologic comment
Suspicious for malignancy	Epithelial, stromal, or lymphoid elements present, most likely malignant, but lacking either in sufficient quantity or significant atypia make a complete diagnosis
Malignant	Includes primary and metastatic lesions, see text

Adapted from Layfield LJ, Baloch Z, Elsheikh T. Standardized terminology and nomenclature for respiratory cytology: The Papanicolaou Society of Cytopathology guidelines. *Diagn Cytopathol* 2016;44:399.

C. **Atypical Cytology.** This diagnosis is rendered when the specimen shows bronchial epithelial cells which can be interpreted as reactive, but in which there is the absence of evidence of an underlying lesion. A repeat aspirate or tissue biopsy is usually suggested. An aspirate which shows markedly reactive bronchial epithelial cells is not diagnostic if the cells are adjacent to ciliated bronchial epithelium (e-**Fig. 8.74**).

D. **Suspicious for Malignancy.** This diagnosis is rendered when rare malignant cells are present, but the quantity is insufficient for a definitive diagnosis of malignancy. This diagnosis usually prompts a repeat diagnostic procedure before definitive surgical treatment.

E. **Positive for Malignancy.** This diagnosis is rendered when both the quality and quantity of malignant cells are sufficient for an unequivocal diagnosis of malignancy. Diagnoses of malignancy are best considered a function of both quality and quantity of atypical cells; either rare markedly atypical cells or an abundance of only minimally atypical cells can suggest malignancy.

IV. **NONNEOPLASTIC CONDITIONS**

A. **Infections**

1. **Viral.** The radiologic correlates to viral infection typically include diffuse pulmonary infiltrates. Cytopathologically, viral changes are best appreciated on bronchial washing and bronchioloalveolar lavage specimens. Ciliocytophthoria, a degenerative change in ciliated epithelial cells, is seen in viral infection.

   The viral cytopathic changes seen in herpesvirus infections include multinucleate and single infected cells that have large nuclei with clear to faintly basophilic centers and peripheralized chromatin; the nuclei are molded with one another. CMV-infected cells have both nuclear and cytoplasmic inclusions that are PAS positive. Adenovirus, which yields a typical "smudged" appearance on the histologic section, shows a polygonal nuclear inclusion and multinucleate cells. Measles shows a characteristic multinucleate giant cell. Parainfluenza viral infection results in multinucleation and eosinophilic cytoplasmic inclusions.

2. **Fungal.** The chest x-ray of patients with fungal infection can exhibit either a mass effect, multiple nodules, or, on occasion, diffuse infiltrates.

   a. The cytologic features of *Pneumocystis jirovecii* are well described. Alveolar casts containing fibrin and the organisms have a bubbly or foamy look on Papanicolaou-stained materials. Romanowsky-stained preparations show a central organism and a clear coat. Methenamine silver stains can highlight the organism, and the stain can be applied to formalin-fixed paraffin-embedded cell blocks, or to cytospins (e-**Fig. 8.75**). Patients taking prophylactic antibiotics for *Pneumocystis* may not have alveolar casts. Their samples may have rare, cup-shaped organisms located within macrophages.

   b. Fragments of *Rhizopus* or *Aspergillus* species (**e-Fig. 8.76**) can be seen in washings, either from cavitary masses or in ABPA. In the latter, concretions of allergic-type mucin or Charcot–Leyden crystals may be noted.

   c. *Histoplasma* infection rarely shows detectable organisms; however, a granulomatous reaction may be present in aspirations of pulmonary masses or of involved lymph nodes.

   d. *Cryptococcus, coccidioidomycosis,* and *blastomycosis* can all induce solitary masses which can be sampled by aspiration. The yeast forms are best appreciated on Romanowsky stains; often the organisms are clear. Again, cell blocks, direct smears, or cytospins can be stained with traditional techniques to better highlight the organisms.

3. Bacterial

   a. The prototypical bacterial infection for which cytologic sampling is pursued is TB. Infection with *M. tuberculosis* can yield both diffuse infiltrates, as in miliary TB, or mass-like lesions, occasionally with cavitation.

   Washings or lavage may be pursued primarily for obtaining material for culture, molecular laboratory test to detect the organism, or antibody-mediated studies. Cytopathologically, washings or lavage fluid can show no significant changes or can exhibit necrosis and acute inflammation. Cavitary lesions can have secondary squamous metaplasia, which may be atypical. Patients with *M. tuberculosis* infection can also have extensive hilar adenopathy, which may sway the less-confident reviewer to a spurious diagnosis of malignancy. Finally, because TB can present as a mass lesion, FNA may be obtained; frequently, multinucleate giant cells are present, again in a setting of acellular necrotic debris and acute inflammation.

   b. Community-acquired bacterial pneumonias are less often sampled. Fluids from such cases exhibit acute inflammation, macrophages, and respiratory epithelial cells. Marked cytologic atypia of pneumocytes may mimic malignancy.

B. Sarcoidosis. Sarcoidosis is a diagnosis of exclusion. FNA from patients with infiltrates and adenopathy is a minimally invasive technique for evaluation. Washings and lavage do not have a high yield for diagnosis. Aspiration of lymph nodes from patients with hilar adenopathy yields rounded nodules of histiocytes (nonnecrotizing granulomas), rare multinucleate giant cells, and a background of mixed chronic inflammatory cells.

C. Pulmonary Alveolar Proteinosis (PAP). Bronchioloalveolar lavage is both diagnostic and therapeutic in patients with PAP. The gross features of PAP cytology specimens are fairly typical in that lavage fluid is white to milky and may have a surface lipid layer. Cytologically, washing samples contain granules and fragments of PAS-positive, diastase-resistant material that is pale on Pap stain and basophilic on Romanowsky stain. The background contains mixed acute and chronic inflammatory cells, with variable numbers of eosinophils.

D. Hemosiderosis. Alveolar hemorrhage from any cause can result in the presence of hemosiderin-laden macrophages, highlighted by iron stain. Detection of hemosiderin pigment in 20% of macrophages on bronchoalveolar lavage reportedly correlates with alveolar hemorrhage. Hemosiderosis requires a combination of radiographic and clinical features and is best diagnosed on open biopsy, after exclusion of other causes of alveolar hemorrhage.

E. Aspiration. Quantitation of lipid-laden macrophages in bronchoalveolar lavage is based on the fact that alveolar macrophages uptake lipid, which may be evaluated by the use of an oil red O stain on ThinPrep or cytospins from bronchoalveolar lavage. These may be quantitated, using quartiles of cytoplasm filled with lipid-laden vacuoles on 100 cells. Increased oil red O index reflects aspiration or lipoid pneumonia. (*Pediatr Pulmonol* 1987;3:86).

V. NEOPLASMS

A. Squamous Cell Carcinoma (SCC), consists of cells with varying degrees of keratinization, inconsistent size and shape, polygonal to amphophilic cytoplasm, and dark pyknotic nuclei.

The background usually shows the so-called dirty necrosis with abundant keratinized cellular debris (e-**Fig. 8.77**).

B. **Adenocarcinoma,** shows cells with fine foamy to vacuolated cytoplasm, and vesicular nuclei with prominent nucleoli. There is typically no background necrosis unless the tumor is large (e-**Fig. 8.78**). Immunohistochemistry can distinguish SCC from adenocarcinoma. Expression of TTF-1 occurs in adenocarcinomas, but not in SCCs. Care must be taken to distinguish between tumor groups and incidentally obtained normal pulmonary epithelial elements which retain TTF-1 expression. In general, SCCs express cytokeratin 5/6, p63, and p40 while adenocarcinomas do not express these antigens. Some poorly differentiated tumors express markers from both subtypes. A diagnosis of adenosquamous carcinoma should not be rendered on cytology unless there is both true glandular formation and discrete keratinization.

C. **Neuroendocrine Carcinoma.** Small cell carcinomas and large cell neuroendocrine tumors must be distinguished from non–small cell carcinomas since they respond differently to chemotherapy.

   1. **Carcinoid tumor (low-grade neuroendocrine carcinoma)** has both polygonal cells with rounded nuclei and spindle cells with elongated nuclei. Nucleoli are not prominent. Aspirate smears can have some nuclear molding and crush artifact, but aspirates should contain some areas where the cells show the morphology of a typical carcinoid. Of note, a Ki-67 immunostain is not recommended to distinguish carcinoid tumor from small cell carcinoma.

   2. **Large cell neuroendocrine tumor** has flattened cohesive groups of cells with large round to polygonal nuclei that have prominent nucleoli and vesicular nuclear chromatin. Cytoplasm is sparse.

   3. **Small cell carcinoma** is composed of cells with only a small amount of cytoplasm. Nuclei show a molding pattern, fine granular chromatin, and streaming. Apoptotic debris and cellular necrosis are prominent (e-**Fig. 8.79**).

D. **Hematopoietic Malignancies.** Both high- and low-grade non-Hodgkin lymphomas occur in the lung, either as solitary pulmonary nodules or associated with adenopathy. The cytologic features are similar to those of lymphomas aspirated at other sites. High-grade lymphomas contain a discohesive single-cell population with fragmented lymphocytes in the background; individual cells have sparse cytoplasm. Prominent chromocenters are present. Low-grade lymphomas are composed of a monotonous mature lymphoid population. For most lymphomas, additional samples should be taken for flow cytometry to characterize the malignant cell population. If the background inflammation is mixed and contains eosinophils, material should be obtained for a cell block to identify the Reed–Sternberg cells of Hodgkin disease or for gene rearrangement studies for T-cell lymphoma.

E. **Mesothelioma** is usually seen in association with a pleural effusion. Cytologically, the cells show variability in size, with those in clusters having scalloped edges. A cell-in-cell arrangement is often present. Enlarged and convoluted nuclei, with or without nucleoli, are typical (e-**Fig. 8.80**). Appropriate immunohistochemical stains to rule out adenocarcinoma should be performed. Mesothelial markers include calretinin, WT-1, D2-40 (podoplanin), and cytokeratin 5/6. Adenocarcinoma markers include MOC-31, BerEp-4, B72.3, or marker specific to pulmonary differentiation such as TTF-1 and NapsinA. BRCA1-associated protein (BAP-1) is lost in mesothelioma. Fluorescence in situ hybridization for homozygous deletion of p16 has been reported as limited to mesothelioma (*Arch Pathol Lab Med* 2018;142:89). Asbestos fibers (e-**Fig. 8.81**) may be seen in bronchioloalveolar lavage specimens from these patients. An iron stain may highlight these as well.

F. **Metastases** to the lung are common and should be evaluated on the basis of the patient's clinical history. The diagnostic approach to tumors of unknown origin presenting as lung metastases is the same as for tumors of unknown origin presenting at other sites (*Semin Oncol* 1993;20:206).

VI. ANCILLARY STUDIES

A. **Flow Cytometry.** Material from pleural effusion and fine needle aspiration of thoracic lymph nodes are pulmonary nodules can be sent fresh for flow cytometry.

B. **Fluorescence in Situ Hybridization (FISH).** FISH assessment for gene rearrangements is currently part of the treatment stratification for lung cancers. FISH studies can be performed on cytospins, direct smears, and formalin-fixed paraffin-embedded tissue.

C. **Sequencing and Gene Expression Classifier Studies.** DNA and RNA sequence analysis, by traditional as well as NGS approaches, can be performed on cytospins, direct smears, and formalin-fixed paraffin-embedded tissue.

SUGGESTED READINGS

Churg A, Green FHY, eds. *Pathology of Occupational Diseases*, New York: Igaku-Shoin; 1988.

Colby TV, Koss MN, Travis WD. *AFIP Atlas of Tumor Pathology. Series III. Tumors of the Lower Respiratory Tract.* Armed Forces Institute of Pathology; 1996.

Colombo JL, Hallberg TK. Recurrent aspiration in children: lipid laden alveolar macrophage quantitation. *Pediatr Pulmonol* 1987;3:86–89.

Fisher A, Antoniou KM, Brown KK, et al. An official European Respiratory Society/American Thoracic Society research statement: interstitial pneumonia with autoimmune features. *J Eur Respir* 2015;46:976–987.

Frankel SK, Cool CD, Lynch DA, et al. Idiopathic pleuroparenchymal fibroelastosis: description of a novel clinicopathologic entity. *Chest* 2004;126:2007–2013.

Katzenstein AA. *Katzenstein and Askin's Surgical Pathology of Non-Neoplastic Lung Disease.* 4th ed. WB Saunders Company; 2006.

Papanicolaou Society of Cytopathology Task Force on Standards of Practice. Guidelines of the papanicolaou society of cytopathology for the examination of cytologic specimens obtained from the respiratory tract. *Diagnostic Cytopathology* 1999;21:61–69.

Pokharel S, Merickel CR, Alatassi H. Parainfluenza virus 3 induced cytopathic effects on lung tissue and bronchoalveolar lavage fluid in a bone marrow transplant recipient. A case report. *Diagn Cytopathol* 2014;42(6):521–524.

Tomashefski TF, Cagle PT, Farver CF, Fraire AE. *Dail and Hammar's Pulmonary Pathology. Vol. 1 Non-neoplastic Lung Disease.* 3rd ed. Springer Verlag; 2008.

Travis WD, Colby TV, Koss MN, Rosado-de-Christenson ML, Müller NL, King TE. *AFIP Atlas of Non-Tumor Pathology. Series I Non-Neoplastic Disorders of the Lower Respiratory Tract.* Armed Forces Institute of Pathology; 2002.

Wick MR, Leslie KG. *Practical Pulmonary Pathology: A diagnostic approach.* 2nd ed. Churchill Livingstone; 2010.

Cardiovascular System

John D. Pfeifer

HEART

I. NORMAL ANATOMY. The normal weight of the **adult heart** is 300 to 350 g (male) and 250 to 300 g (female). Cardiomegaly above a critical weight of 500 g is associated with ischemic changes (see below) and is termed cor bovinum. The normal ventricular thickness is 0.3 to 0.5 cm on the right and 1.2 to 1.5 cm on the left (e-**Fig. 9.1**), measured at the base of the papillary muscles (Fig. 9.1). The heart is composed of three layers: the epicardium (including the serous or visceral pericardium, and the main branches of the coronary arteries), the muscular myocardium, and the endocardium (with an ill-defined subendocardial layer that contains many Purkinje fibers).

Microscopically, the normal myocardium is a functional syncytium of myocardial fibers (cardiac myocytes) that have centrally located nuclei (e-**Fig. 9.1**). Cardiac myocytes are a specialized form of striated muscle; faint dark eosinophilic intercalated discs between the myocytes form the mechanical and electrical couplings. Numerous capillaries with sparse interstitial tissue are found between the myocardial fibers (e-**Fig. 9.1**).

The atrioventricular valves (mitral and tricuspid) are composed of an annulus, leaflets, chordae tendineae, and papillary muscles. The semilunar valves (aortic and pulmonic) are composed of three cusps (each with a sinus), which meet at the three commissures (corpora arantii, e-**Fig. 9.2**). Valves are relatively avascular, and are lined by endothelial cells on a thin layer of collagen and elastic tissue on the atrial/arterial side, a thicker layer of dense collagen on the ventricular side, and loose myxoid connective tissue (zona spongiosa) in between. The fibrous and spongiotic regions are normally of equal thickness (e-**Fig. 9.2**).

The **conduction system** is composed of specialized myocytes, with fewer intercalated discs and higher glycogen content. Masson trichrome, Verhoeff van Gieson, and Alcian blue stains can be used to demonstrate the conduction system (e-**Fig. 9.3**). Exact knowledge of the topographic anatomy and correct sampling techniques are paramount (e-**Fig. 9.4**).

II. GROSS EXAMINATION AND TISSUE HANDLING

A. Endomyocardial Biopsies are usually taken via a right-sided cardiac catheter; the most common indications are monitoring of heart transplant rejection, and grading of Adriamycin toxicity. To avoid sampling errors, a minimum of three, preferably four, samples of myocardium are recommended (e-**Fig. 9.5**). The tissue fragments should be counted and measured during gross examination; their color and consistency should be noted. The tissue should be placed between foam pads or wrapped in filter paper for routine processing. Examination of at least three levels is recommended; some laboratories keep the intervening sections for additional stains if required to assess myocyte damage and fibrosis. Histologically, an adequate biopsy contains at least 50% myocardium, excluding previous biopsy sites (e-**Fig. 9.5**). Occasional cases require fresh frozen tissue or glutaraldehyde fixation for special techniques such as molecular diagnostics or electron microscopy (see below), respectively. Adipose tissue between myocardiocytes is a normal finding and does not indicate ventricular perforation (e-**Fig. 9.5**).

B. Cardiac Valves are often removed because of calcific degeneration or perforation as sequelae of bacterial endocarditis (e-**Fig. 9.2**). Most valves are received in fragments; if possible, the description should include the distribution of vegetations (e-**Fig. 9.6**) and

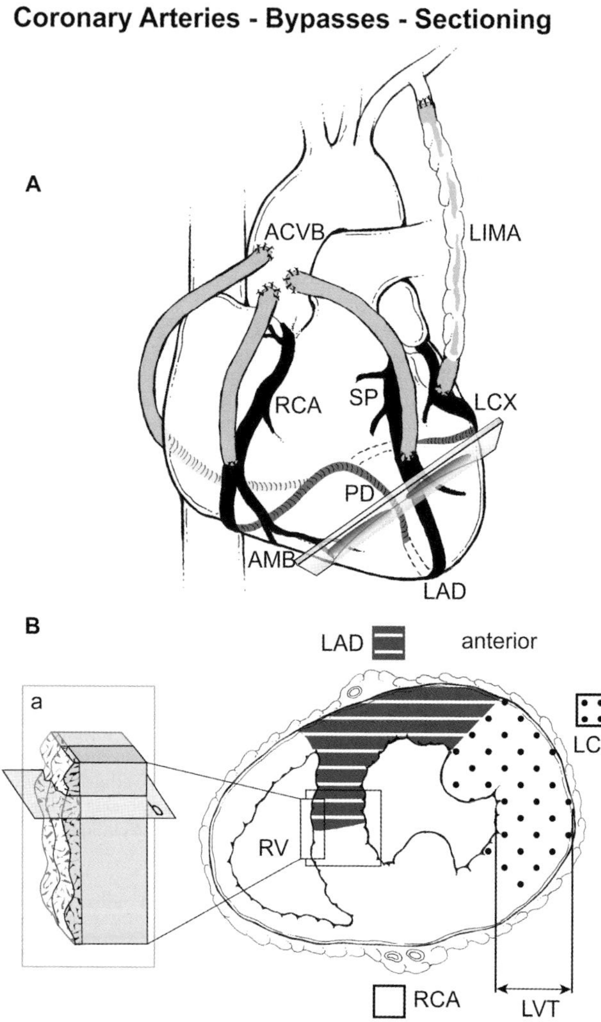

Coronary Arteries - Bypasses - Sectioning

Figure 9.1 Coronary arteries, bypasses, sectioning of the ventricles. **A:** The left coronary artery branches into LCX (left circumflex) and LAD (left anterior descending), the latter supplies the anterior septum via SPs (septal perforators). The RCA (right coronary artery) supplies the AV node (not shown), branches into the AMB (acute marginal branch) and the PD (posterior descending artery). The origin of the PD determines the distribution type (right vs. left). Examples of ACVB (aortocoronary venous bypass) and LIMA (left internal mammary artery) grafts are displayed in gray. **B:** Slice from section illustrated in **A**. The myocardium displays the supplying arteries for mapping of myocardial infarctions. The ventricular thickness (LVT) is measured on the level of the anterior papillary muscle. The large septal square illustrates a section to determine myocyte disarray. The small rectangle close to the RV (right ventricle) illustrates a myomectomy specimen, which is sectioned perpendicular to the endocardial surface; preferred is horizontal (*a*) or vertical (*b*).

presence or absence of nonsurgery related leaflet destruction. In cases of calcific degeneration, slow acid decalcification after fixation may be necessary. Sections are taken from the free edge to the annulus.

Prosthetic valves are typically removed because of thrombosis, anastomotic or valvular leakage, mechanical failure, or infection. Evaluation of the prosthetic valve ring attachment is therefore critical as infective endocarditis typically affects this region. For most mechanical heart valves it is not possible to submit any tissue for histology, unless vegetations are present. For bioprosthetic valves, however, the valve cusp is submitted. Valves from patients treated with the appetite-suppressant drug fen-phen (a combination of fenfluramine and phentermine) show patterns of changes that resemble carcinoid valve disease with superficial layers of myofibroblastic proliferation on otherwise normal valve architecture.

C. **Myomectomy Specimens** from ventricular aneurysm repair or septal myomectomy procedures should be measured, weighed, and sectioned at 3 mm intervals, perpendicular to the endocardial surface (Fig. 9.1). All layers of the heart should be described. For cardiac tumors, appropriate sections should assess the inked specimen resection margins (see below).

D. **Heart Explant Specimens** should be weighed, described, and dissected as outlined (Fig. 9.2). In addition, the valves (circumference or diameter) and walls (Fig. 9.1) should be measured. The septal and ventricular configuration (concentric vs. dilatative ventricular hypertrophy) should be described. Usually the inflow tract of the donor heart is dissected to match the recipient's anatomy; thus, fragments of donor tissue are frequently submitted in the same container.

III. DIAGNOSTIC FEATURES OF COMMON DISEASES OF THE HEART

A. Disorders of the Endocardium

1. **Infective endocarditis** is characterized by bacterial colonization of the valve forming vegetations that are red, irregular (e-**Fig. 9.6**), and composed of granulation tissue and thrombus; their friability explains the propensity for associated septic embolization (e-**Fig. 9.2**). The myocardium is typically not involved. *Staphylococcus aureus* typically produces acute endocarditis, whereas *Streptococcus viridans* produces subacute endocarditis. Several organisms normally found in the oral cavity are also causative, and been referred to as the Gram-negative HACEK organisms (*Haemophilus aphrophilus*, *Actinobacillus actinomycetemcomitans*, *Cardiobacterium hominis*, *Eikenella corrodens*, and *Kingella kingae*). *Staphylococcus epidermidis* also causes infective endocarditis, more common in the setting of prosthetic valves. Healed infective endocarditis leaves residual valve damage, often fenestrations, usually with a hemodynamic jet lesion and adjacent endocardial fibrosis.

2. **Nonbacterial thrombotic endocarditis** (marantic endocarditis) produces small (rarely larger than 0.5 cm), pink, bland, and sterile vegetations attached to the valve surface at the lines of closure (e-**Fig. 9.6**). It is typically seen in cachectic patients with a hypercoagulable state (e.g., Trousseau syndrome).

3. **Libman–Sacks endocarditis** is seen in 4% of cases of systemic lupus erythematosus and is characterized by flat, pale tan, spreading bands of vegetations located on both surfaces of the valves or chordae tendineae (e-**Fig. 9.6**). Affected, in order of frequency, are the tricuspid, mitral, pulmonic, and aortic valves.

4. **Rheumatic heart disease (RHD)** is a sequela of rheumatic fever (RF) caused by *Streptococcus pyogenes* (group A or beta-hemolytic streptococcus). Aschoff nodules (ANs) are a characteristic feature and appear as interstitial collections of plump mononuclear cells with occasional neutrophils arranged in a granuloma-like formation, although the presence or number of ANs does not correlate with clinical course or activity of the rheumatic process. The most characteristic cellular component of ANs is the Aschoff giant cell, which has two or more nuclei with prominent nucleoli; another characteristic feature is the presence of Anitschkow cells, which are mononuclear histiocytes that are often arranged in a palisade around the center of the granuloma. The macroscopic pattern is variable (e-**Fig. 9.6**).

Dissection Techniques of the Heart

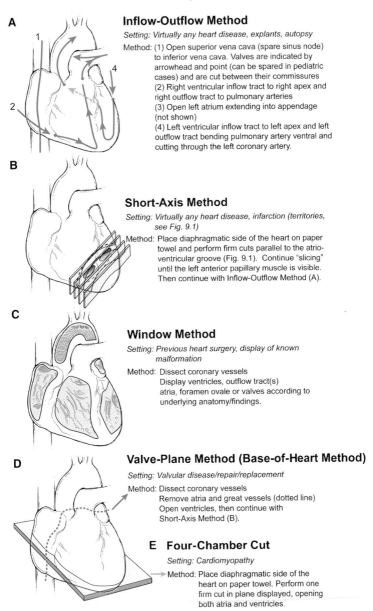

A

Inflow-Outflow Method

Setting: Virtually any heart disease, explants, autopsy

Method: (1) Open superior vena cava (spare sinus node) to inferior vena cava. Valves are indicated by arrowhead and point (can be spared in pediatric cases) and are cut between their commissures
(2) Right ventricular inflow tract to right apex and right outflow tract to pulmonary arteries
(3) Open left atrium extending into appendage (not shown)
(4) Left ventricular inflow tract to left apex and left outflow tract bending pulmonary artery ventral and cutting through the left coronary artery.

B

Short-Axis Method

Setting: Virtually any heart disease, infarction (territories, see Fig. 9.1)

Method: Place diaphragmatic side of the heart on paper towel and perform firm cuts parallel to the atrio-ventricular groove (Fig. 9.1). Continue "slicing" until the left anterior papillary muscle is visible. Then continue with Inflow-Outflow Method (A).

C

Window Method

Setting: Previous heart surgery, display of known malformation

Method: Dissect coronary vessels
Display ventricles, outflow tract(s)
atria, foramen ovale or valves according to underlying anatomy/findings.

D

Valve-Plane Method (Base-of-Heart Method)

Setting: Valvular disease/repair/replacement

Method: Dissect coronary vessels
Remove atria and great vessels (dotted line)
Open ventricles, then continue with Short-Axis Method (B).

E   Four-Chamber Cut

Setting: Cardiomyopathy

Method: Place diaphragmatic side of the heart on paper towel. Perform one firm cut in plane displayed, opening both atria and ventricles.

Figure 9.2 Dissection techniques of the heart.

The valvular disease characteristic of chronic RHD is usually the result of multiple recurrent episodes of acute RF, and typically develops many decades after the initial insult. RHD is the most common cause of mitral stenosis, and in up to 75% of cases the mitral valve is the only valve affected. In 25% of cases the mitral and aortic valve are affected. Progressive fibrosis leads to thickening of the valve and chordae that eventually leads to fusion of the mitral leaflets at the commissures, producing the classic "fish mouth" appearance.

5. **Endocardial fibroelastosis** is an uncommon condition that can result in restrictive cardiomyopathy. Pearl-white fibroelastic thickening, caused by accumulation of collagen and elastic fibers typically in the left ventricular endocardium (e-**Fig. 9.3**), is often associated with aortic valve obstruction. The disease occurs either focally or diffusely in children from birth to age 2 years.

6. **Loeffler endocarditis** is also known as fibroelastic parietal endocarditis with blood eosinophilia. The disease is a component of broader cardiac involvement as part of the hypereosinophilic syndrome (see below).

B. Disorders of the Valves

1. **Myxoid change** is stromal accumulation of glycosaminoglycans as a sign of degeneration (e-**Fig. 9.2**). The layered architecture is preserved; if the architecture is absent or distorted, the differential diagnosis should include RHD. The chordae tendineae are thinned and elongated in myxomatous degeneration, whereas in RHD they are shortened and thickened.

2. **Tricuspid valves** are most commonly removed for insufficiency or infectious endocarditis.

3. **Pulmonary valves** are usually excised because of stenosis due to congenital heart disease (most commonly as a component of tetralogy of Fallot).

4. **Mitral valves** are removed for acquired post-inflammatory stenosis (e.g., RHD) and may show commissural fusion, cusp scarring, and dystrophic calcification (e-**Fig. 9.2**). RHD vegetations are composed mainly of fibrin and are usually no more than 2 mm in size. Cases of mitral insufficiency or myxomatous degeneration show a floppy valve with redundant and ballooned leaflets with abundant myxoid change.

5. **Aortic valves** are removed for stenosis and are typically heavily calcified, sometimes with commissural fusion (senile calcific aortic stenosis), postinflammatory scarring, or calcification due to a congenitally bicuspid valve (present in 1% of the population).

6. **Carcinoid heart disease,** seen in about 50% of patients with carcinoid syndrome, typically affects the heart's right side, particularly the ventricular outflow tract. Tricuspid valve regurgitation (often with stenosis) and pulmonary valve stenosis (often with regurgitation) are common. Gross findings include prominent hypertrophy and plaque-like thickening of the endocardium. Microscopically, the valvular cusps show proliferation of smooth muscle and collagen deposition, without valve destruction. There are no carcinoid tumor cells in the lesion.

C. Disorders of the Myocardium

1. **Myocarditis** is the underlying etiology in about 10% of patients with new-onset cardiac dysfunction. If not fatal, myocarditis often proceeds to dilated cardiomyopathy. Findings in subsequent biopsies, using the first specimen as a reference point, include ongoing/persistent myocarditis, resolving/healing myocarditis (damage substantially reduced), and resolved/healed myocarditis (damage no longer present). The so-called Dallas criteria (*Hum Pathol* 1987;18:619) are often used to categorize myocarditis mainly on histopathologic findings, although it has been suggested that the criteria are no longer adequate. The WHO/International Society and Federation of Cardiology (ISFC) defines myocarditis as a minimum of 14 infiltrating leukocytes per mm^2, preferably T cells, with as many as four macrophages (also known as the Marburg criteria; see *Circulation* 1996;93:841). The diagnosis of *active myocarditis* classically requires the presence of an inflammatory infiltrate (usually lymphocytic) and myocyte necrosis/degeneration or damage not characteristic of an ischemic event; *borderline myocarditis* indicates the absence of necrosis or damage and can be applied to any form of inflammatory infiltrate.

a. **Primary** viral myocarditis accounts for most cases of myocarditis in developed countries. Cardiac involvement typically follows the primary viral infection by several days. The most commonly associated agents are enteroviruses (Coxsackie A and B), adenovirus, and parvovirus B19 (PVB19); less common causes are echovirus, hepatitis C, herpesvirus 6, influenza viruses A and B, and HIV. The infiltrate is composed mainly of lymphocytes with associated myocyte damage (e-**Fig. 9.7**). Eosinophils are typically not seen. Primary viral myocarditis is often divided into four clinical pathologic manifestations: fulminate, subacute, chronic active, and chronic persistent.

   i. **Fulminant myocarditis** has a distinct onset of profound left ventricular dysfunction without dilatation. Biopsy shows multiple foci of active inflammation and necrosis. Patients usually show complete histologic and functional recovery, or die within 2 weeks.

   ii. **Subacute myocarditis** has an indistinct onset. Histologically, there is active to borderline inflammation. While there is typically complete histologic resolution with time, patients often progress to dilated cardiomyopathy.

   iii. **Chronic active myocarditis** also has an indistinct onset with moderate ventricular dysfunction and active or borderline biopsy findings. Ongoing inflammation and fibrosis may result in the development of restrictive cardiomyopathy within 2 to 4 years after presentation.

   iv. **Chronic persistent myocarditis** usually has an indistinct onset without left ventricular dysfunction. Active to borderline inflammation is present, which persists over time. Patients generally continue to have normal left ventricular function.

b. **Eosinophilic myocarditis** can be attributed to eosinophilic syndromes or allergic reactions that result in left ventricular compromise. Eosinophils and myocyte damage are present in the biopsy (e-**Fig. 9.7**). The differential diagnosis of eosinophilia in the myocardium also includes parasitic infection and hematologic malignancies; in an immunosuppressed patient, cytomegalovirus infection should enter the differential diagnosis.

   i. Myocarditis as a component of **hypereosinophilic syndrome (HES)** is classically described as having three stages (acute myocarditis with myocyte necrosis, organizing thrombus, and endomyocardial fibrosis). The cardiac lesions and hypereosinophilia are associated with dense eosinophilic infiltration of other organs. Recently, an *FIP1L1-PDGFRA* fusion gene has been shown to be present in a subset of cases of HES, and genetic testing has become part of the diagnostic algorithm (*Expert Rev Hematol* 2012;5:275).

   ii. The entity sometimes referred to as **hypersensitivity myocarditis** is linked to treatment with methyldopa, antibiotics (penicillin, sulfonamides, streptomycin), anticonvulsants, and antidepressants, and also shows occasional giant cells. The myocardium has little myocyte necrosis and the inflammatory infiltrate is lymphohistiocytic and predominantly perivascular (e-**Fig. 9.7**). In some cases the infiltrate is subendocardial or appears as poorly formed granulomas.

c. **Idiopathic giant cell myocarditis,** traditionally known as Fiedler myocarditis, is associated with autoimmune diseases (e.g., inflammatory bowel disease, hypothyroidism) and is rapidly fatal if untreated. It typically occurs in young, healthy, white adults and presents as congestive heart failure. Diffuse, geographic myocardial necrosis with a mixed inflammatory infiltrate including eosinophils and multinucleated giant cells in the absence of granulomas is typical (e-**Fig. 9.8**). The giant cells have the immunohistochemical profile of histiocytes (*Arch Pathol Lab Med* 2016;140:1429).

d. **Other organisms** associated with myocarditis include bacteria, fungi, spirochetes (especially *Borrelia burgdorferi*), *Rickettsiae*, *Chlamydia*, parasites (including *Toxoplasma gondii* in immunocompromised patients), and helminths (trichinosis).

e. **Chagas disease,** the most form of common protozoal myocarditis, is caused by the hemoflagellate *Trypanosoma cruzi* and is uncommon in the United States.

However, in endemic regions of South and Central America it accounts for 25% of all deaths of 25 to 40 year olds; up to 80% of patients with Chagas disease develop myocarditis. Histologically, myofibers contain parasites with an associated mild chronic inflammatory infiltrate. In the acute phase, dense inflammation with myocyte necrosis and trypanosome amastigotes in myocytes is characteristic, whereas the chronic phase shows interstitial and perivascular lymphoplasmacytic infiltrate without fibrosis.

f. **Secondary myocarditis** can occur in the setting of collagen vascular diseases, RF, drugs, heat stroke, and radiation.

g. **Granulomatous myocarditis** (e-**Fig. 9.9**) can be seen in tuberculosis or sarcoidosis. Cardiac sarcoidosis shows nonnecrotizing granulomas (e-**Fig. 9.9**) in a background of fibrosis and necrosis. Cardiac involvement, though present in 25% of systemic cases of sarcoidosis, is usually patchy and therefore a single negative endomyocardial biopsy does not exclude the disease. The differential diagnosis in cases of suspected cardiac sarcoidosis includes idiopathic giant cell myocarditis, amyloid, Chagas disease, and Fabry disease.

2. **Cardiomyopathy**

   a. **Ischemic cardiomyopathy** is usually secondary to severe coronary artery disease (e-**Fig. 9.10**). Atherosclerotic cardiovascular disease (see below) is by far the most common cause of ischemic cardiomyopathy.

   b. **Hypertrophic cardiomyopathy** is typically seen in healthy individuals less than 30 years old, but can be seen at almost any age. Affected individuals suffer from angina, exertional dyspnea, or sudden cardiac death as a result of diastolic dysfunction due to ventricular thickening. In hypertrophic obstructive cardiomyopathy there is classically asymmetric ventricular septal hypertrophy (with a wall thickness of 15 to 30 mm), with associated fibrous endocardial plaques and mitral valve thickening. Microscopically, disarray of myofibers (e-**Fig. 9.11**), myofiber hypertrophy, basophilic degeneration, and interstitial fibrosis are characteristic, although nonspecific.

   Currently, over 450 disease-causing mutations in 16 genes encoding for myocardial contractile proteins have been implicated in hypertrophic cardiomyopathy, a spectrum of genetic changes that makes so-called next generation sequencing (see Chapter 58) a useful approach for characterizing the underlying genetic abnormality in individual patients (*Gene* 2016;577:227). However, many causal mutations have limited implications in risk stratification and prognostication, and so the role of DNA sequencing for genetic screening remains unsettled (*Eur J Clin Invest* 2010;40:360).

   c. **Dilated cardiomyopathy**, also known as congestive cardiomyopathy, presents as cardiac failure due to progressive cardiac dilatation with systolic dysfunction. Hypertrophy (increased weight with normal or reduced wall thickness) and marked dilatation of all chambers is typical (e-**Fig. 9.12**). Histologic examination shows nonspecific abnormalities; in about 50% of the cases, leukocytic infiltrates are present in endomyocardial biopsies. A significant number of cases are thought to be postviral, or associated with alcohol use or chemotherapeutic agents. Pheochromocytoma is also associated with dilated cardiomyopathy. Dilated cardiomyopathy occurring in the peripartum period (up to 6 months after delivery) is known as peripartum cardiomyopathy.

   About 90% of familial cases show autosomal dominant inheritance, and 5% to 10% are X-linked. In addition to the genes affected by hypertrophic cardiomyopathy, additional mutations in cytoskeletal, nuclear envelope, and mitochondrial proteins have been found (*Genome Medicine* 2017;9:20).

   d. **Restrictive (obliterative) cardiomyopathy** is uncommon in developed countries. The ventricles are normal or slightly enlarged and are not dilated; in contrast, the atria exhibit relative bilateral dilatation. Patchy or interstitial fibrosis is found histologically (e-**Fig. 9.13**). The eosinophilic form shows an eosinophil-rich myocardial infiltrate, whereas the noneosinophilic form (more common in the

United States) shows nonspecific findings. Restrictive cardiomyopathy is typically caused by endomyocardial fibrosis or hemochromatosis, but is often idiopathic. Genetic causes have also been identified (*J Biomed Sci* 2017;24:56).

e. Infiltrative cardiomyopathy is descriptive for a broad panel of metabolic diseases, and can be assigned to any disorder that restricts ventricular filling.

   i. Cardiac amyloidosis histologically shows amorphous, eosinophilic, extracellular material (e-**Fig. 9.14**). Cardiac amyloidosis is associated with restrictive features due to associated decreased ventricular compliance and so presents with diastolic dysfunction. Grossly, the myocardium appears stiff, and rubbery or waxy. The diagnosis of amyloid is confirmed by demonstrating apple-green birefringence with polarized light using a Congo red stain and/or electron microscopy (e-**Fig. 9.14**), or by immunohistochemistry (e-**Fig. 9.15**).

   ii. Hereditary hemochromatosis is a homozygous autosomal recessive disorder resulting from *HFE* gene mutations. The mutation results in unregulated uptake of iron in the small intestine, leading to iron deposition in the liver (hepatomegaly), pancreas (diabetes mellitus), skin (hyperpigmentation), or heart (dilated or restrictive cardiomyopathy). In the heart, myocytes and interstitial macrophages contain abundant brown pigment (e-**Fig. 9.16**), which can be demonstrated to be iron by a Prussian blue stain, but there is little correlation between the amount of cardiac iron and systolic dysfunction. Increased cardiac iron must be distinguished from lipofuscin; the latter is more finely granular, derived from normal intracellular lipid peroxidation, and is not stained by Prussian blue (e-**Fig. 9.16**). Iron overload is not specific for hereditary hemochromatosis but can also be seen in the setting of thalassemia, multiple transfusions, hemosiderosis, or hemolytic anemia.

   iii. Other infiltrative cardiomyopathies include those associated with hypereosinophilic syndrome (see above), endocardial fibroelastosis, and mitochondrial myopathies.

f. Arrhythmogenic right ventricular cardiomyopathy is also known as right ventricular dysplasia, parchment right ventricle, and Uhl anomaly. This uncommon variant of familial cardiomyopathy shows replacement of the myocardium by adipose and fibrous tissue, predominantly in the inferior and infundibular wall, without associated coronary artery sclerosis. Mutations in a number of different genes have been shown to underlie the disease (*J Am Coll Cardiol* 2013;61:1945; *J Med Genet* 2013;50:280) and so genetic testing is likely to become part of the diagnostic workup.

g. Drug/radiation-induced cardiomyopathy is caused by drugs such as Adriamycin and cyclophosphamide and shows primarily subcellular changes that are best seen by electron microscopy (*Cancer Treat Rev* 2004;30:181).

   i. Adriamycin (doxorubicin) toxicity is characterized by dose-dependent changes, predominately in the subendocardial region. It frequently occurs after lifetime doses above 500 mg/m^2. Vacuolization of myocytes (mainly due to marked dilatation of the sarcoplasmic reticulum) is initially present (e-**Fig. 9.17**), followed by the appearance of typical "adria cells" that show loss of cross striations, myofilamentous bundles, and accompanying homogeneous basophilic staining (corresponding to ultrastructural fragmentation of sarcomeres). There is no accompanying inflammation. Since the microscopic features are not specific for Adriamycin toxicity, clinical correlation is required (*Env Health Perspect* 1978;26:181; *Int J Card* 2007;117:6).

   ii. Cyclophosphamide toxicity may produce hemorrhagic necrosis, interstitial hemorrhage, extensive capillary thrombosis, fibrin deposition, and necrosis of myocardial fibers.

   iii. Radiation enhances the changes seen with chemotherapy. Constrictive pericarditis, myocardial fibrosis, and coronary artery lesions are also associated with radiation therapy.

3. Myocardial ischemia—ischemic heart disease

a. The appearance of an acute **myocardial infarct** is dependent on the age of the infarct (e-**Fig. 9.18**). Following acute ischemia, the histologic changes include waviness of fibers (after 1 to 3 hours), progressing to contraction band necrosis (after 4 to 12 hours) (e-**Fig. 9.19**), and infiltration by neutrophils (after 2 to 24 hours). In cases of reperfusion, contraction band necrosis can be seen after 18 to 24 hours as the cells begin to lose cross striations and nuclear detail. Total coagulative necrosis can be seen by 24 to 72 hours.

b. **Chronic ischemic heart disease** culminates in diffuse myocardial atrophy (brown atrophy) with patchy perivascular and interstitial fibrosis, with progressive ischemic necrosis. The heart is small with chocolate-colored myocardium that shows excessive lipofuscin deposition within the fibers.

c. **Microscopic arteriopathy** is a term used to designate the changes in peripheral coronary arteries that undergo sclerotic changes (e-**Fig. 9.20**) resulting in a small lumen (greater than 75% reduction in cross-sectional area). The disease is typically seen in chronic hypertension or with cocaine-induced cardiomyopathy, but will to some degree occur in chronic heart transplant rejection where it becomes the rate-limiting step to long-term survival.

D. Disorders of the Pericardium

1. **Acute pericarditis** (e-**Fig. 9.21**) is idiopathic in 90% of cases, but can be caused by viruses (Coxsackie B, echoviruses, influenza, mumps, Epstein–Barr virus) or bacteria (*Staphylococcus aureus, Streptococci,* or *Haemophilus influenza*). Acute serous pericarditis can be secondary to acute RF, connective tissue disorders (e.g., systemic lupus erythematosus), uremia, metastatic malignancy, and renal transplantation. In contrast, acute fibrinous or serofibrinous pericarditis can be secondary to myocardial infarction (typically after 1 to 3 days), uremia, chest radiotherapy, RF, systemic lupus erythematosus, cardiac surgery, pneumonia, pleural infection, and cardiac trauma. Caseous pericarditis is usually due to *M. tuberculosis* infection. Healed acute pericarditis usually results in a focal pearly thickened epicardial plaque, also known as a "soldier's plaque."

2. **Chronic pericarditis** can lead to constrictive pericarditis where the heart is encased by a thick layer of fibrous tissue. Constrictive pericarditis can follow caseous pericarditis or radiotherapy, but is usually idiopathic.

3. **Neoplasms.** Although primary neoplasms of the pericardium are very rare (including mesothelioma, germ cell tumors, and angiosarcoma), pericardial involvement is present in up to about 10% of patients with disseminated malignancy.

4. **Pericardial effusions.** Effusions can be as large as 500 mL in some settings, such as congestive heart failure and hypoproteinemia. However, in acute cardiac tamponade, rapid accumulation of as little as 200 to 300 mL can cause cardiac compression and death.

IV. NEOPLASMS OF THE HEART.
The four most common cardiac primary tumors (and tumor-like conditions) are all benign and account for 70% of cardiac neoplasms. Primary malignancies of the heart are very rare; involvement of the heart by a malignancy is far more likely to represent metastasis by lung carcinoma, breast carcinoma, melanoma, lymphoma, leukemia, renal cell carcinoma, and choriocarcinoma. In cases of metastatic spread to the heart, the pericardium is often involved.

A. Cardiac Myxoma
is most common primary tumor of the heart. In the sporadic form, the tumor typically occurs in middle-aged women, and is grossly a spherical, soft grey-white, gelatinous, lobulated tumor 1 to 10 cm in maximal dimension, typically attached by a stalk to the left atrium near the fossa ovalis (e-**Fig. 9.22**). In familial cases (e.g., Carney complex and its subsets NAME syndrome [Nevi, Atrial myxoma, Myxoid neurofibroma, and Ephelides] and LAMB syndrome [Lentigines, Atrial myxomas, Mucocutaneous myxomas, and Blue nevi], all caused by mutations in the *PRKAR1A* gene), the mean age of patients is mid-twenties, and the tumor is more often attached to the right atrium or is multicentric. Microscopically, myxomas consist of plump spindled

or stellate cells in abundant loose myxoid stroma (**e-Fig. 9.22**). Heterologous elements including cartilage, foci of ossification (petrified myxoma), or gland formation (glandular myxoma) can be seen, but have no prognostic significance (**e-Fig. 9.22**).

B. Papillary Fibroelastoma occurs typically on the ventricular surface of the semilunar valves or the atrial surface of the AV valves. The tumor accounts for 75% of all valvular tumors, and can be up to 7 cm in greatest dimension. In children the right side is predominantly affected. The branching avascular papillae are composed of fibroelastic myxoid stroma and are lined by hyperplastic endothelium (**e-Fig. 9.22**).

C. Lipomas typically have a subendocardial location in the left ventricle.

D. Rhabdomyoma presents as a single (10% of cases) or multiple (90% of cases) well-circumscribed gray-white firm myocardial nodule up to 6 cm in size that often protrudes into the ventricle. The tumor is often discovered in the first year of life, and is the most common cardiac tumor in the pediatric age group. Patients usually present with heart failure or arrhythmias. Most cases of cardiac rhabdomyoma have clinical or radiographic signs of tuberous sclerosis complex, or a family history of the disease.

Microscopically, the tumor is composed of mixtures of round and polygonal cells with glycogen-rich vacuoles (**e-Fig. 9.22**) that are separated by strands of cytoplasm radiating from the center of the cell (so-called "spider cells"). Rhabdomyoma is mitotically inactive, noninvasive, and non-metastasizing; some tumors even regress spontaneously after the first year of life. Tumors not associated with tuberous sclerosis complex have a generally good prognosis. Rhabdomyoma cells are immunopositive for vimentin, desmin, actin, and myoglobin; focal HMB45 positive cells can also be present.

E. Intramural Cardiac Fibroma usually occurs as a single, white, rubbery lesion (**e-Fig. 9.22**). It is usually a component of Gorlin syndrome (also known as nevoid basal cell carcinoma syndrome). The tumor cells are typically immunopositive for vimentin and smooth muscle actin, indicating myofibroblastic origin. Immunoreactivity for the muscle-specific markers desmin and myoD1 is absent.

F. Other Benign Tumors include mesothelial/monocytic incidental cardiac excrescences (also known as cardiac MICE; **e-Fig. 9.21**), calcified amorphous tumor of the heart (also known as cardiac CAT), lipomatous hypertrophy of the atrial septum, mesothelioma of the atrioventricular node, adenomatoid tumor, epithelioid or histiocytoid hemangioma, paraganglioma (extra-adrenal pheochromocytoma), schwannoma, and granular cell tumor.

G. Angiosarcoma is the most common primary malignant tumor of the heart. It typically involves the right atrium as a large mass with intracavitary extension, and may also infiltrate the myocardium. Primary angiosarcoma of the heart is typically more poorly differentiated than elsewhere (**e-Fig. 9.22**).

H. Other rare primary cardiac sarcomas include Kaposi sarcoma, leiomyosarcoma, liposarcoma, and rhabdomyosarcoma (covered in more detail in Chapter 44).

V. CARDIAC TRANSPLANTS

A. The most sensitive method for the evaluation of **cellular rejection** is microscopic examination of an adequate myocardial biopsy. Often the sample will be taken from a previous biopsy site and show healing foci of ischemic injury with varying degrees of inflammatory infiltrates, changes which should not be confused with acute rejection. The revised and original grading scheme for acute cellular rejection (Fig. 9.3) refers to the histologic findings (**e-Fig. 9.23**); however, the presence or absence of myocyte necrosis should always be documented (*J Heart Lung Transpl* 2005;24:1710).

B. Antibody Mediated Rejection (AMR, also known as humoral or vascular rejection) occurs in 10–20% of cardiac transplants, and is associated with hemodynamic compromise, development of cardiac allograft vasculopathy (see below), poor overall graft survival, and death in 20% to 50% of patients. A working formulation for standardization of the pathologic diagnosis, grading, and reporting of AMR has been developed (*J Heart Lung Transplant* 2013;32:1147) which has been shown to correlate with an increased risk of mortality (*J Heart Lung Transplant* 2016;35:320). Specific vascular and cardiomyocyte changes associated with AMR in endomyocardial biopsies alone may not

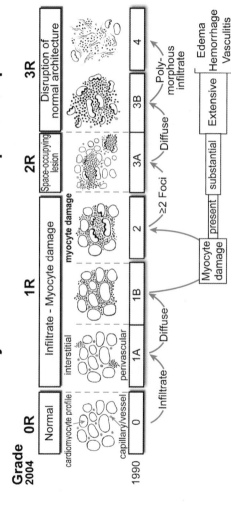

Figure 9.3 Grading of cellular rejection in heart transplant biopsies. The grading is illustrated from left to right. Comparison of original (1990) and revised grading (2004) schemes is schematically illustrated (see also e-Fig. 9.23). *Open circles* represent cardiomyocyte profiles, *small dots* represent vessels or inflammatory infiltrate. The main diagnostic feature of each grade is provided. The diagnostic features required for the 1990 grading are provided below the scheme. (Note: Diagnosis is based on the highest grade findings present; see *J Heart Transplant* 1990;9:587, *J Heart Lung Transpl* 2005;24:1710, *Heart Transpl Pathol* 2007;131:1169.)

be a reliable method for diagnosis. Strong staining of the endothelium of small vessels and the myocardial capillary network (e-**Fig. 9.24**) by immunohistochemistry for the complement component C4d, together with the presence of CD68 positive intravascular macrophages, has been shown to correlate more strongly with AMR. The diagnosis of AMR therefore rests on a combination of histopathologic findings (light microscopic features and identification of diffuse capillary C4d immunostaining and CD68 positive intravascular macrophages) and clinical findings (clinical evidence of anti-donor [HLA] antibodies and graft dysfunction).

Given that rejection is one of the major causes of allograft failure, and that rejection at present can only be diagnosed by endomyocardial biopsy, there is substantial interest in biomarkers of rejection that can be measured via non-invasive techniques. Although it recently has been shown that differential expression of a panel of miRNA measured from serum can be used to identify patients with rejection (*Eur Heart J* 2014;35:3194), this approach is not yet in routine clinical use.

C. **Quilty Effect** (e-**Fig. 9.25**) refers to the presence of a dense subendocardial lymphocyte infiltrate (*Am J Cardiov Pathol* 1988;1:139), composed of predominately B cells. Quilty A lesions are limited to the endo/subendocardium, while Quilty B lesions extend into underlying myocardium where there is often associated myocyte damage (*Curr Opin Cardiol* 1997;12:146). There is no consensus as to the pathogenesis or clinical significance of Quilty B lesions since up to 20% of posttransplant biopsies show this finding (also known as cyclosporine effect). Quilty lesions have no known adverse prognostic effect, and are not associated with EBV infection responsible for posttransplant lymphoproliferative disorders. Quilty effect is therefore classified as one of four nonrejection findings.

Given the location of Quilty B lesions within the myocardium, and the potential for associated myocyte damage, it is often difficult to distinguish the lesions from conventional cellular rejection. However, since Quilty effect is characterized by a collar of T cells surrounding a central aggregate of B cells, immunostains for CD3 and CD20 can be used to help classify problematic cases (e-**Fig. 9.26**). It has recently been demonstrated that a compact network of follicular dendritic cells is also present in the center of Quilty lesions (*Am J Surg Pathol.* 2006;30:1008) which can be highlighted by an immunostain for CD21 (e-**Fig. 9.27**).

D. **Ischemic Injury** is the second nonrejection finding. It presents either early (up to 6 weeks posttransplant) or late, and is related to allograft coronary disease. Ischemic injury must be differentiated from preservation injury, which develops as a result of the lack of organ perfusion between harvest and implantation. Preservation injury is a common incidental finding in endocardial biopsies during the week or two following transplantation and is characterized by necrosis of the most superficial regions of the endocardium with associated overlying organizing fibrin (e-**Fig. 9.28**). Similarly, artifacts of endomyocardial biopsy processing that simulate contraction band necrosis (e-**Fig. 9.19**) must not be confused with true ischemic injury.

E. **Infection and Lymphoproliferative Disorders** are the two other non-rejection findings in biopsies, characterized by diffuse infiltration by small to medium-sized lymphocytes in a pattern resembling rejection (*J Heart Lung Transpl* 2005;24:1710).

Posttransplant lymphoproliferative disorder (PTLD) is an EBV virus–related proliferation of B cells. The infiltrates express CD19 and CD20, and show clonal immunoglobulin light chain expression. Polymerase chain reaction (PCR) for EBV and/or in situ hybridization studies for EBV transcripts are useful ancillary tests in difficult cases.

F. So-called **transplant arteriopathy** or **cardiac allograft vasculopathy** is characteristic of chronic rejection. It features concentric luminal narrowing of small vessels by intimal thickening and medial proliferation with relative preservation of the internal elastic lamina, a pattern thought to represent an accelerated form of atherosclerosis. In cases with complete vascular obstruction ischemic damage can be found, although ischemic events are clinically silent due to the lack of cardiac re-innervation after transplantation.

VESSELS

I. **NORMAL ANATOMY.** The luminal endothelial cell layer defines vessels and **arteries** have three layers (e-**Fig. 9.20**), the intima (composed of the endothelium, internal elastic lamella, and subendothelial connective tissue), media (smooth muscle), and adventitia (connective tissue). Venous vessels have the same three layers, but a thinner media and a thicker adventitia.

Endothelial cells are characterized by immunoreactivity for CD34, CD31, vimentin, endothelin, and von Willebrand factor. Endothelium also stains for Factor VIII related antigen and Ulex europaeus I lectin, both stronger in blood vessels in comparison with lymphatic vessels. The smooth muscle cells of the media express desmin. Depending on the anatomic site, pericytes and smooth muscle or glomus cells are located along the outside of the vessel; these cells show immunoreactivity for actin, vimentin, and myosin.

The size of arterial vessels is typically defined in relation to vessels in the kidney. The aorta is categorized as a large artery, the renal and lobar arteries as medium-sized arteries, and the arcuate and interlobular arteries as small arteries (Fig. 9.4). The next smallest arterial vessels, arterioles, are defined by a media that has two to five layers of smooth muscle cells, or as having a luminal radius that equals the wall thickness.

Vascular Tree and Distribution of Typical Vasculitides

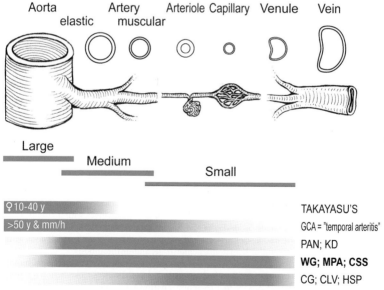

Figure 9.4 Overview of the vascular tree and typical vasculitides. CG, cryoglobulinemia; CLV, cutaneous leukocytoclastic vasculitis; CSS, Churg–Strauss syndrome; GCA, giant cell arteritis = temporal arteritis; HSP, Henoch–Schönlein purpura; KD, Kawasaki disease; MPA, microscopic polyangiitis; PAN, panarteritis nodosa; TA, Takayasu arteritis; WG, Wegener granulomatosis. Boldface type indicates ANCA-positive. See also e-**Figs. 9.20** and **9.29**.

II. **GROSS EXAMINATION AND TISSUE HANDLING. Temporal artery biopsies** are typically about 2 to 3 cm long. Because arteritis can have a patchy distribution with so-called skip areas (see below), proper tissue handling is essential to ensure a maximum diagnostic yield from the biopsy. The external aspect of the vessel should be inked (which is used to ensure that the microscopic sections include the entire wall); the vessel should then be serially sectioned at 3 mm intervals. After processing, embedding of the vessel segments should result in tissue sections with complete ring-like profiles that have an inked external surface. At least three levels should be examined. Orienting the vessel segments in agar prior to processing (*Ann Diagn Pathol* 2001;5:107) is a simple way to ensure that proper orientation is achieved during embedding.

Although **embolectomy** specimens are easy to gross, the submission of all tissue can have tremendous clinical impact, because the pathologist may ascertain the exact source of an embolus (e.g., endocarditis, atrial myxoma) in a minute piece of tissue.

III. **DIAGNOSTIC FEATURES OF COMMON DISEASES.** Vascular diseases affect all organs and contribute to the histopathologic presentation of a variety of diseases.

A. **Congenital and Genetic Diseases.** A wide variety of congenital defects and inherited diseases result in structural abnormalities of the heart, valves, and systemic vessels, or degenerative changes over time. Inherited diseases include abnormalities of fatty acid metabolism, glycogen storage diseases, lysosomal enzyme deficiencies, and even familial causes of amyloidosis (*Pediatr Int* 2017;59:525). Mitochondrial myopathies (a heterogeneous group of maternally inherited diseases that results from mutations in the proteins encoded by the mitochondrial genome) are another cause of a wide variety of cardiac arrhythmias and functional abnormalities (*Clin Sci (Lond)* 2017;131:1375).

In most of these disorders, the surgical pathologic evaluation of endomyocardial biopsies or autopsy specimens by immunohistochemical, molecular genetic, and/or electron microscopic approaches is primarily used to confirm the diagnosis. Genetic testing is of increasing importance in this respect; the clinicopathologic features of the disease dictate whether germline testing performed on peripheral blood is appropriate, or whether testing should be performed on cardiac tissue itself. Genetic testing is increasingly used to determine the risk that the disease will occur in the patient's family members.

B. **Atherosclerotic Cardiovascular Disease** is a progressive degenerative inflammatory disease characterized by the accumulation of lipids (both intracellular and extracellular), macrophages, T cells, proteoglycans, collagen, and calcium in arterial vessels. Major risk factors are hypertension, obesity, diabetes, and smoking. Atherosclerosis is the leading cause of acute coronary artery syndromes (men more affected than premenopausal women; approximately one in three men will suffer a cardiac event secondary to atherosclerosis before the age of 60). Atherosclerosis is also responsible for significant disease in large vessels outside of the heart.

1. **Coronary vessels.** The American Heart Association (AHA) has described the microscopic features of atherosclerosis in detail (*Circulation* 1994;89:2462; *Circulation* 1995;92:1355). The AHA scheme is as follows: Grade 1, isolated macrophages or foam cells; Grade 2, intracellular lipid accumulation; Grade 3, grade 2 lesions along with small extracellular lipid pools; Grade 4, grade 2 changes with a core of extracellular lipid; Grade 5, lipid core and fibrous cap, or multiple lipid cores in fibrous layers that are calcific or fibrotic; Grade 6, more common grade 4 or 5 lesions with a surface defect, and/or hematoma/hemorrhage, and/or thrombosis.

Atherosclerotic plaques with time can lead to significant cross-sectional luminal narrowing, traditionally classified as Grade 1, less than 25% cross-sectional luminal narrowing; Grade 2, 25% to 50% luminal narrowing; Grade 3, 50% to 75% luminal narrowing; and Grade 4, greater than 75% cross-sectional luminal narrowing (75% cross-sectional luminal narrowing is critical stenosis that has an impact on blood flow). However, the most significant sequela of coronary atherosclerosis is plaque rupture with associated thrombosis which is often associated with sudden death (*Cardiovasc Diagn Ther* 2016;6:396).

Of note, it has recently it has become clear that clonal hematopoiesis of indeterminate potential (CHIP) is a significant risk factor for coronary heart disease (*N Engl J Med* 2017;377:111).

2. Aorta. Atherosclerotic disease involving the aorta also features chronic inflammation with formation of atherosclerotic plaques. However, atherosclerosis in the aorta is complicated by the formation of aneurysms, in which by definition the vessel has at least a 50% greater than normal dilatation.

In the aorta, as well as other large arteries, early lesions show a thickened intima with foam cells and scattered lymphocytes in a fatty streak. Atheromatous plaque progression is characterized by collection of extracellular lipid with inflammation, but without significant fibrosis and without significant changes in the media. Increasing fibrosis around the lipid leads to intimal thickening and progressive degenerative changes in the media. The advanced lesions that result in abdominal aortic aneurysms show a constellation of findings including severe atherosclerosis, degeneration of the media, adventitial inflammation, fibrosis of the vessel wall, dystrophic calcification, and nonorganized mural thrombus.

C. Vasculitides. Vasculitis is a noninfectious inflammatory disease of the vessel wall and surrounding tissue. The Chapel Hill classification system for vasculitis based on the size of the vessels (Fig. 9.4) is widely used (*Arthritis Rheum* 1994;37:187).

1. Large vessel vasculitides

  a. Giant cell arteritis (also known as temporal arteritis). As originally proposed by the American College of Rheumatology (ACR), three of the following five diagnostic criteria are required for a diagnosis of giant cell arteritis: over 50 years of age, recent localized headache, temporal artery tenderness, ESR ≥50 mm/hr, and a temporal artery biopsy demonstrating vasculitis (e-**Fig. 9.29**). It is worth noting that up to 60% of patients with clinical features of giant cell arteritis show no evidence of vasculitis by arterial biopsy (*Baillieres Clin Rheumatol* 1991;5:387).

    Classically, there are four key diagnostic features of the vasculitis associated with giant cell arteritis: transmural inflammation, giant cells in close relation to disrupted elastic lamellae, intimal thickening, and marked intimal edema. Giant cells are not required for the diagnosis, but typically are present if a substantial or granulomatous inflammatory infiltrate is present. Noncontiguous foci of inflammation, so-called skip areas, are occasionally present; patches of arteritis can be less than 0.3 mm long, which emphasizes the importance of microscopic examination of multiple tissue levels (*Arch Ophthalmol* 1976;94:2072).

    The diagnosis of **healed** (e-**Fig. 9.29**) or **subacute cranial arteritis** is an indication for prolonged steroid therapy, and so is an important differential diagnosis. Focal aggregates of lymphocytes and/or macrophages in the media, irregular fibrosis and scarring of the media, breaks of the internal elastic lamella (involving up to 25% of the circumference), and irregular intimal fibrosis are the histologic hallmarks. Since the media does not contain blood vessels in normal arterial vessels, medial neovascularization is a useful indicator of previous inflammation.

    Normal changes in the arteries of the elderly can complicate diagnosis. However, arteriosclerosis typically does not include inflammation, and the associated intimal and medial fibrosis is concentric and not irregular. While the internal elastic lamella may show fragmentation, long breaks are uncommon.

  b. Takayasu arteritis. Clinical findings and vascular distribution are necessary to distinguish Takayasu arteritis from giant cell arteritis because both diseases show identical morphologic features. In more than 80% of cases, Takayasu arteritis affects women in the age range of 10 to -40 years. The aorta and typically the left mid to proximal subclavian artery are affected, although in 50% of patients the pulmonary arteries and abdominal aorta are involved. In contrast, giant cell arteritis occurs in patients over 50 years of age and typically involves the external carotid artery branches.

2. Medium vessel vasculitides

a. Polyarteritis nodosa is a rare systemic, necrotizing vasculitis that is not associated with glomerulonephritis. The lesions are segmental, and may be only partially circumferential. The inflammation may cause weakening of the arterial wall, with subsequent aneurysmal dilatation and localized rupture.

b. Kawasaki disease is febrile illness of childhood of unknown etiology that is characterized by a self-limited acute vasculitic syndrome. Microscopically, the vasculitis consists of an acute necrotizing arteritis similar to polyarteritis nodosa. Differentiation from polyarteritis nodosa is based on the distinctive clinical picture and age at presentation.

3. Small vessel vasculitides.
This group of diseases is subclassified based on the presence or absence of anti-neutrophil cytoplasmic antibodies (ANCA) (*Arch Pathol Lab Med* 2017;141:223). Since cytoplasmic ANCA (c-ANCA) mainly recognize proteinase 3 and perinuclear ANCA (p-ANCA) mainly recognize myeloperoxidase, the terms PR3-ANCA and MPO-ANCA, respectively, are also in common use (*BMJ* 2012;344:e26). ANCA-associated small vessel vasculitides are the most common vasculitides in adults.

a. ANCA-positive. There are three ANCA-positive small vessel vasculitides: granulomatosis with polyangiitis (formerly known as Wegener granulomatosis), microscopic polyangiitis, and eosinophilic granulomatosis with polyangiitis (previously known as Churg–Strauss syndrome) (*Clin Med* 2017;17:60).

The absence of granulomas defines microscopic polyangiitis. When granulomas are present, the distinction between granulomatosis with polyangiitis and eosinophilic granulomatosis with polyangiitis is made based on the presence of asthma and eosinophilia.

b. ANCA-negative. There are three main ANCA-negative small vessel vasculitides: Henoch–Schönlein purpura, cryoglobulinemia, and so-called non-ANCA small vessel diseases.

The presence of IgA dominant immune deposits in small vessels is indicative of Henoch–Schönlein purpura (also known as immunoglobulin-A vasculitis), the most common vasculitis in children (**e-Fig. 9.29**); the genetics of the Henoch–Schönlein purpura have recently been characterized, which may assist diagnosis in difficult cases (*Autoimmun Rev* 2018;17:301). The absence of IgA deposits, together with the presence of serum cryoglobulins, is diagnostic of cryoglobulinemia. In the absence of both IgA and cryoglobulins, the differential diagnosis includes various non-ANCA small vessel vasculitides including paraneoplastic small vessel vasculitis, inflammatory bowel disease vasculitis, and immune complex small vessel vasculitis (a category which itself includes lupus vasculitis, rheumatoid arthritis, Goodpasture syndrome, Sjögren disease, drug-induced immune complex vasculitis, Behçet disease, and infection-induced immune-complex vasculitis). The diagnostic criteria for this group of vasculitides have been well described (*Am Fam Phys* 2002;65:1615; *N Engl J Med* 1997;337:1512).

D. Amyloid Angiopathy. The deposition of waxy, extracellular, amorphous, weakly eosinophilic material in the absence of an inflammatory reaction, without intimal myofibroblasts or collagen deposits, is the hallmark of amyloid angiopathy.

IV. NEOPLASMS OF THE VESSELS

A. Benign

1. Leiomyoma is the most common benign tumor of veins, and usually arises in the peripheral veins. Leiomyomas that arise in the inferior vena cava have a prominent luminal component, and often represent extension of a uterine leiomyoma in the setting of intravascular leiomyomatosis.

2. Rare benign neoplasms of the large arteries include inflammatory pseudotumor and benign fibrous histiocytoma. Paragangliomas occur within the aortic adventitia.

3. Benign lesions of the endothelium are covered in the chapter on soft tissue tumors (Chapter 44).

B. Malignant

1. Leiomyosarcoma is the most common malignant neoplasm of veins, and is thought to arise from the smooth muscle cells of the media (**e-Fig. 9.30**). The tumor usually shows extension into the adjacent soft tissues; only rarely is the tumor confined to the vascular lumen. Most cases arise in the inferior vena cava in women (the female to male ratio is over 4:1) in their sixth decade. Microscopically, the tumor has the same morphologic features as leiomyosarcomas that occur at other sites.

2. Aortic intimal sarcoma is the most common malignant neoplasm of large arteries, and is thought to arise from the intima. By definition the tumor is luminal (**e-Fig. 9.30**), although some cases show focal extension into or through the media. Most cases arise within the abdominal aorta in patients in their seventh decade. Microscopically, the tumor is poorly differentiated and shows myofibroblastic or fibroblastic differentiation, although rare cases show specific histologic differentiation such as angiosarcoma or osteosarcoma. Cytologically, the tumor cells are usually spindle-shaped with marked atypia and pleomorphism.

An analogous rare tumor, intimal pulmonary sarcoma, involves the pulmonary arteries, usually in patients in their fifth decade who present with symptoms suggestive of recurrent pulmonary emboli. As with aortic intimal sarcoma, a subset of cases has the morphology of a specific sarcoma type.

ACKNOWLEDGMENT

The author thanks Joe K. M. Lennerz for his contributions to the prior editions of this chapter, especially the excellent figures and e-Figures.

SUGGESTED READINGS

Buja L, Butany J. *Cardiovascular Pathology*. 4th ed. Philadelphia, PA: Academic Press; 2016.
Miller DV, Revelo MP. *Diagnostic Pathology. Cardiovascular*. 2nd ed. Philadelphia, PA: Elsevier; 2018.
Silver MD, Gotlieb AI, Schoen FJ. *Cardiovascular Pathology*. 3rd ed. Philadelphia, PA: Churchill Livingstone; 2001.

10 Mediastinum

Louis P. Dehner

I. **GROSS ANATOMY.** The mediastinum is an anatomic region in the thoracic cavity and is generally divided into superior, anterior, middle, and posterior compartments and is bounded by the pleura laterally. However, a more recent CT-based approach has reduced the number of compartments from four to three: prevascular (anterior), visceral (middle), and paravertebral (posterior) compartments (*J Thorac Oncol* 2014;9(suppl 2):597, *J Thorac Imaging* 2015;30:247). Generally, the first rib defines the superior border and the diaphragm as its inferior border. The sternum, ribs, and thoracic vertebrae (T1 through T11-12) constitute the skeletal confines of the mediastinum. The thymus, heart and great vessels, lungs, and esophagus are the most obvious organs which occupy the anterior (thymus), middle (heart), and posterior (esophagus and aorta) mediastinum. The aortic arch and the proximal segment of the aorta (ascending and proximal aorta) are located in the superior mediastinum which is bounded by the manubrium sterni anteriorly and thoracic vertebrae 1 through 4. The embryological aspects of the mediastinum are basically those of the organs and structures which occupy the compartment.

The definition of the mediastinum also relates to the structures and organs with observable pathology on imaging studies and the accompanying differential diagnosis. For instance, the anterior mediastinum or prevascular compartment is the site of the thymus and lymph nodes with their various pathologies including Hodgkin and non-Hodgkin lymphoma, thymoma, germ cell neoplasms, infectious processes, as well as metastatic carcinoma, melanoma, and less frequently sarcoma and mesothelioma. Most mediastinal tumors (70% to 80%) in adults arise in the anterior mediastinum. The pathology of the posterior mediastinum is dominated by a variety of neurogenic–neuroblastic neoplasms and bronchoenteric developmental cysts, and is the most commonly involved compartment in children under 15 years of age (greater than 50% of cases). Overall, 50% to 60% of extrapulmonary thoracic tumors, exclusive of metastatic neoplasms, are malignant representing either lymphoma or thymoma whereas the remainder are benign (*Semin Thorac Cardiovasc Surg* 2004;16:201).

II. **GROSS EXAMINATION, TISSUE SAMPLING, AND HISTOLOGIC SLIDE PREPARATION**

A. **Fine-Needle Aspiration Biopsy** (FNA). FNA is generally performed as an image-guided or endoscopically directed procedure on suspected pathology in the anterior or middle mediastinum. Specimens are processed in the same manner as other FNA specimens, and are commonly examined for adequacy so that the results can be transmitted contemporaneously to the procedure. Given the broad range in pathologic processes in the anterior and middle mediastinum, an advanced level of experience is recommended for FNA interpretation of specimens from these sites.

One of the more common specimens is a lymph node with the differential diagnosis of an infectious and/or granulomatous process, metastasis, or lymphoma. Metastasis, usually a carcinoma of the lung (or squamous cell carcinoma of the head and neck, papillary thyroid carcinoma, or renal cell carcinoma) accounts for over 50% of diagnoses. Non-Hodgkin lymphoma (NHL), T-lymphoblastic lymphoma, mediastinal large B-cell lymphoma (MLBCL), and Hodgkin lymphoma (HL) are the most common primary malignant neoplasms of the mediastinum accounting for greater than 50% of all cases (*West J Med* 1999;170:161). Both large B-cell lymphoma and classic HL of the nodular sclerosis subtype have a considerable fibrous component which may limit the opportunity to obtain a sufficiently cellular FNA specimen for diagnosis.

B. Biopsy. On biopsy, the mediastinum offers similar challenges as the mesentery and retroperitoneum. A small, slender needle biopsy, with or without an accompanying aspiration, is often the starting point. The background fibrosis with or without lymphocytes, macrophages, and lymphocytes may suggest a possible lymphoma or represent nothing more than a nonspecific inflammatory reaction. A biopsy with extensive necrosis suggests a high-grade malignant process, but raises the issue of whether there is sufficient viable tissue for a reliable immunohistochemical work-up without the distraction of often nonspecific staining associated with the necrosis. Even in the presence of suspected neoplastic cells, morphologic detail may be compromised by compression artifact.

Clinical information such as the age, sex, location of the mass in the chest, and past medical history should necessarily be incorporated into the assessment of diagnostic possibilities before launching into an expensive round(s) of ancillary studies.

1. Fibrosis with or without inflammation. The anterior mediastinum is especially prone to undergo fibrosis in response to any number of pathologic insults whether it is fibrosing mediastinitis, lymphoma, or invasive carcinoma. In the presence of granulomas, an infection like histoplasmosis, HL, or sarcoid is in the differential diagnosis. Discrete nodules of small lymphocytes, plasma cells, and eosinophils with large pale cells should raise the possibility of HL and rarely Langerhans cell histiocytosis (LCH) (*Pediatr Blood Cancer* 2013;60:1759). If the biopsy is composed of fibrosis and scattered inflammatory cells, it may be necessary to recommend a rebiopsy.

2. Lymphocytic infiltrate with minimal fibrosis. The biopsy may represent an otherwise normal but hyperplastic thymus, especially in a child. The immature cortical T-cells are immunoreactive for TdT, CD99, CD1a, and CD5, whereas mature medullary T-cells are reactive for CD3 and CD5. Immature cortical T-cells have the same immunophenotype as T-lymphoblastic lymphoma in most cases, but widespread distribution of cytokeratin (CK7, CK5/6, CK19) is helpful in the identification of a type B1 thymoma (see below); however, CK is occasionally not expressed in the latter neoplasm (*Virchow Arch* 2014;465:313).

3. Mixed lymphohistiocytic infiltrate with or without fibrosis. If the biopsy is from the anterior mediastinum, lymphoma, both HL and MLBCL (especially in patients less than 50 years of age) are worthy diagnostic considerations. If the patient is a male and 50 years old and the infiltrate is largely composed of small lymphocytes with or without granulomas, the diagnosis may be a seminoma; B1 thymoma, lymphoblastic lymphoma, or Castleman disease are other possibilities.

4. Largely necrotic and/or hemorrhagic biopsy. An infectious process in the appropriate clinical setting should be considered, but in most cases the underlying pathology is a high-grade neoplasm. In an adult over 50 years of age with a large anterior to middle mediastinal mass, the tumor is likely of pulmonary origin and small-cell carcinoma should be excluded (CAM 5.2, chromogranin, synaptophysin, and CD56). If the patient is a male less than 40 years old, a malignant germ cell tumor (GCT) as either a primary tumor or a metastasis from a testicular GCT (a rare occurrence) is possible; immunostains for OCT 3/4, SALL 4, CD117, and PLAP are helpful in this setting.

5. Malignant round and/or epithelioid cell neoplasm. In a child or adolescent, lymphoblastic and rarely Burkitt lymphoma, neuroblastoma, Ewing sarcoma/primitive neuroectodermal tumor, embryonal rhabdomyosarcoma (possibly as one of several primitive sarcomatous patterns of pleuropulmonary blastoma [PPB]), NUT-midline carcinoma, malignant rhabdoid tumor, desmoplastic small round cell tumor (arising from the pleura), and poorly differentiated synovial sarcoma (as a pleuropulmonary SS or metastasis) are some of the various candidates in addition to several others (Table 10.1). Malignant round cells with or without rhabdoid morphology are seen in melanoma, mesothelioma, and thoracic sarcoma (*Medicine* [Baltimore] 2017;96:e6436, *Mod Pathol* 2017;30:797).

C. Resection. Surgical resection of mediastinal contents is usually restricted to thymic related mass lesions in the anterior mediastinum, the thymus gland in cases of myasthenia gravis (MG), or germ cell neoplasm (which may or may not be associated with the thymus).

TABLE 10.1 Immunohistochemical Evaluation of Malignant Predominantly Round Cell Neoplasms

	THY	THCA	MLBCL	HL	MGCT	NSCC	NUTMLC	NET-C	SARC	MESO	MM	T-LBL
CK (CAM 5.2)	+	+	−	−	+	+	+	+	±	±	−	−
CK7	+	+	−	−	+	+	±	±	±	±	−	−
CK5/6	+	+	−	−	±	±	+	−	±	+	−	−
CD5	+ (A type)	+	−	−	−	−	−	−	−	−	−	+
VIM	−	−	+	+	±	−	−	−	+	+	+	+
CD45/CD43	−	−	+	±	−	−	−	−	−	−	−	±
NUT	−	−	−	−	−	−	+	−	−	−	−	−
CD30	−	−	+	+	+	−	−	−	−	−	−	−
PAX5	−	−	+	+	−	−	−	−	−	−	−	−
OCT3/4	−	−	−	−	+	−	−	−	−	−	−	−
SALL4	−	−	−	−	+	−	−	−	−	−	−	−
CD117	−	+	−	−	+ (sem)	−	−	−	±	−	−	−
TTF1	± (A type)	−	−	−	−	+	−	±	−	−	−	−
p63/p40	+	+	−	−	−	±	+	−	±	−	−	−
PAX8	+	+	−	−	−	−	−	−	±	−	−	−

CD57	+ (B types)	–	–	–	–	–	–	–	–	–	–	–	–	–	–
CD99	–	–	–	–	–	–	–	–	–	–	–	±	–	–	+
N1ICD	–	–	–	–	–	–	–	–	–	–	–	–	–	–	+
CHR/SYN	–	–	–	–	–	–	–	–	–	–	+	–	–	–	–
S100	–	–	–	–	–	–	–	–	–	–	–	–	–	+	–
SOX10	–	–	–	–	–	–	–	–	–	–	–	–	–	+	–
BAP1	–	–	–	–	–	–	–	–	–	–	–	–	–	+	–
GLUT1	–	+	–	–	–	–	–	–	–	–	–	–	+	–	–
CALR	–	–	–	–	–	–	–	–	–	–	–	±	+	–	–
WT1	–	–	–	–	–	–	–	–	–	–	–	–	+	–	–
D2-40	–	–	–	–	–	–	–	–	–	–	–	–	+	–	–

BAP1, BRCA1-associated protein; CALR, calretinin; CHR/SYN, chromogranin/synaptophysin; GLUT1, glucose transporter 1; HL, Hodgkin lymphoma; MESO, mesothelioma; MGCT, malignant germ cell tumor; MLBCL, mediastinal large B-cell lymphoma; MM, malignant melanoma; N1ICD, Notch1 intracellular domain; NET-C, neuroendocrine tumor-carcinoma; NSCC, non–small-cell carcinoma; NUT, nuclear protein of testis; NUTMLC, NUT-midline carcinoma; SARC, sarcomatoid carcinoma; SEM, seminoma; T-LBL, T-lymphoblastic lymphoma; THCA, thymic carcinoma; Thy, thymoma; TTF1, thyroid transcriptional factor; VIM, vimentin; WT1, Wilms tumor.

Zhang K, Deng H, Cagle PT. Utility of immunohistochemistry in the diagnosis of pleuropulmonary and mediastinal cancers: a review and update. *Arch Pathol Lab Med* 2014;138(12):1611–1628; Du MJ, Shen Q, Yin H, Rao Q, Zhou MX. Diagnostic roles of MUC1 and GLUT1 in differentiating thymic carcinoma from type B3 thymoma. *Pathol Res Pract* 2016;212(11):1048–1051.

An enlarged substernal adenomatous thyroid or parathyroid adenoma may also present in the anterior superior mediastinum (*Ann R Coll Surg Engl* 2015;97:259). The other compartments with resectable specimens include foregut cysts of the middle or posterior mediastinum (most commonly a bronchogenic cyst) and enteric duplication cysts of the posterior mediastinum, as well as the entire morphologic spectrum of neurogenic neoplasms inclusive of neuroblastoma, schwannoma, and paraganglioma (as discussed below).

A thymic resection may be represented by nondescript fibroadipose or adipose tissue which upon sectioning fails to demonstrate any mass lesion (*Thorac Surg Clin* 2011;21:191). On the other hand, a mass lesion may be clearly evident by its size, shape, and weight; the latter three characteristics should be noted upon the initial gross examination before any sectioning takes place. The external surface should be described as to whether it is smooth and/or glistening, or irregular by virtue of apparent fibrosis or attached other tissues; the latter may reflect the presence of adhesions between the mass and contiguous structures such as the pericardium, lung, or pleura which may be included as part of the resection specimen. Because surgical margins are important in pathologic staging, the surface of the tumor should be marked in such a manner that the resection margins can be identified microscopically. If the superior and inferior poles of the specimen can be identified, the specimen can be bisected along that plane and the surface exposed in order to describe the salient features including any apparent capsule or pseudocapsule; circumscription or lack thereof; diffuse or lobulated appearance of the mass; uniform or heterogeneous exposed surface which demonstrates a solid, solid and cystic, or cystic mass with or without hemorrhage, necrosis, or calcifications; and any identifiable portions of attached tissues from possibly another organ(s). The selection of blocks for microscopic section should include a thorough sampling of the margins; sections of the apparent tumor should include any regional variations in the gross features. It is helpful to take a gross photograph so that it can be labeled for the mapping of blocks as to their location.

If the mass is predominantly cystic, the differential diagnosis is teratoma, thymic cyst, or cystic thymoma. A solid, or solid and cystic mass may represent a thymoma, thymic carcinoma, teratoma, seminoma, or mixed germ cell neoplasm, HL, Castleman disease, MLBCL, LCH, myeloid sarcoma (acute myeloid or monocytic leukemia), or localized sclerosing–fibrosing mediastinitis.

III. MEDIASTINAL SOFT TISSUES
A. Inflammation (Mediastinitis)

1. **Acute and chronic inflammation.** Acute mediastinitis with a purely neutrophilic reaction is usually a consequence of a contiguous infection, rupture-perforation of the esophagus, penetrating trauma, congenital duplication, or foregut cyst (*Thorac Surg Clin* 2009;19:37). A peritonsillar abscess, suppurative thyroiditis, periodontal abscess, and post-sternotomy infection, notably by methicillin-resistant *Staphylococcus aureus*, are other causes. In addition to the acute inflammatory reaction, the tissues may have a necrotizing appearance especially in those cases with the spread of an infection from the head and neck region into the mediastinum as in acute descending necrotizing mediastinitis (*Infection* 2016;44:77). With the passage of time, acute inflammation is accompanied by a mixed inflammatory response with macrophages, fibroblastic reaction, and microvascular proliferation.

2. **Chronic fibroinflammatory process (fibrosing–sclerosing mediastinitis).** This uncommon but well-documented clinicopathologic entity comes to attention with a persistent cough and fever in young- to middle-age adults (*Semin Respir Infect* 2001;16:119, *Medicine* [Baltimore] 2011;90:412). A mass lesion is usually present in the right paratracheal or subcarinal region, associated with punctuate calcifications in some cases. Less frequently, the presentation is a diffusely infiltrative process which involves more than one compartment. A needle or wedge biopsy is the usual type of specimen for pathologic evaluation.

An abnormal host response to the antigens of *Histoplasma capsulatum* is thought to account for cases in regions endemic for the infection. It has been estimated that one-third of cases of mediastinal fibrosis are an autoimmune or autoinflammatory processes such as IgG4-related disease (*Int J Rheumatol* 2012;2012:207056, *Clin Rev Allergy Immunol* 2017;52:446, *Medicine* [Baltimore] 2018;97:e10935). A post-radiation reaction is another cause of fibrosing mediastinitis (*Ann Diagn Pathol* 2017;27:43). Diffuse fibrosis of the thymus has been reported but its relationship to other fibroinflammatory process such as IgG4-related disease is uncertain (*Am J Surg Pathol* 2010;34:211).

There are several microscopic stages through which this fibroinflammatory process evolves, from a reactive fibroblastic stage with an edematous background resembling nodular fasciitis, to a dense hyalinized collagenous stage with thickened blood vessels showing similar hyalinized features (e-**Fig. 10.1**). A dispersed population of lymphocytes and plasma cells is usually present throughout the biopsy. Granulomas are not identified in most cases despite the association with *Histoplasma*. Dystrophic calcifications may or may not be present. A similar pathologic process occurs in the lung as pulmonary hyalinizing granulomas. Biopsies with a dense lymphoplasmacytic infiltrate and storiform fibrosis should be viewed with the possibility of IgG4-related disease (*Annu Rev Pathol* 2014;9:315).

The differential diagnosis includes classic HL, NHL, inflammatory myofibroblastic tumor, calcifying fibrous pseudotumor, and fibromatosis (desmoid tumor) (Table 10.2).

3. Granulomatous mediastinitis. A number of infectious etiologies are responsible for a granulomatous inflammatory reaction in the mediastinum. It is generally the case that other sites in the thoracic cavity including the lungs and regional lymph nodes also harbor the particular infection, which is usually tuberculous or fungal in nature. Active infectious granulomas show the presence of caseous necrosis; hyalinized granulomas with or without dystrophic calcifications are generally features of an inactive infection. The two most common causative organisms are *Mycobacterium tuberculosis* or *Histoplasma capsulatum*; other rare causative fungal organisms include *Cryptococcus, Blastomyces, Coccidioides, Rhizopus* group, and Aspergillus (*Cardiovasc Pathol* 2014;23:354). Sarcoidosis typically involves hilar lymph nodes without direct involvement of the mediastinal soft tissues, except in rare cases (*Respiration* 2010;79:341). Classic HL of the nodular sclerosis type may have a prominent granulomatous reaction which can overshadow the presence of isolated Reed–Sternberg cells. Epithelioid granulomas may obscure the presence of a seminoma in the mediastinum (*J Thorac Dis* 2018;10:E98).

B. Neoplasms. Soft tissue or mesenchymal neoplasms, unrelated to the heart or lungs but presenting within the thoracic cavity in one or more of the mediastinal compartments, are exceedingly uncommon, representing 2% to 6% of all mediastinal tumors (*Virchows Arch* 2015;467:487, *Virchows Arch* 2015;467:501). Virtually, every soft tissue neoplasm more commonly seen in peripheral anatomic sites and retroperitoneum has been reported in the mediastinum (*Histopathology* 2015;67:755). With the exception of

TABLE 10.2	Immunohistochemical Phenotypes of Fibroinflammatory Lesions of the Mediastinum				
	CD15	**CD30**	**ALK1**	**Smooth Muscle Actin**	**Factor IIIa**
Fibrosing mediastinitis	–	–	–	±	–
Hodgkin lymphoma	+	+	–	±	–
Inflammatory myofibroblastic tumor	–	–	+	+	–
Calcifying fibrous pseudotumor	–	–	–	±	+
Mediastinal large B-cell lymphoma	–	+	–	–	–
Fibromatosis (desmoids)	–	–	–	+	–

neurogenic tumors of the posterior mediastinum, most soft tissue tumors present in the anterior and middle compartments.

1. Benign tumors. Lipoma and schwannoma are the two most common benign tumors arising, respectively, in the anterior and posterior mediastinum. Lipomatous involvement of the thymus results in the so-called **thymolipoma** whose pathogenesis as a hamartoma or neoplasm remains uncertain (see below). Myelolipoma, lipoblastoma, angiomyolipoma, and hibernoma are other fatty tumors infrequently presenting in the mediastinum (*J Pediatr Surg* 2011;46:E21, *Ann Thorac Surg* 2013;95:1431, *Case Rep Radiol* 2016;2016:1378143).

Vascular anomalies may present as a solid or cystic lesion. Cystic vascular lesions, whether a lymphatic, venous, or lymphovenous malformation, are referred to as a lymphangioma or hemangioma (*Thorac Surg Clin* 2009;19:91, *Ann Thorac Surg* 2011;92:404). A venous malformation (cavernous hemangioma) presents more often as a mass, whereas a lymphatic malformation may be confined to the mediastinum or thymus where its pattern is one of infiltration into and through the surrounding soft tissues, thymus, and/or into contiguous areas in the neck, axilla, or abdominal cavity (*Am J Clin Pathol* 2014;142:683). Glomus tumor, likely another vascular malformation, has been reported in the mediastinum (*Virchows Arch* 2016;469:541).

2. Sarcomas. Any sarcomatous-appearing neoplasm of the thoracic space with spindle and/or round cell features should be questioned as a possible sarcomatoid carcinoma, a metastasis from an organ-related or soft tissue primary site in the chest, an extrathoracic primary malignant neoplasm, or a rare primary or more often metastatic melanoma (*Korean J Radiol* 2012;13:823, *Acta Cytol* 2005;49:424). Malignant peripheral nerve sheath tumor, synovial sarcoma, and leiomyosarcoma are the most common spindle cell sarcomas presenting in the mediastinum, but each is rare in this site. Other sarcomas that occur are Ewing sarcoma/primitive neuroectodermal tumor, desmoplastic small round cell tumor, angiosarcoma, liposarcoma (LPS) including dedifferentiated LPS with its spindle cell sarcoma pattern, clear cell sarcoma, malignant PEComa, dendritic cell sarcoma, myxofibrosarcoma, low-grade fibromyxoid sarcoma, and alveolar soft part sarcoma.

Rhabdomyosarcoma (RMS) in the thoracic space has several potential sources including metastasis, a GCT, or as one pattern in the complex primitive multipatterned sarcoma which characterizes PPB (*Ann Oncol 2002*;13:323, *Pediatr Dev Pathol* 2015;18:504). Most intrathoracic RMSs in children less than 6 years old occur in the context of a PPB, but RMS has been reported in the anterior mediastinum in adults (*Hum Pathol* 1994;25:349).

IV. MEDIASTINAL CYSTS AND NEOPLASMS. Cysts and neoplasms that present in one or more compartments of the mediastinum have a varied pathology and distribution between adults and children. In the adult, the pathology in the case of a solid mass and/or lymphadenopathy may be an infection, a neoplasm arising in the lung with spread into the mediastinal soft tissues, metastasis from a carcinoma arising in the head and neck (thyroid, salivary gland), or a primary carcinoma of the kidney, pancreas, ovary, or testis. Cysts and neoplasms arising in the lung or heart and great vessels are generally not included in the discussion of lesions originating in the mediastinum.

The location and pathologic types of primary mediastinal tumors vary between adults and children. In adults, there is a predilection for the anterior mediastinum (50% to 70% of cases), but in children it is the posterior mediastinum (35% to 45%). In terms of specific types of pathology, the following distribution reflects the age-related differences: thymic, 35% to 40% in adults (children, 5% to 8%); HL-NHL, 10% to 15% in adults (children, 25% to 30%); GCTs, 10% to 15% in adults (children, 15% to 20%); neurogenic, 5% to 10% in adults (children, 40% to 50%) and miscellaneous including cysts, 10% to 15% in all age groups (*J Surg Oncol* 2003;85:23, *Pediatr Hematol Oncol* 2012;29:141). Virtually, the entire repertoire of soft tissue neoplasms has been reported in the mediastinum in addition to those included in the WHO classification (Table 10.3), including INI1-deficient sarcomas, mesothelioma, desmoplastic small round cell tumor, NUT-midline carcinoma,

TABLE 10.3 WHO Classification of Tumors of the Mediastinum[a]

Thymoma

Type A thymoma, including *atypical variant*	8581/3[a]
Type AB thymoma	8582/3[a]
Type B1 thymoma	8583/3[a]
Type B2 thymoma	8584/3[a]
Type B3 thymoma	8585/3[a]
Micronodular thymoma with lymphoid stroma	8580/1[a]
Metaplastic thymoma	8580/3
Other rare thymomas	
Microscopic thymoma	8580/0
Sclerosing thymoma	8580/3
Lipofibroadenoma	9010/0[a]
Thymic carcinoma	
Squamous cell carcinoma	8070/3
Basaloid carcinoma	8123/3
Mucoepidermoid carcinoma	8430/3
Lymphoepithelioma-like carcinoma	8082/3
Clear cell carcinoma	8310/3
Sarcomatoid carcinoma	8033/3

Adenocarcinomas

Papillary adenocarcinoma	8260/3
Thymic carcinoma with adenoid cystic carcinoma-like features	8200/3[a]
Mucinous adenocarcinoma	8480/3
Adenocarcinoma, NOS	8140/3

NUT carcinoma	8023/3[a]
Undifferentiated carcinoma	8020/3
Other rare thymic carcinomas	
Adenosquamous carcinoma	8560/3
Hepatoid carcinoma	8576/3
Thymic carcinoma, NOS	8586/3
Thymic neuroendocrine tumors	
Carcinoid tumors	
Typical carcinoid	8240/3
Atypical carcinoid	8249/3
Large cell neuroendocrine carcinoma	8013/3
Combined large cell neuroendocrine carcinoma	8013/3
Small cell carcinoma	8041/3
Combined small cell carcinoma	8045/3
Combined thymic carcinomas	

Germ cell tumors of the mediastinum

Seminoma	9061/3
Embryonal carcinoma	9070/3
Yolk sac tumor	9071/3
Choriocarcinoma	9100/3
Teratoma	
Teratoma, mature	9080/0
Teratoma, immature	9080/1
Mixed germ cell tumors	9085/3

(continued)

TABLE 10.3 WHO Classification of Tumors of the Mediastinum[a] (*Continued*)

Germ cell tumors with somatic-type *solid* malignancy	9084/3
Germ cell tumors with associated hematological malignancy	9086/3[a]
Lymphomas of the mediastinum	
Primary mediastinal large B-cell lymphoma	9679/3
Extranodal marginal zone lymphoma of mucosa-associated lymphoid tissue (MALT lymphoma)	9699/3
Other mature B-cell lymphomas	
T-lymphoblastic leukemia/lymphoma	9837/3
Anaplastic large-cell lymphoma (ALCL) and other rare mature T- and NK-cell lymphomas	
ALCL, ALK-positive (ALK+)	9714/3
ALCL, ALK-negative (ALK–)	9702/3
Hodgkin lymphoma	9650/3
B-cell lymphoma, unclassifiable, with features intermediate between diffuse large B-cell and classical Hodgkin lymphoma	9596/3
Histiocytic and dendritic cell neoplasms of the mediastinum	
Langerhans cell lesions	
Thymic Langerhans cell histiocytosis	9751/1
Langerhans cell sarcoma	9756/3
Histiocytic sarcoma	9755/3
Follicular dendritic cell sarcoma	9758/3
Interdigitating dendritic cell sarcoma	9757/3
Fibroblastic reticular cell tumor	9759/3
Indeterminate dendritic cell tumor	9757/3
Myeloid sarcoma and extramedullary acute myeloid leukemia	9930/3
Soft tissue tumors of the mediastinum	
Thymolipoma	8850/0
Lipoma	8850/0
Liposarcoma	
Well-differentiated	8850/3
Dedifferentiated	8858/3
Myxoid	8852/3
Pleomorphic	8854/3
Solitary fibrous tumor	8815/1
Malignant	8815/3
Synovial sarcoma	
Synovial sarcoma, NOS	9040/3
Synovial sarcoma, spindle cell	9041/3
Synovial sarcoma, epithelioid cell	9042/3
Synovial sarcoma, biphasic	9043/3
Vascular neoplasms	
Lymphangioma	9170/0
Hemangioma	9120/0
Epithelioid hemangioendothelioma	9133/3
Angiosarcoma	9120/3

TABLE 10.3	WHO Classification of Tumors of the Mediastinum[a] (*Continued*)

Neurogenic tumors	
Tumors of peripheral nerves	
Ganglioneuroma	9490/0
Ganglioneuroblastoma	9490/3
Neuroblastoma	9500/3
Ectopic tumors of the thymus	
Ectopic thyroid tumors	
Ectopic parathyroid tumors	
Other rare ectopic tumors	

[a]Modified from Travis WD, Brambilia E, Burke AP, Marx A, Nicholson AG, eds. *WHO Classification of Tumours of Lung, Pleura, Thymus and Heart.* 4th ed. Lyon, France: IARC Press; 2017. Used with permission.

lipoblastoma, and Ewing and Ewing-like sarcomas. Several of the latter neoplasms are principally seen in young individuals.

A. Thymic Neoplasms. This category of neoplasms includes thymoma, thymic carcinoma, carcinoid, and neuroendocrine carcinoma (Table 10.3). These tumors arise from the thymic epithelium. Within the category of thymic neoplasms, approximately 80% to 85% are thymomas, followed by thymic carcinomas (10%), and pure neuroendocrine tumors (5%). Familiarity with the normal thymus provides insight into some of pathologic aspects of thymoma.

1. Thymoma. Thymoma presents in the anterior mediastinum with rare examples of tumors arising from the pleura, lung, and lower neck, typically in adults between 40 and 70 years (2% to 5% in children). When MG is the clinical presentation, a thymoma is found in 40% to 50% of cases, and 15% of thymomas are accompanied by MG (*Eur J Cancer* 2015;51:2444). There are several other paraneoplastic manifestations of thymomas (*Mayo Clin Proc* 1993;68:1110).

Grossly, thymoma is typically a circumscribed and encapsulated mass, measuring from a few centimeters to 10 cm, surrounded in part by fat often containing microscopic remnants of involuted thymus. A pale tan cut surface often demonstrates a lobular appearance created by intersecting fibrous bands between the lobules of tumor. Though less apparent grossly, a fibrous capsule is invariably present. Sections to include the capsule and the peripheral surgical margins are important in pathologic staging and reporting (*Pathol Res Pract* 2015;211:2, *Histopathology* 2017;70:522).

Thymomas are neoplasms which tend to maintain to a greater or lesser degree the overall architectural and mixture of cell types which are present in the normal thymus (e-**Figs. 10.2** and **10.3**). Most thymomas have a multilobular growth pattern which is accentuated by the presence of fibrous bands that enclose the epithelial islands (e-**Fig. 10.4**). In the past, thymomas were differentiated on the basis of the prominence of the lymphocytic and/or epithelial elements. This descriptive classification was systematized in the World Health Organization (WHO) classification into a series of letter designations which denote the morphology (i.e., type) and in turn correlate with the prognosis (Table 10.3), although pathologic staging in some studies is the more significant determinant of outcome. There is also some correlation between the WHO type and locally aggressive behavior with invasion into or through the capsule. Types A, AB (e-**Fig. 10.5**), and B1 demonstrate invasive features in approximately 10%, 40%, and 45%, respectively, whereas types B2 and B3 (e-**Fig. 10.6**) are invasive in 70% and 85% of cases, respectively. Though uncommon, type A (e-**Fig. 10.7**) or spindle cell thymoma may demonstrate invasive behavior (*Am J Clin Pathol* 2010;134:793). Thymic carcinoma, or type C, is regarded as a separate and distinct entity from thymoma, and for this reason not all clinical series of thymic neoplasms include type C; neuroendocrine carcinoma (or thymic carcinoid as it was initially designated) is classified separately from thymic carcinoma.

Regardless of the pathologic type, thymic neoplasms tend to have macroscopic features of a solid, circumscribed mass that is apparently well encapsulated. Gross or microscopic evidence that the capsule has been invaded, or that the tumor has extended through the capsule into surrounding tissues of the mediastinum, should be noted. If the thymoma has invaded the lung, pleura, pericardium, or great vessels, this finding is usually documented at the time of surgery with or without biopsy confirmation.

Some additional challenges in the pathologic diagnosis of a thymoma include the distinction of a type A or spindle cell thymoma from a soft tissue neoplasm like a solitary fibrous tumor or monophasic synovial sarcoma (*Appl Immunohistochem Mol Morphol* 2011;19:329) (**e-Fig. 10.7**); spindle cell thymoma may have a papillary or pseudopapillary and adenomatoid patterns. Type B3 thymoma and thymic carcinomas are not always readily differentiated from each other in a biopsy, but MUC1 expression in thymic carcinoma has been reported as a useful differential marker (*Virchow Arch* 2011;458:615). Most thymic carcinomas are devoid of immature T-lymphocytes.

Although most thymomas are classifiable into one of the five basic pathologic types of thymoma excluding thymic carcinoma (Table 10.4), there are a few morphologic patterns worth noting (*Am J Clin Pathol* 2016;146:132). The spindle cell pattern of type A can also be seen in conjunction with type B. B1 to B3 thymomas are characterized by the emergence of the epithelial pattern as the number of lymphocytes diminishes from B1 to B3. Type B1 thymoma with its prominent lymphocytic population is problematic in that the immature cortical thymocytes are immunoreactive for TdT, CD1a, and CD99; T-lymphoblastic lymphoma has the identical immunophenotype so caution is required to avoid misclassification, and immunostains for cytokeratin to demonstrate the epithelial cells are required. B3 thymoma is composed of relatively bland-appearing epithelial cells in sheets or with some architecture; the epithelial component may have atypical features which can be worrisome for thymic carcinoma but this concern can be addressed with the differential staining for MUC1 and GLUT-1 (*Pathol Res Pract* 2016;212:1048) (Table 10.5).

TABLE 10.4	Classification of Epithelial Thymic Neoplasms (A, B1, B2, B3, AB and Thymic Carcinoma)		
Type	**% Total**	**% Invasive**	**Microscopic Features**
A	8	10	Spindle to ovoid epithelial cells with diffuse or hemangiopericytoma-like pattern, no lymphocytes
B1	16	45	Resembles normal thymus with cortex-like features of immature thymocytes and scattered epithelial cells, with or without Hassall's corpuscles
B2	28	70	Lobules of large polygonal epithelial cells separated by immature T-lymphocytes
B3	11	85	Lobules of large polygonal epithelial cells in sheets with a minimal lymphocytic component; presence of mild epithelial atypia may raise the possibility of thymic carcinoma.
AB	31	40	Lobules with mixed patterns of type A (lymphocyte poor) and type B (lymphocyte rich) patterns with small spindled- to ovoid-shaped epithelial cells; overall, lymphocytes more numerous than in type A; type A and B equally represented or one pattern may dominate over the other.
Thymic carcinoma	5	5	Any pattern of carcinoma with squamous, lympho-epithelial, clear cell, myoepidermoid, basaloid, sarcomatoid, papillary, and mucinous features

TABLE 10.5 Comparative Immunohistochemistry of Epithelial-Epithelioid (Round Cell) Neoplasm of the Mediastinum

	CK7	CK5/6	p63/p40	TTF1	CAL/WT1	INI1	CD30	CD117	CD20	SALL4	MUC1	GLUT1
Thymoma	+	+	+	–	–	R	–	–	–	–	–	–
Thymic carcinoma	+	+	+	–	–	R	–	+	–	–	+	+
Squamous carcinoma of lung	±	+	+	–	–	R	–	–	–	–	–	–
Seminoma	±	–	–	–	–	R	±	+	–	+	–	–
Yolk sac tumor	+	–	–	–	–	R	–	+	–	+	–	–
Mesothelioma	+	+	–	–	+	R	–	–	–	–	–	+
Hodgkin lymphoma	–	–	–	–	–	R	+	–	±	–	–	–
Mediastinal B-cell lymphoma	–	–	–	–	–	R	+	–	+	–	–	–
Malignant rhabdoid tumor[a] (MRT)	+	±	–	–	–	NR	–	–	–	–	–	–

[a]SMARCA/BR16 1–deficient thoracic sarcoma has overlapping histologic features in common with MRT, but variable positivity for CK, SOX2, SALL4.

NR, not retained (nonstaining nuclei); R, retained (positive nuclear).

Zhang K, Deng H, Cagle PT. Utility of immunohistochemistry in the diagnosis of pleuropulmonary and mediastinal cancers: a review and update. *Arch Pathol Lab Med* 2014;138(12):1611–1628; Du MJ, Shen Q, Yin H, Rao Q, Zhou MX. Diagnostic roles of MUC1 and GLUT1 in differentiating thymic carcinoma from type B3 thymoma. *Pathol Res Pract* 2016;212(11):1048–1051; Yoshida A, Kobayashi E, Kubo T. Clinicopathological and molecular characterization of SMARCA4-deficient thoracic sarcomas with comparison to potentially related entities. *Mod Pathol* 2017;30(6): 797–809.

TABLE 10.6 Clinicopathologic Staging of Thymoma

Stage	Qualifying Features	5-Year Survival (%)
T1a (I)	Completely encapsulated without invasion of capsule	95–100
T1b (II)	Gross invasion into surrounding soft tissues or mediastinal pleural and/or microscopic invasion into capsule	80–85
T2 (III)	Gross invasion of pericardium, lung, and great vessels (established by biopsy or excision or intraoperative confirmation)	60–70
T3 (IVa)	Dissemination to pericardium and/or pleura without contiguous spread as in stage III	40–50
T4 (IVb)	Distant site metastasis (lung, skin, bone, liver)	25–30

The pathologic staging of thymomas has been more or less systematized in the wake of many proposed systems (*Pathol Res Pract* 2015;211:2, *Am J Surg Pathol* 2015;39:427, *Hum Pathol* 2018;73:7). T1 thymoma is one that fails to show any capsular invasion or extension into the mediastinal fat without mediastinal pleural involvement (T1a) or with pleural invasion (T1b) (Table 10.6). The difficulty resides in the ability to identify the mediastinal pleura (some T categories have a stage O without capsular invasion); another problem is assessment of tumor beyond the capsule when small islands of thymus or thymoma reside adjacent to the capsule. Invasion into the pericardium alone qualifies as T2, whereas invasion into the network of major vessels, phrenic nerve, and/or chest wall is T3. Although thymoma is known for locally aggressive behavior with dissemination to the pleura, extrathoracic metastases occur especially in the case of B3 or atypical thymoma; lymph nodes, liver, soft tissue (a challenge in the absence of history), bone, and skin are some of the distant metastatic sites. The presence of CD1a and CD99 lymphocytes in the background is a clue to the diagnosis of metastatic thymoma in a biopsy of suspected metastasis.

Thymectomy for MG is a long-standing therapeutic approach to this autoimmune disorder in which patients have antibodies against A-ChR (85%) or MuSK (5%) (*Clin Rev Allerg Immunol* 2017;52:108, *Semin Thorac Surg* 2016;28:561). A thymoma, often microscopic with type A features, is present in 10% to 20% of cases; follicular lymphoid hyperplasia (FLH) is present in 50% to 60% of resected thymuses without a thymoma (*Clin Neurol Neurosurg* 2013;115:432). Women less than 50 years of age are more likely to have FLH in the resected thymus and generally have a therapeutic response to surgery, whereas older patients are more likely to have a thymoma or an atrophic thymus and less likely to have a response.

Some important pitfalls regarding thymoma follow:

a. Because the lymphocytes in a thymoma are immature T-lymphocytes, they can be mistaken for lymphoblasts as in lymphoblastic lymphoma. These cells are immunopositive for CD1a and CD99.

b. While putative thymomas can measure only 1 to 2 mm in greatest dimension (microthymoma), caution is warranted in thymic resections in cases of MG; residual involuted thymus must be excluded.

c. Sharply angulated predominantly lymphoid lobules surrounded by fibrous stroma and widened perivascular spaces containing individual and small aggregates of lymphocytes are characteristic features of thymoma.

d. Ectopic thymomas can present in the neck or on the pleura, and are primary tumors in both sites.

e. When a lymphocyte-rich thymoma metastasizes, the lymphocytes may be present in the metastatic focus.

f. Primary thymic hyperplasia can resemble type B1 thymoma. However, the presence of lymphoid follicles with germinal centers in the medulla is a useful differentiating feature in thymic hyperplasia (though not present in all cases).

g. Pathologic staging of thymic carcinoma does not reliably predict the behavior of the tumor in the same sense as thymoma, because the carcinoma has a great potential to metastasize that is not necessarily correlated with pathologic stage.

h. A thymoma may be a purely cystic mass. Thymomas with liquefied, degenerated, and necrotic material within cystic spaces present the problem of demonstration of viable tumor to confirm the diagnosis.

i. A multicystic or multilobular thymic lesion may represent a multilocular thymic cyst, cystic thymoma, HL, mature cystic teratoma, or seminoma–germinoma.

j. A small biopsy of an anterior mediastinal mass especially in an adolescent or young adult may consist of thymic tissue which is normal thymus and not a thymoma.

k. Thymomas can present on the pleura and in the lung as apparent primary tumors, but these are also favored sites for recurrent and metastatic disease (*Cases J* 2009;2:9149, *Arch Pathol Lab Med* 1997;121:79, *Am J Surg Pathol* 1995;19:304).

2. Thymic carcinoma. Thymic carcinoma constitutes less than 10% of all primary thymic epithelial neoplasms, and because these tumors often have a solid, squamoid appearance, the distinction from a primary squamous cell carcinoma of the lung can be difficult, although some assistance may be provided by imaging findings. CD5, PAX8, and CD117 are expressed more often in thymic carcinomas than poorly differentiated non–small-cell carcinoma of the lung. Virtually, the entire morphologic spectrum of carcinomas has been reported as a type of primary thymic carcinoma, but most have a resemblance to nonkeratinizing squamous cell carcinoma (*Semin Diagn Pathol* 1999;16:18) (e-**Figs. 10.8** and **10.9**).

a. NUT-midline carcinoma presents in the mediastinum in 3% to 4% of cases, and its poorly differentiated features with squamoid and/or round cell features with a rhabdoid or Ewing-like appearance can be perplexing if it is not considered in the differential diagnosis (*Am J Surg Pathol* 2012;36:1222, *Mod Pathol* 2014;27:1649). These tumors are immunoreactive for p63, pankeratin, EMA, CD99 (uncommon), and CD45RO (rare). The tumor harbors the translocation t(15;19)(q14;p13.1) which produces the *BRD4-NUT* fusion as well as a few variant transcripts (*Nat Rev Cancer* 2014;14:149).

   Not all carcinomas involving the thymus represent a primary tumor. Direct extension of a primary carcinoma of the lung is the most common scenario, but other malignancies that show metastasis to the thymus include primary carcinomas of breast, thyroid, kidney (clear cell and papillary types), and GCTs.

3. Neuroendocrine neoplasms (NENs). NENs of the mediastinum are classified in the same manner as their pulmonary counterparts (see Table 10.3). In aggregate, they constitute 5% or less of all thymic neoplasms.

a. Carcinoid or low-grade NE tumor has the familiar trabecular and/or rosette-like patterns with essentially no mitotic activity or necrosis. In contrast, the atypical carcinoid is characterized by necrosis and/or mitotic activity with 2 to 10 mitoses per 2 mm^2 (e-**Fig. 10.10**). Nuclear enlargement with some pleomorphism may be seen as a patchy feature.

b. Large-cell neuroendocrine carcinoma (LCNEC) constitutes 5% or less of all thymic epithelial neoplasms. Cushing syndrome is one of the known clinical presentations, also as a manifestation of multiple endocrine neoplasia type I. These tumors are typically large and have usually invaded into the surrounding mediastinal tissues. The histologic features (e-**Fig. 10.10**) are those of neuroendocrine carcinomas elsewhere including organoid profiles and/or rosette-like formations of tumor cells with nuclear enlargement, hyperchromatism, and mitotic figures in virtually all microscopic fields. Nested and/or trabecular profiles are commonly associated with foci of necrosis, but not in all cases. Necrosis is commonly located within the center of nests with a palisade of tumor cells at the periphery. It is worth noting that rosette-like profiles are seen in thymoma and MLBCL. The combination of thymoma and neuroendocrine carcinoma patterns in the same tumor suggests that the latter neoplasm is fundamentally derived from thymic epithelium. Other patterns of carcinoma including small-cell carcinoma may accompany LCNEC.

c. Small-cell carcinoma presents in the mediastinum, but given the fact that most of these tumors are biopsied and the patient is generally managed nonoperatively, there is little opportunity to pursue the question of lung versus thymus as the primary site (unless the tumor is well demarcated and potentially resectable). It is estimated that 1% to 2% of extrapulmonary small-cell carcinomas present in the thymus (*Cancer* 2006;107:2262).

d. Thymic cyst is one of several types of mediastinal cysts (Table 10.7). Primary thymic cysts are divisible into unilocular and multilocular types. The unilocular cyst is lined by a simple cuboidal to columnar epithelium (*Int Med Case Rep J* 2015;8:215), whereas the multilocular cyst is usually lined by squamous epithelium, often in association with accompanying attenuated thymus. The surrounding fibrous stroma often has a rich network of blood vessels and inflammatory cells, usually lymphocytes. Lymphoid hyperplasia may be seen as well (*Int J Surg Pathol* 2017;801:1177). Pseudoepitheliomatous hyperplasia may be seen in multilocular cysts, which may raise the question of a thymic carcinoma, but careful inspection shows that the squamous epithelium is reactive.

Mediastinal cysts exclusive of those arising in the thymus have a diverse histogenesis including pericardial, foregut-bronchoenteric duplication cyst (middle and posterior mediastinum), vascular anomaly (lymphangioma and hemangioma), and Müllerian derived cyst (Hattori cyst). The epithelium in the latter cyst is ciliated like the bronchogenic cyst, but usually presents in the posterior rather than the anterior or middle mediastinum and is immunoreactive for WT-1, PAX8, and ER/PR. Other entities that occasionally enter into the differential diagnosis are a teratoma, microthymoma, HL, and seminoma.

e. Other types of pathology in the thymus are detected as simply enlargement or a mass. True hyperplasia of the thymus consists of an enlarged gland with accompanying respiratory symptoms, typically in an infant or young child (*Ann Thor Surg* 1989;47:741). Hemorrhage may occur into the thymus or into a cyst in the thymus; except for the size, the gland is otherwise unremarkable with preservation of the cortex and medulla. Another setting of thymic enlargement in the absence of a cyst or neoplasm is Graves' disease with FLH, similar to MG.

Thymolipoma (TL) is a presumed neoplasm composed of lobules of mature adipose tissue among islands of corticomedullary thymus (*Mod Pathol*

TABLE 10.7	Cysts and Cystic Lesions of the Mediastinum
Bronchogenic cyst (50%–60% of cases)	Thyroglossal duct cyst
Enteric duplication (foregut) cyst	Neuroenteric cyst
Pericardial (coelomic) cyst	Aneurysmal bone cyst (chest wall)
Echinococcal cyst	Multilocular thymic cyst
Thoracic duct cyst	Cystic thymoma
Pancreatic pseudocyst	Cystic adenomatoid tumor
Mullerian (Hattori) cyst	Pleuropulmonary blastoma (type I or II)
Neuroenteric cyst	Cystic teratoma
Parathyroid cyst	

Modified from Thacker PG, Mahani MG, Heider A, Lee EY. Imaging evaluation of mediastinal masses in children and adults: practical diagnostic approach based on a new classification system. *J Thorac Imaging* 2015;30:247.

1995;8:741; *Ann Diagn Pathol* 2000;4:236). TL presents across a broad age range, but is clustered in the second through fourth decades. In most cases, symptoms relating to a mass are the mode of presentation, but MG and inflammatory myopathy are other less common manifestations. Variant pathologic findings include thymoma, liposarcoma, striated muscle, sebaceous glands, and hemangioma-like foci (*Virchows Arch* 2014;464:489).

B. **Germ Cell Tumors** (GCTs). The mediastinum, typically the anterior or prevascular compartment, is the most common extragonadal primary site for this group of neoplasms accounting for 10% to 15% of all GCTs (*Adv Anat Pathol* 2007;14:69). GCTs represent approximately 15% to 20% of all primary mediastinal neoplasms. The distribution of tumor types in the mediastinum is the following: mature teratoma (45% to 55%), seminoma (35% to 40%), malignant mixed (15% to 20%), yolk sac tumor (YST) (10% to 15%), and embryonal carcinoma (1% to 2%) (*Cancer* 1997;80:699). There are rare examples of choriocarcinoma (*Am J Surg Pathol* 1997;21:1007).

Primary malignant GCTs of the mediastinum have a marked male predilection (80% or more of cases) whereas mature and immature teratomas do not have a similar male preference. Metastatic GCTs from the testis, more commonly than the ovary, can present as an apparent primary mediastinal neoplasm.

1. **Mature cystic teratoma** (MCT) presents over a broad age range from the neonatal period into early adulthood. Among mediastinal cysts, MCTs account for approximately 15% of cases. Though the most prominent gross feature is one or more cysts, solid areas may be present as well and should be sampled to exclude any malignant GC elements such as YST. Cysts lined by various types of differentiated epithelia, neuroglia, adipose tissue, and bone and/or cartilage are the various mature somatic tissues in these tumor (e-**Figs. 10.11** and **10.12**). Immature neuroepithelium should be carefully evaluated for the presence of YST. Rarely, an MCT may rupture resulting in a substantial inflammatory reaction. The pericardium and lung are other rare sites of MCT.

2. **Seminoma (germinoma)**, unlike teratoma, can present a diagnostic dilemma from other somewhat similar appearing round cell neoplasms of the anterior mediastinum. Sheets of uniform polygonal tumor cells with a central round nucleus and clear cytoplasm, accompanied by lymphocytes and granulomas, is the classic microscopic appearance regardless of primary site. However, the lymphocytes and/or granulomas may obscure the underlying pathologic process (e-**Fig. 10.13**). The differential diagnosis can include MLBCL, HL, sarcoidosis, and primary or metastatic clear cell carcinoma. Immunohistochemistry can be helpful in most cases since mediastinal seminoma has a distinctive phenotype including positivity for CAM 5.2 (70% to 80%), SALL4 (100%), SOX17 (90% to 95%), CD117 (more than 70%), CD30 (variable), and OCT3/4 (90% to 100%) (Tables 10.1 and 10.5). However, some immunophenotypic differences between the mediastinal and testicular seminoma have been described (*Hum Pathol* 2015;46:376).

3. **Yolk sac tumor** (YST), like mature teratoma, presents in the mediastinum as a single-patterned GCT that histologically can be spindle cell sarcoma–like, hepatoid, tubulopapillary, solid reticular–microcystic; with perivascular pseudorosettes, mucoid-myxoid extracellular material, or Shiller–Duval bodies; and/or necrotic (*Am J Surg Pathol* 1986;10:151, *Int J Surg Pathol* 2014;22:677, *Am J Surg Pathol* 2014;38:1396). YST expresses glypican-3, SALL4, and α-fetoprotein; the latter immunostain is often accompanied by high background staining. YST may be one of several GCT patterns in a malignant mixed GCT.

C. **Lymphoid Neoplasms.** Lymphomas of all categories account for approximately 15% of all mediastinal neoplasms overall, but for 50% to 60% of malignancies in the mediastinum (*Histopathology* 2009; 54:69). In one study of the nodal distribution of HL and NHL, approximately 10% of all lymphomas involved the mediastinum (*Medicine* [Baltimore] 2015;94:e987).

1. **Hodgkin lymphoma (HL)** accounts for 75% to 80% of mediastinal lymphomas where nodular sclerosis is the most common subtype with a predilection for

adolescent and young adult females (*Adv Anat Pathol* 2016;23:285) (e-**Figs. 10.14** and **10.15**). The pathologic diagnosis can be especially challenging because of the fibrosis and the paucity of RS cells. Either fibrosis or only a portion of a nodule may be represented in a needle biopsy. Otherwise, the diagnosis is straightforward in most cases.

2. **Lymphoblastic lymphoma (LL)** includes both precursor T- and B-cell NHL and both express TdT. Most cases of LL are precursor T-cell neoplasms, and a mediastinal mass is present in greater than 80% of cases (*Crit Rev Hematol Oncol* 2017;113:304). The less common B-LL infrequently presents as a mediastinal tumor, but more often with skin, soft tissue, and bone involvement. CD1a, CD3–CD5, CD7, and CD8 are typically expressed in T-LL, but these neoplasms can have a mixed lineage phenotype.

3. **Mediastinal large B-cell lymphoma** (MLBCL), like HL, has a predilection for adolescent and young adult females and is a specific subtype of diffuse LBCL. The large pleomorphic lymphoid cells have somewhat lobulated nuclei, prominent nucleoli, and clear cytoplasm; the tumor cells create formless sheets, or are separated into small nests by strands of collagen. Like RS cells, the large cells express CD30, in addition to CD19, CD20, CD79a, and PAX5. A small subset of mediastinal lymphomas are so-called grey zone lymphomas whose histologic features and immunophenotype overlap with PMLBCL and classic HL (*Semin Hematol* 2015;52:57).

4. **Burkitt lymphoma**, comprising 50% to 60% of NHL in children, presents in the mediastinum in only 5% of cases (*Pediatr Radiol* 2003;33:719, *J Pediatr Hematol Oncol* 2009;31:428).

5. **Castleman disease(s)** in its classic unicentric type (CUT) presents as a solitary, well-circumscribed, often lobulated mass consisting of matted lymph nodes that has a gross resemblance to NS-HL. CUT has a wide distribution, with 10% of all cases presenting in the anterior mediastinum (*Radiology* 1998;209:221). The presence of a peripheral capsule and incomplete fibrous septa between the lymphoid nodules are features that overlap with thymoma. The hyaline vascular type is the more common pathologic type (90% or more of cases); it features a penetrating small blood vessel extending into follicular dendritic cells in a germinal center, which is in turn surrounded by concentrically arranged mantle zone lymphocytes (e-**Fig. 10.16**).

Multicentric CD (MCD) is almost always symptomatic, and occurs in association with HHV-8 in less than 50% of cases and/or HIV. Follicular hyperplasia and plasma cell expansion resemble the plasma cell variant of CUT. MCD is one of several HHV8-positive disorders, including various types of lymphoma (*Am J Surg Pathol* 2017;41:795).

D. **Neurogenic and Neuroblastic Neoplasms** in aggregate account for 20% to 25% of all mediastinal neoplasms. In children, approximately 50% of all mediastinal masses arise in the posterior mediastinum, and 50% or more of these are neurogenic. In contrast, only 10% of all mediastinal tumors in adults are neurogenic, and virtually all present in the posterior mediastinum (*Thorac Surg Clin* 2009;19:47). Neuroblastoma (NB), intermixed ganglioneuroblastoma (GNB), and ganglioneuromas are the most common types in children, whereas in adults, schwannoma, neurofibroma, and ganglioneuroma are the most commonly encountered tumors (*Semin Thorac Cardiovasc Surg* 2004;16:201, *Pediatr Blood Cancer* 2010;54:895).

1. **Neuroblastoma** presenting in the posterior mediastinum represents 15% to 20% of all neuroblastic tumors in children, including all anatomic sites. These tumors tend to have favorable stages (stage 1, 2), histology (poorly differentiated NB, low mitotic karyorrhectic index [MKI], diffuse or intermixed pattern GNB; e-**Fig. 10.17**), and biologic markers (nonamplified *MYCN* and no aberrations in chromosomes 1p and 11q) (Table 10.8).

2. **Ganglioneuroma** (GN) is often detected incidentally as a paraspinal, posterior mediastinal mass in later childhood and into adulthood. These stromal predominant tumors contain generally mature ganglion cells as scattered individual or small

TABLE 10.8 Pathologic Types of Neuroblastic Tumors

Type	Histologic Features
Undifferentiated NB (UF)	High-grade malignant round cell neoplasm with high MKI and need for immunohistochemistry to differentiate from other malignant round cell tumors
Poorly differentiated NB (UF or FH on basis of age and MKI)	Malignant cells smaller than undifferentiated NB, with neurofibrillary processes, variable rosettes, low or high MKI, and absence of neuromatous or schwannian stroma
Diffuse or intermixed ganglioneuroblastoma (FH)	Individual nests or lobular foci of neuroblasts with prominent neurofibrillary processes, ganglion cell differentiation, and neuromatous stroma
Nodular GN (UH)	Distinct nodules of poorly differentiated neuroblasts with high or low MKI in a ganglioneuroma
Maturing ganglioneuroma (FH)	Microscopic foci of neuroblasts in an otherwise mature ganglioneuroma
Mature ganglioneuroma (FH)	Absence of neuroblasts

FH, favorable histology; MKI, mitotic karyorrhectic index; NB, neuroblastoma; UF, unfavorable histology.

collections of cells. Small nests of neuroblastic cells (ranging from poorly differentiated neuroblasts to intermediate stages of ganglion cell maturation) and GN are features of intermixed favorable histology ganglioneuroblastoma, which is a histologically favorable neuroblastic tumor in contrast to nodular GNB whose nodules are composed of poorly differentiated NB with high MK1.

3. Paraganglioma (PG) is a neoplasm of the para-aortic sympathetic chain ganglia and is differentiated from NE tumors (*Am Surg* 2017;83:e153, *Am Thorac Surg* 2017;163:e413). The aortopulmonary PG arises in and around the pulmonary trunk and ascending aorta. PG has a nested pattern of usually bland-appearing small round cells. Though generally immunoreactive for SYNAP and CHR, these tumors may be positive for vimentin but not for CAM 5.2, a pattern of immunoreactivity that is unlike the NENs.

V. HETEROTOPIA AND ECTOPIA. There are several types of tissues which are not usually found in the mediastinum but are normally found in the neck or abdomen. Heterotopias primarily consist of parathyroid and thyroid glands. The prevalence of ectopic parathyroid gland in individuals with hyperparathyroidism is approximately 15% (*Exp Clin Endocrinol Diabetes* 2012;120:604). An ectopic inferior parathyroid is found most commonly in association with the thymus, whereas a superior parathyroid is most often found in the tracheoesophageal groove or behind the esophagus. Supernumerary parathyroid glands (an excess of the usual four glands, which is encountered in 10% or so of autopsies) are usually found in the thymus or carotid sheath.

Pancreatic heterotopia, found in less than 1% of abdominal surgeries but more commonly at autopsy, is usually present in the stomach and proximal small intestine (*Radiographics* 2017; 37:484). It is also rarely reported in the mediastinum, and there is even a report of an adenocarcinoma arising in mediastinal ectopic pancreas (*J Thorac Imaging* 2007;22:256, *Ann Diagn Pathol* 2012;16:494). Supradiaphragmatic caudate lobe of the liver is another rare type of heterotopia (*World J Gastroenterol* 2014;20:5147).

"Heterotopic" neoplasms presenting in the mediastinum, usually posterior, are chordoma and meningioma as extra-axial tumors (*Virchows Arch* 2001;439:196, *Hum Pathol* 1995;26:1354). In addition, the range of tissues in a teratoma also formally represent heterotopia.

Ectopic thyroid is identified in about 1% of cases, usually the neck, often in the setting of a thyroglossal duct cyst, but also in the mediastinum. An enlarged thyroid gland may extend into the anterior superior mediastinum as a cervico-mediastinal goiter (*Int J Surg* 2016;28[Suppl]:S47).

SUGGESTED READINGS

Myers JL. Mediastinum. In: Goldblum JR, Lamps LW, McKenney JK, Myers JL, eds. *Rosai and Ackerman's Surgical Pathology*. 11th ed. Philadelphia, PA: Elsevier; 2018:457–500.
Suster S, Moran CA. *Diagnostic Pathology. Thoracic*. Philadelphia, PA: Elsevier-Amirsys; 2012.
Travis WD, Brambilia E, Burke AP, Marx A, Nicholson AG, eds. *WHO Classification of Tumours of Lung, Pleura, Thymus and Heart*. 4th ed. Lyon, France: IARC Press; 2015.

Serosal Membranes
Jon H. Ritter, Horacio M. Maluf, and John D. Pfeifer

I. INTRODUCTION. The serosal membranes are derived from the mesoderm, and form the visceral and parietal surfaces of the pleural cavity, peritoneal cavity, pericardium, and tunica vaginalis testis. Histologically, the serosal membranes consist of a single layer of flat mesothelial cells that rest on a basement membrane, below which is a poorly delimited connective tissue layer. The parietal surfaces of the serosal membranes are perforated by numerous narrow stomas, the so-called lymphatic lacuna, that connect with the extensive lymphatic plexus which drains the enclosed cavities. By electron microscopy, mesothelial cells show characteristic long slender surface microvilli; their demonstration can be used to support a mesothelial origin for a neoplasm that is indeterminate by other histopathologic methods.

II. SPECIMEN PROCESSING

A. Biopsy samples, from procedures performed for diagnosis or in the context of staging procedures, are usually small tissue fragments in the range of 1 to 5 mm in maximal dimension. Documentation of the number and size of the fragments is important to ensure that they are adequately represented on the slides.

B. Excision specimens, from procedures performed for benign or malignant diseases, include tissue from pleural decortication procedures (stripping procedures to remove thick visceral pleural peels that encase the lung and decrease ventilatory function), debulking procedures, and resections. The aggregate size of the tissue should be described, as well as its color and texture. The presence of gross lesions should also be documented. Gross abnormalities should be thoroughly sampled.

III. NONNEOPLASTIC LESIONS OF THE SEROSAL MEMBRANES

A. Acute Serositis

1. Acute pleuritis is usually infectious in origin and is most commonly associated with pneumonia. Gram positive bacteria are most commonly isolated, although a wide variety of pathogens can be responsible. Spontaneous bacterial pleuritis occurs occasionally in patients who have cirrhosis. Autoimmune pleuritis, though sterile, can produce clinical and pathologic findings that resemble infectious pleuritis.

2. Acute peritonitis is usually associated with a perforated viscus. When due to gastric, biliary, or pancreatic rupture, it has a chemical etiology; when due to intestinal rupture, a bacterial one. Spontaneous bacterial peritonitis also occurs, usually in children, immunocompromised patients, or patients who have cirrhosis. Localized acute peritonitis is a feature of pelvic inflammatory disease.

3. Acute pericarditis can have an infectious etiology or can be a manifestation of autoimmune disease.

B. Granulomatous Serositis can present in a number of different patterns; studding of the serosa by innumerable small nodules can be especially worrisome clinically for disseminated tumor.

1. Infectious. Although special stains can often demonstrate the offending pathogen, microbiologic cultures are a more sensitive and specific method for identification of the organism. Common causes include mycobacteria, fungi (including *Histoplasma*, *Cryptococcus*, and *Coccidioides*), and parasites (including *Schistosoma*, *Echinococcus*, and *Ascaris*).

2. Noninfectious etiologies include a reaction to foreign material from a prior surgical procedure (such as starch granules and sutures) or from a perforated organ. In women, additional causes include retrograde introduction of foreign material through the fallopian tube (e.g., douche fluid, lubricants, radiographic contrast agents), and spillage of amniotic fluid from Cesarean section.

Peritoneal granulomas can form as a response to implants of keratin produced by a neoplasm of the female reproductive tract, including mature cystic teratoma, endometrioid adenocarcinoma with squamous differentiation (of either endometrial or ovarian origin), squamous cell carcinoma of the cervix, or even atypical polypoid adenomyoma of the uterus. Microscopically, laminated deposits of keratin (sometimes including so-called ghost squamous cells) are present in the granulomas, but in the absence of viable tumor, these granulomas have no prognostic significance.

3. Autoimmune causes include Crohn disease and sarcoidosis.

4. Meconium peritonitis in a neonate can lead to a serosal granulomatous reaction.

C. **Mesothelial Hyperplasia** is commonly seen in response to chronic serosal injury. Microscopically, hyperplasia has a number of different patterns, including solid, tubular, trabecular, papillary, or tubulopapillary, and often shows limited extension into the underlying connective tissue (e-Fig. 11.1). The hyperplastic cells are often arranged in linear, parallel, or thin layers in associated organizing fibrinous tissue. Cytologically, mild to moderate nuclear pleomorphism is present, and mitotic figures and occasional multinucleated cells can be identified.

Given its architectural and cytologic features, mesothelial hyperplasia can be difficult to distinguish from well-differentiated papillary mesothelioma (WDPM). Papillary mesothelial hyperplasia has scant connective tissue in the cores and is usually accompanied by inflammatory cells. The distinction from epithelioid mesothelioma is based on the presence of invasion, cellularity, growth pattern, and cytologic atypia (Table 11.1). Knowledge of the clinical setting can be used to guide the diagnosis, although it is well

TABLE 11.1	Reactive Mesothelial Hyperplasia Versus Epithelioid Malignant Mesothelioma	
Histologic Features	**Mesothelial Hyperplasia**	**Malignant Mesothelioma**
Stromal invasion	Absent	Present (the deeper the more definitive; can be highlighted with a pan-cytokeratin immunostain)
Cellularity	Confined to the pleural surface with maturation and decreased deep cellularity (so-called zonation); not in the stroma	Dense; lack of maturation from the surface; stromal reaction
Papillae	Simple; lined by single cell layer	Complex, with tubules and cellular stratification
Vascularity	Capillaries are perpendicular to the surface	Paucity of vessels, without orientation
Necrosis	Rare (note that necrosis may be present within pleural exudates)	Necrosis of tumor area is usually a sign of malignancy
Cytologic atypia	Confined to areas of organizing effusion	Present in any area, but many cells are deceptively bland and relatively monotonous
Mitoses	Mitoses may be plentiful	Many mesotheliomas show few mitoses (however, atypical mitoses favor malignancy)

Adapted from Husain AN, Colby TV, Ordóñez NG, et al. Guidelines for pathologic diagnosis of malignant mesothelioma 2017 update of the consensus statement from the International Mesothelioma Interest Group. *Arch Pathol Lab Med* 2018;142:89 and Travis WD, Brambilla E, Burke AP, Marx A, Nicholson AG. *WHO Classification of Tumours of the Lung, Pleura, Thymus and Heart*. Lyon, France: IARC Press; 2015.

recognized that slowly growing mesothelioma can initially present as a lesion that cannot be distinguished from mesothelial hyperplasia.

D. **Metaplasias** are predominantly a feature of the peritoneal serosal surfaces in women.

Most originate from the so-called secondary Müllerian system, which by convention includes the pelvic and lower abdominal mesothelium and underlying mesenchyme. The close embryologic relationship of the mesothelium in these areas and the Müllerian ducts (which arise from invaginations of coelomic epithelium) provides an explanation for the fact that many of the metaplasias produce tissues that are a normal component of the female reproductive tract.

1. **Endometriosis** is thought to arise via a metaplastic process, through retrograde implantation of menstrual endometrium (the so-called metastatic theory), or as a developmental anomaly (e-**Fig. 11.2**). Rare cases of pleural endometriosis has been reported, as have cases of endometriosis in men who have been treated with long-term estrogen therapy (usually in the setting of adenocarcinoma of the prostate).

2. **Endosalpingiosis** typically occurs in women during their reproductive years. Microscopically, multiple dilated cysts lined by a single layer of fallopian tube-type epithelium are present. The lack of endometrial type stroma distinguishes endosalpingiosis from endometriosis.

3. **Endocervicosis,** consisting of benign glands with an endocervical type epithelium, and **squamous metaplasia**, are both rare. Both occur in women, and are primarily metaplasias of the peritoneal mesothelium.

4. **Ectopic decidual reaction** is an incidental finding in women who are pregnant or on high-dose progestogen therapy. Most lesions are not evident grossly, but when they are, they consist of small gray-white nodules which may be hemorrhagic, and often stud the peritoneal surfaces. Microscopically, the metaplasia involves the sub-mesothelial stroma, and consists of large epithelioid cells with prominent cell borders and abundant amphophilic cytoplasm (e-**Fig. 11.3**) morphologically identical to the cells comprising the decidual reaction characteristic of the fallopian tube, cervix, and upper vagina in pregnant women. Diagnostic difficulty can arise on the rare occasions when the decidual cells assume a signet-ring cell appearance.

5. **Walthard nests,** usually found on the serosal surfaces of the fallopian tube or in the mesovarium as yellow-white nodules, are usually only several millimeters in greatest dimension. They may show cystic change, and are usually lined by mesothelial cells that have undergone transitional (urothelial) metaplasia.

6. **Disseminated peritoneal leiomyomatosis** (leiomyomatosis peritonealis disseminata) is an uncommon multifocal proliferation of smooth muscle-like cells. Although the exact cause of the disease is unknown, it is thought to represent a hormone-induced metaplasia of the multipotential submesothelial mesenchymal cells of the peritoneum. Grossly, it appears as widely scattered nodules that often suggest metastatic malignancy. Microscopically, the lesion is characterized by cytologically bland, benign spindle cells centered in the submesothelial connective tissue (e-**Fig. 11.4**). A conservative approach to treatment is indicated, since the condition tends to spontaneously regress.

E. **Fibrosis**

1. **Pleura**

   a. **Reactive pleural fibrosis** is usually a consequence of prior inflammation or surgery. Often the fibrosis is associated with formation of dense adhesions. Because reactive mesothelial cells are entrapped within the fibrous tissue, careful microscopic examination with knowledge of the clinical history is required to avoid over-interpretation as mesothelioma.

   b. **Pleural plaques,** which primarily occur on the parietal pleura of the thoracic cavity, are raised, discrete, white to gray-white lesions that range from several millimeters to over 6 centimeters in diameter. When pleural plaques are bilateral, they are almost always related to prior asbestos exposure, even very low fiber levels. Causes of unilateral plaques include asbestos, as well as any process that features chronic pleural effusions. Microscopically, they consist of paucicellular dense collagenous connective tissue with a basket-weave pattern, sometimes associated with overlying organizing fibrinous deposits. Asbestos bodies are essentially never seen within the plaques. Mesothelial cells are not a prominent component of the lesion; any significant cellularity in a putative pleural plaque should raise concern for desmoplastic mesothelioma. Finally, since mesothelioma and plaques may occur in the same individual, it is not uncommon for blind biopsies to sample plaques; in this setting, additional biopsies are indicated if there is strong clinical suspicion for a pleural malignancy.

  c. **Diffuse visceral pleural fibrosis** has a number of etiologies. It is a feature of several occupational exposures (e.g., silicosis), and occurs as an advanced hypersensitivity reaction, as a component of connective tissue diseases, and as a sequela of bacterial pneumonia (especially as a result of empyema). Grossly, diffuse visceral pleural fibrosis may be difficult to distinguish from desmoplastic mesothelioma. Microscopically, the fibrosis does not infiltrate the subjacent soft tissue and has a zonated appearance, with more cellular areas near the surface while deeper tissue tend to be more paucicellular; mesothelioma has the reverse pattern. Nonetheless, careful microscopic examination, often accompanied by immunohistochemical studies, can be required to exclude mesothelioma.

2. **Peritoneum**

  a. **Reactive peritoneal fibrosis** is usually a consequence of recurrent bouts of peritonitis (often associated with long-term peritoneal dialysis), decompensated cirrhosis, or surgery, and is often associated with formation of dense adhesions. As is true with reactive pleural fibrosis, reactive mesothelial cells entrapped within the fibrous tissue must not be overinterpreted as mesothelioma.

  Sclerosing peritonitis (also known as sclerosing encapsulating peritonitis, or "abdominal cocoon") is a related lesion that manifests as diffuse sheets of white thickened visceral peritoneum that encase the small bowel and also involve the diaphragmatic, hepatic, and splenic peritoneum. Known etiologies include peritoneal dialysis, infections, autoimmune disorders, therapy with the beta adrenergic blocker practolol, and the carcinoid syndrome. Many cases are idiopathic.

  b. **Localized plaques,** composed of dense hyalinized fibrous tissue, are frequent incidental findings on the splenic capsule (often referred to as "sugar coating").

F. **Cysts**

  1. **Emphysematous bulla** are the most frequent cystic lesion involving the pleural cavity.

  2. **Peritoneal inclusion cysts** characteristically occur in the peritoneal cavity in women of reproductive age (although they also rarely occur in males, and also rarely occur in the pleural cavity). They are usually incidental findings at the time of surgery, although multicystic inclusion cysts are typically associated with lower abdominal pain and often form a palpable mass adherent to the pelvic organs that can grossly be indistinguishable from a cystic ovarian tumor. Most cases (but not all) are associated with a history of previous abdominal surgery, endometriosis, or pelvic inflammatory disease, and there is a high rate of recurrence (*Obstet and Gynecol Surgery* 2009;64:321; *Arch Gynecol Obstet* 2018;297:1353).

  Grossly, the lesions consist of single or multiple, thin-walled, translucent, unilocular cysts. Microscopically, they consist of numerous thin-walled cysts lined by a single layer of bland, flat to cuboidal mesothelial cells. The septa and walls between the cysts are composed of loose fibrovascular connective tissue. The constitutive cells are immunophenotypically identical to those of other mesothelial cell lesions. Cases in which the mesothelium has bland cytologic features with no significant atypia have an indolent course (*Cancer* 1989;64:1336), although very rare cases may progress to conventional malignant mesothelioma (*Am J Surg Pathol* 1988;12:737; *J Surg Oncol* 2002;79:243). However, cases in which the cysts are lined, even focally, by markedly atypical mesothelial cells and/or that harbor areas of conventional malignant mesothelioma are best considered low-grade mesotheliomas from the outset.

3. So-called **pericardial cysts** are the most common cysts associated with the pericardium. They can achieve dimensions of 15 cm or more. Microscopically, they are lined by bland mesothelial cells.

G. **Splenosis** is an incidental finding, and usually represents implantation of splenic tissue as a result of traumatic splenic rupture. Grossly, innumerable red-blue nodules ranging from several millimeters to over 5 cm in diameter are scattered widely through the abdomen.

H. **Eosinophilic Peritonitis** arises in the context of a variety of medical diseases including childhood atopy, autoimmune disorders (especially collagen vascular diseases), and the hypereosinophilic syndrome. It also occurs in association with lymphoma and metastatic carcinoma. Other causes include a ruptured hydatid cyst, and in association with peritoneal dialysis.

IV. BENIGN NEOPLASMS

A. **Adenomatoid Tumor** is of mesothelial origin, and usually arises in the peritoneum, also rarely from the pleura. It most commonly involves the serosal surfaces of the uterus or fallopian tubes, or paratesticular regions. Grossly, the tumor usually forms a tan 1 to 2 cm well-circumscribed nodule. Microscopically, the tumor is composed of tubular and slit-like spaces lined by a single layer of flattened cuboidal cells with bland cytology (e-**Fig. 11.5**). The cells are immunopositive for cytokeratin, calretinin, WT1, and vimentin, but negative for factor VIII-related antigen and CD31 expression, a profile that can be used to distinguish the lesion from vascular tumors. Adenomatoid tumor is clinically asymptomatic and complete excision is the appropriate management.

B. **Calcifying Fibrous Tumor** is a rare benign tumor that predominantly occurs in the visceral pleura of women with a median age of 39 years, and in extrathoracic sites in children and young adults. Grossly, the tumor is firm, gritty, and well circumscribed with an average size of 5 cm. Microscopically, the tumor is unencapsulated but circumscribed, and may entrap adjacent structures. It is composed of bland fibroblasts in hypocellular, hyalinized pattern; dystrophic calcification and variable numbers of psammomatous calcifications are present. About 10% to 15% of cases recur locally after excision, but the tumor does not metastasize.

V. MALIGNANT PLEURAL NEOPLASMS. The WHO classification of tumors of the pleura is shown in Table 11.2.

A. **Mesothelial**

1. **Diffuse malignant mesothelioma** (DMM). The WHO recommends the terminology DMM when referring to malignant neoplasms arising from mesothelial cells. The association of the tumor with asbestos exposure is well established. There is usually a long latency period between asbestos exposure and the onset of mesothelioma, usually 30 to 40 years. Non-asbestos causes include other types of mineral fibers, therapeutic radiation exposure (which carries up to a 30-fold relative risk), chronic inflammation, and carbon nanotubes (*Arch Pathol Lab Med* 2018;142:753). Recently it has been shown that germline mutations in *BAP1* define a familial cancer syndrome characterized by malignant mesothelioma, uveal melanoma, clear cell renal cell carcinoma, intrahepatic cholangiocarcinoma, and possibly other tumors (*Nature Genetics* 2011;43:1022). The lifetime risk of malignant mesothelioma in patients who carry a *BAP1* germline mutation is unclear, as is the interaction with risk factors such as asbestos exposure.

Patients with mesothelioma usually present with dyspnea, chest wall pain, and a significant pleural effusion. Constitutional symptoms include weight loss, malaise, chills, sweats, weakness, and fatigue. While the tumor may begin as multiple small nodules on the parietal and visceral pleura, it eventually encases the lung, invades the soft tissue of the chest wall, and often extends into the mediastinum with encasement of the pericardial sac and other midline structures. DMM of the pleura remains a lethal disease with essentially 100% disease specific mortality, although it is noteworthy that patients with germline *BAP1* mutations have a markedly improved survival. Selected early stage cases may benefit from extrapleural pneumonectomy

TABLE 11.2 WHO Histologic Classification of Tumors of the Pleura

Mesothelial tumors

Diffuse malignant mesothelioma
  Epithelioid mesothelioma
  Sarcomatoid mesothelioma
  Desmoplastic mesothelioma
  Biphasic mesothelioma

Localized malignant mesothelioma
  Epithelioid mesothelioma
  Sarcomatoid mesothelioma
  Biphasic mesothelioma

Well-differentiated papillary mesothelioma

Adenomatoid tumor

Lymphoproliferative disorders

Primary effusion lymphoma

Diffuse large B-cell lymphoma associated with chronic inflammation

Mesenchymal tumors

Epithelioid hemangioendothelioma
  Angiosarcoma

Synovial sarcoma

Solitary fibrous tumor
  Malignant solitary fibrous tumor

Desmoid-type fibromatosis

Calcifying tumor

Desmoplastic small round cell tumor

From: Travis WD, Brambilla E, Burke AP, Marx A, Nicholson AG. *WHO Classification of Tumours of the Lung, Pleura, Thymus and Heart.* Lyon, France: IARC Press; 2017.

and aggressive adjuvant therapy, although the role for therapy other than supportive care is controversial.

Several histopathologic types of diffuse mesothelioma have been described. Recognition of the various types is not only important for diagnosis, but also because in most series the sarcomatoid and desmoplastic variants have a poorer prognosis than epithelioid mesothelioma, while biphasic tumors have an intermediate survival. It has also been shown that certain histologic subtypes of epithelioid mesothelioma have a more favorable (with abundant myxoid change) or less favorable (with pleomorphic features) prognosis. However, accuracy of histologic typing is critically dependent on strict application of diagnostic criteria (*Arch Pathol Lab Med* 2017;141:89; *Arch Pathol Lab Med* 2018;142:747).

Comprehensive genomic analysis of pleural mesotheliomas has identified four molecular subtypes (epithelioid, sarcomatoid, biphasic-epithelioid, and biphasic-sarcomatoid). The recurrent genetic abnormalities include mutations in a specific group of genes, gene fusions, and splice alterations, results that suggest genetic analysis may help in the development of individualized therapy (*Nature Genetics* 2016;48:407).

Immunohistochemically, mesothelioma expresses calretinin, WT1, cytokeratin 5/6, and D2-40; a panel of these markers can be used to support a mesothelial origin for a serosal tumor. CEA (monoclonal), Ber72.3, MOC-31, and BG8 are the markers most commonly used to support a diagnosis of carcinoma (Table 11.3). A wider panel of markers makes it possible to distinguish mesothelioma from carcinoma of pulmonary or extrapulmonary origin in most cases (*Hum Pathol* 2002;33:953; *Am J Surg Pathol* 2002;27:1031).

TABLE 11.3	Immunohistochemistry of Epithelioid Malignant Mesothelioma	
Marker	Sensitivity (%)	Specificity (%)
Mesothelium		
Calretinin	>90	90–95
CK5/6	75–100	80–90
WT1	70–95	~100
Podoplanin (D2-40)	90–100	>85
Adenocarcinoma of the lung		
MOC-31	95–100	85–98
BerEP4	95-100	>80
BG8 (Lewis Y)	90-100	>90
B72.3	~100	~100
Claudin 4	~100	~100
Monoclonal carcinoembryonic antigen	80–100	>95
Squamous cell carcinoma of the lung		
p40 or p63	~100	>90
Claudin 4	95	~100
MOC-31	~100	>90
BG8 (Lewis Y)	80	>90
BerEP4	85–100	80

Adapted from *Hum Pathol* 2002;33:953; *Am J Surg Pathol* 2002;27:1031; *Arch Pathol Lab Med* 2018;142:89; and Travis WD, Brambilla E, Burke AP, Marx A, Nicholson AG. *WHO Classification of Tumours of the Lung, Pleura, Thymus and Heart.* Lyon, France: IARC Press; 2017.

Despite exhaustive study, no markers are available to reliably distinguish reactive from malignant mesothelial proliferations (*Histopathology* 2009;54:55; *Arch Pathol Lab Med* 2016;140:318), an observation that suggests a diagnosis of DMM based strictly on effusion cytology samples is difficult, since definitive stromal invasion cannot be definitively identified in such specimens. The use of immunohistochemistry is, however, often used to confirm the presence of invasion in problematic cases. Pancytokeratin, S100, laminin, and collagen IV are the most useful markers for identifying invasion into tissues and fat.

The recent AJCC staging scheme for diffuse pleural malignant mesothelioma (Amin MB et al., eds. *AJCC Cancer Staging Manual*, 8th ed. New York: Springer, 2017) incorporates changes in the definition of T categories, N groupings, and overall stage. Reporting should follow suggested guidelines (for example, see the College of American Pathologists Protocol for the Examination of Specimens From Patients With Malignant Pleural Mesothelioma, at http://www.cap.org).

a. **Epithelioid mesothelioma,** as its name implies, has an epithelioid morphology, usually consisting of rather bland cells with abundant eosinophilic cytoplasm, although in some cases the cells have more anaplastic features. Architecturally, sheet-like, microglandular (adenomatoid), and tubulopapillary patterns are common (e-**Figs. 11.6** and **11.7**). Psammoma bodies are occasionally encountered.

b. **Sarcomatoid mesothelioma** is composed of spindle cells that have a haphazard distribution (e-**Fig. 11.8**). Some cases resemble fibrosarcoma, others have a pattern that resembles undifferentiated pleomorphic sarcoma. Immunohistochemically, sarcomatoid mesothelioma is less likely to express cytokeratin 5/6; areas of chondrosarcomatous or osteosarcomatous differentiation may show positive staining for actin, desmin, vimentin, and/or S100. Many cases retain expression of calretinin. The potential overlap of histologic and immunohistologic features of sarcomatoid mesothelioma with sarcomatoid carcinoma and various soft tissue sarcomas highlights the necessity for correlation with clinical and radiographic findings.

c. Desmoplastic mesothelioma. By definition, this type of sarcomatoid mesothelioma consists of scattered atypical cells in a storiform or nonspecific pattern in more than 50% of the tumor, set in a dense collagenous background. This subtype is the most likely to be misdiagnosed as organizing pleuritis in small biopsy specimens; invasion of adipose tissue is the best criterion for differentiating desmoplastic mesothelioma from organizing pleuritis.

d. Biphasic mesothelioma. This subtype contains a combination of the other patterns, in most cases a combination of the epithelioid and sarcomatous patterns (e-**Fig. 11.9**). By definition, each component should comprise at least 10% of the tumor.

2. WDPM is a very rare type of mesothelioma that occurs in a wide range of patients, though most patients are elderly. An association with asbestos exposure has been suggested but not formally established. Patients usually present with dyspnea or a recurrent pleural effusion, but rarely with chest pain. At presentation, the tumor may be either solitary and localized, multifocal, or widespread.

Microscopically, the tumor features fibrovascular cores (that often have a myxoid stroma) covered by a single layer of bland, cuboidal to flattened mesothelial cells. The cells have small, round nuclei without atypia or mitoses. The presence of even superficial invasion warrants diagnosis of the tumor as WDPM with invasive foci. Similarly, the presence of significant nuclear atypia, architectural complexity, or solid areas raises the differential diagnosis of an epithelioid mesothelioma with a papillary pattern. These distinctions are important, since when strictly defined, WDPM has an indolent course with prolonged patient survival.

3. Localized malignant mesothelioma is very rare. It presents as a circumscribed nodular lesion attached to the parietal or visceral pleura, and is usually less than 10 cm in greatest dimension. It is usually discovered incidentally on imaging studies. Microscopically, the tumor has architectural patterns that are identical to DMM. Some cases are cured by surgical excision. It is interesting to note that recurrent tumors often metastasize in a pattern more typical of sarcomas, without spread along the pleura surfaces.

B. Mesenchymal

1. Epithelioid hemangioendothelioma is a low-grade malignant neoplasm of endothelial cells that can develop at virtually any anatomic site. Primary cases arising from the serosal surfaces occur, albeit rarely (*Int J Surg Pathol* 2006;14:257).

Microscopically, the lesion is characterized by cords, short strands, and solid nests of bland, round to slightly spindled endothelial cells that have an epithelioid or histiocytoid morphology and a low mitotic rate (e-**Fig. 11.10**). Endothelial differentiation is evident by the formation of intracytoplasmic lumina (said to "blister" the cells), but distinct vascular channels are rarely formed. The neoplastic cells are classically embedded within a chondroid-like to hyalinized stroma. Immunohistochemically, epithelioid hemangioendothelioma typically expresses a variety of vascular antigens including CD31, CD34, ERG, and *Ulex Europaeus* antigen; expression of von Willebrand factor is more variable. Of note, 25% to 30% of cases show focal cytokeratin expression, which can lead to an incorrect diagnosis of metastatic signet ring cell carcinoma. Most cases harbor a translocation which creates a *WWTR1-CAMTA1* gene fusion; a minority harbor a *YAP1-TFE3* gene fusion. In problematic cases, electron microscopy can even be used to confirm the tumor's vascular origin by the demonstration of Weibel–Palade bodies.

2. Solitary fibrous tumor is classically considered a pleural tumor, though it is now recognized to occur at virtually any anatomic location. Most cases, in fact, occur in extrapleural sites. The tumor is most common in patients between 20 and 70 years old. It is classified as a tumor of intermediate (rarely metastasizing) biologic potential (see Chapter 44). Most cases harbor a characteristic *NAB2-STAT6* gene fusion which results from an intrachromosomal inversion of chromosome 12.

Grossly, pleural solitary fibrous tumors can be over 20 cm in greatest dimension, although most tumors are less than 8 cm. The tumor is usually well circumscribed although not encapsulated, and has a firm white cut surface which may show hemorrhage and areas of myxoid degeneration. Microscopically, the tumor is composed of bland plump spindled cells with a so-called patternless architecture that surround branching blood vessels of the type typically associated with hemangiopericytoma (e-**Fig. 11.11**). The cellularity often varies within individual tumors, and the background stroma can show areas of myxoid change or fibrosis. Immunohistochemically, the tumor cells express CD34, STAT-6, and CD99. In a subset of tumors, the cells also show immunoreactivity for smooth muscle actin, BCL2, and epithelial membrane antigen; focal immunoreactivity for desmin, cytokeratin, and/or S100 may even be present. Significant cytokeratin expression should raise concern for sarcomatoid mesothelioma or carcinoma.

Malignant solitary fibrous tumors show an increased mitotic rate (≥4 mitoses per 10 high power fields), areas of necrosis, increased cellularity, and focal marked cytologic atypia, usually with infiltrative margins (*Am J Surg Pathol* 1998;22:1501). However, the clinical behavior of an individual tumor is not absolutely correlated with its histologic features.

3. **Desmoplastic small round cell tumor** (DSRCT) was originally described as a peritoneal tumor (see the section on malignant peritoneal tumors below). However, it is now recognized that the tumor arises at a wide variety of sites outside the peritoneum, including the pleura (though primary pleural DSRCT is very rare).

4. **Synovial sarcoma.** Both monophasic and biphasic primary pleural synovial sarcomas occur. Patients with biphasic tumors tend to be younger (third decade of life) than patients with monophasic tumors (fifth decade of life). The tumor is usually localized at presentation. Tumors that arise in the pleura have the same pathologic features as those that arise in the soft tissue.

C. Lymphoid

1. **Primary effusion lymphoma** is a subtype lymphoma that has a distinct clinical pathologic setting, presenting as an effusion without an associated tumor mass. It is defined by the presence of human herpesvirus 8 (*Adv Cancer Res* 2001;80:115) and most patients are immunocompromised; most cases arise in the setting of HIV AIDS. Immunohistochemically, primary effusion lymphoma almost always expresses CD45 but usually lacks expression of pan-B-cell antigens, although occasional cases express pan-T-cell markers.

2. **Diffuse large B-cell lymphoma associated with chronic inflammation (pyothorax-associated lymphoma)** is an EBV-associated lymphoma that is also known as pyothorax-associated lymphoma. It usually presents as a pleural mass in elderly individuals, and as the name implies, it occurs in patients who have a longstanding history of chronic inflammation, usually in the setting of pulmonary tuberculosis or tuberculous pleuritis. Immunohistochemically, representative B-cell markers other than CD20 are frequently negative, while aberrant expression of T-cell markers such as CD2 is present (*Adv Anat Pathol* 2005;12:324).

D. **Secondary Neoplasms.** Although virtually any type of carcinoma can metastasize to the pleural serosal surfaces, secondary involvement is usually due to a peripheral adenocarcinoma of the lung. In western countries, the ovary, large intestine, pancreas, breast, thyroid, and stomach are as a group the second-most common site of origin for metastatic tumors. Leukemias and lymphomas form the third most common group of tumors that secondarily involve the pleura. Since metastases to the thoracic cavity vastly outnumber mesotheliomas, metastatic malignancy must always enter into the differential diagnosis of a pleural tumor.

VI. **MALIGNANT PERITONEAL NEOPLASMS.** The WHO classification of tumors of the peritoneum is shown in Table 11.4.

TABLE 11.4 WHO Histologic Classification of Tumors of the Peritoneum

Mesothelial tumors	**Tumor-like lesions**
Adenomatoid tumor	Mesothelial hyperplasia
Well-differentiated papillary mesothelioma	Peritoneal inclusion cyst
Malignant mesothelioma	Transitional cell metaplasia
Epithelial tumors of müllerian type	Endometriosis
Serous borderline tumor/atypical proliferative serous tumor	Endosalpingiosis
	Histiocytic nodule
Low-grade serous carcinoma	Ectopic decidua
High-grade serous carcinoma	Splenosis
Others	Others
Smooth Muscle tumors	**Secondary tumors**
Leiomyomatosis peritonealis disseminata	Metastatic carcinoma
Tumors of uncertain origin	Low-grade mucinous neoplasm associated with pseudomyxoma peritonei
Desmoplastic small round cell tumor	
Miscellaneous primary tumors	Metastatic sarcoma
Solitary fibrous tumor Malignant solitary fibrous tumor	Gliomatosis
Pelvic fibromatosis	
Inflammatory myofibroblastic tumor	
Calcifying fibrous tumor	
Extragastrointestinal stromal tumor	
Endometrial stromal tumors	

From: Kurman RJ, Carcangiu ML, Herrington CS, Young RH. *WHO Classification of Tumours of Female Reproductive Organs.* Lyon, France: IARC Press; 2017.

A. Mesothelial

1. WDPM is often discovered incidentally; about 80% of cases occur in women, usually of reproductive age. Grossly, the tumor is typically a solitary to multifocal, gray to white, nodular to papillary mass less than 2 cm in greatest dimension. Microscopically, papillary fronds with a fibrous core are covered by a single layer of bland cuboidal to flattened mesothelial cells.

When the diagnosis is restricted to lesions with bland cytologic features and no invasion, WDPM has an indolent course (*Cancer* 1990;65:292). However, those cases that show evidence of invasion of organ walls or fat (emphasizing the need for thorough microscopic sampling) are associated with progressive disease and a worse prognosis, and so should be classified as DMM.

2. DMM arising in the peritoneum is rare; the ratio of pleural to peritoneal mesothelioma is approximately 10:1 in the United States. In men (in whom 80% of cases occur), the tumor is associated with occupational exposure to asbestos. In women, no association has been established, although the demonstration that asbestos fibers are present in commercial brands of talcum powder commonly used by women for personal hygiene is noteworthy (*Int J Occup Environ Health* 2014;20:318).

a. The **epithelioid** type is most common (e-**Fig. 11.12**); tubular, papillary, and solid are the most common subtypes, in that order. Rare cases, designated the deciduoid type, have a morphology that resembles an exuberant ectopic decidual reaction (*Am J Surg Pathol* 2002;24:285). Immunohistochemically, peritoneal epithelioid mesothelioma expresses the same profile of markers as does pleural epithelioid mesothelioma.

b. **Sarcomatoid** and **biphasic** types are very uncommon in the peritoneum.

B. **Epithelial Tumors of Müllerian Type.** The architectural and cytologic features of these tumors are identical to those of their counterparts that arise within the ovary, fallopian tube, endometrium, and cervix. Their morphology is thought to represent another manifestation of the close embryologic relationship between the mesothelium and the secondary Müllerian system.

The criteria for diagnosis of a tumor as of primary peritoneal origin include the following. The ovaries must be of normal in size, or enlarged only as a result of a benign process, and the extraovarian involvement must be greater than the surface involvement of either ovary. Ovarian involvement must be absent, confined to the ovarian surface epithelium without stromal invasion, or involve the cortical stroma with a maximal tumor dimension of less than 5 × 5 mm (*Cancer Res* 2000;60:1361). Finally, the fallopian tubes (especially the fimbria) must show no evidence of a primary tumor. From a practical perspective, the distinction of a primary peritoneal carcinoma from an ovarian or tubal carcinoma has little importance since the tumors are staged the same, and the clinical behavior and treatment are essentially the same.

1. **Primary peritoneal carcinoma** occurs virtually only in women; the mean age of affected patients is the seventh decade. The most common type is serous adenocarcinoma (e-**Fig. 11.13**), but clear cell adenocarcinoma (e-**Fig. 11.14**), endometrioid adenocarcinoma, transitional cell carcinoma, and even squamous cell carcinomas occur.

2. **Primary peritoneal borderline tumors** (tumors of low malignant potential) are diagnosed by the same criteria as for their borderline counterparts arising in the ovary. Serous borderline tumors are by far the most common histologic type.

C. **Uncertain Origin. DSRCT** was originally described as a peritoneal tumor that arises in young men in their second or third decade. However, the spectrum of disease is now known to include primary tumors arising at a wide variety of sites outside the peritoneum, including the pleura, extremities, viscera, bone, and brain, in patients of all ages.

Microscopically, the tumor is a primitive sarcoma with a growth pattern that includes variably sized sheets and nests of cells separated by a strikingly desmoplastic stroma (e-**Fig. 11.15**). Cytologically, the individual cells are small, round, and have minimal cytoplasm. Immunohistochemically, the cells show unique multilineage differentiation, including immunoreactivity for cytokeratins, EMA, vimentin, desmin, and neuron-specific enolase.

The t(11;22) translocation that produces an *EWSR1-WT1* gene fusion is characteristic of the tumor. Demonstration of the translocation by molecular genetic techniques, or the encoded fusion protein by immunohistochemistry, can be used to aid diagnosis.

D. Other rare tumors of the peritoneal surface include solitary fibrous tumor, inflammatory myofibroblastic tumor, calcifying fibrous tumor, and extragastrointestinal stromal tumor.

E. **Secondary Neoplasms**

1. **Carcinomas** from virtually any primary site can metastasize to the peritoneal serosal surface. By far, the most common group of metastatic tumors in women is epithelial tumors of the reproductive tract, including the ovary, fallopian tube, endometrium, and cervix. Other tumors that commonly secondarily involve the peritoneum are carcinomas of the breast, pancreas, and biliary tract; upper and lower gastrointestinal tract; lung; and sarcomas arising in the female reproductive tract.

2. **Pseudomyxoma peritonei** is the clinical term used to designate masses of jelly-like mucus in the pelvis and abdomen. The tumor producing the mucus originates from

a low-grade mucinous neoplasm of the appendix in the vast majority of cases; less commonly, the stomach, pancreas, or hepatobiliary tract are the sites of origin (*Anat Pathol* 1997;2:198). It has been shown that classification of pseudomyxoma peritonei based on the cytologic features of the neoplastic epithelium (e-**Fig. 11.16**) provides important prognostic information (*Am J Surg Pathol* 1995;19:1390). Cases in which the epithelium shows only mild atypia, which are classified as low-grade mucinous carcinoma peritonei, have the best prognosis. Cases in which the epithelium is frankly malignant, which are classified as high-grade mucinous carcinoma peritonei, are more often associated with metastatic spread to lymph nodes and liver, and have a much poorer prognosis. The presence of signet ring cells confers an even worse prognosis and should be reported.

In all cases of presumed pseudomyxoma peritonei, the surgeon should be instructed to excise the appendix, regardless of its appearance. Even if grossly normal, the appendix should be entirely submitted for microscopic examination. The surgeon should also be instructed to evaluate the pancreas, hepatobiliary tract, stomach, and intestines for any evidence of a primary neoplasm.

VII. MALIGNANT PERICARDIAL NEOPLASMS. The WHO classification of tumors of the pericardium is shown in Table 11.5.

A. Mesothelial. By definition, the diagnosis of primary DMM of the pericardium is reserved for those cases in which there is no tumor outside the pericardium except for lymph node metastases. Histologically, DMM of the pericardium has the same histologic types as tumors arising from the pleura. The development of pericardial mesothelioma is also associated with asbestos exposure, though the association is weak.

B. Germ Cell Tumors. Intrapericardial germ cell tumors are rare, but occur over a wide age range, from neonates to the elderly. Intrauterine presentations are increasingly being recognized in second and third trimester gestations due to the widespread use of prenatal ultrasound examination. Germ cell tumors of the pericardium, as with extragonadal germ cell tumors at other sites, are thought to arise from germ cells that lodge in midline structures early in embryogenesis along the normal route of migration from the yolk sack to the gonad.

Teratomas account for the vast majority of pericardial germ cell tumors. Over 75% of cases occur in children under 15 years old. Teratomas can achieve remarkable sizes, up to 15 cm in greatest dimension. Grossly, they usually have a lobulated, smooth surface. Histologically, the vast majority are mature teratomas that resemble their counterparts arising in the gonads or mediastinum, in which case the differential diagnosis includes a bronchogenic cyst. While teratomas are benign, tumors that contain other germ cell elements (e.g., embryonal carcinoma, choriocarcinoma, endodermal sinus tumor) are malignant. They are exceedingly rare, and most cases arise in adults.

TABLE 11.5 WHO Histologic Classification of Tumors of the Pericardium

Solitary fibrous tumor
    Malignant solitary fibrous tumor

Angiosarcoma

Synovial sarcoma

Malignant mesothelioma

Germ cell tumors
    Teratoma, mature
    Teratoma, immature
    Mixed germ cell tumor

From: Travis WD, Brambilla E, Burke AP, Marx A, Nicholson AG. *WHO Classification of Tumours of the Lung, Pleura, Thymus and Heart.* Lyon, France: IARC Press; 2017.

C. Other rare tumors of the pericardium include solitary fibrous tumor and a variety of sarcomas (the most common of which are angiosarcoma and synovial sarcoma).

D. Secondary Neoplasms. Metastases are the most common tumor of the pericardium. In a significant percentage of cases, a biopsy (often performed to establish the cause of pericarditis or life-threatening tamponade), provides the first evidence that the patient has a malignancy. The most common primary tumors that metastasize to the pericardium, in decreasing order of frequency, are carcinoma of the lung, breast, and thyroid; lymphoma; and sarcoma. Although lymphatic or hematogenous spread is the most common route of involvement, direct extension (e.g., by pleural mesothelioma or malignant thymoma) also occurs.

VIII. MALIGNANT TUNICA VAGINALIS TESTIS NEOPLASMS

A. Mesothelioma occasionally arises from the tunica, and rarely, even from hernia sacs. Grossly, the tumor forms nodules or papillary excrescences. The association with asbestos exposure is unclear.

    1. Malignancy mesotheliomas are most commonly of the epithelioid type, usually of papillary or tubulopapillary architecture. The sarcomatoid variant is rare.

    2. WDPM is also rare. As with cases arising in the pleura, the tumor features fibrovascular cores covered by a single layer of bland, cuboidal to flattened mesothelial cells that have small, round nuclei without atypia or mitoses. The presence of any stromal invasion warrants classification of the tumor as a malignant.

B. Epithelial Tumors of Müllerian Type have been reported.

C. Secondary Neoplasms. The tunica, as well as the lining of hernia sacs, can be involved by metastatic carcinoma. In some cases, the involvement of the tunica or hernia sac is the first manifestation of metastatic disease.

SUGGESTED READINGS

Churg A, Cagle PT, Roggli VL. *Tumors of the Serosal Membranes. AFIP Atlas of Tumor Pathology, Series 4.* Arlington, VA: American Registry of Pathology; 2006.

Travis WD, Brambilla E, Burke AP, Marx A, Nicholson AG. *WHO Classification of Tumours of the Lung, Pleura, Thymus and Heart.* Lyon, France: IARC Press; 2015.

Kurman RJ, Carcangiu ML, Herrington CS, Young RH. *WHO Classification of Tumours of Female Reproductive Organs.* Lyon, France: IARC Press; 2014.

SECTION **III**

GI Tract

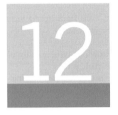

The Esophagus
Deyali Chatterjee

I. **NORMAL ANATOMY.** The esophagus, an approximately 25 cm long tubular structure that connects the pharynx to the stomach, is anatomically divided into cervical, thoracic (upper, mid, and lower), and abdominal segments. More commonly, for descriptive purposes in relation to disease processes, the esophagus is arbitrarily divided into proximal, middle, and lower thirds. It ends at the gastroesophageal junction (GEJ) just below the diaphragm, which is the junction of the tubular esophagus and the saccular stomach. The GEJ may not coincide with the histologic squamocolumnar junction, which is called the Z-line.

By endoscopy, the esophagus begins approximately 16 cm distal to the incisors and extends to approximately 35 to 40 cm. The esophageal mucosa is composed of stratified squamous epithelium, which overlies paucicellular but vascular lamina propria and is delimited by thin muscularis mucosae, which easily thickens and duplicates in response to pathologic processes involving the surface epithelium. The deeper submucosa also has a rich vascular network as well as submucosal glands connected to the lumen by ducts. The muscularis propria is composed of striated muscle in the proximal third, smooth muscle in the distal third, and a mixture of both in the middle third. The outer surface is called adventitia; there is no serosa.

II. **GROSS EXAMINATION AND TISSUE HANDLING**

A. **Endoscopic Biopsy.** When processing the specimen, it is important to record pertinent clinical history and endoscopic findings. Biopsies are typically small fragments of mucosal tissue in the range of 1 to 5 mm in greatest dimension that do not need to be inked or subdivided. Important gross descriptors are the number, the size, and the size range of the biopsy fragments. In cases where numerous fragments are present, an estimate for the number and the dimensions in aggregate should be given (documentation of the number and size is important to ensure that the biopsies are adequately represented on the slides). Routine microscopic examination of endoscopic biopsies entails examination of three hematoxylin and eosin (H&E)-stained slides, each with two to three levels of the tissue.

B. **Endoscopic Mucosal Resection (EMR)** is undertaken for superficial malignant and premalignant lesions. Operatively, the mucosa is lifted by injecting saline in the submucosa, and the lesion is then snared. The specimen can be in a single fragment, but is often in multiple fragments. All dimensions are recorded and the mucosal surface described. Inking of the margins is a matter of choice since cautery artifact will be noted at the time of microscopic evaluation for deep and mucosal margins, and since ink may actually artifactually extend along nonmarginal mucosa. The entire specimen is serially sectioned and entirely submitted. At least three H&E levels are evaluated initially.

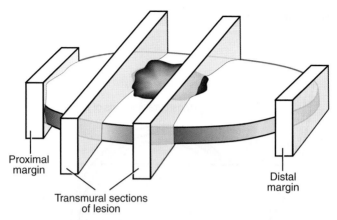

Figure 12.1 Sectioning of endoscopic mucosal resection specimens.

C. **Endoscopic Submucosal Dissection (ESD)** is more effective than EMR in removing superficial tumors. Operatively, the lesion is resected along the submucosal plane
en-bloc and ideally pinned out and oriented by the endoscopist. The specimen should
be inked in different colors to indicate the base and the oriented mucosal margins. It is
sectioned serially at 2 to 3 mm intervals, and blocked systematically, on edge, to evaluate
both lateral and base margins histologically (Fig. 12.1).

D. **Esophagectomy.** Esophagectomy specimens consist of esophagus, proximal stomach,
and attached soft tissue with lymph nodes. The radial soft tissue margins are inked and
the specimen opened longitudinally, avoiding transection of the lesion if possible. The
specimen is pinned flat for fixation. The pertinent gross measurements include the overall length and diameter of the esophagus and stomach; three-dimensional measurements
of the lesion, distance from the surgical margins, and the location of the epicenter of the
lesion in relation to the GEJ; and measurement of other mucosal abnormalities.

The standard sections (Fig. 12.2) should include a shave or *en face* section of the
proximal esophageal margin (often submitted for frozen section and assessed intraoperatively) and distal stomach margin. A few full thickness sections of the lesion at its
deepest point of invasion including the inked adventitial (radial) margin should also be
taken. Perpendicular sections of tumor with closest proximal or distal margins, if applicable, should be submitted to include the entire close margin. In instances of preoperative radiation and/or chemotherapy, the lesion may be difficult to visualize grossly and
only a shallow ulcer or induration may be present; in such cases, the entire area should
be serially sectioned and submitted for histologic examination, with mapping. All lymph
nodes identified in the attached soft tissue need to be submitted.

III. **NONNEOPLASTIC PROCESSES**

A. **Glycogenic Acanthosis.** This incidental finding is endoscopically characterized by
single or multifocal mucosal white nodules or plaques. Microscopically, glycogenic
acanthosis is seen as a thickened squamous epithelial layer with clear cytoplasm (due to
glycogen accumulation) that extends to within one cell layer of the basement membrane.

B. **Gastric Heterotopia.** Also known as the "inlet patch," this lesion is a well-circumscribed,
small (<2 cm) patch of gastric mucosa in the upper esophagus. Histologically, oxyntic
mucosa is usually present, which is often inflamed, and may rarely harbor *Helicobacter
pylori* or intestinal metaplasia (e-**Fig. 12.1**).

C. **Other Heterotopias.** Other ectopic tissues have been described in the cervical esophagus
including thyroid and parathyroid. Sebaceous glands may rarely be seen at all levels of
the esophagus. Pancreatic heterotopia/acinar metaplasia is very common at the GEJ.

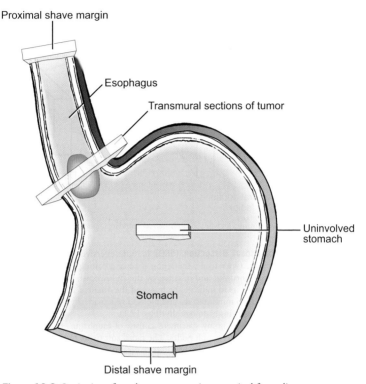

Proximal shave margin

Esophagus

Transmural sections of tumor

Uninvolved stomach

Stomach

Distal shave margin

Figure 12.2 Sectioning of esophagectomy specimens excised for malignancy.

D. **Webs and Rings.** Mostly asymptomatic, or causing dysphagia or symptoms of esophagitis, these are folds of mucosa with mild reactive changes such as parakeratosis. Webs are eccentric folds in upper esophagus associated with iron deficiency anemia (Plummer–Vinson syndrome). Schatzki rings (lower esophagus and GEJ) are complete circumferential folds composed of mucosa and submucosa.

E. **Achalasia.** Primary (neurodegenerative disorder) or secondary (Chagas disease, diabetic neuropathy, amyloidosis, etc.) achalasia leads to a lack of peristalsis, coupled with incomplete relaxation of the lower esophageal sphincter. Patients present with dysphagia. Histologically, there is loss of myenteric ganglion cells and inflammation of myenteric nerves. Other changes include squamous hyperplasia, florid lymphocytic esophagitis, periductal and submucosal gland inflammation, and atrophy.

F. **Reflux Esophagitis.** In patients with gastroesophageal reflux disease (GERD), the distal esophagus may have a range of appearances from minimal erythema to ulceration. Histologically, the damage from GERD is seen as intraepithelial inflammation with reactive changes (e-**Figs. 12.2** to **12.4**) characterized by an increased thickness of the basal layer, elongation of the papillae with vascular congestion, and basal spongiosis (intercellular edema). In severe cases, erosions can be seen as well.

G. **Eosinophilic Esophagitis (EoE).** EoE is characterized clinically by esophageal dysfunction (commonly presenting as dysphagia), and endoscopically by felinization of the esophagus (stacked, concentric rings) with ridges or furrows. It affects the proximal esophagus more than the distal esophagus. The histologic findings in EoE may overlap with PPI-responsive eosinophilia and reflux esophagitis. Therefore, a therapeutic trial of PPI is given for 6 weeks to evaluate histologic response before the diagnosis can be established. Dietary exclusion and/or corticosteroids usually lead to remission. Microscopically there is an eosinophil predominant inflammation (>15 intraepithelial eosinophils/hpf) with eosinophilic microabscesses and degranulation. The inflammation has a full thickness distribution, and is associated with marked basal hyperplasia and fibrosis of lamina propria (e-Figs. 12.5 to 12.7).

H. Eosinophilic Gastroenteritis. Commonly affecting the stomach and small intestine, there may also be some involvement of the esophagus. Unlike EoE, which affects only the esophagus, correlation with gastric and small intestinal biopsies is necessary to establish this diagnosis.

I. Lymphocytic Esophagitis. This is characterized by increased intraepithelial lymphocytes, particularly peripapillary, associated with reactive changes such as spongiosis. It is associated with a variety of conditions such as reflux, *Helicobacter pylori* gastritis, celiac disease, Crohn disease, esophageal lichen planus, graft-versus-host disease, and so forth.

J. Esophagitis Dissecans Superficialis (Sloughing Esophagitis). In this condition, there is sloughing of large fragments of esophageal squamous mucosa, with some degree of intraepithelial splitting, which on endoscopy appears as whitish strips of pseudomembranes in the mid to distal esophagus. It causes dysphagia, odynophagia, and heartburn. It has been reported to be associated with medications such as NSAIDs, but also particularly associated with polypharmacy, hot beverages, chemical irritants, heavy smoking, and chronic debilitation. By histology, there are long detached fragments of superficial squamous epithelium with "mummification" (appearance of "ghost" nuclei due to poor uptake of hematoxylin).

K. Epidermoid Metaplasia/Leukoplakia. Endoscopically seen as white plaques, histologically there are flattened rete pegs, and compact hyperorthokeratosis overlying a prominent granular layer. Associations with esophageal dysmotility, smoking, alcohol, and squamous cell carcinoma (particularly in the upper esophagus) have been reported.

L. Infectious Esophagitis
   1. *Candidiasis* is classically seen as white exudative patches over the length of the esophagus with relatively normal appearing intervening mucosa. Histologically, there is a necroinflammatory background with yeast and pseudohyphae present in the superficial epithelial layers (e-Figs. 12.8 and 12.9). PAS and GMS stains highlight infiltrative fungal organisms (e-Fig. 12.10).

   2. Herpes Simplex Virus (HSV) usually affects immunocompromised patients and presents as shallow ulcerations. The characteristic microscopic diagnostic features are Cowdry A intranuclear viral inclusion bodies (eosinophilic round bodies), ground-glass nuclei, nuclear molding, multinucleated giant cells, and ballooning degeneration of infected cells at the edge of ulcer (e-Figs. 12.11 to 12.13). Cytologically, HSV type I (most common), type II, and *Varicella zoster* are indistinguishable, and immunohistochemical staining is used for distinction.

   3. Cytomegalovirus (CMV) usually presents with multiple discrete areas of ulceration in the distal and mid-esophagus in immunocompromised patients. Granulation tissue from the ulcer base (as opposed to the edge in HSV) is the best location for identifying viral cytopathic change in endothelial and stromal cells. CMV viral cytopathic change characteristically consists of nucleomegaly and cytomegaly associated with large eosinophilic nuclear and/or cytoplasmic inclusions that can be seen on routine H&E-stained sections. Immunohistochemical staining for CMV can highlight or confirm the presence of virus.

M. Radiation Esophagitis. Acute inflammation and ulceration is associated with bizarre epithelial and stromal cells, but the cells have a preserved N:C ratio and only rare mitotic activity is present (e-Figs. 12.14 to 12.16).

N. Chemical and Drug Injury. Different chemicals have characteristic crystalline shapes and colors that can be identified in H&E-stained sections embedded in the ulcer bed, which can suggest the etiology. For example, iron pill esophagitis is recognized as an erosive injury with characteristic brown crystalline iron material embedded in the ulcer bed (an example of pill esophagitis can be seen in **e-Figs. 12.17** and **12.18**). Kayexalate crystals are refractile, nonpolarizable, lightly basophilic on H&E (and red on PAS/ alcian blue staining), and display a characteristic mosaic pattern resembling fish scales. Sevelamer crystals are nonpolarizable rusty-yellow or eosinophilic, broad crystals.

O. Chronic GVHD. This manifests in the esophagus as webs, strictures, or concentric rings due to submucosal fibrosis.

IV. PRENEOPLASTIC AND NEOPLASTIC CONDITIONS

A. Barrett Esophagus. This condition is thought to occur in a background of long term acid reflux. A diagnosis of Barrett esophagus (as defined by American College of Gastroenterologists) entails endoscopic finding of salmon-colored mucosa extending into the tubular esophagus ≥1 cm proximal to the GEJ, with biopsy confirmation of intestinal metaplasia (with goblet cells). Known risk factors of Barrett esophagus are male gender, age over 50 years, Caucasian race, tobacco usage, and central obesity. Barrett esophagus portends an increased risk for development of adenocarcinoma through the dysplasia–carcinoma sequence. The histologic features for identification of grades of dysplasia and early carcinoma are as follows:

No dysplasia: Intestinal metaplasia itself can give rise to mild nuclear enlargement and atypia, however, they are usually basally located and show surface maturation (monolayered cells with polarized basal nuclei). The architecture of the glands is normal (**e-Figs. 12.19** to **12.23**).

Low-grade dysplasia: The surface appears similar to underlying glands (i.e., there is loss of maturation) with nuclear enlargement, hyperchromasia, stratification, occasional mitotic figures, and loss of mucin. There is mild crowding of glands. An abrupt transition between dysplastic and nondysplastic zones is a helpful clue, if present (**e-Figs. 12.24** and **12.25**).

High-grade dysplasia: There are markedly enlarged and hyperchromatic cells, with loss of polarity and readily identifiable mitosis. Glands may show more crowding and some cribriforming (**e-Figs. 12.26** and **12.27**).

Intramucosal carcinoma: Architectural abnormality with extensive back-to-back microglands, syncytial growth, or single cells in the lamina propria are present. Desmoplasia may be mild, or may not be present. The glandular lumina may contain necrotic debris. Due to frequent duplication of muscularis mucosae in chronic mucosal injury and neoplastic conditions, evaluation of the depth of invasion can be difficult (**e-Figs. 12.28** to **12.30**). Unlike the colon, intramucosal adenocarcinoma of the esophagus has the potential to metastasize, therefore distinction of high-grade dysplasia and intramucosal carcinoma is critical.

Indefinite for dysplasia is somewhat of a "catch all" category which should ideally be reserved for cases with severe inflammation in which features of low-grade dysplasia versus reactive changes seem uncertain (**e-Fig. 12.31**).

Cases of Barrett esophagus with no dysplasia or indefinite for dysplasia are followed up endoscopically. Additionally, low-grade dysplasia is also ablated, and high-grade dysplasias or intramucosal carcinomas undergo local resection such as EMR or ESD, in addition to ablation.

B. Adenocarcinoma. This is a malignant epithelial neoplasm with glandular differentiation which predominantly arises from Barrett mucosa in the lower esophagus. Similar to adenocarcinomas of the entire gastrointestinal tract, these are graded into well differentiated (>95% of the tumor composed of glands), moderately differentiated (50.95%), and poorly differentiated (<50%) (**e-Figs. 12.32** to **12.40**).

C. Squamous Cell Carcinoma. A malignant epithelial neoplasm with squamous differentiation, it is characterized by sheets or nests of cells with opaque eosinophilic cytoplasm displaying prominent intercellular bridges and/or evidence of keratinization. Histologically, these tumors are graded as well-differentiated when these features are conspicuous, often with identification of extracellular keratin pearls; they are graded as poorly differentiated when there are more basal-like cells (high N:C ratio), frequent mitosis, and necrosis. Cases with moderate differentiation have intermediate features (e-Figs. 12.41 to 12.43).

Squamous cell carcinomas progress through an in situ component graded as low- or high-grade intraepithelial neoplasia (the latter is also called squamous cell carcinoma in situ, or high-grade dysplasia) based on <50% or >50% involvement of the thickness of the squamous layer, respectively. Risk factors include ethnic and dietary factors, tobacco and alcohol consumption (whose effects are synergistic), ionizing radiation, and Plummer–Vinson syndrome. It is most commonly found in the middle third of the esophagus, followed by the lower, then upper third.

Variants of squamous cell carcinoma include **verrucous carcinoma** (usually at the GEJ, associated with reflux; it grossly presents as an exophytic mass, shows a very well-differentiated histology with a pushing border, and invades locally with a very low chance of metastasis); **spindle cell carcinoma** (also called sarcomatoid carcinoma, carcinosarcoma, or metaplastic carcinoma, it has a biphasic morphology with conventional squamous cell carcinoma and a high-grade spindle cell component, sometimes with heterologous differen-tiation); and **basaloid squamous cell carcinoma** (occurring mainly in the upper esophagus in older males, it has a high N:C ratio and basophilic cytoplasm). Other carcinomas of the esophagus include **adenosquamous carcinoma**, and salivary gland-type carcinomas such as **mucoepidermoid carcinoma** and **adenoid cystic carcinoma.**

For any type of carcinoma of the esophagus, the chances of regional lymph nodal involvement are greater with increased depth of invasion. The term "superficial esoph-ageal carcinoma" is used for tumors invading into mucosa and submucosa. According to NCCN guidelines, recommended treatment for this group of tumors is endoscopic removal (resection and ablation) provided there are no suspicious lymph nodes on endo-scopic ultrasound imaging. For higher stage cancers, the options to treat are neoadjuvant chemoradiation followed by surgery, surgery alone, or definitive chemoradiation.

D. Neuroendocrine Neoplasms (NEN). These are tumors that exhibit diffuse neuroendo-crine differentiation. The diagnosis is suspected on characteristic cytologic (round nuclei with granular chromatin) and histologic features, and confirmed by immunohistochem-istry for neuroendocrine markers such as synaptophysin and chromogranin. The classi-fication of gastroenteropancreatic NEN (WHO 2017) is based on architecture (nests, cords, trabeculae, and other organoid formations) into **well-differentiated neuroendo-crine tumors (NET)** with characteristic architecture present, and **poorly differentiated neuroendocrine carcinomas (NEC)** with no organoid architecture. NET are graded into three categories based on mitotic index and/or Ki-67 proliferative index (G1–G3) (Table 12.1). Based on cell size and N:C ratio, NEC are subclassified into small cell type and large cell type (e-Figs. 12.44 and 12.45). Please note that this new classification is not reflected in the WHO 2010 Classification of Tumors of the Esophagus (Table 12.2).

Because of variation in field sizes in different microscopes, the specified area needs to be translated to the number of high power fields (HPF) according to the specific microscope used. Per CAP recommendation, mitotic rate should be reported as number of mitoses per 2 mm^2, by evaluating at least 10 mm^2 in the most mitotically active part of the tumor (e.g., for a microscope that has a field diameter of 0.55 mm, 42 HPF [10 mm^2] should be counted, and the result divided by 5 to determine the number of mitoses per 2 mm^2, to assign the tumor grade). Only clearly identifiable mitotic figures should be counted; hyperchromatic, karyorrhectic, or apoptotic nuclei are excluded.

TABLE 12.1 Grading of Neuroendocrine Tumors of the Esophagus

Grade	Mitotic Rate (per 2 mm^2)	Ki-67 index (%)
Well-differentiated neuroendocrine tumor, G1	<2	<3
Well-differentiated neuroendocrine tumor, G2	2–20	3–20
Well-differentiated neuroendocrine tumor, G3	>20	>20

TABLE 12.2 2010 WHO Classification of Tumors of the Esophagus

Epithelial tumors	Neuroendocrine carcinoma (NEC)
Premalignant lesions	Large cell NEC
	Small cell NEC
Squamous	Mixed adenoneuroendocrine carcinoma
Intraepithelial neoplasia, low-grade	
Intraepithelial neoplasia, high-grade	**Mesenchymal tumors**
Glandular	Granular cell tumor
Dysplasia, low-grade	Hemangioma
Dysplasia, high-grade	Leiomyoma
Carcinoma	Lipoma
Squamous cell carcinoma	Gastrointestinal stromal tumor
Adenocarcinoma	Kaposi sarcoma
Adenoid cystic carcinoma	Leiomyosarcoma
Adenosquamous carcinoma	Melanoma
Basaloid squamous cell carcinoma	Rhabdomyosarcoma
Mucoepidermoid carcinoma	Synovial sarcoma
Spindle cell (squamous) carcinoma	**Lymphoma**
Verrucous (squamous) carcinoma	**Secondary tumors**
Undifferentiated carcinoma	
Neuroendocrine neoplasms	
Neuroendocrine tumor (NET)	
NET G1 (carcinoid)	
NET G2	

From: Bosman FT, Carneiro F, Hruban RH, Theise ND, eds. *WHO Classification of Tumours of the Digestive System*. Lyon, France: IARC Press; 2017. Used with permission.

Ki-67 index is reported as percent positive tumor cells in area of highest nuclear labeling ("hot spot"). "Eye-balling" is discouraged, especially for tumors with a Ki-67 index close to grade cut-offs; instead it is recommended that a manual count be performed on a print of a camera-captured image of the hot spot. It has also been recommended that a minimum of 500 tumor cells be counted to determine the Ki-67 index, with a notation if less cells are available for counting. Of note, the grade assigned based on Ki-67 index is typically higher than that based on mitotic count, and the case is assigned to the higher of the two if both methods are performed.

Mixed neuroendocrine–nonneuroendocrine epithelial neoplasm (MiNEN) is a relatively new term used to encompass the group of neoplasms composed of at least two separate histologic entities, one with neuroendocrine differentiation and one without. Mixed adenoneuroendocrine carcinoma (MANEC) is a subgroup in which the two components of the tumor are adenocarcinoma and high-grade neuroendocrine carcinoma. The diagnostic criteria were previously restricted to only those cases in which either component represented at least 30% of the lesion, but recent studies have shown a prognostic significance of the high-grade malignant component even if it represents <30% of the tumor. Consequently, it is currently recommended that the histologic components be reported, specifying the percentage of each component, even when the percentage of one component may not reach a cut-off of 30%.

E. **Benign Epithelial Neoplasms.** **Squamous papillomas** are not very common lesions in the esophagus, and usually present as small polyps in distal esophagus, with some association with GERD. Histologically, they are composed of bland polypoid squamous mucosa with fibrovascular cores (e-**Fig. 12.46**). A subset can be linked to HPV infection, especially in association with laryngeal papillomatosis, and there are rare reports of associated high-grade dysplasia, and synchronous or metachronous carcinomas.

F. Mesenchymal Neoplasms.

1. **Granular cell tumors** (GCT) are rare, although the esophagus is the commonest gastrointestinal site for this neoplasm. There is a female and African-American predominance, and typically the tumor presents as an incidental submucosal lesion. Microscopically, GCT is composed of circumscribed, unencapsulated nests and sheets of closely packed cells with abundant granular amphophilic cytoplasm which are S100 and PASD positive. The nuclei are small and pyknotic. The overlying epithelium can show pseudoepitheliomatous hyperplasia (e-**Figs. 12.47** to **12.49**). Rare cases with cytologic atypia, mitosis, and metastasis have been reported.

2. **Giant fibrovascular polyp** is a rare, sausage-shaped pedunculated lesions in upper esophagus with a smooth or lobulated surface and bulbous tip, histologically corresponding to an unremarkable squamous epithelium covering a fibrovascular and adipose tissue core. Because of its size, endoscopic removal is often not complete and may lead to recurrences, therefore an esophagectomy is often required for complete removal.

3. **Leiomyoma** is the most common spindle cell neoplasm of the esophagus. It usually occurs in a relatively young population (median age 35 years) with a male predominance. It usually presents as an intramural, well-circumscribed nodule in the middle to distal esophagus. The firm white-grey cut surface microscopically shows whorls of benign smooth muscle cells which stain positively for desmin and SMA.

4. **GIST (gastrointestinal stromal tumor)** is rare in esophagus (see Chapter 13 for a more complete discussion).

5. **Other mesenchymal tumors** such as rhabdomyoma, hemangioma, lipoma, glomus tumor, rhabdomyosarcoma, synovial sarcoma, and so forth have been reported but occur at a very low frequency in the esophagus.

G. Other Neoplasms.
These are also rare, but should be kept in the differential when encountering an unusual neoplasm, and accordingly, immunohistochemical stains to exclude these entities should be included in the panel.

1. **Melanoma.** Primary melanoma of the esophagus occurs as a pigmented, polypoid lesion in the middle to distal esophagus.

2. **Lymphoma.** Primary lymphoma of the esophagus is rare. The most common type is diffuse large B cell lymphoma, though MALT lymphoma and T cell lymphomas have been described.

3. **Metastasis.** Though uncommonly a site for metastatic disease, breast, lung, and melanoma are the most common malignancies to metastasize to the esophagus.

V. STAGING AND REPORTING.
In the most recent staging scheme for epithelial cancers of the esophagus and esophagogastric junction (Amin MB et al., eds. *AJCC Cancer Staging Manual.* 8th ed. New York: Springer, 2017), due to the unique lymphatic anatomy of the esophagus, stage groupings are not based on an orderly increase in T category and number of involved lymph nodes. Of note, sarcomas and GISTs of the esophagus are staged using the AJCC schemes for soft tissue sarcoma of the trunk and extremities and GIST, respectively.

Reporting follows suggested guidelines (e.g., see the College of American Pathologists Protocol for the Examination of Specimens From Patients With Carcinoma of the Esophagus, at http://www.cap.org).

ACKNOWLEDGMENT

The author thanks Danielle H. Carpenter and Elizabeth M. Brunt, authors of the previous edition of this chapter.

Cytopathology of the Esophagus

Cory Bernadt

I. INTRODUCTION. Indications for esophageal cytologic examination include a suspected neoplasm, an infection, or for surveillance of Barrett esophagus. Mucosal abnormalities are best sampled with endoscopic brushing for circumferential sampling; endoscopic ultrasound-guided fine needle aspiration (EUS-FNA) may be employed to sample targeted mucosal lesions, intramural masses, and for staging of esophageal carcinoma via transmural sampling of paraesophageal lymph nodes. EUS-FNA is the accepted nodal staging modality for esophageal cancer and has a 81% to 97% sensitivity, 83% to 100% specificity, and 83% to 97% accuracy for malignancy (*Ann Thorac Cardiovasc* Surg 2003;9:2).

II. INFECTION/REACTIVE ATYPIA. Brushings are employed in the setting of infection, usually in a patient with esophagitis, erosions, or ulcers. As in other squamous epithelial sites, reactive and reparative atypia are characterized by cohesive two-dimensional sheets of cells that have slightly enlarged nuclei, smooth nuclear contours, and conspicuous nucleoli. Features worrisome for dysplasia such as marked nuclear crowding or a single-cell distribution pattern are lacking. A background of acute inflammation and some debris is typically present. Gastroesophageal reflux disease is not generally an indication for brushings, but some reactive atypia related to epithelial repair may be noted.

Reactive atypia is also present in radiation esophagitis. However, radiation esophagitis will also show the features characteristically present after radiation therapy, such as large bizarre cells, multinucleation, and biphasic cytoplasm.

A. Candidal Esophagitis displays pseudohyphae and yeast form (e-**Fig. 12.50**). Oral contamination should be excluded, especially in the absence of inflammation.

B. Herpetic Esophagitis (almost always HSV-1) shows herpes viral cytopathic effect characterized by ground glass chromatin, thick nuclear membranes, multinucleation, and nuclear molding (e-**Fig. 12.51**). Cowdry type A viral inclusions (distinct eosinophilic nuclear inclusions surrounded by a clear halo and a thick nuclear membrane are present) (e-**Fig. 12.52**).

C. CMV Esophagitis demonstrates significantly enlarged mononuclear cells with a large intranuclear inclusion separated from a thickened nuclear membrane by a clear halo. Occasional cytoplasmic granular inclusions are also present.

III. BARRETT ESOPHAGUS. Cytologic diagnosis relies on the identification of goblet cells within sheets of benign glandular cells. The goblet cells exhibit a single large cytoplasmic vacuole that displaces the nucleus creating a crescent-shaped nucleus. The diameter of the vacuole is at least three times the width of a normal columnar cell (*Am J Clin Pathol* 1988;89:493; *Hum Pathol* 1997;28:465).

Dysplasia in Barrett esophagus. Brushing cytology as a screening tool offers the advantage of sampling a wider area of abnormal mucosa as compared with biopsy. The presence of dysplasia and malignancy is evaluated based on architectural irregularities, cell cohesion, and cytologic atypia. As interobserver discrepancy is high, any dysplasia identified in cytology specimens should be confirmed by biopsy (*Hum Pathol* 1997;28:465). Dysplastic changes are categorized as low-grade and high-grade; high-grade lesions contain more severe cytologic atypia including an increased nuclear:cytoplasmic ratio, nuclear enlargement, hyperchromasia, and nuclear contour irregularity. Cytology has excellent specificity and good sensitivity for the detection of high-grade dysplasia, but poor sensitivity for the detection of low-grade dysplasia (*Diagn Cytopathol* 2003;29:130; *Endoscopy* 2010;42:800).

IV. NEOPLASMS

A. Intramural Neoplasms include gastrointestinal stromal tumor, schwannoma, and leiomyoma. Findings include microfragments composed of spindle shaped cells with oval to spindled nuclei, fine chromatin, and delicate cytoplasm. The distinction among these low-grade spindle cell neoplasms rests on immunohistochemistry (*Am J Clin Pathol* 2003;119:703).

   GCT, which may present as a circumscribed or infiltrative process, is characterized by squamous hypertrophy of the overlying mucosa. The tumor cells themselves are polygonal with granular, eosinophilic cytoplasm. Immunoreactivity for S-100 may be helpful in establishing the diagnosis (*J Gastrointest Cancer* 2008;39:107).

B. **Adenocarcinoma.** The specimen is highly cellular consisting of haphazardly arranged three-dimensional clusters and abundant isolated atypical cells (**e-Fig. 12.53**). Nuclear atypia and pleomorphism are marked. Necrosis may be present. The distinction from high-grade dysplasia is difficult by cytomorphology alone, and the distinction requires excisional biopsies to provide histologic architecture to determine submucosal invasion (*Hum Pathol* 1997;28:465; *Endoscopy* 2010;42:800).

C. **Squamous Cell Carcinoma.** Well-differentiated squamous cell carcinoma displays abundant isolated cells with hyperchromatic and pyknotic nuclei, keratinized cytoplasm with sharp cytoplasmic borders, spindle and tadpole shaped malignant cells, and necrosis (**e-Fig. 12.54**). Poorly-differentiated squamous cell carcinoma shows crowded groups and isolated cells with enlarged nuclei and coarsely clumpy chromatin; distinction from poorly differentiated adenocarcinoma may be difficult due to lack of keratinization.

D. **Secondary Tumors and Metastases.** The most common form of secondary tumor spread to the esophagus is by direct extension of a thyroidal, pulmonary, or laryngeal carcinoma. Rarely, hematogenous metastases to the esophagus have been reported, usually arising from the stomach, breast, larynx, or pancreas. The diagnostic workup rests on recognition of cytomorphology not native to the esophagus coupled with immunohistochemical studies.

ACKNOWLEDGMENT

The author thanks Julie Kunkel, author of the previous edition of this section.

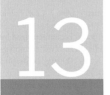

The Stomach

Iván González and Deyali Chatterjee

I. NORMAL ANATOMY. The stomach, a distensible, J-shaped organ, is traditionally divided into five anatomic regions: cardia, fundus, body, antrum, and pyloric canal. The cardia is an ill-defined region distal to the Z-line (squamocolumnar junction) of the gastroesophageal junction (GEJ) and is currently thought to be more likely metaplastic than embryologic in development. The fundus is the region that curves lateral and superior to the level of the GEJ. The remainder of the stomach up to the incisura angularis is the body. The pylorus begins at the incisura angularis, and comprises the antrum (featuring more flattened and firmly anchored mucosa than the fundus or body) and more distally the pyloric canal (an anatomic sphincter surrounded by thickened smooth muscles, controlling passage of food into the duodenum). The stomach ends at the pyloric sphincter.

The mucosal lining is of three types. Cardiac mucosa is composed of only mucus secreting glands (**e-Fig. 13.1**). Oxyntic mucosa, lining the fundus and body, has a predominance of gastric parietal (oxyntic) cells which produce acid and intrinsic factor; a lesser number of chief (zymogenic/peptic) cells which produce pepsinogen; and scattered histamine secreting enterochromaffin-like (ECL) cells (**e-Fig. 13.2**). Antral mucosa is restricted to the pylorus, and in addition to mucus cells, harbors gastrin-producing G cells scattered within the gastric glands which have a distinctive fried-egg appearance (**e-Fig. 13.3**). The surface of the entire gastric mucosa is lined by a special mucous epithelium called foveolar epithelium. The mucus neck cells harbor the regenerative cells of the stomach.

The lamina propria of the stomach normally contains sparse inflammatory cells including lymphocytes, plasma cells, eosinophils, and mast cells. The muscularis mucosae, submucosa, and serosa of the stomach are histologically similar to those of the intestines. The muscularis propria is thickened as compared with the rest of the digestive tract, and consists of three layers of muscle, with addition of an inner oblique layer to the two other commonly present layers (arranged as middle circular and outer longitudinal).

II. GROSS EXAMINATION AND TISSUE HANDLING

A. Smaller specimens can come in the form of endoscopic biopsies, endoscopic mucosal resections, and endoscopic submucosal dissection (the latter two are discussed in Chapter 12). The handling of polypectomy specimens is discussed in Chapter 14.

B. Gastrectomy (often including a portion of the duodenum or esophagus) may be partial or total. The serosal surface should be examined for evidence of tumor penetration and the area overlying the tumor inked (**e-Fig. 13.4**). After opening longitudinally along the greater curvature without transecting the tumor (**e-Fig. 13.5**), the specimen should be pinned on a corkboard (with the mucosal surface facing out) and fixed in formalin overnight to ensure well-fixed and oriented sections. Standard measurements include the length of the greater and lesser curvatures, diameter/circumference at the resection margins, and wall thickness. If a tumor is grossly identified, its location, shape, dimensions, and distance from the margins should be recorded. The tumor should be cross-sectioned and an estimate of the depth of invasion recorded (**e-Fig. 13.6**). The presence of any other mucosal abnormalities should also be noted. The tumor should be entirely submitted if it is small; larger tumors should be sampled at least one section per centimeter, including the deepest invasion and relationship of tumor to uninvolved mucosa. Sections from other mucosal lesions, and uninvolved antrum and body, should also be submitted. The distance of tumor from the radial margins (lesser/greater curvature margin) should be measured. If the tumor is distant from the margins, a single shave section from the proximal and distal margins is adequate; however, if the tumor approaches the margins, radial sections demonstrating the relationship of tumor to margin are preferred. A careful lymph node dissection should be performed; all perigastric lymph nodes are considered regional lymph nodes.

If a previously diagnosed adenocarcinoma cannot be confirmed by a grossly visible lesion, careful examination of the gastric mucosa should be performed to identify subtle mucosal alterations including erosions and effacement of folds. Multiple sections should be taken of any of the abnormalities noted, and a diagram of the sections constructed for later reference. In resections after neoadjuvant therapy, the entire tumor bed should ideally be submitted to assess accurately for residual tumor.

In resections after neoadjuvant therapy where there is no gross abnormality, and especially if the preoperative diagnosis was Lauren diffuse-type gastric adenocarcinoma, the entire proximal and distal margins need to be submitted, and one section every centimeter of the length of the specimen should be sampled with mapping to determine the microscopic extent of the tumor.

In prophylactic gastrectomy specimens for *CDH1* mutation there are usually no gross abnormalities. It is recommended that the entire stomach should be submitted for microscopic examination. With adequate documentation by photographs and accurate mapping, at least the entire mucosa should be submitted.

III. DIAGNOSTIC FEATURES OF NONNEOPLASTIC CONDITIONS OF THE STOMACH

A. **Chronic Gastritis** has an increased lymphoplasmacytic infiltrate in the lamina propria, and in many cases is attributable to *H. pylori*. What constitutes clinically significant chronic inflammation is subjective, but is generally agreed to be a cluster of at least five plasma cells in the lamina propria or lymphoid follicles with germinal centers (e-**Fig. 13.7**). The classification and scoring of gastritis, including the updated Sydney system, lacks universal acceptance. Gastritis is labeled as "active" (active chronic gastritis) in the presence of neutrophils in the lamina propria and/or infiltration into the epithelium, in addition to chronic inflammation (e-**Fig. 13.8**). It is often seen in the setting of active *Helicobacter* infection, especially if there are also reactive lymphoid aggregates in the lamina propria (chronic follicular gastritis), but patchy or focal activity may also be seen with inflammatory bowel disease, especially in children with Crohn disease (e-**Fig. 13.9**).

Helicobacter organisms, most commonly *H. pylori,* and less commonly *H. heilmannii,* can best be identified on routine H&E stain in gastric pits near foci of exocytosis or surface mucin (e-**Fig. 13.10**). However, if needed, immunohistochemical stains can be used to enhance detection of the organisms (e-**Fig. 13.11**). Histochemical stains like Giemsa and Warthin–Starry (e-**Fig. 13.12**) also highlight the organisms. The chance of finding organisms diminishes in the absence of active inflammation, and in regions of intestinal metaplasia. In addition, in patients on proton pump inhibitors, antral inflammation is milder and *H. pylori* may relocate deeper in the oxyntic glands. Finally, treatment with other antibiotics, while not eradicating the organism, may nonetheless hinder the ability to detect *H. pylori*. After treatment for *H. pylori,* neutrophils disappear within 6 to 8 weeks; however, the lymphoplasmacytic infiltrate can persist for longer (up to a year in the body, and 2 to 4 years in the antrum). Lymphoid follicles and intestinal metaplasia may remain indefinitely.

B. **Atrophic Gastritis** is a form of chronic gastritis that can be a consequence of *H. pylori* gastritis, or occur in the setting of an autoimmune process (e-**Fig. 13.13**). Associated findings include intestinal metaplasia and ECL cell hyperplasia (e-**Figs. 13.14 to 13.16**). Dysplasia, adenocarcinoma, and neuroendocrine tumors (NETs) may develop in this background. Table 13.1 summarizes the clinicopathologic features distinguishing autoimmune from nonautoimmune atrophic gastritis. Atrophic fundic/body mucosa may resemble antral mucosa on H&E stain, hence knowledge of the location of the biopsy site is important. If necessary, a positive gastrin immunohistochemical stain can confirm the antral origin of a biopsy.

TABLE 13.1	Clinicopathologic Features of Autoimmune Metaplastic Atrophic Gastritis (AMAG) and Nonautoimmune/Environmental Metaplastic Atrophic Gastritis (EMAG)	
	AMAG	**EMAG**
Patient population	Mainly older white women	Universal
Etiology and pathogenesis	Autoantibodies to parietal cells and intrinsic factor	*Helicobacter Pylori*, other environmental factors
Clinical manifestations	Hypochlorhydria, achlorhydria, pernicious anemia	Abdominal pain, dyspepsia, upper GI bleeding
Gastric involvement	Body and fundus only	Mainly antrum, or multifocal
Microscopic findings	Chronic gastritis, progressive destruction of fundic glands, intestinal metaplasia, pyloric metaplasia, ECL cell hyperplasia	Chronic gastritis, intestinal metaplasia, pyloric metaplasia if body is involved
Serum gastrin level	Elevated	Normal or low
Tumor development	Carcinoid, adenocarcinoma	MALT lymphoma, adenocarcinoma

ECL, enterochromaffin cell–like; GI, gastrointestinal; MALT, mucosa-associated lymphoid tissue

C. **Focally Enhanced Gastritis** is a pattern of inflammation where there are foci of inflammatory activity separated by relatively normal appearing mucosa. In the pediatric setting, it appears to be more predictive of inflammatory bowel disease.

D. **Lymphocytic Gastritis** is rare, and defined as prominent lymphocytic infiltration of the surface foveolar epithelium (>25 lymphocytes per 100 epithelial cells) that should be present away from lymphoid follicles (e-**Fig. 13.17**). Associated conditions include *H. pylori* gastritis, celiac disease, Crohn disease, HIV infection, syphilis, or drugs such as olmesartan. In the proper clinical context a lymphoma should be excluded.

E. **Collagenous Gastritis** is rare, and characterized by an irregular thickened collagen layer (average thickness of 30 to 40 microns) below the luminal surface epithelium, with a variable intraepithelial lymphocyte count (e-**Fig. 13.18**). It can be associated with similar conditions as lymphocytic gastritis.

F. **Eosinophilic Gastritis** is usually a component of eosinophilic gastroenteritis, where there is marked eosinophilic infiltrate in the lamina propria. Currently there is no standardization regarding the absolute number of eosinophils required for diagnosis, but the infiltrate is usually associated with eosinophilic cryptitis, microabscesses, and degranulation (e-**Fig. 13.19**). It may involve any layer of the stomach wall. Approximately half of cases are associated with peripheral eosinophilia, and often associated with history of atopy and food allergies. It is important to exclude certain medications and inflammatory conditions such Crohn disease and parasitic infections, which can also result in eosinophilic infiltrates.

G. **Granulomatous Gastritis** can be seen in Crohn disease, sarcoidosis, foreign body reaction, drugs (including antacids), infections (such as mycobacteria, fungus, parasites, or occasionally *H. pylori*), vasculitis, and in association with a neoplasm. Rarely, granulomatous gastritis is idiopathic (e-**Fig. 13.20**).

H. **Ischemic Gastritis** is a very rare acute event with a high mortality. It has been reported in the setting of systemic hypotension, celiac axis stenosis, post radiologic embolization, and vasculitis. The histologic findings are nonspecific with ulceration, necrosis, and hemorrhage (e-**Fig. 13.21**).

I. **Infectious Gastritis.** A number of bacterial (e.g., mycobacteria, *Treponema pallidum*), viral (e.g., cytomegalovirus [CMV], Epstein–Barr virus [EBV]), fungal (e.g., *Candida, Histoplasma, Mucoraceae*), and rarely parasitic (e.g., *Cryptosporidium, Giardia, Strongyloides, Anisakis*) organisms can infect the stomach (e-**Figs. 13.22 and 13.23**). Some infections can be associated with eosinophilic infiltrates and granulomas.

J. **Reactive Gastropathy or Chemical Gastritis** is characterized by foveolar hyperplasia with tortuous gland outlines, regenerative epithelial changes with decreased mucin, and smooth muscle fibers within the lamina propria. It usually involves the antrum (e-**Fig. 13.24**). Inflammation is typically mild to absent, but erosion may be present. It can be associated with bile reflux or with medications, particularly NSAIDs.

K. **Ménétrier Disease** is endoscopically characterized by diffuse giant gastric folds mainly involving the body and fundus in adults, but the antrum can be involved in children. The histologic findings include marked foveolar hyperplasia with cystic dilatation, which may extend to submucosa; hypertrophy of the muscularis mucosae; and atrophy of oxyntic glands. Clinically, patients present with protein-losing gastropathy and may have GI bleeding. In children, it can be associated with some infections and is usually self-limited; in contrast, adult Ménétrier disease usually does not regress. Treatment with anti-TGF-α therapy is very effective (since the pathogenesis of the disease is driven by excessive secretion of TGF-α).

L. **Parietal Cell Hyperplasia** endoscopically presents with enlarged mucosal folds in the body and fundus. Histologically, there is both hyperplasia and hypertrophy of parietal cells. There may be cytoplasmic vacuolation and protrusion of apical cytoplasm into dilated glands, sometimes filled with inspissated eosinophilic material. It is seen with hypergastrinemia, either primary (Zollinger–Ellison syndrome) or secondary (chronic proton pump inhibitor or antacid use) (e-**Figs. 13.25 and 13.26**).

M.**Gastric Antral Vascular Ectasia (GAVE),** also known as watermelon stomach because of its endoscopic appearance, is characterized by dilatation of mucosal capillaries in the gastric antrum with or without fibrin thrombi (e-**Fig. 13.27**), with associated mucosal smooth muscle fibers. Similar changes can be seen in portal hypertension. However, portal hypertensive gastropathy involves the body and fundus and does not classically show fibrin thrombi (e-**Fig. 13.28**).

N. **Mucosal Calcinosis.** Calcifications are usually found incidentally in mucosal biopsies from patients with renal failure from patients who are organ transplant recipients (e-**Fig. 13.29**).

O. **Mucosal Siderosis (Pseudomelanosis)** results from iron deposition in the mucosa in patients taking ferrous sulfate (surface mucosa, e-**Fig. 13.30**) or in patients with hemochromatosis (full thickness or deep, e-**Fig. 13.31**). In **iron pill gastritis** there may be mild inflammation or erosions, associated with surface iron deposits (e-**Fig. 13.32**).

P. **Xanthelasma or Xanthoma** presents as small, sessile, yellow mucosal nodules, commonly in the body and fundus that are characterized by collections of lipid-laden foamy macrophages in the lamina propria, often in a background of chronic gastritis. This lesion is significant for its potential confusion with poorly differentiated signet ring cell adenocarcinoma on biopsy (e-**Fig. 13.33**). In problematic cases, the diagnosis can be clarified by immunohistochemical stains; positivity for pancytokeratins and CDX2 is seen in most adenocarcinomas, whereas positivity for CD68 and CD163 favors a xanthoma.

Q. **Graft Versus Host Disease** occurs in the setting of allogeneic bone marrow transplantation, and commonly involves the skin, GI tract, and liver. Rarely, it may occur in the setting of solid organ transplant or blood transfusion. Irrespective of the duration of transplantation, acute GVHD presents with nausea, vomiting, anorexia, diarrhea, crampy abdominal pain, or GI bleeding, and manifests as increased epithelial apoptosis, primarily in the regenerative compartment of the mucosa; a paucity of inflammatory cells in the lamina propria; and crypt dropout in more severe cases. It is histologically graded throughout the gastrointestinal system on a 4-tier scale as follows: grade 1—increased intraepithelial apoptosis, with at least 2 apoptotic bodies per biopsy fragment (e-**Fig. 13.34**); grade

2—apoptotic crypt abscess or single gland dropout (e-**Fig. 13.35**); grade 3—two to three confluent crypt loss (e-**Fig. 13.36**); and grade 4–extensive crypt loss.

IV. DIAGNOSTIC FEATURES OF COMMON GASTRIC POLYPS

A. **Hyperplastic Polyps (HPs)** are composed of elongated, dilated, branching foveola with or without cystic change, in association with inflamed edematous lamina propria. These polyps can show surface erosions, regenerative changes, and intestinal metaplasia (e-**Fig. 13.37**). HPs are usually associated with an underlying inflammatory disorders of the stomach. Most polyps are less than 1 cm in diameter, although rarely they can be very large. They occur most commonly in the antrum. Although foci of dysplasia or invasive carcinoma can rarely be present, the association of HP is greater with a synchronous malignant neoplasm elsewhere in the stomach.

B. **Fundic Gland Polyps** are composed of cystically dilated glands lined by parietal and chief cells which may be hyperplastic or attenuated (e-**Fig. 13.38**). They are usually multiple. The polyps can be syndromic and associated with familial adenomatous polyposis (FAP) where there is germline mutation of the *APC* gene; gastric adenocarcinoma and proximal polyposis of the stomach (GAPPS); or *MUTYH*-associated polyposis (MAP). The polyps can also be sporadic, caused by activating mutations of the beta-catenin gene. A third group of fundic gland polyps can be associated with long-term use of PPI. A significant proportion of syndromic (but not sporadic) fundic gland polyps are associated with low-grade dysplasia; however, high-grade dysplasia and invasive carcinoma are exceedingly rare.

C. **Gastric Adenoma,** or gastric polypoid dysplasia, is a true neoplasm and a precursor to gastric cancer. It can be present throughout the stomach, and in 80% of cases is solitary. The epithelial lining is of two major types: intestinal type (containing at least focal goblet cells and/or Paneth cells) and gastric foveolar type. The intestinal type is more likely to show an association with background mucosal pathology (chronic gastritis and intestinal metaplasia) and to harbor high-grade dysplasia and foci of adenocarcinoma within the polyp (e-**Fig. 13.39**).

D. **Pyloric Gland Adenoma** is commonly located in the gastric body and occurs much more frequently in females. At least a third are associated with autoimmune metaplastic atrophic gastritis. Similar lesions are also reported from sites that are prone to pyloric metaplasia such as the gallbladder. Histologically, it is composed of compactly arranged pyloric-type mucus glands, some of which are cystically dilated and can have low- or high-grade dysplasia. These adenomas show *GNAS* mutations.

E. **Oxyntic Gland Adenoma** is composed of anastomosing cords and irregularly branched tubules predominantly composed of chief cells, but also includes scattered parietal cells.

F. **Hamartomatous Polyps** can be sporadic or syndromic. Syndromic cases and seen in patients with Peutz–Jeghers syndrome, juvenile polyposis syndrome, PTEN hamartoma tumor syndrome (including Cowden syndrome), and Cronkhite–Canada syndrome. Sporadic polyps are usually solitary and have a benign course. The histologic features of many of these polyps, including gastric Peutz–Jeghers polyp, are often reminiscent of hyperplastic gastric polyps, and the accurate diagnosis requires correlation with relevant clinical and endoscopic findings (e-**Fig. 13.40**).

G. **Inflammatory Fibroid Polyp** is most commonly found in the gastric antrum and consists of a submucosal collection of bland spindle cells, which are characteristically CD34 positive and c-kit negative, in a background of dilated vascular channels and mixed inflammation which often contains abundant eosinophils (e-**Figs. 13.41** to **13.43**).

H. **Polypoid Foveolar Hyperplasia** is considered to be a regenerative lesion, but can also be a precursor to HPs. Grossly, the findings are usually a sessile 1 to 2 mm lesion in the antrum. Microscopically, there is simple hyperplasia of the foveolar epithelium, without cystic change.

I. **Gastritis Cystica Profunda/Polyposa** is a form of mucosal prolapse in which gastric pits are herniated into the submucosa or deeper portion of the wall, with variable hyperplastic change and cystic dilatation. This occurs most commonly at the gastric side of gastroenteric anastomoses, but can also develop in the absence of any gastric surgery.

J. **Polypoid Gastritis** consists of well-circumscribed nodules usually less than 0.5 cm in diameter, most commonly located in the antrum. Microscopically, there is localized expansion of lamina propria by mixed inflammatory cells and reactive lymphoid aggregates.

V. DIAGNOSTIC FEATURES OF COMMON NEOPLASMS OF THE STOMACH

A. **Adenocarcinoma.** Grossly, gastric adenocarcinoma is classified by the Bormann classification in four distinct types: type I (polypoid carcinoma), type II (fungating carcinoma), type III (ulcerating carcinoma), and type IV (diffusely infiltrating carcinoma). Types I and III are commonly located in the antrum and lesser curvature, and type II in the greater curvature, frequently in the corpus. Type IV carcinomas are associated with a greater depth of invasion, and when greater than 50% of the stomach is affected, it correlates with the morphologic description of linitis plastica.

Gastric adenocarcinomas have classically been divided microscopically according to the Lauren classification into intestinal, diffuse, and mixed types. Intestinal-type adenocarcinomas (gland-forming) develop in the elderly, are more common in the proximal stomach in a background of intestinal metaplasia and dysplasia, and have been associated with certain risk factors such as chronic *H. pylori* infection, atrophic gastritis, and dietary factors such as smoked food and food rich in salt. WHO categories papillary and tubular belong to this category (Table 13.2). Diffuse-type adenocarcinomas (WHO terminology: poorly cohesive carcinomas) occur in a relatively younger population in otherwise unremarkable background mucosa; are characterized by loss of cell cohesion; diffusely infiltrate the gastric wall without clear gland formation; and are more likely to

TABLE 13.2	WHO Histologic Classification of Gastric Tumors
Epithelial tumors	Neuroendocrine carcinoma (NEC)
Premalignant lesions	Large cell NEC
	Small cell NEC
Adenoma	Mixed adenoneuroendocrine carcinoma
Intraepithelial neoplasia (dysplasia), low grade	EC cell, serotonin-producing NET
Intraepithelial neoplasia (dysplasia), high grade	Gastrin-producing NET (gastrinoma)
Carcinoma	**Mesenchymal tumors**
Adenocarcinoma	Glomus tumor
Papillary adenocarcinoma	Granular cell tumor
Tubular adenocarcinoma	
Mucinous adenocarcinoma	Leiomyoma
Poorly cohesive carcinoma (including signet ring cell carcinoma and other variants)	Plexiform fibromyxoma
Mixed adenocarcinoma	Gastrointestinal stromal tumor
Adenosquamous carcinoma	Kaposi sarcoma
Carcinoma with lymphoid stroma (medullary carcinoma)	Leiomyosarcoma
	Synovial sarcoma
Hepatoid carcinoma	**Lymphomas**
Squamous cell carcinoma	**Secondary tumors**
Undifferentiated carcinoma	
Neuroendocrine neoplasms	
Neuroendocrine tumor (NET)	
NET G1 (carcinoid)	
NET G2	

From: Bosman FT, Carneiro F, Hruban RH, Theise ND, eds. *WHO Classification of Tumours of the Digestive System.* Lyon, France: IARC Press; 2017. Used with permission.

have a genetic basis (e.g., e-cadherin/*CDH1* mutations) than an environmental association. In many cases the cells of diffuse-type gastric adenocarcinoma are of signet ring morphology (e-**Figs. 13.44** and **13.45**). A subset of cases is hereditary, with inactivating germline mutations of the *CDH1* gene. Prophylactic total gastrectomy is the standard of care for asymptomatic patients, and the entire stomach should be submitted for histologic processing because almost all cases will harbor multiple foci of signet ring cell adenocarcinoma which are often grossly inapparent.

Another variant of gastric carcinoma is gastric carcinoma with lymphoid stroma, also known as medullary carcinoma or lymphoepithelioma-like carcinoma. More than 80% of cases are associated with EBV infection. The prognosis is considered better than for other gastric adenocarcinomas. This variant commonly seen in younger Caucasian/Hispanic males, and the tumor is located in the cardia/body. The tumor frequently shows a CpG island methylator phenotype (and so is microsatellite unstable) and is likely to respond to PD-L1 blockade therapy.

Other rare variants include mucinous adenocarcinoma (with extracellular mucin comprising at least 50% of the tumor volume), squamous cell carcinoma, adenosquamous carcinoma, and hepatoid adenocarcinoma.

The Cancer Genome Atlas Research describes four major subtypes of gastric cancer, based on their genetic alterations:

1. **Chromosomally unstable (CIN) subtype.** The CIN subtype is the most common subtype, associated with intestinal-type morphology and more commonly located in the GEJ and cardia. Most of the cases show overexpression of p53 consistent with *TP53* mutation. Other mutations associated involve the *ARID1A, KRAS, PIK3CA, ERBB2,* and *APC* genes. Phosphorylation of the epidermal growth factor receptor (i.e., EGFR, pY1068), consistent with amplification of *EGFR,* is present in most of the cases.

2. **Microsatellite instability (MSI) subtype.** The MSI subtype is associated with an older age of presentation and has a female predilection. The main cause of MSI is hypermethylation of the *MLH1* promoter. The MSI subtype can be further divided in MSI-high or -low, depending on the level of MSI. MSI-high tumors morphologically present as intestinal type and have a better prognosis than MSI-low tumors. MSI gastric cancers are also associated with mutations in the *PIK3CA, ERBB2, ERBB3,* and *EGFR* genes.

3. **Genomically stable (GS) subtype.** The GS subtype presents as diffuse-type morphology, and typically in younger patients. Compared with CIN it has a lower frequency of TP53 mutations and aneuploidy. Some of the cases are associated with mutations in the *CDH1* and *RHOA* genes (37 and 15%, respectively). Germline mutations of *CDH1* are associated with hereditary diffuse gastric cancer and a dismal prognosis.

4. **EBV-positive subtype**. This subtype is the least common subtype. The tumors are more frequently located in the fundus and body, and have a male predilection. They are associated with less lymph node involvement and lower mortality.

   Overexpression of ERBB2 (HER2) has been detected in 24%, 12%, and 7% of CIN, EBV-positive and MSI subtypes, respectively. Immunohistochemistry is the first line of evaluation, and FISH testing is recommended for tumors with a score of 2+ (equivocal). If ERBB2 is overexpressed, trastuzumab (Herceptin) is added to the standard chemotherapy regimen, which improves overall survival by a few months. Overall, gastric cancers with overexpression of HER2 are associated with a poor prognosis.

B. NETs. Gastroenteropancreatic neuroendocrine neoplasms (NENs) are discussed in detail in Chapter 12. In the stomach, well-differentiated NETs occur in three distinct settings:

1. **Type I gastric NETs** occur in the setting of autoimmune gastritis (e-**Fig. 13.46**) in which secondary hypergastrinemia induces ECL cell hyperplasia. The cutoff between nodular ECL cell hyperplasia and gastric NET is 0.5 mm. The prognosis of Type I gastric NET is excellent.

2. **Type II gastric NETs** are rare, and occur in association with Zollinger–Ellison syndrome or in patients with multiple endocrine neoplasia (MEN). Metastasis occurs in

about 30% of cases, but the prognosis is still much better than type III, where there is a 70% chance of metastasis with tumors more than 2 cm.

3. Type III gastric NETs are sporadic, solitary, and can occur anywhere in the stomach (in contrast to types I and II, which are usually multiple and occur predominantly in the body) (e-**Fig. 13.47**).

C. **Gastrointestinal Stromal Tumor (GIST)** is the most common mesenchymal neoplasm of the stomach, small, and large intestines. It presents overall with an equal gender predilection, and mostly in patients over 50 years of age. GISTs are more frequent in the stomach (60% to 70%) followed by the small intestine (20% to 30%), extragastrointestinal (10%), colorectal (5%), esophagus (<5%), and others (gallbladder, pancreas, and appendix, together <1%). Grossly GISTs are typically well-circumscribed and unifocal with a median size of 5 cm, and generally submucosal based. Most of the cases on cut surface are firm and tan-white to pink with focal areas of hemorrhage, necrosis, and/or cystic change.

Morphologically, GISTs are divided into spindle cell type (70% to 75%) (e-**Fig. 13.48**), epithelioid cell type (20% to 25%) (e-**Fig. 13.49**), and mixed cell type (5% to 10%). In some cases, especially after treatment, GISTs can have a decrease in cellularity and the stroma can show myxoid, hyalinized, and sclerotic changes as well as areas of calcification (e-**Fig. 13.50**). In the small intestine, the stroma often shows prominent collagen fibers, so-called skeinoid fibers. Spindle cell GISTs are composed of uniform and elongated cells with nuclei featuring evenly dispersed chromatin and inconspicuous nucleoli; eosinophilic fibrillar cytoplasm; and an overall pattern that is organized as intersecting fascicles. In the stomach, spindle cell GISTs often have perinuclear vacuoles that indent the nucleus at one pole. Epithelioid cell GISTs are composed of cells with abundant eosinophilic to clear cytoplasm arranged in nests and sheets. In some cases, binucleated, multinucleate, and bizarre nuclei may be present.

Using immunohistochemistry, 95% of GISTs have diffuse and strong positivity with c-kit (CD117), with a pattern of staining that includes cytoplasmic (e-**Fig. 13.51**), membranous (e-**Fig. 13.52**), or paranuclear dot-like (e-**Fig. 13.53**). It is important to note that c-kit expression by immunohistochemistry is independent of underlying c-kit mutations. C-kit negative GISTs are usually of epithelioid morphology and harbor *PDGFRA* mutations. DOG1 is expressed in 95% of the cases by immunohistochemistry, and more importantly is positive in all epithelioid cases with *PDGFRA* mutations. Other antibodies expressed by GISTs include CD34 (60% to 70%), smooth muscle actin (SMA) (30% to 40%), and desmin (5%). Expression of S-100 and cytokeratins is rare in GISTs.

The differential diagnosis of GIST varies depending on the predominant pattern including: leiomyoma and leiomyosarcoma (negative for C-kit and DOG1, positive for desmin and SMA), schwannoma (negative for C-kit and DOG1, positive for S-100), fibromatosis (negative for C-kit and DOG1, positive for beta-catenin), inflammatory myofibroblastic tumor (negative for C-kit and DOG1, positive for ALK and CD34), and other soft tissue tumors (e-**Figs. 13.54** and **13.55**).

Most GISTs harbor a mutation in the *Kit* gene (75% to 80%), followed by *PDGFRA* (5% to 8%), *BRAF* (7% to 15%), succinate dehydrogenase (*SDH*) (2%), *KRAS* (1%), and familial syndromes including NF-1 (<1% each). *Kit* and *PDGRFA* mutations are tyrosine kinase activating mutations which stimulate downstream events that regulate cell proliferation, adhesion, motility, and survival. Imatinib, a tyrosine kinase inhibitor, is used to treat *Kit* and *PDGFRA* mutated GISTs.

Mutations associated with *Kit* affect more commonly exons 11 and 9; exon 11 mutations include duplications, deletions, and substitutions. Deletions in codons 557 and 558 are associated with tumors with a larger size (>5 cm), higher mitotic index, and a poor survival rate (23% 5-year relapse-free survival), while tumors single nucleotide substitutions have a smaller size (<5 cm) and 50% 5-year relapse-free survival. Tumors with the exon 9 mutation A502-Y503 have a more aggressive behavior and male predominance.

GISTs with *PDGFRA* mutations are usually of gastric location (90%); mutations usually affect exons 14 and 18. Exon 18 mutation have been shown to be resistant to imatinib treatment although they have an excellent prognosis (75% 5-year survival rate). Exon 14 mutations are only found in gastric tumors that have an epithelioid morphology.

BRAF mutated GISTs are usually of spindle cell morphology and resistant to imatinib treatment; clinical trials with dabrafenib are in process for these cases.

SDH-deficient GISTs mostly occur in the stomach, with a predilection for pediatric and younger patients. Typically, the tumor is multinodular or bilobed with an epithelioid or mixed morphology. SDH deficient tumors commonly present with lymphovascular invasion and lymph node metastasis, and are resistant to imatinib. SDH-deficient tumors are characterized by overexpression of IGF1R, which manifests as an increased mitotic index and larger tumor size. Germline mutations in *SDH* are associated with the Carney–Stratakis syndrome characterized by multifocal gastric GISTs and paragangliomas. In contrast, the Carney triad is associated with nongermline mutations in *SDH* and is defined by gastric GIST, paragangliomas, and pulmonary chondromas.

A number of nomograms have been developed to risk stratify GISTs. A new risk-classification has been proposed based on molecular findings: low risk (mutations in *PDGFRA* exon 12, *Kit* exon 13, or *BRAF*), intermediate risk (mutations in *Kit* exon 17, or *PDGFRA* exon 14 or exon 18 D842V), and high risk (mutations in *Kit* exon 9 or 11, or *PDGFRA* exon 18 non-D842V).

D. Marginal Zone B-cell Lymphoma of Mucosa-Associated Lymphoid Tissue (MALT) Type is an extranodal lymphoma composed of morphologically heterogeneous small B-cells (e-**Figs. 13.56** and **13.57**). Up to one-third of gastric MALTs may show plasmacytoid differentiation. The gastrointestinal tract is the most common site for MALT lymphoma (50% of cases) and the stomach is the most common gastrointestinal site (85% of cases).

Table 13.3 describes characteristics useful in distinguishing MALT lymphoma from chronic gastritis. Gastric MALT lymphomas are typically immunopositive for CD20 (e-**Fig. 13.58**), CD79a, CD21, and CD35, but immunonegative for CD5, CD10, and CD23. Some gastric MALT lymphomas are CD43 positive (e-**Fig. 13.59**). Demonstration of light chain restriction is helpful in discriminating MALT lymphoma from reactive lesions. Gastric MALT lymphomas have been associated with *H. pylori* infection, however the chance of detecting *H. pylori* decreases with progression to lymphoma, and some seropositive individuals will be negative for *H. pylori* in histopathologic studies. The most common recurrent cytogenetic abnormality in gastric MALT is t(11;18) which has also been associated with resistance to *H. pylori* eradication therapy. MALT lymphomas tend to be indolent, slow to disseminate, and responsive to radiation therapy. Even involvement of multiple sites and the bone marrow do not portend a worse prognosis. However, if solid areas or sheets of large cells are present, the tumor is more appropriately diagnosed as diffuse large B-cell lymphoma. Some of the MALT lymphomas can show a transformation to diffuse large B-cell lymphoma.

VI. STAGING AND REPORTING. The most recent AJCC staging manual (Amin MB et al., eds. *AJCC Cancer Staging Manual.* 8th ed. New York: Springer, 2017) has separate staging systems for primary carcinomas of the stomach (which includes high-grade neuroendocrine carcinoma) and well-differentiated NETs of the stomach. Of note, GIST and sarcoma of the stomach are staged using the AJCC schemes for GIST and soft tissue sarcoma, respectively.

Reporting follows suggested guidelines (e.g., see the College of American Pathologists Protocol for the Examination of Specimens From Patients With Carcinoma of the Stomach, at http://www.cap.org).

ACKNOWLEDGMENT

The authors thank Kathryn M. Law and Elizabeth M. Brunt, authors of the previous edition of this chapter.

TABLE 13.3	Comparison of Histologic Features Between MALT Lymphoma and Chronic Gastritis	
Histologic Feature	MALT Lymphoma	Chronic Gastritis
Lymphoid follicle	Frequent	May be present
Follicular colonization	May be present	Absent
Interfollicular lymphocytes	Small to intermediate in size, irregular nuclear contour, monocytoid	Small and round, mature
B lymphocytes (positive for CD20)	Predominant, present in lymphoid follicles and interfollicular spaces, may coexpress CD43	Sparse, usually limited to lymphoid follicles, do not coexpress CD43
T lymphocytes (positive for CD3)	Variable in number, scattered	Predominant, diffusely involve the lamina propria and interfollicular spaces
Plasma cells	Variable in number, usually seen beneath the surface lining epithelium, show light chain restriction	Usually prominent, diffusely present in the lamina propria, lack light chain restriction
Lymphoepithelial lesion	Usually prominent, the infiltrative lymphoid cells are B cells and form clusters, glandular destruction evident	Rare and inconspicuous, the infiltrative lymphoid cells are T cells and individually distributed, glandular destruction not evident
Helicobacter pylori microorganisms	May be present	May be present
Infiltration of muscularis mucosae by lymphoid cells	May be present	Absent

MALT, mucosa-associated lymphoid tissue.

Cytopathology of the Stomach

Cory Bernadt

I. **INTRODUCTION.** The indications for cytologic sampling of the stomach include the presence of an inflammatory process or a neoplasm. Mucosal lesions can be sampled by endoscopic brushing cytology, and intramural lesions by endoscopic ultrasound-guided fine needle aspiration (EUS-FNA). EUS-FNA of subepithelial lesions of the upper gastrointestinal tract, including the stomach, is a safe but only moderately effective method of tissue diagnosis with a pooled diagnostic rate of 59.9% (*Surg Endosc* 2016;30:2431).

II. **INFLAMMATORY PROCESSES.** Antral mucosa brushing cytology with Papanicolaou stain is a sensitive, accurate, and simple procedure for investigating the presence of *Helicobacter pylori* infection in cases of gastritis. The bacteria present as curved and S-shaped rods with basophilic staining properties (*World J Gastroenterol* 2005;11:2784). Brushing cytology shows at least comparable sensitivity (88% to 95%) compared with histology, with the advantage of rapid results, high specificity, and low cost (*Acta Cytol* 2000;44:1010; *Acta Cytol* 2008;52:597).

III. NEOPLASMS

A. Adenocarcinoma

1. The smear of **intestinal-type adenocarcinoma** is hypercellular, consisting of haphazardly arranged three-dimensional cell groups and atypical single cells. The malignant cells show nuclear enlargement, hyperchromasia, and irregular nuclear membrane contours (e-**Fig. 13.60**). A necrotic, dirty background is often present.

2. The cytologic diagnosis of **diffuse-type adenocarcinoma** is difficult due to scarcity of the malignant cells; when present, the characteristic signet ring cells demonstrate an intracytoplasmic vacuole that indents the nucleus into a concave shape (e-**Fig. 13.61**), with associated nuclear hyperchromasia. The differential diagnosis of the atypical cells in diffuse-type adenocarcinoma includes histiocytes and goblet cells (*Diagn Cytopathol* 2006;34:177).

B. GIST.

The smear shows microfragments and sheets of spindle cells with moderate to high cellularity (e-**Fig. 13.62**), intact single spindle cells, and abundant stripped nuclei. The spindle cells have spindle to oval nuclei, fine chromatin, and abundant delicate cytoplasm with indistinct borders (e-**Fig. 13.63**). Nuclear atypia, mitosis, and necrosis may be identified occasionally. The epithelioid variant demonstrates large epithelioid cells with round nuclei and distinct cell borders. GIST cannot be graded based on cytologic specimens. Immunostains are required for a definitive diagnosis to exclude other submucosal spindle cell neoplasms that possess similar cytomorphology (*Cancer* 2001;93:269; *Am J Clin Pathol* 2003;119:703).

C. NETs.

The cytomorphology of NETs is identical to that of the tumors at other sites. The smears are cellular and composed of loosely cohesive clusters and isolated cells with characteristic salt-and-pepper chromatin. Focal and variable endocrine atypia are easily identified.

D. Malignant Lymphoma.

The cytomorphology varies among the subtypes of gastric lymphoma. In general, the smears show numerous isolated lymphoid cells exhibiting different degrees of atypia and monotony (the detailed cytomorphology of different lymphomas is discussed in the cytology section of Chapter 41). Precise diagnosis and classification require ancillary studies, which can be applied to EUS-FNA material (*Am J Clin Pathol* 2006;125:703).

ACKNOWLEDGMENT

The author thanks Julie Kunkel, author of the previous edition of this section.

14 | The Intestines, Appendix, and Anus

Deyali Chatterjee

I. NORMAL ANATOMY

A. Gross Anatomy.

The small intestine is approximately 6 m long and divided into the duodenum, jejunum, and ileum. The duodenum, a C-shaped portion of the proximal small intestine, begins distal to the gastric pylorus and is approximately 25 to 30 cm in length. Apart from the first part (which contains the duodenal bulb, and ends at the superior duodenal flexure), it is retroperitoneal. The second part is the descending part, the third part is the inferior/ horizontal part, and the fourth part is the ascending part which ends at the duodenojejunal flexure. The jejunum marks the entry of small intestine into the peritoneal cavity. The intraperitoneal portion of the small intestine is connected to the posterior abdominal wall by the mesentery. The demarcation of the jejunum and ileum is not clearly defined, and arbitrarily the jejunum constitutes the proximal third of the intraperitoneal portion. The ileum ends at the ileocecal valve.

The large intestine is approximately 1.5 m long, and consists of the cecum, colon (ascending, transverse, descending, and sigmoid), and the rectum. Portions of it lie against the posterior abdominal wall (ascending colon, descending colon, and rectum). The transverse and sigmoid colon are connected to the posterior abdominal wall by a mesocolon. The cecum is an outpouching of the large bowel at the junction of ileum and right colon, and is not directly connected to the posterior abdominal wall and does not have its own blood supply, therefore it is considered as entirely intraperitoneal.

The **appendix** is a tubular organ that extends from the cecum. Its length is variable, from 2 to 20 cm, with an average diameter of 0.4 cm. It has its own blood supply via the mesoappendix (which connects the appendix to the lower end of small bowel mesentery).

The **anal canal** is the terminal 3 to 4 cm of the gastrointestinal tract.

B. Normal Histology

1. The small and large intestines, including appendix, are composed of four structural layers, which from the luminal aspect, are:

   Mucosa. Epithelial component associated with the lamina propria. The muscularis mucosae separates the mucosa from the submucosa.

   Submucosa. Loose fibrovascular tissue, with a nerve plexus containing prominent ganglion cells (Meissner's plexus).

   Muscularis propria. Inner circular and outer longitudinal smooth muscle fibers, separated by a nerve plexus (myenteric/Auerbach's plexus).

   Adventitia and adjoining soft tissue, which in areas that are not connected to the posterior abdominal wall are covered by visceral peritoneum (serosa).

2. **The small intestine** is lined throughout its length by villous mucosa. The individual villus is a slender, fingerlike projection with a variable villous-to-crypt ratio (greatest in duodenum and proximal jejunum) ranging from 3:1 to 5:1 (**e-Fig. 14.1**). Shortened and broadened villi are commonly seen in the proximal duodenal mucosa overlying Brunner's glands. The epithelium consists predominantly of tall, columnar absorptive cells that have basally situated nuclei, eosinophilic cytoplasm, and apical microvilli giving the appearance of a "brush border." Other predominant cell types of the intestine include mucin-secreting goblet cells, basal/crypt/stem cells, Paneth cells, and endocrine cells; the granules of Paneth cells are refractile, eosinophilic, and supranuclear, while the granules of endocrine cells are smaller, eosinophilic but non-refractile, and infranuclear.

Within the first and second parts of the duodenum are abundant submucosal mucous glands called Brunner's glands. The lamina propria contains mixed inflammatory cells including plasma cells, but neutrophils are restricted to vascular channels. Lymphoid aggregates are distributed throughout the small and large intestinal mucosa and submucosa. Confluent and dense lymphoid tissue is normally seen in the terminal ileum and constitutes the grossly recognizable Peyer's patches. Intraepithelial lymphocytes (IELs) are mostly CD8+ T lymphocytes scattered within the surface epithelium throughout the intestines. Normally they are more abundant in the crypts than at the tips, and nowhere are these more than one per five enterocytes. However, increased IEL density may be seen in the epithelium overlying lymphoid aggregates.

3. **The large intestine** is lined by non-villous mucosa with a flat surface, and there are evenly spaced, nonbranching crypts arranged perpendicularly to the lumen and extending from the surface to the muscularis mucosae (e-**Fig. 14.2**). Paneth cells may be seen until the mid-transverse colon. Goblet cells are more numerous, particularly in the left colon. The lamina propria has more muciphages (mucin-containing macrophages) in the left colon. In the distal rectum, the crypts may be slightly dilated or tortuous, and may not reach down to the muscularis mucosae.

The appendix mucosa has prominent lymphoid aggregates, which often have well-formed germinal centers. The appendix also has a poorly developed muscularis mucosae that may be interrupted by lymphoid aggregates.

The anus begins after the rectum crosses the puborectalis sling. The mucosa lining the upper portion of the anal canal is a direct extension of the rectal mucosa. The mucosa lining the middle portion of the anal canal (the so-called anal transitional zone [ATZ], a 0.5- to 1-cm segment above the dentate line) has the features of both metaplastic squamous mucosa and urothelium (multilayered transitional epithelium). Submucosal and intramuscular anal glands open into the ATZ via anal ducts that are also lined by ATZ epithelium. The mucosa of the distal anal canal, which extends from the dentate line to the anal verge (mucocutaneous junction), consists of specialized nonkeratinizing squamous mucosa with melanocytes. It is distinguished from the perianal skin by the lack of skin appendages. The columnar mucosa in the upper part has vertical folds, called columns of Morgagni, which are separated by sinuses of Morgagni. The anal columns connect at the distal end by horizontal mucosal folds, called anal valves, corresponding to the dentate line (e-**Fig. 14.3**). The muscularis propria of the large intestines continues down into the anus and functions as the internal sphincter. The anus has an additional outer layer of skeletal muscle which functions as the external sphincter.

II. GROSS EXAMINATION AND SPECIMEN HANDLING

A. **Endoscopic Biopsy.** When processing the specimen, it is important to record pertinent clinical history and endoscopic findings. Biopsies are typically small fragments of mucosal tissue in the range of 1 to 5 mm in greatest dimension that do not need to be inked or subdivided. Important gross descriptors are the number, the size, and the size range of the biopsy fragments. In cases where numerous fragments are present, an estimate for the number and the dimensions in aggregate should be given (documentation of the number and size is important to ensure that the biopsies are adequately represented on the slides). Routine microscopic examination of endoscopic biopsies entails examination of three hematoxylin and eosin (H&E)-stained slides, each with two to three levels of the tissue.

B. **Suction Biopsy** of the rectum, which makes possible sampling of the submucosa, is used for evaluation of Hirschsprung disease. After processing, the tissue is serially sectioned in its entirety, but initially only every third level is H&E-stained; if no ganglion cells are identified in these slides, the remaining sections are stained and examined.

C. **Polypectomy** specimens should be described and measured. The need for inking of the resection margin is a controversial topic; in practice, it is often difficult to do since the stalk retracts and thus may be hard to identify grossly (although the cauterized base can be easily identified microscopically). The specimen is bisected or serially sectioned depending on its size, and entirely submitted. Sectioning should follow the vertical plane of the stalk to maximize the evaluation of the polypectomy margin. At least three H&E levels are examined.

D. **Endoscopic Mucosal Resection (EMR)** is performed for sessile lesions or lesions that are larger and not amenable to polypectomy. Operatively, the mucosa is lifted by injecting saline in the submucosa, and the lesion is then snared. The specimen can be in a single fragment, but is often in multiple fragments. All dimensions are recorded and the mucosal surface described. Inking of the margins is a matter of choice since cautery artifact will be noted at the time of microscopic evaluation for deep and mucosal margins, and since ink may actually artifactually extend along non-marginal mucosa. The entire specimen is serially sectioned and entirely submitted. At least three H&E levels are evaluated initially.

E. **Endoscopic Submucosal Dissection (ESD)** is a more effective method than EMR for removing superficial tumors. Operatively, the lesion is resected along the submucosal plane en bloc and ideally pinned out and oriented by the endoscopist. The specimen should be inked in different colors to indicate the base and the oriented mucosal margins. It is sectioned serially at 2 to 3 mm intervals, and blocked systematically, on edge, to evaluate both lateral and base margins histologically (Fig 12.1).

F. **Bowel Resection**

1. **Neoplastic.** Tumor resections include:

a. **Segmental resection** of a portion of small or large bowel.

b. **Ileocolectomy/right colectomy,** involving terminal ileum and right colon.

c. **Low anterior resection (LAR),** involving distal sigmoid and rectum, with partial mesorectal excision.

d. **Abdominoperineal resection (APR),** involving distal sigmoid, rectum and anus, performed for distal rectal or anal cancers, usually after neoadjuvant therapy. It often involves **total mesorectal excision (TME),** where the surrounding mesorectal soft tissue, up to the plane between the visceral and the presacral fascia, is excised.

e. **Total colectomy,** involving the terminal ileum to distal sigmoid or upper rectum.

For all resections for neoplasms, the portion of resected bowel is oriented and the length and diameter (or circumference), are measured. The width of the mesentery/mesocolon is also measured, if present. The external surface of the bowel is inspected for tumor involvement, perforation, or adhesions. For TME specimens, the grossly observable intactness of the mesorectal fascia is evaluated as "complete," "near complete," or "incomplete" prior to opening the bowel (Table 14.1). The bowel is opened longitudinally along the antimesenteric border, unless this would mean cutting through the tumor.

The maximal size of the tumor and the distance to the proximal, distal, and radial resection margins, or to the closest margin in unoriented specimens, are documented. After fresh tissue is collected for biobanking (if needed), the specimen is pinned out on a corkboard (mucosal side up) and fixed by submerging in 10% formalin overnight, such that the mucosal aspect faces the formalin. The tumor is then sectioned and blocks for microscopic examination are taken to include the area of deepest tumor penetration, possible serosal or adjacent organ/structure involvement (including omentum, particularly for tumor in transverse colon), to demonstrate the relationship to adjacent grossly nonneoplastic mucosa, and to demonstrate the radial margin. The entire tumor is submitted if the lesion is relatively small (arbitrarily assumed to be less than 3 cm), otherwise, at least one block per cm of the greatest extent of the tumor should be submitted. If the inked radial margin cannot be included in the tumor sections, one separate radial margin section should be submitted. Additional sections include proximal and distal resection margins; if tumor approximates the margin, the margin should be inked and multiple sections perpendicular to the margin submitted. Sections from any additional gross lesions (such as separate polyps) should also be submitted. If the appendix is present, it is handled as an appendectomy specimen as described below.

TABLE 14.1 Assessment Parameters for Completeness of Mesorectum[a]

Incomplete

Little bulk to the mesorectum

Defects in the mesorectum down to the muscularis propria

After transverse sectioning, the circumferential margin appears very irregular

Nearly Complete

Moderate bulk to the mesorectum

Irregularity of the mesorectal surface with defects greater than 5 mm, but none extending to the muscularis propria

No areas of visibility of the muscularis propria except at the insertion site of the levator ani muscles

Complete

Intact bulky mesorectum with a smooth surface

Only minor irregularities of the mesorectal surface

No surface defects greater than 5 mm in depth

No coning toward the distal margin of the specimen

After transverse sectioning, the circumferential margin appears smooth

[a]The entire specimen is scored based on the worst area.
From: Washington K, Berlin J, Branton P. *Cancer Protocols and Checklists, Colon and Rectum*. Washington, DC; CAP (College of American Pathologists); 2001; 19. Used with permission.

The mesentery and soft tissue are also dissected for lymph nodes (many nodes are located along large vessels), and the number and size range of identified nodes are recorded. Small lymph nodes can be submitted in toto without sectioning. Larger nodes are serially sectioned and the cut surfaces examined; if metastatic carcinoma is grossly appreciated (as evidenced by a white and hard cut surface), one representative section from each grossly positive node should be submitted. If the cut surfaces of the nodes are tan, soft, homogeneous, and lack gross evidence of metastasis, the entire node should be submitted for microscopic evaluation. Although a minimum of 12 nodes is required by established staging criteria, all nodes that can be found should be submitted. If a grossly involved node is situated close to or abutting the radial margin, perpendicular sections from the inked radial margin to the lymph node should be taken. It is important to remember that tumor within a lymph node, as well as a tumor deposit, less than 1 mm from the radial margin is considered as positive margin as well.

For a suspected neoplastic appendix or on discovery of an incidental mucinous lesion, the specimen should be submitted in its entirety.

2. Nontumor Bowel Resections

a. **For polyposis** specimens, pinning and gross examination are similar as for tumor specimens. Sampling focuses on the largest lesions, lesions with a distinct or worrisome gross appearance (including firmness, ulceration, and adherence to the wall), and flat and/or depressed areas of mucosa. Lymph nodes should be well-sampled since it is an indirect way to exclude micro-invasive carcinoma.

b. Resections for **inflammatory bowel disease (IBD)**, particularly for ulcerative colitis (UC), require sequential sections spaced every 10 cm. The sections should include transition regions between normal-appearing and diseased segments, distal and proximal margins, and representative inflammatory polyps. Any focal lesions (such as areas with raised mucosa), fistula tracts, and strictures should be sampled. The appendix, if present, is handled as an appendectomy specimen, as described below. Representative lymph nodes are submitted, but there is no need for extensive sampling unless a carcinoma is suspected or identified.

c. For **appendectomy** specimens, the length, diameter, surface appearance, and dimensions of the specimen, including the mesoappendix, are recorded. One half of the longitudinally bisected tip, the proximal margin, and two cross-sections are submitted in a single cassette, to include the mid-portion and any possible perforation.

d. **Miscellaneous resections.** In resections for suspected **ischemic** disease, the mesenteric vessels should be carefully examined and sampled to evaluate for thrombosis, embolization, or vasculitis. For penetrating **traumatic** injuries, inspection for possible entry and exit wound sites is performed. It is also important to grossly and microscopically examine the proximal and distal resection margins for tissue viability. When proctectomy or rectosigmoid resection is performed for **Hirschsprung** disease, the distal margin is usually indicated by the surgeon. Sequential sections every 1 to 2 cm from distal to proximal should be submitted to achieve an accurate estimation of the aganglionic region. For **diverticular disease**, a few well-oriented sections to demonstrate diverticula, especially those which appear grossly suspicious for diverticulitis, are sampled. Mucosa in between the diverticula that appears abnormal, such as granular, ulcerated, or polypoid, should be sampled as well to rule out segmental colitis associated with diverticulitis. In bowel perforations, radial sections on edge are needed to demonstrate transmural necrosis. For **ostomy takedown** specimens, representative radial sections from the ostomy edge to include the thin rim of skin as well as adjacent intestine, and a shave section of the proximal intestinal end, should be taken. **Hemorrhoidal excision** normally requires only one section.

III. DIAGNOSTIC FEATURES OF NONNEOPLASTIC CONDITIONS OF THE SMALL INTESTINE

A. Congenital Anomalies

1. **Heterotopic gastric mucosa** typically presents as a small nodule or sessile polyp in the duodenal bulb and consists of full-thickness oxyntic mucosa (e-**Fig. 14.4**).

2. **Heterotopic pancreas** presents as a mass lesion anywhere outside pancreas, but most commonly in the upper gastrointestinal tract, usually buried in the submucosa, and is composed of ducts and acini, with or without islets.

3. **Meckel diverticulum** results from persistence of the proximal portion of the vitelline duct and is always located on the antimesenteric border of the ileum, approximately 2 inches in length, and 2 ft from the ileocecal junction. It is lined by all the usual layers of the intestines, and associated heterotopic pancreatic tissue or gastric mucosa is common (e-**Figs. 14.5** and **14.6**).

4. In children with cystic fibrosis, the mucus can appear thick and inspissated.

B. Noninfective Malabsorptive Disorders

1. **Celiac disease,** also known as gluten-sensitive enteropathy, celiac sprue, or nontropical sprue, is an immune-mediated disorder secondary to hypersensitivity to gluten proteins in wheat, barley, and rye. Classic histologic features include villous atrophy, crypt hyperplasia, increased IELs, a dense lamina propria lymphoplasmacytic infiltrate, and enterocyte damage (flattening and/or cytoplasmic vacuolization). Villous atrophy ranges from partial blunting or broadening to complete flattening, but the overall thickness of the mucosa may not be reduced significantly due to crypt hyperplasia (e-**Figs. 14.7** and **14.8**). The Marsh–Oberhuber classification scheme is based on the range of biopsy appearances that can be seen in this condition, but the classification is not used in routine practice. Essentially, an increased number of IELs in villous tips is an important diagnostic feature even in absence of villous atrophy, especially in early, latent, or partially treated celiac disease. Although the increase is defined as >40 lymphocytes per 100 enterocytes, a formal count or immunostaining for T lymphocytes is usually unnecessary since lymphocytosis is typically diffuse.

The histologic differential diagnoses for celiac disease are broad, and listed in Table 14.2. Therefore, histologic features are integrated with clinical tests (antitissue transglutaminase and antiendomysial tests) to establish the diagnosis of celiac disease. HLA-DQ2 or HLA-DQ8 confer a higher risk.

TABLE 14.2 Conditions That Can Mimic Gluten Sensitive Enteropathy

Tropical sprue

Autoimmune enteropathy

HIV enteropathy

Common variable immunodeficiency

Viral enteritis

Giardiasis

Bacterial overgrowth

Infectious enteritis

Food allergies

Crohn disease

Zollinger–Ellison syndrome

Systemic autoimmune diseases

Dermatitis herpetiformis

Nonsteroidal anti-inflammatory drugs, and other drugs

Helicobacter pylori infection (peptic duodenitis)

2. **Refractory sprue** refers to unresponsiveness to a gluten-free diet or relapse of symptoms despite gluten restriction. It is histologically indistinguishable from classic celiac disease. Patients usually do not have a positive serology, but share the HLA-DQ2 or HLA-DQ8 alleles.

3. **Collagenous sprue** is characterized by villous flattening and subepithelial collagen deposition. Refractory sprue can sometimes progress to collagenous sprue, and medication injury is also considered an important etiology (e.g., olmesartan-associated injury).

4. **Autoimmune enteropathy** shares many clinical and histopathologic features with celiac disease, but often involves both the small and large intestines. A biopsy typically exhibits villous flattening and dense lamina propria lymphoplasmacytic infiltrates (e-**Figs. 14.9** and **14.10**). In contrast to celiac disease, intraepithelial lymphocytosis and crypt hyperplasia may not be evident, and neutrophils may be more numerous. Apoptotic bodies are conspicuous in some cases, and so is a complete lack of goblet cells and/or Paneth cells. A disease association with other autoimmune conditions and endocrine abnormalities is often found, but there are no strong specific serologic correlations with anti-goblet cell antibodies, anti-enterocyte antibodies, or other serologic markers. A clinical response to steroids may help establish the diagnosis.

5. **Eosinophilic gastroenteritis** involving the small intestine exhibits histologic features similar to those described for eosinophilic gastritis (e-**Fig. 14.11**). There may or may not be villous blunting, but IELs are usually not increased. Parasitic infestations, food allergy including cow's milk protein intolerance, a drug reaction, connective tissue disorders, and a neoplasm should be excluded.

6. **Common variable immunodeficiency** is characterized by the absence of lamina propria plasma cells (e-**Fig. 14.12**). Other features may include a variable degree of villous blunting, intraepithelial lymphocytosis, increased apoptosis, and lymphoid aggregates. Infectious agents, particularly *Giardia*, should be searched for in these biopsies.

7. **Pediatric enteropathies** have a poor outcome and often require small bowel transplant. Of the well characterized histologic entities, **microvillus inclusion disease** is an autosomal recessive disorder caused by mutations in the *MYO5B* gene, which codes for a cytoskeletal protein involved in membrane protein trafficking in

epithelial cells. There is villous atrophy with no inflammatory reaction, loss of a normal brush border on the luminal surface of the enterocytes, and a bubbly vacuolated appearance in the apical cytoplasm. Consequently, a PAS stain demonstrates loss of the sharp linear pattern of brush-border staining, replaced by an apical cytoplasmic blush. Immunohistochemical stains that highlight the brush border, such as CD10 or CEA, may also be used. Definitive diagnosis is made on identifying apical microvillous inclusions on electron microscopy. In patients with **tufting enteropathy**, another autosomal recessive disorder with *EpCAM* mutation, there is disorganization of surface enterocytes with focal crowding (resembling tufts). In **enteroendocrine cell dysgenesis**, mutations in the gene *NEUROG3* lead to lack of enteroendocrine cells, evident on H&E and chromogranin immunostains in an otherwise normal small and large bowel biopsy.

8. **Lymphangiectasia**, either primary (congenital) or secondary (due to obstruction), may present as a localized mass lesion or diffusely involve the bowel (e-**Fig. 14.13**). The presence of secondary lymphangiectasia is concerning for an unsampled underlying mass lesion as the source of obstruction, which should be mentioned in the report.

9. **Abetalipoproteinemia and hypobetalipoproteinemia** have defects in apoB containing lipoproteins, and feature lipid accumulation in enterocytes giving rise to a clear or foamy appearance. The normal villous architecture is well preserved. A similar appearance can be produced by ingestion of a fatty meal close to the time of endoscopy.

10. **Small bowel bacterial overgrowth (SBBO)** is usually due to underlying medical conditions, such as diabetes, post-surgery, or other causes of gastroparesis. The biopsy findings are non-specific, and vary from normal to severe chronic active inflammation resembling Crohn disease (CD).

11. **Amyloid deposition**, particularly in the mucosa, can give rise to malabsorption and diarrhea. Dense eosinophilic extracellular deposits in the lamina propria and muscularis mucosae, as well as around submucosal vessels, can be identified on H&E. Characteristic staining with Congo red stain is confirmatory.

12. **Eosinophilic gastroenteritis** is characterized by eosinophilic infiltration of one or more segments of the GI tract, associated with peripheral eosinophilia, allergies, or asthma. Typically it occurs in children and young adults and it is often associated with gastric disease. In the small bowel, the villous architecture is often intact, and the dense infiltrate includes many degranulated forms, eosinophilic crypt abscesses, and/or intraepithelial infiltration with or without ulceration.

C. Infectious Diseases

1. **Tropical sprue** simulates celiac disease, but may involve the entire small intestine with more severe disease distally. Clinical history, including any travel history, is important in establishing the diagnosis.

2. **Giardiasis** (*Giardia lamblia*) often does not induce significant mucosal damage, but may be associated with a variable non-specific inflammatory response. The organisms appear as pear-shaped structures near the luminal surface (e-**Fig. 14.14**). The organisms can be highlighted by trichrome and Giemsa stains, but special stains are often not necessary.

3. **Whipple disease** (*Tropheryma whippelii*) commonly involves the duodenum and jejunum, and exhibits distended villi due to lamina propria accumulation of foamy macrophages stuffed with the diastase-resistant, PAS-positive (e-**Fig. 14.15**), rod-shaped bacterium (actinomycete). Diagnosis can be confirmed by immunohistochemical staining, PCR, or electron microscopy.

4. **Cryptosporidiosis** is characterized by uniform, spherical, 2- to 4-μm bodies attached to the brush border that appear bluish on H&E stain (e-**Fig. 14.16**).

5. **Strongyloidiasis** (*Strongyloides stercoralis*) is diagnosed by identification of larvae, eggs, and rarely adult worms embedded in small intestinal crypts, in a background of inflamed mucosa, with particularly prominent eosinophils (e-**Fig. 14.17**).

6. ***Mycobacterium avium-intracellulare* complex (MAC)** involves the small and large bowel in severely immunocompromised patients. The lamina propria shows massive infiltration by bacilli-loaded histiocytes that can appear as foamy macrophages.

7. ***Mycobacterium tuberculosis*** of the gastrointestinal tract most commonly involves the peritoneum, ileocecal junction, ileum, and jejunum. Associated mesenteric adenopathy is common. Histologically, caseating, often confluent granulomas are present. Older granulomas may be hyalinized and calcified. Acid fast stains rarely detect organisms, especially in immunocompetent individuals, so the diagnosis mainly relies on culture. PCR can also be used for diagnosis.

8. **Viral gastroenteritis** is more common in children, or sometimes in immunocompromised adults. The common etiologic agents are adenovirus, rotavirus, coronavirus, astrovirus, Norwalk virus, and echovirus. Most of these viruses are not associated with inclusions. Biopsy findings vary from increased inflammation to increased apoptosis, and small bowel biopsies may show villous distortion such as fusion, broadening, and blunting, with reactive and degenerative epithelial changes.

9. ***Clostridium perfringens*** causes segmental necrotizing enteritis related to food poisoning.

D. Reactive Conditions

1. **Gastric mucin cell (foveolar) metaplasia** occurs in response to duodenal injury, most commonly by gastric acid (peptic duodenitis), and involves the duodenal bulb most frequently (e-**Fig. 14.18**). It may also impart a nodular appearance to the mucosa.

2. **Gastric pyloric metaplasia** occurs in response to chronic small bowel injury, involves commonly the terminal ileum, and is usually seen in the setting of IBD or chronic NSAID use (e-**Fig. 14.19**).

3. **Pseudomelanosis** consists of an accumulation of various types of pigmented material within macrophages in the lamina propria, and has been attributed to a variety of factors and a variety of diseases.

E. Medication-Associated Injuries

1. NSAIDS: ulcers, active inflammation, pyloric gland metaplasia, and diaphragm disease (multiple mucosal webs that result in luminal narrowing).

2. Immunotherapy: various histologic abnormalities from active inflammation to mimicking celiac disease, IBD, or autoimmune enteropathy.

3. Olmesartan and other angiotensin II receptor antagonists: sprue-like enteropathy.

4. Mycophenolate: increased crypt apoptosis.

5. Colchicine: increased crypt apoptosis, "ring" (metaphase) mitosis, and epithelial pseudostratification and loss of polarity.

6. Kayexalate: erosions, associated with lightly basophilic and refractile (but not polarizable) crystals with a mosaic pattern.

F. Radiation Injury is subdivided into acute and chronic forms. In acute radiation enteritis/colitis, there is villous blunting with or without ulceration, associated with epithelial atypia and increased apoptosis. In chronic radiation injury, there is ulceration, mucosal ischemic changes, or stricture formation. Stromal cells may show reactive atypia.

G. IBD, in particular, CD, can affect any part of the small bowel, manifesting as transmural inflammation, strictures, fistula formation, or granulomas. The distal terminal ileum can be affected in UC (backwash ileitis), however, duodenal involvement in UC has also been reported.

H. Ischemic Disorders. The intestines have a rich anastomosing network of blood vessels, but ischemic injury can still occur when there is a severe compromise in blood flow. The demarcation between uninvolved and involved segments is often sharp. In arterial occlusion, the mesenteric vessels are usually pale, in contrast to venous thrombosis where the mesentery is congested and hemorrhagic. Early changes include submucosal congestion, hemorrhage, and edema. The mucosa shows loss of epithelium (withering), and within hours there is a neutrophilic infiltrate (reperfusion injury). There may also be congestion, hemorrhage, and hyalinization of the lamina propria. A serosal fibrino-inflammatory response is associated with perforation. Mesenteric vessels may show secondary thrombi due to stasis and congestion, therefore clinically significant thrombi are those with evidence of organization.

I. **Graft-Versus-Host Disease (GVHD)** can involve the small bowel as part of isolated upper GI involvement, or more commonly as part of both upper and lower GI involvement. The latter case, the disease is usually more severe in the colon than the small bowel. The diagnostic criteria are discussed in the section on the large intestine below.

IV. **DIAGNOSTIC FEATURES OF POLYPS AND NEOPLASMS OF THE SMALL INTESTINE.** The WHO classification scheme of tumors of the small intestine is given in Table 14.3. Revised staging schemes for neoplasms of the small intestine have recently been published (Amin MB et al., eds. *AJCC Cancer Staging Manual.* 8th ed. New York: Springer, 2017), as have suggested reporting guidelines (e.g., the College of American Pathologists Protocol for the Examination of Specimens From Patients With Carcinoma of the Small Intestine, available at http://www.cap.org).

A. **Brunner's Gland Hyperplasia, Hamartoma, and Adenoma** may actually be variants of the same process and consist of expanded lobules of benign Brunner's glands separated by delicate fibrous septa. They are typically located in the submucosa, but penetration into the mucosa is common. Cystic degeneration may occur, which has been termed Brunner's gland cyst.

B. **Associated With Polyposis/Hereditary**

1. **Peutz–Jeghers syndrome,** an autosomal dominant inherited syndrome (germline mutations of *STK11/LKB1*), is characterized by GI polyposis (anywhere, but most commonly involving the small intestine) and mucocutaneous pigmentation. The hamartomatous polyps are characterized by an arborizing network of smooth muscle fibers supporting benign-appearing mucosa that may be hyperplastic (**e-Fig. 14.20**). Sporadic polyps of the same type may be encountered less commonly. Because syndromic polyps carry an increased risk of cancer, they should always be assessed for dysplasia.

2. **Juvenile polyps** occur in the small intestine in polyposis syndromes such as juvenile polyposis syndrome, PTEN hamartoma tumor syndrome (Cowden syndrome), and Cronkhite–Canada syndrome, which are discussed in the section on the large intestine below.

3. **Adenomas** associated with familial adenomatous polyposis (FAP) and MUTYH-associated polyposis most commonly involve the duodenum, the vicinity of the ampulla of Vater, and occasionally the ileum. Small bowel adenomas may also occur in Lynch syndrome (LS), but there is no particularly strong association with duodenal involvement.

C. **Ampullary Adenomas** can be divided into intestinal type adenomas and pancreatobiliary adenomas.

D. **Adenocarcinoma** of the small intestine is rare, accounting for only 2% of all primary GI tumors despite the fact that the small intestine constitutes about 75% of the length and about 90% of the mucosal surface of the GI tract. Adenocarcinoma of the small intestine is morphologically indistinguishable from colorectal adenocarcinoma, but more cases show CK7 positivity, and some cases may lack CK20 expression.

E. **Ampullary Carcinoma** arises in the vicinity of the ampulla of Vater and can be either intestinal type (more common) or pancreaticobiliary type. The former has a more favorable outcome than the latter, although the overall survival of ampullary carcinoma is better than that of pancreatic ductal carcinoma (which probably reflects differences in resectability). However, distinguishing the site of origin is sometimes a challenge.

F. **Neuroendocrine Tumor (NET)** accounts for one-third of small intestinal tumors. Duodenal NETs are derived from endocrine cells of the foregut and tend to be <2 cm in greatest dimension and asymptomatic. Gastrin producing NETs are associated with ZES (Zollinger–Ellison Syndrome) in 40% to 50% of cases. Distal jejunum and ileal NETs are derived from cells of the midgut; 25% to 30% are multifocal, and clinically they are more aggressive than proximal NET.

TABLE 14.3 WHO Histologic Classification of Tumors of the Small Intestine

Epithelial tumors

Adenoma
 Tubular
 Villous
 Tubulovillous

Dysplasia (intraepithelial neoplasia), low grade

Dysplasia (intraepithelial neoplasia), high grade

Hamartomas
 Peutz–Jeghers polyp
 Juvenile polyp

Carcinoma

Adenocarcinoma
 Mucinous adenocarcinoma
 Signet-ring cell carcinoma

Squamous cell carcinoma

Adenosquamous carcinoma

Medullary carcinoma

Undifferentiated carcinoma

Neuroendocrine neoplasms

Neuroendocrine tumor (NET)
 NET, G1 (carcinoid)
 NET, G2

Neuroendocrine carcinoma (NEC)
 Large cell NEC
 Small cell NEC

Mixed adenoneuroendocrine carcinoma (MANEC)

EC cell, serotonin-producing NET

Gangliocytic paraganglioma

Gastrinoma

L-cell, glucagon-like peptide and PP/PYY-producing NETs

Somatostatin-producing NET

Mesenchymal tumors

Lipoma

Leiomyoma

Gastrointestinal stromal tumor

Leiomyosarcoma

Angiosarcoma

Kaposi sarcoma

Others

Malignant lymphomas

Burkitt lymphoma

B-cell lymphoma, unclassifiable, with features intermediate between diffuse large B-cell lymphoma and Burkitt lymphoma

TABLE 14.3	WHO Histologic Classification of Tumors of the Small Intestine (*Continued*)

Diffuse large B-cell lymphoma

Immunoproliferative small intestinal disease (includes α-heavy chain disease)

Follicular lymphoma

Marginal zone lymphoma of mucosa-associated lymphoid tissue (MALT lymphoma)

Mantle cell lymphoma

T-cell lymphoma

Enteropathy-associated T-cell lymphoma (EATL)

Secondary tumors

WHO, World Health Organization; EC, enterochromaffin cell; L-cell, an intestinal enteroendocrine cell; PP, pancreatic polypeptide; PYY, polypeptide YY; MALT, mucosa-associated lymphoid tissue.
From: Bosman FT, Carneiro F, Hruban RH, Theise ND, eds. *WHO Classification of Tumours. Pathology and Genetics. Tumours of the Digestive System.* Lyon, France: IARC Press; 2017. Used with permission.

Microscopically, small intestinal NET are similar to NET arising elsewhere (e-Fig. 14.21).

G. **Gangliocytic Paraganglioma** is a rare tumor, and most commonly occurs in the second portion of the duodenum. It is a circumscribed lesion centered on the submucosa. The lesion is composed of three components that are arranged haphazardly: nests of epithelioid neuroendocrine cells resembling a paraganglioma, ganglion cells, and spindle shaped Schwann cells with neuromatous stroma (e-Fig. 14.22). Rare cases of metastasis have been reported.

H. **GIST** of the small intestine accounts for 30% to 40% of all GISTs of the GI tract, and tends to be more aggressive than its gastric counterpart.

I. **B-cell Lymphomas.** Diffuse large B-cell lymphoma is the most common type, although extranodal marginal-zone lymphomas of mucosa-associated lymphoid tissue (MALT) are also common. Immunoproliferative small intestinal disease (IPSID) is a distinct type of extranodal marginal zone B-cell lymphoma (MALT lymphoma), typically seen in young adults in Middle Eastern and Mediterranean countries. About half of patients exhibit characteristic α-heavy chain paraproteinemia without associated light chains (α-heavy chain disease). Patients present with malabsorption and diarrhea. Some patients progress to diffuse large B-cell lymphoma. Both endemic and sporadic forms of Burkitt lymphoma can involve the small intestine.

J. **Enteropathy-Associated Intestinal T-cell Lymphoma** typically develops in the setting of refractory sprue and ulcerative jejunitis or jejunoileitis, and most commonly affects the jejunum. It is characterized by dense infiltration of atypical T lymphocytes in association with epithelial destruction.

V. DIAGNOSTIC FEATURES OF NONNEOPLASTIC CONDITIONS OF THE LARGE INTESTINE

A. Neuromuscular Disorders

1. **Hirschsprung disease** is usually a congenital disorder, and affects approximately 1 in 5,000 live births (mainly males). There is lack of ganglion cells in bowel nerve plexuses usually associated with hypertrophic Schwannian nerve fibers. In classic Hirschsprung disease, also known as short-segment disease (75% to 80% of cases), the affected segment is the distal sigmoid and rectum. In approximately 10% of cases, the lack of ganglion cells extends proximal to the splenic flexure (long-segment disease), and rarely, the entire bowel is devoid of ganglion cells (total bowel aganglionosis). Rarely, Hirschsprung disease is zonal.

This condition results from failure of migration of neural crest-derived ganglion cell precursors to the bowel wall during embryogenesis, and has been linked to several mutations (most commonly involving the *RET* proto-oncogene) and genetic polymorphisms. Classical Hirschsprung disease is usually sporadic and frequently associated with other neural crest disorders, but other forms show familial aggregation.

The aganglionic distal segment is narrow and hypertonic, whereas the upstream segment is dilated due to the functional obstruction. A blind rectal suction mucosal biopsy, or a mucosal biopsy with jumbo forceps is commonly used for diagnosis. In normal rectum, a cluster of up to 5 ganglion cells is present for every 1 mm length. Since hypertrophic nerve fibers are also present (e-Fig. 14.23), supportive evidence can be obtained by demonstration of acetylcholinesterase-positive nerve twigs in the muscularis mucosae and lamina propria in frozen sections by use of the histochemical stain, or by the use of calretinin immunohistochemical stain on permanent sections. It is important to recognize that the 10 to 25 mm of rectum immediately above the pectinate line normally has a paucity of ganglion cells and prominent nerve fibers, therefore multiple serial sections should be examined before rendering a definitive diagnosis.

2. Other causes of primary **pseudo-obstruction syndrome** encompasses a heterogeneous group of neuromuscular disorders characterized by colonic inertia and constipation. Diagnosis is challenging. There may be histologic clues in nerves or muscle fibers of the muscularis propria that require careful evaluation with special stains and clinical correlation. Four major categories include the myopathic form (degeneration and fibrous replacement of smooth muscle, with or without cytoplasmic inclusions), neuropathic form (qualitative and quantitative changes in ganglion cells and nerve fibers), mesenchymopathic form (defects of interstitial cells of Cajal; CD117 immunohistochemistry can be helpful), and with abnormalities of neurohormonal peptides (paraneoplastic cause of intestinal dysmotility, e.g., from VIP producing neuroblastoma).

In **hypoganglionosis**, there is a decreased number of ganglion cells per ganglion (2 or less per ganglion, or one or fewer ganglia per millimeter). Hypertrophic nerve twigs associated with Hirschsprung disease are typically lacking. At least two forms of **hyperganglionosis**, also referred to as intestinal neuronal dysplasia, are recognized; in this disorder, the number of ganglion cells per ganglia is increased to 8 or more. In ganglioneuromas (localized) or ganglioneuromatosis (diffuse), ectopic ganglion cells in the lamina propria are noted.

Mitochondrial disorders show both myopathic and neuropathic changes.

B. Ischemic Bowel Disease. Ischemic injury is more common in the colon than in the small bowel. The splenic flexure and sigmoid colon have "watershed" zones that are particularly prone to ischemic injury because they have a limited collateral network (they represent the junction of the area perfused by the superior and inferior mesenteric arteries). The rectum is rarely involved. The causes of ischemia are enumerated in Tables 14.4 and 14.5 gives the histopathologic differential diagnosis of ischemic colitis.

In occlusive disease, ischemia is strictly segmental, and uniform within the affected region. In contrast, nonocclusive cases show patchy often widespread distribution, which is variable in severity. The mucosa is the most susceptible part of the bowel to ischemic injury. In acute ischemia, there is surface epithelial degeneration, necrosis, and sloughing, with the appearance of "withering" crypts. Empty spaces within the mucosa bound by basement membrane may represent the only remnants of intestinal crypts ("crypt ghosts"). The deepest portion of the crypts, however, may be architecturally intact, with reactive changes in the epithelium. In addition, there is usually congestion and hemorrhage in the lamina propria. In some cases a pseudomembrane is present, erupting from the dying crypts and covering the luminal surface. In most cases, the changes do not affect the muscularis propria, but there may be subtle findings of early ischemic necrosis with cell shrinkage and pyknotic nuclei within the muscularis propria layers (e-Fig. 14.24). Submucosal edema is common. In contrast, sudden complete occlusion may cause transmural infarction. With time, subsequent reperfusion leads to neutrophilic infiltration.

Chronic ischemia results in transmural fibrosis, including hyalinization of the lamina propria. Strictures, with intestinal obstruction, are common (e-Figs. 14.25 and 14.26).

TABLE 14.4	Causes of Intestinal Ischemia

Occlusive ischemia

Luminal: such as thrombosis (as in hypercoagulable states), embolism (as in athero-emboli or tumor emboli)

Mechanical obstruction: such as hernia, volvulus, torsion, intussusception

Mural (arterial): as in atherosclerosis, dissecting aneurysms

Mural (venous): portal pylephlebitis, idiopathic myointimal hyperplasia of mesenteric veins, enterocolic phlebitis, mesenteric phlebosclerosis

Nonocclusive ischemia, such as in systemic hypotension, cardiac failure, vasoconstrictor drugs, hypoxemia

Infections, such as Pig Bel (acute segmental necrotizing enterocolitis in adults, due to Clostridium perfringens type C); neonatal necrotizing enterocolitis, and other infections

Vasculitidies and vasculopathies

Microvascular insufficiency other than vasculitis, such as with capillary thrombi (as in disseminated intravascular coagulation, or thrombotic thrombocytopenic purpura), sickle cell disease, amyloidosis, diabetes, chronic radiation injury

Neonatal necrotizing enterocolitis (NEC) is a special form of ischemic bowel disease that has a high mortality rate, and typically occurs in the first week of life in premature infants. It classically affects the terminal ileum and the right colon with gangrenous necrosis. Pneumatosis intestinalis and segmental absence of the muscularis propria may be seen.

C. **IBD,** an idiopathic chronic inflammatory process with a genetic predisposition, refers to CD and UC. The diseases are characterized by chronicity and architectural alterations of the crypts, as well as basal plasmacytosis, basal lymphoid aggregates, mucosal atrophy, Paneth cell metaplasia (defined as the presence of Paneth cells beyond the mid transverse colon), and pyloric metaplasia. Crypt architectural distortion is more pronounced in UC than CD and may manifest as branching, shortening, irregular shape, irregular spacing, size variation, and disarray (e-Figs. 14.27 and 14.28). Pyloric metaplasia is more common in the small bowel in CD, but also occurs in the colon in UC (e-Fig. 14.29).

The lamina propria in IBD is usually densely infiltrated by mixed inflammatory cells, predominantly lymphocytes and plasma cells, but eosinophils can be abundant. Because of crypt shortening, a bandlike inflammatory infiltrate is often seen in the space above the muscularis mucosae, a finding referred to as basal plasmacytosis; lymphoid aggregates may also be present in this space in some cases. Active disease is defined by exocytosis of neutrophils into the crypts (cryptitis) and crypt lumens (crypt abscesses)

TABLE 14.5	Differential Diagnosis of Histologic Findings of Mucosal Ischemic Colitis

C. difficile colitis

Enterohemorrhagic *E. coli*

NSAID damage

Crohn colitis

Radiation colitis

Collagenous colitis

Amyloidosis

Kayexalate injury

Modified from Iacobuzio-Donohue CA, Montgomery EA. *Gastrointestinal and Liver Pathology.* New York; Churchill-Livingstone; 2005: 332. Used with permission.

(**e-Fig. 14.30**). An increased number of neutrophils in the lamina propria raises a concern of infectious colitis. In some institutions, the inflammatory activity is graded as minimal, mild, moderate, or severe. In the absence of neutrophilic infiltration, the disease is characterized by crypt architectural distortion and is referred to as inactive. Treated IBD may be associated with normal histologic findings. CMV inclusions have been described in steroid-refractory UC (**e-Fig. 14.31**).

1. **CD** may involve any portion of the GI tract. Roughly 40% of patients have small bowel disease only, about 40% have small and large bowel involvement, and about 20% have colonic disease only. Based on the clinical behavior and pattern of disease, CD is divided into three categories: inflammatory, fistulizing, and fibrostenotic. Grossly, the involved bowel segment typically has a rigid, strictured, or thickened wall with creeping fat. Upon opening, the segment usually grossly maintains its cylindrical shape (**e-Fig. 14.32**). The mucosa may show cobble-stoning due to linear and transverse ulcers with intervening edematous mucosa. Deep fissuring ulcers and fistula tracts are common. The muscle layer is thickened.

   The microscopic hallmark of CD is transmural inflammation with a lack of homogeneous involvement and so-called skip lesions (areas of active disease separated by normal bowel) are present. In resection specimens, lymphoid aggregates may be present in all layers of the bowel wall, but are characteristically located in the subserosal fat along the vasculature in a "necklace" pattern (**e-Fig. 14.33**). Granulomas, seen in up to 40% of cases, may be found in the mucosa, submucosa, and subserosa. In the mucosa, the granulomas are typically small, well-formed, non-necrotizing, and lack multinucleated giant cells (**e-Fig. 14.34**). A diagnostic pitfall is the so-called crypt granuloma, which represents a pericryptal histiocytic response to mucin from ruptured crypts (**e-Fig. 14.35**) that occasionally includes foreign body–type giant cells. Granulomas within the muscularis mucosae can be overlooked because of similarity to smooth muscle bundles. In the subserosa, granulomas can be larger, can contain giant cells, and are frequently associated with lymphoid aggregates (**e-Fig. 14.36**).

   It should be emphasized that CD is a clinical diagnosis. While supportive histopathologic findings in mucosal biopsies include a lack of uniformity of involvement of all fragments, or a lack of uniformity within of a given fragment, focal colitis is not specific for CD. Focal colitis is also commonly seen in other conditions including infectious colitis, drug toxicity (particularly with nonsteroidal anti-inflammatory drug [NSAID] treatment), and partially treated UC. Consequently, it is prudent to avoid labeling a patient with CD at the first biopsy, but rather to give a descriptive diagnosis (such as focal active colitis) and to provide a differential diagnosis. Appropriate clinical and genetic workup, and subsequent biopsies, usually resolve the diagnostic dilemma.

2. **UC** classically involves the entire colon but not the small bowel, and has a tendency to be more severe distally. In some cases, the disease involves only the rectum (ulcerative proctitis), or presents as left-sided colitis with discontinuous involvement of the cecum (cecal patch), ascending colon, and/or appendix. Grossly, the affected colon often has a thin and flaccid wall that flattens upon opening. The mucosa loses its normal folds and is granular, friable, erythematous, and ulcerated (**e-Fig. 14.37**). Microscopically, the disease is characterized by diffuse crypt architectural distortion and inflammation. In contrast to CD, crypt architectural distortion is more dramatic, and inflammation is usually limited to the mucosa and immediate submucosa. In severe active disease with broad-based ulcers, the inflammatory infiltrate extends into the submucosa and the muscularis propria in the ulcerated areas. Interestingly, in children with UC, the disease may be inhomogeneous at initial presentation. Treated UC may also show inhomogeneous involvement with rectal sparing, or completely normal mucosa, which may potentially be confused with CD.

   Fulminant colitis is more commonly seen in UC. Usually the patients have pancolitis with extensive infiltration of the mucosa with inflammatory cells, mucosal denudation, and granulation tissue. The inflammation may extend to involve the muscularis propria and can cause necrosis.

TABLE 14.6	Gross and Histologic Features Distinguishing Ulcerative Colitis from Crohn Disease	
Feature	**Ulcerative Colitis**	**Crohn Disease**
Distribution	Diffuse, continuous	Focal (skip), segmental
Depth of involvement	Mucosa, submucosa	Transmural
Mucosal appearance	Irregular ulcers, friable, atrophy	Cobblestoning
Bowel wall	Thin	Thickened or normal
Creeping mesenteric fat	Absent	Common
Stricture	Usually absent	Maybe
Fistula	Usually absent	Maybe
Fissuring	Usually absent	Common
Ileal involvement	<10% (backwash)	Common
Upper GI involvement	Usually no	Maybe
Rectal involvement	100%	~15%
Anal involvement	5–10%	~75%
Well-formed granuloma	Absent	Common
Transmural lymphoid aggregates	Absent	Common

GI, gastrointestinal.

Backwash ileitis may be seen in severe pancolitis, presumably due to reflux of colonic contents. It is characterized by mild but active inflammation in the distal few centimeters of the terminal ileum with relative preservation of the normal villous architecture. (e-**Figs. 14.38** and **14.39**). Table 14.6 summarizes the gross and histologic features that help distinguish UC from CD.

3. **Indeterminate colitis** is not a distinct entity, and the diagnosis should be applied only to cases that are truly difficult to classify histologically and clinically. Most cases will eventually evolve into UC or CD. The diagnosis is usually rendered because of insufficient clinical, radiologic, or endoscopic data, and because of prominent overlapping pathologic features. Fulminant colitis that lacks specific diagnostic features may also belong in this category.

4. **Dysplasia** is associated with the extent and duration of IBD and is a recognized precursor of adenocarcinoma. In surveillance biopsies for IBD, the presence of dysplasia should be reported as either negative, or graded as indefinite, low grade, or high grade. Grade is based on architectural complexity of the crypts, as well as surface epithelial cytologic atypia and maturation defects. Conventional low-grade dysplasia simulates a tubular adenoma, while high-grade dysplasia is identical to adenocarcinoma in situ or intraepithelial carcinoma (e-**Fig. 14.40**). However, in some cases where there is abundant inflammation and ulceration, it may be challenging to separate inflammatory or reactive atypia from dysplasia, either in the crypts or the surface epithelium, and these cases usually fall in the category of indefinite for dysplasia.

IBD-associated dysplasia can be flat or raised. Colectomy is recommended for flat dysplasia. Raised dysplasia in IBD is classified into "adenoma-like" (which resembles sporadic adenomas and is amenable to complete endoscopic resection), and "nonadenoma-like", which consists of patches, plaques, carpet-like lesions, or other broadbased masses, that cannot be endoscopically resected. Colectomy is warranted in the latter cases. Morphologic subtypes of dysplasia include intestinal (conventional), hypermucinous/villous, and serrated dysplasia. The biologic behavior of the latter two is not well known.

5. Pouchitis refers to inflammation of the ileal pouch created after a total colectomy, usually for UC. Active pouchitis shows mixed neutrophilic and lymphoplasmacytic infiltrates in the ileal mucosa, and erosions or ulcerations in more severe cases. Chronic changes, such as villous architectural distortion, villous atrophy, and pyloric metaplasia, may be seen in long-term disease. An important differential diagnosis is recurrent CD in a case previously diagnosed as UC. Re-evaluation of a previous colectomy specimen may be necessary if granulomas, a fistula, a sinus tract, or a fissuring ulcer are detected in a pouch.

D. **Diversion Colitis** refers to an inflammatory response in the blind segment, usually the rectum (Hartmann pouch) following ileostomy or colostomy formation. The process is thought to be caused by a deficiency of short-chain fatty acids because the ostomy procedure excludes the rectum from the fecal stream. The classic findings are a granular, friable mucosa with marked lymphoid hyperplasia and cryptitis (e-**Fig. 14.41**). The features can mimic IBD, and therefore interpretation of the biopsy findings in the clinical context is important.

E. **Microscopic Colitis** is a clinical term that includes **lymphocytic colitis** and **collagenous colitis**; these entities share watery diarrhea and normal endoscopic findings clinically, and surface epithelial damage, inflammation, and intraepithelial lymphocytosis microscopically (e-**Fig. 14.42**). The microscopic findings are non-specific in that a focal increase in the number of IELs may be seen in IBD, infectious colitis, gluten-sensitive enteropathy, GVHD, and human immunodeficiency virus (HIV) infection, as well as in areas adjacent to lymphoid aggregates.

The key feature of collagenous colitis is the additional presence of a thickened collagen layer in the subepithelial region, which can be inhomogeneous (e-**Fig. 14.43**). The thickness of the collagen layer is variable but should be >10 μm. Small capillaries and scattered inflammatory cells are typically entrapped within the collagen layer. Evaluation requires well-oriented sections; in difficult cases, a trichrome stain may be helpful. The differential diagnosis includes mucosal fibrosis, which involves the full thickness of the mucosa and may be seen in ischemic colitis, a healed ulcer, and radiation colitis.

By definition, a large number of neutrophils should not be present in either form of microscopic colitis. However, neutrophilic cryptitis or crypt abscesses can be seen in some patients, but should be far less prominent than the lymphocytic infiltration. In patients with collagenous colitis, focal architectural disarray and Paneth cell metaplasia can be seen, findings that can be misinterpreted as IBD.

F. **Diverticular Disease (Diverticulosis),** acquired outpouchings of the mucosa and submucosa through defects in weakened muscularis propria, occurs throughout the colon but is more common in the sigmoid colon (e-**Fig. 14.44**). Approximately 10% of cases become inflamed (diverticulitis), leading to abscess formation, perforation, and fistula formation. On biopsy, diverticular disease–associated segmental colitis (inflammation of the interdiverticular mucosa) may be difficult to distinguish from IBD due to crypt architectural distortion and active inflammation.

G. **Radiation Colitis** occurs following radiation therapy, usually for prostatic or cervical cancer. Biopsies are uncommon in the acute phase, but show apoptotic activity, nuclear atypia, mucin depletion, and decreased mitotic activity. Chronic radiation colitis is characterized by telangiectasias of the mucosal capillaries, lamina propria hyalinization, and atypical stromal fibroblasts. Inflammatory cells are sparse (e-**Fig. 14.45**).

H. **Infectious Colitis.** Most infections in the gastrointestinal tract are self-limited. Biopsies are performed in the setting of chronic or debilitating diarrhea, or in the setting of immunocompromise. A knowledge of the clinical presentation, including underlying diseases, travel and drug history, and endoscopic findings aid the work up of infectious etiology to a great extent.

1. **CMV** infection is symptomatic in immunocompromised patients, and usually presents with diarrhea, abdominal pain, fever, and weight loss. It can also lead to steroid-refractory IBD by superinfection. Endoscopic and histologic findings vary, and the biopsy findings may range from acute inflammation with crypt abscesses and

ulceration, to minimal inflammation with increased crypt apoptosis. Typical viral inclusions (nuclear and/or cytoplasmic, predominantly in endothelial and stromal cells) can be hard to find, but when suspected an immunohistochemical stain can be useful.

2. **Adenovirus** more commonly infects children, but is also seen in similar settings in adults as CMV infection. Typical viral inclusions (nuclear, predominantly in epithelial cells) can be hard to find, but immunohistochemistry can be useful in the right clinical setting.

3. **Acute (self-limited) colitis** is usually caused by bacterial infections such as *Campylobacter, Salmonella,* or *Aeromonas*. There is a neutrophilic infiltrate in the lamina propria, with or without cryptitis or crypt abscess, but in contrast to chronic colitis there is no glandular architectural distortion, basal lymphoplasmacytosis, or Paneth cell metaplasia.

4. **Yersinia** organisms preferentially infect the ileum, right colon, and appendix, with prominent mesenteric adenopathy, more commonly in immunocompromised individuals and in those with iron overload. Both suppurative and granulomatous inflammation are seen. Cultures, serologic studies, and PCR are helpful in confirming the diagnosis.

5. ***Clostridium difficile*–related colitis** manifests after prior exposure to oral antibiotic therapy, and is the most common nosocomial gastrointestinal infection. Involvement can be diffuse or patchy, and although the primary site is the colon, the small bowel or appendix may also be involved. Histologically, the classic manifestation is pseudomembranous colitis featuring ballooned crypts with rupture ("volcano" lesions), intercrypt necrosis, and a "pseudomembrane" composed of fibrin, mucin, and neutrophils (e-**Figs. 14.46** and **14.47**). The differential diagnosis of pseudomembranous colitis includes other types of infectious colitis (such as with *Shigella* or enterohemorrhagic *E. coli*), and ischemic colitis. PCR testing is confirmatory.

6. **Intestinal spirochetosis** manifests as a fuzzy blue line (due to the presence of spirochetal organisms) at the luminal border of the colonic mucosa, with no significant associated inflammation (e-**Fig. 14.48**). It usually affects homosexual and immunocompromised individuals. Immunohistochemistry is preferred, but other stains that can also assist in diagnosis are Alcian blue, PAS, or silver impregnation stains such as Warthin–Starry.

7. **Fungal infections** of the GI tract usually affect the immunocompromised, and are often part of a disseminated process. There is usually variable neutrophilic and granulomatous inflammation. The organisms are often seen on H&E stain, and their presence can be confirmed with GMS or PAS stains. ***Candida*** is identified by budding yeasts, pseudohyphae, or hyphae. Fungal hyphae in **aspergillosis** radiate outward from a zone of ischemic necrosis. In **mucormycosis**, there are broad, ribbon-like, pauci-septate hyphae that branch at various angles. ***Histoplasma*** organisms are small, ovoid, usually intracellular yeast forms in macrophages infiltrating the mucosa and submucosa. **Cryptococci** show round to oval yeast forms with narrow-based budding, and considerable variation in size. There is often a halo effect seen on H&E stain due to the organisms capsule, which can be highlighted with mucicarmine or Alcian blue stains.

8. **Parasitic infections** of the GI tract preferentially occur in tropical/subtropical climates, or in immunocompromised patients, and common examples with diagnostic features on biopsies include the following:

   a. ***Entamoeba histolytica*** commonly involves the cecum and right colon, classically forming flask-shaped ulcers, with undermining of adjacent normal mucosa. Organisms may be found in the associated necro-inflammatory debris and resemble macrophages with round eccentric nuclei, and may show ingested red cells. Amoebae can be distinguished from macrophages in that they are PAS and trichrome positive, and CD68 negative.

b. ***Giardia lamblia*** organisms appear as pear-shaped binucleate trophozoites at the luminal surface in small intestinal biopsies, without tissue invasion or significant associated inflammation.

c. ***Cryptosporidium parvum*** most commonly affects the small bowel, and the 2 to 5 μm basophilic spherical organisms protrude from the apex of the enterocytes, lining the crypts or the surface.

d. Helminthic infections include hookworms, roundworms, and whipworms.

9. **HIV enteropathy** is an entity without clear pathogenesis, and can only be diagnosed after all opportunistic infections are excluded. Patients present with chronic diarrhea, which improves with initiation of HAART. Small intestinal biopsies show mild villous blunting, and the colonic mucosa shows increased apoptosis.

I. **GVHD** commonly affects the skin, GI tract, and liver. Histologic hallmarks in the intestinal tract include a paucity of inflammatory cells in the lamina propria, apoptosis, and crypt dropout (**e-Figs. 14.49 and 14.50**). The common differential diagnoses of these histologic findings include cytomegalovirus infection, and drugs such as mycophenolate mofetil (**e-Fig. 14.51**).

Histologic grades do not always match the clinical course, and histologic features are not entirely specific with a broad differential diagnosis that includes drug injury (in particular, mycophenolate mofetil), cytoreductive therapy for bone marrow transplant, or proton pump inhibitor therapy (in the stomach); infections, particularly CMV; primary immune disorders; or vigorous bowel preparation (although in this situation, the apoptosis is located more at the surface in contrast to the deeper crypts in GVHD). Commonly, both upper and lower GI tract are involved. However, if involvement is limited to only upper GI sites, the prognosis is better.

The histologic grades are as follows. Grade 1: Scattered apoptotic cells in crypts, at least 2 per biopsy piece; Grade 2: Apoptotic crypt abscess, or loss of individual crypts; Grade 3: Loss of two or three contiguous crypts; Grade 4: Contiguous crypt loss involving more than 4 crypt spaces.

Chronic GVHD is a multisystem disease, and primarily a clinical diagnosis. The esophagus is the most commonly affected site, with ulcers and submucosal fibrosis; in the colon, chronic changes resemble UC.

J. **Drug-Induced Colitis** presents with a wide spectrum of histologic findings. NSAID agents are the most common medications that induce injury and can be associated with diaphragm disease in the small intestine, and lymphocytic infiltrates, apoptosis, and microscopic colitis in the large intestine. Kayexalate, cocaine, and amphetamines are among the agents that are associated with ischemic colitis. Excessive laxative use can cause melanosis coli (**e-Fig. 14.52**). Agents used for bowel preparation may cause mucosal edema, hemorrhage, surface epithelial detachment, neutrophilic cryptitis, and increased apoptotic activity.

VI. **DIAGNOSTIC FEATURES OF POLYPS AND NEOPLASMS OF THE LARGE INTESTINE.** The WHO classification scheme of tumors of the colon and rectum is given in Table 14.7. Revised staging schemes for neoplasms of the large intestine have recently been published (Amin MB et al., eds. *AJCC Cancer Staging Manual*. 8th ed. New York: Springer, 2017), as have suggested reporting guidelines (e.g., from the College of American Pathologists, available at http://www.cap.org).

A. **Inflammatory Polyps** are polypoid projections of non-neoplastic epithelial and stromal components admixed with inflammatory cells. **Inflammatory pseudopolyps** represent areas of inflamed and regenerating mucosa, and project above the level of the surrounding mucosa, which is frequently ulcerated. Occasionally, pseudosarcomatous stroma is present, particularly in eroded or ulcerated areas, characterized by bizarre or multinucleated stroma cells simulating sarcoma (**e-Fig. 14.53**). **Prolapse-type inflammatory polyps** develop from traction and other peristalsis induced trauma, which induce localized ischemia and repair. Depending on the location, they are referred to as inflammatory cloacogenic polyps of the ATZ, inflammatory cap polyps and cap polyposis (with surface granulation tissue), colitis cystica polyposa (**e-Fig. 14.54**), or diverticular

TABLE 14.7	2010 WHO Histologic Classification of Tumors of the Colon and Rectum

Epithelial tumors

Adenoma
  Tubular
  Villous
  Tubulovillous

Dysplasia (intraepithelial neoplasia), low grade

Dysplasia (intraepithelial neoplasia), high grade

Serrated lesions
  Hyperplastic polyp, 3 subtypes (see text)
  Sessile serrated adenoma/polyp
  Traditional serrated adenoma

Hamartomatous
  Cowden associated polyp
  Juvenile polyp
  Peutz–Jeghers polyp

Carcinomas

Adenocarcinoma
  Cribriform comedo-type adenocarcinoma
  Medullary carcinoma
  Micropapillary carcinoma
  Mucinous carcinoma
  Serrated adenocarcinoma
  Signet-ring cell carcinoma

Adenosquamous carcinoma

Spindle cell carcinoma

Squamous cell carcinoma

Undifferentiated carcinoma

Neuroendocrine Neoplasms

Neuroendocrine tumor (NET)
  NET G1 (carcinoid)
  NET G2

Neuroendocrine carcinoma (NEC)
  Large cell NEC
  Small cell NEC

Mixed adenoneuroendocrine carcinoma

EC cell, serotonin-producing NET

L-cell, glucagon-like peptide and PP/PYY-producing NETs

Mesenchymal tumors

Lipoma

Leiomyoma

Gastrointestinal stromal tumor

Leiomyosarcoma

Angiosarcoma

Kaposi sarcoma

Lymphomas

B-cell lymphoma, unclassifiable, with features intermediate between diffuse large B-cell lymphoma and Burkitt lymphoma

Burkitt lymphoma

Diffuse large B-cell lymphoma

Mantle cell lymphoma

Marginal zone lymphoma of mucosa-associated lymphoid tissue (MALT lymphoma)

Secondary tumors

EC, enterochromaffin cell; L-cell, an intestinal enteroendocrine cell; MALT, mucosa-associated lymphoid tissue; PP, pancreatic polypeptide; PYY, polypeptide YY; WHO, World Health Organization.
From: Bosman FT, Carneiro F, Hruban RH, Theise ND, eds. *WHO Classification of Tumours. Pathology and Genetics. Tumours of the Digestive System.* Lyon, France: IARC Press; 2017. Used with permission.

disease-associated polyps. The classic histologic feature of prolapse-induced inflammatory polyps are fibromuscular hyperplasia of the lamina propria, architectural distortion and reactive changes in the crypts, and variable inflammation (e-**Fig. 14.55**). **Inflammatory myoglandular polyp** is rare and likely hamartomatous in origin, and shows splaying of the fibers of the muscularis mucosae with surface inflammation and erosion.

B. Hamartomatous Polyps

1. Juvenile polyps can be sporadic (mostly in the rectosigmoid), usually in children. Juvenile polyposis syndrome is diagnosed when (a) there is a positive family history, (b) polyposis involving the entire GI tract, or (c) three or more colonic juvenile polyps. Histologically, the findings include cystically dilated glands with edema and inflammation (e-**Figs. 14.56** and **14.57**). Syndromic patients have an increased risk of GI cancers.

Peutz–Jeghers syndrome is discussed in the small intestine section above.

2. Cowden syndrome is mostly related to *PTEN* gene mutations, and GI manifestations include hamartomatous polyps in the stomach, small, and large intestines. Polypoid ganglioneuromas are the lesion most specific for Cowden syndrome. In patients with

Cowden syndrome, the lifetime risk of development of colorectal adenocarcinoma is increased by 10%.

3. Cronkhite–Canada syndrome is a non-hereditary polyposis syndrome of unknown etiology; it is associated with other ectodermal anomalies. The polyps occur throughout the GI tract except the esophagus, and resemble juvenile polyps.

C. Hyperplastic Polyps (HPs) are the most common type of polyp in colon. They are typically small (usually <5 mm) and feature a serrated or sawtooth luminal configuration (e-**Fig. 14.58**). The serration is most prominent at the upper portion of the crypts and along the luminal surface, whereas the lower crypt portion remains narrow and proliferative. A thickened basement membrane may be seen. Three morphologic types of HP have been described: microvesicular (with frequent *BRAF* mutations), goblet cell rich (with frequent *KRAS* mutations), and mucin-poor (molecular features not well characterized).

D. Sessile Serrated Adenoma/Polyp (SSA/P) most commonly arises in the right colon, and is usually >5 mm in size. The crypts have a prominent serrated epithelium which extend to the base; the crypts are also dilated, flask-shaped, L-shaped, or branched (e-**Figs. 14.59** and **14.60**). The overall architecture is distorted and the proliferative zone is altered in these polyps. About 80% of SSA/P polyps carry *BRAF* mutations, which supports the hypothesis that microvesicular HPs are early precursors of SSA/P. SSA/P also show a high rate of DNA methylation (CpG island methylator phenotype/CIMP) leading to a high level of microsatellite instability (MSI) by transcriptional silencing of the *MLH1* gene. Cytologically, SSA/P are lined by bland epithelial cells, but some polyps can show cytologic dysplasia which is of two main types. "Serrated dysplasia" is characterized by cytologic features that include eosinophilic cytoplasm, vesicular chromatin, and prominent nucleoli. Conventional adenomatous dysplasia resembles cytologic changes of a tubular adenoma (e-**Fig. 14.61**). SSA/P that have dysplastic features are referred as SSA/P with cytologic dysplasia. The current recommendation for SSA/P is complete removal of the lesion. Follow-up for polyps less than 10 mm without cytologic dysplasia is 5 years; for polyps more than 10 mm, or multiple polyps less than 10 mm is 3 years; and for polyps larger than 10 mm and multiple, or for polyps with dysplasia is between 1 and 3 years.

E. Traditional Serrated Adenoma (TSA) tends to be left-sided, and mostly located in the distal colon. These polyps are characterized by a villiform architecture, serration, eosinophilic cytoplasm, cytologic dysplasia, and the presence of so-called ectopic crypt foci within the villi. An ectopic crypt focus is defined as a small abortive crypt with loss of the normal relation between the base of the crypt and the muscularis mucosae (e-**Fig. 14.62**). *BRAF* mutations are present in one-third of cases, *KRAS* mutations are present in approximately 25%, *MGMT* loss in about 20%, and *APC* mutations and *TP53* mutations at variable frequency. Hypermethylation is noted in a lower percentage of cases as compared with SSA/P. The current recommendations are for complete removal and surveillance as with conventional adenoma every 3 to 5 years.

    Serrated polyposis syndrome is viewed as a precancerous syndrome and is defined as at least 5 serrated polyps proximal to the sigmoid colon, 2 of which are >1 cm in maximal dimension; any number of polyps proximal to the sigmoid colon in a patient with a first-degree relative having hyperplastic polyposis; or more than 30 serrated polyps of any size throughout the colon. *BRAF* mutation and loss of MLH1/PMS2 expression is thought to have a role in cancer development.

F. Conventional Adenoma is categorized as a tubular adenoma if the villous component accounts for <25% of the lesion, as a villous adenoma if >75% is villous, and as a tubulovillous adenoma if the villous component is between 25% and 75% (e-**Fig. 14.63**). By definition, adenomas contain at least low-grade dysplasia characterized by nuclear stratification, nuclear enlargement, elongation, and hyperchromasia associated with cytoplasmic mucin depletion. High-grade dysplasia is characterized by nuclear rounding, loss of polarity, prominent nucleoli, and increased mitosis including atypical mitosis (e-**Fig. 14.64**). Paneth cells, neuroendocrine cells, and squamous cell clusters may occur in adenomas. Guidelines for surveillance are as follows:

Every 5 to 10 years for 1 to 2 adenomas <1 cm; every 3 years for an adenoma >1 cm, 3 to 10 adenomas, or an adenoma with villous features or with high-grade dysplasia; and less than 3 years for >10 adenomas (with additional consideration of a familial syndrome for the latter).

In **invasive adenocarcinoma arising in a polyp,** the size of invasive focus, distance of the invasive focus to the polypectomy margin (e-**Fig. 14.65**), histologic grade, and the presence or absence of lymphovascular invasion should be reported since these data are important in determining whether segmental resection should be performed. A diagnostic pitfall for adenocarcinoma arising in a polyp is pseudoinvasion, in which adenomatous elements are entrapped or herniated into the submucosa usually secondary to torsion; pseudoinvasion is commonly associated with hemosiderin granules (e-**Figs. 14.66** and **14.67**). Features that aid in the distinction of pseudoinvasion from true invasion include a lack of overt malignant histology, presence of lamina propria inflammatory cells around the entrapped elements, lack of a desmoplastic response, and lack of direct contact with submucosal muscular vessels. When in doubt, deeper levels of the problematic area may help clarify the diagnosis.

G. Adenomatous Polyposis Syndromes

1. **FAP** is an autosomal dominant disorder caused by germline mutations of the *APC* gene located at 5q21. A minimum of 100 colonic adenomas is required for the diagnosis, but an attenuated form with a reduced number is not uncommon. Adenomas of the upper GI tract, particularly in the ampullary region, and fundic gland polyps are also common findings in FAP patients. Progression to colonic adenocarcinoma approaches 100% by mid-life if prophylactic colectomy is not performed (e-**Fig. 14.68**).

2. **Gardner and Turcot syndromes** are considered variants of FAP. In addition to adenomas of the GI tract, extra-GI tumors are seen in these patients including osteoid osteoma, epidermal cysts, and intra-abdominal fibromatosis (desmoid tumor) for the former; and tumors of the central nervous system for the latter.

3. ***MUTYH*-Associated Polyposis** has a presentation similar to attenuated FAP, but there is no *APC* gene mutation. Instead, patients have biallelic mutations in the human *MUTYH* (Muty homolog) gene that is located on the short arm of chromosome 1. The disease is an autosomal recessive disorder and the colorectal polyps are of different histologic phenotypes. Duodenal and gastric polyps may also occur.

4. **LS/hereditary nonpolyposis colorectal cancer syndrome (HNPCC)** is an autosomal dominant disorder with an increased risk of colorectal cancer as well as an increased risk of other epithelial malignancies including of the endometrium, ovary, stomach, small intestine, upper urinary tract, and other sites. It is caused by defects in the DNA mismatch repair (MMR) genes including *MLH1, MSH2, MSH6,* and *PMS2* that lead to MSI. Defects in MMR can be evaluated indirectly by immunohistochemical stains for DNA MMR proteins, by DNA-based molecular analyses (commonly PCR) for MSI, or directly by DNA sequence analysis of the MMR genes themselves.

Immunohistochemical analysis is used in many centers to identify the most likely mutated MMR genes; the MMR proteins are normally found in all human tissues, thus loss of nuclear staining may represent the presence of a genetic abnormality. The commonly tested proteins are MLH1, MSH2, MSH6, and PMS2. MLH1-PMS2 and MSH2-MSH6 form dimers, the latter member of each pair regulating expression of the former. Thus, if there is a mutation in *MSH6*, expression of both MSH2 and MSH6 proteins will be lost. However, the loss of expression has different implications for each protein pair. If there is loss of MSH2 and MSH6, or of MSH6 alone, the patient is more likely to have LS and therefore should be further referred for genetic counseling. On the other hand, loss of MLH1 and PMS2 can be due to sporadic mutations as well as a rare form of LS, so additional testing for *BRAF* mutation is indicated; the presence of a *BRAF* mutation indicates a sporadic mutation rather than

LS. Immunohistochemistry for the MMR protein is currently recommended for all patients with colorectal cancer.

H. **Adenocarcinoma** is graded based on the percentage of gland formation as with other sites in the GI tract, as well-, moderate-, or poorly differentiated, and per WHO, is grouped into a two-tier grading scheme of low grade (well- and moderately differentiated) and high grade (poorly differentiated). Prognostic factors other than TNM stage include the presence of tumor deposits, status of the circumferential margin, presence of lymphatic invasion, large vessel invasion, and perineural invasion; tumor regression is an additional prognostic factor for neoadjuvant treated rectal carcinoma.

Similar to other sites of the GI tract, mucinous carcinoma and signet-ring cell carcinoma of the colon are defined as >50% of the tumor bulk consisting of a mucinous component or signet-ring cells, respectively. In poorly differentiated mucinous carcinoma, signet-ring cells can be numerous (e-**Fig. 14.69**). Medullary carcinoma consists of sheets of poorly differentiated or undifferentiated tumor cells with a syncytial growth pattern and a pushing border. Characteristically, there is a marked inter- and intratumoral lymphocytic infiltrate, and Crohn-like lymphoid aggregates may be present at the periphery in some cases. These variants of colorectal adenocarcinoma are frequently associated with DNA MMR deficiency leading to MSI and may have a more favorable prognosis despite their high-grade appearance. Although MSI tumors tend to be right-sided, mucinous, or poorly differentiated, they cannot be reliably distinguished on histologic features alone.

EGFR is overexpressed in 60% to 80% of colorectal cancers, and has been associated with increased risk of metastasis and poor survival. Epigenetic upregulation appears to be the predominant mechanism of activation in colorectal cancers; *EGFR* gene amplification and point mutations are less commonly seen. Anti-EGFR monoclonal antibodies (cetuximab and panitumumab) are routinely used to treat patients with advanced disease; *KRAS*, *NRAS*, and to a lesser extent *BRAF* mutations, as well as *HER2* amplification, are predictors of resistance to anti-EGFR therapy. Therefore, testing for these mutations is also now being routinely performed in advanced colorectal tumors. *BRAF* mutation testing has additional value in MLH1 deficient colorectal cancers as a means to differentiate sporadic MLH1 deficient cancers from hereditary MLH1 deficient cancers.

I. **Neuroendocrine Neoplasms**

1. **Well-differentiated NET** is most frequently located in the rectum, followed by the cecum (e-**Fig. 14.70**). It is commonly asymptomatic. Most tumors are grade 1. Of note, rectal NETs are immunopositive with prostatic markers such as prostatic acid phosphatase.

2. **Poorly differentiated neuroendocrine carcinoma (NEC)** of the large intestine is most common in the right colon, and is frequently associated with overlying adenomatous epithelium or an associated adenocarcinoma (MANEC/mixed adenoneuroendocrine carcinoma).

J. **GIST** of the colorectum accounts for less than 5% of all GISTs and is most commonly seen in the rectum (e-**Fig. 14.71**). Colonic GISTs tend to have an aggressive biologic behavior, and tumors with mitotic activity can recur and metastasize despite a small size of <2 cm.

K. **Schwannomas** are thought to arise from the myenteric plexi, and in the GI tract can involve the colon and rectum, but less commonly than the stomach. GI schwannomas have a discontinuous cuff of reactive lymphoid cells at the periphery of the lesion, and typically lack nuclear palisading, Verocay bodies, and hyalinized vessels that are typical features in tumors that arise in the central nervous system or peripheral soft tissue.

L. **Leiomyoma** is the most common mesenchymal tumor of the colon. It arises from the muscularis mucosae and presents as a well-demarcated nodular expansion in the submucosa. It is typically hypocellular, lacks cytologic atypia, and lacks c-kit expression (e-**Fig. 14.72**).

M.**Submucosal Lipoma** can be associated with hyperplastic change in the overlying colonic mucosa (e-**Fig. 14.73**).

N. Ganglioneuroma and Ganglioneuromatosis feature a bland Schwann cell proliferation with nerve fibers that expand the lamina propria, with individual or nests of ganglion cells embedded in a spindle cell background (e-**Figs. 14.74** and **14.75**). The lesion can occur as sporadic and solitary, as ganglioneuromatous polyposis (multiple polyps in upper and lower GI tract in Cowden syndrome), or as diffuse ganglioneuromatosis that may involve the deeper aspects of the bowel wall (as in MEN2B or NF1).

O. Mucosal Perineuriomas are benign nerve sheath tumors composed of bland spindle cells expanding the lamina propria, presenting incidentally at colonoscopy as a small sessile lesion. They have a female predominance and a predilection for the rectosigmoid. In most cases, they are associated with a serrated polyp that shows a BRAF V600E mutation. Immunohistochemically, they are positive for EMA, and negative for S100, SMA, desmin, and c-Kit.

P. Mucosal Schwann Cell Hamartomas are incidentally detected small polypoid lesions in the sigmoid colon and rectum, composed of S100 positive bland spindle cells that entrap glands and have an irregular border with the adjacent lamina propria.

Q. Miscellaneous Polypoid Lesions. Pneumatosis coli is a characterized by gas accumulation in colonic wall. It most commonly affects the sigmoid colon. Microscopically, cystic spaces surrounded by histiocytes and giant cells are seen (e-**Fig. 14.76**). **Endometriosis, pseudolipomatosis**, and **xanthomas** can also present as polypoid lesions.

VII. DIAGNOSTIC FEATURES OF COMMON NONNEOPLASTIC AND NEOPLASTIC CONDITIONS OF THE APPENDIX

A. Nonneoplastic

1. **Acute appendicitis** predominantly occurs in children and young adults. The pathogenesis usually involves luminal occlusion (such as by a fecalith, lymphoid hyperplasia, polyp, or tumor, or parasites such as *Enterobius vermicularis*) followed by bacterial infection. Diverticulosis, IBD, or other infections are rare causes. Microscopically, early lesions reveal only mucosal involvement; later, acute appendicitis is characterized by transmural neutrophilic infiltration (e-**Fig. 14.77**). Abscess formation, gangrenous necrosis, and perforation may ensue. When inflammation is predominantly located in the mesoappendix and the serosa it is called periappendicitis, and other causes of peritonitis should be sought clinically.

2. **Fibrous obliteration of the appendiceal lumen** occurs as a reactive process subsequent to prior acute appendicitis, or as a component of aging. The obliteration occurs by proliferation of bland spindle cells in a collagenous and myxoid background, and starts at the tip. Lesional cells include fibroblasts, Schwann cells, axons, and few inflammatory cells confined to the mucosa.

3. **Cystic fibrosis** involving the appendix is characterized by thick, eosinophilic, inspissated mucoid material in the lumen and in the dilated crypts (e-**Fig. 14.78**).

4. **Polyps** of the appendix are histologically similar to those of the colorectum, but tend to be sessile.

B. Neoplastic. The WHO classification of tumors of the appendix is given in Table 14.8. Revised staging schemes for neoplasms of the appendix have recently been published (Amin MB et al., eds. *AJCC Cancer Staging Manual.* 8th ed. New York: Springer, 2017), as have suggested reporting guidelines (e.g., from the College of American Pathologists, available at http://www.cap.org).

1. **Low-grade appendiceal mucinous neoplasm (LAMN).** The lining mucinous epithelium shows conventional low-grade dysplasia, and may be flat or villous in configuration. In contrast to an adenoma, the neoplastic epithelium rests on fibrous tissue with no underlying lamina propria or muscularis mucosae (e-**Fig. 14.79**). The lesion has a pushing front, and can extend through the full thickness of the wall, but no desmoplasia is present; the lesion can also be associated with acellular mucin. Fibrosis and hyalinization of the wall is common. Rarely, the lining epithelium can show high-grade dysplasia, in which case the lesion is termed as **high-grade appendiceal mucinous neoplasm (HAMN)**. Staging of these tumors is based on the depth of location of either the epithelium or acellular mucin. The tumors are considered to be

TABLE 14.8 WHO Histologic Classification of Tumors of the Appendix

Epithelial tumors	Neuroendocrine neoplasms
Premalignant lesions	Neuroendocrine tumor (NET)
Adenoma	NET G1 (carcinoid)
Tubular	NET G2
Villous	Neuroendocrine carcinoma (NEC)
Tubulovillous	Large cell NEC
Dysplasia (intraepithelial neoplasia), low grade	Small cell NEC
	EC cell, serotonin-producing NET
Dysplasia (intraepithelial neoplasia), high grade	Goblet cell carcinoid
	L-cell, glucagon-like peptide and PP/PYY-producing NET
Serrated lesions	
Hyperplastic polyp	Tubular carcinoid
Sessile serrated adenoma/polyp	**Mesenchymal tumors**
Traditional serrated adenoma	Neuroma
Carcinoma	Lipoma
Adenocarcinoma	Leiomyoma
Mucinous adenocarcinoma	Leiomyosarcoma
Low-grade appendiceal mucinous neoplasm	Kaposi sarcoma
Signet-ring cell carcinoma	**Lymphomas**
Undifferentiated carcinoma	**Secondary tumors**

EC, enterochromaffin cell; L-cell, an intestinal enteroendocrine cell; MALT, mucosa-associated lymphoid tissue; PP, pancreatic polypeptide; PYY, polypeptide YY; WHO, World Health Organization.
From: Bosman FT, Carneiro F, Hruban RH, Theise ND, eds. *WHO Classification of Tumours. Pathology and Genetics. Tumours of the Digestive System.* Lyon, France: IARC Press; 2017. Used with permission.

low-grade malignant neoplasms, and spread along the peritoneal surfaces and recurrences clinically recognized as pseudomyxoma peritonei can occur. These tumors usually do not spread to lymph nodes or distant organs.

2. **Adenocarcinoma** of the appendix, particularly mucinous adenocarcinoma, is distinguished from LAMN by the presence of an invasive growth pattern and associated desmoplastic reaction.

3. **Pseudomyxoma peritonei** is a clinical diagnosis characterized by accumulation of mucin within the peritoneal cavity caused by neoplastic mucin-secreting cells. Appendiceal lesions are responsible for the vast majority of the cases, although mucinous tumors of other sites can rarely cause a similar clinical picture. Based on the histology of the neoplastic cells in the peritoneum, several terms are used. **Peritoneal adenomucinosis/low-grade pseudomyxoma peritonei/disseminated peritoneal adenomucinosis (DPAM)** is defined by the presence of mucin containing a low cellularity of epithelium that has low-grade cytologic atypia. **Peritoneal mucinous carcinomatosis/high-grade pseudomyxoma peritonei** are terms used for peritoneal mucinous tumors with higher cellularity and features of marked cellular atypia. The appropriate nomenclature for peritoneal mucinous neoplasia remains controversial. Surgical debulking with hyperthermic intraoperative peritoneal chemotherapy (HIPEC) and early postoperative intraperitoneal chemotherapy (EPIC) is the current management for pseudomyxoma peritonei.

4. **Neuroendocrine neoplasms** in the appendix are mostly well differentiated, and most are diagnosed incidentally. They commonly occur at the tip of the appendix. Approximately 75% are less than 1 cm in diameter and almost never metastasize.

5. **Goblet cell carcinoid,** which is exclusive to appendix, is a neoplasm in which each neoplastic cell shows a mixed endocrine–exocrine differentiation. The

tumor typically diffusely infiltrates the appendiceal wall with relative sparing of the mucosa. The hallmark of the tumor is the presence of small, tight, round or oval clusters of tumor cells exhibiting a goblet or signet-ring morphology with a small compressed nucleus and conspicuous intracytoplasmic mucin (e-**Figs. 14.80** and **14.81**). Tumor nests also recapitulate crypt morphology, and thus the term "crypt cell carcinoma" has also been used for these tumors. The cells show a low Ki67 proliferation index, low mitotic count, and only mild to moderate cytologic atypia. Fused or cribriform glands, single-file structures, diffusely infiltrating signet ring cells, or sheets of tumor cells are interpreted as a carcinomatous growth pattern, and when present the tumor is termed adenocarcinoma ex goblet cell carcinoid.

6. **Tubular carcinoids** are small neoplasms characterized by discrete tubule formation by bland cuboidal epithelial cells, rarely containing a few goblet cells or Paneth cells, within abundant stroma (e-**Fig. 14.82**). Tubular carcinoid behaves in a benign fashion. These cells stain with synaptophysin and may be weakly positive for chromogranin, but they stain for CEA and glucagon unlike classic NETs.

VIII. **DIAGNOSTIC FEATURES OF COMMON NONNEOPLASTIC AND NEOPLASTIC CONDITIONS OF THE ANUS.** A lesion is considered anal when its epicenter is less than 2 cm from the dentate line proximally, and devoid of cutaneous appendages distally. A perianal lesion is defined as one which is located within a 5 cm radius of the anus, and that is completely visualized with gentle traction on the buttocks.

A. **Nonneoplastic**

1. **Congenital malformations** include anal atresia, anorectal agenesis, and imperforate anus. Genetic factors are most important in their pathogenesis, and usually they are associated with other anomalies in other organ systems. These malformations are often accompanied by fistula formation.

2. **Hemorrhoids** are characterized by dilated thick-walled submucosal vessels, often with thrombi, with hemorrhage into the surrounding connective tissue. Internal hemorrhoids are located proximal to the dentate line, and external hemorrhoids are located distal to the dentate line. Normally the anal submucosa has arteriovenous anastomoses which serve a protective role during defecation; undue elevations of intra-abdominal pressure cause prolapse of these vessels resulting in vascular congestion. Early cases are treated conservatively, but in severe cases surgical excision is performed.

3. **Anal tag** is a fibroepithelial polyp (a benign polypoid projections of squamous epithelium and underlying subepithelial connective tissue) histologically identical to a skin tag (acrochordon). Surgical resection is performed in symptomatic cases.

4. **Inflammatory cloacogenic polyp** is a type of mucosal prolapse presenting as a sessile 1 to 2 cm polyp on the anterior wall, usually in middle-aged patients. Histologically there is fibrosis of the lamina propria, thickening of muscularis mucosae with some extension into the lamina propria, hyperplasia of the mucosa (often with a villous configuration, and often containing areas of ATZ [mixed rectal and squamous] epithelium), and surface erosion (e-**Fig. 14.83**).

5. **Anal fissures** start as mucosal tears that usually occur in the posterior midline, extending from the dentate line to the anal verge. Fissures develop due to poor healing of the tear from ischemia caused by reactive spasm of the internal anal sphincter. Histologic features are those of non-specific inflammation and granulation tissue. If conservative management fails, anal dilatation, internal sphincterotomy, or fissurectomy are performed.

6. **Anal abscesses and fistulas** can be idiopathic, or associated with CD, carcinoma, or hidradenitis suppurativa. Histologic features are those of nonspecific inflammation, and granulation tissue, often with a foreign body giant cell reaction to fecal material.

7. **Infections** of the anal canal are mostly sexually transmitted by unprotected anal intercourse, mostly involving men who have sex with men (MSM). Herpes simplex

TABLE 14.9 WHO Histologic Classification of Tumors of the Anal Canal

Epithelial tumors

Premalignant lesions

Anal intraepithelial neoplasia (dysplasia), low grade

Anal intraepithelial neoplasia (dysplasia), high grade

Bowen disease

Perianal squamous intraepithelial neoplasia

Paget disease

Carcinoma
  Squamous cell carcinoma
  Verrucous carcinoma
  Adenocarcinoma
  Mucinous adenocarcinoma

Neuroendocrine neoplasms

Neuroendocrine tumor (NET)
  NET G1 (carcinoid)
  NET G2

Mixed adenoneuroendocrine carcinoma

Nonepithelial tumors

Secondary tumors

WHO, World Health Organization.
From: Bosman FT, Carneiro F, Hruban RH, Theise ND, eds. *WHO Classification of Tumours. Pathology and Genetics. Tumours of the Digestive System.* Lyon, France: IARC Press; 2017. Used with permission.

virus (HSV) type 2 and *Treponema pallidum* (syphilis) infect the squamous epithelium. HSV produces vesicles and ulceration, and viral cytopathic effect is evident in the form of multinucleation with smudged chromatin. Syphilis is commonly associated with a chronic inflammatory infiltrate rich in plasma cells, and may show granulomatous inflammation. Immunohistochemical stains can be used to detect both of these infections. *Chlamydia trachomatis* (lymphogranuloma venereum) and *Neisseria gonorrhoeae* (gonorrhea) infect the columnar epithelium, and histologically show overlapping features with CD with cryptitis, crypt abscesses, and sometimes granulomas. PCR identification of the pathogen's DNA is the gold standard for diagnosis.

8. IBD, both CD and UC, commonly involves the anus.

B. **Neoplastic.** The WHO classification of tumors of the anal canal is given in Table 14.9. Revised staging schemes for neoplasms of the anal canal have recently been published (Amin MB et al., eds. *AJCC Cancer Staging Manual.* 8th ed. New York: Springer, 2017), as have suggested reporting guidelines (e.g., from the College of American Pathologists, available at http://www.cap.org).

1. **Hidradenoma papilliferum** is a benign sweat gland tumor that exclusively occurs in women. It can occur in the anal region and is histologically identical to its vulvar counterpart. Other adnexal tumors can also be rarely seen.

2. **Granular cell tumor** can affect the perianal region, although in the GI tract, it is most common in the esophagus.

3. **Squamous neoplasms**. Risk factors include anal-receptive intercourse, heavy smoking, a history of sexually transmitted diseases, HIV-positive status, and immunosuppression.

  a. **Anal squamous intraepithelial lesion (SIL),** also known as anal intra-epithelial neoplasia (AIN), or anal squamous intraepithelial neoplasia (ASIN), refers to a spectrum of squamous dysplasia strongly associated with high-risk serotypes of HPV (e.g., HPV-16, HPV-18). ASIN is the nomenclature used by WHO, and is graded as ASIN-L (low grade) or ASIN-H (high grade). Ki67 and p16 can be used to aid grading (e-**Fig. 14.84**). Perianal squamous intraepithelial neoplasia (PSIN), previously known as Bowen disease, is characterized by full thickness dysplasia of the squamous epithelium.

b. Condyloma acuminatum, also known as genital warts, is usually caused by low-risk serotypes of HPV (e.g., HPV-6 and HPV-11). It features a papillomatous proliferation of the squamous epithelium with parakeratosis and viral cytopathic (koilocytic) changes (e-**Fig. 14.85**). Sometimes it can be associated with high-risk serotypes (e.g., HPV-16, HPV-18) and ASIN-H.

c. Squamous cell carcinoma accounts for about 80% of anal carcinomas, and HPV DNA is present in approximately 90% of cases. The current WHO classification scheme recommends the generic term squamous cell carcinoma for diagnosis of these tumors, with description of the presence of basaloid features, mucinous features, and keratinization (and adjacent intraepithelial neoplasia) as needed. The primary treatment is chemoradiation.

4. Anal adenocarcinoma can be seen as extension from a rectal adenocarcinoma, or infrequently as a primary carcinoma arising in the perianal glands, pre-existing fistulas, or sinuses, usually in elderly males. The neoplastic glands are usually deeply situated without evidence of mucosal surface involvement, and are CK7 positive and CK20 negative. This is a slowly growing, well-differentiated tumor with glandular formation, bland cytology, and mucin production, but nonetheless adenocarcinomas are more aggressive than are SCC (e-**Fig. 14.86**). The treatment is similar to that of rectal adenocarcinoma.

5. Paget disease of the anus can be primary (rare) or secondary in association with distal adenocarcinoma of the rectum (about 50% cases); perianal Paget disease can also result from direct extension of perineal Paget disease. Histologically, it is identical to extramammary Paget disease that occurs at other sites (e-**Fig 14.87**). Primary Paget disease stains for GCDFP, CEA, EMA, and low molecular weight keratins. Cases that are associated with rectal adenocarcinoma are CK20 and CDX2 positive, but GCDFP negative. Melanoma and pagetoid SCC are the primary differential diagnoses.

6. Melanoma of the anus usually presents as a polypoid mass near the dentate line. It is histologically identical to melanomas seen in other cutaneous and mucosal sites (e-**Fig. 14.88**). Treatment determining somatic mutations that are commonly tested for include *BRAF* and *KIT* mutations.

IX. MISCELLANEOUS LESIONS OF THE MESENTERY

A. Mesenteric Fibromatosis is the most common primary tumor of the mesentery, and most often occurs in the mesentery of the small intestine. Most cases are sporadic, with mutations in *CTNNB1* (which encodes β-catenin), and rarely, with somatic mutations in *APC*. A subset of cases is associated with FAP related to germline mutations in *APC*. Men are affected more commonly than women. Grossly, the lesion is well-circumscribed, and usually measures >10 cm in greatest dimension.

Histologically, spindle cells are dispersed in a densely collagenous stroma, and myxoid change of the stroma can be present. The borders of the lesion are infiltrative despite the well-circumscribed gross appearance. Immunohistochemically, the tumor cells show nuclear β-catenin and smooth muscle actin positivity. Patients with Gardner syndrome show similar histologic findings, even though the myxoid stroma can be more prominent.

Due to the infiltrative nature of the lesion, complete excision is difficult, and recurrence is common. The clinical course is more aggressive in Gardner syndrome patients; in fact, fibromatosis is the second most common cause of death in this patient group.

B. Sclerosing Mesenteritis is in the differential diagnosis of mesenteric fibromatosis. The lesion is usually solitary and most often arises from the mesentery of the small intestine, although in some cases diffuse involvement by multiple masses may occur. A subgroup of cases represents IgG4-related disease, manifesting as storiform fibrosis with a dense lymphoplasmacytic infiltrate, an elevated number of IgG4-positive plasma cells, and obliterative phlebitis. Non IgG4-related cases usually show widespread fat necrosis. By immunohistochemistry, the tumor cells are smooth muscle actin positive but nuclear β-catenin negative.

C. **Inflammatory Myofibroblastic Tumor (IMT)** involves the mesentery and omentum as the most common non-pulmonary sites. Most common in children and young adults, IMT is multinodular or lobular with a rubbery, tan-white cut surface. A variety of histologic patterns can be seen in different lesions or within a single tumor. One common pattern resembles nodular fasciitis with spindle to stellate shaped cells embedded in a myxoid stroma. Other tumors show spindle cells arranged in a fascicular growth pattern. Prominent lymphoid aggregates or lymphoplasmacytic infiltrates are seen in many cases. Immunohistochemistry is variably positive for smooth muscle actin and desmin. Since rearrangements of the *ALK* gene are characteristic of the tumor, immunostains for the ALK protein are helpful, but are positive in only up to 60% of cases.

ACKNOWLEDGMENT

The authors thank ILKe Nalbantoglu and Elizabeth Brunt, authors of the previous edition of this chapter.

15 The Liver

Lulu Sun, Ta-Chiang Liu, and Elizabeth M. Brunt

I. **NORMAL ANATOMY.** The largest solid organ of the body, the mass of the adult liver is 1,200 to 1,600 g. The right, left, and caudate lobes are subdivided into segments based on inflow blood supply (e-**Fig. 15.1**). The liver has dual inflow supply, with approximately two-thirds from the low pressure, low O_2 portal vein, and one-third from the systemic pressure, high O_2 hepatic artery. Pressure equalization occurs in the sinusoids, along with the nutrient and O_2 gradient from portal tracts to terminal hepatic venules. The venous return is via the left, right, and middle hepatic veins which join the inferior vena cava. Bile duct blood supply is entirely from the hepatic artery plexuses.

Microscopically, the hepatic cords are lined by reticulin fibers and separated by sinusoids. The parenchyma is subdivided into acinar units of Rappaport which reflect an oxygen/nutrient gradient from most (zone 1) to least (zone 3), respectively; zone 2 is an ill-defined area in between. The anatomy of Rappaport's units underlies many pathologic processes. The lobule, often used interchangeably with acinus, is a term based on the concept of the hexagon in which hepatic cords radiate from the central vein toward the portal tracts. Each portal tract is a fibrous matrix that contains a branch each of the hepatic artery, portal vein, and bile duct, and a poorly visualized lymphatic (e-**Fig. 15.2**). Larger portal tracts contain visualizable autonomic nerve fibers. Inflammatory cells are typically lacking, or are few in number. The parenchyma is separated from the portal tract at the *limiting plate.*

II. **GROSS EXAMINATION AND SPECIMEN HANDLING**

A. **Needle Core Biopsy.** Specimen handling depends on the indication for liver biopsy. After measuring and description of the number of cores, liver biopsies may be wrapped in lens paper and fixed overnight or processed after several hours of fixation; use of sponge pads is strongly discouraged because of the angular artifacts created during sectioning. Protocol special stains and six additional unstained sections are recommended for medical liver biopsies at initial preparation. Stains include 3 H&E, a stain for collagen (trichrome or picrosirius red), reticulin, periodic acid Schiff after diastase (PAS-D), and modified Perls' for iron. Additional stains that must be available include copper or copper binding protein (rhodanine, orcein, or Victoria blue; orcein is also useful to differentiate passive septa of collapse from active elastic fiber deposition in fibrosis); and Verhoeff van Gieson for vessel wall architecture *(Semin Diagn Pathol* 2006;23:190).

1. **Tumor.** Processing of guided biopsies for diagnosis of space-occupying lesions requires understanding the imaging differential diagnoses. If greater than three cores have been provided, placement of cores with tumor into two cassettes will allow greater numbers of studies, as needed. It is best to begin with three levels for H&E.

2. **Immunocompromised patients.** Biopsies from immunocompromised patients (typically solid organ or bone marrow transplant patients) may or may not require rush processing; clear communication with the submitting clinicians can assist so that fixation, grossing, and processing are tailored to the specific clinical needs.

3. **Medical liver biopsy.** The reason(s) for the liver biopsy, that is, diagnosis or confirmation; grading and staging of hepatitis; or other possible medical questions should be clearly understood prior to sign out.

4. **Frozen section.** Indications for frozen sections of liver core or wedge biopsies include donor liver evaluations for quantity of steatosis and/or portal inflammation; acute fatty liver of pregnancy (AFLP) for microvesicular steatosis detection by oil red O

stain (from sections of liver biopsies at any stage of processing prior to xylene clearing, cut onto charged slides). Evaluation of intraoperatively encountered lesions is done from fresh tissue submitted on saline-moisturized gauze; cores are best sectioned with as little handling as possible. Wedge biopsies may require bread loafing prior to sectioning. Frozen artifact creates spaces that may be challenging to distinguish from fat, thus conservative estimates of the degree of steatosis are recommended from frozen sections. If electron microscopic examination is expected for a potential metabolic disease, additional fresh tissue should be fixed in 3% buffered glutaraldehyde.

5. Miscellaneous. Iron and copper tissue quantitation can be performed in reference laboratories directly from tissue in the paraffin block.

B. Wedge Biopsy or Excision. Wedge biopsy is not typically recommended for the evaluation of diffuse liver parenchymal diseases as the subcapsular parenchyma contains fibrous extensions for 3 to 5mm that may mimic fibrosis (e-**Fig. 15.3**). The subcapsular regions tend to show parenchymal collapse; elastosis may occur in this location as well as a result of chronic ischemia. Wedge excisions for superficial, circumscribed lesions are managed similarly to resections, described below.

C. Segmentectomy, Lobectomy, or Partial Hepatectomy are performed for large lesions that are not amenable to wedge excision. The surgery may or may not follow anatomic boundaries, and thus prior to sectioning it is important to understand the procedure that was done; review of the imaging studies and reports is invaluable. After the type of surgery, mass, and dimensions of the specimen are recorded, the resection margin is inked, the appearance of the capsule noted, and the specimen is sliced in the axial plane at about 0.5 cm increments. Gross examination of the lesion(s) and nonlesional liver parenchyma should include color(s) (nutmeg; tan; bile-stained; hemorrhagic; yellow), viability (necrotic, nonnecrotic), texture (firm; hard; soft; spongy), and presence of nodularity. If a tumor has been preoperatively embolized via transarterial chemoembolization (TACE), the percentage of tumor necrosis grossly should be assessed; however, only after complete submission and evaluation microscopically can it be adequately reported. Tumor sections (at least three) should demonstrate relationship of lesions to liver parenchyma, grossly visible vessels or ducts, margins (if close), and any variable areas within the tumor. Sections of nonneoplastic liver and inked resection margin(s) are submitted to evaluate underlying liver disease, vascular alterations, and margin status. One nontumor section of uninvolved liver should be submitted and evaluated by routine special stains.

D. Total Hepatectomy (Explant), performed for end-stage chronic liver disease, fulminant hepatic failure, or metabolic disorders, with or without primary liver carcinoma, is followed by orthotopic liver transplantation (OLT). Radiology reports must be consulted prior to processing the specimen to ensure that radiographically detected lesions are adequately sampled. The total weight, dimensions of each lobe, and capsule appearance are recorded. The hilum is completely removed, bread loafed, and submitted *in toto* proximally to distally without dissection. If a TIPS stent has been placed, no attempt should be made to remove it as the spring-opened wires are not protected; rather, the hilar tissue should be dissected away. The liver is then placed on the cutting board facing up, and sectioned axially cephalad-caudad in about 0.5 cm increments. Each slice is carefully examined fresh and after fixation (especially in cirrhotic livers) for bulging, large, or discolored nodules (which are all gross features of dysplastic nodules [DNs], or small HCC) that require documentation which includes location, number, size, color, and relation to the capsule or hilum. For lesions previously ablated, the entire lesion should be submitted in order to document any residual viable tumor. For lesions not treated prior to OLT, only appropriate sections that adequately demonstrate what the lesion is and its relations to capsule and vessels need to be submitted. In all explanted livers, two random sections from the both left and right lobes are submitted. Only one of these sections is necessary for the 4 routine special stains described above. Native and donor gallbladders are evaluated and sections submitted as for routine cholecystectomy specimens.

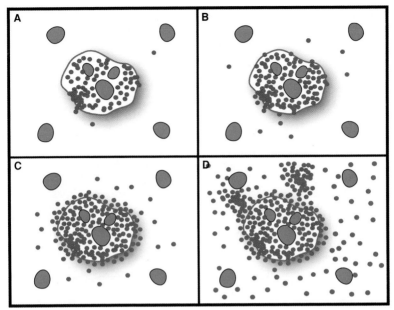

Figure 15.1 Ludwig and Batts: staging of chronic hepatitis. Stage 1 **(A)**; stage 2 **(B)**; stage 3 **(C)**; stage 4 **(D)**.

III. DIAGNOSTIC FEATURES OF COMMON NONNEOPLASTIC CONDITIONS

Approach to the liver biopsy. Knowledge of the clinical information is essential. The adequacy of the biopsy should be assessed, and is based on the nature of the question(s) being asked. Grading and staging chronic hepatitis ideally involve a 1.5 cm core, and up to 11 portal tracts; <5 portal tracts is not optimal *(Semin Diagn Pathol* 2006;23:132).

Grading and staging. Grading and staging schema were initially developed for comparisons of treatment for autoimmune and "nonA–nonB hepatitis" trials, but they quickly transitioned to apply to diagnostic evaluation in all forms of chronic hepatitis *(Hepatology* 2000;31:241). All systems share the assessment of portal and lobular necroinflammation for grade and amount and locations of fibrosis for stage (Figs. 15.1 and 15.2). One published system *(Am J Surg Pathol* 1995;19:1409) is simple to apply and communicate clinically; this system can be applied for any form of chronic hepatitis. It is important to note that none of the methods for staging chronic hepatitis are meant for cholestatic or vascular diseases, or alcoholic or nonalcoholic fatty liver diseases.

Fibrosis and cirrhosis. Patterns of collagen deposition and parenchymal architectural remodeling are frequently suggestive of the precedent injury: hepatitic, biliary, vascular, alcoholic, and so forth. Viral hepatitis and alcoholic hepatitis differ as the former is initially and predominantly portal-based, and the latter is centered in zone 3, is perisinusoidal initially, and results in nodules the size of the acinus (e.g., micronodular cirrhosis). The portal–portal fibrosis of the chronic biliary diseases often result in cirrhotic remodeling with maintenance of the terminal hepatic venule in its central location; a "jig-saw" pattern is therefore suggestive of biliary disease.

A. Infectious Liver Diseases

1. Viral hepatitis refers to one of the hepatotropic viruses: HAV, HBC, HCV, HDV (with superinfection or coinfection with HBV), and HEV.

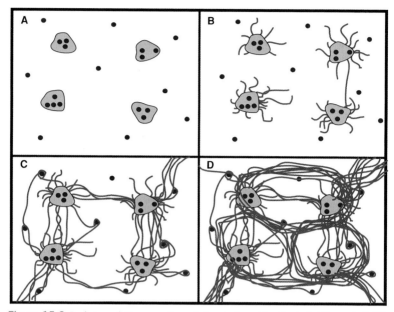

Figure 15.2 Ludwig and Batts: grading of chronic hepatitis. Grade 1 (**A**); grade 2 (**B**); grade 3 (**C**); grade 4 (**D**).

a. Acute viral hepatitis is commonly diagnosed clinically by serologic and clinical tests. Pathologists, therefore, have relatively little experience with this form of liver disease. Histopathologically, acute viral hepatitis is characterized by simultaneous hepatocyte injury and regeneration, chronic inflammation and macrophages, and focal or extensive parenchymal collapse, but no fibrosis. The changes include swollen hepatocytes (hydropic degeneration), apoptotic (acidophil) bodies, lobular spotty necrosis, lobular greater than portal inflammation, sinusoidal cell reaction (Kupffer cell and endothelial cell hypertrophy), and bi- and multinucleated hepatocytes. Collectively, these findings result in "lobular unrest" and "disarray" (e-**Fig. 15.4**). The inflammatory infiltrates consist predominantly of mononuclear cells, with occasional plasma cells and eosinophils. In severe cases, confluent bridging, submassive (panacinar), or massive (multiacinar) hepatic necrosis may occur (e-**Fig. 15.5**). Submassive hepatic necrosis is most often in zone 3, but some diseases such as HAV result in zone 1 hepatic necrosis. The ductular reaction, a form of regenerative response, may be accompanied by mononuclear or polymorphonuclear cells. Trichrome and reticulin stains may be confusing as the reticulin collapse may be extensive and the collapsed sinusoids may seemingly react with the stains for collagen (e-**Fig. 15.6**). In these cases, the orcein stain for elastic fibers is helpful, as elastic fibers are only found in true fibrosis (e-**Fig. 15.7**), but not in collapse. Zone 3 canalicular cholestasis may be present; if prominent, a diagnosis of acute cholestatic hepatitis is given (e-**Fig. 15.8**). Careful evaluation of portal tracts will exclude biliary obstruction (see below).

Fulminant hepatic failure, complete resolution, or smoldering infection of chronic hepatitis with its sequelae are the possible outcomes for acute viral hepatitis. HAV may trigger autoimmune hepatitis (AIH), and additionally may have zone 1 confluent or bridging necrosis and numerous plasma cells, or may resemble cholestatic obstructive hepatitis. HAV does not become chronic. Both HAV and HEV may result in fulminant hepatic failure; the latter is associated with fulminant hepatic failure in pregnancy. Rare cases of HEV in renal transplant settings have been reported to become chronic. HBV, HCV, and HDV may evolve to chronic hepatitis. The differential diagnoses for acute viral hepatitis includes AIH, Wilson disease, AFLP, drug-induced liver injury (DILI), and rarely, ischemic hepatitis. Cryptogenic acute hepatitis, for which no clinical cause is found, is reported as such (e-Fig. 15.9).

b. Chronic viral hepatitis, defined clinically by persistently elevated abnormal liver tests (alanine and aspartate transaminases > alkaline phosphatase) for more than 6 months, is caused by HBV, HCV, or HDV co-infection with HBV, and is histologically characterized by mononuclear cell infiltrates rich in T lymphocytes, predominantly in the portal tracts. Plasma cells, macrophages, and eosinophils are also present, in fewer numbers. There commonly are varying degrees of interface activity (previously referred to as piecemeal necrosis) (e-Fig. 15.10), lobular activity with acidophil bodies (e-Fig. 15.11), spotty necrosis, and portal-based fibrosis (e-Fig. 15.12).

Some features are characteristic of the specific types of chronic viral hepatitis. Chronic HBV is recognized by the presence of ground glass intracytoplasmic inclusions; this is HB S Ag in expanded smooth endoplasmic reticulum (e-Fig. 15.13). HB S Ag IHC has three patterns: membranous, cytoplasmic, and inclusion (e-Fig. 15.14); intranuclear inclusions require HB C Ag IHC for identification (e-Fig. 15.15). In HBV and HDV-coinfected cases, the necroinflammation tends to be more severe, and delta antigen can be demonstrated in nuclei by immunostaining.

The portal lymphoid aggregates of HCV are not pathognomonic because they may occur in HBV and AIH, but they are common and suggestive (e-Fig. 15.16). Steatosis is common in HCV in zone 1; if in zone 3, it is most likely due to pre-existing host factors (metabolic such as diabetes or obesity, or alcoholic). Acidophil bodies, bile duct injury, and sinusoidal lymphocytosis may occur in HCV; the latter resembles phenytoin toxicity or Epstein–Barr viral infection. HCV genotype 3 often has marked, panacinar macrovesicular steatosis. Crystalline material is often present in substances present in IV drugs and may be seen microscopically as foreign, polarizable material with sharp edges within portal macrophages.

c. Epstein–Barr virus hepatitis is characterized by a sinusoidal infiltrate of atypical lymphocytes in a "beads on a string" pattern (e-Fig. 15.17). The diagnosis can be confirmed by in situ hybridization for viral RNA and serologic tests.

d. Cytomegalovirus hepatitis in medically immunocompromised patients commonly induces microabscesses surrounding infected cells that have characteristic intranuclear and/or intracytoplasmic viral inclusions (e-Fig. 15.18). Thus, microabscesses should prompt immunostaining if inclusions are not evident. CMV infection in immunocompetent patients may show only microgranulomas, but in this setting viral inclusions are not usually present. Multinucleation of hepatocytes, and viral inclusions can occur in neonatal infection.

e. Adenovirus hepatitis, uncommon in immunocompetent hosts, causes nonzonal foci of coagulative necrosis with a minimal inflammatory response. Nuclei of infected hepatocytes are hyperchromatic and smudgy, with chromatin margination (e-Fig. 15.19). Confirmation is by immunohistochemical staining.

f. Herpesvirus hepatitis includes pyknotic debris and nonzonal "punched out" necrosis with a negligible inflammatory response. Nuclear ground glass (Cowdry A) viral inclusions with chromatin margination can be found in syncytial nuclei at the periphery of necrosis, or in other cells within the liver (e-Fig 15.20). Immunohistochemistry is confirmatory. Rapid diagnosis and treatment may be lifesaving.

2. Bacterial infections involve the liver in various ways: space-occupying abscess; toxic cholangitis (e.g., toxic shock syndrome); granulomatous inflammation

(*Mycobacterium* species); and peliosis (bacillary angiomatosis in AIDS). Sepsis may result in microabscesses, zone 3 canalicular cholestasis, and/or ductular cholestasis (e.g., cholangitis lenta) (**e-Fig. 15.21**).

3. Fungal infections are most likely due to systemic infections such as candidiasis, aspergillosis, and histoplasmosis. The biopsy may show granulomatous inflammation, organisms, other features of sepsis, or DILI. Stains for fungal elements may be necessary to appreciate organisms.

4. Parasitic infections, including hydatid cyst, amebic abscess, and schistosomiasis, each with characteristic histopathologic features, require a high index of clinical and pathologic suspicion for diagnosis.

B. Metabolic and Toxic Liver Diseases

1. Alcoholic liver disease (ALD) encompasses a histopathologic spectrum of findings including mixed large and small droplet fatty liver, alcoholic hepatitis, alcoholic steatohepatitis, alcoholic foamy degeneration, and alcoholic cirrhosis. Steatosis, steatohepatitis, and cirrhosis may be indistinguishable from nonalcoholic fatty liver disease (NAFLD). Steatosis, reversible with abstinence, is predominantly macrovesicular and initially involves zone 3. The hallmarks of alcoholic hepatitis are hepatocytes with Mallory–Denk bodies (MDB) and satellitosis (neutrophilic infiltration around hepatocytes containing MDB), commonly embedded in dense pericellular fibrosis (**e-Fig. 15.22**). When steatosis is also present, steatohepatitis is diagnosed. Megamitochondria may be readily apparent. The pattern of fibrosis in alcoholic hepatitis/steatohepatitis is characteristic; it begins in zone 3 as perisinusoidal/pericellular collagen deposition and eventually there is dense "chicken-wire" fibrosis that may involve the entire acinus (**e-Fig. 15.23**). Canalicular cholestasis may be seen. Perivenular fibrosis is common. Obliteration of the terminal hepatic venule occurs in severe alcoholic hepatitis and results in sclerosing hyaline necrosis, a feature of poor prognosis (**e-Fig. 15.24**). Alcoholic cirrhosis is typically micronodular. Obliterated outflow veins may be found, as may copper in periseptal hepatocytes. Steatosis is variably present in ALD.

2. NAFLD refers to the spectra of histologic entities ranging from steatosis (NAFL) to steatohepatitis (NASH) to cirrhosis with or without NASH, and includes hepatocellular carcinoma (HCC) occurring in the background of cirrhosis or pre-cirrhotic NAFLD. Some forms of NAFLD may resemble some of the histologic findings of milder forms of ALD. NAFLD occurs in a broader spectrum of patients, including children. By definition, the process is confined to subjects who are not "heavy" drinkers but who commonly have many or all features of Metabolic Syndrome (obesity, hypertension, abnormal glucose tolerance, and dyslipidemia) *(Clin Liv Dis* 2010;14:591*).* NAFLD is also noted in lean individuals, and may be a result of a variety of medications (*JAMA* 2015;313:2263). Unlike alcoholic hepatitis, however, a diagnosis of nonalcoholic steatohepatitis (NASH) requires the presence of steatosis; canalicular cholestasis is uncommon, the MDB are less prominent, and central sclerosing hyaline necrosis has not been reported. Minimum features of adult NASH are zone 3 macrosteatosis, hepatocyte ballooning, and lobular inflammation. Ballooning may be confirmed with use of CK8/18 immunostaining, which highlights clumped positivity of keratins and loss of reactivity throughout the cytoplasm in contrast with diffuse reactivity in cytoplasm in "nonballooned" hepatocytes (**e-Fig. 15.25**). Portal inflammation may be present in all forms of NAFLD, but if disproportionate, should raise concern of a second process such as HCV. Megamitochondria and lipogranulomas are commonly noted. Pediatric NAFLD may show greater steatosis, less zone 3 zonality, and more portal inflammation and fibrosis than adult NASH. The pattern of fibrosis in adult NASH resembles that of ALD in that it is zone 3 perisinusoidal initially. Progressive fibrosis includes periportal fibrosis, bridging, and cirrhosis. As with ALD, steatosis may be absent in cirrhosis resultant from NASH; "burnt-out" NASH is considered the most likely cause of "cryptogenic"

TABLE 15.1 Histologic Methods of Semiquantitative Evaluation of NAFLD

	NASH CRN	SAF/FLIP Algorithm
Patient Population	Adults + Children	Adults
Applicable to	All NAFLD	All NAFLD
Grade	NAFLD Activity Score (NAS): S+LI+B = 0–8 • Unweighted scores for each lesion • Dx correlates, but is not derived by score	• Steatosis is not a component of activity • Activity: LI+B • Steatosis + Activity + Fibrosis = $S_xA_xF_x$ Algorithm for diagnosis
Details of Scoring	Steatosis: 0: <5% 1: 5–33% 2: 34–66% 3: >67% LI: 0: 0 1: <2/20x 2: 2–4/20x 3: >4/20x Ballooning: 0: None 1: Few 2: Many, Prominent Fibrosis Stage 0: none 1a: Zone 3 perisinusoidal, delicate 1b: Zone 3 perisinusoidal, dense 1c: Portal only 2: 1a or 1b + periportal 3: Bridging 4: Cirrhosis	Steatosis: 0: <5% 1: 5–33% 2: 34–66% 3: >67% LI: 0: 0 1: <2/20x 2: >2/20x Ballooning: 0–2 0: 0 1: Clusters, reticulated cytoplasm 2: Enlarged hepatocytes Fibrosis Stage F0: 0 F1: Zone 3 perisinusoidal (all), or portal only F2: Zone 3 + periportal F3: Bridging F4: Cirrhosis

cirrhosis; however, other considerations include burned-out AIH and burned-out alcoholic cirrhosis (e-**Fig. 15.26**).

Grading and Staging NAFLD (Table 15.1). The NAFLD Activity Score (NAS) (*Hepatology* 2005;41:1313), validated and developed for therapeutic trials, is the unweighted sum of scores for steatosis, lobular inflammation, and ballooning. The numeric NAS and the diagnosis are separately reported, as they reflect different properties. (*Hepatology* 2011;53:810) The fibrosis score is based on trichrome stain. A newer system more widely applied in Europe than in the United States is referred to as the FLIP algorithm (*Hepatology* 2014;60:565). This method correlates a numeric score with diagnosis. The two methods are detailed and compared in Table 15.1.

3. **Glycogenic hepatopathy** is an uncommon complication of diabetics due to poor glycemic control; hepatocytes are distended by excess glycogen as in other forms of glycogen storage disease. Steatosis and megamitochondria may be noted (e-**Fig. 15.27**). **Diabetic hepatosclerosis** is manifest by nonzonal dense perisinusoidal fibrosis; steatosis is rare or not present. Alkaline phosphatase may be elevated (e-**Fig. 15.28**).

4. **Iron overload** is most commonly genetically driven and rarely dietary. Hereditary iron overload is complex, and may be polygenic. The current definition is an inborn

error of metabolism resulting in low levels or low activity of the liver-derived protein hepcidin, the master iron regulator, with resultant iron loading of parenchyma of the liver, pancreas, heart, and endocrine organs. Production of hepcidin by hepatocytes is at least partially under the control of *Hfe, HJV, Tfr2,* and *HAMP* genes; levels of serum iron, systemic inflammation or infection, and ER or nutrient stress initiate gene function. *Hfe* mutation (homozygous C282Y, the most common form of hereditary hemochromatosis [HH]) results in mid-life onset; *HJV, Tfr2,* and *HAMP* mutations result in more severe disease and at younger ages. **Ferroportin-associated hemochromatosis** is unique in that hepcidin production is normal, but due to *FPN* autosomal dominant mutation(s) iron absorption from the gut is not regulated; the phenotype is similar to classic C282Y HH with liver cell iron overload. **Ferroportin disease**, on the other hand, is due to loss of iron export function of ferroportin and iron accumulation in the reticuloendothelial system, that is, hepatic Kupffer cells. ALD, anemia of chronic disease, and the above types of HH suppress hepatocellular hepcidin with resultant hepatocyte iron overload; so-called secondary forms of iron overload from aberrant macrophage loading (i.e., ferroportin disease, hemophagocytic syndrome) result in macrophage and sinusoidal lining cell (SLC) iron accumulation. Hepatocellular iron deposition, regardless of genotype, initially occurs in the pericanalicular region of hepatocytes. With loading, the iron can be seen in a gradient from zone 1 to panacinar hepatocytes. Eventually, biliary epithelium and the SLC will also contain iron granules. Large iron-laden Kupffer cell aggregates and siderotic nodules are not uncommon, and are the last to release iron in phlebotomy therapy. In iron-loaded cirrhosis, iron-free foci are clonal, DNs; HCC is also iron-free. Ferroportin disease and secondary iron overload are characterized by preferential panacinar SLC iron loading prior to hepatocellular accumulation.

Many systems exist for histopathologic iron grading (*Semin Liv Dis* 2005;25:392), the most common of which is based on magnification required for discrete granule visualization; more complex methods include separation of cell types with iron overload (e-**Fig. 15.29**). The diagnosis of primary hemochromatosis, however, requires mutational analysis and cannot be made by histologic analysis alone. Iron quantification can be done from FFPE tissue if enough tissue is present; this may be used to guide phlebotomy but is not necessary.

Hemochromatosis carries a significant risk of HCC. **Porphyria cutanea tarda** is associated with hemochromatosis, steatosis, iron overload, hepatitis C infection, cirrhosis, and also carries a risk of HCC. High ferritin levels are characteristic in NAFLD, and may result in liver biopsy due to a clinical concern of hemochromatosis. **Neonatal "hemochromatosis"** is a complement-mediated alloimmune maternal–fetal disorder with giant cell hepatitis that results in intrauterine demise and may or may not have liver and pancreas iron overload (*Hepatology* 2010;51:2061).

5. **α1-Antitrypsin deficiency,** the most common genetic pediatric liver disease, may also manifest as liver disease in adults and is characterized by accumulation of intracytoplasmic eosinophilic globules of varying sizes and shapes in zone 1 hepatocytes, easily demonstrated by PAS-D (e-**Fig. 15.30**). The diagnosis is confirmed by characteristic immunohistochemistry with "peripheral rim" positivity of the larger globules. Serum electrophoresis (PI) phenotyping is necessary for further diagnosis. The hepatocyte globules signify a Z allele, or other rare alleles of M or S. Homozygosity for PI*ZZ is a risk for HCC, with or without cirrhosis. Whether heterozygosity is causative or enhances progression of underlying liver disease remains a debate (*Semin Diagn Pathol* 2006;23:182), but enrichment of MZ phenotypes in liver transplant candidates is recognized. The two most common adult diseases reported to coexist with α1AT deficiency alleles are chronic viral hepatitis and fatty liver disease. In infants under 12 weeks of age, globules may not be easily detected; however, the disease is included in the differential diagnosis of cholestatic infants with giant cell or neonatal hepatitis (e-**Fig. 15.31**). Biliary atresia and Alagille syndromes are mimics. Diagnosis thus rests with PI

phenotyping. Long-standing cholestasis may result in intra- and extrahepatic duct loss and/or narrowing, thus care to exclude α1AT prior to a surgical procedure is warranted in neonates. α1AT globules may also occur in benign and malignant liver neoplasms, regardless of the subject's phenotype. The differential diagnosis of non-α1AT globules includes polyglucosan inclusions in polypharmacy; Lafora bodies; cyanamide therapy; HBSAg; adaptation; and fibrinogen inclusions. The majority of these latter inclusions are not as zonally restricted or as heterogeneous in size as α1AT globules. α1AT deficiency in the liver is cured by liver transplant, and does not recur; however, globules may appear in an allograft liver from a previously unknown donor liver with deficiency alleles.

6. **Wilson disease,** an autosomal recessive disease, is the result of over 500 mutations of a biliary copper transporter; copper can accumulate in the liver, brain, cornea, and kidney. More common in young patients, Wilson disease can present at any age. Clinical features may mimic AIH; other features include Coombs negative hemolysis and aberrant ratios of AST/ALT or Alk Phos/Bili. Recent studies have shown these to be more reliable than reliance on serum ceruloplasmin. Hemolysis may result in pigmented gallstones. Neurologic and/or psychiatric manifestations may be concurrent or primary manifestations, particularly in fulminant cases. Hepatic histology is as protean as the clinical disease. Wilson disease can be queried by either the clinician or pathologist for otherwise unexplained liver histologic features of macro- or microsteatosis, chronic hepatitis (i.e., interface activity), cirrhosis, or submassive necrosis, particularly in a young adult. Hepatocytes may be enlarged with granular cytoplasm. Periportal glycogenated nuclei and MDB are common. Atypical lipofuscin and iron deposition may be present. Excessive copper may not be visible by staining as it largely remains diffusely intracytosolic; diagnostic testing requires quantitation from the paraffin block (>250 μg/g dry weight). Chronic cholestatic diseases of childhood and adults also result in copper deposits in the eyes (Kayser–Fleischer rings) and in periportal/periseptal hepatocytes, but the increase in copper does not reach the requisite quantitative levels of Wilson disease (*Semin Diagn Pathol* 2006;23:182). In cirrhosis due to Wilson disease, hepatocytes may be oncocytic secondary to increased numbers of mitochondria; copper is heterogeneously present, with some negative and some diffusely positive nodules. Ductular reaction and marked parenchymal extinction can be noted in fulminant failure of Wilson disease.

7. **Glycogen storage diseases, or glycogenoses,** are characterized by abnormal accumulation of glycogen in hepatocytes giving rise to a pale, distended, and mosaic appearance. PAS stains and electron microscopy may help confirm the diagnosis.

8. **Lysosomal storage diseases,** the most common of which is Gaucher disease, are characterized by distended Kupffer cells. The cytoplasm of "Gaucher cells" is finely striated as with "wrinkled tissue paper."

9. **Hematologic disorders: Lymphoma, leukemia, mastocytosis, hemophagocytic syndrome, and sickle cell disease.** Lymphoma and leukemia are discussed further below. Macrophage activation syndrome (MAS) is a form of hemophagocytic lymphohistiocytosis (HLH) (e-**Fig. 15.32**), characterized by Kupffer cell erythrophagocytosis that occurs in systemic processes such as malignancy, viral infection, or collagen vascular disease. Serum ferritin levels and triglycerides are elevated; other clinical features include cytopenias, fever, and splenomegaly. Portal and parenchymal CD8+ lymphocytes are common. Liver involvement by systemic mastocytosis results in hepatomegaly and rarely cirrhosis. Portal infiltrates contain abundant mast cells; a high index of suspicion is helpful. Sickle cell disease may result in acute or chronic, direct or indirect liver injury. A minority of patients have acute sickle hepatic crisis with tender hepatomegaly and jaundice; the histologic features range from perivenular sinusoidal microthrombi to hepatic vein thrombosis, ballooning, focal necrosis, and canalicular bile stasis. Cirrhosis may occur from the long-term management of patients as well as repeated episodes of ischemia; sickled cells, erythrophagocytosis, and pigment may be seen in Kupffer cells (e-**Fig. 15.33**).

10. **Reye syndrome** (e-**Fig. 15.34**) and other mitochondriopathies are more common in children than adults. The liver shows pauciinflammatory microvesicular steatosis. Ultrastructural examination highlights mitochondrial alterations. Similar changes occur in alcoholic foamy degeneration.

11. **Total parenteral nutrition (TPN)** results in steatosis or steatohepatitis in adults, and cholestasis with a ductular reaction and fibrosis in children. In both, bridging fibrosis and cirrhosis may occur.

12. **Amyloidosis** commonly involves portal tract arteries and may be inconsequential, and can occur as the result of several disease entities (*Clin Liver Dis* 2004;8:915). However, hepatic involvement is terminal when amyloid extensively replaces the sinusoids and results in compression and atrophy of the hepatocytes (e-**Fig. 15.35**). Hepatomegaly and jaundice are clinical clues. Trichrome stain shows the characteristic gray color of amyloid; Congo red or thioflavin T highlight the amyloid when fluoresced. Amyloid may also result in small or large globular deposits within the sinusoids without compromise of liver function.

13. **Cystic fibrosis** has hepatic manifestations in about 20% of patients. CF may present as a mimic of biliary atresia or neonatal hepatitis, or later as portal hypertension due to bile duct mucus plugging and fibrosis. The histologic hallmarks are dense eosinophilic inspissated mucous in dilated ducts, cholangitis, ductular reaction, chronic inflammation, and fibrosis (e-**Fig. 15.36**). Focal biliary fibrosis occurs in up to 70% of adults and may warrant liver transplant.

14. **Drug induced liver injury (DILI) and toxin-induced liver injury,** commonly in the differential for unexplained liver test elevations, can be direct (predictable, intrinsic) or indirect (unpredictable, idiosyncratic). Direct toxicity involves agents known to produce liver damage in a dose-dependent manner; methotrexate, antibiotics, and chemotherapeutic agents are examples. Indirect toxicity is immune-mediated and dose-independent; granulomatous and eosinophilic inflammation typify this type of injury. Acute injury may lead to cholestatic hepatitis, bland cholestasis, interlobular duct damage, acute hepatitis, and massive necrosis. Chronic injury may assume the form of chronic hepatitis, granulomatous hepatitis, steatosis, steatohepatitis, vascular injury, fibrosis, cirrhosis, or neoplasia. With the advent of precision medicine therapeutics, clinicians and pathologists alike are being exposed to greater numbers of liver-related complications and must be mindful of the newer medications as possible sources of injury. A continually updated online dataset of DILI is maintained by the NIH for queries of all reported drug injuries (available at https://livertox.nih.gov).

C. Autoimmune Hepatitis (AIH) and Bile Duct Disorders

1. **AIH** is a chronic relapsing inflammatory disease that most often presents in females in adolescence or postmenopausal ages, and is associated with hypergammaglobulinemia (IgG) and high titers of antinuclear and anti-smooth muscle antibodies in adults, and anti-liver-kidney microsomal type 1 antibodies in girls. The disease may be triggered by a prior viral or drug-induced hepatitis. The diagnosis is one of exclusion and is made after exclusion of metabolic diseases, and after negative viral serologies have been demonstrated (*J Hepatol* 2015;62(1 Suppl):S100); remission is clinically defined by reduction/normalization of serum transaminase levels and IgG. The majority of cases respond to immunosuppression and can avoid liver transplantation, thus appropriate diagnosis is necessary and includes liver biopsy evaluation (*Clinical Liv Dis* 2014;3:19). Although many features are common microscopically, none is considered pathognomonic and the findings are best interpreted in context with clinical features. In cases highly suggestive at low power, there is a dense portal and lobular mononuclear cell infiltrate enriched in plasma cells; eosinophils are not uncommon (e-**Fig. 15.37**). Marked interface hepatitis, centrilobular confluent or bridging necrosis, and hepatitic rosetting are present. Giant cells may be present. Emperipolesis, hepatocyte engulfment of lymphocytes, is noted most often in zone 1. Fibrosis, even advanced fibrosis, is common even at presentation. Cholestasis is rare but may be seen in severe non-cirrhotic AIH with necrosis or with cirrhosis. AIH may

rarely present as fulminant hepatic failure. Likewise, mild chronic hepatitis and/or cirrhosis may be the initial findings. AIH cirrhosis is a risk factor for HCC. Simple scoring systems developed to predict probability of AIH are rarely applied in clinical settings, but can serve as guidelines (*Curr Gastroenterol Rep* 2012;14:25). AIH can recur, or appear *de novo* in allograft livers.

2. **Primary biliary cholangitis (PBC)**, previously known as primary biliary cirrhosis, is a progressive cholestatic disease of middle-aged women that results in the destruction of the smallest intrahepatic bile ducts. IgM and serum cholesterol are elevated, along with cholestatic liver tests. The early stage (Table 15.2) has mixed chronic portal inflammatory infiltrates and the pathognomonic *florid duct lesion* consisting of granulomatous or lymphocytic infiltration of duct epithelium (e-Fig. 15.38). The granulomas in PBC are epithelioid, may be portal or lobular, and present in any stage of disease. Stains for fungal and acid-fast organisms are appropriate at the time of initial diagnosis. The process is inhomogeneously distributed throughout the liver, but ductular reaction, interface hepatitis, features of chronic cholestasis, and "biliary piecemeal necrosis" develop with

TABLE 15.2	Nakanuma's Proposal for Scoring and Staging Primary Biliary Cholangitis
Score	Fibrosis
0	No fibrosis
1	Fibrosis extends beyond portal tracts; occ incomplete septa
2	Bridging
3	Cirrhosis
	Bile Duct Loss
0	Bile ducts present in all portal tracts
1	Bile ducts absent in <1/3 portal tracts
2	Bile ducts absent in 1/3–2/3 portal tracts
3	Bile ducts absent in >2/3 portal tracts
	Chronic Cholestasis (Orcein Granules)
0	Negative
1	Positive in periportal hepatocytes, <1/3 portal tracts
2	Positive in variable #'s of periportal hepatocytes, 1/3–2/3 portal tracts
3	Positive in many periportal hepatocytes, >2/3 portal tracts

Stage	Total Score: Fibrosis + Bile Duct Loss + Orcein
1 (no progression)	0
2 (mild progression)	1–3
3 (moderate progression)	4–6
4 (advanced progression)	7–9

Stage *If No Orcein Present*	Fibrosis + Bile Duct Loss
1 (no progression)	0
2 (mild progression)	1–2
3 (moderate progression)	3–4
4 (advanced progression)	5–6

Modified from: Nakanuma Y, Zen Y, Harada K, et al. Application of a new histological staging and grading system for primary biliary cirrhosis to liver biopsy specimens: Interobserver agreement. *Pathol Int* 2010;60:167.

progression, with eventual bridging and septal fibrosis, and biliary cirrhosis. Chronic cholestasis is characterized by periportal/periseptal edema, ductular reaction, MDB, lobular foam cells, periportal copper deposition (e-**Fig. 15.39**), and cholestatic rosettes. Nodular regenerative hyperplasia (NRH)-like parenchymal features may occur in any stage of PBC and may explain the clinical findings of noncirrhotic variceal bleeding. The classic staging systems for PBC (Scheuer, Ludwig) included the initial portal injury (stage 1), periportal activity or ductular reaction (stage 2), bridging fibrosis (stage 3), and cirrhosis (stage 4). A newer method (Nakanuma) takes into account the heterogeneity of lesions, and progressive loss of ducts and copper deposition with progressive disease to derive a final summation for severity (*Pathol Int* 2010;60:67). Orcein granule deposits have been shown to correlate with clinical outcome (Table 15.2).

Autoimmune cholangiopathy (AIC) and AMA-negative PBC with or without ANA positivity are synonymous terms for seronegative PBC that is otherwise clinically and histologically identical to PBC (and is distinct from overlap syndrome, discussed below).

3. **Primary sclerosing cholangitis (PSC),** an idiopathic progressive fibro-obliterative disorder of the extra- and intrahepatic biliary tree, primarily affects young men, and leads to biliary strictures and ectasias, and cirrhosis. PSC is closely associated with concurrent ulcerative colitis. The definitive diagnosis of PSC rests on imaging by MRCP or ERCP; liver biopsy may be suggestive (features of chronic cholestasis) or confirmatory (periductal fibrosis), but is not the diagnostic test (see below). Fibrous cholangitis (so-called onion-skin fibrosis) involving large and/or small bile ducts, duct damage, ductular reaction, and chronic cholestasis are typical findings (e-**Fig. 15.40**). PSC inhomogeneously progresses to cirrhosis and is staged according to the portal changes (Table 15.3). Cholangiocarcinoma occurs in up to 10% of cases of PSC, but correctly identifying precursor lesions of dysplasia in the large ducts remains a clinical challenge. Currently, carefully selected and protocolized patients with PSC and cholangiocarcinoma undergo neoadjuvant therapy and months of surveillance prior to orthotopic liver transplant.

Small duct PSC involves only the small intrahepatic ducts, and may be the same disease as idiopathic adulthood ductopenia (IAD). Small duct PSC does not carry a risk of cholangiocarcinoma unless evolution to large duct PSC occurs.

TABLE 15.3 Banff Scheme for Grading Acute Liver Allograft Rejection

Global Assessment	Criteria
Indeterminate	Portal inflammatory infiltrate that fails to meet the criteria for the diagnosis of acute rejection
Mild	Rejection infiltrate in a minority of the triads that is generally mild and confined within the portal spaces
Moderate	Rejection infiltrate expanding most or all of the triads
Severe	As above for moderate, with spillover into periportal areas and moderate to severe perivenular inflammation that extends into the hepatic parenchyma and is associated with perivenular hepatocyte necrosis

4. **Overlap syndrome** refers to cases of clinical and/or histopathologic AIH with the simultaneous presence of diagnostic features of PBC. Overlap features of AIH may also occur with PSC, or less often, viral hepatitis. Correlation with clinical and serologic findings is essential but treatment is based on the dominant histologic finding.
5. **Secondary biliary cirrhosis** results from any cause of mechanical obstruction of the biliary tree. The common causes in adults are lithiasis, tumors, external compression from nodes, and stenosis; in children, the common causes are biliary atresia and choledochal cysts. Infiltrative disorders (e.g., amyloidosis, lymphomas) less often result in changes of secondary biliary cirrhosis.

Histologically, large duct obstruction causes both portal and lobular changes. Initially, there is rounding of portal tracts due to edema; later pericholangitis (ductular reaction with neutrophils) with or without ascending cholangitis is found, occasionally with bile plugs in dilated ducts. In zone 3, feathery degeneration and canalicular cholestasis are noted. With increased pressure, intra-parenchymal bile infarcts occur (e-Fig. 15.41); these nonzonal pink-tan clusters are due to membrane saponification by cholate salts. Long-standing obstruction leads to portal and periductal fibrosis or cirrhosis indistinguishable from PSC. Biliary atresia with extensive lobular injury may simulate neonatal or giant cell hepatitis.

6. **Idiopathic adulthood ductopenia (IAD)** is, by definition, paucity of intrahepatic bile ducts as defined by a ratio of <0.5 interlobular ducts to portal tracts (the normal range is 0.9 to 1.8). This poorly understood condition is pauciinflammatory, insidious in presentation and progression, and rarely familial. Immunostains for keratins 7 or 19 aid in identifying hypoplastic or absent ducts and periportal progenitor cells. Unlike extrahepatic biliary atresia or obstruction, ductular reaction (i.e., proliferation of the progenitor cell compartment) is typically absent in IAD. In pediatric patients, duct paucity may be syndromic (Alagille syndrome) or nonsyndromic; the latter is associated with other causes of neonatal hepatitis and carries a poor prognosis. In adults, the diagnosis requires exclusion of PBC, PSC, chronic allograft rejection, GVHD, sarcoidosis, and untreated Hodgkin disease.

7. **Miscellaneous duct disorders**

   a. **Sepsis** may affect the liver as periportal cholangiolar bile plugs without concurrent interlobular duct inspissated bile and inflammation; this has been referred to as cholangitis lenta. The affected cholangioles may be infiltrated by neutrophils.

   b. **Toxic shock syndrome and other severe extrahepatic bacterial infections** commonly result in intrahepatic canalicular and cholangiolar cholestasis. With septic shock, ischemic changes will be noted as well. Toxic shock syndrome may expand the portal tract and infiltrate the interlobular duct with neutrophils.

   c. **IgG4 sclerosing cholangitis** presents most often in adult men and is more commonly associated with autoimmune pancreatitis, retroperitoneal fibrosis, and chronic sclerosing sialadenitis than its idiopathic counterpart. Grossly, the involved ducts may appear to be involved by tumor due to marked expansion.

D. **Major Vascular Disorders of the Liver**

1. **Venous outflow obstruction** can result from cardiac disease (congestive heart failure) or large vessel disease (occlusion of large hepatic veins or the IVC, i.e., Budd–Chiari syndrome). Both involve zone 3 sinusoidal dilatation (congestion) and may show red cell extravasation into the space of Disse, ultimately with hepatocyte loss, cord atrophy and withering, and fibrous replacement. Ductular reaction may be extensive. Cardiac sclerosis/cirrhosis with reverse lobulation has become uncommon with better medical management. Caudate lobe hypertrophy is a feature of Budd–Chiari syndrome due to separate venous drainage.

2. **Sinusoidal obstruction syndrome (SOS)** occurs unpredictably following pre-conditioning for bone marrow transplant. Formerly referred to as veno-occlusive disease (VOD), the process has been renamed to reflect the fact that the location of initial injury is the sinusoids, which are denuded. Downstream, debris is deposited in the outflow vein branches, which results in subendothelial fibrosis of outflow veins. In the BMT setting, the onset of acute SOS is soon after BMT; abdominal swelling and elevated bilirubin herald SOS, and hepatocyte necrosis in zone 3 is a recognized feature in this setting. Verhoeff van Gieson stain is helpful in visualization of affected veins in the area of necrotic hepatocytes (e-Fig. 15.42). Some cases of changes related to chronic outflow vein injury have been reported in BMT biopsies that are related to dosage of radiation and have resulted in findings similar to SOS, although the injury is less dramatic and nonfatal; the small outflow veins have shown sclerosis (*Histopathology* 2016;68:996).

Following chemotherapy regimens containing oxaliplatin for hepatic colorectal metastases, a type of sinusoidal injury that in some ways mimics SOS occurs. Grossly, the disease is characterized by a "blue liver." Microscopically, seemingly randomly scattered foci of ectatic sinusoids, some nearly peliotic, may be seen. Hepatocyte anisonucleosis in H&E-stained sections is a diagnostic clue (e-**Fig. 15.43**). Obliterated outflow veins are much less common in oxaliplatin-induced sinusoidal injury. Recovery is more common than not, and pretreatment regimens are now decreasing the prevalence of this type of injury.

3. **Noncirrhotic portal hypertension** (idiopathic portal hypertension), usually the result of pre-sinusoidal causes, may also be due to hepatic causes such as schistosomiasis, sarcoidosis, or congenital hepatic fibrosis. Clinically, normal liver synthetic function is maintained in IPH.

   a. **NRH** is a condition related to aberrant flow that commonly results in noncirrhotic portal hypertension. The parenchyma is diffusely nodular, but without fibrosis. The nodularity is appreciated at low magnification and best demonstrated by reticulin stain (e-**Fig. 15.44**), which highlights the regenerative cords outlined by atrophic cords. Nearby terminal hepatic veins may take on the form of a crescent moon.

   b. **Hepatoportal sclerosis** is due to intrahepatic portal vein injury and scarring. The extrahepatic portal vein is patent, at least initially. The parenchyma shows a variety of alterations: abnormally approximated portal tracts, periportal enlarged vessels in direct contact with hepatic cords, and multiple ectatic sinusoidal structures that resemble angiomatoid structures. Portal and/or sinusoidal fibrosis may be present. Portal veins may be inapparent or show marked wall thickening with luminal narrowing (e-**Fig. 15.45**).

4. **Portal vein thrombosis (PVT)** may result in subtle or gross parenchymal atrophy characterized by approximation of vascular structures (i.e., the infarct of Zahn). Biliopathy may also result from PVT.

5. **Osler–Weber–Rendu Syndrome (hereditary hemorrhagic telangiectasia)** is an autosomal dominant disorder that results in multisystem angiodysplasias. Of the four known genetic subtypes, liver lesions are found in the HHT 2 group (*alk1* gene mutations); final diagnosis rests with fulfillment of 3 of 5 Curacao criteria which include hepatic AVMs as well as family history (*J Med Genet* 2011;48:73). Nosebleeds are common. The hepatic malformations may be insidious and range from ischemic biliopathy, to focal nodular hyperplasia (FNH) with high output cardiac failure, to noncirrhotic portal hypertension. Hepatic lesions include intraparenchymal thick-walled veins with adherent arteries, scattered dilated sinusoids, and abnormally sized portal tracts with extruded dilated vascular channels. Commonly, grossly observed subcapsular enlarged vessels are present.

6. **Ischemic "hepatitis"** is a consideration in fulminant hepatic failure. Ischemic hepatitis is strongly associated with sudden onset of low cardiac output, as with massive myocardial infarction. The lesion is rarely biopsied, but may be encountered in a work-up of fulminant hepatic necrosis. Zone 3 confluent or massive hepatic necrosis is present; if older than a few days, scattered inflammation and ductular reaction at the periphery of the necrotic areas can be seen.

E. Miscellaneous Hepatic Lesions

1. **Granulomas** of various sizes can be noted in liver biopsies. Underlying etiologies are as variable as the morphology of the granulomas. Stains for infectious organisms and evaluation under polarized light are useful in the evaluation of true epithelioid types. Considerations specific to liver include PBC, sarcoidosis, DILI, HCV, fungal or mycobacterial infections, foreign bodies, common variable immunodeficiency (pediatric cases), and hepatocellular adenoma (HCA); rarely, granulomatous hepatitis is a *bona fide* clinico-pathologic diagnosis.

2. **Pregnancy** is associated with liver pathology including various mitochondrial alterations. Viral hepatitis of any cause may occur in pregnancy. **AFLP** occurs in the late third trimester and is potentially fatal to both mother and fetus; emergent delivery is the treatment. While the histologic hallmark is zone 3 or diffuse microvesicular steatosis, oil red O stain on a frozen section may be required since hepatitic features

and extra-medullary hematopoiesis may be present. Endophlebitis is common. The affected hepatocytes appear swollen, and the microsteatosis gives an appearance of cytoplasmic reticulation (e-**Fig. 15.46**). Pre-eclampsia/eclampsia and **HELLP syndrome** (hemolysis, elevated liver enzymes, and low platelets) may cause zone 1 hemorrhage, necrosis, and fibrin deposition. Liver rupture is a potentially fatal complication of pregnancy.

3. **Ductal plate malformation (DPM), aka hereditary fibropolycystic disease**, results from developmental arrest with persistence of the embryologic ductal plate which assumes an anastomosing ringlike structure outlining the periphery of the portal tracts (e-**Fig. 15.47**). DPM may further manifest as von Meyenburg complexes (which are noted as irregularly ectatic tubular structures embedded within and extending from portal tracts); congenital hepatic fibrosis; or Caroli syndrome or disease.

   a. **Congenital hepatic fibrosis** (e-**Figs. 15.48** and **15.49**), a lesion of ARPKD, is a significant cause of noncirrhotic portal hypertension with maintained liver synthetic function in children, adolescents, or young adults. The abnormal portal tracts are expanded, have an increased number of aberrant duct profiles located within, and peripherally show hypoplastic or absent portal veins and numerous hypertrophic hepatic artery branches. Bridging fibrous bands are noted but portal-central relationships are maintained. Inspissated bile-stained material may be noted in ectatic ductal structures. Little to no inflammation is seen. There is no communication with the extrahepatic biliary tree.

   b. **Caroli disease, with autosomal recessive inheritance,** is characterized by cystic dilatation of the larger intrahepatic ducts, and is accompanied by recurrent bacterial cholangitis and intra-hepatic choledochal lithiasis. The process may involve the entire organ, or be segmental or lobar. When associated with congenital hepatic fibrosis, it is termed Caroli syndrome. This form of ARPKD does communicate with the extrahepatic biliary tree. Grossly, the numerous cysts are transected by fibrous bands. Involved ducts are embedded in fibrous stroma with marked chronic inflammation with or without polymorphonuclear leukocytes. Adenocarcinoma and HCC have been reported.

   c. **Polycystic liver disease (ADPKD)** is a potentially debilitating process due to progressive hepatic enlargement from massive cystic replacement and expansion within the otherwise normal parenchyma (e-**Fig. 15.50**). Unlike renal cystic disease, liver function is maintained but transplantation may be needed for quality of life. The cysts do not communicate with the biliary tree. Cysts are lined by columnar or cuboidal epithelium; collapsed cysts show hyalinized changes. Intraluminal bile-tinged fluid may be present; in previously manipulated cysts, changes of infection or abscess may be seen. Von Meyenburg complexes commonly co-occur. Other organs that may be involved with similar cysts include the pancreas and ovaries; colonic diverticula, cardiac valve complications, and inguinal hernias also occur. Intracranial aneurysm of the middle cerebral artery can be life threatening, but is the least common of the associations.

   d. **Choledochal cyst,** commonly due to aberrant pancreaticobiliary ductal junction with subsequent dilatation, requires complete excision due to its rare association with biliary carcinoma, the risk of which increases with age. Microscopic evaluation shows wall thickening with fibrosis, mixed chronic inflammation, and rarely foci of intact epithelial cell lining which may show metaplastic changes. Biliary intraepithelial neoplasia likewise is noted with increasing age.

4. **Ascending cholangitis** is typically diagnosed clinically. Histologically, intraluminal neutrophils are present within the interlobular bile ducts. Other features of biliary obstruction have been described (e-**Fig. 15.51**).

IV. TRANSPLANTATION PATHOLOGY

   A. **Donor Liver Evaluation** is performed on frozen sections to evaluate steatosis, or portal inflammation and fibrosis in an HCV donor. For the former, percentages of the core involved by large droplet steatosis are estimated; the presence of >30% macrovesicular steatosis is commonly accepted as a cut-off potentially associated with poor graft function in the immediate posttransplant period. Pitfalls of frozen artifacts include the minute spaces in hepatocytes and sinusoidal spaces that may be misinterpreted as large fat vacuoles. The use of oil red O stain is discouraged as it results in an overestimation of steatosis. For HCV-positive donors, portal inflammation, lobular activity, and fibrosis as seen in H&E-stained sections are documented. Coagulative necrosis is a worrisome finding in donor biopsies, and is worth both verbal communication and written documentation.

B. **Preservation/Reperfusion Injury** is related to harvesting, transportation, and reperfusion of the graft. The relevant findings are located in zone 3; specifically hepatocyte ballooning and cholestasis. Frank necrosis may occur in more severe cases. Resolution is expected within 2 weeks.

C. **Humoral (Hyperacute) Rejection** rarely occurs with current patient management paradigms. Historically, humoral rejection was associated with coagulative and hemorrhagic necrosis or portal/periportal edema, neutrophilic portal infiltrates, prominent ductular reaction, portal vein endothelial cell hypertrophy, portal eosinophilia, and eosinophilic central venulitis (*Liver Transpl* 2014;20:1244–1255).

D. **Acute (Cellular) Rejection** is directed primarily at antigens on duct epithelium and venous endothelium. It can occur anytime immunosuppression is reduced or discontinued, but is most common between 5 and 30 days after transplantation. The classic histologic triad consists of mixed portal chronic inflammation, bile duct damage, and endotheliitis. The portal infiltrates consist of lymphocytes admixed with eosinophils, histiocytes, plasma cells, and occasional neutrophils. Bile duct damage is characterized by inflammatory intercalation into ductal epithelium; it may be accompanied by cytoplasmic vacuolization and other cytologic alterations. However, nuclear pyknosis and cytoplasmic eosinophilia are signs of ischemic injury (e-**Fig. 15.52**). Endotheliitis is defined as subendothelial lymphocytic infiltration with lifting, detachment, and sloughing of endothelial cells; attachment of lymphocytes to the luminal aspect of the endothelium is insufficient for diagnosis (e-**Fig. 15.53**). Endotheliitis most frequently involves portal veins, but central veins can be similarly affected. Centrilobular necrosis is sufficient for a diagnosis of severe rejection.

Centers differ in treatment thresholds, thus careful description and standard evaluation is recommended for optimal clinical communication. Acute rejection may be graded using the Banff schema recommended by an international panel (Table 15.3).

E. **Chronic Rejection (CR)** is a misleading moniker as the characteristic feature, specifically loss of bile ducts, may occur any time after transplantation. The diagnostic criteria are: (1) bile duct loss affecting >50% portal tracts, or (2) obliterative arteriopathy by foamy histiocytes. Biliary epithelial senescence with eosinophilic cytoplasm and nuclear hyperchromasia is considered an early feature of CR. The arterial lesions mainly involve large and medium size vessels and are rarely seen in small vessels sampled by percutaneous biopsy. Therefore, the diagnosis of CR (Table 15.4) is primarily based on the evaluation of bile ducts and has been divided into early and late stages (*Hepatology* 2000;31:792). The early stage typically shows perivenular hepatocyte dropout and central perivenulitis (e-**Fig. 15.54**); the late stage features duct loss in ≥50% of portal tracts with variable perivenular fibrosis (e-**Fig. 15.55**). Portal inflammation and ductular reaction are typically insignificant in the late stage as the progenitor cell compartment is lost along with the ducts, a useful feature that can be used to distinguish CR from recurrent HCV.

F. **Late Complications of Allograft Livers.** So-called "*de novo* **autoimmune hepatitis**" **(DNAIH)** is a plasma-cell rich portal and lobular hepatitis frequently accompanied by central necrosis. **Idiopathic post-transplant chronic hepatitis (IPTH)** has been described in 10% to 50% of long-term liver allograft survivors, and is a diagnosis of exclusion. It shows predominantly mononuclear portal inflammation with interface hepatitis, although features resembling central perivenulitis can also be seen. Bile duct damage and endothelial inflammation are absent to minimal. Progression to bridging fibrosis or cirrhosis has been reported, especially in pediatric patients. Both DNAIH and ITPH may be forms of alloimmune-mediated rejection.

TABLE 15.4	Banff Criteria for Chronic Liver Allograft Rejection (CR)	
Structure	Early CR	Late CR
Small bile ducts	Degenerative changes involving a majority of ducts: Eosinophilic transformation of the cytoplasm; increased nuclear to cytoplasmic (N/C) ratio; nuclear hyperchromasia; uneven nuclear spacing; ducts only partially lined by biliary epithelial cells Bile duct loss in <50% of portal tracts	Degenerative changes in remaining bile ducts Loss in ≥50% of portal tracts
Terminal hepatic venules and zone 3 hepatocytes	Intimal/luminal inflammation Lytic zone 3 necrosis and inflammation Mild perivenular fibrosis	Focal obliteration Variable inflammation Severe (bridging) fibrosis
Portal tract hepatic arterioles	Occasional loss involving <25% of portal tracts	Loss involving >25% of portal tracts
Other	So-called "transition" hepatitis with spotty necrosis of hepatocytes	Sinusoidal foam cell accumulation; marked cholestasis
Larger perihilar hepatic artery branches	Intimal inflammation, focal foam cell deposition without luminal compromise	Luminal narrowing by subintimal foam cells Fibrointimal proliferation
Large perihilar bile ducts	Inflammation damage and focal foam cell deposition	Mural fibrosis

G. **Technical Complications** usually occur during the first few months after transplantation. Hepatic artery or PVT or stricture may cause zone 3 hepatocyte necrosis, but infarction is rare. Ischemic damage of the biliary tree is a sign of hepatic artery complication, with protean manifestations including abscess, cholestasis, obstructive changes, stricture, or loss of the bile ducts. Thus, CR cannot be diagnosed without demonstration of a patent hepatic artery. Hepatic vein thrombosis or stricture results in changes of venous outflow obstruction. Stenosis or obstruction of the bile duct anastomosis causes morphologic changes similar to those of biliary obstruction or biliary cirrhosis.

H. **Recurrent Diseases.** Most diseases recur in the transplanted liver but the timeframe and severity vary; diagnosis is complicated by the fact that recurrent diseases share histopathologic features with rejection or technical complications.

Histologic evidence of recurrent HCV initially is acidophil bodies; portal and lobular chronic inflammation occur later. Overlapping features with mild acute rejection include bile duct damage, endotheliitis, and mixed infiltrates, thus a final diagnosis should include, if possible, description of the balance of damage due to hepatitis versus rejection. HBV recurrence is documented by protocol evaluation of HB S and C Ag testing on every follow-up allograft biopsy (e-Fig. 15.56).

Fibrosing cholestatic hepatitis (FCH) (e-Fig. 15.57) is a rare but progressive disease seen in both recurrent hepatitis B and C, with rapidly rising bilirubin that may result in graft loss. FCH's histologic features include marked portal and periportal perisinusoidal fibrosis with ductular reaction, canalicular cholestasis, and nonzonal hepatocyte ballooning; the latter may be the earliest clue to diagnosis. Inflammatory changes are generally mild. In FCH-B, HB S and C Ag are highly expressed in reinfected hepatocytes.

PBC and PSC may recur several years after transplantation. Even with granulomatous duct lesions, recurrent PBC is difficult to diagnose. Recurrent PSC needs to be distinguished from technical complications due to hepatic artery or biliary stricture, or biliary obstruction. Recurrent steatosis and steatohepatitis are a challenge to distinguish from *de novo* occurrence due to persistence of the patient's metabolic syndrome and/or the medications utilized for allografts. Recurrent HCC or cholangiocarcinoma are typically rapidly lethal complications.

I. **Acute GVHD** (e-**Fig 15.58**) following bone marrow or stem cell transplantation shows duct damage, and less frequently endotheliitis. Hepatitic forms of GVHD may co-exist. The differential diagnosis includes viral infection and DILI.

J. **Chronic GVHD** typically occurs after 100 days and simulates ischemia or ductopenic CR. Skin and GI GVHD are commonly concurrent.

V. **DIAGNOSTIC FEATURES OF COMMON NEOPLASTIC AND TUMOR-LIKE CONDITIONS.** The most current World Health Organization (WHO) histologic classification of tumors of the liver and intrahepatic bile ducts is given in Table 15.5.

The most common tumor type in noncirrhotic livers is **metastasis**; colorectal, pancreatic, renal, pulmonary, and breast carcinomas frequently metastasize to the liver, and melanoma and neuroendocrine tumors may as well. Metastases usually present as multiple nodules in contrast to the single nodules of primary liver tumors. Metastases to a cirrhotic liver are very uncommon.

A. **Epithelial Tumors**

1. **Benign hepatocellular tumors**

   a. **FNH** is a common nonneoplastic lesion. It is not caused by oral contraceptive use, but instead is a polyclonal regenerative response to a local vascular injury. FNH has no malignant potential. The nodularity of the lesion underlies the original moniker of focal cirrhosis. Rarely larger than 5 to 7 cm, FNH is well-demarcated, nonencapsulated, and characterized by a central stellate scar with branches radiating into the nodular mass (e-**Fig. 15.59**); the stalk of FNH contains large, thick-walled vessels. Ductular reaction and copper are present in periseptal parenchyma; normal bile ducts are absent. The architecture may be a challenge to appreciate on biopsy of the periphery of the lesion. The hepatocytes of the lesion resemble those of the surrounding parenchyma, or may be steatotic. Altered TGFβ signaling results in a characteristic "map-like pattern" of glutamine synthetase by IHC; this may also be challenging to discern on a peripheral sample in a needle biopsy (e-**Fig. 15.60**). FNH may occur within cirrhosis. FNH can also be syndromic, multiple, and/or associated with hemangiomas, HCAs, hereditary hemorrhagic telangiectasia, and CNS vascular lesions.

   b. **HCA** is a rare benign neoplasm almost always present in noncirrhotic livers. HCA is significantly more common in women of reproductive age than in children or men, and occurs in a "stimulated" liver; associations include prolonged use of oral contraceptives, anabolic/androgenic steroid use, and metabolic disorders including GSD types 1 and 3, galactosemia, tyrosinemia, alcohol use, and obesity (with or without diabetes). HCA arising in the setting of metabolic disorders has an increased risk of transformation into HCC. HCA is usually solitary; when more than 10 adenomas are present, the condition is referred to as adenomatosis. Although distinguishable by gross evaluation and handheld examination on a microscopic slide, HCA is difficult to distinguish microscopically from the surrounding uninvolved liver by H&E morphology. The tumor consists of bland hepatocytes in sheets or 1 to 3 cells/cord thick, with minimal nuclear pleomorphism and sparse to no mitotic figures. Small unaccompanied arteries and sinusoidal vessels are present, but portal tracts and bile ducts are absent. Granulomas, steatosis, or steatohepatitis with MDB may be present. Variably sized blood vessels, some of which may show fibromyxoid intimal thickening, may be present at the boundary with nontumor liver. HCAs are now classified into eight subtypes according to molecular studies. These subtypes have distinguishing clinical phenotypes, and most can be ascertained by IHC. The subtypes carry different risks of malignant progression or bleeding (*Gastroenterology* 2017;152:880).

      i. **HNF1α-inactivated HCAs** (34% of adenomas) are due to genomic or somatic bi-allelic inactivating mutation of this tumor suppressor gene that results in

TABLE 15.5	WHO Histologic Classification of Tumors of the Liver and Intrahepatic Bile Ducts

Epithelial masses and neoplasms tumors: hepatocellular

Benign

Hepatocellular adenoma
   HNF1α–Mutated
   β-catenin activating
   Inflammatory, gp130 mutated
   Unclassified
Focal nodular hyperplasia

Malignancy-associated and premalignant lesions

Large cell change (formerly "dysplasia")
Small cell change (formerly "dysplasia")
Dysplastic nodules
   Low grade
   High grade

Malignant

Hepatocellular carcinoma, NOS
Early hepatocellular carcinoma
Hepatocellular carcinoma, fibrolamellar
Hepatocellular carcinoma, scirrhous
Hepatocellular carcinoma, sarcomatoid
Lymphoepithelial-like hepatocellular carcinoma
Hepatoblastoma, epithelial variant
Undifferentiated carcinoma

Epithelial tumors: biliary

Benign

Bile duct adenoma (peribiliary gland hamartoma and others)
Microcystic adenoma
Biliary adenofibroma

Premalignant lesions

Biliary intraepithelial neoplasia, grade 3 (BilIN-3)
Pre-invasive intraglandular neoplasms of the peribiliary glands
Intraductal papillary biliary neoplasm with low- or intermediate-grade intraepithelial neoplasia
Intraductal papillary biliary neoplasm with high-grade intraepithelial neoplasia
Intraductal tubulopapillary neoplasm of bile duct
Mucinous cystic neoplasm with low- or intermediate-grade intraepithelial neoplasia
Mucinous cystic neoplasm with high-grade intraepithelial neoplasia

Malignant

Intrahepatic cholangiocarcinoma
Intraductal papillary biliary neoplasm with an associated invasive carcinoma
Intraductal tubulopapillary neoplasm of bile duct with an associated invasive carcinoma
Mucinous cystic neoplasm with an associated invasive carcinoma

Malignancies of mixed or uncertain origin

Calcifying nested epithelial stromal tumor

Carcinosarcoma

Combined hepatocellular-cholangiocarcinoma

Hepatoblastoma, mixed epithelial-mesenchymal

Malignant rhabdoid tumor

(*continued*)

TABLE 15.5 WHO Histologic Classification of Tumors of the Liver and Intrahepatic Bile Ducts (*Continued*)

Mesenchymal tumors

Benign

Angiomyolipoma (PEComa)
Cavernous hemangioma
Infantile hemangioma
Inflammatory pseudotumor
Lymphangioma
Lymphangiomatosis
Mesenchymal hamartoma
Solitary fibrous tumor

Malignant

Angiosarcoma
Embryonal sarcoma (undifferentiated sarcoma)
Epithelioid hemangioendothelioma
Kaposi sarcoma
Leiomyosarcoma
Rhabdomyosarcoma
Synovial sarcoma

Germ cell tumors

Teratoma
Yolk sac tumor (endodermal sinus tumor)

Lymphomas

Secondary tumors

From: Bosman FT, Carneiro F, Hruban RH, Theise ND, eds. *WHO Classification of Tumours. Tumours of the Digestive System.* Lyon, France: IARC Press; 2017. Used with permission.

loss of liver fatty acid binding protein (LFABP-1) expression in the tumor. By IHC normal liver is positive for LFABP, but the steatotic HNF1α-inactivated HCA is negative (e-**Figs. 15.61** and **15.62**). HNF1α mutated adenomas are characterized by steatosis, are more likely to be multiple than the other subcategories, and have a low risk of malignant progression.

ii. **β-Catenin exon 3-mutated HCAs (7%)** show nuclear and cytoplasmic β-catenin by IHC as well as diffuse expression of upregulated glutamine synthetase. β-catenin-activated adenomas may be characterized by borderline histology including cellular atypia and pseudoacinar architecture, and are more common in men than the other types of HCA. b^ex3^HCA are associated with a higher risk of progression to HCC.

iii. **β-Catenin exon 7/8-mutated HCAs (3%)** have weak activation of β-catenin with no β-catenin nuclear staining, and are not associated with a high risk of malignant transformation. Glutamine synthetase stains in a variety of patterns, and identification of this subgroup using IHC alone is challenging.

iv. **Inflammatory HCA (34%),** defined by constitutive activation of the JAK/STAT pathway by various gene mutations, have overexpression of the inflammatory markers SAA and CRP by IHC. Formerly termed "telangiectatic FNH," inflammatory HCA have been shown to be true adenomas by a variety of assays, and are associated with obesity and alcohol use. Clinically, they may be associated with anemia, fever, and inflammatory syndrome resulting from uncontrolled production of cytokines. Inflammatory HCA are often hemorrhagic, have foci of sinusoidal dilatation and peliosis, and have clusters of abnormal vessels; chronic inflammatory infiltrates are common along fibrovascular septa with periseptal ductular reaction (e-**Fig. 15.63**). Inflammatory

HCA may be confused with FNH by imaging and initial gross and microscopic evaluation, but glutamine synthetase staining is not "map-like."

v. b^ex3^IHCA (6%) are β-catenin^ex3^ mutated adenomas with inflammatory infiltrates.

vi. b^ex7,8^IHCA (4%) are β-catenin^ex7,8^ mutated adenomas with inflammatory infiltrates.

vii. Sonic hedgehog HCAs (5%) (*Hepatology* 2018; doi:10.1002/hep.29884) have constitutive activation of the sonic hedgehog pathway, with a gene fusion between *INHBE* and *GL1*. These are associated with a higher risk of clinical bleeding and often contain hemorrhagic foci. Sonic hedgehog HCAs show reactivity for PTGDS (prostaglandin D synthase) diffusely (from 40% to 100% of tumor reactivity), as well as decreased reactivity with LFABP by IHC.

viii. Unclassified adenoma (<7%), is without specific genotypic or phenotypic features.

2. Premalignant lesions DN, a well-defined premalignant lesion arising in the background of cirrhosis (*Semin Liver Dis* 2005;25:133, *Clin Liver Dis* 2015; 19239), is diagnosed by the presence of a nodule with abnormal architecture, clonal hepatocytes with an increased N/C ratio, and nuclear atypia. DNs are usually multiple in livers with chronic liver disease or cirrhosis. Additional features include gross differences from surrounding nodules including bulging above the background, expansile growth with pushing borders, small cell change (nuclear crowding and sinusoidal alignment), resistance to iron accumulation in an otherwise iron-loaded cirrhosis (e-**Fig. 15.64**), clear cell change or deep eosinophilia, and the presence of isolated artery branches. Unlike HCC, DNs do not have cords >3 nuclei thick or stromal invasion. Macroregenerative nodules with intralesional portal tracts are considered low-grade DN. DN may contain small foci of nonencapsulated HCC within them referred to as "nodule-in-nodule" (N-I-N).

DNs are rarely >2 cm in size. When the lesion is <0.1 cm, it is termed a dysplastic focus. Large cell change, although associated with the presence of HCC, is not itself considered premalignant. Large cell change is characterized by cellular and nuclear enlargement with nuclear atypia, but a normal N/C ratio. Small cell change, on the other hand, is strongly associated with progression to HCC.

3. Malignant epithelial neoplasms

a. HCC more common in middle aged and older men, usually but not exclusively occurs in chronic liver disease with cirrhosis. Chronic hepatitis C and B infection account for up to 85% of HCC; alcohol abuse is the most significant nonviral cause. HH carries a significant risk and tobacco use is an additive factor. Obesity and the associated complications of diabetes and steatohepatitis are also risks, and multiple risk factors increase the overall risk. Increasingly, noncirrhotic NASH is seen with HCC.

HCC is usually encapsulated in cirrhotic livers, but not in noncirrhotics. Prior to the advent of advanced imaging for screening, several grossly observable types of HCC were documented: the single nodular type, the multifocal/multicentric type, the diffuse (cirrhotomimetic) type, and the uncommon pedunculated type. Tumor nodules are soft, fatty (yellow) or green (bile) stained, and bulge above the cut surface. Central necrosis is not rare, particularly in TACE or radio frequency ablation (RFA) treated HCC. With advanced screening in known cirrhotics, detected tumor nodules are often small (<1 to 2 cm) and subtle. The differential diagnoses are affected by knowledge of background liver disease: if cirrhotic, considerations include high-grade DN versus HCC; if not cirrhotic, considerations include metastasis versus HCA versus HCC. IHC can be helpful.

Microscopically, HCC assumes a variety of patterns: trabecular, pseudoglandular, acinar, compact, or scirrhous. Unattached, "floating" trabeculae are characteristic. Mixed patterns are common, particularly with increased tumor size. Cell plates are broader than >3 nuclei, a feature useful in distinguishing DN from early HCC. Isolated arteries noted within the tumor can be detected with trichrome, αSMA, and CD34 immunohistochemistry, but can also be seen in HCA. HCC receives blood solely from systemic arteries, thus CD34-positive tumor sinusoidal endothelium contrasts with CD34-negative sinusoids of nontumor liver. Reticulin stain highlights widened cell plates and shows fragmentation, reduction, or foci of loss (e-**Fig. 15.65**). Tumor cells may have any characteristic of nonneoplastic liver cells, for example, intranuclear inclusions; eosinophilic or basophilic cytoplasm; small droplet, large droplet, or microvesicular steatosis; clear cell change; MDB; PAS-D inclusions; fibrinogen inclusions; and HB S Ag. Mitoses may be easily seen. Bile production by tumor cells, once distinguished from bile within entrapped hepatocytes, is a useful marker to identify the tumor as hepatocellular. Stromal invasion is diagnostic of HCC, and vascular invasion is an important parameter for diagnosis and tumor staging. Both are difficult to unequivocally determine in biopsies.

The appropriate immunohistochemistry panel for HCC first depends on the query of HCC versus metastasis or HCC versus HCA versus DN. For the former, gender and age-based panels for the work-up of liver metastases are published elsewhere. Polyclonal CEA and CD10 IHC are reactive with canaliculi in benign and malignant hepatocytes; the less differentiated HCCs will show greater membrane reactivity with pCEA. Cytoplasmic pCEA is considered a marker of adenocarcinoma (e.g., cholangiocarcinoma) (e-**Fig. 15.66**). In an iron-loaded liver, both HCC and DN are iron-free. Arginase-1 and HepPar-1 (aka, "Hepatocyte") are markers of enzymes of the urea cycle. Lack of reactivity, particularly in poorly differentiated HCC, does not exclude a diagnosis of HCC. TTF-1 may be positive in the cytoplasm of HCC, but is dependent on the antibody clone utilized. The oncofetal protein glypican-3 (GPC-3) may be useful when positive; the reactivity is inhomogeneous in a cytoplasmic, membranous, and/or canalicular pattern in up to 70% to 80% of HCCs, but is negative in HCA, although a small fraction of dysplastic and cirrhotic nodules have been reported as immunopositive. Glutamine synthetase, positive only around central veins in non-neoplastic liver, is commonly diffusely positive in HCC (e-**Fig. 15.67**), and heat shock protein 70 (HSP70) is positive in the majority of HCC. Some investigators advocate the use of a panel of GPC-3, glutamine synthetase, and HSP70 to distinguish DN from HCC, with two-thirds of these markers positive in HCC (*J Hepatol* 2009;50:746). The presence of >2% positive keratin 19 (K19) tumor cells in HCC has been proposed as a poor prognostic marker in HCC. Loss of K7 or K19 positive ductular reaction at the periphery of an encapsulated hepatocellular neoplasm signifies the diagnostic stromal invasion of HCC.

Other variants of HCC are listed in Table 15.5. By international consensus, **early HCC** is a low-grade, low-stage, small HCC (*Hepatology* 2009;49:658) that has grossly and microscopically indistinct borders with the surrounding cirrhotic liver, and may be difficult to distinguish from a high-grade DN. Early HCC may be fatty. Nodules of encapsulated HCC that are distinct from the background are not categorized as independent early HCC since they represent biologically advanced tumors.

b. Fibrolamellar HCC (FL-HCC) occurs in noncirrhotic livers and remains less common than HCC in all age groups. The tumor is distinguishable from classical HCC by the unique somatic *DNAJB1-PRKACA* fusion transcripts, the protein product of which can be detected by FISH assay. FL-HCC is characterized by large eosinophilic polygonal tumor cells with prominent nuclei and nucleoli in a background of paucicellular lamellar fibrous bands. FL-HCC may bear resemblance to FNH by imaging and gross examination. Some of the tumor cells may contain cytoplasmic pale bodies due to the presence of fibrinogen (e-**Fig. 15.68**). The presumed better prognosis of FL-HCC has not borne out in large studies; surgical resectability remains the key prognostic factor, and lack of background chronic liver disease plays a large role. Modes of spread (i.e., peritoneal and lymph node) differ from classical HCC.

The primary distinction in biopsy is with the scirrhous variant of HCC; morphology of the hepatocytes is key in this regard. Tumor cells are reactive with various progenitor cell markers such as NCAM, EpCAM, and CD133; K7 expression is common, and CD68 is common in the lysosomes of the tumor cells. However, as with non-FL HCC, basic morphology remains the cornerstone of the diagnosis. Clinical information and serum markers may be helpful: in contrast to HCC, serum AFP is rarely elevated in FL-HCC; however, vitamin B12, vitamin B12 binding capacity, and serum carcinoembryonic antigen may be elevated in FL-HCC.

B. Epithelial Malignancies of Mixed Cellular Origin

1. **Combined hepatocellular-cholangiocarcinoma (cHCC-CCA).** Primary liver carcinomas with both hepatocytic and cholangiocytic differentiation can be referred to as cHCC-CCA according to recent international consensus terminology (*Hepatology* 2018; doi: 10.1002/hep.29789). These are tumors that contain areas of both typical HCC and typical intrahepatic cholangiocarcinoma (iCCA), which may be admixed or found as separate areas within the same tumor. The HCC component can have any/all of the possible cytologic and architectural features of HCCs, and the iCCA component should clearly be an adenocarcinoma with malignant glands. cHCC-CCAs are to be distinguished from collision tumors between separate HCC and iCCA. Diagnosis should be based on routine H&E histology; immunostains for the HCC and iCCA components are supportive but not essential for diagnosis. Although data are scarce about cHCC-CCAs, available data suggest that they are aggressive, with worse outcomes than traditional HCC. cHCC-CCA, intermediate cell carcinoma and cholangiocarcinoma may occur in combination with each other; each may or may not have features of progenitor cells.

2. **Intermediate cell carcinoma** is a type of primary liver carcinoma composed of monomorphic populations of tumor cells that are phenotypically neither classic HCC nor classic iCCA, The tumor cells are smaller than normal hepatocytes and may be arranged in trabeculae, cords, solid nests, or strands in a background of desmoplastic or hyalinized stroma. Well-defined glands are not seen, but the tumor is easily mistaken for iCCA. Tumor cells may be cuboidal to oval-shaped, and atypia and mitoses are uncommon. Tumor cells stain variably with mixed hepatocytic and cholangiocytic markers.

3. **Cholangiolocarcinoma (CLC, aka cholangiolocellular carcinoma)** may conceptually be considered the malignant counterpart of the ductular reaction with tubular, anastomosing, "antler-like" architecture of the epithelial component. Most arise near a portal tract and are embedded in dense stroma. CLC may be a component of HCC, iCCA, cHCC-CCA, or intermediate cell carcinoma. Luminal EMA and pCEA distinguish CLC from the cytoplasmic reactivity of these IHC markers in iCCA.

C. Hepatoblastoma, a primary malignant blastomatous neoplasm of several cell lineages,

is rare but is nonetheless the most common liver tumor of children. Up to 80–90% of cases present by 5 years; prematurity and low birth weight are associations. Most present as symptomatic masses in the right lobe.

1. **The wholly epithelial type** consists of 4 subtypes: fetal, mixed fetal and embryonal, macrotrabecular, and small cell undifferentiated (SCUD). Fetal cells, resembling adult hepatocytes but smaller in size, contain variable amounts of cytoplasmic fat and glycogen giving rise to an alternating light-and-dark pattern (e-**Fig. 15.69**). Embryonal cells have a higher N/C ratio and may form nests, rosettes, or small tubules. The macrotrabecular subtype has a growth pattern reminiscent of HCC.

2. **The mixed epithelial-mesenchymal (MEM) type**, with or without teratoid features, contains malignant mesenchymal components such as cartilage and osteoid in addition to the epithelial elements.

3. **Hepatoblastoma, NOS,** is the final category.

The outcome of hepatoblastoma has improved significantly with the improved ability to shrink tumors prior to surgical extirpation. Chemotherapy induces a variety of predictable tumoral alterations. Hepatoblastoma staging systems are based on pretreatment features and postresection findings.

D. Tumors of Biliary Origin

1. Benign

a. Biliary cysts, whether solitary or as components of the DPM (described above), are lined by a single layer of benign, flattened, cuboidal or columnar biliary-type epithelium surrounded by a variable amount of fibrous tissue.

b. von Meyenburg complex (e-Fig. 15.70) represents persistence of the ductal plate; it is a common finding in normal livers, and may dilate to be the origin of solitary cysts or cysts of polycystic livers. The von Meyenburg complex is usually adjacent to a portal tract and appears as dilated duct-like structures within mature fibrous stroma.

c. Ciliated foregut cyst (e-Fig. 15.71), while rare, may be found by imaging or incidentally during surgery. It is subcapsular and often in segment 4. The lining is composed of ciliated pseudostratified columnar epithelium lying on a basement membrane.

d. Bile duct adenoma/peribiliary gland hamartoma is composed of closely packed, well-formed, and relatively uniform small ducts that form a 1 to 20 mm diameter, sharply demarcated nodule (e-Fig. 15.72). Careful microscopic examination is necessary to exclude the angulated architecture, desmoplastic stroma, cytologic atypia, mitotic activity, and evidence of invasive growth that are indicative of cholangiocarcinoma or metastatic adenocarcinoma.

2. Premalignant (*Histol Histopathol* 2017;32:1001–1015)

a. Biliary intraepithelial neoplasia, grade 3 (Bil-IN3) is a precursor of iCCA. It is characteristically flat dysplasia with multilayering of nuclei and micropapillary intraluminal projections. The morphologic findings are identical to Bil-IN3 of extrahepatic ducts.

b. Intraductal papillary biliary neoplasm (IPNB) are precursors of iCCA. This category of neoplasms has replaced lesions previously known as biliary papilloma and papillomatosis (e-Fig. 15.73). Synchronous or metachronous IPNBs may develop throughout the biliary system. IPNBs are classified as low, intermediate, or high grade based on cellular and nuclear features; the parallels with pancreatic intraductal lesions are many, and up to one-third are mucin producing. Most of the intrahepatic papillary neoplasms are lined by biliary epithelium, although intestinal, oncocytic, or gastric type may also be present. Ducts may be massively expanded by the villous growth and distinction with MCN requires thorough evaluation of surrounding stroma (e-Fig. 15.74). Invasive carcinoma may be found in association with IPNB; perineural invasion is common. Intraductal tubulopapillary neoplasm (IPTN) is a rare neoplasm of tightly packed glands.

c. Mucinous cystic neoplasm, (formerly known as biliary cystadenoma) occurs in women, and does not communicate with the biliary tree. The lesion consists of cystic dilated structures lined by a layer of mucin-producing columnar cells on a spindled-type mesenchymal (ovarian-like) stroma (e-Fig. 15.75). The stroma is diagnostic, but may be sclerotic. Low- or high-grade intraepithelial neoplasia raise the concern of potential progression to carcinoma. Thus, clinically, the recommendation is for complete excision. For pathologists, the recommendations are that numerous sections be evaluated; the use of frozen section for evaluation of these lesions is to be discouraged. Cases associated with an invasive carcinoma occur in older patients.

3. Malignant Intrahepatic Biliary Neoplasms

a. iCCA is a nonencapsulated mucin-secreting adenocarcinoma usually arising in noncirrhotic livers. Cirrhosis or chronic liver disease cannot be used as evidence to exclude the diagnosis, however. The tumor is characterized by three growth patterns that may co-exist: mass-forming, periductal, or intraductal. It is the mass-forming pattern that results in the prominent desmoplastic background with the characteristic firm, white or gray gross appearance.

The tumor is an adenocarcinoma with a variety of architectural patterns resembling canals of Hering, or cholangioles, or bile ducts of varying sizes, or peribiliary glands. In larger iCCA, the central areas may be mostly stroma and paucicellular while the peripheral regions may show a growth pattern that replaces and incorporates portal tracts. Greater than 90% express keratins 7 and 19, and about 40% also express keratin 20; most cases are also positive for expression of CEA (using a monoclonal antibody) and CA19-9. iCCA may be indistinguishable from metastatic ductal adenocarcinoma of the pancreas by histologic and immunohistochemical evaluation. iCCA involving only the peribiliary glands may be challenging to distinguish from reactive atypia.

The prognosis of iCCA is dismal due to the lack of effective treatments. The exceptions are small peripheral iCCAs found incidentally, the mucinous intraductal growth iCCAs that are completely resected, and the highly selected cases of perihilar cholangiocarcinoma arising in PSC treated with protocolized neoadjuvant chemotherapy and liver transplantation.

b. **Cystadenocarcinoma** occurs in men as commonly as in women, and no spindled stroma is present in the wall. These tumors likely arise from IPN within a markedly dilated duct rather than from MCN. Current data support a prognosis superior to that of iCCA.

E. Tumors of Mesenchymal Origin

1. **Mesenchymal hamartoma** is an uncommon childhood tumor, usually of the right lobe, characterized by a gelatinous mass of bile ducts in a ductal plate pattern; mesenchymal cells; vessels; cystic spaces in a loose, edematous, or myxoid stroma with admixed clusters of liver cells; and extramedullary hematopoiesis (e-**Fig. 15.76**). MH may result in cardiopulmonary complications if not resected. Transition into embryonal (undifferentiated) sarcoma (UES) occurs, but is very rare.

2. **Cavernous hemangioma** (e-**Fig. 15.77**), the most common benign tumor of the liver, becomes clinically relevant when greater than 4 cm in maximal dimension. Hemangiomas may increase or rupture during pregnancy. Grossly, tumors are sponge-like and appear well-circumscribed. Microscopically, parenchymal extensions are not uncommon. Organization and fibrosis with time are common, and malignant transformation does not occur.

3. **Infantile hemangioma (IH)** is the most common benign mesenchymal liver tumor of infants and children. Girls are more commonly affected than boys; symptoms may include heart failure or hemangiomas of other organs. IH is characterized by small vascular channels lined by a single layer of plump endothelial cells (e-**Fig. 15.78**) in scant stroma with trapped ducts.

4. **Epithelioid hemangioendothelioma (EHE)** is a low-grade malignancy. The epithelioid tumor cells have abundant eosinophilic cytoplasm, and may be difficult to discern initially as they are arranged as single cells or small clusters of cells in a dense or myxoid fibrous stroma, and may occasionally be dendritic or spindled. Some tumor cells contain an intracytoplasmic vascular lumen simulating signet-ring-cell carcinoma (e-**Fig. 15.79**). Sinusoidal growth of the tumor cells at the periphery of the lesion is characteristic, often accompanied by hepatocyte atrophy. The tumor may grow into and occlude outflow veins. The tumor cells express at least one endothelial marker such as CD34, CD31, or factor VIII–related antigen.

5. **Angiosarcoma,** a highly aggressive tumor, is the most common mesenchymal malignancy of the liver. The characteristic feature of the tumor is a sinusoidal growth pattern by hyperchromatic, plump, malignant endothelial cells with little associated stromal response (e-**Fig. 15.80**). Solid growth patterns of what initially appear to be epithelial cells may pose diagnostic challenges, but immunostains demonstrate the vascular nature of the tumor.

a. **Small vessel neoplasm** is a recently recognized neoplasm of adults with poor demarcation within a stroma-poor background that appears to infiltrate through the parenchyma. The lesion is negative for p53 and GLUT-1, and has a low proliferative rate by MIB-1.

6. **Kaposi sarcoma** consists of a pure spindle-cell proliferation with slit-like spaces containing extravasated red cells, and is restricted to patients with human immuno-deficiency virus (HIV).

F. **Staging.** The most recent staging system for HCC and fibrolamellar variant of HCC is that of the 2017 Tumor, Node, Metastasis (TNM) American Joint Committee on Cancer staging classification (Amin MB et al., eds. *AJCC Cancer Staging Manual.* 8th ed. New York: Springer, 2017). Of note, there is a separate staging system for iCCA and combined hepatocellular-cholangiocarcinoma (both of which are staged according to the system for intrahepatic bile ducts), and for sarcomas of the liver (which are stage according to the system for soft tissue sarcoma of the abdomen and thoracic visceral organs).

Reporting should follow recommended guidelines (e.g., College of American Pathologists Protocol for the Examination of Specimens From Patients With Hepatocellular Carcinoma, or from Patients With Carcinoma of the Intrahepatic Bile Ducts, available at http://www.cap.org).

Cytopathology of the Liver

Hannah R. Krigman

I. **INTRODUCTION.** Fine needle aspiration (FNA) of the liver is typically prompted by the presence of a mass and can be achieved via percutaneous ultrasound or CT-guided FNA; lesions in the left lobe can be aspirated by endoscopic ultrasound-guided FNA (EUS-FNA) (*Gastrointest Endosc* 2002;55:859). Hepatic FNA is a very safe procedure; fatal complications are rare, hemorrhage being the most common which occurs at a rate of 0.006 to 0.031% (*Radiology* 1991;178:253). The sensitivity for malignancy ranges from 76% to 95%, with a specificity close to 100% (*Diagn Cytopathol* 2002;26:283, *Diagn Cytopathol* 2000;23:326).

As with all aspirates, during interpretation it is critical to bear in mind the intervening tissue the needle must pass through, which may be a source of confusion and misdiagnosis. Examples complicating hepatic FNA interpretation include benign or malignant cells originating from the pleura, peritoneum, and lung. Familiarity with and recognition of normal hepatic elements, including bile ductular cells, Kupffer cells, and endothelial cells, are also crucial to avoid a false-positive diagnosis of malignancy (*World Journ of Surg Onc* 2002;2:1). Reactive hepatocytes in particular may pose a diagnostic challenge in the distinction from a well-differentiated HCC (*Arch Pathol Lab Med* 2002;126:670).

II. **BENIGN NONNEOPLASTIC MASSES.** Hydatid cysts, abscesses, granulomas, bile duct adenoma/von Meyersburg complexes, FNH, and regenerative nodules are examples of benign non-neoplastic masses.

A. The aspirate of an **abscess** shows abundant neutrophils and necrotic debris (e-**Fig. 15.81**). Amebic abscesses contain more necrotic debris and fewer inflammatory cells. Culture and special stains are usually necessary to identify microorganisms (e-**Fig. 15.82**).

For cases of suspected abscess, it is always necessary to rule out the presence of a necrotic or infected neoplasm by extensive sampling and careful cytologic evaluation for viable tumor cells which may be obscured by the inflammation. In the instance of suspected tumoral necrosis or well-differentiated hepatocellular carcinoma, rebiopsy with attention toward the periphery of the lesion should be recommended, such that the interface of the lesion and surrounding normal parenchyma may be examined (*Radiology* 1997;203:1).

B. In the case of **hydatid cyst**, the aspirated fluid may be clear or turbid. Laminated cyst walls, scolices, and hooklets are observed; a neutrophilic background is sometimes present. Although aspiration of a hydatid cyst poses a risk of anaphylactic reaction, successful procedures are the norm (*Diagn Cytopathol* 1995;12:173).

III. VASCULAR LESIONS

A. The aspirate of a **hemangioma** usually shows abundant blood. Scattered stromal fragments with bland elongated spindle cells are characteristic (*Diagn Cytopathol* 1998;19:250). Cell block preparations are helpful to identify the vascular channels.

B. Aspirates of **EHE** are paucicellular, containing single cells and small tissue fragments, and display a spectrum of cytomorphology from small bland-appearing epithelioid and spindle cells, to malignant large tumor cells. The epithelioid cells have abundant cytoplasm and may contain characteristic intracytoplasmic lumina or sharply defined intranuclear cytoplasmic inclusions (*Acta Cytol* 1997;41:5).

C. In **angiosarcoma**, the aspirate shows abundant blood in which there are isolated cells and loose clusters of cells. The malignant cells are spindle-shaped to epithelioid, and have hyperchromatic nuclei and abundant but ill-defined cytoplasm. Necrosis is present. Scattered malignant cells may show hemosiderin-laden cytoplasm or erythrophagocytosis (*Diagn Cytopathol* 1998;18:208). Vasoformative structures such as intracytoplasmic lumina, microacinar lumen formation, and vascular channels are identified inconsistently (*Anat Path* 2000;114:210).

IV. FOCAL NODULAR HYPERPLASIA AND HEPATOCELLULAR ADENOMA. These entities typically occur in distinct clinical scenarios as a solitary nodule and as such require clinical, pathologic, and radiologic correlation for the correct diagnosis. In both cases the diagnosis rests on evaluation of the presence or absence of cytologically benign liver elements; it is therefore critical that only lesional tissue is sampled.

A. Aspirates of **FNH** show both abundant benign hepatocytes and benign biliary epithelial cells (*Acta Cytol* 1989;33:857).

B. **HCA** aspirates consist of benign hepatocytes *without* biliary epithelial cells (*Acta Cytol* 1989;33:857).

V. HEPATOCELLULAR CARCINOMA. The most characteristic and specific features are thickened hepatocyte trabeculae rimmed by spindle shaped endothelial cells (e-Fig. 15.83), hepatocyte tissue fragments with well-defined traversing capillaries (e-Fig. 15.84), increased cellular nuclear:cytoplasmic ratio (e-Fig. 15.85), and frequent atypical naked nuclei (e-Fig. 15.86) (*Diagn Cytopathol* 1999;21:370; *Cancer* 1999;87:270). Poorly differentiated HCC demonstrates loose nests, three-dimensional fragments, and occasional gland-like structures of malignant hepatocytes with marked pleomorphism, macronucleoli, necrosis, and numerous mitoses (*Cancer* 2004;102:247). Features that favor hepatocytic origin include polygonal shaped cells with centrally placed nuclei, abundant granular cytoplasm, and bile pigment (e-Fig. 15.86). However, the distinction from cholangiocarcinoma and metastatic adenocarcinoma is challenging and may require immunostains.

The **fibrolamellar variant** of HCC has a distinct cytomorphology which includes poorly cohesive clusters of cells and singly dispersed large monotonous cells with abundant granular cytoplasm, a low nuclear:cytoplasmic ratio, prominent nucleoli, and intracytoplasmic hyaline globules. Fragments of lamellar collagen bands with benign spindle shaped cells are present. The thickened trabeculae typical of classic HCC are not identified (*Diagn Cytopathol* 1999;21:180).

VI. CHOLANGIOCARCINOMA. The aspirate is composed of cells arranged in crowded sheets, three-dimensional clusters, acinar structures, or as singly dispersed cells. The malignant cells (e-Figs. 15.87 and 15.88) show a high nuclear:cytoplasmic ratio, irregular nuclear membranes, prominent nucleoli, and occasional intracytoplasmic mucin (*Cancer* 2005;105:220). Poorly differentiated carcinoma displays marked nuclear pleomorphism and necrosis.

Combined hepatocellular-cholangiocarcinoma is a biphenotypic tumor arising from the canal of Hering cells with features of HCC and cholangiocarcinoma. The tumor bridges these two entities both morphologically and immunohistochemically. These tumors (e-Fig. 15.89) are cytologically malignant but usually require immunostains for correct categorization as the malignant cells exhibit of spectrum of differentiation from hepatoid to glandular (*Acta Cytol* 1997;41:1269).

VII. METASTATIC MALIGNANCY. Metastasis from an extrahepatic primary tumor is the most common malignancy of the liver (*Diagn Cytopathol* 2000;23:326). The most common

primary tumors that metastasize to the liver are adenocarcinomas arising from the colon (**e-Fig. 15.90**), lung, pancreas, breast, and kidney. Comparison with the primary malignancy in cases of metastases is essential for diagnosis, as is appropriate immunohistochemical characterization. Carcinomas with polygonal cell morphology, such as neuroendocrine tumors, renal cell carcinoma, adrenocortical carcinoma, and others must be differentiated from HCC on the basis of their immunoprofile (*Arch Pathol Lab Med* 2007;131:1648).

ACKNOWLEDGMENT

The author thanks Julie Kunkel, an author of the previous edition of this section.

16 The Gallbladder and Extrahepatic Biliary Tree

Lulu Sun and Ta-Chiang Liu

I. NORMAL ANATOMY. The gallbladder, comprising the fundus, body, and neck, is covered by serosa, except the portion in the liver fossa that merges with liver parenchyma. The lining mucosa, a layer of folded columnar epithelium and lamina propria of loose connective tissue, directly rests on the muscularis propria, which consists of longitudinally oriented to irregularly arranged bundles of smooth muscle with overlying subserosa and serosa. No muscularis mucosae or submucosa is present. Secretory mucous glands in the neck and extrahepatic bile ducts are arranged in a lobular pattern (e-Fig. 16.1).

The extrahepatic ducts include the right and left hepatic ducts, which join to form the common hepatic duct in the porta hepatis; where the common hepatic duct is joined by the cystic duct, the common bile duct is formed. A single layer of columnar cells lines the ducts and rests directly on dense connective tissue; from proximal to distal there is a variable periductal smooth muscle fiber investment intermingled with collagen bundles.

II. GROSS EXAMINATION

A. Cholecystectomy is most commonly performed for cholelithiasis. After the gallbladder is measured and opened longitudinally, the following should be described: serosal, mural, and mucosal appearances; cystic duct integrity; and consistency, quantity, and color of stones. Full-thickness sections should be submitted from the fundus, body, neck, and duct; the cystic duct margin should also be submitted, as well as any lymph nodes. For a suspicious lesion, the overlying serosal surface or hepatic bed should be inked, the lesion breadloafed, and sections taken to demonstrate relevant anatomic relationships.

The gross finding that the gallbladder wall is uniformly firm with an associated flattened mucosal surface suggests the diagnosis of a so-called "porcelain" gallbladder. After the specimen is photographed, at least one section per centimeter should be submitted (if not the entire specimen) to exclude adenocarcinoma (e-Figs. 16.2 and 16.3). If adenocarcinoma is suspected or known, a careful search for lymph nodes should be undertaken, with all lymph nodes entirely submitted for microscopic examination.

B. Biopsy of the common bile duct is performed for stricture or overt neoplasm during endoscopic retrograde cholangiopancreatography (ERCP). The number and dimensions of specimens should be recorded to ensure that the biopsy fragments are adequately represented; inking is not needed. At the time of initial histologic sectioning, preparation of three H&E stained slides together with six additional unstained slides avoids refacing the block if subsequent deeper levels or special stains are required for diagnosis.

C. Frozen Section. Evaluation of bile duct margins by frozen section during pancreatoduodenectomy, or liver resections for bile duct adenocarcinoma, is often performed. The tissue should be frozen in its entirety, oriented in the frozen section block to obtain *en face* sections, and cut deeply to obtain sections that represent the entire margin so that small foci of tumor are not missed by inadequate sampling. The tissue that remains after frozen section should be submitted for evaluation by permanent sections, which helps assure adequate sampling.

III. DIAGNOSTIC FEATURES OF COMMON NONNEOPLASTIC CONDITIONS

A. Cholecystitis is associated with cholelithiasis in more than 90% of cases. Acute cholecystitis is characterized by full-thickness edema, congestion, and an associated fibrinopurulent serosal exudate. Hemorrhage, transmural necrosis (gangrenous cholecystitis), and/or perforation may occur (e-Figs. 16.4 and 16.5).

Chronic cholecystitis is variably characterized by mural hypertrophy or atrophy with fibrosis and chronic inflammation (e-**Fig. 16.6**). Intestinal, pyloric, or foveolar surface metaplasia may occur. Rokitansky–Aschoff sinuses, which are herniations of the lining mucosa into the muscle layers, are common. Adenomyoma represents exaggerated herniations in the fundus accompanied by muscular hypertrophy and may appear as a gross deformity (e-**Figs. 16.7** to **16.9**). Both xanthogranulomatous cholecystitis (due to rupture of Rokitansky–Aschoff sinuses) and mucosal ulceration from stones may be transmural with associated bile extravasation and accumulation of foamy macrophages. Acalculous cholecystitis may be acute or chronic. Follicular cholecystitis may be associated with primary sclerosing cholangitis (PSC) (e-**Fig. 16.10**).

B. Cholesterolosis (strawberry gallbladder) is characterized by yellow mucosal specks grossly, and lipid-laden macrophages in the lamina propria microscopically (e-**Fig. 16.11**). It is an incidental finding of no clinical significance.

C. Choledochal Cyst, a form of fibropolycystic disease, results in fusiform or spherical dilatation of the common bile duct. Following photographic documentation, the entire lesion should be submitted for microscopic examination to exclude biliary intraductal neoplasia or adenocarcinoma (e-**Fig. 16.12**).

D. Biliary Atresia is a congenital process in which the extrahepatic ducts and gallbladder may be completely absent or replaced by fibrous cords with no or only a very small lumen.

E. PSC involving the extrahepatic biliary system is an idiopathic disease diagnosed by cholangiography (discussed in more detail in Chapter 15).

F. Secondary Sclerosing Cholangitis, histologically indistinguishable from PSC, has a variety of obstructive and nonobstructive etiologies, including tumors, toxins, ischemia, and infections (including AIDS cholangiopathy).

IV. DIAGNOSTIC FEATURES OF COMMON NEOPLASMS AND PRECURSOR LESIONS (Table 16.1)

A. Adenoma is a single, small, and incidentally found polypoid lesion and is characterized by a tubular, papillary, or tubulopapillary architecture. A pyloric- or intestinal-type epithelium is more common than a biliary-type epithelium; squamous morules, Paneth cells, and neuroendocrine cells may be present. By definition, all adenomas are low grade, but larger adenomas may harbor foci of high-grade intraepithelial neoplasia or invasive carcinoma and thus should be entirely submitted for microscopic examination.

B. Biliary Intraepithelial Neoplasia (BilIN) is a classification nomenclature introduced in 2010 by the World Health Organization (WHO). BilIN-1 and BilIN-2 (low- and intermediate-grade lesions) are incidental and without established clinical significance. BilIN-3 may be associated with invasive carcinoma, and thus, if present in the gallbladder, thorough sampling (including of the cystic duct and margin of excision) is necessary to exclude invasive carcinoma. If no invasive carcinoma is present, and the surgical margin of the cystic duct is not involved, cholecystectomy is considered curative. A distinguishing characteristic between BilIN-3 and reparative atypia is the abrupt transition noted in the former (e-**Fig. 16.13**) compared with the gradual alterations and heterogeneous, widespread epithelial involvement of the latter. In addition, *p53* expression is more extensive in BilIN than in reactive atypia.

C. Intraluminal papillary neoplasms of the gallbladder and extrahepatic bile ducts are currently termed **intracystic papillary neoplasms** and **intraductal papillary neoplasms**, respectively.

   1. Intracystic papillary neoplasms have a biliary rather than pyloric lining, architectural complexity and atypia, and frequent mitoses. These lesions are stratified into low and high grade; the latter may be associated with adenocarcinoma, most commonly tubular. In the gallbladder, the differential diagnosis is adenoma.

   2. Intraductal papillary neoplasms of the extrahepatic bile ducts share the epithelial types characteristic of pancreatic intraductal papillary mucinous neoplasms (IPMNs), including pancreatobiliary, intestinal, oncocytic, and gastric. Intraductal papillary neoplasms can manifest as recurrent and multifocal lesions involving the entire biliary tree and can also be associated with invasive adenocarcinoma.

TABLE 16.1	2010 WHO Histologic Classification of Tumors of the Gallbladder and Extrahepatic Bile Ducts

Epithelial tumors
Premalignant lesions
Adenoma
  Tubular
  Papillary
  Tubulopapillary
Biliary intraepithelial neoplasia, grade 3 (BilIN-3)
Intracystic (gallbladder) or intraductal (bile ducts) papillary neoplasm with low- or intermediate-grade intraepithelial neoplasia
Intracystic (gallbladder) or intraductal (bile ducts) papillary neoplasm with high-grade intraepithelial neoplasia
Mucinous cystic neoplasm with low- or intermediate-grade intraepithelial neoplasia
Mucinous cystic neoplasm with high-grade intraepithelial neoplasia
Carcinoma
Adenocarcinoma
  Adenocarcinoma, biliary type
  Adenocarcinoma, gastric foveolar type
  Adenocarcinoma, intestinal type
  Clear cell adenocarcinoma
  Mucinous adenocarcinoma
  Signet-ring cell carcinoma
Adenosquamous carcinoma
Intracystic (gallbladder) or intraductal (bile ducts) papillary neoplasm with an associated invasive carcinoma
Mucinous cystic neoplasm with an associated invasive carcinoma
Squamous cell carcinoma
Undifferentiated carcinoma
Neuroendocrine neoplasms
Neuroendocrine tumor (NET)
  NET G1 (carcinoid)
  NET G2
Neuroendocrine carcinoma (NEC)
  Large cell NEC
  Small cell NEC
Mixed adenoneuroendocrine carcinoma
Goblet cell carcinoid
Tubular carcinoid

Mesenchymal tumors
Granular cell tumor
Leiomyoma
Kaposi sarcoma
Leiomyosarcoma
Rhabdomyosarcoma

Lymphomas

Secondary tumors

3. **Mucinous cystic neoplasm (MCN)** has replaced the term *cystadenoma*. More common in the extrahepatic ducts than in the gallbladder, MCN may grow to 20 cm in maximal dimension. As in its hepatic counterpart, the lesion contains estrogen receptor- and progesterone receptor-positive mesenchymal stroma. As with papillary neoplasms, MCN lesions may be associated with invasive adenocarcinoma.

D. The classification of **adenocarcinomas of the gallbladder and cystic duct** is shown in Table 16.1.

   1. Adenocarcinoma of the gallbladder may grossly result in mural induration and mimic chronic cholecystitis, or grow as an intraluminal polypoid lesion (**e-Fig. 16.14**). In order of decreasing frequency, the common subtypes are biliary, intestinal (tubular or goblet), and gastric foveolar (**e-Fig. 16.15**). Staging is according to depth of invasion into the gallbladder wall and extent of spread to neighboring lymph nodes and structures, including the liver (Amin MB et al., eds. *AJCC Cancer Staging Manual*. 8th ed. New York: Springer; 2017); of note, the American Joint Committee on Cancer (AJCC) staging scheme for the gallbladder does not apply to well-differentiated neuroendocrine tumors or sarcomas. It is important to document whether the tumor is located on the free peritoneal side (T2a) or the hepatic side (T2b) of the gallbladder, as the latter carries a worse prognosis. The number of involved lymph nodes, rather than location, determines the nodal category (N1 = 1 to 3 involved nodes, N2 = 4 or more involved nodes). Histologic grade is an independent prognostic factor for overall and disease-specific survival and should be reported.

   2. Biliary adenocarcinomas may contain mixed cell types including intestinal, goblet, and neuroendocrine cells. The tumors composed of intestinal-type cells are usually CK20 and CDX2 immunoreactive; the goblet cell variant may also have Paneth and neuroendocrine cells. The gastric foveolar type is usually well-differentiated (**e-Figs. 16.16** and **16.17**).

E. **Adenocarcinomas of Extrahepatic Bile Ducts** have been reclassified by the AJCC as perihilar or distal (Fig. 16.1), and each has its own staging scheme (Amin MB et al., eds. *AJCC Cancer Staging Manual*. 8th ed. New York: Springer; 2017). Of note, the AJCC staging schemes for the perihilar and distal bile ducts do not apply to well-differentiated neuroendocrine tumors or sarcomas.

F. Perihilar tumors arise proximal to the cystic duct and account for 60% of adenocarcinomas; T staging is based on depth of invasion through the bile duct wall and into adjacent structures. Distal tumors arise between the junction of the cystic duct and common bile duct and the ampulla of Vater and account for 30% of adenocarcinomas (**e-Fig. 16.18**); T staging is based on tumor depth (measured from the basement membrane

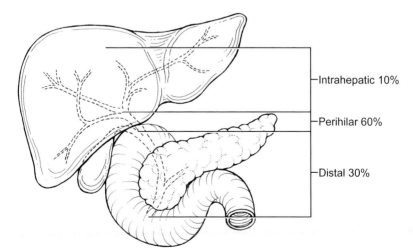

Figure 16.1 Anatomic boundaries for AJCC classification of adenocarcinomas of the extrahepatic bile ducts.

of adjacent normal or dysplastic epithelium), which requires careful sectioning so the deepest tumor invasion can be determined. Grossly, there may be only subtle thickening of the duct wall, and thus thorough sampling is also required to evaluate margins and local extension.

Cytopathology of the Gallbladder and Extrahepatic Biliary Tree

Cory Bernadt

I. GALLBLADDER

A. Inflammatory Lesions. In instances where acute cholecystitis develops into a localized abscess, aspirates typically slow numerous acute inflammatory cells with intermixed necroinflammatory debris. Even when an abscess arises within a necrotic neoplasm, aspirates often show only generic features, and thus it can be challenging to recognize that an underlying neoplasm is present based on the cytopathologic findings alone.

B. Neoplasms. Adenocarcinoma is the most common type of malignancy encountered. On aspiration smears it shows groups and syncytial fragments of cells that have round to oval nuclei, vesicular chromatin, nucleoli, and nuclear membrane irregularities. The overall findings impart an appearance of adenocarcinoma without any particular distinct features (e-**Fig. 16.19**) (*Cytopathol* 2016;6:398).

II. EXTRAHEPATIC BILIARY TREE.
A variety of inflammatory and neoplastic conditions occur in the extrahepatic biliary tree, all of which typically present as strictures with or without an associated mass. Cytopathology can be a valuable method of diagnosis because ERCP provides access to areas involved by a mass or stricture for sampling by brushing (*Cytopathol* 2004;15:74). The specificity of brushing is high, however the sensitivity is more variable (*Arch Pathol Lab Med* 2000;124:387). Ultrasound, computed tomography (CT), and endoscopic ultrasonography (EUS) are all used to guide fine-needle aspiration (FNA) (*Acta Cytol* 2008;52:24).

A. Inflammatory. A variety of inflammatory processes can lead to reactive and inflammatory damage, some of which (primary biliary sclerosis, PSC) have an underlying associated risk for malignancy. Cytopathology has been shown to be helpful for clarifying the nature of an associated stricture or abnormality (*Cancer* 2006;108:231).

1. Reactive. Lithiasis is a common occurrence in the biliary tract and can lead to localized inflammation and/or stricture formation. Bile duct brushing of a benign/inflammatory stricture shows flat sheets of ductal epithelium with minimal crowding and overlap. The nuclei are round to oval with fine chromatin, nucleoli, and minimal pleomorphism (e-**Fig. 16.20**). The background can show granular debris of a postobstructive process. Single atypical cells are not seen. It is important to know whether a stent is in place since stents can cause significant reactive atypia, which can be confused with neoplasia.

2. PSC. Patients with PSC can have multiple strictures throughout the biliary tree that are sampled and followed by bile duct brushing (*Clin Liver Dis* 2010;14:349). When the strictures are inflammatory in nature, they typically show a florid repair appearance consisting of nuclear enlargement, prominent nucleoli, and cellular crowding and overlap with some loss of polarity. Intraepithelial neutrophils can be present (e-**Figs. 16.21** and **16.22**). A spectrum of reactive atypia is present without a distinct second population. Overall, the findings do not meet the criteria required for the diagnosis of carcinoma as detailed later. However, the epithelial atypia present cannot always be clearly categorized, and false-positive diagnoses may occur (*Diagn*

Cytopathol 2005;32:119). In these instances a descriptive diagnosis of epithelial atypia can be appropriate.

B. Neoplastic

  1. Cholangiocarcinoma is most commonly encountered in bile duct brushings, but the advent of EUS FNA is providing more access and better sampling of this neoplasm in the biliary tree. Nonetheless, the lesion's underlying sclerotic nature can present a challenge in obtaining sufficient diagnostic cellular elements (*J Clin Oncol* 2005;23:4561). By means of bile duct brushing, ductal carcinoma can show a number of malignant characteristics, including hypo- or hyperchromasia, nuclear membrane irregularity, nuclear pleomorphism, presence of two-cell population, three-dimensional architecture, high nuclear–cytoplasmic ratio (>50%), nuclear molding, cellular discohesion, and prominent nucleoli (e-**Figs. 16.23** and **16.24**) (*Mod Pathol* 2017;30:273). The application of UroVysion fluorescence in situ hybridization (FISH) (Abbott Laboratories, Abbott Park, IL) to bile duct brushing specimens can assist in the diagnosis (e-**Fig. 16.25**) (*Diagn Cytopathol* 2014;42:351). The aspirate smears obtained by FNA can be variably cellular and show small to intermediate groups arranged as syncytial fragments and flat sheets. The cells show anisonucleosis, and the nuclei possess nuclear membrane irregularities, coarse chromatin, and nucleoli.

ACKNOWLEDGMENT

The authors thank Elizabeth Brunt, Brian Collins, and Julie Kunkel, authors of the previous edition of this chapter.

17 The Pancreas

Deyali Chatterjee and Dengfeng Cao

I. **NORMAL ANATOMY.** The pancreas is located in the retroperitoneum. In adults, the pancreas measures 15 to 20 cm in length and weighs 85 to 120 g. The pancreas is divided into four parts: the head (including the uncinate process), neck, body, and tail. The vascular supply to the pancreas is from branches of the celiac trunk and superior mesenteric arteries. The lymph nodes draining the pancreas consist of two major systems: those ringing the pancreas, and those near the aorta from the level of celiac trunk to the origin of the superior mesenteric artery. Microscopically, the pancreas consists of lobules that include both exocrine and endocrine components.

The vast majority of the exocrine component is the acinar epithelium. The acinar cells are large and polarized, with basally situated nuclei; the apical cytoplasm is eosinophilic due to the presence of abundant zymogen granules, whereas the basal portion is basophilic and contains abundant rough endoplasmic reticulum. The second component of the exocrine pancreas is the duct system that begins with the centroacinar cells. The secretions of the centroacinar cells drain into intercalated ducts, intralobular ducts, interlobular ducts, and then into the main pancreatic duct of Wirsung and the accessory duct of Santorini. The duct system is lined by cuboidal to low columnar cells with no visible cytoplasmic mucin by hematoxylin and eosin (H&E) staining.

The endocrine component, constituting 1% to 2% of the pancreas in adults, is composed of islets of Langerhans and neuroendocrine cells scattered among the acini. The islets of Langerhans contain four major cell types: insulin-secreting β cells (60% to 70%), glucagon-secreting α cells (15% to 20%), somatostatin-secreting δ cells, and pancreatic polypeptide-secreting PP cells.

II. **GROSS EXAMINATION AND TISSUE HANDLING**

A. **Biopsy, Fine Needle Aspiration (FNA), and Brushing Cytology** specimens may be obtained percutaneously, intraoperatively, or via endoscopic procedure such as endoscopic ultrasound (EUS) or endoscopic retrograde cholangiopancreatography (ERCP). Needle core biopsies should be immediately fixed in 10% formalin. The number and the length, or length range, of the biopsies should be recorded. Documentation of the number and length is important to ensure that the biopsies are adequately represented on the slides. Three H&E-stained slides from each block are prepared for microscopic examination. Aspiration smears are processed with alcohol fixation for Papanicolaou staining or air dried for Diff-Quik staining. Brushings are handled by routine liquid-based cytology methods.

B. **Distal Pancreatectomy** specimens consist of the pancreatic tail (usually with attached spleen) and a portion of the pancreatic body. After orientation, each organ should be measured separately. An externally visible mass or lesion should be documented for its size, extent, and location. The proximal and the peripancreatic surface margin should be inked. Before sectioning through the pancreas, the proximal margin is typically taken either as a shave margin or as a series of perpendicular sections, depending on the location of the tumor. The method of sectioning the pancreas depends on personal preference, but the goal is to be able to map the tumor/lesion accurately. One method is to bivalve the pancreas using a probe in the main duct as the guide; another method is to section the pancreas in a breadloaf fashion from proximal to distal. The size and characteristics of any lesions (masses or cysts), along with their relationship to the main duct, spleen, and peripancreatic soft tissue resection margins should be documented. If the lesion is cystic, the cyst contents and the relationship of the cyst to the main duct should be also documented.

If the pancreatic lesion is small, it should be submitted in its entirety. For large lesions (e.g., >5 cm), at least one section per centimeter is recommended. If the lesion is cystic, and no definite solid area indicative of invasive carcinoma is grossly identified, the cyst with the surrounding tissue, extending to the inked posterior surface, needs to be submitted entirely for microscopic examination. One to two representative sections from the spleen are sufficient unless gross abnormalities are detected. Finally, the peripancreatic and splenic hilar soft tissue is searched for lymph nodes; all identified lymph nodes should be submitted in their entirety for microscopic examination.

C. The Whipple Procedure, performed for tumors of the pancreatic head, common bile duct, ampullary, or periampullary region involves excision of a composite specimen usually consisting of the pancreatic head, a portion of the common bile duct, the duodenum, the distal stomach, and the gallbladder. After orientation, the dimension of each organ should be measured. The various surgical margins and surfaces of the pancreas (pancreatic neck, posterior, portal vein groove, and uncinate) should be inked with different colors (preferably in the operating room with the surgeon's aid; frozen section evaluation of the pancreatic neck and bile duct margins is almost always requested intraoperatively at some institutions, and shave sections of these margins are typically taken. The stomach is opened along the greater curvature and the duodenum is opened along the aspect opposite the pancreas to avoid the ampulla. The pancreas can be sectioned based on personal preference, but again, the goal is to be able to map the tumor/lesion accurately. One method is to cut serially along the axial plane; another common method is to bisect the pancreatic head along the plane defined by the pancreatic duct and bile duct using probes as guides. The size, location, and nature of the tumor are recorded, as is the relationship of the tumor to the margins. If the tumor is cystic, its relationship to the main duct is documented. It there is no definite solid area surrounding the cyst, the entire lesion, in relation to the inked surfaces and margins, needs to be sampled entirely for microscopic examination. In general, one section per centimeter of solid tumors is submitted; additional sections should demonstrate uninvolved pancreas and ampulla if they are not already demonstrated in the sampled sections with the tumor. One section from the proximal gastric resection margin, and one from the distal duodenal resection margin should also be submitted. One section from the uninvolved pancreas and one from the uninvolved ampulla are also submitted if not sampled in the tumor sections. All identified lymph nodes in the soft tissue should be submitted for microscopic examination; there is no need to separate the nodes into groups because they are all considered regional. Microscopic examination of a minimum of 12 to 15 nodes has been recommended for Whipple specimens.

III. DIAGNOSTIC FEATURES OF PANCREATITIS

A. Acute Pancreatitis is an inflammatory process in which pancreatic enzymes autodigest the gland. It is most commonly associated with biliary tract disease (such as gallstones) and alcohol abuse. Other associated factors include smoking, drugs, type 2 diabetes, and surgical procedures. The pancreas is swollen and edematous, and hemorrhagic in more severe cases. Chalky white fat necrosis may be evident. Histologically, mild pancreatitis is characterized by interstitial edema and leukocytic infiltration; the pancreatic parenchyma may be well preserved, with only limited necrosis. In severe cases, extensive necrosis and hemorrhage are seen (e-Fig. 17.1). Calcification and secondary infection may occur.

B. Chronic Pancreatitis is an inflammatory process characterized by irreversible destruction of the exocrine components with acinar atrophy, mixed inflammatory cell infiltrates, and fibrosis with relative sparing of the islets of Langerhans (e-Fig. 17.2). Dilatation of the pancreatic ducts with proteinaceous often calcified secretions is characteristic. In later stages, the endocrine component may also be destroyed.

1. **Etiology.** Most cases are associated with chronic alcohol abuse (80%). Other etiologies include bile duct and pancreatic duct obstruction (due to lithiasis),

hyperlipidemia, hyperparathyroidism, autoimmune disorders, and hereditary chronic pancreatitis (due to germline mutations in cationic trypsinogen [*PRSS1*], cystic fibrosis transmembrane conductance regulator [*CFTR*], chymotrypsin C, calcium-sensing receptor, and anionic trypsin [*PRSS2*]) *(Dig Dis* 2010;28:324).

2. **Alcoholic pancreatitis** has as major histologic features including acinar atrophy, fibrosis (initially interlobular, typically uneven), and chronic inflammation. Islets are typically decreased but sometimes they show marked proliferation.

3. **Autoimmune pancreatitis** (AIP) is a distinct type of chronic pancreatitis frequently associated with systemic autoimmune diseases, including inflammatory bowel disease and primary sclerosing cholangitis. AIP may mimic pancreatic cancer radiographically and endoscopically when it presents as a mass lesion in the pancreatic head and/ or with strictures of the pancreatic and common bile ducts. Histologically, AIP shares many features of conventional chronic pancreatitis, but is distinguished by a dense lymphoplasmacytic infiltrate, particularly in the periductal region (e-**Fig. 17.3**), and obliterative phlebitis (e-**Fig. 17.4**). In addition to various autoantibodies, selective elevation of the serum immunoglobulin G4 (IgG4) level helps establish the diagnosis *(Arch Pathol Lab Med* 2005;129:1148; *J Gastroenterol* 2006;41:613). The number of IgG4 plasma cells in the pancreas is typically >10 per high-power field, and >50 per high-power field is highly specific for the diagnosis *(Adv Anat Pathol* 2010;17:303). Patients often respond well to steroid therapy.

A recent study has suggested that AIP can be further divided into type 1 and type 2 diseases *(Am J Surg Pathol* 2011;35:26). Clinically, type 1 disease occurs in older patients with male predominancy. Type 1 AIP is the pancreatic manifestation of IgG4-related systemic disease whereas type 2 is confined to the pancreas; the serum IgG4 level is higher in patients with type 1 disease than in patients with type 2 disease. Pathologically, type 1 and type 2 AIPs share periductal inflammation; however, interlobular inflammation and fibrosis is unique to type 1, and obliterative phlebitis is much more common in type 1 than type 2. The number of IgG4-positive plasma cells in the pancreas is much higher in type 1 disease than type 2 disease. On the other hand, ductular/lobular abscesses and ductal ulceration are much more common in type 2 than type 1 AIP. Type 1 AIP is also known as lymphoplasmacytic sclerosing pancreatitis.

4. **Paraduodenal pancreatitis** is also known as para-ampullary duodenal wall cyst, groove pancreatitis, or cystic dystrophy of the duodenal wall. It most likely arises from the submucosal pancreatic tissue associated with remnants of the minor papilla, and is caused by obstruction of the minor papilla. Three distinct subtypes have been proposed by imaging: solid tumoral, cyst forming, and ill defined *(Am J Surg Pathol* 2017;41:1437). Microscopically the fibroinflammatory process is centered in the groove forming a mass-like lesion. The adjacent duodenal wall typically shows muscularis propria. Within the fibroinflammatory process, there are often dilated ductal structures, and sometimes also an acinar component and islets. The lining of the ducts is often partially denuded and may contain mucinous epithelium and reactive changes (e-**Fig. 17.5**). The cyst wall is composed of inflamed fibrous tissue containing lymphocytes, plasma cells, and neutrophils, and the adjacent pancreatic tissue often shows signs of obstruction including enzymatic concretions and ductal ruptures with associated inflammatory response and multinucleated giant cell reaction.

IV. **CYSTIC LESIONS AND TUMORS OF THE PANCREAS.** Cystic lesions of the pancreas include nonneoplastic and neoplastic types. The former mainly includes pseudocyst, lymphoepithelial cyst, ductal retention cyst, mucinous nonneoplastic cyst, and para-ampullary duodenal wall cyst (paraduodenal pancreatitis). Neoplastic cystic lesions include serous cystic neoplasm, mucinous cystic neoplasm, intraductal papillary mucinous neoplasm (IPMN), intraductal tubulopapillary neoplasm (ITPN), solid pseudopapillary neoplasm, and cystic acinar neoplasm. Pancreatic neuroendocrine tumors (islet cell tumors) can also be cystic. Table 17.1 lists the most recent 2010 WHO classification of tumors of the pancreas.

TABLE 17.1 WHO Histologic Classification of Tumors of the Pancreas

Epithelial tumors

Benign

Acinar cell cystadenoma

Serous cystadenoma

Premalignant lesions

    Pancreatic intraepithelial neoplasia, grade 3 (PanIN-3)

    Intraductal papillary mucinous neoplasm

    Intraductal tubulopapillary neoplasm

    Mucinous cystic neoplasm

Malignant

Ductal adenocarcinoma

Adenosquamous carcinoma

Colloid carcinoma (mucinous noncystic carcinoma)

Hepatoid carcinoma

Medullary carcinoma

Signet-ring cell carcinoma

Undifferentiated carcinoma

Undifferentiated carcinoma with osteoclast-like giant cells

Acinar cell carcinoma

Acinar cell cystadenocarcinoma

Intraductal papillary mucinous neoplasm with an associated invasive carcinoma

Mucinous cystic neoplasm with an invasive carcinoma

Mixed acinar–ductal carcinoma

Mixed acinar–neuroendocrine carcinoma

Mixed acinar–neuroendocrine-ductal carcinoma

Mixed ductal-neuroendocrine carcinoma

Pancreatoblastoma

Serous cystadenocarcinoma

Solid pseudopapillary neoplasm

Neuroendocrine neoplasms

Pancreatic neuroendocrine microadenoma

Neuroendocrine tumors, nonfunctional (grade 1, grade 2)

Neuroendocrine carcinoma (large cell, small cell)

EC cell, serotonin-producing neuroendocrine tumors

Gastrinoma

Glucagonoma

Insulinoma

Somatostatinoma

VIPoma

Mature teratoma

Mesenchymal tumors

Lymphomas

Secondary tumors

From Bosman FT, Carneiro F, eds. *WHO Classification of Tumours of the Digestive System* Lyon, France: IARC Press; 2017. Used with permission.

A. Nonneoplastic Cystic Lesions

1. **Pseudocyst** is the most common cystic lesion of the pancreas and usually develops as a result of pancreatitis or trauma. About two-thirds of pseudocysts are located in the tail. The cyst is lined by granulation or fibrous tissue without an epithelial lining, with a wall thickness ranging from several millimeters to several centimeters (e-**Fig. 17.6**). The cyst content has a high level of amylase.

2. **Lymphoepithelial cyst** is usually lined by the squamous epithelium, typically keratinized, with abundant underlying lymphocytes that occasionally form germinal centers (e-**Fig. 17.7**). The lining epithelium may be of other types such as flat, cuboidal, or transitional. Rarely sebaceous and mucinous cells may be also seen in the wall, but skin adnexal structures are not found.

3. **Ductal retention cyst** (also named simple cyst) is caused by obstruction. Microscopically it is a unilocular cyst lined by a layer of simple epithelium. When the lining epithelium becomes mucinous, it is termed a mucinous nonneoplastic cyst (mucinous simple cyst).

B. Neoplastic Cystic Lesions

1. **Serous cystadenoma** is a benign cystic neoplasm usually found in the body or tail of the pancreas in elderly patients. The vast majority are sporadic but the lesion can be associated with the von Hippel–Lindau syndrome. It is usually multilocular (microcystic cystadenoma), but occasionally unilocular, oligocystic (macrocystic), or even solid. Grossly, the tumor has a spongy appearance with a stellate central scar (e-**Fig. 17.8**) with cysts that are filled with clear serous fluid. Microscopically, the individual cysts are lined by a single layer of flat to cuboidal epithelial cells with pale to clear glycogen-rich cytoplasm (e-**Fig. 17.9**). Focally papillary structures lined with clear cells may be seen. The stroma is typically hyalinized but it may contain calcification, hemosiderin, and cholesterol clefts. The periphery of the tumor may seem infiltrative, extending into the adjacent pancreatic parenchyma. Immunohistochemically, the lining cells are positive for cytokeratin and in most cases are also positive for alpha-inhibin, HIF-alpha, and MUC6 (*Am J Surg Pathol* 2004;28:339; *Semin Diagn Pathol* 2014;31:475) (e-**Fig. 17.10**). The solid variant can mimic metastatic clear cell renal cell carcinoma. Rarely carcinoma may arise from serous cystadenoma (*Am J Surg Pathol* 2012;36:305).

   Serous cystadenocarcinoma is exceedingly rare in the pancreas and is morphologically indistinguishable from serous cystadenoma. The diagnosis is established by the presence of distal metastasis, but vascular invasion and invasion into adjacent structures have been used for diagnosing serous cystadenocarcinoma. The existence of this entity is controversial, because some reported metastatic serous cystadenomas may represent separate primary serous cystadenomas in a different organ.

2. **Mucinous cystic neoplasm** (MCN) tends to occur in the tail or body of the pancreas, predominantly in women about 50 years of age with a female:male ratio of 20:1. The neoplasm is a solitary, multilocular (rarely unilocular) cystic mass filled with mucin (e-**Fig. 17.11**) or mucin admixed with necrotic material. The cysts typically do not communicate with the ductal system but it rarely does so (*Anticancer Res* 2017;37:7017). The cyst lining, which may be partially denuded, consists of tall columnar mucin-producing cells with characteristic underlying ovarian-type stroma (e-**Fig. 17.12**). The ovarian-type stroma surrounding the cysts is the defining feature of MCN and is useful for distinguishing MCN from IPMN. The stromal cells are frequently positive for estrogen receptor, progesterone receptor, and inhibin, and can be luteinized.

   Based on the cytologic and architectural features of the lining epithelium, atypical noninvasive MCN can be divided into two categories: low-grade MCN (with mild and moderate dysplasia) (e-**Fig. 17.13**) and high-grade MCN (with high-grade/severe dysplasia) (*Am J Surg Pathol* 2015;39:3730) (e-**Fig. 17.14**). High-grade/severe dysplasia is characterized by papillary, cribriform, branching, and budding growth patterns; marked nuclear stratification and atypia; mucin depletion; and frequent mitosis (e-**Fig. 17.15**). Up to one-third of MCNs have an associated invasive carcinoma that commonly is of the ductal type and forms tubules and duct-like structures (e-**Fig. 17.16**). Other rare types of invasive carcinoma arising in association with MCN have also been reported including adenosquamous carcinoma, undifferentiated carcinoma, and undifferentiated carcinoma with osteoclast-like giant cells. The prognosis for noninvasive MCN is excellent and surgical resection is curative for almost all patients. The prognosis for those lesions with an invasive component is determined by the extent of invasive carcinoma, stage, and resectability (*Am J Surg Pathol* 1999;23:410). Limited data show that T1a-1b invasive adenocarcinomas demonstrate similar prognosis as MCNs without invasive adenocarcinoma (*Am J Surg Pathol* 2018;42:578). Genetically, MCN is characterized by *KRAS* mutation (the mutation rate increases with increasing cytologic atypia) but no mutation in *GNAS*, *RAF43*, or *PIK3CA* (*Histopathology* 2017;71:591).

The differential diagnosis of mucinous cystic neoplasm mainly includes IPMN. There is ovarian-type stroma in the former but not in the latter (Table 17.2).

3. **Intraductal papillary mucinous neoplasm (IPMN)** is defined as a grossly visible (≥1 cm) epithelial tumor arising in the main pancreatic duct (main-duct-type IPMN) or its branches (branch-duct-type IPMN). IPMN is typically seen in the head of the pancreas but it may diffusely involve the whole organ. Branch-duct-type IPMN tends to involve the uncinate process. Symptomatic patients often have a main-duct-type IPMN whereas most of the branch-duct-type IPMNs are detected incidentally. Histologically, the neoplastic epithelium typically forms papillary fronds lined by mucin-producing columnar cells (e-**Fig. 17.17**). Based on the degree of architectural and cytologic atypia, IPMN can be divided into three categories: low-grade IPMN (with mild to moderate dysplasia, 47%), high-grade IPMN (high-grade dysplasia, 23%), and IPMN with an associated invasive carcinoma (30%) (*Am J Surg Pathol* 2015;39:3730; *HPB (Oxford)* 2016;18:236). Four types of mucinous epithelium can be seen: gastric type, intestinal type, pancreatobiliary, and oncocytic (also known as intraductal oncocytic papillary neoplasm) (e-**Fig. 17.18**); however, recent molecular data have suggested that oncocytic IMPN should be in its own category given its distinct molecular features (see below) (*Virchows Arch* 2016;469:523; *Mod Pathol* 2016;29:1058). These four types of epithelium show distinct mucin profiles by immunohistochemical staining (gastric type MUC1+ variable/MUC2−/MUC6+ variable; intestinal type MUC1−/MUC2+/MUC6−; pancreatobiliary MUC1+/MUC2−/MUC6+ weak; oncocytic type MUC1− variable/MUC2−/MUC6+) (*Am J Surg Pathol* 2010;34:364).

The major determining prognostic factor for surgically resected IPMNs is whether there is an associated invasive carcinoma, which as noted above is seen in approximately one-third of cases, since IPMNs without an associated invasive carcinoma are often cured by surgery.

Two types of invasive carcinomas are seen: colloid (25%, e-**Fig. 17.19**) and conventional ductal (75%, e-**Fig. 17.20**); the former typically arises in association with intestinal-type IPMNs whereas the latter is associated with pancreatobiliary-type or intestinal-type IPMNs. Colloid carcinomas are associated with lower incidence of regional lymph node metastasis, microvascular invasion, and perineural invasion

TABLE 17.2	Distinction Between Intraductal Papillary Mucinous Neoplasm (IPMN) and Mucinous Cystic Neoplasm (MCN)
IPMN	**MCN**
Older women and men	Predominantly middle-aged women
Head	Tail or body
Yes	No
No	Yes

compared with tubular carcinomas (*HPB (Oxford)* 2016;18:236). Rarely, oncocytic carcinoma may arise from oncocytic IPMN. It must be pointed out that the invasive carcinoma may be focal, and therefore IPMNs should be extensively (or, ideally, completely) submitted for histologic examination. Patients with an invasive carcinoma arising in association with an IPMN, except those with an advanced-stage invasive carcinoma, usually do better than those with a ductal carcinoma not associated with IPMN. In addition, patients with an invasive colloid carcinoma arising in association with an IPMN have a better prognosis than those with an invasive conventional ductal carcinoma arising in association with an IPMN (*Ann Surg* 2001;234:313; *Ann Surg* 2004;239:400; *HPB (Oxford)* 2016;18:236).

Recent studies have revealed the molecular profiles of IMPNs. *KRAS* and *GNAS* are mutated in 50% to 60% IMPNs, mainly in the gastric, pancreatobiliary, and intestinal subtypes whereas in the oncocytic subtype these two genes are only rarely mutated (*Pancreas* 2015;44:227; *Spingerplus* 2016;5:1172; *Mod Pathol* 2016;29:1058). Oncocytic IPMNs also show different immunohistochemical profiles from other three subtypes (*Virchow Arch* 2016;469:523). These findings suggest that oncocytic IPMN should be a separate category from the other three subtypes of IPMNs.

4. **Intraductal tubulopapillary neoplasm** (ITPN) is a grossly visible solid nodular tumor obstructing the duct system (*Am J Surg Pathol* 2009;33:1164; *Am J Surg Pathol* 2017;41:313). Approximately half of these tumors involve the pancreatic head, and one-quarter diffusely involve the pancreas (*Am J Surg Pathol* 2017;41:313). Microscopically, the tumor is characterized by intraductal closely packed tubular glands (e-**Fig. 17.21**) and cribriform glands, but papillary structures are also seen in 30% to 40% cases. The cuboidal cells uniformly show moderate- to high-grade nuclear features and have a mild to moderate amount of eosinophilic to amphophilic cytoplasm. More than 50% tumors have an associated invasive carcinoma. ITPNs do not harbor *KRAS* or *BRAF* mutations; in contrast, they harbor mutations in chromatin remodeling genes (32%), or the PIK3CA pathway (27%) (*Mod Pathol* 2017;30:1760). Approximately 20% tumors harbor *FGFR2*-fusions.

5. **Intraductal tubular adenoma, pyloric gland type,** is an uncommon tumor consisting of pyloric-type glandular structures with mild to moderate atypia (*Am J Surg Pathol* 2005;29:607) (e-**Fig. 17.22**). Intraductal tubular carcinoma is characterized by high-grade cytology and can have an associated invasive carcinoma component (*Anticancer Research* 2010;30:4435). Some authors consider intraductal tubular carcinoma as part of the spectrum of ITPN (*Am J Surg Pathol* 2009;33:1164).

6. **Cystic acinar cell cystadenoma** is an extremely rare unilocular or multilocular cystic mass lined by a single layer of cells cytologically resembling acinar cells (*Am J Surg Pathol* 2002;26:698; *Am J Surg Pathol* 2012;36:1579; *Am J Surg Pathol* 2013:37:329). In **acinar cell cystadenocarcinoma**, the cysts are lined by layers of cells that exhibit more cytologic atypia with easily identifiable mitotic figures.

7. **Cystic pancreatic neuroendocrine tumors** are probably more common than previously recognized (8% to 11% pancreatic well-differentiated neuroendocrine tumors are cystic) (*Am J Surg Pathol* 2012;36:1666; *Neuroendocrinology* 2018;106:234). The tumor cells show similar morphologic features as classic well-differentiated neuroendocrine tumors except for cystic structures within the tumor. Prognostically, cystic pancreatic well-differentiated neuroendocrine tumors show similar prognosis as solid-type tumors (*Neuroendocrinology* 2018;106:234).

V. SOLID TUMORS OF THE EXOCRINE PANCREAS

A. **Pancreatic Ductal Adenocarcinoma** (PDAC) accounts for 85% to 90% of pancreatic neoplasms and is most frequently found in the head of the pancreas (60% to 70%), more often in males, and usually in individuals between 60 and 80 years of age. Factors associated with an increased risk include tobacco smoking, dietary factors such as high-fat diet and low intake of fruits and vegetables, chronic pancreatitis, gastrectomy, and diabetes. The highest rates of PDAC are noted among African Americans. In about 10% of cases, there is a positive family history, but in the majority of cases a genetic basis has not been identified. A minority of cases arise in recognized genetic syndromes, which include familial atypical multiple mole melanoma syndrome (FAMMM), Peutz–Jeghers syndrome, Lynch syndrome, hereditary pancreatitis, mutations in *BRCA2,* and mutations in Fanconi anemia complementation genes.

Grossly, PDAC is usually poorly demarcated, firm, and yellowish-grey or white due to its infiltrative growth and associated strong desmoplastic response. Histologic grading is based on the percentage of glandular differentiation, with well-differentiated tumors showing greater than 95% gland formation, moderately differentiated tumors having 50% to 95% glands, and poorly differentiated tumors having 49% or less glands. The Klöppel grading scheme uses a combination of glandular differentiation, mucin production, mitoses, and nuclear pleomorphism, but shows no difference in the predictive value in comparison to glandular differentiation alone. Most tumors are well to moderately differentiated and characterized by glandular structures haphazardly distributed in a desmoplastic stroma (e-Fig. 17.23). In well-differentiated tumors, the neoplastic glands are well formed and usually large or medium sized; however, the neoplastic glands may show rupture or be incomplete, features that are not observed in normal ducts. Mucin production may be evident. The most important histologic features that can be used to distinguish well-differentiated adenocarcinoma from chronic pancreatitis are a haphazard growth pattern (Table 17.3), perineural invasion (e-Fig. 17.24), vascular invasion, and close approximation to muscular vasculature (e-Fig. 17.25). In moderately differentiated adenocarcinoma, there is a mixture of medium-sized duct-like structures and small tubular glands of variable size and shape, including some incompletely formed glands. Cribriform and papillary growth patterns are not uncommon (e-Fig. 17.26); mitotic activity is brisker (typically 6 to 10 per 10 HPFs), and nuclear pleomorphism is more prominent with nuclear sizes varying by more than a factor of 4 in the same gland. Mucin production is usually decreased and irregular in distribution. In poorly differentiated adenocarcinoma, the tumor cells form solid sheets or nests, or infiltrate as single individual cells. Mucin production is abortive. Neoplastic glands, if present, are typically small and irregular, and the tumor cells exhibit marked nuclear pleomorphism and a high mitotic count (often >10 per 10 HPFs). One major differential diagnosis for PDACs is chronic pancreatitis which can clinically, radiographically, and grossly mimic PDCAs; Table 17.3 lists the histologic features that can be used to distinguish PDCA from chronic pancreatitis.

Morphologic variations of PDAC, in addition to the conventional tubular pattern, include the foamy gland pattern (with abundant foamy/microvesicular pale cytoplasm, resembling PanIN-1); large duct pattern (imparting a microcystic/macrocystic appearance); vacuolated pattern (focally, tumor cells have the morphology of adipocytes or signet-ring cells); lobular carcinoma–like pattern (with cords and single-file arrangement); solid nested pattern (mimicking neuroendocrine neoplasm or squamous cell carcinoma); and micropapillary pattern.

Immunohistochemically, PDACs are typically positive for pan-CK, CK7, CK8, CK18, CK19, MUC1, MUC3, MUC4, MUC5AC, CEA, CA125, and CA19.9. CK20 is typically negative or only focally positive. Other markers that are expressed in PDACs

TABLE 17.3	Distinction Between Ductal Adenocarcinoma and Chronic Pancreatitis	
Features	**Ductal Adenocarcinoma**	**Chronic Pancreatitis**
Histologic pattern	Haphazard	Lobular
Ruptured or incomplete glands	Yes	No
Companion muscular vessel	Yes	No
Nuclear pleomorphism	>4:1 in the same glands	Insignificant
Perineural invasion	Yes	No
Angioinvasion	Yes	No
Mitosis	Frequent	Infrequent

include claudin-4, cyclooxygenase (COX)-2, mesothelin, KOC (K homology domain containing protein overexpressed in cancer), S100P, and maspin. These markers may be useful in distinguishing ductal from nonductal pancreatic neoplasms and from benign pancreatic ducts, but are less useful in distinguishing adenocarcinomas of nonpancreatic origin. CDX2 is expressed in benign pancreatic ductal epithelium, and is expressed in approximately a third of PDACs (*PLoS One* 2014;29;9). Approximately 55% of PDACs harbor mutations in *DPC4*, but this is not specific, as loss of DPC4 expression is also observed in cholangiocarcinoma (*Hum Pathol* 2002;33:877) and colonic adenocarcinoma (*Mutat Res* 1999;406:71).

Genetic alterations in pancreatic cancer include losses and gains of large chromosomal regions (such as very high rates of loss at chromosomes 18q, 17p, 1p, and 9p), as well as generalized chromosome instability (an average of five dozen intragenic mutations, although most are believed to be passenger mutations since the genes mutated are individually infrequently involved). Common recurrent genetic alterations include the tumor suppressor genes *CDKN2A*, *TP53*, and *SMAD4/DPC4*, and activation of *KRAS* and *ERBB2/HER2* oncogenes. Microsatellite instability has been identified in 4% PDAC; these tumors are also characterized by wild-type *KRAS*, frequent *BRAF* gene mutations, and the so-called medullary-type histology (see below).

The staging scheme for exocrine cancers of the pancreas (Amin MB, Edge S, Greene F, et al., eds. *AJCC Cancer Staging Manual*, 8th ed. New York: Springer, 2017) is different from that for well-differentiated neuroendocrine tumors arising in the pancreas (see below). Reporting of exocrine tumors should follow suggested guidelines (e.g., see the College of American Pathologists Protocol for the Examination of Specimens From Patients With Carcinoma of the Pancreas, at http://www.cap.org).

Overall, PDAC is associated with a dismal prognosis, and the overall 5-year survival is only 3% to 5%. Resectability is the most important determinant of prognosis; the 5-year survival in patients treated with curative resection is 15% to 25%, but only 10% to 20% of tumors are resectable at the time of diagnosis.

B. Variants of Ductal Adenocarcinoma

1. **Squamous cell carcinoma and adenosquamous carcinoma** constitute approximately 2% of all pancreatic cancers, and may portend a poorer prognosis as compared with conventional PDAC. Adenosquamous carcinoma shows both ductal/glandular and squamous differentiation (e-**Fig. 17.27**). Diagnosis of adenosquamous carcinoma requires at least 30% of the squamous component.

2. **Colloid carcinoma** (mucinous noncystic adenocarcinoma) is mostly associated with IPMN or mucinous cystic neoplasm. Colloid carcinoma is believed to have a better prognosis than conventional ductal adenocarcinoma. Histologically, the tumor is defined by extracellular mucin pools containing suspended neoplastic cells, comprising at least 80% of the tumor.

3. **Hepatoid carcinoma** is an extremely rare tumor in the pancreas. It can occur in a pure form or be associated with ductal adenocarcinoma (*Am Surg* 2004;70:1030; *Int J Surg Pathol* 2018;doi: 10.1177/1066896918783468 [Epub ahead of print]), acinar cell carcinoma, or a neuroendocrine tumor (*Cancer* 2000;88:1582; *Am J Surg Pathol* 2007 31:146; *Gut Liver* 2010;4:98). Morphologically, hepatoid carcinoma consists of large polygonal cells with abundant cytoplasm. Histologically, pancreatic hepatoid carcinomas can be divided into four histologic subtypes: hepatocellular carcinoma like (e-**Fig. 17.28**), with neuroendocrine differentiation (e-**Fig 17.29**), with glandular differentiation (e-**Fig 17.30**), and with acinar differentiation (*Int J Surg Pathol* 2018; doi: 10.1177/1066896918783468 [Epub ahead of print]). Immunohistochemically, the tumor cells are variably positive for hepatocyte-specific antigen (Hep Par1), AFP, glypican-3, arginase, and SALL4. Among them, Hep Par1 is the most sensitive marker. CD10 and pCEA highlight a canalicular pattern, and most cases are also positive for alpha fetoprotein. Prognostically, pancreatic hepatoid carcinomas with pure HCC-like morphology show a better prognosis than other subtypes. Hepatoid carcinoma should be distinguished from metastatic hepatocellular carcinoma.

4. **Medullary carcinoma** is characterized by its distinct morphology that features poor differentiation with limited gland formation, a syncytial growth pattern, and a pushing border (*Am J Pathol* 1998;152:1501). Some cases are also associated with a prominent infiltration by CD3+ T-lymphocytes. Medullary carcinoma arises sporadically or in association with the Lynch syndrome. Immunohistochemically, medullary carcinoma often shows loss of at least one DNA mismatch repair protein (*Hum Pathol* 2006;37:1498). Prognostically, patients with medullary carcinoma do better than those with PDAC.

5. **Signet-ring cell carcinoma** is an extremely rare variant with an extremely poor prognosis. Metastasis from another primary such as gastrointestinal tract should always be excluded.

6. **Undifferentiated/anaplastic carcinoma** histologically exhibits little epithelial differentiation although some or most of the tumor cells express cytokeratin by immunohistochemistry. Morphologically, three variants have been described: anaplastic giant cell carcinoma (e-**Fig. 17.31**), sarcomatoid carcinoma, and carcinosarcoma (e-**Fig. 17.32**). The prognosis for this tumor is extremely poor; the average survival is only 5 months.

7. **Undifferentiated carcinoma with osteoclast-like giant cells** is characterized by the presence of nonneoplastic osteoclast-like giant cells (which are histiocytic in origin) within the tumor (e-**Fig. 17.33**). In most cases there is an associated in situ or invasive adenocarcinoma, or mucinous cystic neoplasm. The prognosis is poor (mean survival is 12 months).

C. **Acinar Cell Carcinoma** accounts for 1% to 2% of adult exocrine pancreatic neoplasms. Most tumors occur in late adulthood but 6% occur in children. Most patients present with nonspecific symptoms but approximately 10% to 15% of the patients develop a paraneoplastic lipase hypersecretion syndrome characterized by subcutaneous fat necrosis, polyarthralgia, and peripheral eosinophilia.

Acinar cell carcinoma frequently presents as a well-circumscribed mass with or without necrosis and cystic degeneration. Microscopically, acinar, nested, and solid patterns are most common, although the tumor may grow in a trabecular or gyriform pattern. Intraductal, papillary, or papillocystic variants have been reported (*Am J Surg Pathol* 2007;31:363). The tumor usually lacks a desmoplastic stroma. The individual tumor cells are monomorphic, typically have basally located nuclei, single prominent nucleoli, and moderate amounts of amphophilic or eosinophilic granular cytoplasm (e-**Fig. 17.34**). Mitotic activity and nuclear pleomorphism are variable. Most acinar cell carcinomas are composed of cells that contain zymogen granules in their cytoplasm which can be demonstrated by PAS stain with diastase or by electron microscopy. The tumor cells also exhibit abundant rough endoplasmic reticulum by electron microscopy.

Immunohistochemically, acinar cell carcinoma cells are reactive with antibodies against trypsin (>95% cases) (e-**Fig. 17.35**), chymotrypsin (>95% cases) (e-**Fig. 17.36**), lipase (approximately 70% of cases), PDX1, and BCL10 (85%) (*Virchows Arch* 2009;454:133; *Am J Surg Pathol* 2012;36:1782). In more than one-third of acinar cell carcinomas, there are scattered tumor cells immunohistochemically positive for chromogranin A or synaptophysin. If more than 30% of the tumor cells show neuroendocrine differentiation by immunostains, the tumor should be designated as a mixed acinar–neuroendocrine carcinoma. Mixed acinar–ductal carcinoma and mixed carcinoma with all three lineages (acinar, ductal, and neuroendocrine) can also occur.

Acinar cell carcinomas are aggressive tumors but their outcome is generally better than stage-matched ductal adenocarcinomas. Staging is the only independent prognostic factor on multivariate analysis (*Am J Surg Pathol* 2012;36:1782).

D. **Pancreatoblastoma** is the most common pancreatic neoplasm of childhood, usually occurring in the first decade of life (mean age: 4 years), although the neoplasm also rarely occurs in adults. Approximately 25% of patients have associated elevated serum alpha-fetoprotein. Pancreatoblastoma is a highly cellular tumor composed of sheets or islands of small monotonous cells divided by cellular stromal bands. The tumor cells predominantly exhibit acinar differentiation and can form small acinar lumina; focal endocrine and ductal differentiation may also be seen. The tumor shares immuno-histochemical and molecular characteristics with acinar cell carcinomas. A histologic hallmark of pancreatoblastoma is the presence of squamoid corpuscles or nests, which are present in virtually every case (e-Fig. 17.37); they serve as a useful feature to distinguish the tumor from other pancreatic neoplasms, particularly acinar cell carcinoma. Squamoid corpuscles consist of an aggregate of plump epithelioid cells, a whorled nest of spindle cells, or a cluster of frankly keratinized squamous cells, and are usually located in the center of the tumor lobules; the cells forming the squamoid corpuscle are usually larger than the surrounding tumor cells. The stroma in pancreatoblastoma may contain heterologous elements such as the bone and cartilage. The stroma in adult patients, however, is often less abundant and less cellular than that in pediatric patients. The prognosis of pancreatoblastoma is better in pediatric patients than that in adults, likely due to an increased frequency of localized and encapsulated tumors in children.

E. **Solid Pseudopapillary Neoplasm** is a tumor of uncertain histogenesis, and is most commonly seen in adolescent girls and young women (mean age 28 years, 90% in women). This tumor can be quite large at the time of diagnosis but is typically well demarcated and may be encapsulated. Grossly, it exhibits variable solid and cystic areas with hemorrhage and necrosis. Microscopically, solid pseudopapillary neoplasm is a cellular tumor consisting of sheets of small relatively uniform tumor cells, sometimes surrounding delicate, often hyalinized fibrovascular cores to form pseudopapillae (e-Fig. 17.38). The tumor cells have eosinophilic or clear vacuolated cytoplasm, indented or grooved nuclei, and inconspicuous nucleoli (e-Fig. 17.39). Intra- and extracellular eosinophilic, diastase-resistant periodic acid–Schiff (PAS)-positive hyaline globules may be evident. Foamy cells, cells with cholesterol crystals, and foreign-body giant cells may be present within the tumor. In necrotic areas, the tumor cells lose their cohesiveness and may undergo cystic degeneration. Mitotic figures are rare.

The most frequently positive immunomarkers in solid pseudopapillary neoplasm are vimentin, neuron-specific enolase (NSE), α1-antitrypsin, α1-antichymotrypsin, progesterone receptor, claudins 5 and 7, galectin 3, cyclin D1, CD56, CD10 (e-Fig. 17.40), nuclear β-catenin (e-Fig. 17.41), and CD99 with a perinuclear dot-like pattern (*Am J Surg Pathol* 2011;35:799). Synaptophysin may be positive in tumor cells but chromogranin A is always negative. Positive CD10 and nuclear β-catenin stains are useful in the distinction from pancreatic endocrine neoplasms. Approximately 50% of solid pseudopapillary neoplasms show c-kit expression by immunohistochemistry without an associated mutation in the *KIT* gene (*Mod Pathol* 2006;19:1157).

Patients with solid pseudopapillary neoplasm usually have an excellent prognosis if the tumor is completely excised, as occurs in 85% to 95% of cases. Approximately 10% to 15% of cases show metastasis, usually to the liver and peritoneum, but metastasis is lethal in only a subset of patients. Rarely, solid pseudopapillary neoplasms have an undifferentiated or sarcomatoid component (*Am J Surg Pathol* 2005;29:512). Biologically aggressive tumors typically show deep extrapancreatic extension, vascular or perineural invasion, significant cellular pleomorphism, nuclear atypia, and increased mitotic activity. In general, solid pseudopapillary neoplasm is considered a low-grade malignancy.

F. **Pancreatic Neuroendocrine Neoplasms** (PanNEN) include well-differentiated neuroendocrine tumors (PanNET, WHO grades 1 to 3, based on the Ki67 index and/or mitotic activity: grade 1 defined as mitotic count ≤2/10 HPFs and Ki67 index <3%; grade 2 as mitotic count 3 to 20/10 HPFs or Ki67 index 3% to 20%; grade 3 as mitotic count >20/10 HPFs or Ki67 index > 20%) and poorly differentiated (WHO grade 3) neuroendocrine carcinomas (PanNEC). PanNECs account for less than 1% of PanNEN, and PanNECs are further divided into small cell carcinoma and large cell neuroendocrine carcinoma. The classification and grading criteria of PanNEN is similar to other gastrointestinal sites (see Chapter 12). Approximately 30% to 40% of PanNETs are nonfunctional (no clinical hormonal syndrome, although serum hormone levels can be elevated). Functional tumors cause clinical symptoms corresponding to the hormones they produce, allowing clinical diagnosis even when the tumor is quite small. Functional tumors are classified based on the clinical syndrome into insulinoma, gastrinoma, glucagonoma, somatostatinoma, VIPoma, or rarely, EC cell type (producing serotonin and causing carcinoid syndrome). Pancreatic neuroendocrine microadenomas (< 0.5 cm in size) are nonfunctional.

PanNETs grow in an organoid fashion including solid, nesting, trabecular, glandular, tubuloacinar, gyriform, and pseudoglandular patterns. Variably hyalinized fibrovascular stroma, sometimes with amyloid deposition, is characteristic (e-Fig. 17.42). The tumor cells are relatively uniform with finely granular amphophilic to eosinophilic cytoplasm and a centrally located round-to-oval nucleus with a characteristic salt-and-pepper chromatin pattern. Other types of cells described include clear cells (e-Fig. 17.43), lipid-rich cells (e-Fig.17.44), oncocytes, and rhabdoid cells (e-Fig. 17.45). Sometimes the tumor cells may be pleomorphic. Necrosis is usually absent. PanNETs are sometimes part of the multiple endocrine neoplasia type I (MEN I) syndrome.

The vast majority of PanNETs are immunohistochemically positive for synaptophysin and chromogranin A. Other markers that are expressed include protein gene product 9.5, CD56, islet-1, and PAX8 (*Am J Surg Pathol* 2010;34:723). PanNECs typically show ill-defined borders; the tumor cells are often arranged in irregular nests or diffuse sheets. There is often extensive necrosis, and the nuclei are high grade with cytologic atypia. Using similar criteria as in the lung, poorly differentiated neuroendocrine carcinomas are further divided into small cell carcinomas and large cell neuroendocrine carcinomas. As noted above, the most recent staging approach to cancers of the pancreas has a separate scheme for neuroendocrine tumors.

VI. PANCREATIC INTRAEPITHELIAL NEOPLASIA (PanIN) is considered a precursor to invasive PDAC. Morphologically, PanIN is a microscopic (typically less than 5 mm in size) papillary or flat epithelial neoplasm confined to the pancreatic duct system. Based on the cytologic and architectural atypia, PanINs are further divided into three categories: PanIN-1 (PanIN-1A, PanIN-1B), PanIN-2, and PanIN-3 (*Am J Surg Pathol* 2004;28:977) (Table 17.4). PanIN1 and PanIN2 are considered low grade and PanIN3 is high grade (*Am J Surg Pathol* 2015;39:1730).

PanIN-1A comprises flat epithelial lesions without atypia. It is composed of tall columnar cells with small and round-to-oval, basal-located nuclei and abundant supranuclear mucin (e-Fig. 17.46). **PanIN-1B** is an intraductal epithelial lesion that has a papillary or micropapillary architecture, but is cytologically identical to PanIN-1A (e-Fig. 17.47).

PanIN-2 may be flat but is usually papillary. By definition, the lesion must have some degree of architectural and cytologic atypia, such as nuclear crowding, enlargement,

TABLE 17.4	Pancreatic Intraepithelial Neoplasia (PanIN) and Corresponding Older Synonyms

Squamous metaplasia: Epidermoid metaplasia, multilayered metaplasia

PanIN-1A (low-grade PanIN): Pyloric gland metaplasia, goblet cell metaplasia, mucinous hypertrophy, mucinous ductal hyperplasia, mucinous cell hyperplasia, mucoid transformation, simple mucinous hyperplasia, flat duct lesion without atypia, flat ductal hyperplasia, ductal hyperplasia grade 1, nonpapillary epithelial hypertrophy, nonpapillary ductal hyperplasia

PanIN-1B (low-grade PanIN): Papillary hyperplasia, papillary ductal hyperplasia, papillary ductal lesion without atypia, ductal hyperplasia grade 2, adenomatous ductal hyperplasia, adenomatoid hyperplasia

PanIN-2 (low-grade PanIN): Atypical hyperplasia, papillary duct lesion with atypia, low-grade dysplasia, any PanIN lesions with moderate dysplasia

PanIN-3 (high-grade PanIN): Carcinoma in situ, intraductal carcinoma, severe ductal dysplasia, high-grade dysplasia, ductal hyperplasia grade 3, atypical hyperplasia.

TABLE 17.5	Distinction Between Pancreatic Intraepithelial Neoplasia (PanIN) and Intraductal Papillary Mucinous Neoplasm (IPMN)	
Features	**PanIN**	**IPMN**
Radiographically detectable	No	Yes
Grossly visible	No	Yes
Grossly visible mucin	No	Yes
Size of involved duct	Usually < 5 mm	Usually > 10 mm
Well-formed papillae	No	Yes
Association with colloid carcinoma	No	Yes

pseudostratification, hyperchromasia, and/or loss of polarity (e-**Fig. 17.48**). Mitotic figures are rare and not atypical. This category represents low-grade dysplasia, and the degree of atypia is insufficient for a diagnosis of PanIN-3.

PanIN-3 is usually papillary or micropapillary, and is only rarely flat. It is a high-grade intraductal lesion and synonymous with carcinoma in situ. True cribriform, budding, or tufting of small clusters of epithelial cells into the lumen, and luminal necrosis should all suggest the diagnosis of PanIN-3. Cytologically, these lesions are characterized by the loss of nuclear polarity, the presence of prominent nucleoli, nuclear membrane irregularities, dystrophic goblet cells, and abnormal mitoses (e-**Fig. 17.49**).

PanIN should not be confused with IPMN, particularly when IPMN extends into small duct branches (Table 17.5). PanIN is a microscopic lesion that is typically <5 mm in size; in contrast, IPMN is a grossly visible lesion usually >10 mm in size (*Am J Surg Pathol* 2004;28:977; *Am J Surg Pathol* 2015;39:1730). The epithelial cells in PanINs have gastric-foveolar differentiation whereas the cells in IMPN have intestinal, gastric-foveolar, pancreatobiliary, and oncocytic differentiation. *GNAS* mutation is seen in 60% IMPNs but is only rarely seen in PanINs (*Am J Surg Pathol* 2015;39:1730). For lesions between 5 and 10 mm in size, it is sometimes difficult to distinguish the entities, but PanINs tend to have short stubby papillary structures whereas the papillae in IPMNs are often long and finger-like (incipient IPMN). The cytoplasmic mucin in IPMNs is typically more abundant than that in PanIN.

On frozen section of pancreatic margins, PanIN-3 lesions should be reported, but the significance of lower-grade PanIN in this context has not been established. However, if the preoperative diagnosis or intraoperative findings suggest IPMN, the presence of PanIN-1 and PanIN-2 lesions should be reported because of the difficulty in differentiating low-grade PanIN from small duct extension by IPMN on frozen sections.

ACKNOWLEDGMENT

The authors thank Hanlin L. Wang, an author of the previous edition of this chapter.

Pancreas Cytopathology

Cory Bernadt

I. **INTRODUCTION.** Cytopathology has an important role in the evaluation of pancreatic lesions. In fact, due to a variety of factors, the cytopathologic sample will frequently be the only diagnostic tissue sample obtained. The advent of EUS-guided FNA has greatly expanded the number and type of cases seen. When an abnormality is identified or suspected, EUS makes it possible to visualize the pancreas by ultrasound, directly visualize the lesion, and then perform an FNA.

By imaging, pancreatic lesions can be broadly categorized into two main categories, solid and cystic. However, heterogeneous lesions with mixed solid-cystic imaging features and other confounding factors that obscure a clear classification also occur. The clinical approach and differential diagnostic considerations vary significantly between these broad categories and thus it is important to ascertain the imaging characteristics of a pancreatic lesion in order to appropriately evaluate and diagnose EUS FNA specimens from the pancreas.

II. SOLID LESIONS
A. Inflammatory
1. **Chronic pancreatitis** can be radiographically indistinguishable from a neoplastic process due to mass-forming fibrosis. This is particularly true for AIP (lymphoplasmacytic sclerosing pancreatitis). Aspirate smears will usually be scant to minimally cellular, show dense fragments of connective tissue with bland spindle cells, and contain fragments of bland ductal and acinar epithelial elements which typically have only minimal reactive cellular changes (e-**Fig. 17.50**). The diagnosis of AIP is difficult by cytology alone, and often leads to an interpretation of "atypical" due to focal-to-marked ductal atypia (*Acta Cytol* 2012;56:228). The presence of underlying chronic pancreatitis does not alter the cytomorphologic findings required for a diagnosis of malignancy (*Diagn Cytopathol* 2005;32:65).

B. Neoplasms
1. **Adenocarcinoma** accounts for the vast majority of pancreatic neoplasms. The majority of patients have disease at clinical presentation that is not resectable and thus EUS FNA provides the definitive diagnosis. The cytopathologic features of adenocarcinoma vary based on the degree of differentiation; individual cases that have a spectrum of differentiation are also encountered.
   a. **Well-differentiated adenocarcinoma** accounts for roughly 20% of aspirates and can be diagnostically challenging. Aspirates show large cohesive fragments with very few background single cells. The main diagnostic features are nuclear enlargement, nuclear membrane irregularities, anisonucleosis (at least 4× size variation), and cellular crowding and overlap (e-**Figs. 17.51–17.53**). However, these features can vary within aspirate smears (*Cancer* 2003;99:44).
   b. **High-grade adenocarcinoma** is less cohesive with numerous single cells and small groups of cells with overlap and crowding. Nuclei are round to oval with evidence of pleomorphism, and have large nucleoli. The cells usually have a moderate amount of granular cytoplasm with only few intracytoplasmic vacuoles (e-**Fig. 17.54**).
   c. **Undifferentiated (anaplastic) carcinoma** is cellular with numerous dispersed single cells that are epithelioid or spindled and show marked pleomorphism, with scattered intermixed bizarre multinucleated giant tumor cells (e-**Fig. 17.55**).
   d. **Undifferentiated carcinoma with osteoclast-like giant cells** shows an undifferentiated pattern with intermixed benign multinucleated giant cells (e-**Fig. 17.56**).
2. **Pancreatic neuroendocrine tumor (PanNET)** presents as a solid mass usually in the body or tail. On aspiration, PanNET is very cellular and characteristically shows a loosely cohesive aspirate with single cells and loose clusters of cells with pseudorosettes (e-**Figs. 17.57** and **17.58**). The individual cells have round to oval nuclei with variable nucleoli, eccentric nuclear placement imparting a plasmacytoid appearance, and neuroendocrine-type chromatin (*Diagn Cytopathol* 2006;34:649). The cytoplasm is generally finely granular or dense but may show vacuolization. Cases with diffuse vacuolization may resemble metastatic renal cell carcinoma (e-**Fig. 17.59**).
3. **Solid pseudopapillary neoplasm** is typically seen in young women and is often solid by imaging. On aspiration, the smears are typically cellular although the cystic component can predominate making diagnosis difficult. Along with a variable cystic background of histiocytes and granular debris, the epithelial elements consist of individual cells and loosely cohesive groups around vascular cores expanded by myxoid

or hyaline material (e-**Fig. 17.60**). The cells are round-to-oval, small, uniform, and have a moderate amount of cytoplasm, which may contain hyaline globules (e-**Fig. 17.61**). Nuclei are eccentrically located and can have grooves and pseudoinclusions (*Am J Clin Pathol* 2004;121:654).

4. **Acinar cell carcinomas** are most often solid but can have a cystic component. On aspiration, these tumors are cellular with a variable pattern that ranges from cohesive fragments to more dispersed single cells. The cohesive fragments tend to be arranged as monolayers with a sheet-like pattern with varying degrees of vascularity. The cells show monomorphic round to oval nuclei, with nucleoli and an even chromatin distribution (e-**Fig. 17.62**). There is typically a moderate amount of granular cytoplasm imparting an acinar appearance, and small groups of cells can be arranged in acinar-like configurations. Stripped naked nuclei are common in the background (*Diagn Cytopathol* 2006;34:367).

III. **CYSTIC LESIONS.** EUS FNA is only one factor in the overall assessment of a cystic pancreatic lesion; a variety of clinical features (age, sex, size, shape, duct findings) and concomitantly measured fluid properties (CEA, enzyme levels) also contribute to the evaluation. The variable cellularity obtained by EUS FNA can significantly limit classification based on the cytomorphologic findings alone (*Surg Clin North Am* 2010;90:399).

A. **Pseudocysts** can be present in the background of known acute or chronic pancreatitis, although the clinical history and imaging findings are not always definitive. On aspiration, a variable to abundant amount of green-brown bile-tinged thick material is obtained which consists of granular debris with variable amounts of intermixed bile pigment, macrophages, neutrophils (usually a more acute phase component), and scant benign ductal and acinar tissue fragments (e-**Fig. 17.63**). The epithelial elements can show a reactive appearance, however, the atypia does not approach the quantitative and qualitative features of adenocarcinoma (e-**Fig. 17.64**).

B. **Serous Cystadenoma,** by aspiration, is predominantly hypocellular. The lining cells that are present are usually grouped as small- to intermediate-sized cohesive flat sheets, and have round nuclei and a moderate amount of cytoplasm which tends to be nondescript. The aspirate alone is often not sufficient for diagnosis (*Cancer* 2008;114:102; *Acta Cytol* 2017;61:27).

C. **Mucinous Cystic Neoplasm and Intraductal Papillary Mucinous Neoplasm.** Cytologically, the neoplasms of this category share a variable amount of extracellular mucin, sheets of glandular epithelial cells with varying degrees of cellularity, and a spectrum of cytologic atypia. These tumors can have varying degrees of complexity of cell groups; papillary configurations can be present in IPMN (e-**Fig. 17.65**). Often MCN cannot be distinguished from IPMN by cytology; however, if subepithelial ovarian-type stroma is present, the distinction can be made (e-**Fig. 17.66**). Invasion cannot be reliably determined based on aspiration smears (*Cancer Cytopathol* 2014;122:40).

ACKNOWLEDGMENT

The author thanks Brian Collins and Julie Kunkel, authors of the previous edition of this section.

SUGGESTED READINGS

Ali SZ, Erozan YS, Hruban RH. *Atlas of Pancreatic Cytopathology With Histopathologic Correlations.* New York: Demos Medical Publishing, LLC, 2009.

Bosman FT, Carneiro F, Hruban RH, Theise ND, eds. Tumors of the pancreas. In: *Pathology and Genetics of Tumors of Endocrine Organs (WHO Classification of Tumors).* Lyon, France: IARC Press; 2010: 279–334.

Chhieng DC, Stelow EB. *Pancreatic Cytopathology.* New York: Springer Science + Business Media, LLC, 2007.

Lloyd RV, Osamura RY, Koppel G, Rosai J, eds. Neoplasms of the neuroendocrine pancreas. In: *WHO Classifications of Tumors of Endocrine Organs.* Lyon, France: IARC Press, 2017; 209–240.

Hruban RH, Pitman MB, Klimstra DS. Tumors of the pancreas. In: *Atlas of Tumor Pathology*, Fourth Series. Washington, DC: American Registry of Pathology; 2007.

Thompson LD, Basturk O, Adsay NV. Pancreas. In: Mills SE, ed. *Steinberg's Diagnostic Surgical Pathology*, 6th ed. Philadelphia, PA: Lippincott Williams & Wilkins; 2015: 1577–1662.

Lamps LW. Pancreas. In: Goldblum JR, ed. *Rosai and Ackerman's Surgical Pathology*, 11th ed. Philadelphia, PA, Elsevier; 2017: 886–935.

Pitman MB, Layfield LJ. *The Papanicolaou Society of Cytopathology System for Reporting Pancreaticobiliary Cytology.* New York: Springer Science + Business Media, LLC, 2015.

18 Breast Pathology

Farhan A. Khan, Neda Rezaei, and Souzan Sanati

I. **INTRODUCTION.** This chapter addresses the most common diseases of the breast, in order of clinical importance, ranging from potentially lethal cancers to common benign changes (**e-Appendix 18.1**). Specific issues important to other specialists will be emphasized, such as correlating histologic with mammographic findings for radiologists, status of surgical margins for surgeons, TNM staging (essential elements of which include: tumor size (T), nodal status (N), and distant metastasis (M) for oncologists, and so on).

II. **SPECIMEN PROCESSING**

A. **General Approach.** The primary goals of grossing in breast pathology are to (1) identify the specimen, and determine its orientation and dimensions; (2) identify the presence, location, and dimensions of lesions (masses, calcifications, etc.); (3) estimate the distance of lesions from surgical margins; and (4) take small samples for more precise microscopic evaluation. Secondary goals include taking samples from various other locations depending on the type of specimen (e.g., nipple, all quadrants, and lymph nodes associated with mastectomies).

There are many methods of grossing breast surgical specimens; all acceptable methods adequately address the goals listed above even if their specific strategies vary. The central element of the basic strategy is a generic grossing template (**e-Appendix 18.2**), which can accommodate specimens of almost any size, ranging from small lumpectomies to large mastectomies. Utilization of the template creates a permanent record (diagram) of the most important features of a specimen (e.g., size, orientation, location of samples, location of mass lesions, distance of lesions from margins). The small amount of extra time required to create the diagram has several additional benefits, including (1) providing relatively precise information on the size and distribution of lesions that are not apparent grossly; (2) enabling better control of margins; (3) assistance in taking additional samples if necessary; and (4) facilitating succinct, comprehensive, and standardized gross dictations.

The main steps of grossing a surgical breast specimen are as follows:

1. **Identification**
2. **Orientation**
3. **Dimensions**
4. **Inking of margins**
5. **Sectioning** into thin slices to facilitate fixation. Small specimens are usually cut (2 to 4 mm thick) into a few slices and entirely submitted in a corresponding number of cassettes for formalin fixation. Larger specimens are usually cut into slices (5 mm thick

and hinged at the bottom to maintain intact orientation), and allowed to fix before submitting samples in cassettes.

6. Fixation in 10% neutral buffered formalin (NBF) for a minimum of 8 to 12 hours. The recommended maximum fixation time is 72 hours.

7. Diagramming of the specimen on the template. Diagrams are more informative and useful than gross dictations alone.

B. Ancillary Information. Most patients with breast pathology present with a clinically or radiologically detected mass and/or a mammographically detected abnormality, often in the form of microcalcification. The manner of presentation often dictates the approach to specimen processing. Because most breast specimens lack natural anatomical landmarks, careful specimen processing, especially margin assessment, is crucial for accurate pathologic interpretation. In addition, evaluation of specimen radiographs represents an integral part of examination of breast specimens, and should be reviewed whenever available. Review provides valuable information as to the nature of the lesion (ill-defined vs. well-defined mass; microcalcification) and location of the lesion(s), and assists planning of the sectioning of the specimen.

C. Specimen Types. Most breast specimens received for pathologic evaluation are in one of the following forms.

1. Needle core biopsies have almost totally replaced fine-needle aspiration (FNA) biopsy specimens for the initial pathologic evaluation of localized breast lesions in most centers. They are obtained to diagnose palpable breast masses or nonpalpable breast lesions detected by screening mammography, such as stellate densities or suspicious microcalcifications. For nonpalpable lesions, biopsy is usually obtained using image guidance (ultrasound-guided, stereotactic, or MRI-guided). Vacuum-assisted biopsies increase the volume of tissue obtained for microscopic examination. If biopsy is performed for calcifications, a radiograph of the specimen is often obtained to confirm that the calcifications have been adequately sampled. After describing the shape, size, and color of the tissue cores, they should be aligned in parallel and placed in a cassette between two sponges (preferable) or wrapped in tissue paper; similar to biopsies from other organs, overstuffing of cassettes should be avoided. Formalin fixation time is absolutely critical, as underfixation and overfixation both may result in altered biomarker results by immunohistochemistry. Current CAP/ASCO guidelines recommend that core needle biopsy samples be fixed in formalin for 6 to 72 hours prior to processing. At least three histologic levels should be obtained from each paraffin block to ensure adequate representation of the lesion(s). As for all other breast specimens, the histologic findings should always be correlated with the clinical and radiologic findings, and, if discrepant (such as when microcalcifications are not seen in original sections of a biopsy performed for microcalcifications), additional deeper sections from the block, and/or radiographic images of the paraffin block need to be examined to resolve the discrepancy.

2. Excisional biopsy/lumpectomy specimens are either oriented or nonoriented. Nonoriented specimens are those in which evaluation of the status of specific margins is not required by the surgeon (such as excisions of benign lesions or malignant lesions with separate margin specimens); nonetheless, these specimens should be inked. Oriented specimens need to be inked differentially to facilitate specific margin orientation. A four ink color approach is useful to orient the margins (the superior, inferior, anterior, and posterior margins will be inked by four different colors); the medial and lateral margins are covered by any ink color, and amputated, sliced, and completely submitted in separate cassettes. Another acceptable approach is to use six ink colors to orient all the margins.

For these specimens, the gross dimensions and weight should be recorded. Then the specimen should be serially sectioned as soon as possible to allow for adequate penetration of fixative. Such sectioning is usually performed perpendicular to the long axis of the specimen; however, sectioning may be influenced by the shape and proximity of the lesion(s) to particular margins. Gauze should be placed between the sections, and the specimen should be fixed in formalin for 6 to 48 hours before submitting samples in cassettes.

a. **If excision is performed for a mass lesion.** The size of the mass (accurate to nearest millimeter), consistency (gelatinous, rubbery, firm, or hard), growth pattern (well-circumscribed, infiltrative, pushing), and distance from margins should all be described. The presence and size of a biopsy cavity should also be noted. For well-circumscribed lesions thought to be benign (such as fibroadenomas), one section per centimeter of the lesion is usually sufficient. Ill-defined and suspicious lesions need to be entirely submitted if possible. If the mass is too large to be completely submitted, at least one section per centimeter of the mass should be submitted. Margins are microscopically examined by submitting a perpendicular section of the mass with each margin (superior, inferior, anterior, posterior). If the margins are distant from the mass, representative shave sections suffice. Medial and lateral margins are usually amputated, sliced, and completely submitted in labeled cassettes (Fig. 18.1). Representative sections of grossly noninvolved breast should additionally be submitted with particular attention to fibrous areas of the breast.

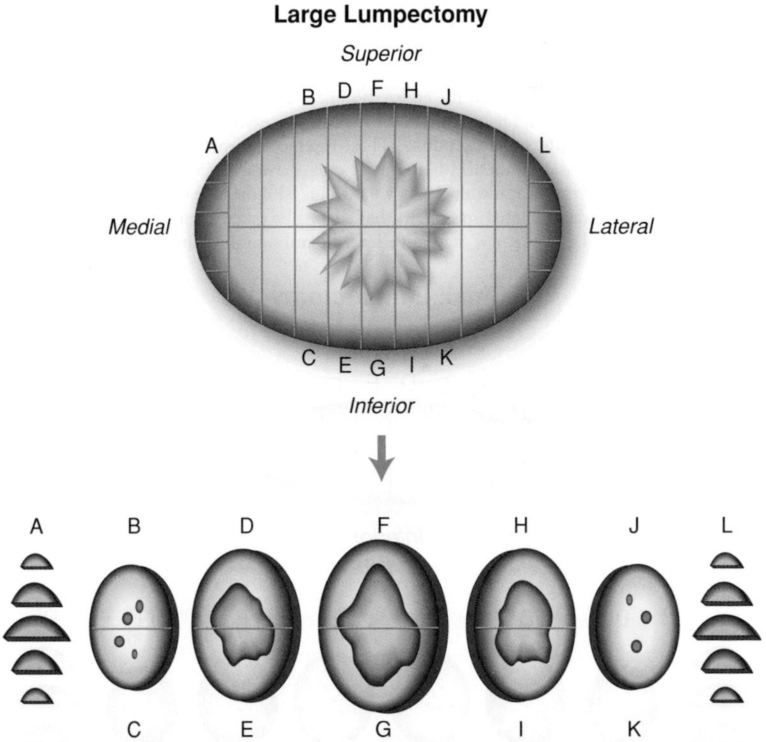

Figure 18.1 Schematic representation of "bread-loafing" and sampling of mass lesions. **A:** The specimen was serially sectioned perpendicular to its long axis, and an irregular mass was identified in the center of the specimen. Sections A and L would be submitted as medial and lateral margins, respectively, that are perpendicularly sectioned and entirely submitted. Given the size of the specimen and the mass, submission of sections B through K would appear to adequately represent the entire mass, as well as the immediately adjacent superior, inferior, anterior, and posterior (deep) margins.

b. If excision is performed for imaging-detected microcalcifications. Most of these specimens show no significant gross pathology. These specimens are usually oriented (by two perpendicular sutures or clips), contain a guiding wire, and are accompanied by a specimen radiograph. Similarly, a surgical clip may have been placed at the area of previous core biopsy. The guiding wire, which is placed at the site of imaging detected abnormality, should be used in conjunction with the specimen radiograph to preferentially sample areas of abnormality, immediately adjacent areas, as well as the margins. For smaller specimens, it is preferable to entirely submit the specimen in consecutive sections, as this facilitates accurate estimation of the extent of disease. In larger specimens, wide sampling of the area of the wire tip and adjacent tissue is advised. If possible, the specimen should be sectioned in a way that facilitates some inference of the three-dimensional aspects of the lesion when histologic sections are evaluated. This can be achieved by labeling the cassette numbers on a generic diagram that can be used to determine the relationship of tissue blocks containing abnormalities with each other (see **e-Appendix 18.2**). If there are multiple lesions, their location and relationship to each other should be documented; in addition to sampling each lesion individually, sections from normal appearing areas in between the lesions can be used to determine whether they represent individual or multiple masses. Representative sections from grossly noninvolved breast with attention to fibrous areas should also be submitted (Fig. 18.2). In situations where gross examination and the initial set of sections do not show a histologic abnormality, the entire specimen, or at least all the fibrous parts of the specimen, should be submitted for microscopic examination.

3. Margin and biopsy re-excisions. These cases range from unoriented flat portions of tissue that should be laid flat in a cassette (shave margin), where the presence of any malignancy seen histologically would thus be indicative of a positive margin; to larger, variably oriented specimens that should be inked preferentially, bread-loafed perpendicular to the new margin (oriented), and submitted in a manner to examine

Small Lumpectomy

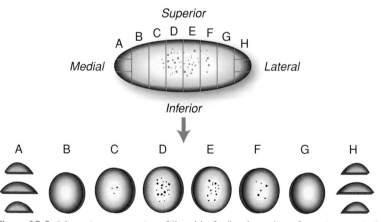

Figure 18.2 Schematic representation of "bread-loafing" and sampling of a specimen excised for microcalcifications. Especially given the scattered widespread distribution of the microcalcifications and their proximity to several margins, the specimen should be entirely submitted for histologic examination. The medial and lateral margins are amputated, perpendicularly sectioned, and entirely submitted. The remaining tissue is serially sectioned and entirely submitted as marked on the diagram.

the new margin. For re-excisions following invasive carcinoma, the status of gross residual disease should be evaluated as well as its relationship to different excision margins; in the absence of gross disease, the specimen need only be representatively sampled. For re-excisions following a diagnosis of in situ carcinoma, the specimen may need to be more widely sampled to detect residual disease and/or associated invasive carcinoma. Complete re-excision of the cavity created by a prior lumpectomy may also be performed; these specimens should be inked with respect to orientation, and serially sectioned as in a lumpectomy. The blood-filled biopsy cavity should be entirely submitted, in particular with respect to new margins to evaluate the residual disease and status of surgical margins.

4. **Mastectomy specimens** range from simple nipple-sparing mastectomy (which removes the breast tissue beneath overlying skin and nipple), to skin-sparing mastectomy (which removes the breast only covered by the nipple–areola complex and a narrow rim of surrounding skin), to simple mastectomy (mastectomy without axillary tissue), to modified radical mastectomy (mastectomy with axillary lymph nodes). Radical mastectomy (modified radical mastectomy with pectoral muscles), is rarely performed in current practice. Mastectomies may be prophylactic or therapeutic. When the specimen is received by pathology it should first be measured and weighed. Then the specimen should be oriented and the surgical margins inked; it should then be serially sectioned perpendicular to the skin at 5 mm intervals from the posterior aspect, packed with gauze, and fixed in formalin overnight. The size of any masses, including their growth pattern, location, and distance from all surgical margins, should be recorded; the same principles discussed above (for excisional biopsy/lumpectomy specimens) also apply to grossing mastectomy specimens. Masses should be entirely submitted if small, in a manner that demonstrates the relationship to the surgical margin. If a mass is predominantly composed of ductal carcinoma in situ (DCIS) with focal microinvasion, submitting the entire mass is required to exclude a larger size of invasive carcinoma. In addition, at least one section of nipple, grossly normal tissue from each of the four quadrants of the breast, skin, and dermal scars from previous biopsies should be submitted for microscopic examination. If the specimen is a modified-radical mastectomy, the axillary tail should be removed and dissected for lymph nodes, which should all be submitted for microscopic evaluation in their entirety (see below). A search for lymph nodes should always be performed even in simple mastectomies and if lymph nodes are found, they should be sampled accordingly. It is important to correlate the gross and microscopic findings with imaging studies to optimize patient care; for nonpalpable lesions, radiographing the specimen with submission of the entire area of radiologic abnormality is recommended.

5. **Mammary implants** should be documented, photographed, and inspected grossly for any evidence of leakage. One or two sections are usually sufficient to evaluate the surrounding fibrous "capsule" that is usually submitted with the implant(s).

6. **Sentinel lymph nodes.** The sentinel lymph node(s) is (are) the first lymph node or group of lymph nodes that drain the breast into the axilla and in most cases they are the first lymph node(s) involved by metastatic carcinoma. Only rarely does cancer "skip" the sentinel node and metastasize to a nonsentinel lymph node. As such, specimens designated as sentinel lymph nodes should be dissected carefully. Intraoperative evaluation (frozen sections and/or touch preparations) is usually limited to lymph nodes grossly suspicious for malignancy; in these situations, intraoperative imprint cytology of the lymph node can provide results at the time of surgery. For permanent sections, each node is serially cut at 2-mm intervals and, in the absence of gross evidence of metastatic carcinoma, entirely submitted for histologic examination. There are many different protocols for microscopic evaluation of a sentinel lymph node, but one common approach involves examination of three hematoxylin and eosin (H&E)-stained sections from each paraffin block. The use of cytokeratin-stained sections if initial H&E sections are negative, especially for lobular carcinoma, is optimal, but not required. In the event of a positive sentinel lymph node, axillary dissection is indicated.

7. Nonsentinel (axillary) lymph nodes. Axillary lymph node dissection may be performed in conjunction with lumpectomy in a patient with a positive sentinel lymph node, or may be performed as part of a modified-radical mastectomy (see above). After carefully dissecting grossly benign appearing nodes from the fat, nodes smaller than 0.4 cm can be submitted intact, whereas larger nodes need to be bisected or trisected and submitted in a manner that permits accurate enumeration (either by submitting them in individual cassettes or by differential inking). If possible, the size of the largest grossly positive node or metastatic deposit should be measured, and the presence of extranodal extension sampled in one section. It is recommended that a minimum of ten lymph nodes should be identified in an axillary dissection (although this number is dependent on the surgical technique and the extent of axillary lymph node dissection during surgery). Attention should also be directed to identification of possible intramammary lymph nodes, which are usually identified in the upper outer quadrant of the breast.

D. Examples of Reporting Template. To demonstrate the organization of a pathology report on breast samples using the discussed diagnostic template (**e-Appendix 18.1**), a few examples are shown in **e-Appendix 18.3**. Other recommended templates for reporting tumors in breast specimens have also been promulgated (e.g., College of American Pathologists Protocol for the examination of specimens from patients with invasive carcinoma of the breast, or for the examination of specimens from patients with DCIS of the breast; available at http://www.cap.org).

III. NORMAL BREAST. An understanding of normal breast histology is essential for accurate histologic evaluation of breast specimens. It should be noted that what constitutes normal varies based on gender, age, menstrual phase, pregnancy, lactation, and menopausal status.

The breast represents a modified skin adnexal structure composed of major lactiferous ducts that originate from the nipple, progressively branching, until eventually inducing grape-like clusters of secretory glands as lobules. Breast development starts during the fifth week of gestation, at which time thickenings of ectoderm appear on the ventral surface of the fetus extending from axilla to the groin (mammary ridges or milk lines). The majority of this thickening regresses as the fetus develops, except an area in the pectoral region. Failure of this regression results in ectopic mammary tissue or an accessory nipple. The most common location for an accessory nipple is the axilla.

The adult female breast consists of a series of branching ducts, ductules, and lobulated acinar units embedded within a fibroadipose stroma. Terminal duct lobular units (TDLUs) are composed of lobules, which are groups of alveolar glands, embedded in loose intralobular connective tissue that connect to a single terminal ductule. These are the structural and functional units of the breast and most pathologic processes arise within them (**e-Figs. 18.1** and **18.2**). The lining throughout the duct/lobular system of the breast is composed of two distinct layers: an inner (luminal) epithelial layer that is cuboidal to columnar, and an outer (basal) myoepithelial layer (**e-Fig. 18.3**). The myoepithelial cells have variable morphologies ranging from flattened**,** to epithelioid with clear cytoplasm, to a myoid appearance**.** Identification of these two cell layers is very important in the assessment of breast lesions as they are almost always preserved in benign lesions, as well as in noninvasive malignant lesions, but are absent in invasive carcinomas. Immunohistochemistry can also be used to identify myoepithelial cells, as myoepithelial cells are usually positive for calponin, p63, CD10, and smooth muscle myosin heavy chain, among other markers (**e-Fig. 18.4**). A panel-based approach of two or more markers is recommended (*Arch Pathol Lab Med* 2011;135:422). In addition, a proportion of luminal epithelial cells almost always expresses estrogen receptors (ER) and/or progesterone receptors (PR). The intralobular stroma is usually sharply demarcated from a denser, collagenized paucicellular interlobular stroma. The proportion of dense stroma to adipose tissue is variable, with younger women having denser connective tissue (which partially explains why mammography is less sensitive in younger individuals). Breast lobules can be classified based on their morphology into three major types. Type 1 lobules are the most primitive and rudimentary, and are usually seen in prepubertal and nulliparous women. Type 3 lobules are the most developed, and are usually seen in parous and premenopausal women. The progression from type 1 to type 3 is accompanied by additional branching and increased number of alveolar buds. Type 1 lobules also predominate in postmenopausal women and premenopausal women with breast cancer (*Dev Biol* 1989;25:643; *Cancer Epidemiol Biomarkers Prev* 1994;3:219; *Breast J* 2001;7:278).

Breast development starts with puberty and cyclic secretions of estrogen and progesterone. The ducts elongate and branch primarily due to estrogen stimulus, and lobulocentric growth advances primarily under the influence of progesterone. In addition, the breast undergoes various physiologic changes during menstruation, pregnancy, and lactation. These physiologic changes should not be mistaken for pathologic processes. Cyclic menstrual changes in the breast tissue are subtle in comparison with other sites such as endometrium. The follicular phase of the menstrual cycle is characterized by simple acini and collagenized stroma, while the luteal phase is characterized by apical snouting of the epithelial cells, prominent vacuolization of myoepithelial cells, and loose edematous stroma. The epithelial cells show peak mitotic activity in the late luteal phase. During pregnancy, there is progressive epithelial cell proliferation resulting in an increase in both the number and size of TDLUs. By late pregnancy, lobular myoepithelial cells become inconspicuous while the cytoplasm of the luminal epithelium becomes vacuolated as secretions accumulate in the expanded lobules. After parturition, florid changes including the frequent presence of luminal cells with atypical nuclei protruding into the lumen (hobnail cells) can be seen which can be alarming (e-Fig. 18.5). Gradually and slowly the lobules involute to their resting appearance.

In postmenopausal women, the lobules undergo involution and atrophy characterized by reduction in size and complexity with an increase in fat (type 1 lobules) (e-Figs. 18.6 to 18.8).

In contrast to women, due to lack of hormonal stimulation, TDLUs do not develop to a significant extent in men, and male breast consists of branching ducts within a fibroadipose stroma.

IV. **INVASIVE BREAST CARCINOMA.** The WHO classification of breast tumors is provided in Table 18.1. Most invasive carcinomas present as a palpable mass and/or as a mammographic abnormality. However, in some cases the primary tumor is occult, and the patient may present with lymph node or distant metastasis. The pathology report should communicate all the diagnostic, prognostic, and predictive findings to a multidisciplinary team of surgeons, oncologists, and other specialists; some findings are strong prognostic factors (histologic type, histologic grade, lymph node status), some determine the likelihood of response to specific treatment (hormonal therapy, Trastuzumab), and some determine the need for additional surgical procedures (margin status). Determination of pathologic stage is vital to determine prognosis and to guide the therapy; the updated 2017 TNM AJCC staging classification scheme for invasive carcinoma and DCIS has recently been published (Amin MB, et al., eds. *AJCC Cancer Staging Manual*. 8th ed. New York: Springer, 2017). In addition to pathologic stage, the prognosis of breast carcinoma is greatly dependent on additional prognostic and predictive factors that are mandatory and should be evaluated and reported for all breast carcinomas, and are most significant in lymph node–negative breast carcinoma.

A. **Prognostic and Predictive Factors**

1. **Histologic subtype.** Histologic typing remains the gold standard for classification of breast carcinoma and provides useful prognostic information. Approximately 75% of invasive breast carcinomas (IBCs) are characterized by lack of unique histologic features and are referred to as invasive "ductal" carcinomas, no special type, or not otherwise specified. These carcinomas are histologically and prognostically very heterogeneous. The remaining IBCs are referred to as "special" subtypes and are characterized by relatively unique/uniform histologic features. Collectively, the special subtypes account for about 25% of all IBCs with the most common subtypes including the so-called invasive lobular, tubular, mucinous, and medullary carcinomas (approximately 15%, 5%, 2% to 3%, and 1% to 2%, respectively) (*Breast Cancer Res* 2008;10:S4). Except for perhaps invasive lobular carcinoma (ILC), all the

TABLE 18.1	World Health Organization 2012 Histologic Classification of Breast Tumors[a]

Epithelial tumors

Microinvasive carcinoma

Invasive breast carcinoma

Invasive carcinoma of no special type (NST)
  Pleomorphic carcinoma
  Carcinoma with osteoclast-like stromal giant Cells
  Carcinoma with choriocarcinomatous features
  Carcinoma with melanotic features

Invasive lobular carcinoma
  Classic lobular carcinoma
  Solid lobular carcinoma
  Alveolar lobular carcinoma
  Pleomorphic lobular carcinoma
  Tubulolobular carcinoma
  Mixed lobular carcinoma

Tubular carcinoma

Cribriform carcinoma

Mucinous carcinoma

Carcinoma with medullary features
  Medullary carcinoma
  Atypical medullary carcinoma
  Invasive carcinoma NST with medullary features

Carcinoma with apocrine differentiation

Carcinoma with signet-ring-cell differentiation

Invasive micropapillary carcinoma

Metaplastic carcinoma of no special type
  Low-grade adenosquamous carcinoma
  Fibromatosis-like metaplastic carcinoma
  Squamous cell carcinoma
  Spindle cell carcinoma
  Metaplastic carcinoma with mesenchymal differentiation
    Chondroid differentiation
    Osseous differentiation
    Other types of mesenchymal differentiation
  Mixed metaplastic carcinoma
  Myoepithelial carcinoma

Rare types

Carcinoma with neuroendocrine differentiation
  Neuroendocrine tumor, well-differentiated
  Neuroendocrine carcinoma, poorly differentiated (small cell carcinoma)
  Carcinoma with neuroendocrine differentiation

Secretory carcinoma

Invasive papillary carcinoma

Acinic cell carcinoma

Mucoepidermoid carcinoma

Polymorphous carcinoma

Oncocytic carcinoma

Lipid-rich carcinoma

Glycogen-rich clear cell carcinoma

Sebaceous carcinoma

Salivary gland/skin adnexal type tumors
  Cylindroma
  Clear cell hidradenoma

Epithelial–myoepithelial tumors

Pleomorphic adenoma

Adenomyoepithelioma
  Adenomyoepithelioma with carcinoma

Adenoid cystic carcinoma

Precursor lesions

Ductal carcinoma in situ

Lobular neoplasia
  Lobular carcinoma in situ
    Classic lobular carcinoma in situ
    Pleomorphic lobular carcinoma in situ
  Atypical lobular hyperplasia

Intraductal proliferative lesions

Usual ductal hyperplasia

Columnar cell lesions—flat epithelial atypia

Atypical ductal hyperplasia

Papillary lesions

Intraductal papilloma
  Intraductal papilloma with atypical hyperplasia
  Intraductal papilloma with DCIS
  Intraductal papilloma with LCIS

Intraductal papillary carcinoma

Encapsulated papillary carcinoma
  Encapsulated papillary carcinoma with invasion

Solid papillary carcinoma (in situ, invasive)

Benign epithelial proliferations (adenomas)

Tubular adenoma

Lactating adenoma

Apocrine adenoma

Ductal adenoma

TABLE 18.1 World Health Organization 2012 Histologic Classification of Breast Tumors[a] (Continued)

Mesenchymal tumors	Fibroepithelial tumors
Nodular fasciitis	Fibroadenoma
Myofibroblastoma	Phyllodes tumor
Desmoid-type fibromatosis	Benign
	Borderline
Inflammatory myofibroblastic tumor	Malignant
Benign vascular lesions	Periductal stromal tumor, low-grade
Hemangioma	Hamartoma
Angiomatosis	**Tumors of the nipple**
Atypical vascular lesions	Nipple adenoma
Pseudoangiomatous stromal hyperplasia	Syringomatous tumor
Granular cell tumor	Paget disease of the nipple
Benign peripheral nerve sheath tumors	**Malignant lymphoma**
Neurofibroma	**Metastatic tumors**
Schwannoma	**Tumors of the male breast**
Lipoma	Gynecomastia
Angiolipoma	Carcinoma
Liposarcoma	Invasive
Angiosarcoma	In situ
Rhabdomyosarcoma	**Clinical patterns**
Osteosarcoma	Inflammatory carcinoma
Leiomyoma	Bilateral breast carcinoma
Leiomyosarcoma	

[a]Condensed from: Lakhani SR, Ellis IO, Schnitt SJ, et al. *WHO Classification of Tumours of the Breast.* Lyon, France: IARC Press; 2017.

special type carcinomas have more favorable prognosis compared with invasive ductal carcinoma, although the degree of improved outcome is variable for different types. Other less common subtypes of IBC that have a favorable prognosis include invasive cribriform and adenoid cystic carcinomas (AdCC). Different experts have used variable criteria for diagnosing special type carcinomas, which is partially responsible for the variable prevalence reported in different studies. For practical purposes, a carcinoma is considered "special type" if more than 90% of the tumor shows special type differentiation. For a carcinoma to be considered "no special type" more than 50% of the tumor should lack special type differentiation. Tumors with special type differentiation in 50% to 90% of the tumor are considered variants or mixed types. Some experts believe that variant/mixed type carcinomas have an outcome intermediate between no special type carcinomas and the pure special type carcinomas (*Am J Surg Pathol* 1991;15:334; *Breast Cancer Res* 2008;10(S4)). The diagnostic features of major histologic subtypes of breast carcinoma (discussed below) are also summarized in Table 18.2.

2. **Tumor size** is one of the most powerful prognostic factors for clinical outcome. The prognostic value of tumor size is independent of axillary lymph node status and is an especially significant determinant in node-negative disease. It is usually determined by taking into consideration the gross findings correlated with the microscopic

TABLE 18.2 Diagnostic Features of Major Histopathologic Types of Invasive Breast Carcinoma

Histologic Type	Incidence (%)	Clinical/Gross Findings	Microscopic Features	Favorable Prognosis	Typical Biomarkers
Invasive lobular carcinoma	5–15	Architectural distortion, density (no distinct mass), multifocal/bilateral	Uniform noncohesive cells, eccentric nuclei, intracytoplasmic lumina, Indian filing, targetoid pattern		ER (+), PR (+), HER2 (−)
Invasive tubular carcinoma	5	Spiculated mass, small size	Angulated tubules with tapered ends, open lumina, dense stroma	Yes	ER (+), PR (+), HER2 (−)
Invasive mucinous carcinoma	2–3	Well-circumscribed lobulated mass, gelatinous cut surface	Tumor cells floating in pools of extracellular mucin	Yes	ER (+), PR (+), HER2 (−)
Invasive medullary carcinoma	1–2	Young women, well-circumscribed mass, no calcifications	Syncytial growth, pushing borders, lympho-plasmacytic infiltrate, high nuclear grade	yes (if pure)	ER (−), PR (−), HER2 (−) (triple negative)
Invasive micropapillary carcinoma	1–2	Similar to IDC, NST	Tumor clusters within empty spaces, reverse polarity, no fibrovascular cores	Higher rate of LN metastasis	Variable
IDC, NST	70–75	Spiculated mass, variable	Variable, devoid of special type histologic features	Variable	Variable
Metaplastic carcinoma	<1%	Larger size	Tumor transformation to non-glandular (squamous) or mesenchymal elements	Lower LN metastasis, poor overall prognosis	ER (−), PR (−), HER2 (−); (triple negative) ER and PR can be positive in glandular elements

IDC, invasive ductal carcinoma; NST, no special type.

examination. In some cases, it may also be helpful to include information about tumor size from imaging studies. In small tumors where the bulk of tumor has been excised by a previous core needle biopsy, it may be best to use the core biopsy in conjunction with radiologic findings to estimate the maximum size of the invasive carcinoma. Although the aggregate volume of multifocal tumors may better correlate with the risk of lymph node metastasis than the size of the largest focus (*Cancer* 2004;100:20), multiple foci of invasive carcinoma are not currently added together and the diameters of the different foci should be individually reported, and only the largest focus of contiguous area of invasion should be used for staging purposes. Only the size of invasive carcinoma (best measured by microscopic assessment), which does not include adjacent DCIS outside the invasive carcinoma, should be used for staging purposes.

3. **Histologic grade** is used to convey the degree of differentiation of tumors. The most widely accepted grading system for IBC is the Elston–Ellis modification of the Scarff–Bloom–Richardson (ESBR) grading system. This grading system is based on three characteristics of the tumor: the degree of gland/tubule formation, nuclear pleomorphism, and mitotic activity (e-**Figs. 18.9** to **18.11**). Variation in these three elements is the basis for this universally accepted grading scheme (*Histopathology* 1991;19:403; *J Clin Oncol* 2008;26:3153) (Table 18.3). A numerical scoring system on a scale of 1 to 3 is given to each variable to ensure that each factor has been assessed individually. The histologic grade is of particular importance for ductal carcinomas of no special type. However, given the strength of histologic grade as a prognostic marker (second only to axillary lymph node status), it should be reported for all carcinomas (*Histopathology* 1991;19:403; *J Clin Oncol* 2008;26:3153; *Histopathology* 1991;19:403). Within each TNM stage grouping, there is a correlation between histologic grade and patient outcome, although a combination of factors, such as a combination of histologic type and grade (*J Clin Oncol* 2008;26:3153), or tumor size, nodal status, and histologic grade (Nottingham Prognostic Index [NPI]) is a better tool to assess the prognosis in any given tumor (*Pathol Oncol Res*

TABLE 18.3	Elston–Ellis Modification of Scarff–Bloom–Richardson Grading System for Invasive Breast Carcinoma		
Tubule Formation			**Score**
	Majority (>75%) of tumor		1
	Moderate (10–75%) of tumor		2
	Little or none (<10%) of tumor		3
Nuclear pleomorphism			
	Small, regular, uniform nuclei		1
	Moderate increase in size and variability		2
	Marked variation		3
Mitotic activity			
Field diameter (mm)	0.44	0.59	0.63
Field area (mm²)	0.152	0.274	0.312
Mitotic count			
	0–5	0–9	0–11	1
	6–10	10–19	12–22	2
	>11	>20	>23	3

Add up the score to reach the total points:
3–5 points: Grade 1 (well-differentiated)
6–7 points: Grade 2 (moderately differentiated)
8–9 points: Grade 3 (poorly differentiated)

2008;14:113). Recently, histologic grade has been incorporated into TNM stage groups by the AJCC to further stratify patients into prognostic stage groups.

4. **Surgical margin.** The distance of tumor from the margin of surgical excision is also important because it is inversely related to the likelihood of local recurrence, especially in tumors removed by lumpectomy. Wide margins with grossly distinct tumors can be adequately measured with a ruler, whereas close margins require microscopic measurement. A margin is considered positive only if the ink that was applied to the margin at the time of gross examination transects tumor cells. The distance of the closest margin, as well as its location, should be reported. The extent of margin involvement can be relayed as focal (less that 4 mm), multifocal (more than one focus), or extensive (5 mm or greater).

5. **Others**

   a. **Mitotic index** (MI) is a measure of the capability of the tumor cells to divide and replicate and is determined by calculating the average number of mitotic figures in a minimum of 10 consecutive high-power fields (HPFs) in the most mitotically active part of the tumor, usually at the periphery of the tumor. Only the clearly identifiable mitotic figures should be counted.

   b. The presence of **lymphovascular space invasion** (e-Fig. 18.12) is an important and independent prognostic factor, particularly in node-negative patients with IBC. The presence of lymphatic channel invasion recognizes a subgroup of node-negative patients who are at increased risk of lymph node metastasis or distant metastasis (*Diagn Pathol* 2011;13:18; *Ann Oncol* 2005;16:1569). There is a high degree of interobserver variability in diagnosing lymphovascular invasion (LVI), and so adherence to strict criteria is recommended in order to reduce this interobserver variability. It is recommended that the focus of LVI should be outside the borders of invasive carcinoma. In addition, identification of an endothelial lining, and lack of conformation of tumor emboli to the shape of vascular space, help to differentiate a vascular space from artifactual stromal clefting. LVI present within lymphatic spaces in the dermis is often correlated with the clinical features of inflammatory carcinoma (diffuse erythema and edema involving one-third or more of the breast). In the absence of the clinical features of inflammatory carcinoma, this finding still remains a poor prognostic factor but is insufficient to classify a cancer as inflammatory carcinoma.

   c. **Skin and nipple involvement.** Skin can directly be involved by underlying invasive carcinoma (with or without ulceration). This usually is seen in association with large tumors, or in tumors that are small but very superficial. In addition, tumor cells from underlying lactiferous ducts of the nipple that are involved by DCIS can percolate through the epidermis without breaking through the basement membrane (Paget disease).

      Recently, gene expression profiling studies have classified breast tumors on the basis of their gene transcription patterns into different types or classes with different prognostic implications (*Nature* 2000;406:747). These new technologies provide important information that can be integrated into routine patient care (see below). Although histologic typing of breast tumors still remains the gold standard for classification of breast carcinoma and provides useful prognostic information, information provided by gene expression profiling assays has recently been incorporated by the AJCC into the information provided by traditional prognostic factors to further classify patients into prognostic stage groups.

B. **Invasive Ductal Carcinoma, No Special Type** is the most common subtype of breast cancer, comprising 70% to 75% of IBCs. This subtype is composed of a heterogeneous mixture of tumors with different morphologies, clinical findings, and patient outcomes. These tumors are devoid of histologic features that would allow categorization of these tumors in a special type category, and usually present as a spiculated mass, with or without calcifications, or as a mammographic abnormality. Grossly, the tumors usually form a hard mass, with a tan-white to gray, gritty cut surface which is a manifestation of dense stromal desmoplasia. The morphology of these tumors is quite heterogeneous with regard to growth pattern, cytologic features, mitotic activity, and extent of associated in situ carcinoma. The growth pattern can be solid, trabecular, in cords, in tubules, or as single cells (e-Figs. **18.13** to **18.25**). Most often, heterogeneity can also be noted within different parts of the same tumor. As mentioned earlier in this chapter, the ESBR grading system is an important prognostic tool for categorizing these tumors into groups with good versus poor outcome.

C. Special Subtypes

1. **ILC** is the second most common type of IBC, and comprises about 15% of all invasive carcinomas with a reportedly increased incidence in patients receiving postmenopausal combined hormone replacement therapy (*Breast Cancer Res* 2004;6:R149). These tumors are associated with a higher rate of multifocality in the ipsilateral breast, and are also more often bilateral than other subtypes. They may present as a palpable mass, but more commonly they present with an area of density or architectural distortion on mammogram. Some tumors do not show any mammographic abnormalities. Grossly, they may either form a mass which is indistinguishable from a mass of invasive ductal carcinoma, or they may only show an area of firm, rubbery breast tissue. Sometimes carcinoma is only revealed upon microscopic examination. Histologically, ILC has a distinct morphology and pattern of infiltration within the stroma. The **classical form** is characterized by small, uniform, noncohesive tumor cells infiltrating in a single "Indian file" pattern and forming linear strands (e-Figs. **18.26** to **18.28**) that may concentrically surround benign epithelial elements (targetoid pattern of growth) (e-Fig. **18.29**). Typically the tumor cells infiltrate without provoking a stromal reaction and without destroying normal architecture. Cytologically the nuclei are small and uniform, and located eccentrically within a cytoplasm that occasionally shows intracytoplasmic lumina (an intracytoplasmic vacuole containing an eosinophilic mucin droplet). Mitotic activity is sparse. Variant forms of ILC differ from the classical type with regards to architecture or cytology. While occasional signet ring cells can be seen in classical lobular carcinoma, in the **signet ring cell variant** the tumor shows a prominent population of signet ring cells (e-Fig. **18.30**). In the **solid** and **trabecular variants** tumor cells are cytologically similar to the classical form; however, they have a different growth pattern of either large sheets (e-Figs. **18.31** and **18.32**), or nests of 20 cells or more which are separated from each other by stroma (e-Fig. **18.33**), respectively. In the **pleomorphic variant** the tumor cells are larger (greater than 4 times the size of lymphocytes), and show more significant pleomorphism and increased mitoses (e-Fig. **18.34**). Most cases of ILC show reduced or absent expression of E-cadherin by immunohistochemistry. As suggested by their higher grade, pleomorphic ILCs do not share the somewhat better outcome (compared to IDC-NST) that characterizes classic ILC. Other differences from IDC-NST include a lower incidence of parenchymal metastasis, and isolated tumor cell (ITC) metastatic patterns in minimally involved axillary lymph nodes (as opposed to the usual finding of tumor cell clusters in the subcapsular sinuses). ILCs have characteristic metastatic spread to certain organs such as the ovary and stomach (where the metastases can resemble primary signet-ring cell carcinoma). Up to 95% of ILCs are immunopositive for ER and PR expression. ILCs typically do not overexpress the *HER2* gene product, except the pleomorphic variant which may show HER2 overexpression.

2. **Tubular carcinoma.** This tumor type constitutes 5% of invasive carcinomas (even higher in screening detected tumors) (*J Clin Oncol* 1999;17:1442), and is associated with limited metastatic potential and an excellent prognosis. As a result of increased use of screening mammography, these tumors present as a nonpalpable mammographic abnormality, or are incidentally found on biopsies for other abnormalities. Grossly, they form a spiculated mass. Microscopically, these tumors are characterized by a haphazard arrangement of angulated tubules with tapering ends and open lumens. The tubules are lined by a single layer of epithelial cells that often

display eosinophilic to amphophilic cytoplasm with apical snouts and oval nuclei, with only mild to moderate nuclear pleomorphism (e-**Figs. 18.35** and **18.36**). A cellular often fibroelastotic stroma is characteristic. The lack of a myoepithelial layer is a helpful feature in distinguishing this tumor from benign sclerosing lesions of the breast (sclerosing adenosis, radial scar, complex sclerosing lesions). ER and PR are expressed in greater than 90% of these tumors (*J Clin Oncol* 1999;17:1442), but they rarely, if ever, overexpress HER2. Axillary lymph node metastasis is uncommon, and if present, occurs only with larger tumors and is limited to the low-axillary lymph nodes; axillary lymph node metastasis is not associated with the same adverse outcome as in IDC, NST tumors (*J Clin Oncol* 1999;17:1442).

3. **Invasive cribriform carcinoma** accounts for <1% of breast carcinomas. The tumor infiltrates in angulated islands and nests with well-defined cribriform spaces (e-**Figs. 18.19** to **18.21**). The nuclei show mild atypia with minimal mitotic activity. They are positive for ER and PR, while negative for HER2 overexpression. A fibroblastic stroma with osteoclast-like multinucleated giant cells can be seen (e-**Fig. 18.21**). The prognosis is excellent.

4. **Mucinous carcinoma.** Depending on the series and stringency of diagnostic criteria, this variant comprises 1% to 6% of all invasive carcinomas. This tumor is also associated with a favorable outcome. Grossly, the tumor is well circumscribed and lobulated, with a soft gelatinous consistency, and a glistening cut surface. Microscopically, the tumor is composed of tumor cell clusters and trabeculae floating within lakes of extracellular mucin (e-**Fig. 18.37**). Nuclear grade characteristically is low to intermediate. These tumors typically are immunopositive for ER (>90% of tumors) and PR biomarkers, and negative for HER2 overexpression (*J Clin Oncol* 1999;17:1442). A significant proportion of mucinous carcinomas show neuroendocrine differentiation (*Mod Pathol* 2004;17:568).

   Mucinous carcinoma should be differentiated from other mucin-producing lesions of the breast. Mucocele-like lesions are characterized by mucin-filled benign ducts and cysts that often rupture and result in extravasation of mucin into surrounding stroma (e-**Fig. 18.38**), sometimes the ducts show proliferative changes, and portions of ductal epithelium may become detached and float within the mucin pool; however, the linear configuration of epithelial cells and presence of myoepithelial cells favors a diagnosis of a mucocele-like lesion. Whenever the distinction between the two is not possible, especially in core needle biopsies, excision should be recommended for definitive evaluation (*J Clin Pathol* 2008;61:11).

5. **Medullary carcinoma.** This tumor comprises 1% to 2% of all invasive carcinomas. There is an association between medullary carcinomas and familial mutations in the *BRCA1* DNA repair gene. Medullary carcinoma is usually diagnosed in younger women and presents with a palpable mass. On mammogram, the tumor is seen as a well-circumscribed mass usually without calcifications. On gross examination, the tumor is a well-circumscribed, soft, tan-brown to gray mass, with a bulging cut surface. Hemorrhage, necrosis, or cystic change may be noted. Microscopically, these tumors are characterized by a syncytial growth pattern in more than 75% of the tumor, an intense lymphoplasmacytic infiltrate, pushing borders, highly pleomorphic nuclei (nuclear grade 2 to 3), and a lack of glandular differentiation (e-**Fig. 18.39**). Tumors that show most, but not all, of the above criteria are recognized as variant/atypical medullary carcinomas. Medullary carcinomas are generally negative for all biomarkers (triple-negative tumors). Pure medullary carcinomas have a favorable outcome; however, variant types do not share this prognostic advantage.

6. **Other rare, but clinically significant subtypes**

   a. **Invasive micropapillary carcinoma.** In a pure form (>75% of the tumor), invasive micropapillary carcinoma accounts for less than 1% of invasive carcinomas; however, it is much more frequently a minor component of IDC, NST tumors. Histologically, this variant is composed of small solid clusters of malignant cells floating within clear stromal spaces (e-**Fig. 18.40**). These cell clusters lack true fibrovascular cores and show reverse polarity (the apical surfaces of the cells are polarized to the outside) (e-Fig. 18.41). The importance of recognizing this variant of invasive carcinoma (as well as mixed tumors with a micropapillary component) is the associated high incidence of axillary lymph node metastasis. It should be noted, however, that when matched for stage, this variant does not necessarily have a worse prognosis than IDC, NST (*Mod Pathol* 1993;6:660; *Breast* 2010;19:231; *Am J Surg Pathol* 2009;33:202).

b. Metaplastic carcinomas are rare and comprise less than 1% of breast carcinomas. They include a heterogeneous group of tumors in which a portion of the malignant cells have undergone transformation into a different cell type: nonglandular epithelial (squamous), or mesenchymal cell (chondroid, osseous, muscle, spindle cell) types. These tumors are similar to invasive ductal carcinomas of no special type with regard to clinical presentation except that they are usually larger at the time of presentation.

Tumors with squamous differentiation show a spectrum of differentiation from well to poorly differentiated. **Low-grade adenosquamous carcinoma**, frequently associated with papillary and sclerosing lesions, is characterized by angulated glands embedded in a cellular stroma composed of cells with low-grade cytologic atypia and focal squamous differentiation (e-Fig. 18.42). In contrast to higher-grade tumors that resemble adenosquamous carcinoma elsewhere, low-grade adenosquamous carcinomas rarely metastasize. **Metaplastic spindle cell carcinoma** includes carcinomas with abundant spindle cell transformation (e-Fig. 18.43). The diagnosis is relatively straightforward when glandular or squamous elements are evident, but when absent, diagnosis may only be made by demonstrating cytokeratin immunoreactivity in the spindle cells. It should be noted that spindle cell carcinoma can be histologically bland and show minimal cytologic atypia (such as in so-called fibromatosis-like spindle cell carcinoma). The key to correct diagnosis is wide sampling of the tumor to identify areas with clear glandular elements, and/or the use of a panel of immunohistochemical markers, particularly high-molecular-weight/basal cytokeratins, myoepithelial markers, and p63 to demonstrate the epithelial nature of the tumor (e-Fig. 18.44) (*Histopathology* 2008;52:45). **Metaplastic carcinomas with heterologous differentiation** are most commonly composed of foci of chondroid or osseous differentiation; however other types of mesenchymal differentiation such as fibrosarcoma, rhabdomyosarcoma, and other sarcomas can also be seen (e-Figs. 18.45 to 18.47). Despite the lower relative rate of lymph node metastasis (considering their larger size at the time of diagnosis), metaplastic carcinomas have a high rate of lymphovascular space invasion and a poor overall prognosis. ER, PR, and HER2 are usually negative, but can be focally expressed in the glandular component.

7. Other rare types of breast carcinoma include, among others, microinvasive carcinoma, secretory carcinoma, AdCC, carcinoma with apocrine differentiation, clear cell/glycogen-rich carcinoma, myoepithelial carcinoma, sebaceous carcinoma, acinic cell carcinoma, and oncocytic carcinoma.

a. Microinvasive carcinoma is defined as extension of cancer cells beyond the basement membrane of TDLUs to an extent less than or equal to 1 mm. Microinvasion is usually seen in association with high-grade DCIS. In this setting, the presence of a dense periductal stromal reaction and periductal lymphoplasmacytic infiltration should prompt the pathologist to search for foci of microinvasion that occur as single cells or small clusters infiltrating outside the confines of TDLUs (e-Figs. 18.48 and 18.49). The focus of invasion should be obvious and care should be taken to avoid interpretation of DCIS involving the lobules (so-called cancerization of lobules), or DCIS involving sclerosing lesions, as microinvasion. In this setting, immunostains for myoepithelial markers and examination of deeper levels of the block can be extremely helpful. If there are multiple foci of microinvasion, the number of foci and the size of the largest focus should be noted; separate individual foci of microinvasion should not be added together.

b. **Neuroendocrine carcinomas** of the breast are morphologically and immunophenotypically similar to neuroendocrine tumors of the lung and GI tract. The majority of primary neuroendocrine carcinomas of the breast are mucinous and solid papillary carcinomas, but well-differentiated neuroendocrine tumors and poorly differentiated small cell carcinomas can occur as well. A metastasis from another source (such as lung and GI tract) should be clinically excluded.

c. **Secretory carcinoma** is an extremely rare tumor accounting for 0.1% to 0.2% cases of invasive breast cancers. The tumor is known to have a favorable prognosis in children and young adults but manifests an aggressive course in older patients. Histologically, it is composed of clusters of tumor cells in microcystic, solid, or tubular architecture with thick PAS-positive intracellular and extracellular secretions and low-grade nuclear atypia. The tumor cells are usually negative for ER, PR, and HER-2, but are positive for S-100 and Mammaglobin (e-**Fig. 18.50**). They harbor the characteristic t(12;15) balanced translocation resulting in an *ETV6-NTRK3* fusion gene.

d. **AdCC** is a rare variant of breast carcinoma accounting for less than 0.1% of cases. Histologically, it is similar to its salivary gland counterpart with epithelial and myoepithelial cells arranged in tubular or cribriform architecture. The neoplastic cells polarize around true glandular spaces and pseudolumina. The true glandular spaces are surrounded by epithelial cells and contain neutral PAS-positive mucin, while pseudolumina result from invaginations of the myxoid Alcian blue positive stromal substance which is surrounded by basal-myoepithelial cells (e-**Fig. 18.51**). By immunohistochemistry, basaloid cells are positive for p63, calponin, and high-molecular-weight keratin, while luminal cells are positive for CD117, CK-7, and CK 8/18. The tumor is generally negative for ER, PR, and HER2, and similar to its salivary gland counterpart, has the characteristic t(6;9)(q22–23;p23–24) translocation. This tumor carries an overall good prognosis with an overall 10-year survival of >90%.

e. **Clear cell/glycogen-rich carcinoma** is composed of a tumor in which >90% of the neoplastic cells have abundant clear cytoplasm. The tumor cells have sharply defined cell borders with polygonal contours and clear cytoplasm (e-**Fig. 18.52**), which contains PAS-positive, diastase-resistant glycogen. Approximately 50% of the tumors are ER positive. This tumor has a prognosis comparable to IDC, NST when tumor grade and stage are comparable.

f. **Carcinoma with apocrine differentiation** is seen in approximately 4% of breast carcinomas. Morphologically, the tumor cells show finely granular eosinophilic cytoplasm, enlarged vesicular chromatin, and prominent nucleoli (e-**Fig. 18.16**), or abundant foamy cytoplasm. The tumor is usually ER/PR negative and androgen receptor (AR) positive while HER2 is overexpressed in roughly half of the cases. Prognosis of these tumors is dependent on the tumor grade and stage.

g. **Inflammatory carcinoma** is a clinical-pathologic entity characterized by diffuse erythema, induration, and tenderness of breast skin associated with nonpitting edema (*peau d'orange*) involving one-third or more of the skin of breast. A breast mass may or may not be evident. Histologically, there is extensive dermal lymphatic invasion by tumor emboli, which is thought to be the underlying mechanism for the clinical picture. A tissue diagnosis is necessary to demonstrate invasive carcinoma in the underlying breast tissue. The presence of dermal lymphatic tumor emboli without the skin changes does not qualify as inflammatory carcinoma.

V. **PATHOLOGY OF TREATED INVASIVE BREAST CANCER.** Neoadjuvant chemotherapy and radiation are increasingly being used in the management of breast cancer, and so it is important to be familiar with radiation-induced changes in normal breast to avoid interpreting them as malignant or premalignant disease. Likewise, familiarity with chemotherapy/radiation-induced changes in tumors is required to evaluate response to treatment.

Posttreatment changes in normal breast tissue usually include lobular atrophy, hyalinization, and nuclear atypia with other nuclear and cytoplasmic degenerative changes. Response to treatment is often categorized clinically as complete, partial, or no response, and is a strong prognostic factor for disease-free and overall survival. During gross examination, careful attention to identifying and evaluating the tumor bed is necessary. In addition, exhaustive sampling of the tumor bed region is necessary before making a diagnosis of complete treatment response. Treatment may affect the morphology of the primary tumor and lymph nodes involved by metastatic disease and produce various histologic changes in tumor morphology including necrosis, chronic inflammation, foamy histiocytic collections, decreased cellularity, cytoplasmic eosinophilia, nuclear alterations, fibrosis, and hemosiderin deposition (e-Figs. 18.53 to 18.55). The detailed morphologic features of postneoadjuvant treated tumor have been described (*Surg Pathol* 2012;5:749). Invasive carcinomas with a minor response may show little change in size; with greater degrees of response, the carcinoma shows decreased cellularity or may show multiple foci of invasion scattered over a larger tumor bed. When evaluating treated carcinomas, the volume of the tumor is determined by the largest focus of contiguous tumor and/or the number of foci involved over the tumor bed, not by the area of tumor bed. Most carcinomas are of the same grade after treatment, but in some cases a change in the grade of tumor occurs. Changes in biomarker status rarely occur after treatment and in most cases are attributed to technical issues in the immunohistochemistry protocol. Many systems have been developed for grading of pathologic response to treatment (*Breast* 2003;12:320; *J Clin Oncol* 2007;25:4414; *Surg Pathol* 2018;11: 213).

Lymph nodes with treatment response usually show fibrous scarring and foamy histiocytic aggregates in the place of previous tumor (complete response), or may show small tumor deposits within an area of fibrosis. A lymph node with complete response should not be reported as "positive for carcinoma."

VI. NONINVASIVE CARCINOMA.
Noninvasive carcinomas have historically been divided into two major categories: ductal and lobular, based on the misconception that they arise from ducts versus lobules, respectively. However, now it is recognized that both of these lesions arise from TDLUs.

A. DCIS encompasses a heterogeneous group of lesions with highly variable clinical presentations, histologic findings, biomarker profiles, genetic abnormalities, and clinical potential. They have in common a monoclonal proliferation of neoplastic epithelial cells confined to the ductal-lobular system, typically in a segmental distribution, without extension through the basement membrane. DCIS is a nonobligate precursor of invasive cancer. It expands and unfolds TDLUs, and it may grow into larger ducts or into adjacent lobules, giving an appearance referred to as cancerization of lobules, or it may even grow further and expand into spheres, a source of the misnomer "ductal" carcinoma. The most common clinical presentation of DCIS is as calcifications seen on mammogram (e-Figs. 18.56 and 18.57) although up to 30% of detected DCIS is not associated with calcifications; in this latter scenario, DCIS is seen as densities and architectural distortions on a mammogram. Less commonly DCIS may present as a mass.

Grossly, most cases of DCIS are not visible. If palpable, they may form a mass with cords of tissue extruding a paste-like material from their cut surfaces (a gross correlation to the material seen on histologic sections as comedonecrosis, see below). Morphologically, DCIS is seen as proliferation of neoplastic cells with variable nuclear cytology, and in a variety of growth patterns which usually grow over and obliterate the luminal space of the ducts and TDLUs. High-grade DCIS may incite a desmoplastic stromal response mixed with chronic inflammation which raises the concern for invasive breast cancer (e-Fig. 18.58). Myoepithelial markers may be useful in such cases as they highlight the myoepithelial layer, thus providing evidence that proliferation has not yet breached the ductal-lobular system. DCIS may become displaced during previous needle biopsy, leading to carcinoma within a biopsy tract that may be confused with invasive breast cancer in the subsequent excisional specimen. DCIS may show a variety of morphologies including apocrine (e-Figs. 18.59 and 18.60) and clear cell (e-Fig. 18.61) differentiation. While familiarity with these morphologic patterns is helpful in recognizing the lesion, most of these morphologic variants do not bear clinical significance independent of their nuclear grade.

For clinical purposes, a few prognostic and/or diagnostic characteristics of in situ carcinomas should be reported in a pathology report. This information may affect the clinical decision making.

1. **Size/extent.** If the lesion is only present on one slide, microscopic measurement of the focus of DCIS will be the most accurate measurement. If the lesion is present on multiple slides, the most accurate measurement is achieved by correlating the microscopic sections containing DCIS with the gross diagram of the breast specimen showing location and relationship of different sections within the specimen (**e-Appendix 18.2**). By correlating the two, an estimate of the size of the lesion can be provided. In rare cases where an accurate size estimate cannot be given, extent of the lesion can be reported as the fraction of slides involved by DCIS.

2. **Nuclear grade.** Based on nuclear features, DCIS is classified into three grades by SBR criteria: low, intermediate, or high-grade (Table 18.4). Low-grade DCIS consists of a proliferation of small, monomorphic, and evenly spaced luminal epithelial cells with homogeneous chromatin distribution and inconspicuous nucleoli. Mitotic counts are usually low (**e-Fig. 18.62**). In contrast, high-grade DCIS consists of a proliferation of highly pleomorphic, less-organized epithelial cells with vesicular or coarse chromatin and prominent/multiple nucleoli. Mitotic counts are high, apoptotic cells are frequent, and comedonecrosis (defined as calcified necrosis in the center of the proliferation) is common (**e-Figs. 18.58 to 18.60, e-Fig. 18.63**). Intermediate-grade carcinomas are lesions with features that fall in between high-grade and low-grade carcinomas (**e-Fig. 18.64**). However, as with invasive carcinomas, DCIS commonly contain areas of multiple histologic grades (*Clin Cancer Res* 2008;14:370).

3. **Growth pattern.** DCIS is extremely diverse histologically, both with respect to nuclear grade and architecture. A variety of different growth patterns can be recognized, although commonly more than one growth pattern is present within a given lesion (**e-Figs. 18.65 and 18.66**). The most common growth patterns include solid, papillary, micropapillary, and cribriform (sieve-like) architectural patterns.

   a. **In the cribriform growth pattern**, the neoplastic cells form punched out spaces with round and rigid extracellular lumens formed by neoplastic cells polarizing around the spaces (**e-Figs. 18.67 and 18.68**).

   b. **The micropapillary growth pattern** is manifested by a proliferation of tufts of neoplastic cells projecting into the lumen of TDLUs. These tufts are characterized

TABLE 18.4 The Criteria for Nuclear Grading of DCIS

	Grade 1 (low)	Grade 2 (intermediate)	Grade 3 (high)
Nuclear pleomorphism	Monotonous	intermediate	markedly pleomorphic
Nuclear size	1.5–2 times the size of a red blood cell or normal ductal-epithelial nucleus	Intermediate	2.5 times the size of red blood cell or normal ductal epithelial nuclei
Chromatin distribution	Diffuse, finely dispersed	Intermediate	Vesicular, irregular chromatin distribution
Nucleoli	Occasional	Intermediate	Prominent, multiple
Mitoses	Occasional	Intermediate	May be frequent
Orientation	Polarized toward the luminal spaces	Intermediate	Not polarized toward luminal spaces

by a lack of fibrovascular cores, a club-shaped end, and proliferation of a mono-morphic, evenly distributed cell population (e-**Figs. 18.69** to **18.71**).

c. **The solid growth pattern** is characterized by a proliferation of sheets of mono-morphic, cohesive cells that fill the lumen of TDLUs. These cells may form pseudorosettes or microacini with polarization of surrounding cells (e-**Figs. 18.72** and **18.73**).

d. **The clinging growth pattern** is recognized by some experts as a distinct growth pattern. It is characterized by a duct lined by a few layers of highly atypical neoplastic cells at the periphery and filled by abundant comedonecrosis (e-**Fig. 18.74**). Some experts consider this growth pattern as a variation of the solid growth pattern with extensive necrosis.

e. **Papillary DCIS** consists of a papillary proliferation characterized by branching fibrovascular cores covered by a monotonous epithelial proliferation showing mild to moderate nuclear atypia (e-**Figs. 18.75** and **18.76**). In contrast to benign papillomas, papillary DCIS has no invested myoepithelial layer (e-**Figs. 18.77** to **18.79**) as demonstrated by a lack of staining with myoepithelial markers such as p63 and calponin. Some markers such as smooth muscle actin (SMA) can highlight the myoepithelial cells, but they can also stain the vascular walls within the fibrovascular cores of papillary DCIS, which should not be overinterpreted as evidence of a myoepithelial layer.

f. **Intracystic papillary carcinoma** (IPC) is considered by most experts as a variant of DCIS that consists of proliferation of monomorphic neoplastic cells within an expanded enlarged cystic space with an outer fibrotic wall (e-**Figs. 18.80** and **18.81**). The intracystic tumor usually shows scattered fibrovascular cores lined by atypical epithelial cells that are not supported by a myoepithelial layer (e-**Figs. 18.82** to **18.84**). Various architectural growth patterns of DCIS, including micro-papillary, cribriform, and solid, may be present within the lesion. Care must be taken to avoid overinterpretation of malignant cells in the fibrous wall as a result of distortion of the wall secondary to fibrosis, or at the site of previous core biopsy, as the criteria for invasive carcinoma require the cells to be outside of the fibrous wall (e-**Fig. 18.85**). The presence of adjacent hemorrhage or hemosiderin-laden macrophages can be a helpful clue to the presence of displaced tumor cells secondary to previous biopsy.

4. **Extent of comedonecrosis.** Comedonecrosis can be seen in any grade DCIS but more commonly is seen in high-grade lesions, and is characterized by calcified necrosis within the center of a duct which is involved by DCIS (e-**Fig. 18.58**). Some studies have shown that abundant comedonecrosis is associated with increased local recurrence following lumpectomy for DCIS.

5. **Skin involvement** (Paget disease). Paget disease of the nipple can be seen when neoplastic cells percolate through the underlying lactiferous ducts to the epithelium without breaching the basement membrane. It is usually associated with underlying high-grade DCIS (e-**Fig. 18.86**). It is important to distinguish the Paget cells within nipple squamous epithelium from other clear cells that occasionally can be seen within the nipple, mainly Toker cells. Toker cells are incidentally found clear cells within the nipple, which are smaller in size compared to Paget cells and do not show significant atypia. A HER2 immunohistochemical stain can be useful in difficult cases, as the cells of Paget disease are positive for HER2 while Toker cells are negative (*Histopathol* 2009;24:367).

6. **Surgical margin status** is of particular importance and has an inverse relationship with the incidence of local recurrence. Since DCIS usually is not grossly visible, margins should be microscopically examined, and the location of the closest margin and its distance from DCIS should be mentioned in the report. As with invasive carcinoma, a margin is considered positive only if carcinoma is present at the inked margin. The extent of involved margin (focal, multifocal, extensive) should be reported. If in situ carcinoma is mixed with invasive carcinoma, the volume of in

situ carcinoma in the tumor (reported as the fraction of total tumor) should be mentioned, as extensive DCIS mixed with invasive carcinoma has a higher rate of local recurrence, particularly when DCIS is close to or present at the margins.

7. Presence of associated microcalcifications should be noted, as DCIS that is first detected by microcalcifications will frequently recur with calcifications.

8. Biomarker status. Assessment of ER/PR status is an essential factor in the evaluation of DCIS for adjuvant hormonal therapy. Although ER/PR status can provide prognostic information, their major clinical value is to assess the likelihood of response to hormonal therapy (see below).

B. Lobular Neoplasia. This term refers to the entire spectrum of atypical epithelial proliferations arising in TDLUs composed of loosely cohesive uniform cells with small nuclei and indistinct nucleoli, which expand TDLUs and grow in a pagetoid fashion underneath the epithelial layer. Traditionally LCIS and atypical lobular hyperplasia only differ in the degree of involvement and expansion of the lobules; however, most authorities now consider such lobular proliferations under the rubric of "lobular neoplasia" or "lobular intraepithelial neoplasia." Many studies show that there is a direct relationship between the extent of the disease and risk of developing IBC.

1. Lobular carcinoma in situ (LCIS) is characterized by a neoplastic proliferation of small, loosely cohesive, uniform cells with homogeneous chromatin and inconspicuous nucleoli. The cells may contain intracytoplasmic vacuoles containing eosinophilic mucin globules (**e-Figs. 18.87** and **18.88**). The proliferating cells fill (and often distend) most of the lobules (greater than 50%) in the involved TDLUs. Although pagetoid extension of neoplastic cells into the major ductal system is usually seen with LCIS, it can also be seen in association with DCIS; such extension undermines the normal epithelial layer and produces a clover leaf–like appearance (**e-Figs. 18.89** and **18.90**). Differentiating LCIS from intermediate and high-grade DCIS is usually straightforward. However, distinguishing LCIS from low-grade DCIS, particularly with a solid growth pattern, can be challenging. In contrast to solid LG-DCIS, the cells of LCIS are usually small and discohesive, and often display intracytoplasmic lumina. The loss of membranous expression of E-cadherin protein by immunohistochemistry has been recognized to be characteristic of lobular carcinoma (cytoplasmic expression may still be evident) (**e-Fig. 18.91**), and retention of expression is characteristic of ductal carcinoma. However, about 10% to 15% of cases of lobular carcinomas retain E-cadherin expression and a minority of ductal carcinomas lose E-cadherin expression; therefore, the two should be distinguished mainly on histologic grounds (*Am J Surg Pathol* 2010;34:1472). Most cases of classic LCIS are managed by steroid hormone receptor antagonists, and most data in the literature do not support re-excision for LCIS present at the surgical margins. In cases where LCIS is diagnosed on core biopsy material and there is sufficient radiologic–pathologic correlation, an excisional biopsy is not recommended.

2. Pleomorphic LCIS is a morphologically distinct variant of LCIS which shares with classic LCIS distension of the TDLUs by discohesive malignant cells; however, as the name indicates, it is composed of poorly differentiated cells with significant nuclear pleomorphism that show nuclear enlargement (greater than 4 times the size of a lymphocyte), 2- to 3-fold nuclear size variation, nuclear membrane irregularity, and prominent nucleoli. Central comedonecrosis and calcifications may be observed (**e-Fig. 18.92**). The main differential diagnosis for pleomorphic LCIS is intermediate or high-grade DCIS, a differential confounded by the not infrequent presence of central comedo-like necrosis in all these lesions. The discohesive nature of neoplastic cells can be very useful in confirming the diagnosis. Similar to classic LCIS, pleomorphic LCIS can also spread along the duct system in a pagetoid fashion. Given the clinical, radiologic, and pathologic similarities of pleomorphic LCIS to DCIS, including the frequent extension into larger ducts, it is managed in a manner similar to DCIS; nevertheless, it is still important to correctly identify pleomorphic LCIS due to the occasional coexistence of ILC that can be focal and quite subtle (e-Fig. 18.28), especially on needle biopsy. In such difficult cases the use of E-cadherin can be potentially useful (*Future Oncol* 2009;5:233). Intraepithelial macrophages can mimic lobular neoplasia; however, microscopic examination at higher magnification can resolve any uncertainty (e-Fig. 18.93).

VII. **THE ROLE OF BIOMARKERS IN BREAST CANCER.** The role of biomarkers in establishing the prognosis and the management of patients with breast cancer cannot be overemphasized. Established biomarkers such as ER and PR have been used both as prognostic factors and predictors of response to endocrine therapy in patients with breast cancer. More recently, human epidermal growth factor receptor 2 (HER2) was added to this list as a prognostic factor (marker of poor outcome), and as a predictor of response to certain chemotherapeutic regimens including trastuzumab (a monoclonal antibody against the HER2 receptor). Currently, evaluation of these biomarkers in patients with invasive carcinoma is considered standard of care. Additional biomarkers have changed breast cancer treatment in the past decade and to some extent have enabled providing individualized therapies to different molecular subgroups. The shift toward an earlier diagnosis of breast cancer due to improved imaging methods and screening programs highlights the need for biomarker discovery to quantify the residual risk of patients to indicate the potential value of novel treatment strategies. With the introduction of high-throughput technologies, numerous multigene signatures have been identified that have the potential to outperform traditional markers (*Endocrine-Related Cancer* 2010;17:R245).

A. **Estrogen and Progesterone Receptors.** The ER belongs to a family of nuclear hormone receptors that function as transcription factors when they are bound to their respective ligands. ERs and PRs are parts of complex signaling pathways which interact with multiple survival and proliferation pathways in the cell and play a critical role in the development and progression of breast cancer. They have proven usefulness as prognostic factors, and more importantly as predictive factors, in the clinical management of breast cancer. There is growing evidence that patients with endocrine-responsive breast cancers benefit less from adjuvant chemotherapy.

Assessment of ER and PR status is an important task in the evaluation of breast cancer and is mandated in every primary carcinoma, as well as metastatic tumors if the result could influence decision making. Approximately 70% to 80% of breast carcinomas are ER/PR positive. Immunohistochemistry is the first-line attempt in evaluating hormone receptor status, although it can be highly affected by a variety of preanalytic factors, including time of tissue fixation and the antigen retrieval method (*J Clin Oncol* 2010;28:2784). The expression of PR is strongly dependent on the presence of ER and is reflective of a functioning ER pathway. Tumors expressing PR but not the ER are uncommon and represent less than 1% of all breast cancer cases in some large series; therefore, re-testing of the ER status in this setting is recommended to eliminate false ER negativity. In rare cases of solely PR-positive tumors, the patients still benefit from endocrine therapy. Recently, quantitative methods using RNA-based assays (see below) have been established for ER and PR quantification. These quantitative assays have potential advantages compared with IHC methods and may become the assays of choice in the future.

Several studies have shown excellent concordance rates between the evaluation of biomarkers on needle core tissue and subsequent excision specimens (*Acta Oncol* 2008;47:38; *Ann Oncol* 2009;20:1948; *Clin Breast Cancer* 2010;10:154; *Cancer Sci* 2010;101:2074). Because of better fixation of the needle core tissue, and the potential for guiding subsequent therapy, immunohistochemical assessment of hormone receptors and HER2 status is best performed on needle biopsy material if available. In cases of negative hormone receptors on core biopsy material, re-evaluation of the excisional specimen may be warranted to exclude a negative result due to tumor heterogeneity. To minimize the effect of preanalytic variables on test results, the American Society of Clinical Oncology/College of American Pathologists (ASCO/CAP) recommended using only 10% NBF as a fixative and controlling the formalin fixation time between 6 and 72 hours.

The American Society of Clinical Oncology/College of American Pathologists (ASCO/CAP) has also recommended an algorithmic approach to assess hormonal status. In order to standardize immunohistochemical evaluation of breast carcinoma, several scoring systems incorporating both intensity and percentage of staining have been established. In general, in order to obtain benefit from hormonal treatment, a sample should demonstrate nuclear staining in at least 1% of tumor cells (**e-Fig. 18.94**) (*J Clin Oncol* 2010;28:2784).

B. **Human Epidermal Growth Factor Receptor 2 (HER2).** ERBB2 protein is a receptor tyrosine kinase which is a member of the epidermal growth factor receptor (EGFR) family of tyrosine kinase proteins; it is a membrane protein that is expressed in all epithelial cells at low levels. The *HER2/neu* oncogene that encodes ERBB2 is involved in the regulation of cell proliferation, survival, motility, and invasion, and is overexpressed in about 20% of breast cancers. ERBB2 amplification is an independent prognostic marker of poor outcome in the absence of adjuvant treatment and has been associated with an increased rate of metastasis, decreased time to recurrence, and decreased overall survival. As a predictive marker, it has been associated with responsiveness to anthracycline-based therapy and trastuzumab. Immunohistochemistry and in situ hybridization are the most common methods to evaluate HER2 status; they determine protein overexpression and gene amplification, respectively. Immunohistochemistry is a simple, rapid, and inexpensive method to assess HER2 protein overexpression on formalin fixed tissues, and as noted above the American Society of Clinical Oncology/College of American Pathologists (ASCO/CAP) has recommended an algorithmic approach whereby cases are initially tested by immunohistochemistry. Positive for overexpression (3+) is characterized by a uniform, intense membranous staining of more than 10% of invasive tumor cells (**e-Fig. 18.95**). A negative result is an IHC staining of 0, defined by lack of any membranous staining, or 1+, weak partial membranous staining (**e-Fig. 18.96**). Equivocal results (2+) are defined as complete membranous staining that is either non-uniform or weak in intensity but with obvious circumferential distribution in at least 10% of invasive tumor cells (**e-Fig. 18.97**), or intense complete membranous staining of 10% or fewer of tumor cells. As with hormone receptors, tissue handling, fixation, and processing can greatly affect immunoreactivity of tissue samples; however, well-calibrated immunohistochemistry can identify the majority of cases as positive or negative. According to this algorithmic approach, indeterminate IHC results (2+) are evaluated by fluorescence in situ hybridization (FISH) to determine gene amplification status (**e-Fig. 18.98**) (*Arch Pathol Lab Med* 2007;131:18; *Arch Pathol Lab Med* 2009;133:775) (since the initial guidelines were published, chromogenic in situ hybridization [CISH] has also been approved by the FDA for the same purpose). There should be a high concordance rate (above 95%) between ERBB2 protein overexpression by immunohistochemistry and gene amplification by FISH/CISH.

C. **Other Immunohistochemical Prognostic Markers.** Among other markers, proliferation markers such as Ki67/MIB1 have been used as markers of poor outcome. Ki-67 is reported as the percentage of tumor cell nuclei that are positive; however, the lack of standardized methodology and specific cut-off values limit its value. *TP53* tumor suppressor gene mutation has also been associated with a worse outcome. Neither test has been recommended as a prognostic marker for routine use.

D. **Multiparameter-Based Markers.** Recent expression profiling studies of breast cancer have indicated the existence of at least four molecularly distinct types of breast cancer, which may originate from different cell types (*Nature* 2000;406:747). These subtypes differ with regard to their patterns of gene expression, clinical features, response to treatment, and outcome, and are termed luminal A, luminal B, HER2, and basal-like.

Luminal A and B cancers (accounting for approximately 70% of breast cancers) are characterized by expression of ER. They also express cytokeratins 8 and 18, typical of the mammary gland. Luminal A tumors are mostly histologically low grade, while luminal B tumors tend to be of higher grade; in general, compared with other subtypes, they have a better prognosis. Some of luminal B cancers may overexpress HER2. Both luminal A and B cancers tend to respond to hormonal therapy, but luminal B cancers show a better response to chemotherapeutic agents than luminal A.

HER2-associated cancers (accounting for 15% of breast cancers) show high expression of HER2 and low expression of ER and ER-regulated genes. They are usually ER- and PR-negative and are more likely to be high grade and involve axillary lymph nodes.

Basal-like cancers show high expression of basal epithelial genes (basal cytokeratins such as CK 5/6 and CK 17) and low expression of ER, PR, and HER2 genes, the reason for calling these tumors triple-negative carcinomas. This subtype is especially common in African-American women, has a poor prognosis, and is the most common phenotype in *BRCA1*-associated breast cancers. These tumors are not amenable to treatment by endocrine therapy or trastuzumab (*Nature* 2000;406:747).

These results demonstrate that although breast cancer shows significant heterogeneity, from a biologic point of view many tumors can be classified into particular groups based on genetic similarities, with gene signatures that correlate with clinical outcome and response to chemotherapy. Based on genomic profiling data, several genomic tests have been developed with the intent of providing even stronger prognostic information. A 70-gene signature has been developed to predict the risk of recurrence within 5 years in node-negative, ER-positive or -negative patients; this test is able to accurately classify tumors into good or poor prognostic categories (*Nature* 2002;415:530; *N Engl J Med* 2002;347:1999), is performed on fresh frozen tissue or formalin-fixed tissue, and is FDA approved for clinical use as a prognostic test. Similarly, a 21-gene signature assay has been designed to predict the risk of distant recurrence in patients with ER-positive early breast cancer (stages I and II) who are receiving tamoxifen; it also predicts the benefit from chemotherapy treatment in node-negative, ER-positive patients. This test is done on formalin-fixed paraffin-embedded tissue and is based on real-time PCR measurement of the expression of 16 genes with known significance in breast cancer; the results are used to calculate a recurrence score (RS) that is predictive of overall survival independent of age and tumor size, which classifies patients into groups with a low (<10%), intermediate (10% to 30%), or high (>30%) risk of 10-year distant recurrence. Another 76-gene assay has been developed for use on node-negative breast cancers (*New Eng J Med* 2009;360:790; *PNAS* 2003;100:10393; *Expert Rev Mol Diagn* 2004;4:169); the 76 genes used in this assay do not overlap with the genes used in 70-gene or 21-gene assays.

Of note, the latest edition of AJCC Cancer staging manual has incorporated tumor-grade, ER, PR, and HER2 biomarker results into tumor staging algorithm to provide further prognostic information by assigning tumors to "Prognostic Stage Groups." For some subsets (ER-positive, HER2-negative, node-negative) breast carcinomas, incorporation of multigene panel assays has also been advocated.

VIII. INTRADUCTAL PROLIFERATIVE LESIONS

A. Intraductal proliferative lesions that **carry an increased risk** include atypical ductal hyperplasia (ADH) and atypical lobule hyperplasia.

1. **ADH** is a term used to describe an intraductal proliferation with some of the cytologic and/or architectural features of low-grade DCIS, which qualitatively or quantitatively falls short of diagnosis of DCIS. Examples of ADH include a duct partially involved by a uniform cell population resembling LG-DCIS (e-Figs. 18.99 and 18.100), or a duct that is focally expanded by a uniform cell population with geometric spaces (e-Figs. 18.101 and 18.102). Quantitatively, there are a variety of arbitrary criteria for distinction of ADH from LG-DCIS (for example, the duct is <2 mm in diameter, or <2 duct spaces are involved) (*Hum Pathol* 1992;23:1095; *Am J Surg Pathol* 1992;16:1133); however, although there is agreement on the importance of the extent of the lesion, there are no widely accepted size cut-offs (e-Fig. 18.103). While a diagnosis of DCIS confers a 10-fold risk of later developing IBC, and ADH confers a 4- to 5-fold risk, they are both on a continuum of the same neoplastic process. A diagnosis of ADH made on a core needle biopsy is usually followed by excision, as studies have shown that depending on the technique of the biopsy and size of the

needle, a follow-up excision is associated with an in situ or invasive carcinoma in 20% to 40% of these cases (*Breast* 2011;20:50; *Adv Anat Pathol* 2003;10:113). It should be noted that a diagnosis of ADH is only conferred to lesions with low-grade nuclear cytology; intermediate and high-grade DCIS should be diagnosed as such regardless of their size.

2. **Atypical lobular hyperplasia (ALH)** differs from LCIS in regard to the degree of lobular involvement and expansion (e-**Figs. 18.104** to **18.106**). ALH and LCIS are also on a continuum of the same neoplastic process. While ALH is associated with 6-fold increased risk of invasive carcinoma, LCIS is associated with 12-fold increase in risk.

B. Several intraductal proliferative lesions **do not carry an increased risk.**

1. **Usual ductal hyperplasia** (UDH) is characterized by proliferation of a heterogeneous epithelial cell population with a tendency to bridge across, fill, and distend duct lumens. Haphazard placement of cells of variable size and shape (both epithelial and myoepithelial), variable spacing of the cells often with prominent streaming and/or swirling, indistinct cell borders, and irregular and usually peripheral secondary spaces are all features of UDH that distinguish it from low-grade DCIS (e-**Fig. 18.107**). Bridges formed in UDH are usually not rigid, and show stretching with central attenuation. Immunohistochemically, UDH is usually positive for high-molecular-weight keratin (e-**Fig. 18.108**) unlike most examples of DCIS. UDH is not a direct precursor of breast cancer; however, if florid, it is a marker of low increased risk of breast cancer (1.5- to 2-fold). UDH is usually not acted upon clinically.

2. **Columnar cell lesions (CCLs).** The enlargement of normal TDLUs by hyperplastic epithelial cells is one of the most common abnormalities of growth in the adult female human breast (*Adv Anat Pathol* 2003;10:113; *Semin Diagn Pathol* 2004;21:18; *Histopathology* 2008;52:11; *Am J Pathol* 2007;171:252). These lesions have been called by many names over the years (*Semin Diagn Pathol* 2004;21:18), but currently they are most commonly referred to as CCLs or columnar cell hyperplasia (CCH). CCHs are often multifocal, bilateral, and up to 100-fold larger than the TDLUs they evolve from. The majority of CCLs are lined by one or two layers of monotonous, crowded columnar epithelial cells (e-**Figs. 18.109** to **18.111**), but many exhibit more diverse histologic features contributing to the complex terminology that has evolved to describe them.

It is currently unknown whether the cytologic atypia occasionally observed in CCLs is associated with significantly higher risk for developing breast cancer than the majority of cases that are without atypia, although in some preliminary studies up to 20% of cases with atypia identified on core biopsies are associated with cancer in follow-up excisions, a worrisome association that has led some authors to advocate follow-up excisions in this setting (*Histopathology* 2008;52:11; *Am J Surg Pathol* 2005;29:734). However, not all studies find a significant relationship between CCH with atypia and cancer. Current guidelines recommend clinical and radiologic follow-up in cases with concordant radiology–pathology correlation where the radiologic abnormality has been excised on core biopsy material.

IX. **COMMON BENIGN ABNORMALITIES.** The breast can be involved by a large number of benign abnormalities. While these findings do not harbor clinical importance in terms of breast cancer risk, they must be distinguished from clinically significant abnormalities.

A. **Fat Necrosis.** Although fat necrosis can result from trauma, most cases are idiopathic, or are secondary to prior surgery or radiotherapy. It can clinically and mammographically mimic invasive carcinoma. Histologically, a cellular inflammatory response composed of foamy macrophages and foreign body giant cells is seen infiltrating the fat (e-**Figs. 18.112** and **18.113**). In later stages, fibrosis and dystrophic calcification may be seen.

B. **Duct Ectasia** usually presents in middle-aged women as pain and nipple discharge, with or without an associated mass lesion. It is characterized by dilation of the major duct system, often with luminal amorphous material and complete filling and distention by intraepithelial foamy macrophages (e-**Fig. 18.114**). There is usually associated fibrosis and periductal chronic inflammation.

C. Microcysts With Apocrine Changes. Cystic dilation of the breast TDLUs (as opposed to the major duct system in duct ectasia) is quite common and can produce marked expansion and, especially when associated with microcalcification or fibrosis, can result in mammographically detectable and/or palpable lesions. Histologically, these cysts are usually lined by flat nonatypical epithelium (e-**Fig. 18.115**). Apocrine metaplasia is a very common change that occurs in these cystic lesions (as well as normal TDLUs), usually as an incidental finding; it is usually found in premenopausal women and is often part of so-called fibrocystic changes. Histologically, apocrine change is characterized by eosinophilic cells with abundant finely granular cytoplasm and rounded nuclei, often with a prominent nucleolus (e-**Fig. 18.116**). A papillary architecture is sometimes evident.

D. Fibroadenoma is a very common benign lesion of the breast that presents as a mass or radiographic abnormality, more commonly in younger women. On mammogram, it usually presents as a round, well-circumscribed mass. Grossly, fibroadenomas are grayish-white, firm, well-circumscribed, lobulated masses. Histologically, they are composed of a biphasic growth of variably cellular spindle-cell stroma with cleft-like (intracanalicular) (e-**Fig. 18.117**) or tubular glandular (pericanalicular) (e-**Fig. 18.118**) growth patterns. The glandular elements are composed of two cell layers: an inner epithelial layer and an outer myoepithelial cell layer (e-**Figs. 18.119** and **18.120**). Some fibroadenomas, especially those arising in the second decade of life, can grow rapidly and appear quite cellular (an appearance that overlaps with benign phyllodes tumor); such lesions have been termed cellular fibroadenomas. Myxoid fibroadenomas display prominent myxoid changes in the stroma and rarely may be a component of Carney syndrome (primary adrenocortical hypercortisolism, skin hyperpigmentation, and a variety of nonendocrine and endocrine tumors). Fibroadenomas may undergo secondary changes such as infarction or prominent hyalinization of the stroma (e-**Fig. 18.121**), with or without calcification (the former is usually seen with pregnancy, whereas the latter is more often seen in elderly patients with a longstanding lesion). In addition, almost all of the epithelial changes that arise in the breast can secondarily develop in fibroadenomas including various metaplasias, epithelial hyperplasia, sclerosing adenosis, DCIS, LCIS, and invasive carcinoma (e-**Figs. 18.122** and **18.123**). Fibroadenomas with epithelial proliferation, sclerosing adenosis, or large cysts have been termed complex fibroadenomas. The main differential diagnosis of fibroadenoma is a benign phyllodes tumor.

Phyllodes tumor is much less common than fibroadenoma, accounting for <3% of fibroepithelial lesions. The main feature distinguishing phyllodes tumor from fibroadenoma is the presence of a characteristic leaf-like architectural pattern produced by extensive branching of the epithelial component. Stromal heterogeneity and hypercellularity is the rule, often with accentuation near the epithelial clefts. Phyllodes tumor can be divided into benign (e-**Fig. 18.124**), borderline (e-**Fig. 18.125**), and malignant (e-**Fig. 18.126**) categories; the first two are only distinguished by the degree of cellular atypia and mitotic activity. A focally infiltrative border can be seen in borderline phyllodes tumor. Malignant phyllodes tumor shows a prominent infiltrative border, unequivocal sarcomatous areas, and stromal overgrowth (areas of stroma devoid of epithelium). Heterologous sarcomatous elements may also be occasionally present in malignant tumors. Overall, about 20% of phyllodes tumors recur (ranging from 17% for benign tumors to 27% for malignant tumors) and 10% metastasize (0%, 4%, and 22% of benign, borderline, and malignant tumors, respectively).

E. Intraductal Papillomas usually show an arborizing growth pattern of fibrovascular cores covered by two layers of cells, one layer of myoepithelial cells with an overlying layer of nonatypical epithelial cells (e-**Figs. 18.127** to **18.129**). Intraductal papillomas are generally categorized into two groups: central papillomas, which are usually solitary papillomas which involve large lactiferous ducts of the nipple; and peripheral papillomas, which are smaller papillomas that involve TDLUs and are usually multiple. Central papillomas generally present as a mass or with nipple discharge. Peripheral papillomas present as incidental findings or sometimes as a mammographic abnormality. Secondary hemorrhagic infarction, squamous or apocrine metaplasia, and extensive sclerosis (sclerosing papilloma) can sometimes be seen (**e-Figs. 18.130** and **18.131**). Intraductal papillomas and related lesions can secondarily be involved by other intraepithelial proliferations including UDH, ADH, DCIS, and LCIS. In the absence of any secondary neoplastic proliferation, primary excision is adequate treatment for papillomas.

F. **Sclerosing Adenosis.** This relatively common lesion is often incidental and admixed with proliferative lesions. However, it can present mammographically with calcification and/or architectural distortion, or clinically as a mass termed "adenosis tumor" or "nodular sclerosing adenosis." Sclerosing adenosis is characterized by a lobulocentric proliferation of tubular glands (adenosis) accompanied by a fibrotic (sclerosing) stromal proliferation (**e-Fig. 18.132**). The fact that the glands/tubules are markedly compressed and often obliterated renders identification of a dual cell layer sometimes difficult (**e-Fig. 18.133**). Accordingly, the main differential diagnosis is invasive (usually tubular) carcinoma, which may be difficult to exclude on small biopsies, especially in areas in which sclerosing adenosis has a pattern mimicking perineural invasion, or is secondarily involved by a neoplastic intraepithelial proliferation such as ADH, DCIS (**e-Figs. 18.134** and **18.135**), or LCIS. Elongated and compressed (as opposed to angulated) tubules, lack of a cellular desmoplastic stroma, and a lobulocentric pattern of growth are useful diagnostic features. If in doubt, immunohistochemical demonstration of myoepithelial cells can additionally exclude an invasive process.

G. **Radial Scar/Complex Sclerosing Lesions** are characterized by a central fibrous/fibroelastotic scar from which a stellate arrangement of benign ducts/lobules radiates (**e-Figs. 18.136** to **18.138**). Associated hyperplastic or neoplastic epithelial proliferations are often identified. In addition to their microscopic pseudoinfiltrative nature, these lesions may also be clinically, radiologically, or grossly confused with invasive carcinoma due to their fibrotic nature and their characteristic stellate/spiculated appearance. Nevertheless, excisional biopsy is still recommended after a diagnosis of radial scar based on a needle biopsy because of the occasional presence of associated unsampled DCIS or invasive carcinoma at the periphery of the lesion.

X. **LYMPH NODE STATUS.** The presence of metastatic tumor deposits in axillary lymph nodes as determined microscopically is a highly unfavorable prognostic feature, as are a high number of involved nodes and (to a lesser degree) a large size of the deposits. Nodal status (N) is so powerful prognostically that it plays a major role in determining therapy.

The pathology report should include the total number of examined lymph nodes, the number of positive lymph nodes, size of metastases, and the presence or absence of extranodal extension by tumor deposits (the presence of extranodal extension is an indicator of tumor recurrence and its presence may dictate additional radiation therapy). According to the AJCC TNM staging system, assessment of the size of metastasis is important in determining the stage: ITCs are clusters of tumor cells smaller than 0.2 mm or less than 200 cells (**e-Fig. 18.139**); micrometastasis is defined as metastatic deposits that measure between 0.2 and 2.0 mm, or greater than 200 cells in one cross-section; macrometastasis is defined as a metastatic focus larger than 2.0 mm. For staging purposes, lymph nodes with a micrometastasis are counted toward total number of positive nodes if at least one lymph node with macrometastasis is present; nodes that only show ITCs should not be counted in the total number of positive nodes. Cancer nodules in axillary tissue without histologic evidence of a classical lymph node are classified as regional lymph node metastasis, unless they are surrounded by breast tissue or DCIS to imply a separate focus of invasive carcinoma.

Histologically, involvement of axillary lymph nodes by metastatic carcinoma is most frequently manifested within the subcapsular sinuses with or without sinusoidal involvement (**e-Figs. 18.140** and **18.141**). However, metastases in ILC most commonly appear as scattered individual tumor cells within the parenchyma and sinusoids. In all of these situations, the size of the largest deposit should be measured and reported.

There are a few pitfalls in the evaluation of axillary lymph nodes for metastatic carcinoma that can lead to overdiagnosis. **Heterotopic epithelial elements** including heterotopic breast tissue are rare findings that can occasionally be seen in axillary lymph nodes (e-Fig. 18.142); the presence of myoepithelial cells and sometimes specialized stroma can be helpful diagnostic features. The heterotopic tissue is subject to all changes that can occur in breast tissue in the mammary gland itself. **Nevus cell aggregates** are capsular aggregates of nevus cells that are infrequently identified in axillary lymph nodes (e-Fig. 18.143); they usually present as nests of epithelioid cells within the lymph node capsule. The diagnosis of nevus aggregates can easily be substantiated by a combination of S-100 and/or HMB45 immunoreactivity and a negative reaction with cytokeratin antibodies.

ACKNOWLEDGMENT

The authors thank Omar Hameed, Josh Warrick, and Craig Allred, authors of the previous edition of this chapter.

Cytology of the Breast

Behzad Salari and Souzan Sanati

I. METHODS OF SPECIMEN PROCUREMENT

A. **FNA** of palpable and nonpalpable breast lesions through mammographic guidance is currently accepted as a cost-effective, reliable, and accurate tool in the primary evaluation of breast lesions. The combination of mammographic features, clinical findings, and cytologic evaluation of breast FNA specimens (the so-called triple test) has considerably decreased the false diagnosis rate of breast cancer.

B. **Ductal Lavage** has been employed as a screening method in women with a personal history of breast cancer, but the sensitivity and accuracy of the approach for detecting premalignant lesions of the breast ductal epithelium has yet to be established (*Clin Lab Med* 2005;25:787; *Am J Surg* 2006;191:57).

II. SPECIMEN ADEQUACY.
There is no uniform criterion (or set of criteria) on which specimen adequacy can be determined, even in the presence of well-preserved and well-visualized breast epithelium (e-Fig. 18.144), without taking into consideration the experience of the aspirator and/or interpreter, clinical presentation, and mammographic findings of the individual mass.

III. DIAGNOSTIC CATEGORIES

A. **Negative for Malignancy.** This diagnosis is generally rendered for benign breast lesions, including inflammatory or infectious lesions that are without clinical or mammographic findings suspicious for malignancy.

B. **Atypical Cytology.** This diagnosis is rendered on cellular lesions showing some degree of nuclear atypia; the cells generally maintain a well-organized pattern (e-Fig. 18.145).

C. **Suspicious for Malignancy.** This diagnosis is rendered when the aspirate shows cells with worrisome cytologic features that fall short of those required for a definitive diagnosis of malignancy.

D. **Positive for Malignancy.** This diagnosis is rendered when both the quality of the cytologic changes and the quantity of the malignant cells are sufficient for an unequivocal diagnosis of malignancy.

IV. CYTOLOGIC FEATURES OF COMMON BREAST LESIONS

A. **Fibroadenoma** is a clinically well-circumscribed nodule with a homogeneous mammographic appearance. Cytologically, it is composed of benign ductal cells arranged in a staghorn pattern with abundant singly dispersed myoepithelial cells (e-Fig. 18.146). Abundant stromal fragments may be seen.

B. **Gynecomastia** is clinically a well-circumscribed and often painful subareolar lesion in a man. The lesion has mammographic and cytologic findings that are similar to those of a fibroadenoma (e-Fig. 18.146).

C. **Fibrocystic Changes** typically present as a palpable, ill-defined lesion which may have mammographically detectable microcalcifications. Cytologically, the lesion is composed of apocrine, ductal cells, mucus, and muciphages in varying amounts (**e-Fig. 18.147**).

D. **Subareolar Abscess** is a clinically painful, palpable subareolar mass typically associated with lactation. Cytologically, it consists of neutrophils and benign anucleate squamous epithelium (**e-Fig. 18.148**).

E. **Ductal Adenocarcinoma** usually presents as a clinically palpable, mammographically suspicious mass which cytologically shows a cellular smear containing large ductal cells which maybe poorly cohesive, without a myoepithelial component. The cells have pleomorphic nuclei, vesicular chromatin, and prominent nucleoli. Individual cells may have intracytoplasmic vacuoles containing inspissated material (**e-Fig. 18.149**).

F. **Lobular Adenocarcinoma** may not be clinically palpable, but presents mammographically as an ill-defined mass lesion. Cytologic preparations show singly dispersed small plasmacytoid cells with vacuolated cytoplasm, often containing inspissated material. The nuclei are uniformly small, round-to-oval, and not much bigger than a neutrophil (**e-Fig. 18.150**).

V. **SPECIAL STUDIES.** Immunocytologic evaluation of ER and PR studies can be performed on cytospin slide preparations. Immunocytologic evaluation of HER2 on cytospin slide preparations is limited due to the requirement of an intact cell membrane for proper assessment. Immunohistochemical evaluation of these markers can also be performed on formalin-fixed paraffin-embedded cell block samples prepared from fine needle aspirates. FISH for *HER2* gene amplification can be performed on cytospin slide preparations or paraffin-embedded cell blocks.

ACKNOWLEDGMENT

The authors thank Lourdes Ylagen, an author of the previous edition of this section.

SUGGESTED READINGS

Amin MB, Edge S, Greene F, et al., eds. *AJCC Cancer Staging Manual*. 8th ed. New York: Springer; 2017.

Dabbs DJ. *Breast Pathology*. 2nd ed. Philadelphia, PA: Elsevier; 2016.

Hoda SA, Brogi E, Koerner FC. *Rosen's Breast Pathology*. 4th ed. Philadelphia, PA: Lippincott Williams & Wilkins; 2014.

Lakhani SR, Ellis IO, Schnitt SJ, et al. *World Health Organization Classification of Tumors: Tumors of the Breast*. 4th ed. Lyon, France: IARC Press; 2012.

Masood S. *Cytopathology of the Breast*. American Society of Clinical Pathology. 1996.

Mckee GT. *Cytopathology of the Breast with Imaging and Histologic Correlation*. Oxford University Press; 2002.

O'malley FP, Pinder SE, Mulligan AM. *Breast Pathology: A Volume in the Foundations in Diagnostic Pathology series*. 2nd ed. Philadelphia, PA: Elsevier Saunders; 2011.

Page DL, Anderson TJ. *Diagnostic Histopathology of the Breast*. Churchill Livingstone; 1987.

Schnitt SJ, Collins LC. *Biopsy Interpretation of the Breast*. 3rd ed. Philadelphia, PA: Lippincott Williams&Wilkins; 2017.

Tavassoli FA. *Pathology of the Breast*. 2nd ed. McGraw-Hill; 1999.

Tavassoli FA, Eusebi V. *AFIP Atlas of Tumor Pathology, Series 4, Tumors of the Mammary Gland*. Silver Spring. ARP press; 2009.

Zakhou H, Wells C, Perry NM. *Diagnostic Cytopathology of the Breast*. Churchill Livingstone; 1999.

Urinary Tract

Medical Diseases of the Kidney

Satoru Kudose and Joseph Gaut

I. MEDICAL RENAL BIOPSY HANDLING AND PROCESSING. Renal biopsy is performed for various reasons, among which is monitoring the status of renal allografts, diagnosis of renal masses, and diagnosis of medical renal diseases. This chapter covers medical renal biopsies; biopsy for diagnosis of renal masses is covered in Chapter 20.

Renal allograft and medical renal biopsies are usually received in transport media allowing distribution of tissue for light microscopy (LM), immunofluorescence (IF), and electron microscopy (EM).

A. Light Microscopy. Three hematoxylin and eosin (H&E), one trichrome, two PAS, and one Jones silver stained section is common practice. Transplant biopsies with seven glomeruli and one artery are required for adequate LM evaluation. No minimum criteria exist for native biopsy evaluation.

B. Immunofluorescence. A minimum of two glomeruli is recommended. A direct immunofluorescence method is routinely used employing a panel of antibodies including anti-IgG, IgA, IgM, C3, C1q, fibrinogen, albumin, and kappa and lambda light chains. It is important to document the staining pattern (linear vs. granular) and distribution (mesangial, loop, or combined).

C. Electron Microscopy. Ultrastructural evaluation of two glomeruli is recommended. EM allows for evaluation of cellular and extracellular abnormalities in the glomeruli, tubules, interstitium, and vessels. EM is very useful in confirming the presence and distribution of electron-dense deposits, which can be located in the mesangium or the glomerular capillary basement membrane. In the basement membrane, electron-dense deposits can be subepithelial, subendothelial, or intramembranous (surrounded by basement membrane).

II. GLOMERULAR DISEASES. Glomerular diseases may be primary or secondary (associated with systemic diseases). Patients can be grouped into those that present with nephrotic syndrome (>3 g urine protein/day), nephritic syndrome (proteinuria + hematuria), rapidly progressive glomerulonephritis, or isolated hematuria. It is important to the pathologist to have access to patient's clinical and laboratory data. For example, minimal change disease, focal segmental glomerulosclerosis, and membranous glomerulonephritis (MGN) usually present with nephrotic syndrome. In contrast, postinfectious glomerulonephritis (PIGN) usually presents with nephritic syndrome.

A. Minimal Change Disease (MCD)/Focal Segmental Glomerulosclerosis (FSGS) are the most common causes of nephrotic syndrome in children and are also common in adults, affecting about 10% to 20% of patients with kidney disease. Primary FSGS may be primary, secondary, or familial (*Am J Nephrol* 2003;23:353). Less than nephrotic range proteinuria may be present in advanced cases. Some patients have concurrent hematuria and hypertension.

The classic findings in MCD (see Table 19.1) are:

LM: Normal appearing glomeruli

IF: Negative

EM: Extensive foot process effacement (e-**Fig. 19.1**).

The diagnostic features of FSGS are:

LM: Segmental sclerosis in some but not all glomeruli. Accurate diagnosis of FSGS depends on the extent of the disease and the number of glomeruli present in the biopsy. Diagnosis may be missed because of sampling error particularly with the smaller-size needles currently used. Notably, even one glomerulus with FSGS is sufficient for diagnosis. The corticomedullary glomeruli are the first to be sclerosed; therefore needle biopsies should opt to sample this region.

IF: Is either entirely negative or has focal and weak mesangial C3 or IgM immunoglobulin deposits.

EM: Shows diffuse (in primary) or focal (in secondary FSGS) foot process effacement (e-**Fig. 19.2**), the degree of which may depend on the degree of proteinuria. Other EM findings in MCD/FSGS include microvillus transformation of foot processes, endothelial cell edema, podocyte detachment, and GBM wrinkling (e-**Fig. 19.2**).

Beyond this classic presentation, light and electron microscopic findings may be similar in MCD and FSGS. For example, glomeruli may appear normal in FSGS and focal foot process effacement may be present in MCD.

Glomerular hypercellularity and enlargement (glomerulomegaly) is thought to represent an early lesion of FSGS (*Kidney Int* 1990;38:115). An FSGS classification scheme describes various histologic patterns with significantly different prognosis (*Am J Kidney Dis* 2004;43:368). The cellular variant is rare (seen in only about 3% of FSGS); the following variants are more frequent: perihilar FSGS (26%), tip lesion (17%), usual type not otherwise specified (NOS) (42%), and collapsing FSGS (11%) (e-**Fig. 19.2**). The tip variant has the best prognosis, collapsing FSGS the worst, with cellular and NOS in between (*Kidney Int* 2006;69:920). Pathologic similarities between MCD and FSGS initially suggested one disease with a spectrum of findings, but FSGS is less likely to respond to steroid treatment and has worse prognosis. Mutations in various podocyte genes (*NPHS1/2, WT1, PLCE1, LAMB2*, etc.) are increasingly identified in MCD/FSGS, especially in young patients resistant to steroid therapy (*J Am Soc Nephrol* 2015;26:1279). Targeted sequencing studies are clinically available.

B. **Collapsing FSGS** is a distinct FSGS variant associated with African ancestry, *APOL1* risk variants (*Clin Kidney J* 2017;10:443), a high incidence of nephrotic syndrome, and rapidly progressive renal failure.

LM: Characterized by segmental/global glomerular capillary collapse and podocyte hypertrophy, often accompanied by microcystic tubular dilatation and interstitial inflammation (e-**Fig. 19.2**). The main difference from usual FSGS is the collapse of the loops versus sclerosis, and podocyte proliferation versus podocyte loss.

IF: Nonspecific.

EM: Shows proliferating podocytes and wrinkled/collapsed capillary loops. First identified in HIV patients, collapsing FSGS was later recognized in association with viruses such as Parvovirus 19 and hepatitis B and C, and with pamidronate chemotherapy (*Semin Diagn Pathol* 2002;19:106).

It is an aggressive and difficult to treat disease (*Semin Nephrol* 2003;23:209), and may also involve the allograft kidney. Pathogenesis involves podocyte cell cycle dysregulation resulting in proliferation and/or proliferation of parietal epithelial cells (*Nat Rev Nephrol* 2014;10:158).

An entity known as **C1q nephropathy** is characterized by predominant C1q deposits and is considered a variant of MCD/FSGS (*Am J Clin Pathol* 1985;83:415). C1q nephropathy is primarily a disease of children and young adults.

TABLE 19.1 Major Glomerular Patterns and Differential Diagnosis on Light Microscopy

Minimal Changes	FSGS	Mesangial Hypercellularity	Thick Loops	Tram-Track	Proliferative	Crescents	Nodular Pattern
Minimal change disease	Primary NOS	IgA-HSP, MCD/FSGS	Membranous	MPGN	Postinfectious GN	Pauci-immune	Diabetes
Thin membrane disease	Secondary NOS		Diabetes	HSP	GN	Anti-GBM	MPGN
Early lupus	Cellular type	Lupus	Alport	Lupus	Lupus	Lupus	Amyloidosis
Early/mild IgA	Perihilar	IgM nephropathy	Amyloidosis		HSP	>50% = crescentic	MIDD
Early diabetes	Tip lesion	C1q nephropathy				<50% = other GN	
	Collapsing	C3 glomerulopathy					

FSGS, focal segmental glomerulonephritis; GN, glomerulonephritis; HSP, Henoch–Schönlein purpura; Ig, immunoglobulin; MCD, minimal change disease; MIDD, monoclonal immunoglobulin deposition disease; MPGN, membranoproliferative glomerulonephritis; NOS, not otherwise specified.

C. Mesangial Proliferative Glomerulonephritis (IgA, IgM, and C3). Mesangial hypercellularity is defined as ≥3 mesangial cells per mesangial region, although many glomerular diseases may have increased mesangial cells (Table 19.1) including variants of MCD and FSGS. Mesangial hypercellularity indicates mesangial immune deposits and/or reactive proliferation.

IgA nephropathy is the most common glomerular disease worldwide, characterized by micro or macrohematuria with variable prognosis (about 30% develop end-stage renal disease [ESRD]). Henoch–Schönlein purpura (HSP) mimics IgA pathologically, but clinically is a systemic disease that presents with skin rash, arthritis, and abdominal pain in addition to nephritis. HSP tends to be self-limiting with only about 18% of patients progressing to ESRD. Both IgA nephropathy and HSP may recur in transplant kidneys.

LM: Mesangial hypercellularity varies from focal to diffuse. Crescents are more commonly seen in HSP compared to IgA nephropathy.

IF: Diagnosis is made by the presence of predominant or co-dominant IgA mesangial deposits (e-**Fig. 19.3**). Mild IgG and IgM deposits may also be present, particularly in HSP, which is thought of as the systemic form of IgA disease.

EM: Shows mesangial/paramesangial deposits and occasionally capillary loop, subendothelial deposits that may extend to the GBM and cause splitting (more common in HSP).

Histologic parameters (MEST-C score) which negatively affect prognosis in IgA disease were established in Oxford Classification (*Kidney Int* 2017;91:1014) and include mesangial hypercellularity (extent ≤ or >50%), endocapillary hypercellularity (presence/absence), segmental sclerosis (presence/absence), tubular atrophy/interstitial fibrosis (extent ≤25%, 26% to 50% or >50%) and crescents (extent 0%, ≤25% or >25%).

Mesangial hypercellularity not infrequently accompanies various types of glomerulonephritis. For example, MCD and/or FSGS with mesangial hypercellularity are generally thought to have a worse prognosis. Focal IgM deposits are seen in some such cases. Rarely, diffuse IgM deposits are detected (which have raised considerable debate whether they represent a separate entity named IgM nephropathy).

Recent studies have clarified the entity known as **C3 glomerulopathy** (*Kidney Int* 2013;84:1079), which may present with mesangial hypercellularity or membranoproliferative glomerulonephritis (MPGN), but is characterized by an isolated deposition of C3 on immunofluorescence with intensity at least 2+ stronger than other reactants. C3 glomerulopathy is classified as dense deposit disease (DDD) when highly osmiophilic ribbon-like or "sausage-string" appearing intramembranous electron-dense deposits are seen, and C3 glomerulonephritis when other types of deposits are seen on EM. Immunofluorescence demonstrates intramembranous and mesangial C3 deposits without significant IgG or C1q staining (e-**Fig. 19.4**). Interestingly, the disease is associated with dysregulation of the alternative complement pathway secondary to defects in complement regulatory proteins (*Nat Rev Nephrol* 2010;6:494; *Kidney Int* 2009;75:1230), or may have an autoantibody that stabilizes C3bBb (C3 nephritic factor) resulting in overactivation of the alternative complement pathway. The deposits in DDD contain alternative and terminal complement pathway components (*Kidney Int* 2009;75:952).

D. MGN is the most common cause of nephrotic syndrome in adults (30% to 50% of cases). It may occur at any age, but accounts for <5% of childhood nephrotic syndrome. Most cases are associated with autoantibody to the phospholipase A2 receptor 1 (PLA2R1), which can be measured in serum (*N Engl J Med* 2009;361:11). Approximately 10% of cases are associated with identifiable causes such as malignancy, autoimmune diseases (e.g., systematic lupus erythematosus), drugs, and infections (hepatitis B, syphilis).

LM: Diffuse thickening of the capillary basement membrane without hypercellularity is seen. In Jones silver stained sections, the basement membrane can show "spikes" projecting from the epithelial side of the basement membrane. Spikes result from the presence of subepithelial electron-dense deposits (silver stain negative) and deposition of basement membrane like material on the sides of the deposits (e-**Fig. 19.5**). Glomeruli appear essentially normal in early stage cases.

IF: Diffuse, granular staining for IgG and C3 is present along the glomerular capillary loops by IF. Other immunoglobulins can be present but have lower intensity staining. Staining for PLA2R on pronase-digested sections and predominant staining for IgG4 over other subclasses support the diagnosis of primary MGN (*Mod Pathol* 2013;26:709).

EM: At early stages, the electron-dense deposits are subepithelial. As the disease progresses, deposition of basement membrane-like material at the sides of the electron-dense deposits occurs so that with time the electron-dense deposits are surrounded by basement membrane and thus becomes intramembranous. The deposits eventually become electron lucent, suggesting resolution (**e-Fig. 19.5**).

E. PIGN and Infection-Associated GN (IAGN). PIGN is a classic complication of streptococcal pharyngitis and presents acutely with nephritic syndrome in children. However, classic PIGN is infrequently biopsied. A large proportion of infectious glomerulonephritides are seen in adults and are associated with other bacterial infections including infectious endocarditis, skin infections, infected shunts, and deep-seated infections (*Kidney Int* 2013;83:792). It is important to recognize cases with active infections since typical immunosuppressive regimens would be contraindicated in this setting.

LM: The pathology of PIGN is characterized by white cells in the glomeruli (predominantly neutrophils in the acute phase), and lymphocytes or macrophages in chronic cases. IAGN typically shows similar histology but may also present with focal endocapillary proliferation, mesangial proliferation, or rarely crescentic glomerulonephritis (*Kidney Int* 2013;83:792).

IF: There are large granular IgG and C3 deposits along capillary loops. Patients in the resolving phases of infection may have deposits that are devoid of IgG, raising the differential diagnosis of a C3 glomerulonephritis (**e-Fig. 19.6**). Such cases are termed glomerulonephritis with dominant C3 (infection-associated); differentiation from C3 glomerulonephritis requires clinical follow-up over months to evaluate for normalization of serum C3 levels (*Kidney Int* 2013;84:1079).

EM: Shows characteristic subepithelial bell-shaped deposits (humps). Erythrogenic toxin type B is thought to be the target antigen for immune complexes that are implanted in the GBM. PIGN, IAGN, and C3 glomerulopathy may all show hump-shaped subepithelial deposits on EM.

F. MPGN. MPGN is a morphologic pattern that was previously classified into three types based on the appearance and location of deposits. Recently, MPGN was reclassified into immune complex mediated (previously type I and III) or complement mediated (*Semin Nephrol* 2011;31:341). Complement-mediated MPGN includes C3 glomerulonephritis (C3GN) and MPGN type II.

Patients with MPGN can present with features of nephrotic and/or nephritic syndrome and most patients have low serum C3. Although MPGN can affect patients of all ages, it is more common in children. Type I is the most common type, followed by types II and III. It is important to note that MPGN type I can be associated with other diseases such as viral hepatitis, so patients should be worked up for secondary causes of MPGN when the pathologic diagnosis is established.

LM: MPGN is characterized by diffuse endocapillary proliferation that results in lobular accentuation (**e-Fig. 19.7**). The glomerular basement membranes are thick, and the capillary lumens are not evident. The Jones silver stain reveals double contours of the capillary loops, also known as "tram-tracking." These findings are more commonly seen in MPGN type I. Cryoglobulinemia can show MPGN pattern but, in addition, has a PAS+ intracapillary deposits (**e-Fig. 19.7**).

IF: MPGN is classified as immune complex mediated when C3 deposition is observed along glomerular capillary walls and mesangium, together with at least one of IgG, IgM, or C1q. If dominant C3 deposition is seen, C3 glomerulonephritis should be considered.

EM: MPGN type I shows mesangial interposition (extension of mesangial cell cytoplasm into the capillary wall) and subendothelial electron-dense deposits. When the mesangial cell cytoplasm extends into the glomerular capillary wall, basement membrane-like material is laid down by the mesangial and endothelial cells, creating a second "new" basement membrane. This process results in the "tram-tracking" observed by light microscopy. The ultrastructural findings of MPGN type III are similar to those of MPGN type I, but with subendothelial and subepithelial electron-dense deposits (e-**Fig. 19.7**). The ultrastructural features of C3 glomerulonephritis were described above.

G. Crescentic Glomerulonephritis (Crescentic GN). The term crescentic GN refers to the presence of cellular crescents in >50% of glomeruli available in a renal biopsy. Glomerulonephritides that most commonly manifests as crescentic GN are classified into pauci-immune, anti-GBM disease (Goodpasture syndrome), and immune-complex types by IF. The usual clinical presentation is a rapidly progressive glomerulonephritis. Patients may have disease limited to the kidneys or systemic disease.

   LM: Cellular crescents and necrotizing glomerular lesions are seen (e-**Fig. 19.8**). In pauci-immune crescentic GN, medullary angiitis may be seen (e-**Fig. 19.9**).

   IF: In anti-GBM disease, termed Goodpasture syndrome when there is pulmonary involvement, glomeruli exhibit smooth linear IgG staining along the capillary basement membrane. Immune-complex glomerulonephritis has a granular staining pattern for one or more immunoglobulins. Pauci-immune glomerulonephritis is negative for all immunoglobulins, and is typically associated with presence of pANCA or cANCA.

   EM: The glomerular changes noted by EM correspond to necrosis, disruption of the GBM, and crescents. Cases of immune complex glomerulonephritis will show electron-dense deposits, while pauci-immune and anti-GBM disease show no electron-dense deposits.

H. Lupus Nephritis (LN). Systemic lupus erythematosus (SLE) is a multisystemic auto-immune disorder with a peak incidence in the second and third decades of life and a female predominance (male:female ratio of 1:9). It is more common in African-Americans. Renal involvement by the disease is relatively common; approximately half of lupus patients develop LN during the first year of the disease. Although this chapter emphasizes the glomerular findings of LN, interstitial, tubular, and vascular lesions can also accompany the glomerular changes. Use of the revised ISN/RPS classification of LN (*Kidney Int* 2018;93:789) is recommended.

   LM: LN can present with various light microscopic patterns (Tables 19.2 and 19.3). With time and/or treatment, the renal lesion can evolve into a different class. Membranous LN can occur in combination with Class III or IV. Mesangial hypercellularity is defined as ≥4 mesangial cells, as in IgA nephropathy. All LN classes should be scored using the modified NIH lupus activity and chronicity scoring system (Table 19.2) in lieu of active/chronic (A/C) designations used previously. The following are considered glomerular active lesions: endocapillary hypercellularity with/without leukocyte infiltration and with substantial luminal reduction; karyorrhexis/neutrophils; fibrinoid necrosis; cellular or fibrocellular crescents; hyaline deposits (e-**Fig. 19.10**). The glomerular chronic lesions are segmental or global glomerulosclerosis, fibrous crescents, and tubular atrophy and interstitial fibrosis.

   IF: A glomerular IgG-positive immunostain is almost universal in LN; the term "full house" is used when IgG, IgA, and IgM, as well as C3 and C1q, immunostains are positive.

I. Diabetes Mellitus (DM). DM is a disorder of carbohydrate metabolism that affects multiple organ systems. In the kidney it increases the propensity to pyelonephritis, papillary necrosis, arteriosclerosis, and glomerular disease. Hyperglycemia in these patients induces biochemical changes in the GBM, nonenzymatic glycosylation of proteins, and hemodynamic changes with glomerular hypertrophy. Diabetic glomerulosclerosis is unlikely to develop in the absence of vascular changes in the eye fundus.

   LM: GBM thickening develops in early stages. Increased mesangial matrix eventually results in diffuse nodular glomerulosclerosis, also known as Kimmelstiel–Wilson disease.

   IF: Immunofluorescence studies are essentially negative. However, glomeruli exhibit nonspecific linear capillary loop staining for IgG and albumin. The identical

TABLE 19.2	ISN/RPS Classification of Lupus Nephritis[a,b]
Class I	Minimal mesangial LN
Class II	Mesangial proliferative LN
Class III	Focal LN (involvement of <50% glomeruli)
Class IV	Diffuse LN (active or inactive diffuse, segmental and/or global endocapillary and/or extracapillary GN involving 50% or more glomeruli)
Class V	Membranous LN
Class VI	Advanced sclerosing LN (90% or more glomeruli globally sclerosed)

Modified NIH Activity Index	Definition	Score
Endocapillary hypercellularity	<25% (1), 25–50% (2), >50% (3) glomeruli	0–3
Neutrophils/karyorrhexis	<25% (1), 25–50% (2), >50% (3) glomeruli	0–3
Fibrinoid necrosis	<25% (1), 25–50% (2), >50% (3) glomeruli	0–3 ×2
Wire loops or hyaline thrombi	<25% (1), 25–50% (2), >50% (3) glomeruli	0–3
Cellular/fibrocellular crescents	<25% (1), 25–50% (2), >50% (3) glomeruli	0–3 ×2
Interstitial inflammation	<25% (1), 25–50% (2), >50% (3) cortex	0–3
Total		*0–24*

Modified NIH Chronicity Index	Definition	Score
Total glomerulosclerosis	<25% (1), 25–50% (2), >50% (3) glomeruli	0–3
Fibrous crescents	<25% (1), 25–50% (2), >50% (3) glomeruli	0–3
Tubular atrophy	<25% (1), 25–50% (2), >50% (3) cortical tubules	0–3
Interstitial fibrosis	<25% (1), 25–50% (2), >50% (3) cortex	0–3
Total		*0–12*

[a]ISN/RPS, International Society of Nephrology/Renal Pathology Society (*Kidney Int* 2018;93:214).
[b]Modified from *Kidney Int* 2018;93:789. Precise definitions for endocapillary hypercellularity and other lesions are being developed but are not yet available. Segmental or global sclerosis with fragmented tuft with surrounding fibrosis and extensive disruption of Bowman's capsule or deposits other that IgM/C3 can be attributed to lupus nephritis for a purpose of scoring.

TABLE 19.3	Summary of Pathologic Findings of Lupus Nephritis		
Class	Light Microscopy	Immunofluorescence	Electron Microscopy
I	Minimal mesangial hypercellularity	Mesangial +	Mesangial deposits
II	Mesangial hypercellularity and increased matrix	Mesangial +	Mesangial deposits
III	Endocapillary and/or extracapillary proliferation in <50% of glomeruli	Mesangial and loop +	Mesangial and subendothelial deposits
IV	Endocapillary and/or extracapillary proliferation in 50% or more of glomeruli	Mesangial and loop +	Mesangial and subendothelial deposits
V	Thick loops and mesangial hypercellularity	Mesangial and loop +	Numerous subepithelial and scattered mesangial deposits

morphology seen in older white hypertensive men who smoke, in the absence of DM, is termed idiopathic nodular glomerulosclerosis (*Hum Pathol* 2002;33:826).

EM: Shows thickening of the GBM and various degrees of mesangial expansion. Electron-dense deposits are not identified by electron microscopy (e-**Fig. 19.11**).

J. Amyloidosis and Other Deposition Diseases. Renal amyloidosis can be primary or secondary. Patients often present with nephrotic syndrome (~50%), peripheral neuropathy (carpal-tunnel syndrome), heart failure, and/or liver disease due to amyloid deposits. There are many different proteins that form amyloid, including AA, AL amyloid, transthyretin (ATTR) and familial types, which confer a different prognosis (e.g., worse for AL amyloid compared with ATTR). Amyloid is composed of polymerized proteins forming beta-pleated sheets and stains red with Congo red.

LM: Varies from GBM thickening to nodular or segmental sclerosis. Amorphous material is often apparent in the mesangium or the capillary loops and is PAS/silver negative. A Congo red stain is diagnostic, showing apple green fluorescence under polarized light (e-**Fig. 19.12**).

IF: May show κ or λ chain restricted staining.

EM: Is characteristic and consists of randomly arranged 4- to 12-nm fibrils (e-**Fig. 19.10B**). EM shows either finely granular or filamentous deposits in the mesangium or the GBM (*Semin Diagn Pathol* 2002;19:116).

In some patients there are deposits of fragments of IgG, IgM, or IgA immunoglobulin heavy chains or light chains that do not form amyloid. In these cases a Congo red stain is negative, and monoclonal immunoglobulin deposition disease (MIDD) (*J Am Soc Nephrol* 2001;12:1482) or proliferative glomerulonephritis with monoclonal IgG deposits (PGNMID) should be considered (*J Am Soc Nephrol* 2009;20:2055).

LM: In MIDD, glomeruli may appear nodular or have nonspecific changes. In PGNMID, membranoproliferative or endocapillary hypercellularity are seen.

IF: Linear, dominant staining for one specific type of immunoglobulin fragment (heavy or light chain) (e-**Fig. 19.13**). For PGNMID, IgG3κ is most commonly deposited in granular pattern.

EM: In MIDD, powdery electron-dense deposits are seen in the subendothelium and in tubular basement membranes, and, in PGNMID, granular nonorganized deposits are seen.

The differential diagnosis of amyloidosis/MIDD includes other nodular GN such as diabetes, and fibrillary and immunotactoid glomerulopathy. The latter two may have overlapping IF, but have wider fibrils on EM (12 to 20 nm for fibrillary and >20 nm for immunotactoid, with the latter forming microtubules) than amyloid (*Kidney Int* 2002;62:1764). Recently, immunohistochemical staining for DnaJ heat shock protein family member B9 (DNAJB9) has been found to be specific for fibrillary glomerulopathy (*J Am Soc Nephrol* 2018;29:51).

In young females with autoimmune disease, a membranous-like staining pattern with C3 may have "masked" monoclonal IgG deposits that are evident only after performing IF on pronase digested FFPE (*Kidney Int.* 2014; 86:154).

K. Alport Syndrome/Thin Basement Membrane Disease. Classic X-linked (X-L) Alport syndrome presents with microscopic or gross hematuria and deafness. Deafness and/or proteinuria are indications of severe disease. Such symptoms are usually absent in young children. Mutations in *COLIV5* cause X-L Alport; *COLIV4* mutations cause autosomal dominant (AD) and *COLIV3* mutations cause autosomal recessive (AR) Alport. 15% of X-L Alport patients have no family history and are thought to represent a new mutation. Patients with AR Alport are clinically similar to X-L Alport; AD Alport is rare. The involved organs in Alport syndrome reflect the sites where these collagen IVα chains are normally expressed (α3, α4, α5 are exclusively found in the kidney, eye, and ear). Renal biopsy is performed for diagnosis as well as assessment of disease progression.

LM: Is not specific; it varies from unremarkable glomeruli, to FSGS, to chronic scarring. Foamy interstitial cells were once thought characteristic of Alport, but they are in fact seen in many types of proteinuria.

IF: Routine stains are negative. Diagnosis of Alport is facilitated by collagen IV chain immunostaining. The α5 chain of collagen IV is distinctly absent in X-L Alport, and it is accompanied by absent α3 and α4 chains in glomeruli (collagen IV monomers are incorporated into basement membrane as triple helices to form the structural meshwork (*Kidney Int* 2004;65:1109); when one chain is mutated, all three chains may degenerate because they become susceptible to enzymatic proteolysis). Typically, women with X-L Alport have mosaic linear staining with collagen IVα5 in the glomeruli or skin (**e-Fig. 19.11**) (*Hum Pathol* 2002;33:836). However some women may have positive staining, making it difficult to distinguish from thin membrane disease (TMD) (see below). A screening test for families with potential X-L Alport is skin biopsy (IVα5 is the only chain found in skin): the diagnostic pattern in men is absent collagen IVα5, and mosaic staining (linear interrupted positivity) in X-L women carriers (**e-Fig. 19.14**).

EM: The cardinal pathologic findings of X-L Alport are seen on electron microscopy and consist of abnormal splitting, widening, or thinning of the GBM with degeneration of collagen IV in the lamina densa known as "bread crumbs" (**e-Fig. 19.14**). The lesions may involve tubular basement membranes as well. However, the specificity of the EM findings is moderate (*Kidney Int* 1999;56:760); for example, young children and in women with Alport nephritis may only manifest uniformly thin GBM and thus be indistinguishable from TMD (*Semin Nephrol* 2005;25:149). About 30% of Alport heterozygotes have uniformly thin GBM, but have collagen IVα3-5 mutations by genetic testing. Others show only GBM lamellation in thin segments. Routine genetic testing is not only technically difficult (several different genes must be evaluated and mutational hot-spots do not exist), but also does not strictly correlate with pathology or prognosis. A good family history of close relatives is very helpful.

TMD is defined as GBM thinning <250 nm in adults and <200 nm in children. These values are approximate as there is no true consensus as to how thin the GBM should be for the diagnosis of TMD. It is also debated as to whether GBM thinning must be diffuse or focal, though most cases have focal GBM thinning involving <50% of loops.

LM: Usually unremarkable.

IF: Routine stains are negative. Collagen IVα3-5 immunostains are positive.

EM: Shows GBM diffuse or segmental thinning without lamellation (**e-Fig. 19.14**).

L. **Miscellaneous Entities Affecting Glomeruli.** In general, various lysosomal storage diseases cause diffuse clear cytoplasmic vacuolization in the podocytes and tubules, without necessarily causing renal impairment. However, Fabry disease can cause progressive renal impairment without overt proteinuria or hematuria. In this disease, electron microscopy reveals characteristic myelin or "Zebra" bodies (**e-Fig. 19.15**), which can also be seen patients taking chloroquine/hydroxychloroquine (*Mod Pathol* 2005;18:733).

III. TUBULOINTERSTITIAL DISEASES

A. **Infectious Processes.** Infectious agents can result in tubulointerstitial nephritis by colonizing the renal parenchyma, or by triggering a systemic immunologic response that will target the renal tubules and interstitium. Bacterial agents are responsible for most cases of **acute pyelonephritis**. Most cases of acute pyelonephritis are ascending infections caused by gram-negative bacteria, particularly *E. coli*. When bacteria reach the kidney using a hematogenous route, *Staphylococcus aureus* is usually the responsible agent. Acute pyelonephritis is characterized by an abundance of neutrophils in the lumen of tubules and the interstitium. Neutrophils are usually accompanied by other inflammatory cells.

Viral agents are also associated with tubulointerstitial nephritis. Polyomavirus and cytomegalovirus (CMV) typically manifest in renal allografts (see below), although they may rarely occur in native kidneys in presence of immunosuppression or ureteral stents.

A granulomatous inflammatory response is usually seen with mycobacterial or some fungal infections. Histochemical stains, AFB, PAS, and silver stains are needed to visualize the microorganisms.

B. **Acute Tubular Injury (ATI).** ATI is the most common cause of acute kidney injury and can be caused by toxins or ischemia. The histologic changes are most prominent in proximal tubules and include simplification (flattening), cell sloughing of the epithelial lining, interstitial edema, and various types of casts as well as regenerative changes including mitotic activity, nuclear enlargement, and prominent nucleoli (**e-Fig. 19.16**). Other findings such as loss of brush borders, cytoplasmic blebbing, and tubularization of glomeruli are also described, although they may not correlate with severity of AKI (*Am J Surg Pathol* 2018;42:625). Historically, the term acute tubular necrosis was used for ATI even though necrosis of the lining epithelium is rare in routine practice. When present, epithelial necrosis tends to be more extensive and confluent in the toxic type of ATN, and patchy in the ischemic type.

C. Acute Interstitial Nephritis. Most cases of acute interstitial nephritis are drug-related; renal manifestations develop approximately 2 weeks after drug exposure. The typical presentation includes fever, skin rash, and eosinophilia, but this triad is only present in approximately one-third of patients. Interstitial eosinophils are the most important histologic clue for diagnosis. Eosinophils are accompanied by other inflammatory cells, mainly lymphocytes, and may be seen only focally (**e-Fig. 19.17**). Tubulitis and tubular injury usually accompany the interstitial changes. If the interstitial inflammatory infiltrate contains nonnecrotizing granulomas, a diagnosis of granulomatous interstitial nephritis is warranted (*Int J Surg Pathol* 2006;14:57). Granulomas raise the differential of drug reaction, sarcoid, and infection.

D. Cast Nephropathy and Light Chain Proximal Tubulopathy (LCPT). Amyloidosis, cast nephropathy, light/heavy chain deposition disease, and LCPT are renal complications of patients with plasma cell neoplasms. Casts are usually located in the collecting ducts, but due to retrograde filling casts may be seen in proximal tubules. Casts are composed of light chains and Tamm–Horsfall protein, and tend to have a fractured appearance. A granulomatous response with multinucleated macrophages and reactive epithelial cells is typically found at the periphery of myeloma casts (**e-Fig. 19.18**); other inflammatory cells, such as neutrophils and lymphocytes, may be part of the inflammatory process. Immunofluorescence studies often exhibit a monoclonal light chain in the casts.

In some cases, light chains are taken up within the proximal tubular cytoplasm and result in LCPT (*J Am Soc Nephrol* 2016; 27:1555). The typical presentation is ATI or Fanconi syndrome. In most cases, light chains crystallize and are visible on LM/EM (**e-Fig. 19.19**).

LM: Tubular injury with intracytoplasmic crystals (crystalline LCPT) or vacuoles (noncrystalline), which are typically fuchsinophilic.

IF: Kappa or lambda light chain restriction of tubular epithelial droplets.

EM: Membrane and non-membrane bound crystals of various shapes and sizes in crystalline LCPT and membrane bound vacuoles containing finely granular material in the noncrystalline form.

IV. VASCULAR DISEASES

A. Vasculitides. The kidney has a dense arterial, venous, and lymphatic network. Vasculitides affect all these vessels, but most commonly the arteries. They are usually classified as large, medium, and small vessel vasculitides based on the predominant vessel size affected. Although this classification is convenient, it is controversial because there is variability in the size of affected vessels (*Arthritis Rheum* 2013;65:1). Vasculitides are also classified by the underlying pathogenetic mechanism as either immune complex mediated or pauci-immune.

Large vessel vasculitis (Takayasu arteritis and giant cell arteritis) and medium vessel vasculitis (polyarteritis nodosa, Kawasaki disease) are uncommonly seen in renal biopsies. Small vessel vasculitis such as anti-GBM disease, granulomatosis with polyangiitis, microscopic polyangiitis, and eosinophilic granulomatosis with polyangiitis typically present as crescentic glomerulonephritis (see above). Immune complex–mediated vasculitides such as lupus and HSP are described in the appropriate sections above.

1. Thrombotic microangiopathy (TMA). TMA is a pattern of injury associated with a multitude of morphologic changes and etiologies. Patients typically present with microangiopathic hemolytic anemia (MAHA) and thrombocytopenia. Entities that can manifest as TMA include diarrhea-associated (classic HUS; *E. coli* 0157:H7), atypical HUS (aHUS), thrombotic thrombocytopenic purpura, eclampsia, preeclampsia, drugs (oral contraceptives, chemotherapy), cryoglobulinemia, idiopathic hypereosinophilia, antiphospholipid syndrome, hereditary deficiency of blood clotting factors, malignancy, and malignant hypertension (HTN) (*J Am Soc Nephrol* 2003;14:1072). Recently, a subset of patients (aHUS) presenting with MAHA was found to have gene variants in complement regulatory genes, most commonly *CFH* (*Kidney International* 2017;91:539). The variants abrogate regulatory capacity of *CFH* resulting in overactivation of the alternative complement pathway, similar to C3GN. Identification of these variants is important diagnostically, prognostically (MCP variants tend to be milder), and therapeutically because eculizumab appears to be an effective therapy, and combined liver–kidney transplantation may be indicated in some patients.

LM: Glomerular fibrin thrombi, congestion, endothelial cell swelling resulting in closure of capillary loops (endotheliosis), and mesangiolysis are acute manifestations of TMA. Duplication of the glomerular basement membranes is seen in the chronic phase. Vessels show mucoid intimal edema, fibrinoid change, fragmented red blood cells, and concentric myointimal hyperplasia ("onion skinning") (e-**Fig. 19.20**). Concentric myointimal hyperplasia is more typical of malignant hypertension-associated TMA. Currently, there is no consensus on which and how many of these features are required for the diagnosis of TMA. Furthermore, these histologic features do not have enough discriminative power to distinguish between TMA associated with different etiologies.

IF: Fibrin thrombi may be seen, but otherwise are noncontributory.

EM: Subendothelial edema, closure of the endothelial fenestrae, and fibrin thrombi (e-**Fig. 19.19**).

2. **Systemic hypertension.** Vascular diseases of the kidney are often associated with systemic hypertension. The most common cause of is idiopathic, which, despite modern pharmacologic therapies, remains a primary cause of renal failure. High blood pressure damages parenchymal arteries causing intimal thickening; the arterioles show characteristic acellular eosinophilic material (hyalinosis) due to increased intravascular pressure and endothelial injury that allows leaking and deposition of plasma proteins. Glomeruli beyond damaged arterioles show signs of ischemia (retraction, wrinkled capillary loops) and eventually undergo segmental and global sclerosis.

A small fraction (5% to 10%) of benign HTN is secondary to specific causes, some of which may be amenable to surgical therapy, that together are known as **renovascular HTN**. Most common is renal artery stenosis due to atherosclerotic aneurysms in older mostly diabetic men. Patients with abdominal or renal artery atherosclerosis may present with acute renal failure or proteinuria due to cholesterol embolism in parenchymal arteries (e-**Fig. 19.17D**). Fibromuscular dysplasia, an idiopathic mural thickening of the renal artery, is seen in young women (*Am J Kidney Dis* 1997;29:167).

V. PATHOLOGY OF THE ALLOGRAFT KIDNEY

A. Processing of Renal Allograft Biopsies.
Renal biopsy is a key component of managing transplant recipients since the clinical diagnosis is changed in about 40% of cases, and therapy in ~60%, of cases following biopsy (*Am J Kidney Dis* 1998;31:S15). Transplant biopsies in most centers are performed when clinically indicated (indication biopsies) or at standardized time intervals (protocol biopsies). Criteria for indication biopsies include proteinuria, acute renal failure, and increased creatinine levels, among others. Adequacy criteria of the renal allograft biopsy were established at the Banff 1997 consensus conference (*Kidney Int* 1999;55:713).

It is recommended that two 16- or 18-gauge needle core biopsies are submitted for pathologic evaluation: one for light microscopy, and one divided for immunofluorescence and electron microscopy. The core for light microscopy is submitted in 10% buffered formalin; the immunofluorescence core should be submitted in refrigerated transport media, and a small fragment from cortex should be submitted for electron microscopy fixed in 2% glutaraldehyde. For light microscopy, 10 glomeruli and 2 arteries are required for definitive diagnosis; 7 to 10 glomeruli and 1 artery are considered marginal, while <7 glomeruli and no arteries are an inadequate sample. The paraffin blocks should be sectioned at 2 to 3 μm thickness; seven slides including three hematoxylin and eosin (H&E) stains, three periodic acid-Schiff (PAS) or silver stains, and one trichrome stain should be prepared (*Kidney Int* 1999;55:713). For immunofluorescence, a minimum of 2 glomeruli is required for the evaluation of glomerular disease; immunofluorescence evaluation for IgG, IgA, IgM, C3, fibrinogen, albumin, and C4d is standard. For electron microscopic evaluation at least 1 glomerulus is recommended.

B. **Transplant Rejection.** Major complications with specific pathologic findings in the allograft biopsy are acute and chronic rejection (which are subdivided into cellular- and antibody-mediated rejection), and recurrent and de novo disease (Table 19.4).

1. **Acute T-cell–mediated (cellular) rejection.** Tubules, arteries, and the interstitium are the principal targets of acute T-cell–mediated rejection. The Banff 2005 updated classification of renal allograft rejection (Table 19.5) is based on histologic scoring of tubular, interstitial, and arterial inflammation (*Am J Transplant* 2007;7:518). Higher grade rejection correlates with worse outcome and requires more aggressive therapy.

Tubulitis is scored in nonseverely atrophic tubules (i.e., tubules with each of the following: reduced caliber by ≥20%, undifferentiated-appearing cuboidal/flat epithelium,

TABLE 19.4 Major Histopathologic Findings in Renal Transplant Biopsies

Rejection	Recurrent Disease	De Novo Disease
Acute T-cell mediated	**Glomerular**	**Glomerular**
- Lymphocytic tubulitis	- FSGS	- FSGS
- Arteritis (endotheliitis)	- Diabetes	- Diabetes
- Interstitial inflammation	- Lupus	- Anti-GBM
	- IgA	- Postinfectious
	- MPGN	- Membranous
	- Membranous	- Other
	- Vasculitis (ANCA, anti-GBM)	
	- Amyloidosis/light chain deposition disease	
Chronic, active T-cell mediated	**Tubulointerstitial**	**Vascular**
- Interstitial inflammation in fibrosis	- Myeloma cast nephropathy	- Thrombotic microangiopathy (drug induced)
- Arterial intimal fibroplasia		- Cholesterol embolism
- Tubulitis		- Renal artery thrombosis
- Interstitial fibrosis		- Renal vein thrombosis
		- Antibody-mediated rejection
Antibody mediated (AMR)	**Vascular**	**Tubulointerstitial**
- Glomerulitis	-Recurrent HUS	- Acute interstitial nephritis usually drug reaction
- Peritubular capillaritis		- Oxalate crystals
- Acute tubular injury[a]		- Calcium phosphate crystals
- Thrombotic microangiopathy[a]		- Acute tubular injury
- Transplant glomerulopathy		- Polyomavirus nephropathy
		Malignancy
		- Malignant lymphoma
		- PTLD

[a]In the absence of another etiology.
Modified from Liapis H, Wang H, eds. *Pathology of Solid Organ Transplantation.* Heidelberg, Germany: Springer; 2011.

TABLE 19.5	Banff Diagnostic Categories for Renal Allograft Biopsies

Active antibody-mediated rejection (require all three criteria)

Acute tissue injury (one or more of the following):
1. Microvascular inflammation (g and/or ptc > 0)[a]
2. Intimal arteritis (v > 0)[a]
3. Acute TMA
4. ATI

Current/recent antibody interaction with endothelium (one or more of the following):
1. C4d+ in peritubular capillaries (C4d2 or C4d3)
2. g + ptc ≥ 2
3. Increased expression of ABMR-associated gene transcripts

Serologic evidence of DSAs[b]

Chronic-active antibody-mediated rejection (require all three criteria)

Morphologic chronic tissue injury (one or more of the following):
1. cg > 0
2. Severe peritubular capillary basement membrane multilayering (EM)
3. Arterial intimal fibrosis of new onset

Current/recent antibody interaction with endothelium as above

DSA evidence as above

Borderline changes: "suspicious" for acute T-cell–mediated rejection

This category is used when no intimal arteritis is present, but there are foci of tubulitis (t1, t2, or t3) with minor interstitial inflammation (i0 or i1) or interstitial inflammation with mild tubulitis (t1)

Acute T-cell–mediated rejection

Grade
IA. Significant interstitial infiltration (>25% parenchyma, i2 or i3) and moderate tubulitis (t2)
IB. Significant interstitial infiltration (>25% parenchyma, i2 or i3) and severe tubulitis (t3)
IIA. Mild to moderate intimal arteritis (v1)
IIB. Severe intimal arteritis comprising >25% of the luminal area (v2)
III. Transmural arteritis and/or arterial fibrinoid change and necrosis of medial smooth muscle cells with accompanying lymphocytic inflammation (v3)

Chronic-active T-cell–mediated rejection

Grade
IA. Significant interstitial inflammation in areas of fibrosis (i-IFTA2 or 3) and moderate tubulitis
IB. Significant interstitial inflammation in areas of fibrosis (i-IFTA2 or 3) and severe tubulitis
II. Chronic allograft arteriopathy (arterial intimal fibrosis with mononuclear cell infiltration in fibrosis, formation of neo-intima)

[a]AMBR, antibody-mediated rejection; cg, Banff chronic glomerulopathy score; DSA, donor-specific antibody; g, Banff glomerulitis score; IFTA, interstitial fibrosis and tubular atrophy; ptc, Banff peritubular capillaritis score.
[b]C4d expression may substitute for DSA; advise testing for non-HLA antibodies.
Modified from Haas M, Loupy A, Lefaucheur C, et al. The Banff 2017 Kidney Meeting Report: Revised diagnostic criteria for chronic active T cell-mediated rejection, antibody-mediated rejection, and prospects for integrative endpoints for next-generation clinical trials. *Am J Transplant* 2018;18:293–307.

and wrinkled and/or thickened tubular basement membrane) (*Am J Transplant* 2018;18:293). The degree of infiltrating mononuclear cells, lymphocytes, and macrophages is graded as mild (t1; ≤4 cells/tubular cross-section), moderate (t2, 5 to 10 cells/tubular cross-section), or severe (t3, >10 cells/tubular cross-section) (**e-Fig. 19.21**).

Interstitial inflammation typically consists predominantly of CD4+ and CD8+ T cells, and macrophages. Involvement of >25% of the nonatrophic parenchyma (i2 or i3), away from subcapsular and perivascular area, is required for diagnosis of acute cellular rejection. If foci of t2 or t3 tubulitis are present with <25% interstitial inflammation (i1) or when t1 tubulitis is present with i2 inflammation, then the specimen is considered borderline or "suspicious" for acute cellular rejection.

Arteritis, or endotheliitis, is the presence of subendothelial or mural mononuclear cell infiltration in the wall of renal parenchymal arteries (e-**Fig. 19.22**). Any size artery may be affected. Arterial inflammation is scored based on the degree of intimal inflammation as follows: mild (v1, <25% luminal diameter), moderate (v2, >25% luminal diameter), and severe (v3, transmural ± fibrinoid necrosis). The presence of even mild endotheliitis is significant and warrants a diagnosis of at least grade IIA rejection (see Table 19.2).

2. Active antibody-mediated (humoral) rejection may occur shortly after implantation, or months to years following transplantation. According to the Banff 2009 and 2013 updates, the diagnosis requires all three of the following (Table 19.5): (1) evidence of interaction between antibody and endothelium [at least one of microvascular inflammation (g + ptc ≥2), linear C4d+ immunostaining of peritubular capillaries (C4d2 or C4d3), or increased expression of validated transcripts associated with endothelial injury], (2) circulating antidonor specific antibodies [or C4d positivity, or gene expression classifier as in (1)], and (3) morphologic evidence of acute tissue injury [microvascular injury (g or ptc >0, with g >0 required in presence of concurrent T-cell–mediated rejection), tubular injury, or TMA that cannot be attributed to other causes] (*Am J Transplant* 2010;10:464; *Am J Transplant* 2014;14:272; *Am J Transplant* 2018;18:293). The earliest feature of acute antibody-mediated rejection may be ATN, but as the lesions develop peritubular capillaritis becomes prominent (e-**Fig. 19.23**). Peritubular capillaritis is defined as dilation of cortical peritubular capillaries by marginating inflammatory cells (*Am J Transplant* 2008;8:753). A minimum of 10% of peritubular capillaries must be involved (normally, peritubular capillaries contain no more than two mononuclear cells), graded by the maximum number of cells present (ptc1, <5; ptc2, 5 to 10; ptc3, >10).

C4d staining is considered present when linear and circumferential staining is seen in either cortical or medullary peritubular capillaries, and is graded by extent (C4d1, <10%; C4d2, 10 to 50%; C4d3, >50%). Immunofluorescence is considered the gold standard for C4d evaluation (*Kidney Int* 1993;44:411) (e-**Fig. 19.24**). Based on current Banff classification, a biopsy may be diagnosed as AMR even in the absence of C4d staining. Clinical features of AMR with or without C4d are similar (*Curr Opin Organ Transplant* 2013; 18:319).

3. Chronic active T-cell (cellular) rejection (TCMR). Repeated graft injury from episodes of cellular rejection may manifest as nonspecific tubulointerstitial fibrosis (IFTA). A recent update to the Banff classification specifies interstitial inflammation within areas of interstitial fibrosis (i-IFTA), graded as >25% (i-IFTA1), 25% to 50% (i-IFTA2), and >50% (i-IFTA3), as critical to the diagnosis of chronic active TCMR (*Am J Transplant* 2018;18:293). Cases with i-IFTA2 or 3 plus moderate tubulitis are classified as Grade IA while cases with severe tubulitis are Grade IB. Grade II is defined by chronic allograft arteriopathy, defined as fibrointimal hyperplasia (thickening of the intima) (*Kidney Int* 1999;55:713). Elastin staining may help to distinguish transplant arteriopathy from arterial thickening due to hypertension since the stain will highlight intimal proliferation with multilamination in hypertension, a finding absent in transplant arteriopathy.

4. Chronic active antibody-mediated rejection. Diagnosis of chronic active antibody-mediated rejection requires all three of the following: circulating anti-donor specific antibodies, evidence of interaction between antibody and endothelium (as in active AMR), and evidence of chronic tissue injury. Chronic tissue injury requires either transplant glomerulopathy (cg > 0), peritubular capillary basement membrane multilayering on EM (at least one with ≥7 layers, and another with ≥5 layers) or arterial intimal fibrosis, in the absence of another attributable cause. Transplant glomerulopathy is characterized by mesangial expansion and hypercellularity with a lobular appearance resembling MPGN, and glomerular basement membrane duplication. Subendothelial edema, GBM multi-lamellation, and endothelial fenestrae closure are typical electron microscopic findings (e-**Figs. 19.25** and **19.26**). Glomerular basement membrane duplication (cg) is scored by an extent of involvement in the most severely affected glomerulus (cg1, <25%; cg2, 25% to 50%; cg3, >50% of glomerular tuft). Chronic TMA shows similar histopathology and should be excluded.

C. Recurrent Glomerular Disease occurs in up to 36% of cases with a mean interval of 5 years, and is currently the third leading cause of graft loss. The most common recurrent glomerular diseases are focal segmental glomerulosclerosis (10% to 50%), IgA nephropathy (13% to 46%), DDD (80% to 100%), MPGN type I (20% to 25%), MGN (10% to 30%), antineutrophil cytoplasmic antibody (ANCA) vasculitis (17%), diabetes (8% to 30%), and amyloid (5% to 30%). DDD and FSGS have the highest rates of graft loss at 15% to 30% and 13% to 20%, respectively.

D. De Novo Disease includes glomerular, malignant, tubulointerstitial, and infectious diseases. Combined de novo and recurrent glomerular disease accounts for over 15% of diagnoses in transplant biopsies.

1. De novo glomerular disease. A variety of de novo glomerular diseases can be seen (Table 19.4), and glomerulonephritis in the post-transplant setting is more likely to be recurrent than de novo. MGN is considered to be the most common de novo glomerular disease after transplant (~2%), although FSGS and IgA nephropathy are also common (*Clin J Am Soc Nephrol* 2014;9:1479). These diseases manifest similarly to their native counterparts, and are generally distinguished from recurrence by an absence of documented disease prior to transplant.

2. Posttransplant lymphoproliferative disease (PTLD) is a rare de novo disease following renal transplant. Both native and transplant kidneys are typically enlarged. Monoclonal or polyclonal B-lymphocyte proliferations can occur, and in most cases are associated with Epstein–Barr virus.

3. Calcineurin inhibitor (CNI) toxicity. The CNIs (e.g., cyclosporine, tacrolimus) have markedly improved short-term allograft survival but are nephrotoxic.

  a. Patients with **acute CNI toxicity** typically present with signs of acute renal failure which manifests on renal biopsy as isometric vacuolization of the proximal tubular epithelial cells and/or ATN. The changes are reversible with decreased exposure to the offending agent. Importantly, isometric vacuolization and ATN are nonspecific findings requiring clinical correlation. Osmotic nephrosis, for instance, may also produce isometric vacuolization.

  b. Chronic CNI toxicity, in contrast to acute CNI toxicity, is irreversible (*Transplantation* 1989;48:965). Biopsy findings include stripe or skip interstitial fibrosis and arteriolar hyalinosis (e-**Fig. 19.27**). Subendothelial beaded arteriolar hyalinosis is particularly characteristic, but since arteriolar hyalinosis may also occur secondary to hypertension or diabetes, clinical correlation is warranted. Tubulointerstitial calcium deposits are also part of CNI toxicity.

4. Infection. Infectious agents may be encountered, albeit rarely, in the transplant renal biopsy. The opportunistic fungi *Candida, Aspergillus, Cryptococcus,* and *Zygomycetes* account for approximately 5% of all renal transplant infections (*Transpl Infect Dis* 2001;3:203). White blood cell casts, granulomatous inflammation, and crescentic glomerulonephritis are all seen in association with fungal infections, typically occurring within 6 months posttransplantation.

Viral infections, most commonly polyomavirus (BK and JC) infections, may also be encountered. The polyoma BK virus is a DNA virus that causes respiratory infections with high prevalence during childhood. Respiratory infection follows hematogenous spread, reaching organs like the kidney, where it remains dormant in the collecting system; with immunosuppression, the virus reactivates and causes polyomavirus nephropathy (PVN). Polyoma virus typically infects distal tubules and collecting ducts, manifesting histologically as homogeneous intranuclear inclusions, clumped nuclear chromatin, or bubbly inclusions (e-**Fig. 19.28**). These infected cells can lyse and cause denudation of the basement membrane. PVN is staged by extent of interstitial fibrosis and extent of tubular cross-section with evidence of viral infection by cytopathic effect or immunohistochemistry (IHC) in the entire core (pvl1, <1% of tubular cross-section; pvl2, 1% to 10%; pvl3, >10%). PVN is considered to be class 1 if pvl and interstitial fibrosis ci score ci ≤1, and class 3 if pvl = 3 and ci ≥ 2) (*J Am Soc Nephrol* 2018:29:680). Cells with these features in urine cytology specimens are known as decoy cells because of their similarity to malignant cells.

CMV infects the renal allograft, causing characteristic intranuclear and cytoplasmic inclusions, but is rare due to CMV prophylactic therapy applied as a standard practice.

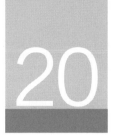

20 Surgical Diseases of the Kidney

NORMAL ANATOMY

In the adult, the normal kidney weight is 115 to 155 g for women and 125 to 170 g for men. Anatomically, the kidneys are composed of an outer cortex and an inner medulla that has 8 to 18 pyramids. The base of each pyramid is at the corticomedullary junction, and the apex forms a papilla where the collecting ducts open into the renal pelvis. The minor calyces receive the papillae, and in turn join to form the major calyces that are the dilated upper portion of the ureter in the renal pelvis. Histologically, the components of the kidney include glomeruli, tubules, blood vessels, and interstitium.

Congenital Anomalies and Polycystic Renal Disease (Renal Ciliopathies)

Louis P. Dehner and Joseph Gaut

Congenital anomalies of the kidney and urinary tract (CAKUT) are seen by the pathologist as a resected multicystic mass from the abdomen of an infant, a resected portion of the ureteropelvic junction (UPJ) in a child with obstruction, or explanted kidney(s) in the case of hereditary polycystic kidney disease (PKD).

It is estimated 20% to 30% of congenital anomalies are CAKUTs. They are present in 3 to 6 per 1,000 live births, and these various anomalies are responsible for 30% to 50% of cases of chronic renal failure in children (*Birth Defects Res Pt C* 2014;102:374; *Nat Rev Nephrol* 2015;4:720). The most common CAKUT is UPJ obstruction, representing 20% of cases. Both syndromic and nonsyndromic forms of CAKUT are recognized, as well as more than 20 single-gene causes (*Fetal Pediatr Pathol* 2014;33:293).

I. DEVELOPMENTAL ABNORMALITIES

A. **Renal Dysplasia** (RD) is one of several anomalies in normal renal development, which also includes renal hypoplasia (RH) and unilateral agenesis (*Pediatr Nephrol* 2007;22:1675; *Birth Defects* Res 2017;109:1204); the incidence is 1:1,006 live births. There are many morphologic expressions of RD, basically defined by the absence of normal nephronogenesis and in its wake the presence of immature or primitive tubules as small, rounded structures with and without accompanying cyst formation; pale myxoid spindle cell stroma containing abortive, fetal-appearing glomeruli (some cases); and small nodules of immature cartilage (10% to 30% of cases) (e-**Figs. 20.1** and **20.2**). The tubules are often surrounded by collarettes of spindle cells, one of the characteristic findings in RD. Foci of dysplasia may also be interspersed as islands in a background of more normal-appearing renal parenchyma, which reflects the stage in renal development when the interaction of the ureteric bud and metanephric ridge is disrupted in the complex mesodermal and epithelial interaction (*Cold Spring Harb Perspect Biol* 2012;4:2008300).

Obstructive and nonobstructive types of RD are generally recognized. Unilateral multicystic RD is the most common type and is associated with an atretic thread of ureter or no identifiable remnant at all. Multiple variably sized, smooth-walled cysts convey only a vague sense of a kidney since the renal pelvis is often not identifiable (e-**Fig. 20.3**). Bilateral lower urinary tract obstruction (posterior urethral valves or atresia as in prune belly syndrome) results in bilateral hydroureters and hydronephrosis with interruption in nephronogenesis and RD (*Fetal Pediatr Pathol* 2013;32:13).

Nonobstructive RD is bilateral with an intact lower urinary tract, and is in most cases a manifestation of several syndromes (*Curr Opin Pediatr* 2016;28:209). Affected infants are more often encountered in the setting of the oligohydramnios sequence (OS) and pulmonary hypoplasia. Bilateral RD is second to bilateral renal agenesis as a cause of OS.

Segmental RD presents as an upper pole cystic or multicystic structure and a duplex collecting system.

B. **Renal Hypoplasia** (RH) is a primary defect in growth and development since the microscopic features of RD are often present in these kidneys. The weight of the affected kidney is less than two SDs below the expected mean (*Pediatr Res* 2010;68:91). Germline mutations in *HNF1*β, *PAX2, EYA1, S1X1,* and *SALL1* have been detected in 15% of those cases with dysplasia (*J Am Soc Nephrol* 2006;17:2864). These kidneys are small and have a reduced number of nephrons.

C. **Polycystic Kidney Disease** (PKD) is one in a group of single-gene mutation disorders resulting in defective ciliary function termed ciliopathies (*N Engl J Med* 2011;364:1533) (Table 20.1). The other principal renal ciliopathy is nephronophthisis (NPHP), but there are many other ciliopathies associated with renal manifestations, commonly RD (*Pediatr Nephrol* 2018;28:683; *J Pediatr Genet* 2017;6:18). The pathology of the renal ciliopathies is usually encountered in explanted kidneys as surgical specimens or perinatal autopsy as in the case of the Meckel–Gruber syndrome.

1. **Autosomal recessive PKD (**ARPKD**)** results from mutations in the *PKHD1* gene which encodes polyductin/fibrocystin. ARPKD is characterized in the neonate or infant by symmetrical enlargement of the kidneys with retention of the reniform contours and otherwise normal renal pelvises and ureters (e-**Fig. 20.4**). Because of the small size of the cysts, they are often not readily apparent by gross examination. The kidneys instead have a spongiform appearance throughout. The cysts are present in the collecting ducts, measure 1 to 2 mm, and are concentrated in the medulla, where they are fusiform and have a radial orientation through the cortex and medulla (e-**Fig. 20.5**). A single layer of cuboidal epithelium lines the cysts.

   The pathologic findings in the kidneys of older children and adults are not particularly well documented, but their sizes are often appropriate for age or somewhat atrophic. Medullary cysts are present, but are less conspicuous than in the infant kidney; there is also interstitial fibrosis with tubular atrophy in the cortex and arteriolonephrosclerosis (*Clin Nephol* 2017;88:292).

   Those who survive into adolescence and adulthood may develop end-stage renal disease (ESRD), but they are at risk for hepatic complications from congenital hepatic fibrosis (portal hypertension) and/or intrahepatic bile duct cysts (Caroli disease) complicated by cholangitis in some cases.

2. **Autosomal dominant PKD** (ADPKD) results from mutations in *PKD1* (85% of cases) or *PKD2* (15% of cases) genes encoding polycystin-1 and polycystin-2, respectively. ADPKD is manifested by massively enlarged kidneys with macrocysts bulging from beyond the normal contours of the kidneys (e-**Fig. 20.6**). Smaller cysts are typically present in both kidneys, and are detectable by ultrasonography in the prenatal and newborn period in infants in affected kindreds (Table 20.1). The cysts are known to enlarge rapidly, and less than 5% of nephrons are involved in the development of the rounded cysts which occur along the entire length of the nephron with the formation of cortical and medullary cysts. The individual cysts measure from a few millimeters to several centimeters (e-**Fig. 20.7**). Columnar, cuboidal, and an inconspicuous flattened epithelium, often with patchy micropapillary hyperplasia, line the cysts (e-**Fig. 20.8**). A thickened basement membrane surrounds the cysts. Interstitial fibrosis, chronic inflammation, and arteriolar thickening are present in the end-stage kidneys.

TABLE 20.1 Renal Ciliopathies—ARPKD, ADPKD, and NPHP

	ARPKD	ADPKD	NPHP
Gene	*PKHD1*-fibrocystin (6p 12.3-p12.2)	*PKD1*-polycystin-1 (16p 13.3) (85% of cases) PKD2-polycystin-2 (4q21)(15% of cases)	*NPHP1*-nephrocystin-1 (2q 12.3)(20% of cases); 24 other genes (20% of cases); 60% genes unknown
Incidence	1:2,000–10,000 live births	1:400–1,000 live births	1:50,000–1,000,000 (AR)
In utero/infant presentation	Enlarged, cystic (<10 mm) kidneys, second trimester; OS	Unilateral or bilateral renal cysts, OS rare; PKD1, earlier and more cysts with severe disease	Infantile type (*NPHP2*) with nephromegaly and corticomedullary cysts; OS
Features in neonates and later childhood	Symmetrical, enlarged kidneys, pulmonary hypoplasia (os) 50–70% survive beyond the newborn period	Later childhood with multiple, bilateral cysts, varying sizes and extending beyond the normal contour of the kidneys, thin cortex	Juvenile type—normal or small kidneys, echogenic, loss of corticomedullary differentiation, ESRD (13 yrs)
Location of renal cysts	Collecting ducts (macrocysts in older children)	Cysts develop along the entire length of the renal tubule	Corticomedullary junction cysts, tubular basement membrane disruption, and thinning or thickening, inflammatory tubulointerstitial fibrosis
Extrarenal findings	Bile duct plate abnormality with congenital hepatic fibrosis and/or nonobstructive fusiform dilatation of bile ducts (Caroli disease) or isolated cysts, biliary microhamartoma (von Meyenburg complex)	Hepatic cysts (portal) variable size with or without bile duct plate abnormality (80% by 30 yrs) Pancreatic cysts (10%, only *PKD1*) Mitral prolapse (25%) Cerebral artery aneurysm (20–30% FH; 10% no FH) Endocardial fibroelastosis Ovarian cysts Bronchiectasis (30–40%) Seminal vesicle cysts (30–40%)	50% with only NPHP Portal fibrosis without bile duct plate defect (non-*NFHP1*) Developmental delay Visual difficulty
Complications	ESRD, portal hypertension, and cholangitis Pancreatic ductal cysts	ESRD, 2% <40 yrs, 50% >60 yrs Nephrolithiasis (20–30%) Hypertension (50–70%) Urinary tract infection (30–50%)	ESRD, 60% between 5 and 15 yrs

ADPKD, autosomal dominant polycystic kidney disease; AR, autosomal recessive; ARPKD, autosomal recessive polycystic kidney disease; ESRD, end-stage renal disease; FH, family history; NPHP, nephronophthisis; OS, oligohydramnios sequence; yr, year.
J Am Soc Nephrol 2009;20:23; *Am J Med Genet Pt C* 2009;15C:296; *Clin J Am Soc Nephrol* 2017;12:1974; *WIREs Dev Biol* 2014;3:465; *Pediatr Nephrol* 2016;31:113; *Clin Perinatol* 2014;41:543; *Am J Nephrol* 1991;11:252; *Am J Kidney Dis* 2016;67:792; *Nephrology* 2018;doi:10.1111/nep.13393; *Curr Opin Pediatr* 2015;27:201.

Any intracystic gross irregularities or parenchymal lesions should be thoroughly sampled to rule out renal cell carcinoma (RCC). Whether the cystic kidneys are intrinsically prone to develop RCC or as a complication of chronic renal dialysis remains an unresolved question (*Lancet Oncol* 2016;17:1419).

ADPKD and tuberous sclerosis complex (TSC), specifically *PKD1* and *TSC2*, may present together as a contiguous gene deletion syndrome since only 100 base pairs separate these two genes on chromosome 16p. In this setting, multiple cysts measuring less than 1 cm are detected in the first year of life with a marked increase in the size and number with cortical thinning (*Pediatr Radiol* 2015;45:386). One or multiple lesions, most commonly angiomyolipomas (AML), are also present.

D. **Nephronophthisis** (NPHP) is a collective designation for a group of predominantly AR disorders caused by more than 25 mutations of genes encoding primary ciliary proteins which have in common corticomedullary cysts with enlarged kidneys and OS in the infantile type (Table 20.1). Disruption of the renal tubules, and tubulointerstitial fibrosis with tubular basement membrane duplication with variable chronic inflammation are the rather nonspecific microscopic findings, but the diagnosis of NPHP should be considered in a child who presents with ESRD.

E. **Autosomal Dominant Tubulointerstitial Kidney Disease** (ADTKD), previously known as medullary cystic disease (MCD), is defined by at least four disorders, each with a unique mutation, *MUC1* (1q22), *UMOD* (16p 12.3), *HNF1*β (17q12), and *REN* (1q32.1). However, as many as 40% to 50% of cases do not as yet have a detectable mutation. *MUC1*-ADTKD is seemingly the most common of these disorders, presents as slowly progressive chronic kidney disease; may have corticomedullary cysts, interstitial fibrosis, tubular atrophy and microcyst formation; and progressive loss of glomerular basement membrane. The overall size of the kidney is normal or small. *UMOD*-ADTKD is characterized by childhood hyperuricemia, gout, small kidneys with corticomedullary cysts, and interstitial fibrosis. *HNF1*β-ADTKD, unlike the previous two disorders, is associated with these manifestations: pancreatic dysplasia, early onset diabetes, gout, bilateral renal cortical cysts, multicystic dysplastic kidneys (MDK), hypoplasia, and unilateral agenesis. Tubulointerstitial fibrosis is uncommon as the only features of *HNF1*β-ADTKD. *REN*-ADTKD is also accompanied by hyperuricemia, interstitial fibrosis, and tubular atrophy with or without chronic inflammation.

F. **Renal Tubular Dysgenesis** (RTD) occurs as both a genetic disorder (AR; mutations in renin–angiotensin system genes) and an acquired disorder (twin–twin transfusion syndrome, maternal ACE-inhibitors, AT2-receptor blockers, NSAIDs) characterized by renal hypoperfusion when it occurs in utero with anemia. There is also detective ossification of the skull. In addition to mutations in the renin–angiotensin cascade, it has been observed in the fetal alloimmune disorder, the so-called neonatal hemochromatosis. Otherwise normal fetal kidneys in the presence of OS, placental massive perivillous fibrosis, histiocytic intervillositis, absence of proximal renal tubules, and glomerular cysts are the range of findings in this AR, usually fetal disorder which has been identified in less than 1% of fetal autopsies.

G. **Medullary Sponge Kidney** (MSK) is a somewhat enigmatic disorder which is usually detected after several episodes of nephrolithiasis, but is seen in association with various malformation conditions and Wilms tumor (WT). Hereditary transmission is suspected though has not been established. Radial linear streaking of the medullary papillae corresponds to ectasia of the intramedullary collecting ducts.

H. **Syndromic Associated Cysts** of the kidney are manifestations of the ciliopathies and are represented by multicystic RD in Meckel–Gruber, Joubert, and Bardet–Biedl syndromes as some examples (*Pediatr Nephrol* 2013;28:863; *J Pediatr Genet* 2017;6:18).

The other syndromic category includes those hereditary disorders with autosomal dominant inheritance, von Hippel–Lindau disease (VHL) and TSC. In VHL, scattered, small cysts are present in both kidneys, but generally do not attain a size to transform the kidneys into an enlarged, polycystic organ. A low cuboidal to clear cell epithelium lines the cysts. With proliferation, an intracystic clear cell RCC develops cysts (*Semin Diagn Pathol* 2018;35:184). Countless small cysts (1 to 2 mm) and complex cystic and solid lesions in the hundreds are present in both kidneys and many of these are RCCs measuring 1 to 3 cm or less. Approximately 70% of those with VHL by age 60 have developed one or more RCCs.

TSC with renal involvement is present in 60% to 80% of affected adults with cysts, AMLs, oncocytoma, and RCC. Cysts and/or AMLs are present in 40% of children by 6 years old and in 75% by age 18. Unlike the VHL cysts with their somewhat nonspecific appearance, cuboidal cells with abundant eosinophilic cytoplasm line the renal cysts which are generally larger than those in VHL. Epithelial stratification with and without papillary proliferation of the eosinophilic tubular epithelium is also seen.

I. **Acquired Cystic Disease** (ACD) is a complication of chronic renal dialysis and is seen in 50% of those on dialysis for 3 or more years. The kidneys contain multiple cysts, but they do not attain the size of those in ADPKD. A low cuboidal and/or flattened epithelium (e-**Fig. 20.9**) lines the cysts; a more complicated papillary epithelial proliferation raises the differential diagnosis of microscopic papillary RCC. High-grade microcystic RCC with oxalate crystals is the specific histologic pattern in the setting of ACD (*Am J Surg Pathol* 2006;30:141).

J. **Simple Renal Cyst** is a common incidental finding in adults on imaging studies of the abdomen. The cyst(s) usually arises in the cortex. When these cysts are present at autopsy, they are often multiple with clear fluid enclosed in a translucent membrane, often in the presence of arterionephrosclerosis. The lining epithelium is often inconspicuous.

K. **Glomerulocystic Kidney** (GCK) is a pattern of cystically dilated Bowman spaces with diminutive glomerular tufts involving the cortical and deeper glomeruli in various congenital disorders, as well as in primary GCK disease. One of the more common settings is in association with ARPKD, but it is also associated with other ciliopathies, TSC, and as an acquired lesion in the wake of hemolytic-uremic syndrome.

ACKNOWLEDGMENTS

The authors thank Johann D. Hertel, Peter A. Humphrey, and Helen Liapis, authors of the previous edition of this chapter.

SUGGESTED READINGS

Harris PC, Torres VE. In: Adam MP, Ardinger HH, Pagon RA, et al., eds. *GeneReviews®* *[Internet]*. Seattle, WA: University of Washington, Seattle; 1993–2018. 2002 Jan 10 [updated 2018 Jul 19].

Patil A, Sweeney WE, Avner ED, Pan C. Childhood polycystic kidney disease. In: Li X, ed. *Polycystic Kidney Disease [Internet]*. Brisbane: Codon Publications; 2015.

Sweeney WE, Avner ED. In: Adam MP, Ardinger HH, Pagon RA, et al., eds. *GeneReviews®* *[Internet]*. Seattle, WA: University of Washington, Seattle; 1993–2018. 2001 Jul 19 [updated 2016 Sep 15].

Pediatric Renal Neoplasms

Louis P. Dehner and Mai He

I. **INTRODUCTION.** An abdominal mass centered upon the kidney is not always a neoplasm. For example, unilateral MDK has an incidence of 1:1,000 to 4,300 live births, compared with WT with 1 case per million children less than 15 years old (*Curr Urol Rep* 2015;16:67). Congenital hydronephrosis may also present as a mass-like lesion.

However, in terms of primary renal neoplasms in children, WT predominates all others and accounts for 85% to 90% of all kidney tumors before 20 years of age. It is estimated that WT accounts for 5% to 6% of all malignancies in children, but 7% to 8% of all malignancies in children and adolescents present in the kidney as a reflection of the other malignant non-WTs including RCC.

II. **GROSS EXAMINATION AND TISSUE SAMPLING.** Renal tumors, with some exceptions, are large relative to the size of the uninvolved kidney especially in a child. In addition to the size, the tumor is often soft to very friable (since there is relatively little stroma in the background of tumor) with or without hemorrhage and/or substantial necrosis. Weight and external dimensions should be recorded. Perirenal soft tissue attached to the capsule varies from case to case and its sampling is important to determine the status of the all important surgical margins; any disruption on the external surface may represent sites of tumor rupture which should be confirmed by a review of the surgical report. The ureter and hilar blood vessels should be identified and palpated to determine whether the renal vein is free of a tumor thrombus; the margins of these structures should be sampled. The external surface should be inked so that the margins can be identified microscopically. Bisection of the kidney reveals the mass and its relationship to the renal hilum and to the contiguous kidney, and the presence or absence of a capsule; dimensions of the tumor should be obtained at this time. Gross illustrations of the bisected specimen are desirable to label for block locations. The critical microscopic sections are those obtained from the capsule, surgical margins, and the renal hilum to document the pathologic stage, and additional sections of the tumor to ascertain for the presence or absence of anaplasia. A large soft tumor often bulges beyond the edges of the specimen so that the microscopic section may not demonstrate the capsule or peripheral margins; this problem can be addressed by overnight fixation of the other bisected half of the specimen prior to submitting sections of the margins of resection. Lymph nodes from the hilum should be sought, but lymph nodes may have been sampled and submitted separately. The various findings are brought together in a report according to cooperative research groups (Table 20.2) or standardized templates (e.g., see the College of American Pathologists Protocol for the Examination of

TABLE 20.2	Wilms Tumor Staging According to Children's Oncology Group (COG) and International Society of Pediatric Oncology (SIOP)	
Stage	**COG (Prechemotherapy)**	**SIOP (Postchemotherapy)**
I	Tumor is limited to the kidney and is completely resected	Tumor limited to the kidney or surrounded with fibrous pseudocapsule if outside the normal contours of the kidney, the renal capsule or pseudocapsule may be infiltrated with the tumor, but it does not reach the outer surface, and it is completely resected (resection margins "clear")
	Renal capsule intact, not penetrated by the tumor	The tumor may be protruding (bulging) into the pelvic system and "dipping" into the ureter, but it is not infiltrating their walls
	No tumor invasion of veins or lymphatics of the renal sinus	The vessels of the renal sinus are not involved, but intrarenal vessel involvement may be present
	No nodal or hematogenous metastases	Fine needle aspiration or percutaneous core needle biopsy ("tru-cut") do not upstage the tumor. The presence of necrotic tumor or chemotherapy-induced changes in the renal sinus/hilus fat and/or outside of the kidney should not be regarded as a reason for upstaging a tumor.
	No prior biopsy Negative margins	

TABLE 20.2	Wilms Tumor Staging According to Children's Oncology Group (COG) and International Society of Pediatric Oncology (SIOP) (Continued)	
II	The tumor extends beyond the kidney but completely resected	The tumor extends beyond the kidney or penetrates through the renal capsule and/or the fibrous pseudocapsule into the perirenal fat but is completely resected (resection margins "clear")
	The tumor penetrates the renal capsule	The tumor infiltrates the renal sinus and/or invades the blood and lymphatic vessels outside the renal parenchyma but it is completely resected
	The tumor in lymphatics or veins of the renal sinus	The tumor infiltrates adjacent organs or vena cava but is completely resected
	The tumor in the renal vein with the margin not involved	
	No nodal or hematogenous metastases	
	Negative margins	
III	The residual tumor or nonhematogenous metastases confined to the abdomen	Incomplete excision of the tumor which extends beyond resection margins (gross or microscopic tumor remains postoperatively)
	Involved abdominal nodes	Any abdominal lymph nodes are involved
	Peritoneal contamination or tumor implant	Tumor rupture before or intraoperatively (irrespective of other criteria for staging)
	Tumor spillage of any degree occurring before or during surgery	The tumor has penetrated through the peritoneal surface
	Gross residual tumor in the abdomen	Tumor implants are found on the peritoneal surface
	Biopsy of the tumor (including fine needle aspiration) prior to removal of the kidney	The tumor thrombi present at resection margins of vessels or ureter, transsected or removed piecemeal by the surgeon
	Resection margins involved by the tumor or transection of the tumor during resection (i.e., piecemeal excision of the tumor)	The tumor has been surgically biopsied (wedge biopsy) prior to preoperative chemotherapy or surgery
		The presence of necrotic tumor or chemotherapy-induced changes in a lymph node or at the resection margins should be regarded as stage III
IV	Hematogenous metastases or spread beyond the abdomen	Hematogenous metastases or spread beyond the abdomen
V	Bilateral renal tumors	Bilateral renal tumors
	Each side's tumor should be substaged separately according to the above criteria	Each side's tumor should be substaged separately according to the above criteria

Am Soc Clin Oncol Educ Book 2014;215–223.

Specimens From Patients With Wilms and Other Pediatric Renal Tumors at http://www.cap.org).

For WT, under most COG protocols, surgery is performed before chemotherapy except in those patients with an initially unresectable tumor. Some of the potential problems in the assessment of pretreated tumor specimens include a completely necrotic mass, and remnants of nephrogenic rests and hypocellular stroma with no discernible gross or microscopic tumor (*J Clin Pathol* 2010;63:102). ISOP staging reflects some of the problems encountered in the pretreated WT (Table 20.2).

III. CLINICAL, PATHOLOGIC, AND MOLECULAR ASPECTS OF RENAL NEOPLASMS IN CHILDREN. WT is not the only unique renal tumor of childhood; other pediatric tumors include clear cell sarcoma of the kidney (CCSK), malignant rhabdoid tumor, classic and cellular mesoblastic nephroma, cystic nephroma, and ossifying renal tumor of infancy (ORTI). WT and these various childhood neoplasms are rare in adults, but are well documented (*Expert Rev Anticancer Ther* 2011;11:1105).

A. Wilms Tumor (nephroblastoma) presents in approximately 600 children per year before the age of 10 years (90% of cases) in the United States, and most commonly between 3 and 5 years (65% to 70% of cases) with a slight male predilection, and more often in African Americans and less often in Asian children. Children with bilateral tumors and/or a syndromic association are generally younger than the average. In children over 10 years of age with a renal tumor (5% of all cases), WT accounts for 75% of neoplasms, but 15% of cases are RCCs and the remaining 10% represent other pediatric renal tumors. A unilateral solitary mass is present in 85% of cases, with unilateral multifocal lesions in another 10% of cases, and bilateral tumors in 5% to 8% of cases. Approximately 5% to 10% have a nonsyndromic genitourinary tract malformation (5%) or one of several malformational or overgrowth syndromes. The risk of WT varies among these disorders, especially in those with *WT1* (11p13) mutations; in Denys–Drash it is >90%, in WAGR it is 30%, and in Fraiser it is 8%. Mosaic-variegated aneuploidy, Perlman syndrome, and Fanconi anemia have risks of WT in 25% to 35% of affected children. Isolated or syndromic-associated hemihypertrophy is present in approximately 6% of WT cases. The *WT2* imprinted focus (11p15) is associated with the Beckwith–Wiedemann syndrome (BWS) with a 5% risk of WT. In addition to germline mutations in *WT1* and *WT2*, mutations in *FWT1* and *FWT2* (present in 1% of those with familial WT) and *DICER1* are associated with WT. Sporadic WTs are accompanied by somatic biallelic inactivation of *WT1* in 5% to 10% of cases. Somatic mutations in exon 3 of the *CTNNB1* gene (encodes β-catenin) in 10% to 15% of WTs and inactivation of *WTX* in almost one-third of tumors are additional events.

WTs with diffuse anaplasia have 17p (TP53) loss or mutations. Other cytogenetic abnormalities in WTs include gains in 1q, 2, 7q, 8, 12, and 15 and losses in 1p, 7p, 16q, and 22q. Loss of heterozygosity of chromosomes as 1p and 16q in favorable histology WT is correlated with a poor outcome.

The gross features of WT (e-**Fig. 20.10A–C**) can vary to a considerable degree on the basis of the composition of histologic findings (e-**Fig. 20.11A–E**), secondary changes in the form of necrosis and/or hemorrhage, and cystic formations. WT is usually a well-circumscribed mass with a well-formed capsule or pseudocapsule that serves as the boundary between the tumor and residual uninvolved kidney; WT does not infiltrate into the residual kidney but rather has a pushing border. The typical cut surface has a glistening mucoid, grey-tan appearance (e-**Fig. 20.10A**).

An extremely friable WT is often accompanied by blastemal predominant features of relatively uniform compact primitive round cells with or without faint lobulation and scattered miniature neoplastic tubules or rosettes (e-**Fig. 20.11B**). Infiltration of adjacent parenchyma can be seen on occasion; similar infiltration is present in cases of adrenal or hilar neuroblastoma (NB). WTs with a predominant stromal component (fibromyxoid or rhabdomyomatous elements) (e-**Fig. 20.11E**) have a gross resemblance to a leiomyoma and classic mesoblastic nephroma. In addition to the blastema, epithelial differentiation includes tubules, papillary profiles and abortive immature glomerular structures (e-**Fig. 20.11D**); squamous, mucinous, and primitive neuroepithelial structures are other types of epithelial formation. Primitive spindle cell mesenchyme and rhabdomyomatous differentiation are the principal types of stroma. Heterologous elements such as cartilage, adipose tissue (also seen in intralobar nephrogenic rests [ILNRs]), pigmented neuroepithelium, and other tissue types are features of the so-called teratoid WT (also seen in hepatoblastoma). It is probably fair to say

TABLE 20.3	Comparative Risk Assessment Categories of Children's Oncology Group and International Society of Paediatric Oncology	
	Surgery Followed by Chemotherapy (COG)	Chemotherapy Followed by Surgery (SIOP)
Low-risk tumors	Mesoblastic nephroma Cystic partially differentiated nephroblastoma	Mesoblastic nephroma Cystic partially differentiated nephro-blastoma Completely necrotic WT
Intermediate-risk tumors	WT without anaplasia WT with focal anaplasia	WT-epithelial, stromal, mixed, regressive, and focal anaplasia
High-risk tumors	WT with diffuse anaplasia Clear cell sarcoma of kidney Malignant rhabdoid tumor	WT, blastemal type WT with diffuse anaplasia Clear cell sarcoma of kidney Malignant rhabdoid tumor

J Clin Pathol 2010;63:102.

that no two WTs have identical pathologic features given the many variations that are typical of WTs.

1. **The presence or absence of favorable or unfavorable histology** in a WT is based on the absence or presence of enlarged (three times the size of other tumor nuclei) hyperchromatic nuclei and bizarre mitotic figures (Table 20.3) (e-**Fig. 20.12**). An unfavorable WT is one in which the nuclear changes are present in different areas of the tumor (diffuse) rather than in a limited focus (focal). If anaplasia is present in an invasive focus beyond the circumscribed mass, within the renal sinus, or tumor thrombus, or in metastatic sites, the tumor qualifies as unfavorable histology. A needle biopsy with anaplasia is also regarded as unfavorable histology.

Following chemotherapy in initially unresectable WT, biopsied or partially resected (usually bilateral) nephroblastomas are categorized according to histologically observed treatment effect (summarized in Table 20.5). Most tumors will fall into the "intermediate" grade with subtotal necrosis and classic triphasic elements observed in the remaining viable tumor; under current protocols, these patients receive an additional 6 weeks of chemotherapy. Less frequently, tumors may show complete necrosis in which case no additional chemotherapy is given. Biopsy specimens demonstrating worrisome histologic features such as predominance of blastemal elements or anaplasia after initial treatment are switched to more aggressive chemotherapeutic regimens.

An entirely different risk assessment approach on the basis of the microscopic findings is followed by SIOP since most cases receive preoperative chemotherapy, in contrast to surgery followed by chemotherapy typical of COG protocols (Table 20.3).

2. **Precursor nephrogenic lesions** of WT are represented by perilobar nephrogenic rests (PLNR) and the less common intralobar nephrogenic rest (ILNR). They are usually identified by microscopic examination except in those cases of hyperplastic NR which form mass lesions, usually less than 5 cm in maximal dimension. PLNRs are located at the periphery of the renal lobule, whereas the ILNR may occur in any location in the kidney, but more often centrally (Table 20.4). Unlike the PLNR which are discrete foci separate from the renal parenchyma (e-**Fig. 20.13A)**, ILNR has poorly defined margins and commingles with normal renal tissue resulting in indistinct margins (e-**Fig. 20.13B**).

Immature dysplastic-appearing tubules and glomeruli with and without a sclerotic stroma are the features of PLNR; these foci are found most commonly beneath the

TABLE 20.4 Features of ILNR and PLNR

	ILNR	PLNR
Location	Random (usually central)	Periphery
Composition	Stroma usually predominant Blastemal and epithelial cells usually present	Blastemal and/or epithelial Stroma poor or sclerotic
Wilms tumor histology	Triphasic/stromal Ectopic mesenchymal elements (+)	Blastemal/epithelial Ectopic mesenchymal elements (−)
Sex	Predominantly male	Predominantly female
Age at diagnosis	Early	Late
Associated anomalies	Genitourinary malformations (WAGR/Denys–Drash)	Overgrowth syndromes (BWS/hemihypertrophy)
Chromosome	11p 13	11p 15
Gene	Loss of WT1 expression	Loss of IGF2 imprinting
Interethnic variations	Common in East Asian and white	Predominantly white, rare in East Asian

J Pediatr Hematol Oncol 2007;29:590.

capsule as isolated or discontinuous foci, or as contiguous foci. When PLNR evolves into a hyperplastic rest and forms a mass lesion, the distinction from WT is a challenge especially in a biopsy. However, the resected hyperplastic rest does not form a distinct capsule and abuts the adjacent uninvolved kidney unlike WT (e-Fig. 20.13C).

ILNR is composed of tubules which may be cystic, fibrous stroma, and cartilage and adipose tissue; this lesion has a vague resemblance to RD.

The presence of multiple NRs or WTs in one kidney is one type of nephroblastomatosis; these patients are at risk for similar lesions, if not WT, in the contralateral kidney. In diffuse hyperplastic perilobar nephroblastomatosis, the kidneys are not only enlarged, but are extensively replaced by bulging contiguous nodules. It is generally unnecessary to biopsy these lesions since the imaging features are regarded as diagnostic. In the absence of a response to chemotherapy, these lesions are resected by a kidney-sparing procedure. Overall, NRs, usually microscopic, are found in 40% of unilateral WTs with the following types: PLNR (25%), ILNR (9%), both types (5%), and nephroblastomatosis (1%). Based upon the type of NR, WT has been divided into two types: type I (ILNR) and type II (PLNR) (*Pediatr Nephrol* 2013;28:13). Type I WT has a high rate of *WT1* germline mutation as well as *CTNNB1* mutation, presents in children less than 3 years old, and is often manifested by bilateral tumors. Type II WT has wild type *WT1*, presents in children 3 years of age or older, may be unilateral or bilateral, and may be accompanied by overgrowth syndromes such as BWS (Table 20.4).

WT may have two somewhat unusual presentations; one with cystic changes in the background of an otherwise typical-appearing WT. These changes are often secondary in nature with cystic necrosis and hemorrhage, but not in all cases where epithelial-lined cysts are found in the background of an otherwise typical WT. The other unique gross presentation is a WT with a botryoid or polypoid mass projecting into the renal pelvis, and even extending into the ureter and bladder (*World J Surg Oncol* 2013;11:102). These central tumors may be accompanied by ILNR.

a. **Both cystic partially differentiated nephroblastomas** (CPDN, e-Fig. 20.14) and **cystic nephroma** (CN, e-Fig. 20.15) have identical gross features as a sharply demarcated multicystic lesion whose differentiation one from the other is based upon the presence nephroblastic elements in the septa of CPDN (*J Pediatr Surg*

2003;38:897). No masses or nodules are present in CPDN, but if present, then the tumor should be regarded as a cystic WT.

  b. **Extrarenal or heterotopic nephrogenic and nephroblastic tissues** are rare but well documented in the soft tissues of the lumbosacral, inguinal, and scrotal regions as a small nodule(s) composed of immature tubules, glomeruli, and nephrogenic blastema in varying proportions; these tumors are also reported in the ovary, adrenal, uterus, and teratomas (*Pediatr Dev Pathol* 2011;14:244). They are predominantly nephroblastic lobules forming a large mass with histologic features of favorable histology WT, but small nodules in virtually the same anatomic sites have been generally interpreted as WT.

B. **Metanephric Tumors** are a presumably related group of tumors whose pathologic features range from a purely epithelial (metanephric adenoma [MA]), to an exclusively spindle cell (metanephric stromal tumor [MST]) morphology, to a mixed epithelial and stromal pattern (metanephric adenofibroma) (*Clin Lab Med* 2005;25:379). The demonstration of *BRAF* V600 mutation in MAs and MSTs has served to further support the pathogenetic relationship of these tumors beyond their overlapping pathologic features (*J Surg Pathol* 2016;40:719).

  1. **Metanephric stromal tumor (MSTs)** occurs throughout childhood, but most commonly in infancy (e-**Fig. 20.16**). This tumor was considered a mesoblastic nephroma (MN) at one time (see below), but is now regarded as a distinct entity. MST is usually solitary, unencapsulated, solid or cystic, and extends out from the renal medulla. The cut surface is firm and myomatous-appearing like the classic MN (see below). The tumor is composed of spindled to stellate cells with indistinct cytoplasm, and at low magnification has a distinctly nodular appearance on the basis of alternating areas of hypocellularity and hypercellularity. Bands of tumor cells extend outward to entrap the adjacent glomeruli and tubules, resulting in cysts. The tumor has epithelial embryonal epithelium and juxtaglomerular hyperplasia-like MN; although the spindle cells extend into the adjacent kidney, the distinguishing features of the MST from MN include concentric cuffs of spindled cells around blood vessels and renal tubules ("collarettes"), and angiodysplasia of arterioles with epithelioid transformation of smooth muscle. Heterologous elements such as cartilage and glial tissue are infrequent findings (*Am J Surg Pathol* 2000;24:917).

  2. **Metanephric adenofibroma** (MAF) occurs in both children and adults (e-**Fig. 20.14**). In children, the tumor has been reported as early as 5 months of age. MAF is centrally located and has a spindle cell stroma resembling MST as well as the epithelial nodules of MA. The peripheral stromal component merges with normal renal parenchyma in a manner similar to ILNR, MST, and MN (see section on adult tumors below) (*Am J Surg Pathol* 2001;25:433).

  3. **Metanephric adenoma** (MA) occurs most frequently in adults, although the tumor is reported in children as young as 5 years of age and may be multifocal (see section on adult tumors below). Epithelial predominant WT and papillary RCC are the other tumors in the differential diagnosis. Importantly, MA does not have the well-formed fibrous pseudocapsule of WT, but for that matter neither does a hyperplastic NR. Like WT, MAs are positive for WT1, CD57, and CDH17. Unlike WT, mitoses are rare and there is no pseudocapsule, blastemal component, or vascular invasion. Immunohistochemical stains are helpful in distinguishing MA (CK7+, AMACR-) from papillary RCC (CK7+, AMACR+), but not for distinguishing MA from an epithelial predominant WT (*Mod Pathol* 2006;19:218).

C. **Cystic Nephroma** (CN) is a distinctive neoplasm of early childhood with multilocular cystic features in common with CPDN, but it is associated with germline or somatic mutation in *DICER1* unlike CPDN. This tumor is present in 10% of children with pleuropulmonary blastoma (PPB). Only 2% to 3% of all renal neoplasms in children are CNs and most are diagnosed before 3 years of age. Grossly, the tumor is a sharply demarcated multilocular cyst, measuring up to 6 cm, distinct from the uninvolved kidney. The septa are composed of a variable cellular fibrous stroma, with or without small renal tubules or cysts which lack any associated nephroblastic stroma or tubules resembling those of nephrogenic rests or WT. The cysts are often lined by cuboidal or hobnail-like cells. CN is different from a similar appearing cystic and solid (spindle cell) neoplasm that occurs predominantly in women over 20 years of age and is known as mixed epithelial and spindle tumor (*Arch Pathol Lab Med* 2009;133:1483). Rarely, CN can undergo malignant progression to renal anaplastic sarcoma whose histologic features are virtually identical to the type II or type III PPB.

D. Mesoblastic Nephroma (MN) designates two tumor types, classic and cellular types, and may represent two distinct neoplasms with overlapping clinical features and some pathologic similarities (e-**Fig. 20.17**). However, cellular MN has a more diverse, even primitive cellular appearance and has the same translocation t(12;15) as congenital infantile fibrosarcoma (CIF) (*Pathology* 2016;48:47) (e-**Fig. 20.17C,D**). Like CIF, cellular MN has the potential to metastasize to the lung, liver, and brain. Both tumor types are unencapsulated solitary masses. The surface of classic MN has a more trabeculated surface–like MST and is rarely hemorrhagic, whereas the cellular MN has a uniform, mucoid surface and may be quite hemorrhagic as seen in CIF. Intersecting fascicles of spindle cells infiltrate from the mass into the adjacent renal parenchyma with entrapment of tubules and glomeruli in classic MN; individual embryonal appearing tubules and cartilage are included in the range of histologic features in classic MN. In contrast, cellular MN is usually sharply demarcated from the adjacent kidney in the absence of a capsule. Plump to small spindle cells with or without the formation of fascicles, readily identifiable mitotic figures, patchy foci of necrosis in some cases, and hypercellularity in excess of classic MN are the features of cellular MN. In a minority of MNs, both classic and cellular features may be present. Involvement of the renal sinus is seen in MNs.

Complete nephrectomy is the recommended treatment and positive surgical margins are managed with adjuvant chemotherapy. The recurrence rate ranges from 5% to 10% and is more common in cellular MN. Both tumor types together constitute 3% to 5% of all primary renal tumors in children; 70% are diagnosed at or before 3 months of age and virtually all cases by 2 years of age. WT and MN represent 90% of all renal tumors in children less than 12 months of age with the remainder as either MRT or CCSK (*J Pediatr Hematol Oncol* 2017;39:103; *J Pediatr Surg* 2004;39:522).

E. Rhabdoid Tumor of the Kidney (RTK) is a highly aggressive malignant neoplasm of infancy, accounting for 2% of all pediatric renal tumors (e-**Fig. 20.18**). Most patients present at less than 1 year of age with metastatic disease, and almost all patients are diagnosed by 3 years of age. Approximately 10% to 15% of RTKs are associated with rhabdoid tumors (atypical rhabdoid/teratoid tumor) of the central nervous system; these children likely have the rhabdoid predisposition syndrome with a germline mutation in *SMARCB1/INI1* (chromosome 22q11) (*Pediatr Dev Pathol* 2015;18:49). Inactivation of this gene results in the failure of nuclear staining for INI1 (BAF 47). Grossly, the renal tumor is pale tan, unencapsulated, and arises from the renal medulla (e-**Fig. 20.18A**). Multicentric or bilateral tumors are considered metastatic lesions. Sheets of discohesive tumor cells with large vesicular nuclei, prominent nucleoli, and abundant eccentric cytoplasm with large eosinophilic inclusions are the classic features (e-**Fig. 20.18**), but there are variant patterns of small cells and spindle cells whose presence can be demonstrated more effectively with vimentin and/or cytokeratin immunostains. CD99 is consistently expressed. RTK is the archetype of a family of INI1-deficient tumors (*Am J Surg Pathol* 2011;35:e47); the other INI1-deficient kidney tumor is renal medullary carcinoma (RMC).

F. Clear Cell Sarcoma of the Kidney (CCSK) represents 4% of pediatric renal tumors and is the second most common kidney neoplasm. It is a primitive mesenchymal neoplasm with a reported t(10;17) translocation in 10% of cases, or internal tandem duplication of *BCOR* in 80% to 90% of cases (*Fetal Pediatr Pathol* 2018;37:128). *BCOR* ITD is also found in primitive mesenchymal tumor of infancy and undifferentiated sarcoma of infancy. CCSK usually presents between the ages of 1 and 4 years, but is also seen in very early infancy (including stillborns) and rarely occurs in adults. It is a high-risk neoplasm with a tendency for metastases (lung, bone, brain, and soft tissue) and late recurrence. Boys are affected more often than girls.

Grossly, the tumor is unilateral, solitary, well circumscribed, and located in the renal medulla. Its cut surface is typically tan-grey and mucoid, although the surface may have a firm, whorled appearance (e-Fig. 20.19A). Cysts are often present. Microscopically, areas with classic histology contain nests and cords of uniform polygonal to spindled cells that have ovoid nuclei with finely granular to vesicular chromatin, inconspicuous nucleoli, and indistinct cytoplasm in a background of clear extracellular matrix. A delicate, arborizing fibrovascular network separates groups of tumor cells. The tumor interface is well circumscribed, but the tumor may extend a short distance into the adjacent parenchyma, entrapping tubules that may become cystic or have epithelial metaplasia. Almost all tumors have at least focal classic histology; however, numerous variant histologies are recognized and may predominate (e-Fig. 20.19B–H) including myxoid, sclerosing, cellular, epithelioid, palisading, spindle cell, pericytomatous, storiform, and anaplastic patterns. CCSK tumor cells are positive for vimentin as well as Cyclin-D1 and CD117, but neither is specific for CCSK (*Hum Pathol* 2017;67:225).

G. **Ossifying Renal Tumor of Infancy** (ORTI) is a rare neoplasm of uncertain histogenesis which is diagnosed throughout the first year of life, has a male predilection, and has a preference for the left kidney (*Pediatr Dev Pathol* 2017;20:511). The calcified tumor arises from the renal papilla and projects into the renal pelvis. In addition to the osteoid matrix with epithelioid osteoblasts, a stroma with blastemal and spindle cell features is present. The stromal and osteoblastic cells express vimentin and nuclear WT1, whereas the osteoblasts are immunoreactive for EMA and STAB2 (nuclear).

H. **Pediatric** RCC represents about 5% to 6% of primary neoplasms of the kidney in children and is second only to WT in the first two decades of life. The overall incidence of RCC has continued to increase in the United States, especially in the 20- to 24-year age group (*J Urol* 2014;191:1665). The average age at diagnosis is 11 to 14 years with a nearly equal distribution of males and females. The types and distribution of renal cell neoplasms are quite different between adults and children (Table 20.5). Higher-stage disease, histologic grade, and larger tumors in children are some significant differences between the pediatric and adult RCCs (*J Urol* 2015;193:1366).

1. **Microphthalmia transcription factor (MiTF) or translocation family of RCCs** (tRCC) includes those tumors with fusion transcripts including *TFE3* (Xp11.2) and *TFEB* (6p21.1). There are several fusion partners with Xp11.2 including the two

TABLE 20.5	Types of Renal Cell Neoplasms in Children and Adults		
Adults[a]	**No (%)**	**Children**[b]	**No (%)**
CcRCC	703 (20)	tRCC	56 (47)
pRCC	142 (14)	unRCC	25 (21)
Onco	76 (8)	pRCC	20 (17)
unRCC	37 (4)	RMC	13 (11)
chRCC	29 (3)	chRCC	4 (3)
mulRCC	13 (1)	Onco	1 (<1)
cdRCC	3 (<1)	ccRCC	1 (<)
RMC	1 (<1)		
Total	1,004 (~100)		120 (~100)

ccRCC, clear cell renal cell carcinoma; cd, collecting duct carcinoma; ch, chromophobe; mul, multilocular; onco, oncocytoma; p, papillary; RMC, renal medullary carcinoma; t, translocation; un, unclassified.
[a]*J Urol* 2008;17:439.
[b]*Cancer* 2015;121:2457.

most common at chromosome 17q25 (same fusion transcript as alveolar soft part sarcoma) and at chromosome 1q2. Approximately 15% of children with Xp11.2 RCCs have a history of prior cytotoxic therapy. Both tRCCs are also known to occur in adults.

Grossly, both tumors present as a solitary mass, measuring up to 10 cm and have a grey-tan to brown appearance, with or without cystic and/or hemorrhagic features. The histologic features of the Xp11.2 RCC include papillary and nested patterns with clear to more acidophilic cytoplasm, sharply defined cell borders, vesicular nuclei, and prominent nucleoli (e-**Fig. 20.20**). Psammoma bodies are found in 50% to 60% of cases. These tumors can be quite variable in their histologic features, so that from a morphologic perspective the differential diagnosis often includes PRCC or ccRCC; it is the presence of a second population of smaller tumor cells arranged around eosinophilic nodules of basement membrane–like material which is the essential clue to the correct diagnosis.

These tumors have some overlap in their immunophenotype which is not surprising, but the nuclear overexpression of TFE3 and TFEB unequivocally discriminates between these tumors (Table 20.6). TFEB RCC, unlike TFE3 RCC, does not have an epithelial phenotype, but strongly expresses Mel A and HMB-45 which is weakly or not expressed in TFE3 RCC.

2. **Renal medullary carcinoma (RMC) and VCL-ALK RCC**, the latter a more recently reported entity (see below), have in common that they occur in children, adolescents, and young adults with sickle cell trait (*Pediatr Blood Cancer* 2015;62:1694; *J Oncol Pract* 2017;13:414). RMC is another tumor type in the family of SMARCB1 (INI1-deficient) neoplasms whose archetype is malignant RTK (*Adv Anat Pathol* 2014;21:394). RMC presents as a large infiltrating mass which appears to arise from the renal medulla, but oftentimes this soft, necrotic tumor has invaded and replaced a substantial proportion of the kidney (e-**Fig. 20.21A**). Microscopically, solid sheets, cords, cribriform nests, and microcystic (yolk sac–like) patterns are seen in

TABLE 20.6	Differential Immunohistochemical Staining of TFE3 and TFEB Translocation Renal Cell Carcinomas	
	TFE3	**TFEB**
TFE3	+	−
TFEB	−	+
CD10	+	+ (focal)
AMACR	+	±
Mel A	±	+
HMB-45	±	+
AE1/AE3	±	−
VIM	±	+ (weak)
EMA	±	−
CK7	±	−
CATHK	+ (PRCC) − (ASPSCR1)	±
CD117	−	+
RCC	+	±
CAM 5.2	+	+
PAX 8	+	±

an otherwise monotonous round cell neoplasm with high-grade features; the tumor cells have variably prominent eosinophilic or rhabdoid inclusions that can be easily demonstrated by vimentin and/or cytokeratin immunostaining (e-**Fig. 20.21B**). There is loss of INI1 nuclear reactivity.

3. **VCL-ALK RCC** is in another renal tumor associated with the sickle cell trait, mainly in children between the ages of 6 and 14 years (*Am J Surg Pathol* 2014;38:858). As the name implies, it is characterized by an *ALK* rearrangement. Grossly, the tumor measures up to 8 cm and can have focal necrosis. Microscopically, the tumor is largely composed of round cells with some interposed spindle cells. The tumor cells have resemblance to those of RMC but lack cytoplasmic inclusions; in their place, the cells have intracytoplasmic vacuoles which are EMA positive. The vesicular nuclei have smaller nucleoli than those of RMC and MRT. Immunohistochemical staining reveals CAM 5.2, AE1/AE3, PAX 8, and noncircumferential ALK-1 positivity. The following stains are nonreactive: CD10, RCC, Mel A, HMB-45, and Cath K.

4. **Collecting duct carcinoma**, rare overall and rarer yet in children, is discussed below in regard to its resemblance and differences from RMC and fumarate hydratase (FH)-deficient RCC.

5. **Postneuroblastoma RCC** was initially considered a distinctive subtype of RCC occurring in older children and adolescents with a prior history of NB. More recent data reveal that these tumors are examples of tRCC, oncocytic-chromophobe tumor, and PRCC, and are not recognized as a specific subtype of RCC in the 2016 WHO classification (Moch H, Humphrey PA, Ulbright TM, Reuter VE, eds. *World Health Organization Classification of Tumours of the Urinary System and Male Genital Organs.* Lyon: IARC Press; 2016).

I. **Mesenchymal and Small Cell Neoplasms** are represented by a diverse array of tumors which occur more commonly in the bone or soft tissues of older children and adults (*Semin Diagn Pathol* 2015;32:160).

1. **Neuroblastoma** (NB) is known to invade into the kidney from the adrenal or perirenal–perihilar soft tissues. One series indicated that 20% of abdominal NBs invade into the kidney (*J Pediatr Surg* 1994;29:930). A true intrarenal NB is diminishingly rare and its existence is controversial in some quarters (*Am J Surg Pathol* 2012;36:94). NB can be present in the hilum of the kidney and is difficult to differentiate from WT, or as an intrarenal mass difficult to distinguish from mesoblastic nephroma. Diagnostically, it is important to remember that the primitive tubules of WT resemble the rosettes of NB.

2. **Other malignant round cell neoplasms** as primary tumors of the kidney include Ewing sarcoma-primitive neuroectodermal tumor, desmoplastic small round cell tumor, and poorly differentiated synovial sarcoma (e-**Fig. 20.22**).

3. **Anaplastic sarcoma** of the kidney is a *DICER1*-related neoplasm that is morphologically a complex multipatterned sarcoma with primitive features arising from CN. These tumors have an appearance which is virtually identical to the solid areas of type II or III PPB (*Am J Surg Pathol* 2007;31:1459; *Mod Pathol* 2014;27:1267; *Pediatr Blood Cancer* 2016;63:1272).

4. **Spindle cell tumors** of the kidney have been noted in the context of MN and MST. Other examples include solitary fibrous tumor, EBV-associated smooth muscle tumor, and pericytic tumors including myofibroma and myopericytoma. Renomedullary interstitial cell tumor, though relatively common in adults, is uncommon in children (*Am J Surg Pathol* 2016;40:1693).

5. **Vascular neoplasms** are in general rare in the kidney and usually occur in adults, but an example of kaposiform hemangioendothelioma in a child has been reported.

6. **Angiomyolipoma (AML)** of the kidney is the most common representative of a group of tumors known as PEComas (*Ann Diagn Pathol* 2015;19:359). Approximately 80% of patients with AML have TSC, especially in children. The epithelioid variant of AML is reported in children, and as in adults, has a malignant potential (*Urology* 2014;83:1394).

ACKNOWLEDGMENTS

The authors thank Jason A. Jarzembowski and Frances V. White, authors of the previous edition of this chapter.

SUGGESTED READINGS

Argani P, Beckwith JB. Renal neoplasms in childhood. In: Mills SE, ed. *Sternberg's Diagnostic Surgical Pathology*. 6th ed. Philadelphia, PA: Wolters Kluwer; 2016:2034–2035.
Chintagumpala M, Muscal JA. Presentation, diagnosis, and staging of Wilms tumor. https:www.uptodate.com/contents/presentation-diagnosis-and-staging-of-wilms-tumor.
Fernandez CV, Geller JI, Ehrlich PF, Hill DA, Kalapurakal JA, Dome JS. Renal tumors. In: Pizzo PA, Poplack DG, eds. *Pediatric Oncology*. 7th ed. Philadelphia, PA: Wolters Kluwer; 2016:753–771.
Moch H, Humphrey PA, Ulbright TM, Reuter VE, eds. *WHO Classification of Tumours of the Urinary System and Male Genital Organs*. 4th ed. Lyon: IARC; 2016:48–53.
Popov SD, Sebire NJ, Vujanic GM. Wilms tumor-histology and differential diagnosis. In: van den Heuvel-Eibrink MM, ed. *Wilms Tumor*. Brisbane (AU): Codon Publications; 2016.

Adult Renal Neoplasms

Jennifer K. Sehn and Peter A. Humphrey

I. **GROSS EXAMINATION AND TISSUE SAMPLING.** Renal tissue sampling for tumor includes partial and radical nephrectomies and, less commonly, needle biopsies and fine needle aspirates.

A. **Needle Core Biopsy** of a renal mass is most commonly performed prior to percutaneous ablation (radiofrequency heat ablation or cryotherapy) of the mass, or in cases where other clinical entities such as lymphoma or metastasis are in the differential diagnosis. The cores are usually processed for routine H&E-stained slides. If lymphoma is in the differential diagnosis, additional core(s) should be submitted fresh for lymphoma workup. Histopathologic diagnosis of needle core biopsy tissue from renal masses is highly accurate in establishing a malignant diagnosis (*J Urol* 2008;180:2333). Immunohistochemistry may aid in typing (*Am J Surg Pathol* 2014;38:e35–e49). RCC grade in needle core tissue is often lower than the grade in the whole tumor (*Urology* 2010;76:610).

B. **Partial Nephrectomy.** The surgical resection margin is inked, the specimen is serially sectioned, and the size of the mass and distance to the resection margin are recorded. Sections demonstrating the relationship of the mass to the surgical resection margin and perirenal fat are taken. Intraoperative consultation for gross or frozen section examination of the margin is sometimes requested (*Arch Pathol Lab Med* 2005;129:1505).

C. **Radical Nephrectomy.** A radical nephrectomy includes the kidney; a portion of the ureter, renal vein, and artery; perinephric fat; and the Gerota fascia. The adrenal gland may also be present. Intraoperative consultation is most commonly requested to grossly confirm the presence of a renal or pelvic mass in the nephrectomy specimen (*Arch Pathol Lab Med* 2005;129:1586).

After weighing the entire specimen, the renal hilum is examined to identify the ureter, renal vein, and artery; cross-sections of these margins are taken (Fig. 20.1). The renal vein and ureter are opened longitudinally. The perirenal soft tissue is inked.

The kidney is bivalved longitudinally through the renal pelvis then serially sectioned. The tumor size, location, involvement of calyceal or pelvic mucosa, invasion into

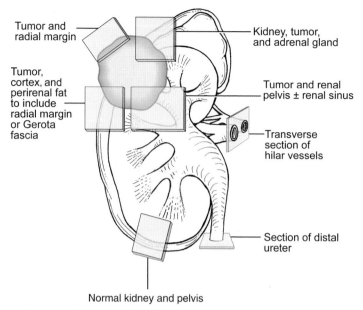

Tumor and
radial margin

Kidney, tumor,
and adrenal gland

Tumor,
cortex, and
perirenal fat
to include
radial margin
or Gerota
fascia

Tumor and renal
pelvis ± renal sinus

Transverse
section of
hilar vessels

Section of distal
ureter

Normal kidney and pelvis

Figure 20.1 Sampling of radical nephrectomy specimen for adult renal tumors. Sections through renal masses should demonstrate the relationship of mass to capsule, peripheral fat, renal parenchyma, and renal pelvis. (Modified from Schmidt WA. *Principles and Techniques of Surgical Pathology*. Menlo Park, CA: Addison-Wesley; 1983.)

perinephric or renal sinus soft tissue, and involvement of the adrenal gland (direct extension or metastasis) are recorded. The uninvolved parenchyma is also examined; color, cortical thickness, additional focal lesions, and renal pelvis are described. One section per centimeter of the tumor, demonstrating its relationship to the capsule/perinephric fat, renal sinus fat, renal pelvis, and renal parenchyma is submitted, as well as sections of any additional lesions, uninvolved renal parenchyma, and adrenal gland (Fig. 20.2) (*Am J Surg Pathol* 2013;37:1505). Nephroureterectomy for urothelial carcinoma is described in Chapter 21.

II. DIAGNOSTIC FEATURES OF COMMON TUMORS OF THE ADULT KIDNEY

A. Renal Cell Carcinoma (RCC). RCC arises from the epithelium of the renal tubules and represents approximately 90% of all renal malignancies in adults.

1. Risk factors. The most important risk factor is tobacco smoking. Additional risk factors include obesity, hypertension, unopposed estrogens, and exposure to arsenic, asbestos, cadmium, organic solvents, pesticides, and fungal toxins. Patients with tuberous sclerosis, chronic renal failure, and ACD of the kidney have an increased incidence of RCC. About 5% of patients with ACD of the kidney develop renal cell tumors (see below). Most RCCs are sporadic, although there are several inherited cancer syndromes that affect the kidney (*Am J Surg Pathol* 2015;39:e1), the most common of which are described below.

a. von Hippel–Lindau (VHL) disease is inherited in an autosomal dominant manner and is characterized by clear cell RCC, hemangioblastomas of the cerebellum and retina, pheochromocytoma, pancreatic neuroendocrine tumors, and inner ear tumors. Typically, renal tumors are multiple and bilateral (**e-Fig. 20.23**). Numerous

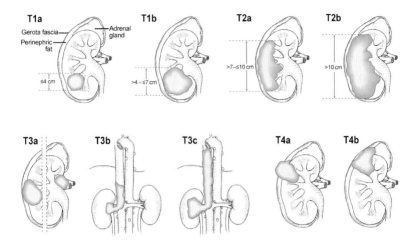

Figure 20.2 Renal cell carcinoma pathologic primary tumor (pT) stages. (Modified from Moch H, Humphrey PA, Ulbright TM, Reuter VE, eds. *WHO Classification of Tumours of the Urinary System and Male Genital Organs.* Lyon, France: IARC Press; 2017.)

renal cysts lined by neoplastic clear cells (**e-Fig. 20.24**) are also characteristic. The disease is caused by germline mutations of the *VHL* tumor suppressor gene on chromosome 3p25.3.

b. **Hereditary papillary RCC** is also inherited in an autosomal dominant manner and is characterized by multiple, bilateral papillary RCCs. Multiple papillary adenomas are frequently seen in the background kidney. The disease is caused by mutations of the *MET* oncogene on chromosome 7q31.

c. **Birt–Hogg–Dubé syndrome** is characterized by cutaneous hamartomas (fibro-folliculomas), pulmonary cysts, and renal tumors. Multiple and bilateral diverse types of renal tumors are present; the chromophobe RCC is most common, but oncocytoma, "hybrid" chromophobe-oncocytic (**e-Fig. 20.25**), papillary, and clear cell tumors can also be seen (*Arch Pathol Lab Med* 2006;130:1867). The syndrome is autosomal dominant with incomplete penetrance. The responsible gene, *FLCN* (encoding the protein folliculin), is located on chromosome 17p11.2.

d. **Tuberous sclerosis complex (TSC)** is an autosomal dominant but variably penetrant disorder characterized by hamartomas and neoplasms of the brain, eyes, skin, kidney, and heart. AML is the most common renal tumor in TSC; oncocytoma and RCC also can be seen (*Am J Surg Pathol* 2014;38:895). Two genes have been implicated in tuberous sclerosis: *TSC1* and *TSC2*, located at 9q34 and 16p13.3, respectively.

e. **Hereditary leiomyomatosis and RCC** is an autosomal dominant disease caused by mutations in the fumarate hydratase (*FH*) gene. Patients are predisposed to cutaneous and uterine leiomyomas, as well as RCC and uterine leiomyosarcoma. Tumors usually have papillary architecture and high-grade cytologic features, including prominent eosinophilic macronucleoli (*Am J Surg Pathol* 2014;38:627).

f. **Hereditary paraganglioma-pheochromocytoma syndrome** is caused by mutations in the genes encoding succinate dehydrogenase (SDH). Renal tumors (SDH-deficient RCC) have been described in patients with mutations in one of four genes encoding subunits of the SDH enzyme (*SDHA, SHDB, SDHC,* or *SDHD*). SDH-deficient gastrointestinal stromal tumors also have been seen in this population.

2. **Clinical diagnosis.** Hematuria, pain, and a flank mass compose the classical triad of presenting symptoms, but in North America most renal tumors are now detected as incidental findings by radiologic studies. Other presentations include weight loss, anorexia, fever, hypercalcemia, erythrocytosis, hypertension, gynecomastia, anemia, and hepatosplenomegaly. Radiologic studies, especially ultrasound and computed tomography (CT), are useful for detection and characterization of renal masses, but up to 15% of renal masses thought to be malignant by radiology are histologically benign, typically oncocytomas or AMLs.

3. **Histologic typing and diagnosis of renal epithelial malignancies.** The 2016 World Health Organization (WHO) classification of neoplasms of the kidney is given in Table 20.7, which represents a significant revision of the prior WHO 2004

TABLE 20.7 WHO Histologic Classification of Tumors of the Kidney

Renal cell tumors

Clear cell renal cell carcinoma

Multilocular clear cell renal neoplasm of low malignant potential

Papillary renal cell carcinoma

Hereditary leiomyomatosis and renal cell carcinoma–associated renal cell carcinoma

Chromophobe renal cell carcinoma

Collecting duct carcinoma

Renal medullary carcinoma

MiT family translocation renal cell carcinomas

Succinate dehydrogenase–deficient renal cell carcinoma

Mucinous tubular and spindle cell carcinoma

Tubulocystic renal cell carcinoma

Acquired cystic disease–associated renal cell carcinoma

Clear cell papillary renal cell carcinoma

Renal cell carcinoma, unclassified

Papillary adenoma

Oncocytoma

Metanephric tumors

Metanephric adenoma

Metanephric adenofibroma

Metanephric stromal tumor

Nephroblastic tumors and cystic tumors occurring mainly in children

Nephrogenic rests

Nephroblastoma

Cystic partially differentiated nephroblastoma

Pediatric cystic nephroma

Mesenchymal tumors

Occurring mainly in children
   Clear cell sarcoma
   Rhabdoid tumor
   Congenital mesoblastic nephroma
   Ossifying renal tumor of infancy

Occurring mainly in adults
   Leiomyosarcoma (including the renal vein)
   Angiosarcoma
   Rhabdomyosarcoma
   Osteosarcoma
   Synovial sarcoma
   Ewing sarcoma
   Angiomyolipoma
   Epithelioid angiomyolipoma
   Leiomyoma
   Hemangioma
   Lymphangioma
   Hemangioblastoma
   Juxtaglomerular cell tumor
   Renomedullary interstitial cell tumor
   Schwannoma
   Solitary fibrous tumor

Mixed epithelial and stromal tumor family

Adult cystic nephroma

Mixed epithelial and stromal tumor

Neuroendocrine tumors

Well-differentiated neuroendocrine tumor

Large cell neuroendocrine carcinoma

Small cell neuroendocrine carcinoma

Pheochromocytoma

Miscellaneous tumors

Renal hematopoietic neoplasms

Germ cell tumors

From Moch H, Humphrey PA, Ulbright TM, Reuter VE, eds. *WHO Classification of Tumours of the Urinary System and Male Genital Organs.* Lyon, France: IARC Press; 2017. Used with permission.

TABLE 20.8 Immunohistochemical Stains in Select Renal Tumors with Clear Cells

Tumor Type	CA IX	CD10	Vim	CK7	CD117	PAX8	HMB-45 Melan-A	EMA	Inhibin	Hale Colloidal Iron
ccRCC	+	+	+	−	−	+	−	+	−	+
chRCC	−	−	−	+	+	+	−	+	−	+
CCP RCC	+ (cup-like)	− (focal)	+	+	−	+	−	+	−	−
Translocation carcinoma	− (weak, focal)	+	+/−	−	−	+	+	−	−	−
Epithelioid AML	−	−	+	−	−	−	−	−	+	−
Adrenal cortex	+/−	−	+	−	−	−	−	−	+	−

−, most tumors are negative; +, most tumors are positive; +/−, tumors may be positive or negative; AML, angiomyolipoma; CA IX, carbonic anhydrase IX; CCP RCC, clear cell papillary RCC; ccRCC, clear cell renal cell carcinoma; chRCC, chromophobe RCC; vim, vimentin.
Modified from *Arm J Surg Pathol* 2014;28:e35–e49, *Arch Pathol Lab Med* 2017;141:1181–1194, and Amin MB, Grignon DJ, Srigley JR, Eble JN, eds. *Urological Pathology.* Philadelphia, PA: Lippincott Williams & Wilkins, 2014.

classification. Many renal neoplasms can be typed based on the examination of H&E-stained slides, though immunohistochemistry also can be helpful in typing or in confirming the diagnosis of metastatic RCC (*Am J Surg Pathol* 2014;38:e35).

a. **Clear cell RCC** is the most common histologic type. Grossly, these tumors often have a variegated appearance (e-**Fig. 20.26**). Bright yellow areas (e-**Fig. 20.27**) are due to the high lipid content of the cells, whereas red and white-yellow regions are due to hemorrhage, fibrosis, and degeneration or necrosis. Calcification and cystic change are fairly common. The cysts can be multilocular (e-**Fig. 20.28**). Histologic sections show round or polygonal cells with clear or eosinophilic cytoplasm and centrally located nuclei. The cells are arranged in nests within a fine vascular network (e-**Fig. 20.29**). The classic vascular meshwork investing alveolar collections of tumor cells is particularly helpful in distinguishing clear cell RCC from other tumor types with clear cytoplasm. In higher-grade tumors, the cytoplasm frequently becomes more eosinophilic. Immunohistochemical stains that are useful in distinguishing clear cell RCC from other tumors with clear cells are summarized in Table 20.8. *VHL* is frequently mutated or deleted in both sporadic and syndromic clear cell RCCs.

WHO/ISUP nucleolar grading (a simplification of the previously utilized Fuhrman nuclear grading) is the most important prognostic factor after staging (Table 20.9; *Am J Surg Pathol* 2013;37:1490). Tumors should be graded according to the highest grade present, even if focal (defined as occupying at least one 400× high-power field) (e-**Figs. 20.30–20.33**). Sarcomatoid or rhabdoid features confer a worse prognosis, as does tumor necrosis (*Am J Surg Pathol* 2016;40:1224).

Clear cell RCC spreads locally into the renal sinus or perinephric fat by direct extension, and by venous invasion into the renal vein and vena cava. Lymphatic spread to lymph nodes can occur. Hematogenous spread to the lungs, liver, and bone is most frequent, although metastasis to unusual sites is a well-known characteristic. Metastasis can develop many years after primary diagnosis. In the appropriate morphologic and clinical context, PAX8 is a useful immunostain in establishing the renal origin for a metastatic carcinoma. However, reactivity for PAX8 must be interpreted with caution, as multiple tumor types arising in other sites (particularly the gynecologic tract) also are positive for PAX8. CD10 and RCC immunoreactivity also can be supportive (*Am J Surg Pathol* 2014;38:e35).

b. **Multilocular cystic neoplasm of low malignant potential** (MCNLMP, formerly multiloculated cystic RCC) is a rare neoplasm consisting of multiple cysts separated by thin septa and lined by clear cells with bland cytologic features (WHO/ISUP grade 1 or 2) (e-**Fig. 20.34**); clear cells should be present within the septa (e-**Fig. 20.35**) but are not permitted to form expansile nodules, in which case a diagnosis of clear cell RCC would be more appropriate (e-**Fig. 20.28**). Calcification is common. MCNLMP shares immunohistochemical and genetic features with clear cell RCC. However, the prognosis in these purely cystic tumors is excellent, with no reported recurrence or metastasis when strictly defined (*Am J Surg Pathol* 2013;27:1469).

c. **Papillary RCC** comprises about 10% of RCCs. Grossly, the tumor is usually tan and friable and is frequently grossly described as necrotic, even when the tumor histologically lacks necrosis. Tumors may be cystic or hemorrhagic and typically

TABLE 20.9	**ISUP/WHO Nucleolar Grading of Renal Cell Carcinoma**
Grade 1	Nucleoli absent or inconspicuous and basophilic at 400× magnification
Grade 2	Nucleoli conspicuous and eosinophilic at 400× and visible but not prominent at 100×
Grade 3	Nucleoli conspicuous and eosinophilic at 100×
Grade 4	Extreme nuclear pleomorphism, sarcomatoid and/or rhabdoid differentiation

have a fibrous pseudocapsule (**e-Fig. 20.36**). Multifocality and bilaterality are more common than for other RCCs. Microscopically, there is a papillary or tubulopapillary architecture composed of papillae with thin fibrovascular cores, which classically harbor aggregates of foamy macrophages (**e-Fig. 20.37**).

There are two types of papillary RCC. Type I tumors have papillae lined by a single layer of cuboidal cells with scant cytoplasm (**e-Fig. 20.37**) that has a basophilic quality. Type II tumors have taller cells with more abundant eosinophilic cytoplasm, higher nuclear grade, and pseudostratified nuclei (**e-Fig. 20.38**).

Immunohistochemical stains can be useful in distinguishing papillary RCC from other types of RCC that can have papillary architecture (Table 20.10). Genetically, there is characteristic trisomy of chromosomes 7 and 17 with loss of chromosome 4, although type II papillary RCC is actually genetically very heterogeneous; chromosomal analysis is therefore not as diagnostically useful (*Am J Surg Pathol* 2017;41:1618). Papillary RCC, especially type I, has a better prognosis than clear cell RCC. WHO/ISUP nucleolar grading is prognostic in papillary RCC and should be applied.

d. Chromophobe RCC accounts for approximately 5% of RCCs. Grossly, chromophobe RCCs are well circumscribed, solid, and beige to light brown (**e-Fig. 20.39**). The tumors are composed of pale polygonal cells with prominent cell borders ("vegetable cells"), irregular/wrinkled nuclear membranes, and perinuclear halos (**e-Fig. 20.40**). The cytoplasm is flocculent (**e-Fig. 20.41**) to eosinophilic (**e-Fig. 20.42**), but may also show clearing. WHO/ISUP nucleolar grading is not applied in chromophobe RCC. Chromophobe RCC has a much better prognosis than clear cell RCC.

Diagnostic difficulty may arise with the eosinophilic variant of chromophobe RCC, where other tumors with eosinophilic or oncocytic features enter into the differential diagnosis. A panel of immunostains and Hale colloidal iron (characteristically diffusely positive in the cytoplasm of chromophobes) can help resolve the diagnostic dilemma (Table 20.11). Genetically, chromophobe RCC shows the loss of multiple entire chromosomes (aneusomy).

e. Hereditary leiomyomatosis and renal cell carcinoma–associated renal cell carcinoma is a recently described rare tumor type in patients with hereditary (germline) mutations in FH. As noted above, HLRCC-associated RCC shows

TABLE 20.10	Immunohistochemical Stains in Select Renal Tumors With Papillary Architecture							
Tumor Type	CA IX	CD10	CK7	AMACR (P504S)	p63	CK 34BE12	TFE3 TFEB	HMB-45 Melan-A
pRCC, T1	−	+	+	+	−	−	−	−
pRCC, T2	−	+	+/−	+	−	−	−	−
CCP RCC	+ (cup-like)	− (focal)	+	−	−	+	−	−
Translocation carcinoma	− (weak, focal)	+	−	+	−	−	+	+
Collecting duct carcinoma	−	+/−	+	−	+	+	−	−

−, most tumors are negative; +, most tumors are positive; +/−, tumors may be positive or negative; CA IX, carbonic anhydrase IX; CCP RCC, clear cell papillary RCC; CK 34BE12, cytokeratin 34betaE12; pRCC, T1, papillary RCC, type I; pRCC, T2, papillary RCC, type II.
Modified from *Am J Surg Pathol* 2014;28:e35–e49; *Arch Pathol Lab Med* 2017;141:1181—1194; and Amin MB, Grignon DJ, Srigley JR, Eble JN, eds. *Urological Pathology*. Philadelphia, PA: Lippincott Williams & Wilkins, 2014.

TABLE 20.11		Immunohistochemical Stains in Select Renal Tumors With Eosinophilic/Oncocytic Cells					
Tumor Type	CA IX	CD10	AMACR	CK7	CD117	HMB-45 Melan-A	Hale Colloidal Iron
ccRCC, eosinophilic variant	+	+	+/–	–	–	–	–
chRCC, eosinophilic variant	–	–	–	+	+	–	+ (diffuse cytoplasmic)
Oncocytoma	–	+/– (focal)	–	–	+	–	– (luminal)
pRCC, eosinophilic variant	–	+	+	+ (focal)	–	–	–
Epithelioid AML	–	–	–	–	–	+	–

–, most tumors are negative; +, most tumors are positive; +/–, tumors may be positive or negative; AML, angiomyolipoma; CA IX, carbonic anhydrase IX; ccRCC, clear cell renal cell carcinoma; chRCC, chromophobe RCC; pRCC, papillary RCC.
Modified from *Am J Surg Pathol* 2014;28:e35–e49; *Arch Pathol Lab Med* 2017;141:1181—1194; and Amin MB, Grignon DJ, Srigley JR, Eble JN, eds. *Urological Pathology*. Philadelphia, PA: Lippincott Williams & Wilkins, 2014.

prominent cherry-red macronucleoli and frequently has papillary architecture. Immunohistochemical staining for loss of FH and/or overexpression of 2-succinocysteine (2SC) is diagnostically useful but not widely available.

f. **Collecting duct carcinoma** is thought to arise from the collecting ducts of Bellini. It accounts for <1% of renal cell tumors. These tumors are centered in the medulla, have tubular or tubulopapillary architecture, and have a surrounding desmoplastic reaction (e-**Fig. 20.43**). The tumor cells are of high nuclear grade and can have hobnail morphology. Immunohistochemical stains are most useful for excluding other types of RCC or urothelial carcinoma, which are the main entities in the differential diagnosis (Table 20.10). Prognosis in collecting duct carcinoma is poor.

g. **Renal medullary carcinoma** is very rare. Tumors in adults are identical to those in the pediatric age group as discussed above.

h. **MiT family translocation RCCs** are defined by translocations involving the *TFE3* gene (at Xp11) or *TFEB* gene (at 6p21). Although rare in adults, they are histologically identical to those in the pediatric age group as discussed above (e-**Fig. 20.44A,B**). A high index of suspicion, particularly in younger adults, is helpful in recognizing these tumors. *TFE3* immunohistochemistry can be useful but is technically difficult; fluorescence in situ hybridization for *TFE3* or *TFEB* gene rearrangements is the most definitive test for this tumor type.

i. **Succinate dehydrogenase (SDH)-deficient RCC** is a recently recognized tumor type in patients with mutations in one of the *SDH* genes. Tumors are well circumscribed and may have cystic areas. The tumor cells have rounded nuclei with even chromatin, and characteristically have eosinophilic cytoplasm with bubble-like cytoplasmic inclusions. Loss of SDHB expression by immunohistochemistry is diagnostic; these tumors also are negative for CK7 and CD117. The tumor's nuclear features may bring neuroendocrine neoplasms (e.g., carcinoid tumor) into the differential diagnosis, but SDH-deficient RCC is negative for chromogranin and synaptophysin expression. Patients also may have hereditary paragangliomas, gastrointestinal stromal tumors, or pituitary adenomas, as mentioned above.

j. Mucinous tubular and spindle cell carcinoma is an uncommon, predominantly low-grade renal epithelial neoplasm that is grossly well circumscribed with light tan, uniform cut surfaces (**e-Fig. 20.45**). Microscopically, elongated tubules are separated by a mucinous stroma (**e-Fig. 20.46**). The tumor cells are cuboidal or spindle shaped with low-grade nuclear features. Uncommonly, necrosis, clear cells, papillations, foamy macrophages, and inflammation can be present (*Am J Surg Pathol* 2006;30:1554). Sarcomatoid or high-grade epithelial components are also uncommon. The immunophenotype shows significant overlap with papillary RCC.

k. Tubulocystic RCC is a rare multicystic renal tumor with a sponge-like gross morphology (*Am J Surg Pathol* 2009;33:384). Histologically, the tumor consists of tubules and cysts in a fibrous stroma, lined by a single layer of cuboidal to hobnail cells with WHO/ISUP grade 3 nucleoli (**e-Fig. 20.47**). These tumors lack intraluminal papillations. Genetic features overlap with papillary RCC. However, tubulocystic RCC usually follows an indolent course with only rare reported metastases and recurrence.

l. Acquired cystic disease–associated RCC occurs in patients with end-stage kidney disease on dialysis (*Am J Surg Pathol* 2006;30:141; *Am J Surg Pathol* 2018;42:1156). The tumor classically has a sieve-like microcystic architecture imparted by intra- or intercytoplasmic vacuoles in large, eosinophilic tumor cells (**e-Fig. 20.48**). Intratumoral oxalate crystals are characteristic and may be abundant. The tumors are typically indolent but may metastasize, particularly if sarcomatoid or rhabdoid features are present. Of note, most carcinomas arising in end-stage kidneys are of more common types (e.g., clear cell, papillary, or chromophobe).

m. Clear cell papillary RCC can arise in ESRD but also in kidneys without end-stage features (*Am J Surg Pathol* 2010;34:1608; *Mod Pathol* 2009;22:S2). Tubuloacinar or papillary architecture is common. The cuboidal tumor cells have clear cytoplasm and characteristically show apical nuclear orientation (**e-Fig. 20.49**). Cup-like staining for carbonic anhydrase IX is classic (**e-Fig. 20.50**). Despite the name, clear cell papillary RCC is genetically unrelated to either clear cell or papillary RCC. Most tumors are low stage at presentation and limited outcome data suggest an extremely favorable prognosis.

n. Unclassified RCC is a diagnosis that should be reserved for tumors that do not fit into other categories. It is a diagnosis rendered in about 5% of RCC cases. Features that place tumors in this group include the following: a combination of different histologic types, mucin production, purely sarcomatoid appearance, presence of epithelial and stromal elements, and lack of identifiable patterns. This designation is linked to a worse prognosis than clear cell RCC (*BJU Int* 2007;100:802).

Sarcomatoid change (**e-Figs. 20.51** and **20.52**) can be associated with a specific type of carcinoma or can overgrow the preexisting carcinoma type and exist in pure form. The percentage of the tumor that is sarcomatoid should be specified as being less than or greater than 50%. Heterologous malignant bone, cartilage, fat, and skeletal muscle, or homologous undifferentiated malignant spindle cells can be seen. Rhabdoid cells (**e-Fig. 20.53**) can be found in about 5% of RCC cases, usually clear cell carcinoma (*Am J Surg Pathol* 2000;24:1329–1338). Both sarcomatoid and rhabdoid features are associated with a poor prognosis.

B. Benign Epithelial Tumors

1. Papillary adenoma of the kidney is the most common benign epithelial neoplasm of renal cells. Grossly, the tumor consists of single or multiple well-defined white nodules in the renal cortex. The tumors have papillary, tubular, or tubulopapillary architecture (**e-Fig. 20.54**), low nuclear grade (**e-Fig. 20.55**), and measure ≤15 mm in diameter. The cytoplasm is scant and noncleared, and nuclear grooves can be present. Psammoma bodies and foamy macrophages are common. Genetic and morphologic features are similar to papillary RCC, but tumors ≤15 mm reportedly do not metastasize.

2. **Oncocytoma** is a benign epithelial neoplasm that comprises approximately 5% of all neoplasms of the renal tubular epithelium. The lesion is more frequent in men, and the peak incidence is during the seventh decade of life. Grossly, the tumors are well circumscribed and the cut surface is typically mahogany-brown (e-**Fig. 20.56**). A central scar (e-**Figs. 20.56** and **20.57**) is seen in up to 33% of cases, generally with larger tumors; such scarring, although characteristic, is not specific for oncocytoma. Hemorrhage is frequent, but necrosis is almost always absent.

Microscopically, these tumors are composed of nests and tubules of polygonal cells that have granular eosinophilic cytoplasm, round nuclei, and single central nucleoli (e-**Fig. 20.58**). Scattered larger cells with atypical nuclei can be seen (e-**Fig. 20.59**). Smaller cells with scant cytoplasm (known as oncoblasts) can also be noted in some cases (e-**Fig. 20.60**). A hyalinized or edematous stromal background is frequent. Extension into perirenal fat and vessels has been described. Rare cases of numerous oncocytic tumors (oncocytosis) have been described. Chromosomal abnormalities in oncocytoma include t(5;11) and loss of chromosomes 1 and 14, but assessment for these abnormalities is not usually necessary. No cases of death due to metastatic disease have been reported. Oncocytoma should be distinguished from eosinophilic or oncocytic variants of RCC; immunohistochemical staining can be helpful, as noted previously (Table 20.9). Great caution should be exercised in diagnosing oncocytoma on renal needle biopsies, as many RCC types can harbor oncocytoma-like areas. In some cases, a biopsy diagnosis of "oncocytic renal neoplasm" is most appropriate.

C. **Metanephric Tumors** (see also the pediatric renal neoplasm section above)

1. **Metanephric adenoma** occurs in children and in adults during the fifth and sixth decades. It is more frequent in women. About 50% of cases are incidental. Tumors are usually well circumscribed and gray to yellow. Hemorrhage, necrosis, calcification, and cyst formation are common. Microscopically, MAs are composed of small, uniform tubules and acini with small lumens (e-**Fig. 20.61**). Papillary formations and psammoma bodies are commonly seen. The cells are uniform with scant cytoplasm, small nuclei, and inconspicuous nucleoli. In the differential diagnosis with papillary RCC, immunoreactivity for WT1 with focal staining for CK7 but negative staining for EMA favor MA.

2. **Metanephric adenofibroma** is more common in men. Grossly, it is solitary and partially cystic. Histologically, its cells are similar to those of an MA but are embedded in a stroma of fibroblast-like spindle cells. Psammoma bodies are also common.

D. **Mesenchymal Tumors**

1. **Leiomyosarcoma** is the most common renal sarcoma; it occurs mainly in adults and affects women and men equally. Leiomyosarcomas can arise from the renal capsule, parenchyma, pelvic muscularis, or the renal vein. They are solid, gray-white, and focally necrotic. Histologically, these tumors are composed of spindle cells with a fascicular growth pattern (e-**Fig. 20.62**). Necrosis, nuclear pleomorphism, and numerous mitotic figures indicate malignancy. Leiomyosarcoma is an aggressive tumor with a 5-year survival rate of 29% to 36%, and most patients die within 1 year of diagnosis. Sites of metastasis include the lung, liver, and bone. Sarcomatoid RCC and urothelial carcinoma are in the differential diagnosis and are significantly more common; diffuse desmin, smooth muscle actin, and h-caldesmon immunoreactivity favor leiomyosarcoma.

2. **Rare primary sarcomas** include rhabdomyosarcoma, angiosarcoma, osteosarcoma, synovial sarcoma, Ewing sarcoma, chondrosarcoma, low-grade fibromyxoid sarcoma, and malignant mesenchymoma.

3. **Angiomyolipoma (AML)** is a benign clonal mesenchymal neoplasm tumor composed of thick-walled blood vessels, smooth muscle cells, and adipose tissue (e-**Fig. 20.63**). This tumor belongs to the perivascular epithelioid cell tumor (PEComa) family. The

mean age at presentation is 45 to 55 years for patients without tuberous sclerosis, and 25 to 35 years for patients with tuberous sclerosis. Patients with tuberous sclerosis tend to have multiple bilateral renal tumors, and can have associated pulmonary lymphangioleiomyomatosis. Tumors are nonencapsulated, yellow to pink masses (e-**Fig. 20.64**). Rarely, AMLs can extend into the renal vein or the vena cava. Vascular invasion and lymph node involvement can be present; however, these features are considered to be evidence of direct extension and multifocality, respectively, rather than metastatic disease.

Microscopically, the smooth muscle cells are generally spindled (e-**Fig. 20.65**) but can appear round or epithelioid in some cases (e-**Fig. 20.66**). The smooth muscle cells often appear to radiate from the outer aspect of thick-walled, hyalinized blood vessels (e-**Fig. 20.67**). Nuclear atypia can be present (e-**Fig. 20.68**). The amount of fat is variable and can be very focal (e-**Fig. 20.66**). Uncommon to rare histologic variants include fat predominant, smooth muscle predominant, lymphangioleiomyomatous (e-**Fig. 20.69**), oncocytoma like, sclerosing type, and AML with epithelial cysts (e-**Fig. 20.70**). Characteristically, AMLs coexpress melanocytic markers such as HMB45 and smooth muscle markers such as smooth muscle actin. Epithelial markers including cytokeratin are always negative. AMLs can be diagnosed in needle biopsy tissue (e-**Fig. 20.71**). Classic AMLs are benign.

4. Epithelioid angiomyolipoma is a potentially malignant mesenchymal neoplasm that presents more commonly in patients with tuberous sclerosis. It is much less common than usual AML. Grossly, these tumors are usually large with tan-gray or hemorrhagic cut surfaces and necrosis. The cells are epithelioid with abundant granular cytoplasm. Multinucleated cells, nuclear pleomorphism, mitotic activity, vascular invasion, necrosis (e-**Fig. 20.72**), and involvement of perinephric fat can be present. These tumors express melanocytic markers with variable expression of smooth muscle markers. Metastases to lymph nodes, liver, lungs, and spine have been reported.

5. Leiomyoma is a benign smooth muscle neoplasm that can arise from the renal capsule, the muscularis of the renal pelvis, or from cortical vascular smooth muscle. Most leiomyomas are found incidentally. Grossly, they are firm well-defined masses, although calcification and cysts can be present. Necrosis should be absent. Leiomyomas are composed of spindled cells arranged in fascicles, with minimal nuclear pleomorphism and no mitotic activity. They demonstrate a smooth muscle immunophenotype, with actin and desmin immunopositivity. The so-called capsulomas that look like leiomyomas originating from the capsule that are HMB-45 positive are thought to be monophasic leiomyomatous AMLs.

6. Hemangioma is a benign vascular tumor that presents in young and middle-aged adults. The tumor is usually unilateral and single, with a red spongy gross appearance. Microscopically, the lesion is characterized by irregular blood-filled spaces lined by a single layer of endothelial cells. No mitoses or nuclear pleomorphism is present.

7. Lymphangiomas are more common in adults and can represent a lymphatic malformation or can develop secondary to urinary tract infections. Grossly, they are cystic, encapsulated lesions that can overgrow the entire renal parenchyma. The cysts are filled with clear fluid and lined by a single layer of flat endothelium.

8. Juxtaglomerular cell tumors are benign renin-secreting tumors that occur in younger individuals and are more common in women. Clinically, the tumor manifests with severe hypertension and hypokalemia. The tumors are solid, well circumscribed, and composed of sheets and papillae composed of polygonal or spindled cells with central regular nuclei, well-defined borders, and granular eosinophilic cytoplasm. Mast cells, hyalinized vessels, and tubular elements are common. The tumor cells are immunoreactive for renin, actin, vimentin, and CD34.

9. Renomedullary interstitial cell tumors (medullary fibromas) are a common incidental finding. Frequently, they are multifocal. They are 1- to 5-mm white nodules located within the renal pyramids. Histologically, they contain small stellate cells in a delicate basophilic stroma. Entrapped renal tubules can be seen (e-**Fig. 20.73**).

10. Hemangioblastomas, schwannomas, and solitary fibrous tumors rarely occur in the kidney and are identical to their counterparts in other anatomic sites.

E. **Mixed Epithelial and Stromal Tumor (MEST) Family** represents a spectrum of biphasic tumors with a combination of spindled stroma, glands, and a variable cystic component, including tumors previously classified as adult cystic nephroma. These tumors also have been referred to as renal epithelial stromal tumors (REST) (*Am J Surg Pathol* 2007;31:489). The tumors occur primarily in perimenopausal women; in men, a history of hormone therapy is typically present. In contrast to pediatric cystic nephroma, adult MEST lack mutations in the *DICER1* gene and are not associated with a tumor syndrome. Grossly, the tumor is mostly solid and cystic. Microscopically, tubules and cysts are lined by cuboidal to flattened or hobnailed epithelium (e-**Figs. 20.74** and **20.75**). The stromal component comprises the septa and solid areas; stroma may exhibit myxoid, smooth muscle, ovarian stromal–like, or collagenous features. Fat can be present. The tumor behavior is benign, except in rare cases that undergo frank malignant transformation.

F. **Neuroendocrine Tumors**

1. **Renal well-differentiated neuroendocrine tumors (carcinoid tumors)** are very rare and present between the fourth and seventh decades. There is a tendency for occurrence in horseshoe kidneys, and there is an association with renal teratomas. Renal carcinoid tumors are solid, lobulated, and well circumscribed, and are histologically similar to carcinoids in other organs (e-**Fig. 20.76**) (*Am J Surg Pathol* 2007;31:1539). Metastases are common (first to regional lymph nodes and subsequently to viscera), but survival is often long.

2. **High-grade neuroendocrine carcinoma,** including small cell carcinoma, can rarely arise in the adult kidney. A primary tumor elsewhere should be clinically and radiologically excluded. Morphology and prognosis is the same as high-grade neuroendocrine carcinoma arising in other sites.

3. **PNETs** are rare primary renal tumors, and are discussed above in the pediatric renal neoplasm section.

4. **Primary renal NB and paraganglioma (extra-adrenal pheochromocytoma)** are very rare.

G. **Hematopoietic and Lymphoid Tumors.** Primary renal lymphomas usually arise in transplanted kidneys and are Epstein–Barr virus (EBV)-associated B-cell lymphoproliferations. Secondary involvement of the kidney by lymphoma is more common (e-**Figs. 20.77** and **20.78**). Plasmacytoma can occur as a manifestation of disseminated multiple myeloma. Diffuse infiltration of the kidney secondary to acute leukemia has also been reported.

H. **Germ Cell Tumors** include choriocarcinomas and teratomas, and are very rare.

I. **Metastatic Tumors** to the kidney include tumors of the lung, breast, gastrointestinal tract, pancreas, ovary, testis, and malignant melanoma. Involvement is usually in the setting of known, widely metastatic disease. Only infrequently does metastatic tumor mimic a primary renal tumor. Most metastases are multiple and bilateral.

III. **HISTOLOGIC GRADING OF RCC** should be reported for all RCCs of clear cell and papillary types, as described in Table 20.7.

IV. **PATHOLOGIC STAGING** of RCCs follows the 2017 American Joint Committee on Cancer (AJCC)/International Union Against Cancer (UICC) TNM staging classification (Amin MB, Edge S, Greene F, et al., eds. *AJCC Cancer Staging Manual*, 8th ed. New York: Springer, 2017). Recent changes include that invasion of the pelvicalyceal system is now considered a T3a disease. Careful examination and sampling of the tumor–renal sinus fat interface is essential for correct classification of T2 versus T3a tumors. It is also important to document whether adrenal gland involvement, when present, is via direct extension from the primary tumor (T4) or represents a separate metastatic focus to the adrenal (M1).

V. **REPORTING OF ADULT KIDNEY CARCINOMA** should follow suggested guidelines (e.g., College of American Pathologists Protocol for the Examination of Specimens from Patients with Invasive Carcinoma of Renal Tubular Origin, available at http://www.cap.org). Notably, it has recently become a requirement to comment on the nonneoplastic renal parenchyma whenever possible (*Am J Surg Pathol* 2013;37:1505).

A. **For a fine needle aspiration (FNA) biopsy,** report the presence or absence of a neoplasm, and the type of neoplasm (by WHO classification).

B. **For a core needle biopsy,** report the histologic type, histologic grade (WHO/ISUP grade), and any additional pathologic findings (such as inflammation and glomerular disease).

C. **For a nephrectomy**, report the procedure (partial or radical nephrectomy), tumor size (largest, if multiple), focality (unifocal or multifocal), histologic type, presence or absence of sarcomatoid or rhabdoid features, WHO/ISUP grade (if clear cell or papillary RCC), presence or absence of tumor necrosis, extent of tumor involvement, margin status, lymph node status (if applicable), and AJCC TNM classification. The adrenal gland, if present, should be reported as uninvolved by tumor, involved by direct invasion, or involved by metastasis. Additional pathologic findings in nonneoplastic tissue 5 mm or more from the mass must be recorded, including glomerular, tubulointerstitial, and vascular disease.

VI. **NONNEOPLASTIC TUMOROUS CONDITIONS** include the maldevelopment and nonneoplastic cystic diseases discussed above. Another important pseudoneoplastic category includes inflammatory masses such as xanthogranulomatous pyelonephritis (XGP), renal malakoplakia, and tuberculosis.

A. **Xanthogranulomatous Pyelonephritis** (XGP) is a subacute to chronic, unilateral inflammatory process that can form a mass in the kidney mimicking RCC clinically, radiographically, grossly, and histologically. This disease most commonly occurs in women from the fourth to the sixth decades of life. XGP typically presents with fever, flank pain, or a tender flank mass, and is frequently related to nephrolithiasis. Urine cultures show common urinary tract pathogens, such as *Escherichia coli* and *Proteus mirabilis,* in up to 70% of cases. If the kidney itself is cultured, an organism can be isolated in 95% of cases.

   Macroscopically, XGP can either be confined to the kidney or extend into the surrounding soft tissue. XGP is typically composed of yellow nodules of varying size replacing the normal renal parenchyma (e-**Fig. 20.79**); the nodules can range in size from a few millimeters to several centimeters. Microscopically, the nodules are composed of lipid-laden macrophages (e-**Fig. 20.80**) that can mimic low-grade clear cell RCC, especially in small tissue samples like needle biopsy specimens. The lesion may also contain reactive and even multinucleated fibroblasts that can mimic a sarcomatoid component in RCC. However, XGP lacks the vascularity typically seen in RCC, and moreover, XGP often exhibits neutrophils, lymphocytes, foreign-body giant cells, plasma cells, cholesterol clefts, and microabscesses. If there is concern for RCC, a panel of immunohistochemical stains can be helpful; the clear cells in XGP will be positive for CD68 and vimentin but negative for epithelial markers such as EMA and cytokeratins.

B. **Renal Malakoplakia** is uncommon but can simulate a primary renal neoplasm when forming a discrete mass. Most patients are women; extrarenal involvement of the urinary bladder, ureter, or retroperitoneum is common. The lesion is bilateral in about one-quarter of cases. Grossly, there may be diffuse multinodular cortical enlargement or a large yellow mass. Abscesses and cystic spaces may also be seen. Microscopically, the hallmark is sheets of macrophages (von Hansemann histiocytes) with intracellular or extracellular Michaelis–Gutmann bodies (e-**Fig. 20.81**). Lymphocytes and plasma cells may also be present, and with time, fibrosis may develop.

C. **Renal Tuberculosis.** The kidney is the most common site of tuberculosis in the genitourinary tract. Grossly, miliary tuberculosis in the kidney is remarkable for numerous very small white nodules, mainly in the cortex. In the ulcerative form of renal tuberculosis, caseating necrosis can involve multiple renal pyramids with associated papillary necrosis, cavitation, and extension of the necrosis into the renal pelvis. In advanced disease, necrotic nodules can also efface the renal cortex.

ACKNOWLEDGMENT

The authors thank Maria F. Serrano, an author of the previous edition of this chapter.

Cytopathology of Renal Neoplasms

Lily Zhang and Souzan Sanati

The role of FNA in diagnosis of renal masses is limited in comparison with many other deep-seated organs, due in part to the success of imaging techniques in correct classification of most renal masses as benign or malignant. For cystic renal lesions, FNA is considered a diagnostic modality only when imaging studies shows equivocal results (Bosniak category 2 and 3). However, since the majority of these cysts require extensive tissue sampling for a definitive diagnosis, the role of FNA in establishing a diagnosis is limited with unacceptably low sensitivity for detection of malignancy. Therefore, due to the high pretest probability of malignancy (5% to 57%) in these lesions, a negative result is best classified as nondiagnostic. However, FNA can be extremely useful when malignant cellular features are identified.

Despite these limitations, FNA of renal masses, under radiologic guidance, can be used as an alternative to core biopsy in evaluating metastatic tumors, benign masses (eliminating the need for a surgical procedure), masses diagnosed in patients who are poor surgical candidates, masses with equivocal radiologic features, and in masses occurring in candidates for partial nephrectomy or tumor ablation procedure.

When the renal pelvis is involved by tumor, cytologic sampling can be performed endoscopically. Since the endoscopic biopsies are usually small, cell block processing is advocated, particularly in low-grade lesions where the architectural features are of diagnostic importance. Cytologic evaluation of ureteral catheterization samples is also useful for detecting high-grade urothelial lesion of the upper urinary tract (*J Urol* 2000;164:1901). In the case of renal abscesses, FNA can have a therapeutic as well as diagnostic role.

I. CYTOPATHOLOGY OF RENAL NEOPLASMS

A. Benign Neoplasms

1. **Angiomyolipoma (AML).** Mature adipose tissue, smooth muscle, and blood vessels are the main components of this tumor (e-**Fig. 20.82**). Identification of adipose tissue in the FNA biopsy is an important clue for diagnosis; however, most AMLs subject to cytologic sampling have a low fat content. The smooth muscle component may have an epithelioid appearance with significant nuclear atypia, and it is important not to misinterpret this finding as a malignant process. Immunostains for HMB45 and Melan-A are used to differentiate AML from RCC since most RCCs are negative for these markers (*Acta Cytol* 2006;50:466).

2. **Oncocytoma** can be solitary or multifocal, and usually has a characteristic radiologic appearance that includes good demarcation, a central scar, and a density similar to the uninvolved renal parenchyma. Cytologic samples are cellular and show numerous singly dispersed large cells and round nests (usually seen on cell blocks) with abundant granular cytoplasm, round nuclei, and distinct cell borders. The nucleolus can be prominent (similar to nucleoli in Fuhrman nuclear grade 2 clear cell RCC), but no necrosis or mitoses are present (e-**Fig. 20.83**). Binucleation and/or multinucleation are common (e-**Fig. 20.84**). The morphology of this tumor has overlapping features with chromophobe RCC and the granular variant

of clear cell RCC; it is therefore prudent to diagnose these lesions as oncocytic neoplasm on cytologic samples if the round-nested architecture is not seen (*Cancer* 2001;93:390).

B. Malignant Neoplasms

1. Clear cell RCC is the most common renal malignancy. FNA samples are usually richly cellular and bloody. The neoplastic cells have abundant vacuolated cytoplasm that may be more noticeable in air-dried, Romanowsky-stained slides (**e-Fig. 20.85**). The tumor cells have abundant wispy cytoplasm with indistinct cell borders. The small cytoplasmic vacuoles are usually located peripherally, and the granular cytoplasm is central. It is not unusual to see naked nuclei from disrupted tumor cells in the background. When tumor microfragments are available, a rich capillary network is seen (**e-Fig. 20.86**). The degree of nuclear abnormality and the presence of prominent nucleoli are dependent on the nuclear grade of the tumor. Application of the Fuhrman nuclear grade to cytology samples is appropriate.

The most common pitfalls which result in a false-positive diagnosis include XGP (in which macrophages can be mistaken for the malignant cells of clear cell RCC) and contamination (with benign cellular elements such as benign hepatocytes and adrenal cortical cells). Caution when making a diagnosis of malignancy on sparsely cellular samples will prevent an overdiagnosis in these situations.

2. Papillary RCC is characterized by papillary structures, foamy macrophages which usually distend fibrovascular cores on sections of cell block (**e-Fig. 20.87**), and psammoma bodies. Some tumors may show higher degree of cytologic atypia (**e-Figs. 20.88, 20.89**). In addition, nuclear pseudoinclusions, nuclear grooves, and cytoplasmic hemosiderin can be identified (*Diagn Cytopathol* 2006;334:797).

3. Chromophobe RCC consists of cells with abundant cytoplasm, well-defined cell borders, and a perinuclear halo. The nuclei show significant size variation and usually show irregular contours and hyperchromasia resulting in a raisinoid appearance, nuclear features that allow for differentiation from oncocytoma. Nuclear grooves and/or pseudoinclusions and necrotic debris can also be present. The cell block can be quite helpful when it demonstrates a trabecular growth pattern; a cell block also provides material for appropriate stains (such as Hale colloidal iron).

4. Urothelial carcinoma is the most common tumor arising in the renal pelvis. It is morphologically similar to urothelial carcinomas arising at other sites. The tumor consists of large elongated cells with dense cytoplasm and occasionally "cercariform" cells. The cytologic findings vary according to the grade; cells from low-grade tumors lack nuclear atypia and may have a spindle shape (**e-Fig. 20.90**).

5. Metastatic tumors. The kidney is a common site for metastatic tumors. The most common origin of metastatic tumors to the kidney is the lung. A history of malignancy in another organ and appropriate use of immunohistochemistry (ideally on sections of cell block) are keys to correct diagnosis.

21

Renal Pelvis and Ureter
Jennifer K. Sehn and Peter A. Humphrey

I. **NORMAL ANATOMY.** The upper tract of the urinary collecting system is composed of the renal calyces, pelves, and ureters. Renal papillae protrude into the minor calyces, which expand into two or three major calyces, which in turn are outpouchings of the renal pelvis, a sac-like expansion of the upper ureter.

The mucosa is normally arranged in folds. The urothelium is three to five cell layers thick in the renal pelvis and five to seven cells thick in the ureter. The lamina propria is composed of highly vascularized connective tissue without a muscularis mucosa; it is absent beneath the urothelium lining the renal papillae and is thinned along the minor calyces. The thickness and amount of muscularis propria in the collecting system within the renal sinus fat can be variable. Ureteral muscularis propria is composed of interlacing bundles of smooth muscle, without inner or outer layers (SE Mills ed., *Histology for Pathologists.* 2nd ed., Philadelphia, PA: Lippincott Williams and Wilkins, p. 839–907, 2007).

II. **GROSS EXAMINATION AND TISSUE SAMPLING.** Tissue samples include ureteroscopic biopsies, needle biopsies, segmental ureterectomy specimens, radical cystectomy/cystoprostatectomy specimens, and radical nephroureterectomy with urinary bladder cuff resection specimens.

  A. **Ureteroscopic Biopsies** should be entirely submitted. Because these are often minuscule, one approach to processing is to submit the biopsy sample for cytology cell block preparation (*Urology* 1997;50:117).

  B. **Needle Core Biopsies** of renal masses, including urothelial carcinoma involving the kidney, should be completely submitted. For microscopic examination, it is recommended that three levels on each of three hematoxylin and eosin (H&E)-stained slides be produced.

  C. **Pyeloplasty Specimens** from ureteropelvic junction (UPJ) obstruction procedures consist of a portion of the distal pelvis with an attached short segment of the ureter. If the specimen is intact, it will be funnel shaped; narrowing and/or angulation of the ureter may be evident. However, usually the specimen will be longitudinally splayed open by the surgeon and consists of a flat, fan-shaped pelvis with the nub of the opened ureter at the "handle" of the fan. The mucosa should be examined to rule out rare mass lesions. Measurements include mural thickness of the pelvis and ureter, and both external and internal diameter of the ureter (the latter at its narrowest point). If present, narrowing and angulation of the ureter should be noted. Submitted sections include serial cross-sections of the ureter and distal pelvis.

  D. **Segmental Ureterectomy** is performed for localized tumors of the ureter. The length and diameter of the intact ureter is recorded, searching for a mass by palpation and visual inspection. The outer aspect of the ureter is inked, and proximal and distal margins are taken. The ureter is then opened longitudinally and assessed for mucosal abnormalities. After overnight fixation in 10% formalin, sections are taken to demonstrate the deepest invasion of any lesion(s). At least one section of the uninvolved ureter should also be submitted.

  E. **Radical Cystectomy/Cystoprostatectomy With Segments of Ureters.** Ureteral margin(s) may be submitted for frozen section for evaluation of carcinoma (particularly carcinoma in situ [CIS]). These are shaved margins and should be submitted as cross-sections.

  F. **Radical Nephroureterectomy With Bladder Cuff.** Gross examination and sampling should document the relationship of the tumor to the adjacent renal parenchyma, peripelvic fat, nearest soft tissue margin, and ureter. Sections of grossly unremarkable kidney, pelvis, and ureter should also be submitted. The important urothelial margin is the urinary bladder cuff, which can be sampled as shave sections.

III. DIAGNOSTIC FEATURES OF COMMON DISEASES

A. Benign Conditions that involve the urothelium in the upper tract have an appearance similar to those in the urinary bladder. Examples are ureteritis (e-Fig. 21.1), pyelitis cystica and glandularis, malakoplakia, nephrogenic adenoma, and squamous metaplasia (e-Fig. 21.2).

B. Ureteropelvic Junction (UPJ) Abnormalities can be seen in biopsies performed for UPJ obstruction (UPJO), which is the most common cause of pediatric hydronephrosis and is usually diagnosed by fetal ultrasound. UPJO can also be seen in adults. Although in a minority of cases, ureteropelvic junction obstruction is due to extrinsic compression by aberrant vessels, most cases are thought to be due to an intrinsic abnormality of the UPJ itself. The pathogenesis of intrinsic UPJO is not well established. Proposed etiologies include abnormal recanalization of the proximal ureter during embryogenesis, persistence of fetal mucosal folds, abnormalities of smooth muscle including disorientation and discontinuity, and abnormal innervation. UPJO initially results in pelvic and calyceal dilatation, followed by progressive obstructive renal damage which results in features of renal dysplasia in patients with end-stage disease. Gross and histopathologic findings reported in UPJO specimens include increased mural thickness, abnormal mucosal folds/fibroepithelial polyps, smooth muscle hypertrophy and disarray (e-Fig. 21.3), attenuation of smooth muscle with increased collagen to smooth muscle ratio, and chronic inflammation. Prognosis is based on concurrent renal biopsy and renal function rather than UPJ findings (*Pediatr Nephrol* 2000;14:820, *Pediatr Develop Pathol* 2006;9:72, *Histopathol* 2007;51:709). Malignancy should also be excluded.

C. Benign Epithelial Neoplasms are rare and include urothelial papilloma, inverted papilloma, villous adenoma, and squamous papilloma.

D. Benign Nonepithelial Neoplasms include the distinctive fibroepithelial polyp (e-Fig. 21.4), which is most frequently seen in the proximal ureter of young males. Microscopically, these are bulbous intraluminal projections of a variably inflamed fibrovascular stroma lined by a normal urothelium. Benign mesenchymal neoplasms such as leiomyoma, hemangioma, neurofibroma, and fibrous histiocytoma are rare.

E. Urothelial Dysplasia in isolated form is rare and displays the same features as in the urinary bladder. More commonly, dysplasia occurs in conjunction with urothelial CIS.

F. Renal Pelvic and Ureteral Cancers are of urothelial type in the vast majority of cases, as in the urinary bladder (*Am J Surg Pathol* 2004;28:1545, *Mod Pathol* 2006;19:494, *Adv Anat Pathol* 2008;5:127). Upper tract tumors differ from those in the urinary bladder in the following ways. Upper tract tumors are less common; have a stronger association with long-term analgesic (such as phenacetin) abuse and urinary tract obstruction; are associated with an increased frequency (up to 65% of patients) of synchronous or metachronous urothelial neoplasms elsewhere in the urinary tract (Murphy WM, Grignon DJ, Perlman EJ. *Tumors of the Kidney, Bladder, and Related Urinary Structures.* Washington, DC: American Registry of Pathology, 2004); and tend to present with higher histologic grade and at higher stage. Also, biopsy of upper tract tumors is more difficult than lower tract tumors. In about one of four cases, small ureteroscopic biopsies of the upper tract will be nondiagnostic due to inadequate tissue (*Am J Surg Pathol* 2009;33:1540).

1. Risk factors. The main risk factor, as for urinary bladder malignancies, is smoking. Other risk factors are analgesics as noted above; occupation in chemical, petrochemical, or plastics industries; exposure to tar, coal, or asphalt; papillary necrosis; thorium contrast exposure; hereditary nonpolyposis colorectal cancer (HNPCC) syndrome (Lynch syndrome II) (*J Urol* 2011;185:1627); and toxins such as aristolochic acid associated with Balkan nephropathy and Chinese herbs nephropathy (*Ann Int Med* 2013;158:469).

2. Clinical features. Most patients are around 70 years of age, and the chief presenting symptoms are hematuria and flank pain. In the majority of patients, there is a prior history of a bladder cancer; many upper tract tumors are detected during the course of clinical surveillance after diagnosis of a bladder tumor.

3. **Histologic typing and diagnosis of upper tract tumors** are accomplished by examination of H&E-stained sections. Typing of upper tract urothelial neoplasia is the same as that for the urinary bladder as defined in the 2016 World Health Organization (WHO) classification of neoplasms (Table 22.1).

4. **Urothelial carcinoma** is by far the most common type of upper tract tumor.

   a. **Gross diagnosis** is possible in resection specimens. Patterns of growth include papillary, polypoid, nodular, ulcerative, and infiltrative. Exophytic tumors can fill and distend the pelvis (e-**Fig. 21.5**), with or without associated hydronephrosis and stones. High-grade invasive tumors can grossly involve soft tissue and/or renal parenchyma (e-**Fig. 21.6**). Extensive renal parenchymal involvement can mimic a primary renal parenchymal neoplasm; in these cases there is often a request for an intraoperative consultation to determine whether the mass is urothelial carcinoma or renal cell carcinoma (RCC), because the distinction alters the extent of surgery. The correct diagnosis can usually be determined by gross examination alone, but in some cases a frozen section may be required. The average size of renal pelvic tumors is just under 4 cm, with a range of 0.3 to 9 cm (*Am J Surg Pathol* 2004;28:1545). Multifocality in the pelvis and ureter is seen in about one-quarter of cases. In the ureter, the tumor may be associated with a stricture and hydroureter.

   b. **Microscopically,** the full range of urothelial carcinoma may be seen, from flat intraepithelial neoplasia, including CIS (e-**Fig. 21.7**); to noninvasive papillary neoplasia, including papillary urothelial neoplasm of low malignant potential; to low-grade papillary urothelial carcinoma (e-**Fig. 21.8**); to high-grade papillary urothelial carcinoma (e-**Figs. 21.9** and **21.10**). The full spectrum of invasive urothelial carcinoma and its variants as found in the urinary bladder can also be found in the upper tract. Of note, unusual histomorphologic variants seem to be more common in the upper tract (*Mod Pathol* 2006;19:494), including carcinomas with micropapillary (e-**Fig. 21.11**), lymphoepithelioma-like (e-**Fig. 21.12**), sarcomatoid (e-**Fig. 21.13**), squamous, clear cell, glandular, rhabdoid, signet-ring, and plasmacytoid features or areas.

   Primary resections performed for renal pelvic urothelial carcinoma show high-grade carcinoma in >70% of cases, with deep invasion (pT2 or greater) in 45% of cases and with lymph node metastases in one-quarter of patients. Cancerization of the distal renal collecting ducts is common in high-grade urothelial carcinoma (e-**Fig. 21.14**). Levels of invasion include lamina propria invasion (e-**Fig. 21.15**); extension into muscularis propria (e-**Fig. 21.16**), renal sinus and hilar fat, and periureteral fat (e-**Fig. 21.17**); and renal parenchymal infiltration. Metastatic sites include lymph nodes, peritoneum, and liver. When the differential diagnosis of a centrally located high-grade carcinoma centers on urothelial carcinoma versus RCC, extensive mucosal sampling can facilitate identification of urothelial CIS, in keeping with a urothelial primary.

   c. **Immunohistochemical studies** are not usually needed but can be useful in the differential diagnosis of urothelial carcinoma versus RCC or collecting duct carcinoma when the diagnosis is not clear by standard gross and microscopic examination. A useful marker panel includes GATA3, p63, high–molecular-weight keratins (e.g., 34βE12), and PAX8. Reactivity for the first three favors urothelial carcinoma, while reactivity for PAX8 supports RCC or collecting duct carcinoma rather than urothelial carcinoma (*Am J Surg Pathol* 2014;33:1017, *Am J Surg Pathol 2014;*38:e35). Of note, up to 23% of upper tract urothelial carcinomas may be PAX8 positive (*Mod Pathol* 2009;22:1218).

   d. **Molecular studies.** The most promising test is fluorescence in situ hybridization (FISH) performed on cells in urine from the upper tract. In this test (offered by several laboratories), fluorescent probes to chromosomes 3, 7, 17, and 9p21 loci are used to detect numerical chromosomal abnormalities associated with urothelial carcinoma (*Expert Rev Mol Diagn.* 2007;7:11). The precise clinical indications for its use for upper tract tumors are not yet established.

5. **Squamous cell carcinoma** is rare, is more common in the pelvis, is frequently associated with nephrolithiasis and/or infection, and often presents with high-stage and high-grade disease (**e-Fig. 21.18**). Pure squamous cell carcinomas should be distinguished from urothelial carcinoma with squamous differentiation.

6. **Adenocarcinoma** is rare and may display enteric, mucinous, and/or signet-ring features. Pure adenocarcinomas should be separated from urothelial carcinoma with glandular differentiation. Intestinal metaplasia, nephrolithiasis, and infection are predisposing factors.

7. **Small cell carcinomas** arising from the renal pelvis are very rare. There may be admixed urothelial carcinoma.

8. **Malignant mesenchymal neoplasms** are rare. The most common is leiomyosarcoma. Exceedingly rare other mesenchymal tumor types include osteosarcoma, rhabdomyosarcoma, fibrosarcoma, angiosarcoma, and Ewing sarcoma.

9. **Hematolymphoid neoplasms** in the ureter and renal pelvis typically are due to secondary involvement.

10. **Miscellaneous neoplasms** rarely encountered include paraganglioma, carcinoid tumor, Wilms tumor, malignant melanoma, and choriocarcinoma.

11. **Secondary (metastatic) malignancies** include carcinomas of the cervix, prostate, colon, breast, and urinary bladder.

IV. **HISTOLOGIC GRADING** should be performed for all carcinomas, with urothelial carcinoma grade being assigned as low grade or high grade, as for the urinary bladder. Pure squamous cell carcinoma and adenocarcinoma may be graded as well differentiated, moderately differentiated, or poorly differentiated.

V. **PATHOLOGIC STAGING** of the ureter and renal pelvis is performed according to the 2017 Tumor, Node, Metastasis (TNM) American Joint Committee on Cancer/International Union Against Cancer (AJCC/UICC) staging classification (Amin MB et al., eds. *AJCC Cancer Staging Manual*, 8th ed. New York: Springer, 2017). It is important to note that different staging schemes exist for neoplasms of renal origin (including RCC) and urothelial carcinoma of the bladder.

Stage is the most important prognostic factor for upper tract carcinoma. Noninvasive carcinomas are classified as pathologic stage pTa (noninvasive papillary neoplasia) or pTis (flat urothelial CIS). Similar to the bladder, pT1 disease involves the lamina propria; pT2, the muscularis propria; pT3, tissue beyond the ureter or pelvis (periureteral fat, renal sinus fat, or renal parenchyma). One important note is that renal pelvic carcinoma extending into the renal collecting ducts does not represent renal parenchymal invasion, which is pT3 disease (**e-Fig. 21.19**). Tumors that invade adjacent organs (other than the kidney) or extend through the kidney into the perinephric fat are pT4. It is worth noting that in the 2017 AJCC staging classification, staging of positive regional lymph nodes has been simplified to pN1 or pN2, such that cases previously classified in the 2010 AJCC scheme as pN3 are now grouped with pN2.

VI. **REPORTING CARCINOMA OF THE URETER AND RENAL PELVIS** should follow recommended guidelines (College of American Pathologists Protocol for the Examination of Specimens from Patients with Carcinoma of the Ureter and Renal Pelvis, available at http://www.cap.org). In addition to histologic type, grade, tumor size and extent, stage, and margin status, pertinent pathologic features that should be reported include the following. For biopsies, the presence or absence of muscularis propria should be specified. For nephroureterectomy or ureterectomy specimens, gross characteristics such as tumor location, focality (unifocal vs. multifocal), gross appearance (papillary, solid/nodule, flat, ulcerated), gross depth of invasion, and distance to margins should be given. Additional gross abnormalities such as other mucosal lesions, renal parenchymal lesions, stones, hydronephrosis, and hydroureter should be documented when present. Microscopically, additional relevant pathologic findings, if present, include lymphovascular space invasion by carcinoma, flat urothelial CIS (focal vs. multifocal), inflammation, renal disease (neoplastic or nonneoplastic), and metaplasias of the urothelium, including keratinizing squamous metaplasia and intestinal metaplasia. A nomogram predicting cancer-specific survival after nephroureterectomy for upper tract urothelial carcinoma uses age, tumor grade, pT stage, and pN stage (*Cancer* 2010;116:3774).

ACKNOWLEDGMENT

The authors thank Dr. Souzan Sanati and Dr. Frances V. White, authors of previous editions of this chapter.

The Urinary Bladder

Jennifer K. Sehn and Peter A. Humphrey

I. **NORMAL ANATOMY.** The wall of the urinary bladder is formed by four layers (**e-Fig. 22.1**). The thickness of the innermost layer, the urothelium, depends on the degree of bladder distension, and the shape of its constituent urothelial cells ranges from smaller cuboidal cells at the base to larger polyhedral cells toward the surface. Umbrella cells, the most superficial cells, have abundant eosinophilic cytoplasm and are often binucleated. Separated from the urothelium by a thin basement membrane, the underlying lamina propria is the second layer. It is composed of loose connective tissue with blood vessels, nerves, adipose tissue, and a variable number of smooth muscle fibers forming a discontinuous muscularis mucosae. The muscularis mucosae may become hypertrophic in patients with long-standing bladder outlet obstruction, causing difficulty in distinguishing thickened muscularis mucosae fibers from the smooth muscle bundles of the muscularis propria (detrusor muscle). Aggregates of the urothelium termed von Brunn nests (**e-Fig. 22.2**) are often seen as invaginations or separate clusters in the lamina propria. The term cystitis cystica is used when these nests become prominent and undergo cystic change (**e-Fig. 22.3**). Cystitis glandularis is similar to cystitis cystica except that the cells lining the cysts are mucin-secreting cuboidal or columnar cells, or true goblet cells, in which case the term cystitis glandularis with intestinal metaplasia is used (**e-Fig. 22.4**). These proliferative lesions, although sometimes seen associated with local inflammation, represent variants of normal histology. Their main importance lies in the fact that they can occasionally cause visible lesions simulating a bladder neoplasm. The third layer, the muscularis propria or detrusor muscle, is composed of large bundles of muscle fibers and is covered by the outermost fourth layer, the adventitial layer, including the perivesical adipose tissue. It is important to note that adipose tissue can also be found in the submucosa and wall (**e-Fig. 22.5**), so identification of fat does not equate to a specific layer of the bladder wall.

II. **GROSS EXAMINATION AND TISSUE SAMPLING OF THE BLADDER.** The most common samples submitted for surgical pathology examination include small biopsies, larger transurethral resection specimens, partial and radical (complete) cystectomies, and cystoprostatectomy specimens.

A. **Biopsy Specimens** are usually obtained without cautery ("cold-cup") and should be immediately immersed in formalin. If multiple biopsies are submitted separately, as in mapping procedures, they should be processed separately. After gross examination, bladder biopsies should be marked with ink or hematoxylin, then placed in a cassette after being put in a fine-mesh envelope, wrapped in lens paper, or sandwiched between sponge pads. After processing, three hematoxylin and eosin (H&E)-stained slides should be prepared, each with a strip of three to four levels.

B. **Transurethral Resection Specimens** are usually obtained with the aid of thermal cautery, often for the transurethral resection of bladder tumors (TURBT). Because of the significant prognostic and therapeutic implications for the presence of muscularis propria invasion by the bladder neoplasms, it is often necessary to process all of the submitted tissue to ensure that such foci of invasion are not overlooked.

C. **Partial Cystectomy Specimens.** Partial or segmental cystectomy is indicated in only a minority of bladder cancer patients, typically those who suffer a first-time tumor recurrence with a solitary tumor, and tumor location that allows for a 1- to 2-cm margin of resection, such as at the dome. Urachal carcinomas at the dome and above, with extension toward the umbilicus, may also be treated by partial cystectomy, as can carcinoma in a bladder diverticulum. Carcinoma in situ (CIS) elsewhere in the bladder (or multifocal tumors) is an absolute contraindication. The specimens usually consist of a sheet-like portion of tissue that should be pinned down and fixed overnight. In addition to describing and sampling any gross tumor as described for cystectomy specimens, the status of the margins is very important; these can be shaved off or sampled by perpendicular sections, depending on their relationship and proximity to the tumor. Frozen section of the mucosal margin may be requested.

D. Total Cystectomy and Cystoprostatectomy Specimens. Radical cystoprostatectomy in men and anterior exenteration in women, along with pelvic lymphadenectomy, are standard surgical approaches for detrusor muscle–invasive bladder carcinoma in the absence of clinically evident metastatic disease. Cystectomy may be performed in some cases for non–muscle-invasive bladder carcinoma if the bladder is nonfunctional (e.g., neurogenic bladder), or for high-grade pT1 carcinoma that is not responsive to intravesical therapy with Bacillus Calmette–Guérin (BCG) or mitomycin. A request to perform frozen sections on the ureteric and urethral margins may be received (*Arch Pathol Lab Med* 2005;129:1585). After orientation and inking of the perivesical soft tissue margins, one of two methods can be used to fix the specimen. The first entails filling the bladder with formalin (through the urethra, or by using a large bore needle through the dome) and fixing overnight; the second entails opening the bladder (usually through the urethra extending upward on the anterior surface) and pinning it flat, then fixing overnight. After opening the bladder, the mucosa is examined for tumors(s) and, if present, the size, location (dome, trigone, anterior, posterior, right or left walls), pattern of growth (exophytic, endophytic, and/or ulcerated), and depth of invasion are recorded. Relationships to pertinent anatomic landmarks (ureteral and urethral orifices, margins) also should be noted. The mucosa of the adjacent bladder should be examined for areas of hemorrhage or discoloration that may represent areas of CIS. In addition to sampling of any tumor(s) (three to four sections of each, or one section per cm), representative sections need to be submitted from the different areas of the bladder including the trigone; posterior, lateral, and anterior walls; and dome (Fig. 22.1), to evaluate for CIS. Only an ulcer or erythematous area may remain in patients who underwent therapy before surgery; in those cases, the abnormal area should be submitted entirely for histologic examination to evaluate for residual tumor cells, which may be very focal. If ureteric and urethral shave margins were not submitted for frozen-section examination, they should be sampled for permanent sections, as should any possible lymph nodes identified in the perivesical fat. In cystoprostatectomy specimens, additional blocks from the prostate and seminal vesicles should be submitted, the extent of which depends on whether a preoperative diagnosis or suspicion of prostatic carcinoma exists (see Chapter 29). When the bladder (with or without the prostate) is removed as part of larger pelvic exenteration specimens (that may include portions of the rectum and/or the gynecologic tract in females), it then becomes imperative to document the presence or absence of involvement of these additional organs by preferentially sampling suspicious areas, as well as by sampling the resection margins of these organs.

III. DIAGNOSTIC FEATURES OF COMMON DISEASES OF THE BLADDER
A. Congenital Malformations
1. **Urachal abnormalities.** The urachus is a vestigial structure that connects the dome of the bladder to the umbilicus; it normally closes by the fourth month of fetal life. Persistence or malformations of the urachus can present in childhood and occasionally in adulthood; they include urachal remnants (e-Fig. 22.6), patent urachus, urachal cysts, and urachal sinuses, all of which can result in secondary infection or development of malignant tumors, most frequently adenocarcinoma (e-Fig. 22.7).

2. **Exstrophy.** This is a rare congenital anomaly characterized by failure of development of the anterior wall of the bladder and abdominal wall, usually resulting in severe urinary tract infection if left untreated.

B. Inflammatory Conditions. Cystitis most frequently has an infectious etiology. There are, however, specific variants of cystitis that produce somewhat characteristic cystoscopic

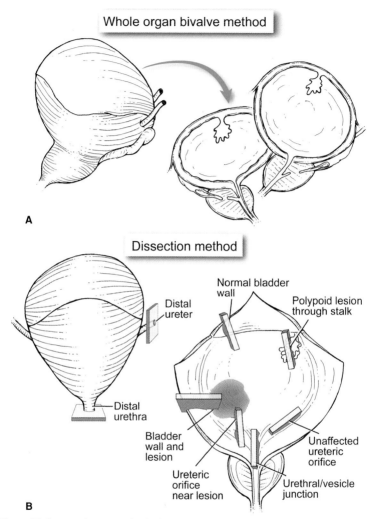

Whole organ bivalve method

A

Dissection method

Distal
ureter

Normal bladder
wall

Polypoid lesion
through stalk

Distal
urethra

Bladder
wall and
lesion

Ureteric
orifice
near lesion

Unaffected
ureteric
orifice

Urethral/vesicle
junction

B

Figure 22.1 Gross dissection of radical cystectomy specimens by whole organ bivalve method
(**A**) and by opening along the urethra and anterior wall, with demonstration of sections to be
taken (**B**). Three to four sections, or complete embedding, of masses should be performed.
(Modified from Schmidt WA. *Principles and Techniques of Surgical Pathology*. Menlo Park, CA:
Addison-Wesley Publishing Co.; 1983; 525.)

and/or microscopic appearances. The latter includes hemorrhagic, granulomatous,
eosinophilic, and interstitial variants, as well as malakoplakia.
 1. **Infectious cystitis.** Acute and chronic cystitis is most frequently secondary to bac-
    terial infection (usually by enteric organisms). The incidence is higher in females,
    and when intermittent urinary obstruction or stasis is present. Biopsy during active

infection is contraindicated, but biopsy may be performed in cases of chronic cystitis to rule out neoplasia, especially CIS. The histopathologic features include a non-specific acute and/or chronic inflammatory infiltrate, occasionally with lymphoid aggregates/follicles (follicular cystitis) (e-**Fig. 22.8**), and a variable degree of lamina propria edema. Of note, similar findings may be seen in the absence of infection, such as following radiation or cytotoxic chemotherapy. Other infections can produce specific histologic findings such as viral inclusions (polyoma and herpes viruses) or granulomas (tuberculosis, fungal infections, and schistosomiasis).

2. **Granulomatous cystitis.** As noted above, bacterial, fungal, or parasitic infections can lead to granuloma formation. The most frequent cause, however, is iatrogenic, either secondary to intravesical BCG therapy for urothelial CIS and/or superficially invasive carcinoma (e-**Fig. 22.9**), or following TURBT (e-**Fig. 22.10**).

3. **Hemorrhagic cystitis.** This is an uncommon side effect of cyclophosphamide therapy that results in extensive ulceration and hemorrhage that, if severe, may require cystectomy. Adenovirus infection (in immunocompromised individuals) may also produce the same pattern.

4. **Papillary and polypoid (bullous) cystitis.** These related forms of cystitis are characterized by finger-like (papillary) or broad (polypoid) projections of edematous, variably inflamed lamina propria covered by reactive nonneoplastic urothelium (e-**Fig. 22.11**). These forms of cystitis are most frequently seen with prolonged indwelling catheter use. The presence of such an inflammatory component in papillary cystitis can help in making the occasionally difficult distinction from a low-grade papillary urothelial neoplasm.

5. **Eosinophilic cystitis.** This is characterized by dense infiltration of eosinophils in the bladder lamina propria (e-**Fig. 22.12**) and/or wall. Such infiltrates are most frequently seen adjacent to invasive urothelial carcinoma, but they also occur in patients with allergic conditions and in patients with parasitic infections, both often in association with peripheral eosinophilia.

6. **Interstitial cystitis.** This is an uncommon inflammatory disorder that predominantly affects middle-aged and elderly women and results in severe intractable symptoms of culture-negative cystitis. Petechial submucosal hemorrhages or ulcers (termed Hunner ulcers) are usually evident cystoscopically. The microscopic features are nonspecific and include a mixed inflammatory infiltrate in the lamina propria, often with an increased number of mast cells that can also involve the muscularis propria (e-**Fig. 22.13**) and nerves. Clinical correlation is required in these cases because the histologic findings are, at most, consistent with the clinical impression of interstitial cystitis.

7. **Malakoplakia.** This is an uncommon form of cystitis characterized by the presence of soft yellowish mucosal plaques composed of inflammatory cells, including abundant epithelioid histiocytes (known as von Hansemann histiocytes) (e-**Fig. 22.14**) that have granular eosinophilic cytoplasm, and characteristic 3- to 10-micron rounded basophilic intracytoplasmic inclusions (Michaelis–Gutmann bodies) that contain iron and calcium, best demonstrated by Prussian blue and von Kossa special stains, respectively. The condition is thought to result from a defect in the ability of histiocytes to degrade phagocytosized bacteria. Control of urinary tract infection can help control the disease.

C. Reactive and Metaplastic Urothelial Lesions

1. **Squamous metaplasia.** This can be of two types: nonkeratinizing and keratinizing. The former is considered a normal finding in the trigone and bladder neck of females, but can rarely be seen in males receiving estrogen treatment for prostate cancer. In contrast, keratinizing squamous metaplasia is more common in males in association with chronic irritation and is considered a significant risk factor for the subsequent development of carcinoma (*Eur Urol* 2002;42:469; *Am J Surg Pathol* 2006;20:883).

2. **Intestinal metaplasia.** In addition to the intestinal metaplasia occasionally seen in cystitis glandularis, intestinal metaplasia in the presence of a chronically irritated

bladder can involve the bladder mucosa and lamina propria in a focal or diffuse manner, resulting in an appearance almost indistinguishable from colonic mucosa. Enteric-type adenomas or carcinomas can arise in a background of intestinal metaplasia, especially when long-standing.

3. Nephrogenic metaplasia (adenoma). This is a benign epithelial proliferation composed of cells resembling renal tubular epithelium (hence the name), which usually arises in the setting of chronic irritation or injury such as infection or calculi (*Adv Anat Pathol* 2006;13:247). The lesion was believed to be metaplastic, but more recent evidence has demonstrated that, at least in renal transplant recipients, nephrogenic metaplasia is derived from shed renal tubular epithelial cells that may attach to areas of prior injury. Although most frequently seen in the bladder, it is also quite common in the urethra, and less so in the ureters and renal pelvis. Nephrogenic metaplasia is usually an incidental finding, but it may also present as a mass lesion simulating cancer. Histologically, papillae (**e-Fig. 22.15**), small tubules (**e-Fig. 22.16**), or cystically dilated tubules (**e-Fig. 22.17**) lined by cuboidal, low columnar, or flattened hobnail cells are seen. The importance of nephrogenic metaplasia lies in the fact that in the bladder it can be confused with adenocarcinoma (especially clear cell adenocarcinoma) and glandular variants of urothelial carcinoma (*Mod Pathol* 2009;22:S37–S52); in the urethra it can be confused with prostatic adenocarcinoma. The immunohistochemical reactivity of nephrogenic metaplasia with cytokeratin 7, alpha-methylacyl coenzyme A racemase (AMACR), PAX2, and PAX8 antibodies, and the lack of reactivity with high–molecular-weight cytokeratin (e.g., 34βE12) and prostate-specific antigen (PSA) antibodies help in distinguishing it from its mimics. Note that PAX8 positivity can be seen in clear cell adenocarcinoma.

4. Urothelial hyperplasia. An increase in the thickness of the urothelium (>7 layers) is usually reactive and most frequently seen secondary to chronic inflammatory conditions. Flat urothelial hyperplasia (**e-Fig. 22.18**) is more common than papillary urothelial hyperplasia, which some authors have also found to be associated with papillary urothelial neoplasms. In the 2016 WHO classification (Table 22.1), the term urothelial proliferation of uncertain malignant potential replaces urothelial hyperplasia (*Eur Urol* 2016;70:106).

5. Pseudocarcinomatous epithelial hyperplasia. This change may be seen after radiation therapy, chemotherapy, or unassociated with either therapy (*Arch Pathol Lab Med* 2010;134:427). The light microscopic appearance is of pseudoinfiltrative nests of urothelium in the lamina propria (**e-Fig. 22.19**), sometimes with squamous metaplasia. Nuclear atypia may be detected, secondary to therapy or irritation/ischemia. The irregular nests and aggregates may appear to wrap around ectatic vessels with fibrin thrombi, which is a useful diagnostic finding.

6. Reactive urothelial atypia. Usually seen in a setting of acute and/or chronic inflammation, reactive atypia may be associated with hyperplastic or thin urothelium. Nuclear enlargement, often with vesicular chromatin and a single prominent nucleolus, is the most prominent finding (**e-Fig. 22.20**). Mitotic figures may be increased and cell crowding may be observed; however, polarity, cell uniformity, and maturation are usually well preserved. Acute or chronic inflammation is often identified.

D. Miscellaneous Nonneoplastic Conditions

1. Endometriosis. Most frequently seen on the serosal aspect of the bladder in women with a previous history of pelvic surgery, foci of endometriosis can also involve the lamina propria or muscularis propria and may be visible cystoscopically. As elsewhere, at least two of the three histologic features of endometriosis—endometrial glands, endometrial stroma, and hemosiderin-laden macrophages—are required for the diagnosis (**e-Fig. 22-21**).

2. Endocervicosis and endosalpingiosis. These are characterized by the presence of glands within the bladder wall, lined by columnar endocervical-type mucinous cells or ciliated tubal epithelial cells, respectively. When both are present with endometriosis, the term "müllerianosis" has been used. Lack of nuclear atypia, mitoses, and a

TABLE 22.1	WHO Histologic Classification of Tumors of the Urinary Tract (Including Bladder)

Urothelial tumors

Infiltrating urothelial carcinoma
  Nested, including large nested
  Microcystic
  Micropapillary
  Lymphoepithelioma-like
  Plasmacytoid/signet-ring cell/diffuse
  Sarcomatoid
  Giant cell
  Poorly differentiated
  Lipid-rich
  Clear cell
Noninvasive urothelial neoplasias
  Urothelial carcinoma in situ
  Noninvasive papillary urothelial carcinoma, high grade
  Noninvasive papillary urothelial carcinoma, low grade
  Papillary urothelial neoplasm of low malignant potential
  Urothelial papilloma
  Inverted urothelial papilloma
  Urothelial proliferation of uncertain malignant potential
  Urothelial dysplasia

Squamous neoplasms

Squamous cell carcinoma (pure)
Verrucous carcinoma
Squamous cell papilloma

Glandular neoplasms

Adenocarcinoma, not otherwise specified (NOS)
  Enteric
  Mucinous
  Mixed
Villous adenoma

Urachal carcinoma

Tumors of müllerian type

Clear cell carcinoma
Endometrioid carcinoma

Neuroendocrine tumors

Small cell neuroendocrine carcinoma
Large cell neuroendocrine carcinoma
Well-differentiated neuroendocrine tumor
Paraganglioma

Melanocytic tumors

Malignant melanoma
Nevus
Melanosis

Mesenchymal tumors

Rhabdomyosarcoma
Leiomyosarcoma
Angiosarcoma
Inflammatory myofibroblastic tumor
Perivascular epithelioid cell tumor
  Benign
  Malignant
Solitary fibrous tumor
Leiomyoma
Hemangioma
Granular cell tumor
Neurofibroma

Urothelial tract hematopoietic and lymphoid tumors

Miscellaneous tumors

Carcinoma of Skene, Cowper, and Littre glands
Metastatic tumors and tumors extending from other organs
Epithelial tumors of the upper urinary tract
Tumors arising in a bladder diverticulum
Urothelial tumors of the urethra

From Moch H, Humphrey PA, Ulbright TM, Reuter VE, eds. *WHO Classification of Tumours. Tumours of the Urinary System and Male Genital Organs.* Lyon, France: IARC Press; 2017. Used with permission.

stromal tissue reaction help distinguish these benign lesions from adenocarcinoma or implants of serous borderline tumor.

3. **Diverticula.** These outpouchings of mucosa through the muscularis propria are mostly due to increased pressure from bladder outlet obstruction, frequently secondary to prostatic hyperplasia. Diverticula may be complicated by inflammation, squamous metaplasia, and lithiasis, and in less than 10% of cases by secondary neoplastic development.

4. **Amyloidosis.** The bladder may rarely be involved by systemic amyloidosis, or by a primary localized form of amyloidosis limited to the bladder.

5. **Ectopic prostatic tissue.** These are usually small polypoid projections most frequently seen in the trigone area. They are composed of benign prostatic epithelium (very similar to the so-called "prostatic urethral polyps" of the urethra).

6. Fibroepithelial polyp. These rare polyps are considered nonneoplastic. They may be acquired or congenital. About one-half are found in neonates and children. Histologically, there is a polypoid configuration, often with club-like or finger-like projections (e-**Fig. 22.22**) (*Am J Surg Pathol* 2005;29:460). The surface urothelial lining is normal and there may be tubular or anastomosing urothelium in the dense fibrous tissue of the polyp fibrovascular core. Degenerative-type stromal cell atypia, without mitotic activity, may be present. These polyps have a broader fibrovascular core than urothelial papillomas and lack the edema and inflammation of polypoid cystitis.

E. Neoplastic Urothelial Lesions. Urothelial neoplasms are the most common neoplasms involving the bladder (Table 22.1). Histologic typing and diagnosis of urothelial abnormalities are accomplished by examination of H&E-stained sections.

1. Flat urothelial lesions with atypia. In addition to reactive atypia discussed above, flat lesions include urothelial dysplasia and urothelial CIS.

    a. Urothelial dysplasia. Dysplasia is an intraepithelial neoplastic urothelial proliferation characterized by variable degrees of loss of polarity, nuclear enlargement, and chromatin clumping (e-**Fig. 22.23**), all of which fall short of the degree seen in CIS. Dysplasia is often identified in patients with urothelial neoplasms. Occasionally it may be difficult to distinguish urothelial dysplasia from reactive atypia; in such situations a diagnosis of atypia of unknown significance may be warranted. Isolated urothelial dysplasia progresses to bladder carcinoma in about 15% of cases (*Cancer 2000*;88:625).

    b. Urothelial carcinoma in situ (CIS). This is a high-grade, often multifocal intraurothelial neoplastic proliferation characterized by the presence of unequivocal malignant urothelial cells within the bladder epithelial lining (Fig. 22.2, e-**Fig. 22.24**). The urothelial proliferation need not involve the entire thickness of the urothelium, and pagetoid and undermining patterns of growth are not uncommon. Another common feature is the discohesive nature of the neoplastic cells that often leads to denudation and a "clinging" pattern of growth in which only scarce malignant cells remain attached to the bladder wall (e-**Fig. 22.25**). CIS cells can also extend into and "cancerize" von Brunn nests (e-**Fig. 22.26**). Rarely, glandular differentiation in the form of columnar cells with apical cytoplasm can be noted in urothelial CIS (*Am J Surg Pathol* 2009;33:1241). In difficult cases, immunostains

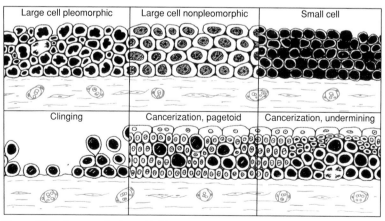

Figure 22.2 Patterns of urinary bladder carcinoma in situ. (From McKenney JK, Gomez JA, Desai S, Lee MW, Amin MB. Morphologic expressions of urothelial carcinoma in situ: a detailed evaluation of its histologic patterns with emphasis on carcinoma in situ with microinvasion. *Am J Surg Pathol.* 2001;25:356–362, with permission).

for p53 and CK20 can be useful in differentiating reactive urothelial atypia from CIS, with mutant pattern of p53 staining (entirely negative or diffusely positive) and full-thickness reactivity for CK20 supporting an interpretation of CIS, in the appropriate morphologic context (*Am J Surg Pathol* 2014;38:1017). Urothelial CIS is often associated with invasive urothelial carcinoma and carries a significant risk of death from bladder carcinoma (*Cancer* 1999;85:2469). CIS cells typically harbor deletion or mutation of *TP53*, a common finding in high-grade tumors across multiple anatomic sites and histologic types.

2. Papillary urothelial neoplasms

a. **Urothelial papilloma.** This uncommon benign neoplasm is composed of delicate papillary urothelial fronds with no or minimal branching or fusion. The constituent cells are identical to normal urothelial cells, and no mitoses are present (**e-Fig. 22.27**). The classic cystoscopic finding is a solitary lesion in a younger patient with hematuria. Papillomas may recur (in up to 80% of cases) or progress to higher-grade disease (in 2% of cases).

b. **Inverted papilloma.** Another uncommon neoplasm, an inverted papilloma has a polypoid or sessile appearance cystoscopically. It is composed of anastomosing islands and cords of bland urothelial cells that invaginate and grow downward in the lamina propria with peripheral palisading, absent to rare mitoses, and no to minimal cytologic atypia (**e-Fig. 22.28**) (*Am J Surg Pathol* 2004;28:1615; *Cancer* 2006;107:2622). These latter two features help distinguish this lesion from other papillary neoplasms that may also occasionally have an inverted growth pattern. Inverted papillomas rarely recur.

c. **Papillary urothelial neoplasm of low malignant potential (PUNLMP).** This neoplasm shares the clinical and endoscopic features of papilloma, but is characterized histologically by occasionally fused papillae and ordered, yet larger, nuclei than are seen in papillomas (**e-Fig. 22.29A, B**). Mitotic figures are rare and basal. Compared with papillomas, PUNLMP has higher recurrence (25% to 35%) and progression rates (up to 4%), and thus close follow-up is warranted.

d. **Noninvasive papillary urothelial carcinoma, low grade.** In contrast to PUN-LMP, this urothelial neoplasm shows frequent branching and fusion of papillae and variations in the nuclear size, shape, and contour (**e-Fig. 22.30**). Mitoses are occasional and may be found at any level. These tumors tend to be larger than papillomas and PUNLMPs and are more likely to be multiple. They are also more likely to recur (64% to 71%) and progress (2% to 10%). In general, low-grade papillary urothelial carcinoma harbors mutations in *FGFR3*, without the additional mutations seen in high-grade or invasive tumors (*Urol Oncol* 2010;28:409).

e. **Noninvasive papillary urothelial carcinoma, high grade.** These are uncommon noninvasive papillary neoplasms; more frequently there is associated invasion. They are characterized by frequent branching and fusion with moderate to marked cytoarchitectural disorder and nuclear pleomorphism (**e-Fig. 22.31**). Mitoses are frequent. Similar to low-grade tumors, these tumors frequently recur (56%) and have a higher propensity for progression to invasive carcinoma (18%).

3. Invasive urothelial neoplasms.

Invasive urothelial carcinomas can have papillary, polypoid, nodular, or ulcerative configurations. Most are cytologically high-grade tumors. Determination of anatomic depth of invasion by carcinoma is vital, because pathologic stage is the single most important prognostic feature; invasion into muscularis propria (muscle wall, detrusor muscle) (**e-Fig. 22.32**) is an ominous finding that makes the patient a candidate for aggressive surgical therapy (radical cystectomy) or radiation therapy, with or without adjuvant chemotherapy.

Recurring mutations identified in muscle wall–invasive bladder cancer have potential for targeted therapy (including mTor, cyclin-D1, Her-2, Ras, and SWI/SNF and histone modification pathways); p53/Rb pathway mutations also are common (*Nature* 2014;507:315; *Urol Oncol* 2010;28:409). Some urothelial carcinomas also have defective mismatch repair, providing an indication for immune checkpoint blockade with PD-1 and PD-L1 inhibitors (*Science* 2017 357:409). Mismatch repair gene mutations may be germline (as in Lynch syndrome) or sporadic.

Numerous histologic variants of invasive urothelial carcinoma have been described (*Mod Pathol* 2009;22:S96), including the following entities in the 2016 WHO classification of urothelial tumors. In addition, high-grade urothelial carcinomas (HGUC) frequently show squamous or glandular differentiation (e-**Fig. 22.33**), which should be distinguished from pure squamous cell carcinoma (SCC) or adenocarcinoma, respectively. Very rare cases of urothelial carcinoma with hCG-positive syncytiotrophoblasts (e-**Fig. 22.34**) have been reported. True syncytiotrophoblasts should be distinguished from the tumoral giant cells of giant cell carcinoma and from osteoclast-like giant cells. Trophoblastic differentiation portends a particularly poor prognosis.

a. Nested variant (including large nested). This variant is characterized by the presence of infiltrating nests and tubules of urothelial carcinoma (e-**Figs. 22.35** and **22.36**). Despite its relatively bland low-grade cytologic features, this variant often has a poor prognosis due to presentation at high stage. Because of its cytoarchitectural features, florid von Brunn nests, cystitis cystica and glandularis, inverted papilloma, nephrogenic adenoma, and paraganglioma are all in the differential diagnosis. Clues that are of aid in establishing the diagnosis are the high-density, nearly confluent nests that can anastomose and invade muscularis propria. Nuclear atypia may be only focally present, and is often found in the deeper aspects of the proliferation. Stromal desmoplasia may be absent. Although the nested variant of urothelial carcinoma has a higher proliferation index than florid von Brunn nests by Ki-67 (MIB-1) immunostaining (8.8% vs. 2.8%), and a higher p53 immunopositivity (4.2% vs. 1.5%), the degree of overlap precludes the use of these markers as diagnostic tools (*Am J Surg Pathol* 2003;27:1243).

b. Microcystic variant. This variant is also deceptively bland and somewhat similar to the nested variant, except for characteristic prominent cystic change (e-**Fig. 22.37**). It is uncommon, accounting for only about 1% of bladder carcinomas. Microscopically, there are variable-sized cysts ranging up to 1 to 2 mm in diameter. The cysts are round to oval and may contain necrotic material or pink secretions. The layer of lining cells may be flattened or denuded. The differential diagnosis includes cystitis cystica and glandularis, and nephrogenic adenoma. Correct diagnosis is achieved by the detection of an association with usual urothelial carcinoma, haphazard and infiltrative growth, and variability in cyst size and shape. In the largest series, 25% of cases had invasion of muscularis propria and 11 of 12 were high grade (*J Urol* 1997;74:722).

c. Micropapillary variant. This rare pattern of urothelial carcinoma resembles serous carcinoma of the ovary, an important differential diagnosis in women. It is characterized by the presence of small nests of cells and filiform papillae that have retracted from the surrounding stroma, with multiple papillae per lacuna (e-**Fig. 22.38**) (*Am J Surg Pathol* 2010; 34:1367). Lymphovascular invasion is common. Admixed invasive usual urothelial carcinoma is detected in a majority of cases. Because the proportion of the tumor that is micropapillary seems to be of prognostic significance, the percentage of the invasive tumor that is micropapillary should be reported (*Adv Anat Pathol* 2010;17:182). This variant is aggressive; muscle wall invasion is commonly detected. Micropapillary-like architecture that is present only in the noninvasive component of a tumor should not be classified as micropapillary carcinoma (Moch H, Humphrey PA, Ulbright TM, Reuter VE, eds. *World Health Organization Classification of Tumours. Tumours of the Urinary System and Male Genital Organs.* Lyon, IARC Press; 2016). It has been argued that early cystectomy should be offered to patients with non–muscle-invasive micropapillary urothelial carcinoma (*Cancer* 2007;110:62). Intravesical therapy is ineffective (*Urol Oncol* 2009;27:3). The 10-year overall survival is 24%.

d. Lymphoepithelioma-like variant. This is characterized by sheets and nests of poorly differentiated malignant cells that grow in a syncytial pattern with an admixed dense lymphoplasmacytic infiltrate (e-**Fig. 22.39**) (*Am J Surg Pathol* 2011;35:474). It may be pure or mixed with usual urothelial carcinoma. There is a tendency for patients to present with muscle wall–invasive disease. The differential diagnosis centers on large cell lymphoma and severe chronic cystitis, including follicular cystitis; immunostains for pan-cytokeratin and CD45 are confirmatory, and Epstein–Barr virus is not present. These are aggressive carcinomas with 26% mortality at 3 years.

e. **Plasmacytoid/signet-ring cell/diffuse variant.** These variants are exceedingly rare and are usually admixed with conventional urothelial carcinoma. However, the diagnosis of urothelial carcinoma in small biopsies composed solely of such variants (e-**Fig. 22.40**) may only be achieved with the help of immunohistochemistry (positive reactivity to cytokeratin with negative reactivity to CD45 and other lymphoid markers). Importantly, CD138 is reactive in plasmacytoid urothelial carcinoma (as in many other carcinomas) and is not helpful in differentiation of this variant from true plasma cells. The differential diagnosis also includes metastatic carcinoma from other sites with similar morphology (e.g., gastric or lobular breast carcinoma, e-**Fig. 22.41A, B**). Notably, GATA3 is not useful in differentiating urothelial versus breast carcinoma (*Am J Surg Pathol* 2014;38:e20).

f. **Sarcomatoid variant** (previously known as carcinosarcoma). This is a biphasic neoplasm displaying histomorphologic and/or immunophenotypic evidence of both epithelial and mesenchymal differentiation (*Am J Surg Pathol* 1994;18:241). Both components share the same clonal origin, as seen in carcinosarcomas of other sites. This variant accounts for <1% of bladder malignancies. Previous radiation and cyclophosphamide treatment are predisposing factors. Grossly, the tumor is often exophytic, polypoid, and deeply invasive into muscularis propria. Microscopically, the growth is typified by a biphasic population of neoplastic cells with the epithelial and mesenchymal components (e-**Fig. 22.42A, B**). The carcinomatous component is usually urothelial (85%) but can be adenocarcinoma, SCC, or small cell carcinoma. The amount of the malignant epithelial element varies and in some cases is only represented by CIS; consequently, apparently pure malignant spindle cell tumors of the bladder should be sampled extensively in an attempt to find epithelial areas. The sarcomatous component is usually an undifferentiated high-grade spindle cell proliferation arranged in fascicles, a storiform pattern, or as a patternless confluence. The most common heterologous element is osteosarcoma, followed by chondrosarcoma (e-**Fig. 22.43**), rhabdomyosarcoma, leiomyosarcoma, liposarcoma, angiosarcoma, or mixtures thereof. The sarcomatous regions are almost always high grade. Immunohistochemical staining of the sarcomatoid variant shows strong, diffuse immunopositivity for pan-cytokeratin, particularly in the identifiable epithelial areas (e-**Fig. 22.42B**), although epithelial membrane antigen (EMA) immunostaining is characteristically weak; however, note that epithelial markers can be negative, especially in the sarcomatoid component. Anaplastic lymphoma kinase (ALK)-1 immunostaining, which typifies inflammatory myofibroblastic tumor (IMT), is negative in sarcomatoid carcinoma. Extraintestinal gastrointestinal stromal tumor also should be considered in the differential; cases with dedifferentiation can be particularly difficult to recognize but often retain immunoreactivity for CD34, c-Kit, and/or DOG-1. Rhabdoid cells rarely may be observed in urothelial carcinoma; less than 10 cases have been reported (*Hum Pathol* 2006;37:16). In children, primary malignant rhabdoid tumor of the bladder is in the differential diagnosis and should be excluded by INI-1 immunohistochemistry. For cases of sarcomatoid carcinoma, the pathology report should include whether the sarcomatoid carcinoma is homologous or heterologous, although to date this does not appear to be of prognostic importance. Surgery and radiation result in 25% survival at 2 years.

g. **Giant cell and poorly differentiated variants.** Giant cell carcinoma is a high-grade variant that is characterized by numerous pleomorphic and bizarre tumor giant cells (e-**Fig. 22.44**); it needs to be distinguished from urothelial carcinoma with osteoclast-like giant cells, which represents an unusual stromal response to invasive carcinoma and may morphologically resemble a giant cell tumor of bone. Outcome is poor, with median survival of 11 months (*Br J Urol* 1995;75:167).

h. Clear cell (glycogen-rich) and lipid-rich variants. The main importance of these rare variants is the fact that they may be confused with clear cell adeno-carcinoma of the bladder (discussed later) or clear cell renal cell carcinoma, and liposarcoma or signet-ring carcinoma, respectively. The lipid-rich (also known as lipoid-cell) variant typically presents at high stage (*Br J Urol* 1995;75:167). The prognostic implication of the glycogen-rich variant is not clear due to the paucity of reported cases. Clear cell variant of urothelial carcinoma should be distinguished from clear cell carcinoma of the müllerian type.

F. Squamous Neoplasms

1. **Squamous papilloma.** This is a very rare papillary lesion that typically presents in elderly women and, unlike condyloma accuminatum (which can also involve the bladder), has not been associated with human papilloma virus infection or with subsequent development of carcinoma (*Am J Surg Pathol* 2006;20:883; *Cancer* 2000;88:1679). Recurrence is rare.

2. **Squamous cell carcinoma (SCC).** In areas of the world where schistosomiasis is endemic (parts of Africa and the Middle East), this type of carcinoma is the most common primary neoplasm of the bladder. Elsewhere, SCC is relatively rare, representing <5% of bladder carcinomas. Other predisposing conditions include chronic cystitis and chronic irritation due to vesical lithiasis or long-term indwelling catheters. Smoking is also a significant risk factor (as for conventional urothelial carcinoma). SCC is represented at a higher percentage in patients with nonfunctioning bladders (50% of carcinomas) or diverticula (20%), and in renal transplant patients (15%). Keratinizing squamous metaplasia is a potential precursor and is a risk factor for subsequent detection of carcinoma; 20% to 42% of patients with keratinizing squamous metaplasia are later diagnosed with carcinoma.

   SCC typically presents as invasive carcinoma, although in a few cases pure squamous cell CIS may be detected (*Am J Surg Pathol* 2006;20:883). Squamous cell CIS is a strong risk factor for subsequent detection of invasive carcinoma, and approximately 45% of patients with in situ disease are diagnosed with invasive squamous cell or urothelial carcinoma within 12 months (*Am J Surg Pathol* 2006;20:883). Grossly, SCCs are often large, solid, necrotic masses that can fill the entire bladder lumen (e-**Fig. 22.45**). Some, however, may be flat and infiltrative with ulceration. Microscopically, the carcinoma must be purely squamous (as opposed to urothelial carcinoma with squamous differentiation), with keratin production and/or intercellular bridges (e-**Fig. 22.46**). Adjacent keratinizing squamous metaplasia strongly supports a diagnosis of SCC; such metaplasia is seen in 20% to 60% of cases of invasive SCC. Histologic variants of SCC of the bladder include the exceptionally rare basaloid variant and the uncommon verrucous variant. Involvement by SCC of adjacent sites (e.g., cervix, anus) should be excluded; human papilloma virus in situ hybridization (HPV-ISH) can be helpful (*Am J Surg Pathol* 2014;38:e20).

   Grading is three tiered (well, moderately, or poorly differentiated), and histologic grade may correlate with stage and outcome. However, stage is the most important determinant of outcome. Many patients with SCC of the bladder present with muscularis propria–invasive disease, and this accounts for the poor outcome for most patients.

3. **Verrucous squamous cell carcinoma.** This variant of SCC is seen almost exclusively in patients with schistosomiasis and appears as an exophytic "warty" mass composed of thickened papillary squamous epithelium with minimal cytoarchitectural atypia and a rounded pushing border. This tumor is considered to be clinically indolent.

G. Glandular and Urachal Neoplasms

1. **Villous adenoma.** An uncommon exophytic papillary neoplasm histologically resembling its colonic counterpart, villous adenoma is usually located in the trigone and, unless associated with an invasive component, does not recur following excision.

2. Adenocarcinoma and urachal carcinoma. Primary adenocarcinomas are rare, representing 2% of malignant bladder neoplasms, and may be of urachal or nonurachal origin. The latter is more common and usually arises in patients with a nonfunctional bladder or with exstrophy. Urachal adenocarcinomas usually arise from the dome or anterior wall of the bladder but may also involve urachal remnants in the anterior abdominal wall. Characteristics of urachal adenocarcinomas that are helpful in differentiating them from nonurachal adenocarcinomas are that their bulk is in the wall rather than the lumen of the bladder; they lack an associated in situ component or cystitis glandularis; and they are sharply demarcated from the surface urothelium. Identification of urachal tumors is important because, unlike nonurachal tumors, surgical management of urachal adenocarcinomas usually includes excision of the median umbilical ligament and umbilicus. Bladder adenocarcinomas (of urachal or nonurachal type) may have different morphologic appearances including enteric (e-**Fig. 22.47A, B**), mucinous (e-**Fig. 22.7**), signet-ring cell, clear cell, and mixed. The main differential diagnosis for most of these patterns is the more common metastasis or secondary extension from another primary tumor site, most notably the prostate and the colon. Clinical correlation is essential for a definitive diagnosis of primary adenocarcinoma. Immunohistochemistry may be helpful, especially when the clinical findings are not helpful or available. Reactivity with PSA and NKX3.1 or β-catenin (in a nuclear pattern) supports a diagnosis of prostate or colon adenocarcinoma, respectively; cytokeratin 20 and CDX-2 immunostains are not useful in this context (*Am J Surg Pathol* 2014;38:e20). Primary adenocarcinoma of the bladder has a generally poor prognosis, with 5-year survival rates ranging from 18% to 47%.

H. Tumors of the Müllerian Type (Clear Cell or Endometrioid Type). These rare tumors arise most commonly in the setting of endometriosis involving the bladder. Clear cell differentiation also may be seen as a variant morphology in urothelial carcinoma (discussed above). Pure clear cell carcinoma is rare in the bladder, though it is seen more frequently in the urethra. Müllerian-type tumors arising in endometriosis are essentially identical to their counterparts in the gynecologic tract.

I. Neuroendocrine Neoplasms

1. Paraganglioma. Derived from bladder paraganglia, paragangliomas are typically found in the muscularis propria and classically are associated with hypertension and/ or headaches, palpitations, and sweating precipitated by micturition. The tumor is composed of cells with abundant amphophilic, clear, or eosinophilic cytoplasm arranged in a diffuse or nested (Zellballen) pattern of growth with an associated thin capillary network (e-**Fig. 22.48**). Nuclear atypia is occasionally prominent. The tumor is frequently immunopositive for neuroendocrine markers and negative for cytokeratin (useful in distinguishing the tumor from nested urothelial carcinoma), whereas the spindle cells surrounding tumor nests (sustentacular cells) are positive for S100 protein. GATA3 is frequently positive in paraganglioma, which may lead to misdiagnosis as urothelial carcinoma (*Mod Pathol* 2013;26:1365). The majority (85% to 90%) of bladder paragangliomas are benign and do not recur following surgical excision. Patients with germline mutation of a succinate dehydrogenase gene (*SDHA, B, C,* or *D*) have a higher risk for malignant paraganglioma (*Am J Surg Pathol* 2013;37:1612). Those patients also are at risk for other tumors, including the recently defined SDH-deficient renal cell carcinoma and SDH-deficient gastrointestinal stromal tumors. Screening for SDH mutations with SDHB immunohistochemistry may be helpful in identifying patients for genetic counseling, germline testing, and clinical surveillance.

2. Small cell (neuroendocrine) carcinoma. This is a rare neoplasm, which is diagnosed even when mixed with other bladder carcinomas (urothelial, squamous, or adenocarcinomas); the presence of any small cell carcinoma component has a significant negative impact on prognosis. As with other bladder carcinomas, hematuria is the most common presentation; however, almost half of patients present with metastatic disease, with or without a paraneoplastic syndrome. Histologically, the tumor cells are identical to small cell carcinoma in other sites (scant cytoplasm, stippled chromatin, and inconspicuous nucleoli with nuclear molding). Admixture with usual urothelial carcinoma is common and is present in about one-half of cases (e-**Fig. 22.49**). The diagnosis can often be confirmed by immunoreactivity with one or more neuroen-docrine markers such as chromogranin, synaptophysin, and CD56, with or without dot-like paranuclear reactivity for cytokeratin. Notably, TTF-1 is reactive in a major subset of all small cell carcinomas and is not informative for determining site of origin. *TERT* promoter mutations, which are common in urinary bladder small cell carcinoma and absent in small cell carcinomas from other sites, may be useful in establishing bladder origin for a small cell carcinoma (*J Hematol Oncol* 2014; 7:47).

3. Rare neuroendocrine tumors. Large cell neuroendocrine carcinomas and well-differentiated neuroendocrine tumors (carcinoid) are rare as primary tumors in the urinary bladder.

J. Melanocytic Tumors. Melanocytic lesions of the bladder are exceptionally uncommon and include melanosis (melanin granules in the urothelial cells) and melanoma. Melanoma of the urinary tract most commonly involves the urethra.

K. Mesenchymal Lesions and Neoplasms

1. Smooth muscle neoplasms. Leiomyomas and leiomyosarcomas represent the most common benign and malignant mesenchymal neoplasms of the bladder, respectively. Leiomyomas usually present as well-circumscribed submucosal masses and are composed of intersecting fascicles of spindle cells with abundant eosinophilic cytoplasm and oval/elongated nuclei with blunt ends. By definition, there should be no significant nuclear atypia (hyperchromasia, nuclear membrane irregularity, or pleomorphism) or evidence of an infiltrative growth pattern. In contrast, leiomyosarcomas (e-**Fig. 22.50**) are infiltrative tumors with nuclear atypia, coagulative tumor cell necrosis, and brisk mitotic activity (usually >5 mitoses per 10 high-power fields). In addition to showing immunoreactivity with one or more smooth muscle markers (actin, desmin, caldesmon), leiomyosarcomas can also be at least focally reactive for cytokeratin and EMA. Myofibroblastic tumors (including IMT) are frequently reactive for smooth muscle markers, a potential diagnostic pitfall. Most patients with leiomyosarcoma develop recurrence and/or metastasis, resulting in mortality in almost one-half of cases.

2. Rhabdomyosarcoma. Embryonal rhabdomyosarcoma is the most common malignant bladder tumor in children. Grossly, most present as polypoid intraluminal masses resembling a cluster of grapes ("botryoid" type), with the remainder being deeply invasive tumors. Histologically, they are mostly composed of small round tumor cells with a variable admixture of spindle cells embedded in a myxoid stroma, often with tumor cell condensation under the surface urothelium, forming the characteristic "cambium layer" (e-**Fig. 22.51 and 22.52**). The latter feature, as well as the identification of rhabdomyoblasts and cross-striations, is particularly useful for diagnosis. Immunohistochemistry can confirm the diagnosis; these tumors are positive for myogenin and myoD1, among other muscle markers. The prognosis of embryonal rhabdomyosarcoma has greatly improved with multimodality treatment, although the alveolar type and the rare rhabdomyosarcomas presenting in adulthood are associated with a worse outcome.

3. Inflammatory myofibroblastic tumor (IMT). The bladder is the most common visceral site for IMT, which more commonly involves abdominal or retroperitoneal soft tissues. The tumors may be large (>10 cm) and infiltrative; they contain elongated spindle or stellate cells resembling tissue-culture fibroblasts, embedded in a myxoid matrix that contains a variable chronic inflammatory infiltrate and extravasated red blood cells (e-**Fig. 22.53**). Although enlarged nuclei with prominent nucleoli and brisk mitotic activity can be observed, the presence of significant nuclear atypia and/or abnormal mitotic figures should suggest an alternative diagnosis such as sarcomatoid carcinoma or leiomyosarcoma. A panel of immunostains including smooth muscle actin, desmin, pancytokeratin (AE1/AE3), p63, cytokeratin 34βE12, and

ALK1 is recommended in the differential diagnosis of sarcomatoid carcinoma, leiomyosarcoma, or IMT (*Am J Surg Pathol* 2014;38:e20). Around two-thirds of IMTs are immunoreactive for ALK1. Fluorescence in situ hybridization for *ALK1* gene rearrangement also may be helpful and occasionally can be positive in cases with negative ALK1 immunostaining. The differential also includes the so-called postoperative spindle cell nodule (a reactive myofibroblastic proliferation), a diagnosis for which clinical history is essential. Recurrences can be seen and the proliferations can be locally aggressive, though only one reported case had metastatic spread; in that case, overt sarcomatous features were also present (*Am J Surg Pathol* 2006;30:1502).

4. Other spindle cell neoplasms. There are other spindle cell neoplasms that can occasionally involve the bladder including hemangioma, granular cell tumor, neurofibroma, solitary fibrous tumor, angiosarcoma, and perivascular epithelioid cell tumor (PEComa). These tumors are histologically identical to their nonbladder counterparts.

L. Other Miscellaneous Neoplasms. As discussed earlier, the bladder can be involved by metastatic carcinomas and those extending from adjacent organs, where clinical data and immunohistochemical findings can help resolve the diagnosis. Hematolymphoid neoplasms can involve the bladder primarily or secondarily (more common) and may present as mass lesions.

IV. HISTOLOGIC GRADING OF UROTHELIAL CARCINOMA is indicated as low grade or high grade, as discussed above. Histologic grade of primary adenocarcinoma or SCC of the urinary bladder can be reported as well-, moderately-, or poorly differentiated.

V. PATHOLOGIC STAGING OF URINARY BLADDER CANCER follows the 2017 American Joint Committee on Cancer (AJCC) staging classification (Amin MB, Edge S, Greene F, et al., eds. *AJCC Cancer Staging Manual*, 8th ed. New York: Springer, 2017) and applies to carcinomas only. Pathologic primary tumor (pT) stage is illustrated in Figure 22.3.

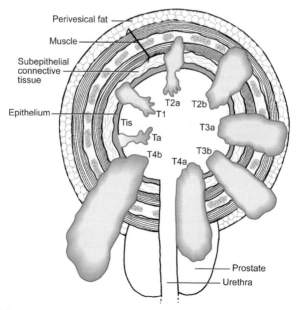

Figure 22.3 Pathologic T-staging of carcinoma of the urinary bladder. (Modified from Greene FL, Compton CC, Fritz AG, Shah JP, Winchester DP, eds. *AJCC Cancer Staging Atlas*. New York: Springer; 2006).

Lamina propria invasion may be very focal and can occur in the fibrovascular cores or at the base of papillary carcinomas, underlying urothelial CIS, or at the edge of an area of inverted growth (e-**Figs. 22.54–22.56**). The nested variant of invasive urothelial carcinoma may be particularly difficult to recognize, as the overlying urothelium may be benign. The extent of invasion in pT1 disease is related to the patient outcome, with a worse prognosis for patients with tumors that invade the muscularis mucosae or deeply into the lamina propria. Some have recommended substaging of "microinvasive" pT1 carcinoma (variously defined as occupying <1 high-power field, invading to a depth of ≤1 mm, or invading above the muscularis mucosae and to a depth of 2 mm or less), but this is not a formal part of the 2017 AJCC system and is not universally reported; there is no established method for estimation that is consistently applicable and reproducible (Moch H, Humphrey PA, Ulbright TM, Reuter VE, eds. *World Health Organization Classification of Tumours. Tumours of the Urinary System and Male Genital Organs.* Lyon, IARC Press; 2016.).

Determination of the type of muscle (muscularis mucosae vs. muscularis propria) invaded by carcinoma can occasionally be difficult because of small tissue sample size, tissue distortion, cautery artifact, poor orientation, fibrosis, inflammation elicited by destructive growth of invasive tumor, or hypertrophy of the normally thin, wispy, and discontinuous muscularis mucosae. The designation of "muscle type indeterminate" is a viable description in some cases. Smoothelin immunohistochemistry has potential for distinction of muscularis mucosae from muscularis propria, though its routine use is not currently recommended (*Am J Surg Pathol* 2010;34:792; *Am J Surg Pathol* 2014;38:e20).

Substaging of pT2 muscularis propria invasion (pT2a, inner half vs. pT2b, outer half) and distinction of pT2 versus pT3 can only be performed on radical cystectomy specimens and not samples from transurethral resections of bladder tumor. Even in cystectomy specimens, it can be a challenge to evaluate extravesical (pT3) invasion because the boundary between muscularis propria and its fat is not well demarcated from perivesical fat. Moreover, this boundary can be distorted, obscured, or obliterated by fibrosis and inflammation associated with infiltrating tumor.

Pathologic stage pT4 bladder urothelial carcinomas invade adjacent organs or the pelvic wall. It is essential to distinguish invasion of a bladder carcinoma into the prostate through the bladder wall versus invasion of the prostatic ducts or stroma via the prostatic urethra. Urethral tumors not in continuity with the bladder mass should be staged and reported separately.

Regional metastasis to true pelvic lymph nodes is categorized as pN1 (single node) or pN2 (multiple nodes); common iliac nodal metastases warrant a pN3 designation. Metastasis to nodes beyond the common iliac group is considered distant metastasis.

VI. REPORTING URINARY BLADDER CARCINOMA follows suggested guidelines (e.g., see the College of American Pathologists Protocol for the Examination of Specimens From Patients With Carcinoma of the Urinary Bladder Cancer Protocol, at http://www.cap.org).

For urinary bladder biopsy and transurethral resections, the histologic type, grade, and depth of invasion are reported. The presence or absence of muscularis propria should also be noted for each biopsy sample. CIS always should be reported, even when present in conjunction with a papillary or invasive neoplasm. If lymphovascular space invasion by carcinoma is seen, it should be reported.

For cystectomy (partial or total), radical cystoprostatectomy, and pelvic exenteration specimens, the following gross features are reported: tumor location, size in three dimensions, growth pattern (papillary, nodular/solid, flat, ulcerated), depth of invasion, involvement of adjacent structures (prostate, vagina, uterus, colon), and relation to surgical margins. Microscopic features that should be reported include the histologic type, grade, extent of invasion, involvement of other structures, lymphovascular invasion, and margin status. Important margins include the ureters, distal urethra, perivesical soft tissue (for cystectomy specimens), and pelvic soft tissue (for exenteration specimens). For regional lymph nodes, the total number examined and number positive for carcinoma should be documented.

Cytology of the Urinary Bladder

Cory Bernadt

I. TYPES OF SPECIMENS

A. **Voided Urine** normally has a mixture of benign urothelial cells and squamous cells. Although the squamous cells are often contaminant from the external genital tract, they can also be derived from areas of squamous metaplasia that often develop in the bladder trigone.

B. **Catheterized Urine** normally has papillary-like clusters of urothelial cells resulting from the mechanical disruption of the urothelial mucosa. They should not be confused with low-grade urothelial carcinoma.

C. **Bladder Washings** are obtained by irrigating the bladder with saline instilled via a catheter, or during cystoscopic evaluation. The cytologic findings in this specimen type are similar to those seen in catheterized urine.

D. **Neobladder or Ileal Conduit Samples** have abundant degenerated cells, some of which are arranged in clusters and have vacuolated cytoplasm. Well-preserved intestinal-type epithelium is rarely present. A variable number of inflammatory cells, macrophages, and bacteria are seen (e-**Fig. 22.57**).

II. THE PARIS SYSTEM FOR REPORTING URINARY CYTOLOGY

A. **Introduction.** The main purpose for the evaluation of urine cytology specimens is to detect HGUC. Recently, the Paris System Working Group introduced a standardized reporting system with specific diagnostic categories and cytomorphologic criteria for the reliable diagnosis of HGUC (*Acta Cytol* 2016;60:185).

B. **Nondiagnostic/Unsatisfactory.** Currently, the Paris System does not contain strict numerical thresholds on cellularity for adequacy. This is largely due to the variety of specimen collection and processing methods. In general, if the urothelial cells are completely obscured by lubricant or inflammatory cells, the specimen is "unsatisfactory." Any atypical cells, regardless of the overall cellularity, represent a satisfactory specimen.

C. **Negative for High-Grade Urothelial Carcinoma (NHGUC).** The majority of urine specimens fall into this category and are typically composed of benign urothelial cells, superficial squamous cells from the external genital tract, and benign glandular cells (from cystitis glandularis). Groups or clusters of urothelial cells that can be seen in both instrumented and noninstrumented urine specimens should be classified as negative, unless the cytomorphology of the cells fits into one of the categories outlined below. In addition, changes that can be attributed to urolithiasis, treatment effect, or polyomavirus (BK virus) should be classified as NHGUC.

D. **Atypical Urothelial Cells (AUCs).** The criteria for AUC include one major and one minor criterion. The major criterion is the presence of nonsuperficial and nondegenerated urothelial cells with an increased nuclear cytoplasmic (N/C) ratio (>0.5). Only one of the following minor criteria is required: (1) mild nuclear hyperchromasia, (2) irregular nuclear membranes, or (3) irregular, coarse, clumped chromatin.

E. **Suspicious for High-Grade Urothelial Carcinoma (SHGUC).** There is severe urothelial atypia, but it falls quantitatively short (very few cells, 5 to 10 cells) of HGUC. The major criterion is the presence of nonsuperficial and nondegenerated urothelial cells with an increased N/C ratio (>0.7) and severe nuclear hyperchromasia. Only one of the following minor criteria is required: (1) irregular nuclear membranes or (2) very dark, irregular, coarse, clumped chromatin (e-**Fig. 22.58**).

F. **High-Grade Urothelial Carcinoma (HGUC).** The necessary morphologic features are the same as those for SHGUC, the only difference being the number of severely atypical cells.

G. **Low-Grade Urothelial Neoplasm (LGUN).** This designation is reserved for specimens that show clusters of urothelial cells with fibrovascular cores. This is a rare finding in urine specimens, and this category should be used in conjunction with NHGUC to clarify the absence of HGUC.

H. Other: Primary and Secondary Malignancies and Miscellaneous Lesions

1. **SCC** can rarely occur as a primary bladder tumor or can arise in adjacent organs (e.g., the uterine cervix) and extend into the bladder. A more common scenario is squamous differentiation within a conventional urothelial carcinoma. Cytologic features that indicate the presence of squamous differentiation include neoplastic cells with a variable amount of dense and eosinophilic cytoplasm, pyknotic nuclei, and bizarre cell shapes (**e-Fig. 22.59**). Parakeratotic and/or anucleated cells are often seen in the background. Poorly differentiated SCC that is nonkeratinizing may be confused with HGUC.

2. **Adenocarcinoma of the bladder** can be primary or metastatic. Although most (87%) of adenocarcinomas of the bladder can be identified as malignant by urine cytology, only 67% will be additionally classified as adenocarcinoma (*Cancer Cytopathol* 1998;84:335). Columnar or cuboidal cell shapes, with cytoplasmic vacuoles within the neoplastic cells, are cytologic features that support the diagnosis of adenocarcinoma.

III. **ANCILLARY TECHNIQUES.** Numerous ancillary techniques have been developed to improve the cytologic detection of urothelial carcinoma. Many of these have greater sensitivity than cytology alone, but suboptimal specificity limits their use. One of the most commonly used technique is the FDA-approved UroVysion test (Abbot Molecular, Des Plaines, IL). It is a multitarget FISH assay that has been approved for the surveillance of patients treated for bladder cancer and as a screening tool in patients with hematuria (*J Mol Diagn* 2000;2:116). This assay combines centromeric probes to chromosomes 3, 7, and 17 with a locus-specific probe to band 9p21. HGUCs are associated with aberrations of chromosomes 1, 3, 7, 9, 11, and 17; deletion of the p16 gene at chromosome 9p21 is an alteration that is commonly present in low-grade urothelial carcinoma. The performance of UroVysion varies widely in the literature with reported sensitivity and specificity for the detection of HGUC to range from 8% to 100% and 29% to 100%, respectively (*Cancer Cytopathol* 2013;121:591). Despite its limitations, UroVysion can be useful in the setting of atypical cytologic findings to guide the urologist in further patient management (*Histopathology* 2011;58:1048).

ACKNOWLEDGMENT

The authors thank Omar Hameed and Rosa M. Dávila, authors of the previous edition of this chapter.

23 Urethra

Jennifer K. Sehn and Peter A. Humphrey

I. NORMAL ANATOMY. The male urethra is divided into three anatomic regions: prostatic (bladder neck to apex of the prostate), bulbomembranous (apex of the prostate to inferior surface of the urogenital diaphragm), and penile (inferior surface of urogenital diaphragm to the urethral meatus). The prostatic portion is lined by the urothelium, the bulbomembranous portion is lined by the pseudostratified or stratified columnar epithelium, and the penile portion shows a transition from the stratified columnar epithelium at its origin to the squamous epithelium at the meatus. The female urethra is lined by urothelium in the proximal one-third, and squamous epithelium in the distal two-thirds.

The urethra has associated periurethral glands. Skene glands are present in females and are concentrated distally. Bulbourethral glands (Cowper glands) and glands of Littre, located in the bulbomembranous portion and along the penile urethra, respectively, are present in males.

II. GROSS EXAMINATION AND TISSUE SAMPLING

A. Urethroscopic Biopsy Tissue Samples should be entirely submitted for histologic examination, and three levels should be examined.

B. Surgical Excision of Urethral Carcinoma. For men, the type of surgery is dependent on the tumor location and extent, and includes transurethral resection (TUR), local segmental excision, partial or radical penectomy, and cystoprostatectomy. TUR chips should be submitted in their entirety. Segmental excision specimens should be sampled to include sections of the proximal and distal margins and area of deepest growth. Urethrectomy (primary or secondary) involves stripping of all or part of the urethra with preservation of the penis, and is performed for patients with primary urethral carcinoma or secondary involvement by bladder carcinoma; sampling should include sections of the proximal and distal margins and area of deepest growth. Gross processing of penectomy and cystoprostatectomy specimens is covered in Chapters 30 and 29, respectively.

For women, local excision of the distal urethra and the adjacent vaginal wall is often sufficient surgical therapy for carcinoma of the urethra; sections of the mass and urothelial, radial soft tissue, and vaginal mucosal margins should be submitted. For proximal urethral cancer in women, cystourethrectomy (anterior exenteration, with excision of part or all of the vagina) is often necessary; sections of the mass demonstrating relationships to adjacent structures and depth of invasion, grossly uninvolved urethra and urinary bladder, and ureteral and radial soft tissue margins should be submitted.

III. DIAGNOSTIC FEATURES OF BENIGN DISEASES

A. Congenital Anomalies

1. **Urethral valves** are mucosal folds lined by the normal urothelium that project into the urethral lumen, causing obstruction, hematuria, or inflammation. Posterior urethral valves are usually seen in men and are associated with bladder neck hypertrophy.

2. **Diverticula** are invaginations of the urethral mucosa usually seen in women as a result of infection, trauma, or obstruction. They are lined by urothelium that may undergo squamous or glandular metaplasia (e-Fig. 23.1).

3. **Fibroepithelial polyp** is a congenital anomaly usually involving the posterior urethra of male infants and young boys. It consists of a fibrous connective tissue stalk lined by urothelium.

B. Inflammation and Infection

1. **Urethritis** is an inflammatory response in the urethra that is usually secondary to sexually transmitted diseases. Diagnosis is made by examination of a urethral smear that

shows neutrophils. Polypoid urethritis is usually seen in the prostatic urethra near the verumontanum, and is the result of inflammation that induces multiple polypoid lesions with edematous stroma, distended blood vessels, and chronic inflammation (e-**Fig. 23.2**).

2. **Caruncle** is a pedunculated or sessile polypoid inflammatory mass in the distal urethra in postmenopausal women showing a mixed inflammatory infiltrate with rich vascularity (e-**Fig. 23.3**).

3. **Malakoplakia** is a rare urethral granulomatous inflammatory process more commonly seen in women, showing histiocytes containing characteristic Michaelis–Gutmann bodies.

4. **Condyloma acuminatum** of the urethra is caused by the human papilloma virus (HPV), usually serotypes 6, 11, 16, and 18. Condyloma acuminatum can primarily involve the urethra, but more commonly arises by direct extension from similar lesions in adjacent sites including the external genitalia, perineum, and anus. Histologically, there is a flat or polypoid proliferation of squamous epithelium (e-**Fig. 23.4**) with koilocytic atypia. Multiplicity and recurrence are common.

C. Metaplasia

1. **Squamous metaplasia** can occur as a response to chronic inflammatory insults secondary to infection, diverticula, calculi, or instrumentation.

2. **Urethritis cystica and glandularis** consists of small cysts lined by urothelial and glandular cells, respectively.

3. **Nephrogenic adenoma** (metaplasia) is rare in the urethra. It occurs at the site of previous damage, often related to a previous surgical procedure. Microscopically, there is a proliferation of tubular and papillary structures, sometimes with cystic change, lined by flattened to cuboidal to hobnail cells with bland nuclear features (e-**Fig. 23.5**). Some cases may be due to implantation and growth of tubular epithelial cells shed from the kidney. Nephrogenic adenoma is immunoreactive for AMACR and negative for p63/34βE12, which can cause diagnostic confusion with Gleason pattern 3 prostatic adenocarcinoma when it involves the prostatic urethra. Reactivity for PAX8 is helpful in confirming the diagnosis of nephrogenic adenoma in this setting.

D. Hyperplasia

1. **Urothelial hyperplasia** is a reactive thickening of the cytologically bland urothelium, and can be flat or papillary. In the papillary form the mucosa can be undulating but still lacks a well-developed fibrovascular core, differentiating it from papillary urothelial neoplasia. In the 2016 World Health Organization (WHO) classification (Table 22.1), urothelial proliferation of uncertain malignant potential is the recommended diagnostic terminology for papillary and flat urothelial hyperplasia.

2. **Prostatic urethral polyp** is seen in the verumontanum in young men and consists of benign prostatic tissue arranged in a polypoid or papillary configuration, with projection into the urethral lumen.

IV. DIAGNOSTIC FEATURES OF NEOPLASTIC DISEASES

A. Benign Neoplasms are exceedingly rare and have the same appearance as in the urinary bladder.

1. **Benign epithelial neoplasms** include villous adenoma, squamous papilloma, and urothelial (including inverted) papilloma.

2. **Benign mesenchymal neoplasms** include leiomyoma and hemangioma.

B. Malignant Neoplasms originating in the urethra are very rare and are carcinomas in the vast majority of cases (*Semin Diagn Pathol* 1997;14:147; *Hematol Oncol Clin North Am* 2012;26:1291). Compared with urinary bladder carcinomas, urethral carcinomas are more often found in women; a much higher percentage are squamous cell carcinomas; there is a greater percentage of high-grade and high-stage tumors; and there is a poorer prognosis. The histologic type of primary urethral carcinomas corresponds to the anatomic site of origin in the urethra. In general, proximal neoplasms (prostatic urethra in men; proximal one-third in females) tend to be urothelial carcinomas, whereas distal tumors (bulbomembranous or penile in men; distal two-thirds in women) are frequently squamous cell carcinomas. Often it is difficult to ascertain the precise site of origin of a urethral carcinoma due to its infiltrative growth and destruction of normal cells. For primary and secondary urothelial neoplasia, the 2016 WHO urinary bladder classification is used for histologic typing (Table 22.1).

1. **Squamous cell carcinoma** is the most common urethral carcinoma in both sexes. HPV infection has a significant role in its etiology; 30% of squamous cell carcinomas in men and 60% in women test positive for high-risk HPV, although HPV identification is not necessary for diagnosis. Grossly, squamous cell carcinoma can be verruciform or scirrhous, often with necrosis (e-**Fig. 23.6**). Microscopically, most are moderately differentiated and deeply invasive. Squamous cell carcinomas of the distal penile urethra frequently invade the corpus cavernosum; more proximal tumors in men may penetrate directly into the urogenital diaphragm, prostate, rectum, and bladder neck. In women, tumors arising in the distal third of the urethra are commonly low-grade squamous cell carcinoma (e-**Fig. 23.7**) or verrucous carcinomas.

2. **Urothelial carcinoma** rarely primarily involves the urethra, but more commonly results from secondary involvement by bladder carcinoma; the so-called secondary involvement can represent direct extension, multifocal disease, and/or lymphovascular invasion. Grossly, carcinoma in situ (CIS) can be erythematous and/or ulcerative; carcinomas can be papillary, nodular, ulcerative, and/or infiltrative. Histopathologically, primary or secondary urothelial tumors can present as pure CIS (e-**Fig. 23.8**), noninvasive papillary neoplasia (e-**Fig. 23.9**), or invasive carcinoma, with or without a papillary component. In men, there is a propensity for high-grade carcinoma (CIS or invasive) to involve the prostate, which can represent in situ duct/acinar spread (e-**Fig. 23.10**) and/or stromal-invasive disease. Immunohistochemical stains can be helpful in differentiating high-grade prostatic adenocarcinoma from urothelial carcinoma involving the prostate, with reactivity for GATA3, p63, and high–molecular-weight cytokeratin (e.g., 34βE12) arguing for urothelial origin versus reactivity for PSA, PSAP, prostein (P501S), and/or NKX3.1 typical of prostatic adenocarcinoma (*Am J Surg Pathol* 2014;38:1017). CIS also can cancerize periurethral glands, which may mimic invasion (e-**Fig. 23.11**).

3. **Adenocarcinoma** is usually seen in the proximal urethra and can originate in a diverticulum. Grossly, the tumor is often infiltrative, with or without an exophytic component, with mucinous, gelatinous, and/or cystic cut surfaces (e-**Fig. 23.12**). Microscopically, glandular metaplasia and urethritis cystica and glandularis are frequently seen in adjacent epithelium. In women, the most common subtype is clear cell adenocarcinoma (40% of cases). In men, enteric, colloid, or signet-ring histomorphologic features are common.

   a. **Clear cell adenocarcinoma** is a rare tumor that is almost always found in women. Histologically, it is similar to müllerian-type clear cell adenocarcinoma of the vagina or uterus. Architectural heterogeneity is common, with solid, tubular, tubulocystic, micropapillary, or papillary patterns (e-**Fig. 23.13**). Hyalinized stroma is often seen, at least focally. Mitotic activity is usually brisk and includes atypical forms. The neoplastic cells show hobnail morphology and have well-defined borders, with amphophilic, acidophilic, or clear cytoplasm containing glycogen. Nuclei are large and hyperchromatic with prominent nucleoli. Clear cell adenocarcinoma should be differentiated from nephrogenic adenoma (metaplasia), which lacks an infiltrative pattern, sheet-like growth, mitotic figures, necrosis, and significant nuclear atypia (*Hum Pathol* 2010;41:594).

   b. **Non–clear cell adenocarcinoma** includes enteric, mucinous (e-**Fig. 23.14**), signet-ring-cell, and not otherwise-specified subtypes. Extension of adenocarcinoma from adjacent organs (e.g., endometrium, cervix, colon) should be excluded.

4. **Paraurethral gland carcinomas** usually develop in paraurethral (Skene glands in females; glands of Littre in males) and bulbourethral (Cowper) glands. Establishing the origin of adenocarcinoma can be difficult because of mucosal ulceration and obliteration of landmarks by the time of diagnosis.

5. Other rare carcinomas include small cell carcinoma, adenosquamous carcinoma, sarcomatoid carcinoma, and lymphoepithelioma-like carcinoma.

6. Melanoma. The urethra is the most common site of primary melanoma of the genitourinary tract (*Am J Surg Pathol* 2000;24:785), but secondary involvement as a result of spread from the glans penis or vulvar lesions is more common (**e-Fig. 23.15**). Melanomas in this site are frequently amelanotic and may cause diagnostic confusion with other lesions including caruncles or fibroepithelial polyps. Evaluation of margin status and the absence of skip lesions are important in determining the prognosis. In contrast to cutaneous melanomas, *BRAF* mutations are infrequent in melanomas arising from mucosal sites, though a subset do harbor mutations in *KIT* and may be amenable to the targeted kinase inhibitor therapy.

7. Hematopoietic neoplasms. Case reports exist of non-Hodgkin lymphoma, mucosa-associated lymphoid tissue (MALT) lymphoma, and plasmacytoma in the urethra.

V. HISTOLOGIC GRADING OF URETHRAL CARCINOMA. For squamous cell carcinoma and adenocarcinoma, well, moderately, or poorly differentiated grades may be applied. Urothelial carcinomas are graded as low or high grade.

VI. PATHOLOGIC STAGING OF URETHRAL CARCINOMA follows the 2017 Tumor, Node, Metastasis (TNM) American Joint Committee on Cancer (AJCC) staging classification for tumors of the male and female urethra (Amin MB, Edge S, Greene F, et al., eds. *AJCC Cancer Staging Manual,* 8th ed. New York: Springer, 2017). Tumor location and pathologic stage are the most significant pathologic prognostic indicators for urethral carcinoma. Proximal tumors have a worse outcome. Pathologic pT stage for noninvasive carcinoma (pTa for papillary neoplasia, pTis for flat CIS) and tumors involving subepithelial connective tissue (pT1) is analogous to staging in bladder and ureter/renal pelvis. In the penile urethra, pT2 tumors involve the corpus spongiosum (erectile tissue surrounding the penile urethra), while pT3 tumors extend into one or both of the corpora cavernosa. For tumors arising in the intraprostatic portion of the male urethra, urothelial carcinoma confined to the periurethral/prostatic ducts (pTis) is to be distinguished from carcinoma invading the prostatic stroma (pT2); tumors invading through the prostate into the periprostatic fat or adjacent organs are pT3 or pT4, respectively. In the female urethra, pT2 represents invasion of the periurethral muscle, with pT3 showing invasion of the anterior vagina. A single regional (inguinal, pelvic, presacral) lymph node metastasis is categorized as N1, regardless of the size of the metastatic deposit (which is a change from the prior 2010 AJCC staging scheme); multiple metastases to regional nodes warrant classification as N2.

VII. REPORTING URETHRAL CARCINOMA. The pathology report of a urethral malignancy should follow recommended guidelines (College of American Pathologists Protocol for the Examination of Specimens from Patients with Carcinoma of the Urethra and Periurethral glands, available at http://www.cap.org) and include the histologic type, histologic grade, anatomic location (proximal vs. distal), extent of involvement (depth and invasion of adjacent anatomic structures, if resected), presence or absence of lymphovascular space invasion and perineural invasion, and pathologic TNM staging for resection specimens. The status of the margins should also be indicated, if applicable, including identification of the number and location of positive sites. Any additional findings such as inflammation, metaplasia, presence of a diverticulum, or presence of a stricture, should also be reported.

A C K N O W L E D G M E N T

The authors thank Dr. Souzan Sanati, an author of the previous editions of this chapter.

Endocrine System

24

Thyroid
Kirk Hill and Rebecca D. Chernock

I. **NORMAL ANATOMY.** The thyroid gland is a bilobed organ in the lower neck surrounding, and in intimate contact with, the trachea. It consists of right and left lobes connected by a small isthmus in the midline (Fig. 24.1). Two functioning cell types, follicular cells and calcitonin-secreting C cells, comprise the thyroid follicle. The follicular component develops from the invaginating tissue from the tongue base (foramen cecum) at 5 to 6 weeks gestation. Through differential embryonic growth and migration, the bilobed gland assumes its definitive location in the neck, and the thyroglossal duct, the structure along the path of its downward migration, undergoes atrophy. The C cells, which comprise 0.1% or less of the total thyroid cell mass, originate from the ultimobranchial body that develops from the fourth branchial pouches; they are distributed in a gradient, being most prominent in the upper lobes.

The normal gland has a relatively firm consistency, is dark brown and glistening, and lacks any obvious nodules. Microscopically, it consists of follicles lined by low cuboidal bland epithelial cells. This follicular epithelium surrounds a central core of eosinophilic colloid. In normal glands, the follicles have only mild variation in size (**e-Fig. 24.1**). The C cells lie within the follicular epithelium and are invested by the basement membrane. They are inconspicuous in normal thyroid.

II. **GROSS EXAMINATION, TISSUE SAMPLING, AND HISTOLOGIC SLIDE PREPARATION**

   A. **Biopsy.** Tissue needle biopsies of the thyroid gland are only very rarely performed because fine needle aspiration is technically easy to perform, has low morbidity, and is effective for triaging lesions for further management (see section cytopathology below).

   B. **Resection.** Hemithyroidectomy and total thyroidectomy are common procedures for the management of thyroid disease. The specimens from both types of procedure are handled in a similar manner. The gland is oriented, if possible, based on the anatomy alone or on markings provided by the surgeon. It is then measured and weighed. The surface is inspected for any disruptions or attached soft tissue which may contain lymph nodes, parathyroid glands, or sequestered thyroid in cases of nodular hyperplasia. The gland should be inked, the lobes sectioned in an axial plane ("bread loafed") at intervals of 3 to 5 mm, and described, clearly indicating masses and their size(s), color, and consistency. For diffuse or inflammatory lesions, three or four sections from each lobe should be submitted for microscopic examination, along with one of the isthmus. A solitary, encapsulated mass should be generously sampled, including the entire circumference of the capsule in relation to the surrounding thyroid tissue because the distinction of adenoma or noninvasive follicular thyroid neoplasm with papillary-like

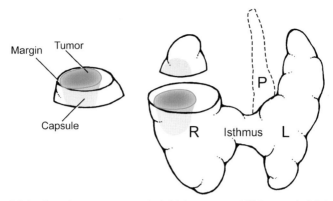

Figure 24.1 Thyroid anatomy/grossing (L, left lobe; P, pyramidal lobe; R, right lobe).

nuclear features (NIFTP) from carcinoma relies on demonstrating invasion. In the case of NIFTP, submission of the entire tumor may be necessary. For a solitary, nonencapsulated or not completely encapsulated mass, at least one section per centimeter should be submitted, and some sections should demonstrate the closest inked margin (Fig. 24.1). For multinodular glands (nodular hyperplasia), sections of each nodule should be submitted, including the edge and/or adjacent soft tissue margin. Any attached perithyroidal soft tissue should be removed and sampled. Lymph nodes or parathyroid glands should be removed and sampled as well, although oftentimes the parathyroid gland(s) are first detected by microscopic examination (the number of parathyroid glands should be recorded).

Prophylactic thyroidectomy is currently recommended in infancy, early childhood, adolescence, or early adulthood for patients with a germline *RET* gene mutation. The specimen often consists of the thyroid gland with no grossly identifiable lesions. Each lobe should be entirely submitted sequentially from superior to inferior to allow thorough examination for C-cell hyperplasia or medullary microcarcinoma.

III. DIAGNOSTIC FEATURES OF COMMON DISEASES

A. Developmental. Residual thyroid tissue can be present anywhere along the path of thyroid migration during development. Carcinomas can rarely develop outside of the thyroid gland in these residual tissue sites.

1. Pyramidal lobe. The most common developmental remnant is a pyramidal lobe, a linear projection of thyroid tissue from the isthmus pointing cranially (Fig. 24.1).

2. Thyroglossal duct cyst. Failure of closure of the thyroglossal duct commonly results in a midline cyst known as a thyroglossal duct cyst (TDC). Excision specimens generally consist of soft tissue (containing the cyst) and the central portion of the hyoid bone. The hyoid bone is excised because remnants of the midline tract pass through it. Failure to resect the bone often results in persistence of the TDC. If a cyst is identified grossly, it should be sampled in a few sections. Microscopically, these lesions have a squamous or respiratory-type lining epithelium without a muscular wall (e-**Fig. 24.2**). TDCs can become infected and inflamed with associated granulation tissue, which may obscure the epithelial lining. Only a subset have thyroid tissue in the cyst wall (approximately 5% do on routine sections, and about 40% on serial sectioning).

3. Lingual thyroid. Thyroid tissue can be present at the base of the tongue at the site of developmental invagination, referred to as lingual thyroid. Microscopically, the thyroid tissue is usually normal.

B. Inflammation (Thyroiditis)

1. **Acute thyroiditis** is caused predominantly by bacteria but rarely can have a fungal origin. It is usually seen in the setting of neck trauma or as spread from infection of adjacent structures. Microscopically, the gland is infiltrated by neutrophils with microabscesses and necrotic foci. Organisms can often be seen with or without special stains. Patients usually recover with antibiotics.

2. **Subacute granulomatous thyroiditis (de Quervain thyroiditis).** Subacute granulomatous thyroiditis or de Quervain thyroiditis is a disease primarily of women and is thought to be due to systemic viral infection. Patients present with fever, malaise, and neck pain. The disease consists of three phases: hyperthyroidism, hypothyroidism, and recovery.

   Grossly, the gland is usually asymmetrically enlarged and slightly firm. Microscopically, in the hyperthyroid phase, there is disruption of the follicles, with depletion of colloid and associated acute inflammation with microabscesses. Aggregates of neutrophils in the follicles are a characteristic feature. Multinucleated giant cells are rare. In the hypothyroid phase, the follicular epithelium may be very scarce, and there is a florid mixed inflammatory response with lymphocytes, plasma cells, and multinucleated giant cells. Finally, in recovery, there is regeneration of follicles with fibrosis. Virtually all patients recover thyroid function after a few months without specific treatment.

3. **Chronic thyroiditis**

   a. **Focal lymphocytic thyroiditis.** Also termed nonspecific thyroiditis or focal autoimmune thyroiditis, this is a common disorder found in up to half of patients in autopsy studies, and is usually discovered incidentally in surgically excised thyroids. It is most common in older women. Patients are asymptomatic but often have a low level of antithyroid antibodies.

      There are no significant gross findings. Microscopically, focal lymphocytic thyroiditis consists of isolated aggregates of lymphocytes between the follicles, occasionally with germinal centers (e-**Fig. 24.3**). The lymphocytes can infiltrate follicles, but there is no significant destruction or damage. The disease is not progressive.

   b. **Hashimoto thyroiditis.** Hashimoto thyroiditis, or **chronic lymphocytic thyroiditis**, is an autoimmune disease with thyroid enlargement and circulating antithyroid antibodies. It occurs most often in middle-aged women and is caused by autoantibodies against thyroglobulin (Tg) and thyroid peroxidase (TPO) that lead to inflammation and destruction of the follicles. There is a familial association, and Hashimoto thyroiditis is often associated with other autoimmune diseases. There is also an association with certain HLA types such as DR3 and DR5. Patients usually present with hypothyroidism. Ultrasound shows an enlarged gland with a hypoechogenic pattern, and anti-Tg and anti-TPO antibodies are present in approximately 60% and 95% of cases, respectively.

      Grossly, the thyroid is diffusely enlarged and firm with a mildly nodular surface. On sectioning, lobulation is accentuated due to fibrosis, and the gland is tan or off-white rather than the usual brown due to the abundant lymphoid tissue. Microscopically, there are sheets of lymphocytes and plasma cells with abundant germinal centers. The follicles are atrophic with minimal colloid. Characteristic Hürthle cell change (oncocytic metaplasia) is present, consisting of large cells with abundant, granular, eosinophilic cytoplasm and large, round nuclei with vesicular chromatin and often prominent nucleoli (e-**Fig. 24.4**). The inflammatory infiltrate may extend into the perithyroidal soft tissue causing adherence of the gland at the time of surgery. Finally, there may be fibrous septa between the lobules, and the follicular epithelium may develop squamous metaplasia.

      A number of variants of Hashimoto thyroiditis occur, including fibrous (sclerosing), fibrous atrophy, juvenile, and cystic forms. Both of the fibrous variants show the same histologic findings, namely retention of a lobulated pattern with extensive and severe fibrosis. Atrophic follicular cells are more scattered but show Hürthle cell change, and there is abundant chronic inflammation with germinal centers. In the fibrous variant, the gland is markedly enlarged throughout. In the fibrous atrophy variant, the gland is small and shrunken. Both of the latter variant forms are associated with marked hypothyroidism and high titers of antithyroid antibodies. A subset of the fibrous variant cases may belong to the spectrum of IgG4-related diseases.

The differential diagnosis for Hashimoto thyroiditis includes Riedel thyroiditis, lymphoma, and papillary carcinoma (PTC). The fibrous variant of Hashimoto thyroiditis may simulate Riedel thyroiditis with an enlarged fibrotic gland. However, the fibrosis is typically limited to the gland itself, whereas in Riedel thyroiditis there is severe adherence of the fibrotic gland to the neck soft tissues. The dense inflammation in Hashimoto thyroiditis can simulate lymphoma, and most thyroid lymphomas do arise in the setting of Hashimoto thyroiditis. The distinction lies in the absence of sheets of atypical lymphocytes, the lack of a strikingly prominent lymphoepithelial pattern with intraluminal lymphocytes, and the lack of clonality of the lymphocytes by flow cytometry or molecular studies. Lastly, the nuclear features of the epithelium in Hashimoto thyroiditis can simulate those of PTC (including nuclear crowding, clear chromatin, and occasional nuclear grooves) and develop frequently in the inflamed follicular epithelium. A true carcinoma arising in Hashimoto thyroiditis should stand out sharply from the neighboring follicular epithelium, as in uninflamed thyroid.

c. Graves disease. Graves disease, also known as diffuse hyperplasia, is an autoimmune condition resulting in excess thyroid hormone production. It causes the majority of cases of spontaneous hyperthyroidism, occurs most often in the third and fourth decades, and is 5 to 10 times more common in women. Thyroid-specific autoantibodies, specifically thyroid-stimulating immunoglobulin (TSI), are present in Graves disease patients. TSI binds to and stimulates thyrocytes through the thyroid-stimulating hormone (TSH) receptor, resulting in thyrotoxicosis. Patients may also develop a characteristic infiltrative ophthalmopathy with proptosis.

Grossly, the thyroid gland is diffusely and symmetrically enlarged. Post-treatment or after long-standing disease, the gland may be somewhat nodular or fibrotic. Microscopically, the gland typically shows a low-power lobular accentuation due to increased septal fibrous tissue. Inflammation varies from almost none to patchy lymphocytic with formation of germinal centers. The follicular epithelium is hyperplastic and has increased amounts of cytoplasm, is convoluted and irregular, and often assumes a papillary appearance. Colloid is decreased or absent and typically has a "scalloped" appearance from clearing at the interface with the follicular epithelium (**e-Figs. 24.5** and **24.6**). Treated cases have a variable morphology often having more abundant colloid. After radioactive iodine treatment, marked nuclear atypia may be present. The differential diagnosis includes PTC when the stellate outlines of follicles resemble papillae. The lack of cytologic changes of PTC and the diffuse gland involvement are keys to the correct diagnosis of Graves disease.

d. Riedel thyroiditis. Originally described as a peculiar hard, infiltrative lesion of the thyroid gland that could be clinically mistaken for malignancy, Riedel thyroiditis is a rare chronic thyroiditis that is now considered to be part of the spectrum of IgG4-related disease. IgG4-related diseases are a collection of disorders affecting various organ systems and characterized by elevated serum IgG4 in a majority of patients, dense lymphoplasmacytic infiltrations with a predominance of IgG4-positive plasma cells in the affected tissue, and storiform fibrosis. Riedel thyroiditis is more common in women, occurs most commonly in the fifth decade, and is commonly associated with other IgG4-related diseases such as those affecting the mediastinum, retroperitoneum, and lung. Patients present with firm thyroid enlargement and local symptoms such as dysphagia, stridor, or dyspnea. Recurrent laryngeal nerve or sympathetic trunk involvement can lead to hoarseness or the Horner syndrome; compression of the large vessels can lead to superior vena cava syndrome. Most patients are euthyroid at presentation, but many subsequently develop hypothyroidism.

Grossly, the thyroid gland is usually received in irregular pieces because the fibrosis makes it difficult to remove surgically. It is tan to white, firm, and may have attached muscle. Microscopically, the characteristic finding is dense and hypocellular eosinophilic and often storiform fibrosis with scattered and patchy aggregates of lymphocytes, plasma cells, neutrophils, and eosinophils, without germinal centers or granulomas. Rare entrapped and atrophic thyroid follicles are seen typically without Hürthle cell change. A characteristic finding is small veins with infiltrating lymphocytes and myxoid intimal thickening (features of occlusive vasculitis). Marked fibrosis extends into and involves the surrounding soft tissue as well. IgG4 immunohistochemistry highlights numerous IgG4-positive plasma cells between atrophic thyroid follicles, and in combination with IgG, shows an increased IgG4:IgG ratio.

The differential diagnosis includes hypocellular anaplastic thyroid carcinoma and the fibrous variant of Hashimoto thyroiditis. The lack of necrosis or markedly atypical cells rules out anaplastic carcinoma. The lack of Hürthle cell change and germinal centers, and the profound degree of perithyroidal fibrosis, rule out fibrous Hashimoto disease.

C. Nodular Hyperplasia. Nodular hyperplasia (clinically termed multinodular goiter) is an extremely common disorder of the thyroid gland. It consists of enlargement of the gland with varying degrees of nodularity. The pathogenesis is complex but has been related either to excess iodine intake with impaired organification or to genetic factors. Iodine deficiency with impaired thyroid hormone synthesis and subsequent TSH stimulation also causes nodular hyperplasia. It is much more common in women than men, and typically presents in middle age as asymptomatic enlargement. Large goiters, however, can cause dysphagia, hoarseness, or stridor, and can extend into the upper mediastinum. A small percentage of patients present with hyperthyroidism (toxic multinodular goiter).

Grossly, the thyroid gland is diffusely but irregularly enlarged. Some glands can attain a weight of several hundred grams. Parasitic nodules that have only a tenuous connection to the gland can develop. On sectioning, the nodules may be semitranslucent, glistening, fleshy, red-brown, tan, and solid or, more commonly, show varying degrees of degeneration with cystic change, hemorrhage, fibrosis, and calcification. Heterogeneity of the nodules is typical (e-**Fig. 24.7**).

The common microscopic appearance is heterogeneous nodules composed of variably sized follicles (e-**Fig. 24.8**). The nodules may be quite cellular with tightly packed follicular epithelium and little colloid, resembling follicular adenomas or carcinomas. Around cystic areas there is often fibrosis with variably sized foci of dystrophic calcification and hemorrhage, with abundant hemosiderin-laden macrophages. Hürthle cell change is common. Pseudopapillary and truly papillary structures (Sanderson polsters) can project into the cystic areas. The surrounding grossly normal thyroid tissue usually demonstrates microscopic nodularity as well.

The differential diagnosis for cellular nodules includes follicular adenoma or carcinoma. Hyperplastic nodules have a fibrous capsule that is not as well developed or continuous as the capsule of adenomas and carcinomas. Follicular adenomas are discrete and well-encapsulated lesions, are microscopically different from the surrounding thyroid tissue, and have a monotonous cell population—all features that are not characteristic of hyperplastic nodules. Papillary areas in nodular hyperplasia show dark, basally oriented nuclei without other nuclear features of PTC.

D. Neoplasms. The World Health Organization (WHO) classification of tumors of the thyroid gland is listed in Table 24.1.

1. Adenoma. Follicular adenomas are benign, encapsulated tumors that are clonal. They are seen mostly in young to middle-aged adults and are more common in women than

TABLE 24.1   WHO Histologic Classification of Thyroid Tumors

Follicular adenoma

Hyalinizing trabecular tumor

Other encapsulated follicular-patterned thyroid tumors
  Tumors of uncertain malignant potential
  Non-invasive follicular thyroid neoplasm with papillary-like nuclear features (NIFTP)

Papillary thyroid carcinoma

Follicular thyroid carcinoma

Hürthle (oncocytic) cell tumors

Poorly differentiated thyroid carcinoma

Anaplastic thyroid carcinoma

Squamous cell carcinoma

Medullary thyroid carcinoma

Mixed medullary and follicular thyroid carcinoma

Mucoepidermoid carcinoma

Sclerosing mucoepidermoid carcinoma with eosinophilia

Mucinous carcinoma

Ectopic thymoma

Mixed medullary and follicular carcinoma

Spindle epithelial tumor with thymus-like differentiation

Intrathyroid thymic carcinoma

Paraganglioma and mesenchymal/stromal tumors
  Paraganglioma
  Peripheral nerve sheath tumors
  Benign vascular tumors
  Angiosarcoma
  Smooth muscle tumors
  Solitary fibrous tumor

Hematolymphoid tumors
  Langerhans cell histiocytosis
  Rosai–Dorfman disease
  Follicular dendritic cell sarcoma
  Primary thyroid lymphoma

Germ cell tumors

Secondary tumors

From Lloyd RV, Osamura RY, Klöppel G, Rosai J, eds. *WHO Classification of Tumours of Endocrine Organs*. Lyon, France: IARC Press; 2017. Used with permission.

men. There is a relationship with previous irradiation or radiation exposure, just as with follicular carcinoma. There is also an association with inherited diseases including the Cowden syndrome. Most follicular adenomas are asymptomatic and are detected by careful physical examination or incidentally by imaging performed for other reasons.

Grossly, follicular adenomas are very well-defined, round to oval lesions with a complete capsule. They are typically very soft and homogeneous with color ranging from gray-white to tan or dark brown depending on the amount of colloid (e-**Fig. 24.9**). Cystic change and hemorrhage are uncommon. Microscopically, they are encapsulated without, by definition, capsular or vascular invasion. They show a monotonous follicular or trabecular arrangement. The microfollicular pattern features trabeculae with only scattered small follicles with colloid. The macrofollicular pattern has prominent, large follicles with abundant colloid. The cells typically have small amounts of eosinophilic cytoplasm and are quite regular with uniform, round nuclei that have condensed chromatin and inconspicuous nucleoli. There is a well-developed and thin capsule (e-Fig. 24.10). As with all endocrine organ tumors, there may be a marked degree of nuclear pleomorphism which is not necessarily an indication of malignancy or aggressive behavior. Mitotic figures are rare.

A number of adenoma variants are recognized, most notably the oncocytic or Hürthle cell adenoma, now considered a separate neoplasm by the WHO, which has cells with abundant granular eosinophilic cytoplasm (due to the accumulation of abundant mitochondria) and vesicular nuclei with nucleoli and pleomorphism (e-Fig. 24.11). Lipoadenoma (with intratumoral fat; e-Fig. 24.12), signet-ring cell adenoma, and follicular adenoma with papillary hyperplasia are other adenoma variants.

Follicular adenomas are benign, so surgical removal is curative. The differential diagnosis includes hyperplastic nodules of nodular hyperplasia, follicular variant of PTC, NIFTPs, and minimally invasive follicular carcinoma. Consequently, it is critical to assess for nuclear features of PTC and thoroughly sample the lesion including sectioning of the entire capsule to look for microscopic capsular penetration or vascular invasion (see Table 24.2).

2. Follicular thyroid carcinoma. Follicular carcinomas account for approximately 10% of thyroid malignancies and are grouped into three types that have vastly different clinical behavior: minimally invasive, encapsulated angioinvasive, and widely invasive. Follicular carcinomas are more common in women than men, occur in middle-aged adults, and usually present as asymptomatic masses. There is some association with iodine deficiency and prior irradiation.

Minimally invasive tumors have an excellent prognosis, and minimally invasive and encapsulated angioinvasive are distinguished from widely invasive follicular carcinomas primarily on the gross appearance. Minimally invasive and encapsulated angioinvasive follicular carcinomas are well encapsulated and, thus, are grossly indistinguishable from follicular adenomas (microscopic evidence of capsular or vascular invasion is necessary to render a diagnosis of carcinoma, as discussed below). In contrast, widely invasive follicular carcinomas are not encapsulated and show extensive invasion of the surrounding gland and/or soft tissue beyond the thyroid (e-Fig. 24.13). Follicular carcinomas are almost always unifocal and have tan to brown, solid cut surfaces.

Microscopically, the growth pattern ranges from well-formed follicles throughout, to solid, to trabecular. The nuclei of follicular carcinoma tend to be round to oval with granular chromatin (e-Fig. 24.14). Mitotic activity is low and necrosis is lacking.

Hürthle (or oncocytic) cell carcinoma shares many histologic features with follicular carcinoma and was previously considered a variant of follicular carcinoma, but is now classified as a separate entity by the WHO because of its distinctive clinical and pathologic features including a different molecular profile and a propensity for

TABLE 24.2	Histologic Features Differentiating the Solitary Benign From the Malignant Follicular Lesion	
Benign	**Malignant**
Complete but delicate capsule	Dense, circumferential fibrosis
Entrapped or sequestered thyroid in/near capsule	Transcapsular "mushrooming" invasion
Juxtaposed or prolapsed thyroid tissue near vessels, but with intact endothelium	Adherence of thyroid tissue to endothelium with associated thrombus

lymphatic invasion with nodal metastases, both of which are uncharacteristic of nononcocytic follicular carcinomas. Hürthle cell carcinoma is composed of oncocytes that have voluminous eosinophilic and granular cytoplasm and nuclei that are characteristically vesicular with prominent, single nucleoli (e-**Fig. 24.15A**).

By immunohistochemistry, follicular carcinomas are positive for thyroglobulin, thyroid transcription factor-1 (TTF-1), and low–molecular-weight cytokeratins, but these are rarely necessary or useful for diagnosis except occasionally to assess distant metastases as thyroid in origin. Characteristic molecular alterations include *RAS* mutations, found in 30% to 50% of cases, and molecular rearrangements in the *PPARγ* gene, most commonly with fusion to the *PAX8* gene, in 20% to 30% of cases. *TERT* promoter mutations, seen in 20% of cases, are associated with more aggressive behavior. All of these molecular alterations may be encountered in follicular adenomas as well, supporting the concept that a subset of follicular adenomas represents precursors to follicular carcinomas.

The differential diagnosis includes follicular adenoma, medullary carcinoma, and poorly differentiated carcinoma. The distinction of follicular carcinoma from adenoma lies in capsular and/or vascular penetration alone (Table 24.2). Capsular invasion is defined as tumor penetration through the capsule not caused by previous fine needle aspiration. This invasion needs to be definitive and classically takes the form of "mushrooming" of the tumor outward (e-**Fig. 24.14**). Vascular invasion is defined as the presence of intravascular tumor cells either covered by endothelium or associated with thrombus (e-**Fig. 24.15B**). Strict adherence to these criteria is necessary to assure that the diagnosis of carcinoma is correct.

The distinction of follicular carcinoma from medullary carcinoma is based on morphology (medullary carcinomas are rarely follicular in their growth patterns and lack true colloid) and immunohistochemical findings (neuroendocrine markers, carcinoembryonic antigen [CEA], and calcitonin are positive in medullary carcinoma but negative in follicular carcinoma, whereas immunohistochemistry for thyroglobulin is positive in follicular carcinoma and negative in medullary carcinoma). Finally, poorly differentiated carcinomas can be similar to widely invasive follicular carcinomas, but the former have cells with less cytoplasm, minimal follicular architecture, marked mitotic activity, and necrosis (see diagnostic criteria below).

Unlike PTC, regional lymph node involvement is extremely rare. Instead, metastasis is via a hematogenous route to lung and bone. Carcinomas that lack vascular invasion (minimally invasive tumors) have a better outcome (<5% long-term mortality) than encapsulated angioinvasive follicular carcinomas. Further, the presence of four or more foci of vascular invasion has been shown to correlate with more aggressive behavior. Widely invasive follicular carcinomas have a poorer long-term mortality approaching 50%.

3. Poorly differentiated thyroid carcinoma. This type of thyroid carcinoma shows evidence of follicular differentiation but fits morphologically and biologically between well-differentiated and anaplastic carcinomas.

Poorly differentiated carcinoma accounts for much less than 5% of cases of thyroid carcinoma in the United States, but between 4% and 7% in Italy and some Latin American countries. It is slightly more common in women, particularly after age 50. Most cases present as sizable asymptomatic masses, with or without pathologically enlarged regional lymph nodes. There is occasionally a history of a long-standing mass with recent, rapid growth.

Grossly, most tumors are large with solid gray to white nodules. Necrosis is common. Extrathyroidal extension is present in some cases, but is much less extensive than in anaplastic carcinomas (e-**Fig. 24.16**). The Turin criteria for the histologic diagnosis of poorly differentiated carcinoma include: (1) a solid, trabecular, or insular growth pattern; (2) lack of well-developed nuclear features of PTC; and (3) one of the following: convoluted nuclei, tumor necrosis, or 3 or more mitoses per 10 high-power fields (e-**Figs. 24.17–24.20**). Most cells have only a small amount of cytoplasm giving the tumor a somewhat neuroendocrine look, although the tumor nuclei typically do not have "salt and pepper" chromatin and often have prominent nucleoli as well as convoluted nuclei (e-**Figs. 24.17–24.20**). Colloid is rare. It is not uncommon for well-formed capsules to be present around some of the nodules. Vascular invasion is often a prominent feature. By immunohistochemistry, the tumors are positive for thyroglobulin, PAX8 and TTF-1, although the thyroglobulin reactivity may be focal.

The differential diagnosis includes medullary carcinoma, the solid variant of PTC, and metastasis (particularly from a neuroendocrine tumor). The mean 5-year survival is approximately 50%.

4. **Papillary thyroid carcinoma.** PTCs show evidence of follicular differentiation and are characterized by distinct nuclear features. The terminology has become somewhat confusing because papillary architecture, although very commonly present, is not necessary for diagnosis. PTC is the most common malignant thyroid tumor (representing 85% to 90% of differentiated thyroid carcinomas) and has been increasing in incidence, but its prognosis is excellent (see below). The commonality of the tumor relative to its indolent behavior makes the appropriate management controversial. The tumors occur across all ages, and women are affected four times more commonly than men. There is a close link with previous radiation exposure, particularly in younger patients.

Grossly, most tumors are tan or white often with infiltrative borders and a firm, sometimes gritty cut surface (e-**Fig. 24.21**). Cystic change is relatively common, particularly in lymph-node metastases, and the bulk of nodal metastatic disease may far outstrip the volume of tumor in the thyroid gland. Microscopically, PTC is diagnosed based on a constellation of architectural and cytologic features (Table 24.3). Architectural patterns include papillary, trabecular, micro- and macrofollicular, solid, and cystic. The stroma around the tumor is often fibrotic or sclerotic. In tumors with follicles, the colloid is typically described as "bright" or "dark" red relative to the normal thyroid. Another very typical feature is the presence of psammoma bodies (small, round, laminated calcifications, e-**Fig. 24.22A**). Psammoma bodies are not pathognomonic but are an extremely typical feature. Distinct nuclear features are necessary for diagnosis and include marked crowding with overlapping of adjacent nuclei, pale or clear chromatin, irregular nuclear contours, grooves (e-**Fig. 24.22B**), and intranuclear cytoplasmic pseudoinclusions where round nodules of cytoplasm overlap the nucleus. Since NIFTP shares these nuclear features, exclusion of NIFTP is important for any encapsulated or circumscribed tumor (see below). Grading is not important because PTC is, by definition, well differentiated although some authors have found that tumors with necrosis and/or mitotic activity higher than 4 per 10 high-power fields are more clinically aggressive. Multifocality is common (present in up to 50% of cases) and may be appreciated grossly.

Although rarely needed for diagnosis, immunohistochemistry in PTC is positive for pancytokeratin, cytokeratin 7, thyroglobulin, PAX8 and TTF-1 but negative for

TABLE 24.3	Diagnostic Histologic Features of Papillary Thyroid Carcinoma
True papillae	
Psammoma bodies	
Dark red colloid	
Crowded nuclei	
Optically clear ("Orphan Annie") chromatin	
Irregular nuclear contours	
Nuclear grooves	
Intranuclear cytoplasmic pseudoinclusions	

cytokeratin 20, calcitonin, CEA, and neuroendocrine markers. Other markers that have been reported to be useful for differentiating the follicular variant of PTC from follicular adenoma include HBME-1, CK19, and galectin 3; however, these markers have not gained widespread acceptance, and the diagnosis ultimately rests on hematoxylin and eosin (H&E) morphology.

The classical type, which has papillary architecture, can be infiltrative or encapsulated. A number of other morphologic variants have been described.

a. **The follicular variant** (e-Fig. 24.23) can be infiltrative or encapsulated with invasion and is composed of follicles throughout without papillae.

b. **Papillary microcarcinoma** is a focus (or foci) <1 cm in maximal diameter (e-Fig. 24.24); papillary microcarcinoma is an extremely common incidental finding and, although capable of metastasizing, the vast majority of these tumors pursue a benign course.

c. **Both a tall cell** (tumor cells at least—two to three times as tall as they are wide in ≥30% of the tumor; e-Fig. 24.25) and a **columnar cell variant** also exist, both of which have been reported to be more aggressive than classic PTC.

d. **The diffuse sclerosing variant** tends to occur in younger patients, shows diffuse involvement of one or both lobes without a dominant mass, and has numerous psammoma bodies, dense lymphocytic infiltration, and stromal fibrosis. Squamous metaplasia is common.

e. **The solid variant** is only diagnosed when nearly all of the tumor is solid, since focal solid areas are common in other variants and classical PTC. The solid variant is more common in younger patients and those with prior exposure to ionizing radiation.

f. **The cribriform–morular variant** is rare but important to recognize as it may be a harbinger of familial adenomatous polyposis (FAP) syndrome in a subset of patients. Tumors are often encapsulated with an admixture of cribriform, papillary, and trabecular/solid growth; show absent colloid; and have squamoid morules. Nuclear features of PTC are present but nuclei are hyperchromatic rather than clear. Beta-catenin positivity supports the diagnosis of the cribriform–morular variant.

g. **The hobnail variant**, characterized by micropapillae lacking true fibrovascular cores comprising at least 30% of the tumor, is a newly characterized more aggressive variant. The carcinoma cells have eosinophilic cytoplasm, apically placed nuclei, decreased nuclear/cytoplasmic ratio, and loss of cellular cohesion.

h. Other rare variants include **oncocytic, Warthin-like, spindle cell, clear cell,** and **PTC with fasciitis-like stroma.**

The prognosis for PTC is excellent, with a 10-year survival approaching 100% for younger patients, and >90% overall. Older patients may have more biologically aggressive tumors.

The most common molecular alteration in PTC is the *BRAF V600E* point mutation found in over half of tumors, more commonly in the classical type and tall cell variant. *RAS* mutations are concentrated in the follicular variant. Chromosomal rearrangements involving the receptor tyrosine kinase gene *RET* are found in approximately 20% to 30% of cases. From 5% to 25% harbor *TERT* promotor mutations that are associated with a more aggressive clinical course.

5. **Noninvasive follicular thyroid neoplasm with papillary-like nuclear features (NIFTP)** is a new entity that was previously classified under the spectrum of encapsulated follicular variant of PTC. A consensus conference convened by the Endocrine Pathology Society renamed this entity due to documented very indolent behavior. Diagnostic criteria are: (1) complete tumor encapsulation or circumscription; (2) no capsular or vascular invasion; (3) follicular growth pattern; and (4) nuclear features of PTC (e-Fig 24.26). Strict criteria are necessary, including examination of the entire tumor capsule to exclude invasion. Further, the following features should not be seen in NIFTP: (1) >30% solid, insular, or trabecular growth; (2) papillary

architecture or psammoma bodies; (3) tall cell or columnar cell variants; (4) tumor necrosis or >3 mitoses/10 high-power fields. This tumor type has a high prevalence of *RAS* mutations.

6. **Anaplastic (undifferentiated) thyroid carcinoma.** Anaplastic carcinomas are extremely aggressive malignant tumors composed, at least in part, of pleomorphic cells that show evidence of epithelial differentiation either by light microscopy, immunohistochemistry, or ultrastructural analysis. They are rare and compromise 2% or less of all thyroid carcinomas in the United States. Anaplastic carcinoma is a tumor of the elderly, with 75% of cases occurring in patients older than 60 years. There is a slight female preponderance. Long-standing goiter is a well-known risk factor. Patients classically present with a rapidly growing neck mass with local signs and symptoms such as hoarseness, dysphagia, pain, vocal cord paralysis, and/or dyspnea.

At surgery, the tumor is usually large, ill-defined, and difficult to excise due to extensive surrounding soft tissue invasion. The cut surface is fleshy and tan-white often with areas of hemorrhage and necrosis. Microscopically, it is typically composed of a variable admixture of sheets of spindle cells, epithelioid cells, and giant cells obliterating the majority of the thyroid gland. The cells have a moderate amount of eosinophilic cytoplasm and almost always show brisk mitotic activity (e-Fig. 24.27). There is often geographic necrosis. On thorough examination, a residual well-differentiated carcinoma, either papillary or follicular, is sometimes identified which indicates transformation from a well-differentiated carcinoma. Predominantly spindled tumors often mimic true sarcomas. Rare variants include paucicellular (which may mimic a benign reactive process), angiomatoid, rhabdoid, lymphoepithelioma-like, and small cell. The prognosis is very poor with a median survival of less than 6 months despite aggressive surgery, radiation, and chemotherapy.

Immunohistochemistry for cytokeratin is positive in approximately 80% of cases, and for epithelial membrane antigen in 30% to 50%. Immunostains are useful for the diagnosis of tumors in which no obvious carcinomatous differentiation is present on H&E in order to confirm that the neoplasm is a carcinoma rather than a high-grade sarcoma. However, lack of staining with epithelial markers does not completely exclude the diagnosis. Nuclear reactivity for PAX8 has been reported in over half of anaplastic carcinomas and may be useful for diagnosis. TTF-1 is only positive in a minority of cases and thyroglobulin is typically negative.

7. **Neuroendocrine neoplasms of the thyroid.**

a. **Reactive (nonneoplastic) C-cell hyperplasia** occurs in aging and a number of other thyroid diseases, most notably hyperparathyroidism and lymphocytic thyroiditis. Although the histology of C-cell hyperplasia is somewhat controversial, a few generalities apply. First, reactive C-cell hyperplasia is usually not identifiable by H&E examination alone. Second, if there are aggregates of C cells greater than 50 in number, in nodules, bilaterally, or diffusely, neoplastic C-cell hyperplasia is favored.

b. **Neoplastic C-cell hyperplasia**, a precursor lesion to medullary carcinoma that is more commonly observed in hereditary cases, is identified in the middle third to upper third of the thyroid lobes where C cells are preferentially located; it is characterized by groups of enlarged, intrafollicular atypical C cells that may begin to obliterate the normal follicular epithelium (e-Figs. 24.28 and 24.29). Neoplastic C cell hyperplasia progresses to medullary carcinoma when C cells extend through the follicular basement membrane into the stroma. Distinction between neoplastic C cell hyperplasia and a small medullary carcinoma can be difficult. Helpful histologic features of microcarcinoma include: (1) nuclear pleomorphism; (2) expansile growth pattern with C cell clusters spilling out of follicles; (3) sclerotic stroma; and (4) amyloid deposition.

c. **Medullary thyroid carcinoma.** Medullary carcinoma, unlike other thyroid carcinomas, has C-cell differentiation and represents a neuroendocrine neoplasm of the thyroid. C cells secrete calcitonin, a peptide that causes increased renal excretion of calcium and inhibits osteoclasts to prevent calcium liberation from the bone. Virtually all patients with medullary carcinoma have an elevated serum calcitonin level.

Medullary carcinoma represents approximately 5% of thyroid tumors. Although the majority of cases are sporadic, up to 20% to 30% are familial and there is a strong association with multiple endocrine neoplasia (MEN) types 2A and 2B, which must always be considered in the workup of patients with medullary carcinoma. The clinical presentation strongly depends on the familial or nonfamilial nature of the tumor. Sporadic tumors present in the fifth or sixth decades of life as a unilateral thyroid mass. A high percentage of patients have associated cervical lymphadenopathy. As an index case, familial cases associated with MEN type 2A are frequently detected at a younger age (mean, third decade), and are multicentric and bilateral. When associated with MEN type 2B, medullary carcinoma occurs in even younger patients (i.e., in early childhood or adolescence).

Grossly, medullary carcinoma is typically circumscribed but unencapsulated, and is tan-yellow to white. Sporadic tumors are solitary, whereas familial tumors are often multifocal and bilateral. Microscopically, medullary carcinoma shows great variability. The typical features are sheets, nests, or trabeculae of cells with moderate to generous amounts of eosinophilic to amphophilic cytoplasm. The nuclei are round to oval with a coarse and somewhat granular neuroendocrine chromatin. Nucleoli are usually not prominent (e-**Fig. 24.30**). A great number of variants have been described including spindle cell, papillary, or pseudopapillary (e-**Fig. 24.31**), plasmacytoid, glandular, giant cell, (e-**Fig. 24.32**), small cell or neuroblastoma-like, paraganglioma-like, and oncocytic. Another characteristic feature is the presence of amyloid, which is formed from the deposition of calcitonin in the peritumoral stroma (e-**Fig. 24.30**). The amyloid is positive by Congo red staining.

Immunohistochemistry is useful to confirm the diagnosis. C cells and medullary carcinoma are usually strongly positive for calcitonin, synaptophysin, chromogranin-A, and CEA, but negative for thyroglobulin. Although the differential diagnosis of medullary carcinoma includes thyroid paraganglioma, intrathyroidal parathyroid adenoma, follicular adenoma, follicular carcinoma, poorly differentiated carcinoma, and oncocytic tumors, all of these tumors can be differentiated by a combination of histology and immunohistochemistry.

Medullary carcinoma (whether sporadic or hereditary) is strongly associated with activating point mutations of the *RET* proto-oncogene. From 30% to 66% of sporadic MTCs are associated with somatic *RET* gene mutations, but all cases of hereditary MTC have germline *RET* mutations. Each specific germline mutation of the *RET* proto-oncogene correlates with/predicts the age of onset and aggressiveness of medullary carcinoma. The M918T mutation, which occurs as a germline mutation in most patients with MEN2B, is also the most common somatic mutation in sporadic carcinomas, and is also associated with the most aggressive clinical course. Clinical trials of tyrosine kinase inhibitors targeting the RET kinase have shown promise in reducing tumor burden in metastatic disease. A significant subset of *RET* mutation negative sporadic tumors harbor *RAS* mutations.

The behavior of medullary carcinoma is highly stage dependent. Patients who do not have metastatic disease are usually cured by total thyroidectomy, and their 10-year survival approaches 100%. Lymph-node metastases are very common, and common distant metastatic sites include the lungs, liver, and bone. The overall 10-year survival for patients with cervical lymph-node metastases is approximately 70% to 80%, and for patients with distant metastases 40% to 50%. Because C-cell hyperplasia and medullary carcinoma may occur early in life in hereditary cases, prophylactic thyroidectomy and central lymph node dissection should be performed as early as possible in MEN type 2B, but may be delayed somewhat in MEN type 2A, depending on the particular *RET* mutation and serum calcitonin levels.

IV. **HISTOLOGIC STAGING AND REPORTING.** The most recent American Joint Committee on Cancer staging classification (Amin MB, Edge S, Greene F, et al., eds. *AJCC Cancer Staging Manual*, 8th ed. New York: Springer, 2017) includes a system for differentiated and anaplastic carcinoma, and a separate system for medullary carcinoma. Of note, there is no AJCC staging system for thyroid carcinomas arising from the TDC, or thyroid carcinomas arising in malignant struma ovarii. Thyroid lymphomas are staged via the Hodgkin and non-Hodgkin lymphoma systems.

Reporting should follow recommended guidelines (e.g., the Protocol for the Examination of Specimens From Patients With Carcinomas of the Thyroid Gland available at http://www.cap.org, which includes guidelines for papillary, follicular, poorly differentiated, anaplastic, and medullary carcinomas).

ACKNOWLEDGMENT

The authors thank Changquing Ma and James S. Lewis, authors of the previous edition of this chapter.

Thyroid Cytopathology

Cory Bernadt

I. **INTRODUCTION.** The advent of widespread use of thyroid FNA has dramatically decreased surgical excision of abnormal clinical lesions for diagnostic purposes. The sensitivity for the detection of lesions requiring surgical management is up to 98%, but specificity lags. The introduction of the Bethesda System for Reporting Thyroid Cytopathology (BSRTC) made possible a more probabilistic approach to the cytology of the thyroid, based on cellularity, colloidal composition, architectural patterns, and nuclear morphology (*Am J Clin Pathol* 2009;132:658). The BSRTC was recently revised due to new data and developments in the field of thyroid pathology (*Thyroid* 2017;27:1341). One of the major changes is revised risks of malignancy (ROM) complicated by the reclassification of the noninvasive follicular variant of PTC as noninvasive follicular thyroid neoplasm with papillary-like nuclear features (NIFTP).

II. **NONDIAGNOSTIC/UNSATISFACTORY**

A. Six groups of well-visualized follicular cells, with each group containing 10 or more cells, preferably on one slide, constitute the minimal adequacy criteria for thyroid FNA. Exceptions include paucicellular samples with marked cytologic atypia; solid nodules with inflammation (i.e., Hashimoto thyroiditis, abscess, or granulomatous inflammation) in which inflammatory cells predominate over a very scant epithelial population; and colloid nodule, in which abundant thick colloid is readily identified in the near-absence of follicular cells. Failure to meet the above criteria makes an aspirate nondiagnostic/unsatisfactory (e-Fig. 24.33).

B. **"Cyst fluid only"** is an important subset of the nondiagnostic category. If only macrophages and noncolloidal cyst fluid are present, and there is a solid clinical/sonographic lesion, the assumption should be made that the lesion has not been adequately sampled. In more reassuring clinical/sonographic cases, cyst fluid only may be consistent with a benign process. It should be clear that "cyst fluid only" requires careful contextual interpretation.

III. **BENIGN.** This is a category with high negative predictive value (0% to 3% malignancy rate on follow up). Smears generally show significant amounts of colloid and variable degrees of cellularity. Benign follicular nodule is the most common pathologic correlate, but the presence of inflammatory cells or fibrous stroma may indicate a thyroiditis.

A. **Benign Follicular Nodules,** the most common diagnosis in thyroid aspirates, are characterized by benign follicular cells and colloid in variable proportions, variably sized follicular groups, Hürthle cells, and macrophages. Abundant colloid and relatively low cellularity are reassuring features of benignity (e-**Figs. 24.34** and **24.35**). However, since the pattern is seen in a constellation of benign proliferations, the underlying process can be diagnosed definitively only upon resection: nodular goiter, hyperplastic nodules, colloid nodules, and nodules in the setting of Graves disease.

B. Thyroiditis

1. **Acute thyroiditis** is rarely sampled given its typical clinical presentation. The aspirate shows predominantly neutrophils and necrotic debris with scattered histiocytes and scant reactive follicular cells. Special stains and culture are required for microorganism identification.

2. **Chronic lymphocytic thyroiditis (Hashimoto thyroiditis).** The aspirate is usually cellular and consists of two major components: (1) a large population of polymorphous lymphocytes, plasma cells, and tingible body macrophages, and (2) scattered, two-dimensional clusters of Hürthle cells with variable nuclear atypia (e-**Fig. 24.36**). Occasional multinucleated giant cells can be identified. Normal follicular cells and colloid are scant (*Diagn Cytopathol*. 1994;11:141).

3. **Subacute granulomatous thyroiditis (de Quervain thyroiditis).** The aspirate can be hypocellular due to fibrosis. Granulomas consisting of cohesive aggregates of epithelioid histiocytes with elongated and kidney-shaped nuclei, granular chromatin, small nucleoli, and abundant pale cytoplasm with ill-defined borders (e-**Fig. 24.37**) are the key diagnostic feature. Multinucleated giant cells and lymphocytes are usually present (*Diagn Cytopathol*. 1997;16:214).

4. **Riedel thyroiditis**. The aspirate is markedly hypocellular, containing microfragments of stroma with bland spindle-shaped cells. Other cellular components are absent.

IV. ATYPIA OF UNDETERMINED SIGNIFICANCE/FOLLICULAR LESION OF UNDETERMINED SIGNIFICANCE (AUS/FLUS). AUS/FLUS is an equivocal category created in recognition of the fact that the cytologic pattern does not always allow discrimination between a benign nodule and a more serious lesion such as a follicular neoplasm or PTC. These specimens contain cells (follicular, lymphoid, or other) with architectural and/or cytologic atypia that does not meet diagnostic criteria for suspicious for a follicular neoplasm, suspicious for malignancy, or malignant (SFM) (e-**Fig. 24.38**). Often these specimens are paucicellular or have other compromising features such as obscuring blood or excessive clotting. This designation should generally comprise 7% to 10% of a cytology laboratory's thyroid interpretations and carries a risk of malignancy of 6% to 30% dependent upon classification of NIFTPs as equivalent to cancer or not. Recent studies have also shown that subclassification of the atypia results in differences in the risk of malignancy (*Cytopathol*. 2017;28:65; *Diagn Cytopathol*. 2016;44:492). For this reason, the 2017 BSRTC recommends subclassification of the atypia into the following categories: (1) cytologic atypia, (2) architectural atypia, (3) cytologic and architectural atypia, (4) Hürthle cell, and (5) atypia, not otherwise specified.

V. FOLLICULAR NEOPLASM/SUSPICIOUS FOR FOLLICULAR NEOPLASM (FN/SFN). FN/SFN yield richly cellular smears with both architectural and cytologic abnormalities, consisting of microfollicle formation with mild nuclear changes (increased nuclear size, nuclear contour irregularity, and/or chromatin clearing) without true papillae or intranuclear pseudoinclusions (e-**Fig. 24.39**). The differential diagnosis includes follicular adenoma, follicular carcinoma, the follicular variant of PTC, and NIFTP. The nonspecificity of the diagnosis underlies use of the phrase "suspicious for follicular neoplasm" although FN and SFN are equivalent monikers in the Bethesda system.

Most patients with this diagnosis will undergo lobectomy or complete thyroidectomy, although only 20% to 30% of lesions will be malignant upon resection (*CytoJournal* 2008;5:6). For this reason, molecular testing may be used to supplement risk assessment rather than proceeding directly to surgery.

VI. FOLLICULAR NEOPLASM, HÜRTHLE CELL TYPE/SUSPICIOUS FOR FOLLICULAR NEOPLASM, HÜRTHLE CELL TYPE (FNHCT/SFNHCT). Hürthle cells are present in both neoplastic and nonneoplastic processes (*Am J Clin Pathol* 1993;100:231). Hürthle cell

neoplasms are cytologically distinct in that they yield hypercellular specimens composed of an almost pure population of Hürthle cells (e-**Figs. 24.40** and **24.41**). The Hürthle cells are often dyshesive single cells with prominent nucleoli, and the background contains an insignificant number of normal follicular cells, lymphocytes, and colloid. As is the case in other follicular neoplasms, the diagnosis of Hürthle cell carcinoma is based on the assessment of capsular and vascular invasion, which cannot be evaluated in cytology specimens. It should also be noted, in further similarity to FN/SFN, that PTC is in the differential diagnosis of FNHCT/SFNHCT.

VII. SUSPICIOUS FOR MALIGNANCY. SFM describes malignant appearing features similar to those in the "malignant" category (see below) but in an insufficient quantity to allow a confident diagnosis of malignancy. The use of this diagnosis is at the discretion of the pathologist and will certainly vary between laboratories and pathologists based on a number of factors including patient population, cytologic preparations, aspiration technique, and so on. Up to 75% of the lesions in this cytologic category are proven malignant at resection; however, the risk of malignancy diminishes if it is recalculated by removing NIFTPs from the malignant category.

VIII. MALIGNANT. This category encompasses cytologic features diagnostic of any of the malignant primary or metastatic tumors that may be seen in the thyroid. When the criteria are appropriately applied, there are very few false positives.

A. **Papillary Thyroid Carcinoma (PTC).** The specimen is richly cellular, consisting of large sheets with occasional papillary structures (e-**Figs. 24.42** and **24.43**). The follicular cells are slightly enlarged and have crowded nuclei. The characteristic nuclear features are fine open chromatin with nuclear membrane prominence, small and peripherally located nucleoli, intranuclear cytoplasmic inclusions, and longitudinal nuclear grooves (e-**Fig. 24.44**). Other associated features include dense cytoplasm, "bubble gum"-like dense colloid, psammoma bodies (e-**Fig. 24.45**), and multinucleated giant cells (*Diagn Cytopathol* 1991;7:462).

B. **Hyalinizing Trabecular Adenoma** is a controversial entity with great similarity to PTC, including the characteristic nuclear features and *RET-PTC* rearrangements. Definitive diagnosis rests upon histologic examination (*Am J Clin Pathol* 1989;91:115).

C. **Poorly Differentiated (Insular) Carcinoma.** The aspirate is richly cellular and composed of monomorphic follicular cells with scant cytoplasm. The follicular cells display insular, sold, or trabecular architecture (e-**Fig. 24.46**). FNAs often lack the mitotic activity and necrosis that are included in the histologic diagnostic criteria (*Cytopathol.* 2016;27:176).

D. **Anaplastic Carcinoma.** The aspirate is highly cellular and contains single cells exhibiting marked nuclear atypia. Necrosis is common. The malignant cells show diverse morphology, including epithelioid (e-**Fig. 24.47**), spindle-shaped, and giant pleomorphic cells (*Acta Cytol* 1996;40:953).

E. **Medullary Carcinoma** typically generates highly cellular specimens predominantly consisting of single cells and loose clusters of cells. The cell morphology is variable, ranging from monotonous with little atypia to highly atypical. The characteristic features are mixtures of plasmacytoid and spindle-shaped cells with characteristic salt-and-pepper chromatin (e-**Fig. 24.48**). Amyloid is usually present, but its distinction from colloid is impossible without a Congo red stain (*Pathologica* 1998;90:5).

F. **Lymphoma.** Most primary thyroid lymphomas develop in the background of Hashimoto thyroiditis. Diffuse large B-cell lymphoma (DLBCL) is the major type, followed by extranodal marginal zone B-cell lymphoma of mucosa-associated lymphoid tissue (*Am J Surg Pathol* 2000;24:623). DLBCL exhibits monotonous large atypical lymphoid cells with irregular nuclear contours, vesicular chromatin, and single prominent nucleoli (immunoblast-like cells) or multiple nucleoli (centroblast-like cells) (e-**Fig 24.49**). Marginal zone B-cell lymphoma shows a heterogeneous population of lymphoid cells with a predominance of small lymphoid cells, and intermixed plasmacytoid cells and immunoblasts; monocytoid cells with abundant pale cytoplasm are frequently seen. Demonstration of light chain restriction by flow cytometry is critical for diagnosis.

G. Metastatic Malignancy. Metastasis to the thyroid is uncommon. The kidney is the most common primary site of metastatic tumors, followed by the lung and breast. In a patient with a history of malignancy, the differential diagnosis for a new thyroid nodule should include metastasis. Comparison of the aspirate with the slides of the primary malignancy, together with immunostains, is critical for diagnosis.

ACKNOWLEDGMENT

The author thanks Michael Hull and Julie Kunkel, authors of the previous edition of this section.

SUGGESTED READINGS

Ali SZ, Cibas, ES. *The Bethesda System for Reporting Thyroid Cytopathology—Definitions, Criteria and Explanatory Notes.* New York: Springer Science + Business Media, LLC; 2010.

Chernock RD, Thompson LDR. Non-neoplastic lesions of the thyroid gland. In: Thompson LDR, Bishop JA, ed. *Head and Neck Pathology*, 3rd ed. Philadelphia, PA: Elsevier; 2019.

Lloyd RV, Osamura RY, Kloppel G, eds. *World Health Organization Classification of Tumours of Endocrine Organs.* 4th ed. Lyon: IARC Press; 2017.

Nikiforov YE, Biddinger PW, Thompson LDR. *Diagnostic Pathology and Molecular Genetics of the Thyroid.* 2nd ed. Philadelphia, PA: Wolters Kluwer Health/Lippincott William & Wilkins; 2012.

Thompson LDR, Chernock RD. Benign neoplasms of the thyroid gland. In: Thompson LDR, Bishop JA, ed. *Head and Neck Pathology*. 3rd ed. Philadelphia, PA: Elsevier; 2019.

Thompson LDR. Malignant neoplasms of the thyroid gland. In: Thompson LDR, Bishop JA, ed. *Head and Neck Pathology*. 3rd ed. Philadelphia, PA: Elsevier; 2019.

25 Parathyroid Glands
Rebecca D. Chernock

I. **NORMAL ANATOMY.** The endodermally derived parathyroid glands develop from the third (inferior parathyroids) and fourth (superior parathyroids) pharyngeal pouches. They produce parathyroid hormone (PTH) which acts to increase serum calcium. They are normally found along the posterior surface of the thyroid gland, but given their complex embryologic development, normal variations in location range from within the substance of the thyroid gland, superiorly to the hyoid bone, inferiorly into the mediastinum, within the thymus gland, or within the pericardium. Furthermore, 2% to 7% of individuals have more than the usual four glands.

Most normal parathyroid glands are from 0.3 to 0.6 cm in largest dimension, and the normal aggregate weight of all glands is 120 to 140 mg. They are brown to yellow-brown, oval, and have a thin capsule. Histologically, they consist of chief (or principal) cells, oxyphil cells, and clear cells. Chief cells have round nuclei with granular chromatin and slightly eosinophilic cytoplasm with perinuclear clearing; oxyphil cells have more abundant brightly eosinophilic and granular cytoplasm; clear cells are the least common and have abundant clear cytoplasm (e-Fig. 25.1). The cells are arranged in sheets, nests, and cords. Occasional pseudoglandular or pseudoacinar foci with central eosinophilic proteinaceous material can also be seen in the normal parathyroid. Intraparenchymal adipose tissue is a normal feature of the parathyroid glands; it is usually scant in children but progressively increases with age to constitute about 50% of the gland by the fifth decade, and plateaus beyond that time (e-Fig. 25.2).

Parathyroid cells are positive by immunohistochemistry for PTH, chromogranin-A, synaptophysin, and cytokeratins, and this immunoprofile is maintained in virtually all pathologic processes. Parathyroid cells are negative for thyroglobulin and thyroid transcription factor-1 (TTF-1).

II. **GROSS EXAMINATION, TISSUE SAMPLING, AND HISTOLOGIC SLIDE PREPARATION**

A. **Fine Needle Aspiration (FNA).** FNA of parathyroid lesions is rarely performed. The two exceptions are, first, when an adenoma arises within the substance of the thyroid gland and thus a biopsy is taken as part of the evaluation of a presumed thyroid lesion, and second, when parathyroid carcinoma presents as a large neck mass.

B. **Biopsy.** Intraoperative biopsies (frozen sections) are frequently performed to confirm that the excised tissue is parathyroid because lymph nodes, thymus, thyroid, and fat may all be mistaken surgically for parathyroid tissue. The tissue should be weighed, but no other special handling is required.

C. **Excision.** The initial step in the gross examination of parathyroid glands is recording their weight and measurement in three dimensions. The glands should be closely examined and if firm, ragged, or irregular, should be inked around their periphery. They should then be sectioned and their color and consistency described. The parathyroid gland should be submitted in its entirety for histologic evaluation. This is usually achievable in one tissue cassette. The larger the parathyroid, the greater the concern for carcinoma and, therefore, large parathyroid glands should also be entirely submitted to exclude this possibility.

III. **DIAGNOSTIC FEATURES OF COMMON DISEASES**

A. **Nonneoplastic**

1. **Abnormal development** of the parathyroid glands rarely occurs. The classic example is DiGeorge's syndrome in which there is failure in the development of several of the

branchial pouches with resulting absence of the thymus and parathyroid glands. Neonates develop hypocalcemia due to lack of PTH. Albright's hereditary osteodystrophy is due to pseudohypoparathyroidism as a result of target organ unresponsiveness to PTH, and neonates present with hypocalcemia, hyperphosphatemia, and blunted responses to PTH.

2. **Parathyroiditis** is a rare and poorly understood condition thought to be autoimmune in nature. It is characterized by extensive infiltration of the glands by lymphocytes. It is usually idiopathic and isolated, but may be associated with a rare autoimmune polyglandular syndrome in which two or more endocrine glands are affected. Between one quarter and three quarters of patients will have circulating antiparathyroid tissue antibodies. Most patients are asymptomatic but may have hypo- or hyperparathyroidism. Histologically, the glands are infiltrated by clusters of lymphocytes, often with germinal center formation (e-**Fig. 25.3**).

3. **Cysts** of the parathyroid glands are relatively uncommon. They occur in the neck and less commonly in the mediastinum. Most patients do not have clinical hyperparathyroidism. Grossly, they are often loosely attached to the thyroid gland, range from microscopic up to as large as 10 cm, have thin walls, and contain watery fluid. Microscopically, they are lined by a cuboidal layer of epithelial cells with round, hyperchromatic nuclei (e-**Figs. 25.4** and **25.5**). The cyst wall consists of fibrous tissue with entrapped islands of parathyroid chief cells.

4. **Hyperplasia** is an increase in the overall mass of parathyroid cells, and accounts for approximately 15% of all cases of primary hyperparathyroidism. Hyperplasia is divided into primary (where there is no known clinical stimulus), secondary (usually due to renal failure or another known metabolic cause), and tertiary (where there is an autonomously increased parathyroid mass in patients who have had secondary hyperparathyroidism and now are on dialysis or have had a renal transplant) (Table 25.1). A significant minority of cases of primary hyperparathyroidism (up to 40%) have been shown to be monoclonal, indicating that some cases represent true neoplasia. However, the clinical and pathophysiologic importance of this finding is unclear.

Approximately 75% of patients with primary hyperparathyroidism are women. Less than 5% present with familial disease (most commonly multiple endocrine neoplasia [MEN] type 1 or 2A, but rarely as an isolated familial hyperparathyroidism or hyperparathyroidism-jaw tumor syndrome). Many patients are asymptomatic and are identified only indirectly through clinical evaluation for other reasons. The symptoms and signs of hyperparathyroidism can be vague such as fatigue, lethargy, nausea, constipation, arthralgia, or anorexia. The classic "bones, stones, and abdominal moans" (osteitis fibrosa cystica, kidney stones, and peptic ulcer disease) presentation is rare, and patients rarely present with a neck mass. Psychological disorders such as depression, psychosis, emotional instability, and confusion are sometimes the presenting symptoms.

In hyperplasia, all of the glands are involved but to varying degrees, leading to asymmetric findings. Grossly, the glands are usually enlarged and are soft and brown, but they may also be nodular or cystic. The total weight is above normal, but is still usually <1 g. Microscopically, all of the glands show similar findings but to different degrees, including increased parenchymal cells in a nodular, multinodular, or diffuse pattern, and a commensurate decrease in fat (e-**Fig. 25.6**). Sometimes a follicular

TABLE 25.1	Classification of Parathyroid Hyperplasia
Primary hyperparathyroidism	No known stimulus
Secondary hyperparathyroidism	Known stimulus such as chronic renal failure, malabsorption, or vitamin D metabolism abnormality
Tertiary hyperparathyroidism	After long-standing renal failure with development of autonomous parathyroid hyperfunction

(pseudoglandular) pattern is present. Cytologic atypia can be seen but is rarely widespread. There is minimal mitotic activity. A rare type of hyperplasia termed "water-clear cell hyperplasia" is sometimes encountered in which all the cells have abundant clear cytoplasm but no adipose tissue is present (e-Fig. 25.7).

The differential diagnosis of hyperplasia includes parathyroid adenoma. Because the histologic features of an adenoma are not consistently different than those of hyperplasia, examination of multiple glands is necessary to distinguish between the two entities. Correlation with the clinical findings is often required to make the distinction. Water-clear cell hyperplasia must be distinguished from metastatic renal cell carcinoma (RCC); RCC will show diffuse nuclear atypia and will be negative for PTH and neuroendocrine marker expression by immunohistochemistry, and while PAX 8 expression may be observed in both RCC and parathyroid tissue it is usually weak and focal in the latter.

   a. **Autotransplantation.** A common surgical approach to hyperplasia is to remove three glands entirely and then a portion of the fourth. Alternatively, all four glands are excised, and a portion of one gland is implanted (usually in the skeletal muscle of the forearm or neck) to facilitate surgery in case of recurrent hyperparathyroidism. Because the cells of a hyperplastic autotransplanted gland can be mitotically active and infiltrate the skeletal muscle imitating a malignant process, clinical history is required for correct diagnosis at autotransplanted sites.

   b. **Parathyromatosis** is a rare condition that presents as a primary or, more commonly, secondary disease in which numerous nests of parathyroid tissue are present throughout the neck and/or mediastinum. When it is a primary condition, it is commonly associated with an MEN syndrome. Secondary parathyromatosis is thought to occur after parathyroid surgery as a result of spillage of cells into the soft tissues which then become hyperplastic. The morphology of the nodules in parathyromatosis is similar to that of the glands in hyperplasia (e-Fig. 25.8).

B. **Neoplasms.** The World Health Organization (WHO) classification of tumors of the parathyroid gland is listed in Table 25.2.

   1. **Adenoma.** Parathyroid adenomas are benign neoplasms composed of chief cells, oxyphil cells, clear cells or a mixture of the three. They occur in approximately 0.1% of the population and account for approximately 85% of cases of hyperparathyroidism. They are more common in women and have a peak incidence in the sixth and seventh decades of life. Adenomas are sometimes (albeit rarely) familial; these cases are usually associated with MEN types 1 or 2 or the uncommon hyperparathyroidism-jaw tumor syndrome. Adenomas involve a single gland (it is controversial as to whether patients with more than one adenoma actually suffer from asymmetrical hyperplasia). Patients present with signs and symptoms related to hypercalcemia (as detailed above). Technetium is concentrated in parathyroid tissue, so technetium sestamibi scans are often used to detect and localize the abnormal gland.

   Grossly, adenomas are rounded, encapsulated, tan to reddish-brown, and have an average weight of 1 g (e-Fig. 25.9). On sectioning, they are soft and homogeneous, although degeneration and cystic change may occur. Microscopically, adenomas are well-circumscribed, thinly or nonencapsulated masses with little stroma and no or very minimal fat, often with a rim of normal appearing parathyroid gland. One cell type usually predominates but a mixture of chief, oxyphil, and clear cells may be present

TABLE 25.2	WHO Histologic Classification of Parathyroid Tumors
Parathyroid carcinoma	
Parathyroid adenoma	
Secondary, mesenchymal, and other tumors	

From: Lloyd RV, Osamura RY, Kloppel G, eds. *WHO Classification of Tumours. Pathology and Genetics of Tumours of Endocrine Organs.* 4th ed. Lyon, France: IARC Press; 2017. Used with permission.

(e-**Figs. 25.10** and **25.11**). The cells are usually arranged in solid sheets although pseudoglandular (pseudoacinar or follicular) areas may be seen (e-**Fig. 25.12**), sometimes containing central eosinophilic material mimicking thyroid follicles. The nuclei are small, round, regular, and hyperchromatic. Nuclear pleomorphism can be seen although it is usually very localized (e-**Fig. 25.13**). Mitotic figures are scarce (1 or fewer per 10 high-power fields). Long-standing adenomas may contain areas of irregular fibrosis, calcification, and hemosiderin deposition.

The differential diagnosis of an adenoma includes parathyroid hyperplasia. As mentioned above, adenomas simply cannot be distinguished from hyperplasia without sampling multiple glands because the morphologic features overlap. If only one gland is provided for evaluation, it is best to diagnose "hypercellular parathyroid consistent with adenoma" to reflect the fact that only one gland was excised, implying that the other glands were not clinically abnormal and that intraoperative PTH monitoring likely confirmed a sufficient drop after the single gland was excised. Adenomas can be distinguished from cellular nodules of thyroid tissue (particularly from patients with nodular hyperplasia of the thyroid) by finding convincing colloid in thyroid lesions, finding a rim of definite parathyroid tissue in adenomas, or by immunostaining for thyroglobulin, PTH, and/or TTF-1.

2. Carcinoma. Parathyroid carcinoma is rare and is estimated to be the cause of <1% of hyperparathyroidism. The average age of patients is between 45 and 55 years, and the sex distribution is roughly equal. The etiology is unknown; the only significant association with any of the familial syndromes that cause other parathyroid disease is with hyperparathyroidism-jaw tumor syndrome. Most patients present with profound hyperparathyroidism and hypercalcemia (with serum calcium levels often >16 mg/dL with secondary nephrolithiasis, renal insufficiency, and bone involvement with osteopenia and/or "brown tumors"), and most have typical nonspecific symptoms of hypercalcemia such as weakness, fatigue, nausea, and depression.

Grossly, parathyroid carcinomas are usually large, poorly circumscribed, and adherent to surrounding tissues, particularly the thyroid gland (e-**Fig. 25.14**). They range from 1.5 to 6.0 cm or larger, and average 6.7 g. Their cut surface is usually gray-white and firm. Microscopically, they usually have a thick, hypocellular, and collagenous capsule with intratumoral fibrous bands (e-**Fig. 25.15**). Capsular invasion by the tumor is common, and invasion through the capsule as tongue-like or mushroom-like extensions is typical (e-**Fig. 25.16**). Carcinoma often extensively invades soft tissue and nearby structures. Vascular and less often perineural invasion may be seen. The growth pattern is usually solid to trabecular, occasionally with areas of necrosis. The individual cells may have clear cytoplasm or be exclusively oxyphilic, but most often they have an intermediate eosinophilic color. Most carcinomas have nuclei that show mild to moderate variability, but occasional tumors will show marked nuclear pleomorphism (e-**Fig. 25.17**). Mitotic activity can be quite low, but most tumors have >5 mitoses per 50 high-power fields.

The differential diagnosis of parathyroid carcinoma is primarily with parathyroid adenoma. Invasion (lymphovascular, perineural, or into surrounding structures) or evidence of metastasis is necessary to render a diagnosis of carcinoma (Table 25.3). Features such as broad fibrous bands, diffuse trabecular growth, increased mitotic activity, necrosis, and clinical adherence to adjacent structures intraoperatively are worrisome for parathyroid carcinoma and, in the absence of invasive growth, may warrant a diagnosis of "atypical adenoma" (it is noteworthy that "atypical adenomas" usually behave in a benign manner). Primary thyroid neoplasms, as well as metastases from RCC or thyroid medullary carcinoma, can be excluded by morphology and immunohistochemistry.

Surgery is the mainstay of treatment, and complete surgical excision at presentation offers the best chance for cure. The 5-year survival is approximately 85%, and 10-year survival is 50%. Patients frequently develop local recurrence and less commonly develop metastases to neck lymph nodes, lung, liver, and bone. Severe hypercalcemia is a cause of significant comorbidity and frequently the cause of death.

TABLE 25.3	Pathologic Features of Parathyroid Carcinoma
Diagnostic Features	**Supportive Features**
Invasion of surrounding structures	Diffuse trabecular growth
Lymphovascular invasion	Broad fibrous bands
Perineural invasion	Increased mitotic activity
Metastasis (regional or distant)	Necrosis
	Intraoperative adherence to surrounding structures

3. **Metastatic tumors.** The parathyroid glands are an uncommon site for metastases, although they are sometimes involved by direct extension from thyroid or laryngeal tumors. The rare metastases from distant sites most commonly arise from breast, kidney, and lung carcinomas or melanoma.

IV. **HISTOLOGIC GRADING, STAGING, AND REPORTING OF PARATHYROID CARCINOMA.** Grading of parathyroid carcinoma based on cytologic features or degree of differentiation has not been found to predict behavior. In addition, the impact on prognosis of tumor size and lymph node status at presentation remains unclear with different studies reporting different results. Despite these uncertainties, the American Joint Committee on Cancer (AJCC) provided TNM definitions in the 8th edition of its cancer staging manual (Amin MB et al., eds. *AJCC Cancer Staging Manual.* 8th ed. New York: Springer, 2017).

For resection specimens, the surgical pathology report should include tumor size in three dimensions and weight, involvement of adjacent structures, and relation to surgical margins. Presence of lymphovascular invasion, perineural invasion, and mitotic rate should also be recorded. The number of regional lymph nodes examined and the number positive for carcinoma should also be reported.

Cytopathology of the Parathyroid Glands

Hannah R. Krigman

I. **INTRODUCTION.** The parathyroid glands are not often sampled intentionally by FNA since adjunct testing (including serum calcium levels, radiolabeled imaging studies [Sestamibi scans], and assessment of aspirated fluid for OTH levels) generally obviate presurgical analysis of parathyroid masses. However, FNA may be used to evaluate the presence of parathyroid tissue in unusual locations, or to evaluate persistent hypercalcemia following excision of parathyroid glands. With the increasing frequency of FNA of thyroid nodules, parathyroid glands are often incidentally sampled during assessment of thyroid nodules. As many as 0.4% of aspirates of thyroid have incidentally sampled parathyroid tissue (*Cancer Cytopathology* 2017;125:674). Rarely, unanticipated parathyroid adenomas are aspirated as thyroid or neck nodules.

II. **CYTOLOGIC FINDINGS.** If not recognized as parathyroid tissue, these samples are most often classified as atypia of undetermined significance (Bethesda Thyroid Class III) or suspicious for follicular lesion (Bethesda Thyroid Class IV) (*Head Neck* 2002;24:157; Ali SZ, Cibas ES, eds. *The Bethesda System for Reporting Thyroid Cytopathology.*2nd ed. Springer; 2018). Direct smears show predominantly two-dimensional groups of 50 to 100 relatively evenly sized cells with granular cytoplasm. Three-dimensional groups, papillary fragments, and microacinar structures may also be seen (**e-Fig. 25.18**). Oxyphilic epithelial change may be seen and is most often misinterpreted as evidence of thyroid differentiation. Nuclei are predominantly round, with finely mottled chromatin (e-**Fig. 25.19**); sometimes nuclear molding and overlap are present. Modest variation in nuclear size may be seen, but this feature has no prognostic importance. Mitotic activity is uncommon. The background often contains stripped nuclei and single cells, macrophages, and colloid-like material. Diff Quik stained fresh smears may show fat vacuoles which are a helpful clue since they are not typically seen in aspirates of thyroid tissue.

Several studies have analyzed the empirically observed differences between thyroid and parathyroid tissue in direct smears. Statistical significance has been assigned to the presence of bare nuclei, cellular three-dimensional fragments, eccentric location of nuclei, and vascular proliferation (*Cancer Cytopathol* 2017;125:674; *Coll Antropol* 2010;34:25; *Korean J of Pathol* 2013;47:466). Many of these features are lost on liquid-based monolayer preparations. A microfollicular pattern is the most common feature when parathyroid aspirates are reviewed on ThinPrep (*Cancer Cytopathol* 2014;122:678). Intranuclear inclusions may be seen in parathyroid adenoma, accordingly, this feature should not be overinterpreted as indicative of papillary thyroid carcinoma in the absence of other features (*Coll Antropol* 2010;34:25).

Differentiation of parathyroid from thyroid in FNA specimens can be problematic. Microacinar groupings of parathyroid cells are an occasional source of error in that they may be misinterpreted as follicular neoplasm/suspicious for follicular neoplasm, especially in the setting of parathyroid adenomas. Follicular groups of parathyroid cells can also be misinterpreted as thyroid follicular cells, although intervening fat should suggest the correct diagnosis. In problematic cases, parathyroid origin can be confirmed with an immunostain for PTH.

Cytologic features do not reliably discriminate among normal parathyroid tissue, hyperplasia, adenoma, or carcinoma.

III. **ADJUNCT DIAGNOSTIC TECHNIQUES.** While quantitation of PTH levels remains a mainstay of perioperative monitoring for parathyroid sampling, assessment of parathormone levels in aspirates has been replaced by molecular assays. Adjunct molecular techniques applied to atypia of undetermined significance or suspicious for follicular neoplasm (commercially available gene expression analysis assays, miRNA analyses, and NGS sequencing assays) all routinely assess for the presence of parathyroid material.

SUGGESTED READINGS

Absher KJ, Truong LD, Khurana KK, Ramzy I. Parathyroid cytology: avoiding diagnostic pitfalls. *Head Neck* 2002;24(2):157–164.

Agarwal AM, Bentz JS, Hungerford R, Abraham D. Parathyroid fine-needle aspiration cytology in the evaluation of parathyroid adenoma: cytologic findings from 53 patients. *Diagn Cytopathol* 2009;37(6):407–410.

DeLellis RA, Nikiforov YE. Thyroid and parathyroid glands. In: Gnepp DR, ed. *Diagnostic Surgical Pathology of the Head and Neck.* 2nd ed. Philadelphia, PA: W.B. Saunders Publishers; 2009.

Dimashkieh H, Krishnamurthy S. Ultrasound guided fine needle aspiration biopsy of parathyroid gland and lesions. *Cyto Journal* 2006;3:6.

Lloyd RV, Osamura RY, Kloppel G, eds. *WHO Classification of Tumours of Endocrine Organs.* 4th ed. Lyon, France: IARC Press; 2017.

Thompson LDR. Benign neoplasms of the parathyroid gland. In: Thompson LDR, Bishop JA, eds. *Head and Neck Pathology.* 3rd ed. Philadelphia, PA: Elsevier; 2019.

Thompson LDR. Non-neoplastic lesions of the parathyroid glands. In: Thompson LDR, Bishop JA, eds. *Head and Neck Pathology.* 3rd ed. Philadelphia, PA: Elsevier; 2019.

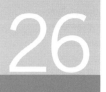

26 The Adrenal Gland and Paraganglia

Louis P. Dehner, Farhan A. Khan, and Mai He

I. INTRODUCTION

A. Development. The adrenal gland is referred to as a composite organ with two distinct embryologic primordia, the adrenogonadal or urogenital ridge (UGR) as paired foci medial to the mesonephros and the neural crest (NC), giving rise respectively to the steroidogenic cortex and the sympathochromaffin medulla. At 4 to 5 weeks (wks) gestation the coelomic epithelium (adrenogonadal primordia) in the UGR is identifiable by the expression of steroidogenic-factor-1 (SF-1), a transcription factor, and by 8 weeks the adrenal anlage from the outer coelom and gonadal anlage (medial) separates (50-52 postconception day) and migrates into the retroperitoneum where it is positioned at the upper pole of the mesonephros (*Curr Topics Dev Biol* 2013;106:239). The cortex become divisible into the outer definitive (DZ) and inner fetal zone (FZ). At 9 weeks the NC cells migrate into the cortex as individual cells and small nests of neuroblasts which remain dispersed in the adrenal until after birth (1 to 1½ years of age) when coalescence occurs and the medulla becomes a formed structure with three distinct lineages: chromaffin, ganglionic-neural, and sustentacular cells (S-100 protein positive Schwann-like cells) (*Am J Pathol* 1990;137:605). The FZ, only present in higher primates, comprises 80% of the fetal adrenal and is steroidogenic throughout gestation where androgenic precursors are produced and converted to estrogen in the placenta for pregnancy maintenance; the FZ undergoes involution by the age of 6 months through apoptosis. The DZ and transition zone (TZ) between the DZ and FZ are the sites of cortisol synthesis; the DZ and TZ differentiate into the outer-zone glomerulosa (ZG) and fascicula by 3 years of age and the zone reticularis (ZR) by 4 years of age (*Endocrinol Metab Clin N Am* 2015;44:243). The definitive zonation of the cortex does not occur until puberty (adrenarche) with the production of androgens by the ZR.

B. Normal Anatomy and Histology. The definitive or adult adrenal glands are located anterior to the upper poles of the kidneys. The glands are pyramidal on the right and crescentic on the left. At birth, the adrenals are disproportionately large because of the FZ and have a combined weight of 6 to 10 g. In adults the normal combined weight generally does not exceed 6 to 8 g. Each adrenal gland is divided into head (most medially), body (middle), and tail (most lateral).

Microscopically, the cortex consists of three zones: the outer ZG (secreting aldosterone), middle ZF (secreting mainly cortisol and minor amounts of sex steroids), and inner ZR (secreting mainly sex steroids) (e-**Fig. 26.1**). The ZG is composed of a thin, usually discontinuous layer of cells in ball-like formations; these cells have less cytoplasm than the cells in the other two cortical zones. The ZF consists of radial cords or columns of cells with abundant lipid-rich cytoplasm. The cells of the ZR have compact, finely eosinophilic cytoplasm with or without lipofuscin pigment.

Normally, the medulla accounts for 10% of the adrenal volume and has a gray-white color. The predominant cell in the medulla is the mature chromaffin cell (pheochromocyte), organized in nests and cords (e-**Fig. 26.2**). The cytoplasm of the chromaffin cells is commonly basophilic but may be amphophilic or even eosinophilic. These cells have indistinct cell borders and usually a single nucleus which is variable in size and hyperchromatism. The chromaffin cells are surrounded peripherally by the sustentacular cells. Rare ganglion cells may be identified in the medulla unlike their obvious presence in normal ganglia (e-**Fig. 26.3**). The major function of the medulla is the synthesis and secretion

TABLE 26.1	World Health Organization Histologic Classification of Tumors of Adrenal Cortex, Medulla, and Extra-adrenal Paraganglia

Cortical tumors	**Extra-adrenal paragangliomas**
Adrenal cortical carcinoma	Head and neck paragangliomas
Adrenal cortical adenoma	Carotid body
Adenomatoid tumor	Jugulotympanic
Sex cord-stroma tumor	Vagal
Leydig cell tumor	Laryngeal
Granulosa cell tumor	**Neuroblastic tumor of the adrenal gland**
Mesenchymal and stromal tumors	Neuroblastoma
Myelolipoma	Ganglioneuroblastoma, nodular
Schwannoma	Ganglioneuroblastoma, intermixed
Hematolymphoid tumor	Ganglioneuroma
Secondary tumor	**Composite pheochromocytoma**
Adrenal Medulla and Paraganglia	**Composite paraganglioma**
Pheochromocytoma	

From: Lloyd RV, Osamura RY, Kloppel G, Rosai J. *WHO Classification of Tumours: Pathology and Genetics of Tumours of Endocrine Organs.* 4th ed. Lyon, France: IARC Press; 2017. Used with permission.

of catecholamines (epinephrine and norepinephrine). The chromaffin cells or pheochromocytes and those of the ZR are immediately contiguous to each other; however, cortical and medullary cells can be found in either compartment (e-**Fig. 26.2**). Though infrequently discussed, there is substantial corticomedullary paracrine interaction which is important in hormone synthesis and response to stress (*Endocr Dev* 2011;20:28).

As a dual organ, the adrenal gland gives rise to tumors of cortical or medullary origin, as well as other types (Table 26.1).

II. **GROSS EXAMINATION OF ADRENAL GLAND SPECIMENS.** The adrenal glands are removed either as part of a radical nephrectomy, or for excision of an adrenal tumor. Biopsies of the adrenal are generally fine needle aspirations (FNAs) or thin needle biopsies to evaluate for the presence of metastatic tumor.

A. **Needle Biopsy.** The entire tissue should be submitted for histologic examination.

B. **Adrenal Gland Removed as Part of Radical Nephrectomy.** After gross examination of the kidney, the gland should be measured and weighed. Then the gland should be serially sectioned at 2 to 3 mm intervals perpendicular to its long axis; the thickness of the cortex and medulla should be noted (e-**Fig. 26.4**). Infrequently, the adrenal may be invaded directly by renal cell carcinoma (RCC) or is the site of discontinuous metastases.

C. **Adrenalectomy for a Primary Pathologic Process.** The first step is to orient the specimen and examine the contour of the adrenal gland. If it is apparent that the gland has been largely replaced by a mass, the periphery should be inked since the margins may be important. If the cortex and medulla maintain their normal relationship to each other, the thickness of each should be recorded. Serial sectioning should be done at intervals appropriate for the pathology. If the disease process is apparently diffuse hyperplasia, the periadrenal soft tissue should be removed and the gland should be measured and weighed. If the adrenal contains a solitary mass or multiple nodules, three dimensional measurements should be obtained. The cut surface of any lesion and its relationship to any identifiable normal tissue should be described, including color, consistency, presence of hemorrhage or necrosis, degree of circumscription, and degree of encapsulation. If any portions of adjacent organs such as liver, kidney, spleen, or abdominal wall are attached (usually for tumors), their appearance and relationship to the gland should be noted. A large, en bloc resection will require numerous sections from the peripheral margins. For diffuse and/or nodular hyperplasia, representative sections are sufficient.

For a neoplasm, the following sections should be taken: tumor (including sections demonstrating the relationship of the tumor to the associated soft tissues and adjacent organs, and relationship of the tumor to uninvolved adrenal gland); the tumor capsule, if present; margins; periadrenal fatty tissue overlying a bulging mass; a representative section from uninvolved adrenal, if any; and regional lymph nodes. The gross description should clearly document the site of the sections. For large specimens, a gross photograph is extremely helpful in that it depicts the specimen at a time when landmarks are still maintained with some anatomic orientation.

D. Neuroblastoma (NB) Specimens. Neuroblastic tumors present some special issues regarding acquisition of neoplastic tissue for a variety of special studies to biologically profile the tumor for children enrolled in a Children Oncology Group (COG) protocol. If the specimen is an adrenal-based NB, then generally the amount of available tumor is sufficient for pathologic diagnosis as well as for all other ancillary studies. The difficulties arise in those cases of NB when only biopsies are obtained prior to chemotherapy in the case of an initially unresectable tumor. Accuracy of tumor subtype is based upon a thorough microscopic examination which may be limited by the amount of well-preserved tumor in the specimen. These small biopsies are often subjected to considerable compression artifact.

A resected primary NB of the adrenal, or extra-adrenal retroperitoneal mass, should be examined fresh if at all possible as discussed in the previous section. The COG reference laboratory requests at least 1 g of snap frozen tumor tissue, but will accept any frozen sample of tumor; the snap freezing should occur as soon as the specimen becomes available following resection. Tumor samples should be labeled "primary" or "metastatic"; involved bone marrow is required as well. Storage at $-70°C$ is preferable to $-20°C$.

Fresh tissue should also be collected for local institutional studies including conventional cytogenetic studies. Snap-frozen fresh tissue should be saved for possible molecular studies. Tumor for fluorescent in situ hybridization can be recovered from formalin-fixed, paraffin-embedded tissue without compromising the quality of results.

III. ADRENAL CORTICAL LESIONS

A. Congenital Abnormalities

1. Heterotopia (adrenal rests) is the most common congenital anomaly of the adrenal and is usually an incidental finding whose features are microscopic foci of cortical tissue or nodule(s) along the path of descent of the gonads, although rare examples of heterotopia have been reported in a wide variety of other anatomic sites. Heterotopias are identified in 1.5% to 2.7% of groin procedures in males; the spermatic cord, inguinal hernia sac, and paraepididymal soft tissues are the three most common sites. Only cortical tissue is identified as a rule and may be organized into a normal-appearing cortex. Medullary tissue is distinctly uncommon since the cortical primordium migrates with the gonad before NC cells have arrived at their destination. Small cortical nodules are relatively common around the adrenal and are external to the capsule. Arising from a heterotopia, there are examples of cortical adenoma in the gastric wall, renal hilum, and within the dura (*World J Gastroenterol* 2013;19:778; *Brain Tumor Pathol* 2010;27:121; *Diagn Pathol* 2016;11:40).

2. Testicular adrenal rest tumors (TARTs) are manifestations of 21-hydroxylase deficiency in 90% of cases. These lesions are detected in 25% of male children with congenital adrenal hyperplasia (CAH) where they are located in the region of the rete testis. TARTs are bilateral and multifocal as nodules separated by fibrous septa; eosinophilic polyhedral cells usually contain abundant lipochrome pigment. Nuclear atypia and fatty metaplasia are other features (*Presse Med* 2017;46:572). The differential diagnosis is Leydig cell tumor (LCT), which is not associated with CAH. Like the adrenal cortex, TARTs are immunoreactive for synaptophysin (LCT is not immunoreactive for synaptophysin); both are immunopositive for expression of inhibin A and CD56. Adrenal rests in and around the ovary are uncommon even in cases of CAH when compared with their frequency in the testis.

3. **Heterotopia in the adrenal gland** includes examples of thyroid or pancreatic cyst in the adrenal.

4. **Fusion** of the adrenal with the liver and kidney is rare but well-documented. The two adrenals may fuse producing a horseshoe or butterfly gland; this anomaly is reported in association with heterotaxy and renal anomalies.

5. **Adrenal cytomegaly** probably represents an acquired process in the adrenal cortex of fetuses and neonates, and possibly is a response to stress. It has been observed in hemoglobin BART and Beckwith-Wiedemann syndrome. Enlarged cortical cells have prominent pleomorphic nuclei.

B. **Adrenal Cortical Nodules (ACN).** ACNs are generally bilateral and discovered as either an incidental lesion(s) on imaging for other indications (since most are nonfunctional) or at postmortem examination, in 4% and 40% to 50% of cases, respectively. Bilateral nodules as incidentalomas may indicate the presence of subclinical Cushing syndrome (CS) (*Endocrine* 2016;51:225). Circumscribed but nonencapsulated nodules consist of fasciculata-type cells with various patterns. Myelolipomatous metaplasia, osseous metaplasia, and secondary changes (hyalinization, calcification, or hemorrhage) may be present. Pigmented nodules are composed of zona reticularis-type cells with lipofuscin or neuromelanin.

C. **Adrenal Cortical Hypofunction** (insufficiency) is divided into primary and secondary types.

1. **Primary adrenal cortical insufficiency** (ACI, Addison disease) is caused by a diverse group of pathogenetic disorders whose end result is deficient production or action of glucocorticoids, with or without deficiency in mineralocorticoids and adrenal androgens (*Lancet* 2014;383:2152). Autoimmune adrenalitis (AIA) in adults (80% of cases) and CAH in children (70% to 75% of cases) are the most common causes in these two age groups. Both cellular and humeral immunity have a role in the AIA with autoantibodies against steroidogenic 21-hydroxylase as the most common finding (*Autoimmun Rev* 2014;13:408). The weight of the combined glands is considerably less than the normal 6 to 10 g. During the active phase of inflammation, the infiltrate is rich in T-lymphocytes, some plasma cells, and macrophages. Small lymphoid nodules may be seen. In the process, the tri-zonal cortex is represented by scattered small collections of residual cortical cells.

2. **Autoimmune polyendocrine syndromes** (APS) are the other disorders associated with AIA (*Autoimmun Rev* 2014;13:85). APS1 and APS2 are the two most thoroughly characterized autosomal recessive disorders, involving the *AIRE* gene and genes within the major histocompatibility complex, respectively.

3. **Other causes of ACI** range over a variety of infections, including meningococcemia (Waterhouse–Friderichsen syndrome), metastatic carcinoma, lymphoma, hereditary iron overload, amyloidosis, medications, and the genetic disorder adrenoleukodystrophy (ALD). The latter X-linked peroxisomal disorder is caused by mutations in *ABCD1* gene (*Nature Rev Endocrinol* 2016;12:606). The first manifestation in childhood is ACI. The cortical nodules are composed of ballooned cortical cells with striated cytoplasm.

4. **Congenital adrenal hypoplasia** (CAHP) is an uncommon condition that is more likely to be encountered in a fetopsy or perinatal autopsy. Its estimated incidence is 1:12,500 live births, compared with the incidence of anencephaly of 1:10,000 live births in the United States. It should be anticipated that 1% to 2% of fetopsies will have evidence of CAHP as defined by combined adrenal weights of less than 2 g at term, or more accurately an adrenal weight over body weight of less than 1:1000. There are three distinct morphologic patterns: cytomegaly type (most common with X-linked inheritance with inactivating deletion mutations in the gene *NROB1 (DAX-1)*; anencephalic type (without CNS or pituitary defects but the cortex is attenuated and the fetal cortex is inconspicuous); and the so-called miniature type with a definitive cortex and an attenuated fetal cortex.

5. CAH is the most common cause of primary AI in children. There are presently seven types of CAH which have autosomal recessive inheritance (*Lancet* 2017;390:2194).

This group of disorders, depending on the particular mutation, occurs in approximately 1:15,000 to 20,000 live births with 21-hydroxylase deficiency accounting for 90% of cases. The weight of the glands is increased 4 to 5 times normal. Marked diffuse hyperplasia of the ZF results from continuous ACTH stimulation, the cells are lipid depleted with their transition into ZR-type cells with compact features. Myelolipomas (MYLs) are described in association with CAH, but the cause and effect relationship is unclear.

6. **Secondary and tertiary adrenal cortical insufficiencies** are due to the failure of the pituitary gland to secrete ACTH (secondary) or of the hypothalamus to secrete CRH (tertiary). The glands are small and the ZF is atrophic, whereas the ZG and medulla are usually relatively normal.

D. **Adrenal Cortical Hyperplasia** is divisible morphologically into diffuse and nodular types. In the prior section on ACI, diffuse hyperplasia was discussed in the context of CAH which is driven by a failure in the feedback mechanism between cortisol synthesis and adrenocorticotropic hormone (ACTH) secretion. The consequence is enlarged glands and hyperfunction with the synthesis of androgenic and/or mineraloid precursors. This section focuses on the other forms of hyperplasia of ACTH-independent and dependent types.

1. **Diffuse hyperplasia** is usually ACTH-dependent presenting with Cushing disease with an ACTH-producing pituitary adenoma (70% to 75% of cases), ectopic ACTH-producing neuroendocrine neoplasm (10%), or cortisol-producing cortical lesions (20%) (*Am J Surg Pathol* 2015; 39:374). Both glands are symmetrically enlarged. The ZF and ZR are expanded with their relative proportions varying from case to case. The ZF is lipid depleted but markedly expanded by a population of cortical cells with abundant eosinophilic cytoplasm (e-**Fig. 26.5**).

2. **ACTH-independent bilateral macronodular adrenocortical hyperplasia** (ABMAH) accounts for 2% or less of cases of CS. It is estimated that 20% to 50% of affected individuals have an *ARMC5* germline mutation (*N Engl J Med* 2013;369:2105). There is intra-adrenal ACTH synthesis with a paracrine effect. Other hereditary disorders accompanied by ABMAH include multiple endocrine neoplasia type I, familial adenomatosis polyposis, McCune–Albright syndrome (MAS), and hereditary leiomyomatosis-RCC. Infants and young children with CS may have MAS with a postzygotic mutation of the *GNAS1* gene (*J Clin Endocrinol Metab* 2014;99:E2029). The adrenal glands together can weigh in excess of 150 g and have distorted, bosselated contours, but in some cases there is asymmetry with only one enlarged gland. The nodules range in size to greater than 4 to 5 cm and are yellowish. Two patterns of nodules include those that are separated by atrophic compressed internodular cortical tissue, and those in which the internodular cortex is also hyperplastic. The nodules are composed of ZF and ZR-type cells or one or the other type cell. Both macro- (>1 cm) and micronodules (<1 cm) with intervening atrophy are composed of hyperplastic ZG-type cells in children with MAS. A solitary microcortical nodule (adenoma) is seen in some cases of MAS.

3. **Micronodular bilateral adrenocortical hyperplasia** (MiBAH) is an uncommon cause of autosomal dominant CS whose clinical onset occurs in children and young adults (*Presse Med* 2018;47:e127). Three categories or groups of MiBAH are recognized. Those with Carney complex (90% of cases) have various extra-adrenal phenotypic manifestations and pigmented MiBAH in virtually all cases with germline mutations in *PRKARIA*, *PDE8B*, and a 2p16 locus; isolated pigmented MiBAH has mutations in *PRKARIA*, *PRKACA*, *PDE11A*, and a 2p16 locus; and isolated nonpigmented, micronodular adrenocortical disease (iMAD) that has mutations in *PDE11A*, *PRKACA*, and at loci at 2p16 and 5q. The combined weight of pigmented MiBAH generally does not exceed 15 to 20 g; the sectioned pigmented nodules measure from 1 to 3 mm with a capsule and are located at the corticomedullary junction. The compact, nonvacuolated cytoplasm contains the brownish pigment lipofuscin. Some nodules may be seen just beyond the capsule. The internodular

cortex is generally atrophic in contrast to the adrenals in iMAD which are normal sized, composed of yellowish to brownish nodules, and show an intervening cortex with hyperplastic features. In some cases of iMAD, the adrenals are pigmented and are indistinguishable from pigmented MiBAH. In the case of *PRKACA* germline amplification, cortical adenoma, hyperplasia, and pigmented nodules have been documented (*Hum Pathol* 2015;46:40).

4. **Adrenocortical hyperplasia** (aldosterone type), as bilateral nodules, is seen in 20% to 30% of those with hypertension and primary aldosteronism. It is estimated that 6% to 13% of the hypertensive population have aldosteronism. Whether hyperplasia is unilateral or an adenoma, the disorder is characterized by aldosterone secretion which is independent of renin, angiotensin II, and sodium status. The size, weight, and overall appearance are variable from case to case, but there is often a dominant nodule with smaller secondary nodules. The formation of nodules alters the overall architecture of the gland. Microscopically, tongue-like projections of the hyperplastic ZG-like cells extend toward and into the ZF.

5. **Adrenogenital syndrome with sex hormone production** is infrequently caused by a cortical adenoma (ACA), but is more often associated with an estrogen-producing adrenocortical carcinoma. Androgen-producing ACA is generally larger than those with CS and is also sharply demarcated from the adjacent cortex. The tumor cells have ZR-like features with compact, eosinophilic cytoplasm.

E. Adrenal Cortical Tumors (ACTs)

1. **Introduction.** A substantial body of observations on the molecular genetics of adrenocortical tumors is available; much of it has evolved with the appreciation that these neoplasms occur in various hereditary syndromes. Most ACTs with the differential diagnosis of adenoma (ACA) versus carcinoma (ACC) are straightforward on the basis of pathologic findings including size, capsular/vascular invasion, and mitotic activity, but some cases require the presence or absence of several histologic features to arrive at a numerical score and with it, the diagnosis of ACA or ACC (*Histopathology* 2014;64:567; *Semin Diagn Pathol* 2013;30:197; *Surg Pathol Clin* 2015;8:725). In a few cases, the pathologic findings are equivocal which results in an equivocal interpretation in cases where the tumor weighs 100 to 200 g and is confined to the gland.

2. **Adrenal cortical adenoma (ACA).** ACA occurs in all age groups, both sexes, and is relatively common (4% to 10%) as an incidental finding on imaging or at autopsy. These tumors are either nonfunctional (nonsecretory) or functional (secretory) with CS (60% to 65% of cases), mineralocorticoid-androgens (20%), combined CS-androgens (4%), estrogen (12%), and aldosterone (4%). Based upon the frequency of so-called incidentalomas, most ACAs are nonfunctional or have undetected aldosterone-production to explain hypertension; approximately 10% of incidental ACAs are functional with subclinical CS.

Grossly, ACA is unilateral, solitary, and encapsulated with a bright yellow to tan coloration with infrequent areas of hemorrhage and necrosis. There is a correlation between size and risk of malignancy (<2% ACC if <4 cm; 6% if 4.1 to 6 cm; 25% if >6 cm) (e-**Fig. 26.6**). ACA usually weighs less than 50 g, but there are exceptional tumors weighing 500 g or more.

   a. *CS-associated ACA* is a well-demarcated nodule with or without a capsule (often without) which merges with adjacent cortex as a bulging nodule. Solid nests and/or alveolar profiles are composed of ZF-like cells; these cells are larger than normal cortical cells and ZR-like cells may be present as well (e-**Fig. 26.7**).

   b. *Primary aldosteronism* in majority of cases is due to an ACA (60% to 70%), generally measuring 2 cm or less in most cases (see above).

   Approximately 90% to 95% of cases are sporadic and the remainder have autosomal dominant inheritance and a defined genetic basis: type I (*CYP11B1/CYP11B2* fusion), type II (*CLCN2*), type III (*KCNJ5*), and type IV (*CACNA-1D*). Somatic mutations are found in 7% of aldosterone-producing adenomas in the P-type ATPase gene family; another somatic mutation is found in *KCNJ5*.

These tumors are unilateral, typically measuring 2 cm or less, have a bright yellow surface, and may or may not have a well-defined capsule (e-**Fig. 26.8**). Those ACAs with a *KCNJ5* mutation are composed of ZF-like, lipid rich cells; ATPase gene family and *CACNA-1D* mutated ACAs have predominant ZG-like features (e-**Fig. 26.9**). Some tumors may display hybrid features. Unlike cortisol-producing ACAs, the adjacent cortex is not atrophic. Spironolactone bodies are present in the cytoplasm as 2 to 6 mm, round to oval eosinophilic bodies which have lamellated, concentric rings in those tumors which have been treated with the aldosterone antagonist.

c. *Additional pathologic features* of ACAs include those rare examples of so-called black adenomas with dark brown to black coloration on the basis of lipofuscin deposition in ZR-like cells; this same pigmentation occurs in pigmented micro-nodular hyperplasia. Lipomatous or myelolipomatous foci are also seen in some cases. A reticulin network typically invests cords of cortical cells unlike most ACCs. Like other benign tumors of the endocrine systems, nuclear enlargement and hyperchromatism may be seen in the ACA, and even isolated mitotic figures. Hemorrhage is seen on occasion, but necrosis and atypical mitotic figures should be viewed with concern especially in an ACT larger than 6 cm and weighing in access of 50 to 100 g. There are reports of "giant" ACAs weighing in excess of 1 kg (*Urology* 2012;80:e25).

d. *Other ACTs* with special microscopic features beyond the usual, more common ACA and ACC include the myxoid and oncocytic neoplasms, and the rare so-called adrenal blastoma.

  i. *Myxoid ACTs* are rare morphologic variants of ACA or ACC with a focal or near diffuse background with a myxoid-mucoid, rich Alcian blue positive stromal mucin. Most myxoid ACTs are ACCs, but several examples of myxoid ACAs have been reported from infancy to adulthood. The myxoid stroma separates the tumor cells into cords, nests, alveolar profiles, pseudoglands (e-**Fig. 26.10**), and trabecular strands. Pseudoglands and alveolar profiles can be especially problematic but like most ACTs, these tumors are immunopositive for SF1, inhibin, melan-A, calretinin, and synaptophysin (e-**Fig. 26.10**). The individual tumor cells may be spindled to epithelioid in contrast to the usual ACA and ACC.

  ii. *Oncocytic ACTs* (oncocytomas) include both benign and malignant types as in other organs (*Int J Surg Pathol* 2014;22:33). Since most tumors are non-functional (80%), they are usually an incidental finding. These tumors have a brownish-yellow appearance, are encapsulated, and have an average size of 8 cm; the latter is problematic since the size overlaps with ACC. A central scar as seen in renal oncocytoma is generally not present. The cytoplasm is mitochondria-rich which accounts for the oncocytic appearance that the tumor cells have in common with extra-adrenal oncocytomas. These tumors are often characterized by large, bizarre cells; despite the presence of these atypical cells, the histologic criteria to differentiate an ACA from ACC are applicable (*Int J Surg Pathol* 2004;12:231; *Ann Diagn Pathol* 2010;14:204). These tumors may have cytoplasmic globules and inclusions like those seen in pheochromocytoma (PCC), which can also be problematic since the latter tumor may also have oncocytic features in rare cases.

3. Adrenal cortical carcinoma (ACC). ACC is a rare neoplasm with an incidence of $1:10^6$ in the United States. The tumor is recognized in all age groups, but it appears to have a bimodal age distribution with one peak in children less than 5 years old and a second peak in adults in the fourth through fifth decades of life. However, many of the cases of ACC in children, especially those diagnosed early in the first decade of life, do not behave clinically as their adult counterparts although the microscopic features associated with ACC in adults are present (see below). ACC occurs in several hereditary syndromes including Li-Fraumeni syndrome (*TP53*), Beckwith-Wiedemann syndrome (*CDKN1C/NSD1*), MEN1 (*MEN*1), and Gardner syndrome (*APC*); however, hereditary cases in aggregate constitute 5% or less of all ACCs.

Most cases present as a functioning neoplasm (50% to 60% of cases), with CS as the most common presentation. Females are more commonly affected than males, and more often have functional ACCs. Approximately 40% to 45% of ACCs are confined to the adrenal and are completely resectable. By the most recent AJCC staging scheme for adrenal cortical carcinoma (Amin MB et al., eds. *AJCC Cancer Staging Manual.* 8th ed. New York: Springer, 2017), only 5% to 10% of tumors are 5 cm or less (T1) whereas 35% to 40% are greater than 5 cm (T2). Over 50% of cases have infiltrated beyond the adrenal (T3) or have already metastasized at presentation in 30% to 35% of cases (T4).

Grossly, hemorrhage and necrosis often provide the background for a soft yellowish to tan neoplasm with or without cystic areas (**e-Fig. 26.11**). However, ACC can have a variety of gross features in terms of coloration and presence or absence of apparent necrosis. Those ACCs less than 5 cm in greatest dimension tend to have a more uniform gross appearance as do ACAs; these are the cases which may prove to be problematic in the histopathologic differential diagnosis between an ACC and ACA, a point that is especially pertinent as it relates to ACTs in children.

Over the past 30 to 40 years, several pathologic systems have been proposed for the assessment of histopathologic features to differentiate an ACA from ACC in adults, but the most durable one is the modified Weiss system to predict malignant behavior: mitotic rate (>5 per 50 hpf), atypical mitotic figures (any number), <25% clear cells, necrosis, and capsular invasion (**e-Fig. 26.12**) (*Semin Diagn Pathol* 2013;30:197; *Histopathology* 2018;72:82). Of note, high power microscopic fields with mitotic activity rather than random fields should be utilized in the assessment. An ACT with at least three features should be diagnosed as an ACC. Once an ACC has invaded into adjacent soft tissues or organs, a major vessel, or metastasized to regional lymph nodes or remote site(s), the diagnosis of ACC is more than apparent.

Immunohistochemistry to corroborate that a particular neoplasm is cortical in nature is infrequently necessary, with the uncommon exception of a dilemma between a cortical and medullary neoplasm (which is usually obvious in most but not all cases), but there are rare examples of composite corticomedullary tumors or ones with ambiguous features. Another example is metastatic RCC to the adrenal which can mimic a primary cortical neoplasm. A more frequent diagnostic challenge is presented by a needle biopsy of a retroperitoneal mass in which the microscopic features consist of dense cords and nests of eosinophilic, epithelioid cells or scattered malignant cells in a background of necrosis with the differential diagnosis of a hepatic, adrenal, or renal neoplasm, as well as perivascular epithelioid cell tumor (PEComa), angiomyolipoma (AML), epithelioid smooth muscle neoplasm, epithelioid mesothelioma, and epithelioid gastrointestinal stromal tumor (Table 26.2). Most adrenal cortical neoplasms are vimentin (70% to 80% of cases), inhibin (85% to 90%), melan-A (85% to 90%), SF-1 (85% to 90%), and calretinin (85% to 90%) immunopositive (*Am J Surg Pathol* 2011;35:678). CAM5.2 is expressed in ACTs whereas the other keratins are nonreactive, and when positive should suggest another diagnosis. There is an overlap of the immunophenotype with ovarian and testicular sex-cord stromal neoplasms, which should come as no surprise since these tumors have similar developmental and functional attributes.

Variants of the classic pattern of ACC includes those neoplasms with oncocytic (rare), myxoid (more commonly ACCs), and sarcomatoid features. In the latter cases, the sarcomatoid pattern has highly pleomorphic, spindle cell sarcomatous features or even rhabdomyosarcomatous differentiation. Sarcomatoid RCC, pancreatic sarcoma, and dedifferentiated liposarcoma are other considerations in the differential diagnosis.

Molecular analysis of ACTs including ACCs has provided considerable insight into tumorigenesis. ACA and ACC share several chromosomal aberrations, but the

TABLE 26.2	Comparative Immunohistochemistry of Adrenal Cortical Tumors and Other Similar Appearing Extra-Adrenal Neoplasms						
	ACT	**HCT**	**RCT**	**PEComa-AML**	**EGIST**	**ESMT**	**EMESO**
VIM	−	−	+[a]	+	−	+	+
CK (AE1/AE3)	±	±	+	−	−	−	+
CK5/6	−	−	−	−	−		+
CK7	−	−	±	−	−	−	+
CK20	−	−	−[b]	−	−	−	−
34βE12	−	+	−	−	−	−	−
EMA	−	−	±	−	−	−	±
HEP-PAR	−	+	−	−	−	−	−
CD10	±[c]	±[c]	+	−	−	−	−
CD34	−	−	−	−	+	−	−
CD117	−	−	−	−	+	−	−
HMB-45	−	−	±[d]	+[d]	−	−	−
MEL-A103	+	−	−[e]	+	−	−	−
INH	+	−	−	−	−	−	−
CAL	−	−	−	−	−	−	+
RCC	−	−	+	−	−	−	−
SMA	−	−	−	+	±	+	−
WT1	−	−	−	−	−	−	+

[a]VIM negative in most chromophobe RCCs and oncocytomas.
[b]CK20 positive in type PAPRCC (*Arch Pathol Lab Med* 2011;135:92).
[c]CD10 canalicular staining (*Arch Pathol Lab Med* 2007;131:1648).
[d]HMB-45 positive in 50% Xp11 translocation RCCs.
[e]MEL-A positive in 90% Xp11 translocation RCCs.
ACT, adrenocortical tumor; AML, angiomyolipoma; CAL, calretinin; CK, cytokeratin; EGIST, epithelioid gastrointestinal stromal tumor; EMA, epithelial membrane antigen; EMESO, epithelioid mesothelioma; ESMT, epithelioid smooth muscle tumor; HCT, hepatocellular tumor; HepPar, hepatocyte antigen; INH, inhibin; MEL, melanoma; PEC, perivascular epithelioid cell tumor, including angiomyolipoma; RCC, renal cell carcinoma antigen; RCT, renal cell tumor; SMA, smooth muscle actin; VIM, vimentin; WT1, Wilms tumor.

number of these is greater in frequency in ACC including gains in chromosomes 5, 7, 13, 16, 19, and 20 and losses at 13 and 22; six foci show high sensitivity and specificity for ACC (5q, 7p, 11p, 13q, 16q, and 22q) (*Endocrin Rev* 2014;35:282). Several susceptibility genes for ACC have been identified, including at 11p15 with high IGF2 and low H19 expression, *TP53* germline inactivating mutation in Li-Fraumeni syndrome, and somatic mutation in sporadic ACCs in the Wnt-β catenin pathway.

4. **Adrenocortical neoplasms in children** have been disproportionately diagnosed as ACCs in the past, especially in young children, because of the presence of pathologic features that are associated with ACCs in adults (*Pediatr Dev Pathol* 2009;12:284). Others have also observed an overall favorable outcome for ACCs in children, especially in those 5 years old or less (*J Pediatr Surg* 2016;51:1795; *Contemp Clin Trials* 2016;50:37). Localized adrenal tumors weighing in excess of 400 g are more likely to behave in malignant fashion since few tumors weighing less than 200 g are malignant, but those between 200 and 400 g are less predictable in behavior (**e-Fig. 26.11**). GLUT1 overexpression in ACTs in children is reported to be correlated with malignant behavior (*Oncotarget* 2017;8:63835). It has been suggested that tumorigenesis of ACTs including ACCs is different in children than in adults (*Hum Pathol* 2012;43:31).

IV. ADRENAL MEDULLARY LESIONS. Major categories of adrenal medullary lesions include medullary hyperplasia, pheochromocytoma (PCC), corticomedullary mixed tumors (CMMTs), and neuroblastic tumors (Table 26.1).

A. Adrenal Medullary Hyperplasia (AMH) is defined as an increase in the mass of medullary cells with expansion of these cells into areas of the gland that normally do not contain pheochromocytes. The normal ratio of cortex to medulla is approximately 10:1 in the adult and is higher in children less than 5 years old. Multiple endocrine neoplasia (MEN type 2A, 2B) is the most common setting of AMH, but it is also seen in association with Beckwith-Wiedemann syndrome, NF1, and somatostatin-rich duodenal well-differentiated neuroendocrine tumor. Several mutations of succinate dehydrogenase (SDH) are associated with familial paraganglioma (PGL) and less often familial PCC. Sporadic examples of AMH are rare.

Diffuse or nodular hyperplasia with multiple nodules is present in both glands in MEN 2A and 2B; nodules when present are less than 1 cm and those in excess of 1 cm are regarded as PCC. AMH unlike PCC is not associated with overproduction of catecholamines. The microscopic distinction between AMH and normal medulla can be difficult, since the hyperplastic medullary cells have a nonnested diffuse appearance like normal medullary pheochromocytes, unlike the cytologically atypical pheochromocytes with nested Zellballen features. AMH is often present adjacent to a PCC.

B. PCC arises from the truncal NC-derived cells which differentiate into chromaffin cells as well as neuroblasts (ganglion cells) and Schwann-like sustentacular cells (*Int J Dev Biol* 2017;61:5). There are rare examples of neoplasms with the combined features of a neuroblastic tumor and PCC reflecting the common NC progenitorship; these tumors are generally referred to as composite PCCs (see below). PCC refers to the intra-adrenal chromaffin neoplasm (80% to 85% of cases), whereas PGL is the designation for those neoplasms with similar morphology to PCC that present in the various extra-adrenal sites of sympathetic and parasympathetic paraganglia (15% to 20% of cases). Approximately 65% to 70% of PCCs and PGLs are initially regarded as sporadic (of these, 8% to 10% show a germline mutation on subsequent testing) and the remaining 25% to 30% of patients have a germline mutation with or without a designated tumor syndromes (Table 26.3). Germline mutations in four genes which encode subunits of SDH are found in PCC/PGL syndromes and in aggregate account for 70% or so of all cases (*J Clin Pathol* 2018;71:95). PCC has been referred to as the "10% tumor": 10% bilateral, 10% extra-adrenal, 10% malignant, and 10% in children. Paroxysmal or persistent hypertension is the most common presentation, but CS and watery diarrhea (vasoactive intestinal peptide) syndrome are reported in a small minority of cases.

A protocol-based examination of PCCs and PGLs has been proposed (*Arch Path Lab Med* 2014;138:182). PCCs range from 2 to 10 cm or greater, have a yellow-tan to dark hemorrhagic appearance, appear multinodular, and weigh between 10 and 100 g (**e-Fig. 26.13**); they may be hemorrhagic and cystic. It is not always clear from the gross examination whether the tumor is arising from the cortex or medulla, especially in those tumors which have largely replaced the entire gland, but remnants of the cortex may be identified microscopically.

Microscopically, a nested/nesting pattern with the formation of so-called Zellballen is the classic morphology of PCC (**e-Fig. 26.14**), but other patterns include trabecular, mixed alveolar and trabecular, solid, diffuse, and rarely spindle cell formations (which are usually focal). A myxohyaline stroma has been noted in those tumors occurring in the setting of von Hippel–Lindau syndrome. The chromaffin cells often have slightly eosinophilic and finely granular cytoplasm, but they may be amphophilic to basophilic or even oncocytic (**e-Fig. 26.14**). A finely vacuolated cytoplasm is present in some cases due to lipid accumulation. Intracytoplasmic periodic acid-Schiff positive, diastase resistant hyaline globules are yet another finding (**e-Fig. 26.15**). Melanin-containing PCCs are rare but well documented. The polygonal cells can vary in size and nuclear detail, with marked nuclear enlargement and hyperchromasia, although less impressive cytologic atypia is often present. Prominent nucleoli and nuclear pseudoinclusions are

TABLE 26.3 Susceptibility Genes for Pheochromocytoma/Paraganglioma in Syndromic and Nonsyndromic Settings

Syndrome	Gene/Chromosomal Location	Pathology[a]
Multiple endocrine neoplasia 1	MEN1/11q13	PCC (rare), pituitary adenoma, pancreatic NE tumors, ACA
Multiple endocrine neoplasia 2	RET/10q11.2	PCC
Neurofibromatosis type 1	NF1/17q11	PCC/head and neck PGLs
von Hippel–Lindau disease	VHL/3p25.3	PCC (bilateral)/abdominal, multiple PGL
Paraganglioma syndrome 1	SDHD/11q23.3	PCC/head, neck, and abdominal PGL
Paraganglioma syndrome 2	SDHAF2 (SDH5)/11q12.2	Head and neck PGL, PCC (−)
Paraganglioma syndrome 3	SDHC/1q23.3	Head and neck PGL, SDH-deficient RCC (rare), SDH-deficient GIST
Paraganglioma syndrome 4	SDHB/1p36.13	PCC/head, neck, thoracic, and abdominal PGL, SDH-deficient RCC, SDH-deficient GIST
Carney–Stratakis	SDHD/11q23.3	PGL, GIST
Carney triad	SDHX (10%)	PGL, gastric epithelioid GIST, lung chondroma
-	TMEM-127/2q11.2	Bilateral PCCs
-	MAX/14q23.3	Bilateral PCCs, PGLs (rare)

[a]Both sympathetic and parasympathetic paragangliomas occur in these various syndromes.
ACA, adrenocortical adenoma; GIST, gastrointestinal stromal tumor; NE, neuroendocrine; PCC, pheochromocytoma; PGL, paraganglioma; RCC, renal cell carcinoma; SDH, succinic dehydrogenase.

additional but inconsistent findings (e-**Fig. 26.16**). Mitotic figures, if seen, are not a definitive indication of malignancy. The stroma may exhibit extensive hyalinization, fibrosis, or rarely amyloid deposition, and the vasculature may be prominent. The periadrenal adipose tissue often has a hibernomatous appearance regardless of the age of the patient (e-**Fig. 26.17**). The chromaffin cells are positive for chromogranin A, synaptophysin, and CAM5.2 in some cases; the tumor cells do not express EMA, melan-A, or inhibin. S-100 labels sustentacular cells that are usually located at the periphery of the nests. SDHx immunostaining of PCCs and PGLs has been utilized in the screening of these tumors in individuals with possible germline mutations (*Lab Invest* 2018;98:414).

Prognostic assessment of an individual PCC which is confined to the gland and without metastasis is an exercise in uncertainty, but has not served to entirely discourage those attempts. A number of morphologic features have been assessed from the architectural pattern (nested vs. diffuse), presence or absence of confluent necrosis, mitotic rate, Ki-67 index, as well as several others including weight (less than or greater than 10 g), but the conclusion that there are no absolute histologic criteria for predicting malignant potential still maintains some currency (*Histopathology* 2011;58:155). It has also been suggested that less well-differentiated, SDHB-negative PCCs are more prone to metastasize. Overall, 10% to 25% of PCCs prove to be malignant as demonstrated by metastasis to bone, lymph nodes, lungs, and liver (e-**Fig. 26.18**). These metastases may occur several years after the initial resection. The most recent AJCC staging scheme for PCCs and PGLs incorporates these uncertainties (Amin MB et al., eds. *AJCC Cancer Staging Manual.* 8th ed. New York: Springer, 2017).

1. **PCC in children** is responsible for hypertension in 2% or less of cases, and as many as 20% of cases are diagnosed in the first two decades of life (*Front Pediatr* 2017;5:155). It is estimated that more than 90% of cases are inherited, in contrast to the adult experience. *SDHB* germline mutations in younger individuals with PCC and/or PGL were more likely to be malignant (*Ann Surg Oncol* 2017;24:3624).

2. **Composite or compound PCC,** a rare variant, is defined in most cases as a PCCs with a ganglioneuroma (GN) (80%), ganglioneuroblastoma (GNB) (20%), NB (<1%), malignant peripheral nerve sheath tumor, or neuroendocrine carcinoma (extremely rare) component (**e-Fig. 26.19**). This variant accounts for 1% to 3% of all PCCs, and these tumors are reported in the clinical settings of NF1 and MEN 2A.

3. CMMT represents a commingling of nests and cords of compact cells with clear to eosinophilic cytoplasm arranged in nests and trabecula, and larger pheochromocytes with granular basophilic cytoplasm and nuclei that often have some pleomorphism and are typically arranged in Zellballen. The coincident ACA and PCC in the same gland are differentiated from a CMMT *(Korean J Intern Med* 2015;30:114).

C. **Neuroblastic Tumors** (also known as peripheral neuroblastic tumors) are embryonal tumors arising from the sympathoadrenal neuroendocrine system, account for 7% to 10% of all childhood malignancies, are the most common extracranial solid malignancy of childhood, and are responsible for 15% of all cancer-related deaths in children. About 600 new cases are diagnosed each year in the United States. Approximately 98% of NBs are diagnosed by 10 years of age, and 85% to 90% are detected before 5 years of age. The abdomen and/or retroperitoneum are the sites of clinical presentation in 65% of cases; 50% of NBs arise in the adrenal medulla. Neuroblastic tumors have a set of basic histopathologic features reflecting the spectrum of differentiation within this group of related neoplasms; these must be integrated into the clinical stage (Table 26.4) and a set of biologic markers to assess the plan of management and projected outcome (*Annu Rev Med* 2015;66:49).

1. **NB** and its pathologic examination and diagnosis can occur in the setting of a bone marrow biopsy, a resected adrenal gland, or a resected extra-adrenal mass, at a variety of sites including the retroperitoneum or mediastinum. The approach to a case of suspected NB has recently been outlined (e.g., College of American Pathologists Protocol for the Examination of Specimens From Patients with Neuroblastoma; available at https://cap.objects.frb.io/protocols/cp-pediatric-neuroblastoma-16protocol-3103.pdf).

   The gross features of a NB are dependent upon anatomic site, treatment with preoperative chemotherapy, and recurrence. Dense fibrosis, calcifications, hemorrhage, and necrosis are some of the apparent gross findings. As with any major resection of a tumor, the status of surgical margins is an important consideration so the external surfaces should be inked before the specimen is sectioned to reveal the mass.

   A well-circumscribed, soft, gray-tan tumor, measuring 2 to 10 cm in dimension, with or without hemorrhage and calcifications, is the common appearance of a poorly

TABLE 26.4	International Neuroblastoma Staging System

Stage	Definition
1	Localized tumor confined to the primary site with gross complete excision, with or without microscopic residual disease, negative lymph nodes
2	Localized tumor with incomplete gross excision or positive ipsilateral lymph nodes but negative contralateral lymph nodes
3	Unresectable unilateral tumor infiltrating across the midline (positive or negative lymph nodes) or localized unilateral tumor with positive contralateral lymph nodes
4	Tumor disseminated to distant lymph node groups, bone, bone marrow, liver, skin, and/or other organs (except as defined in 4s)
4s	Localized tumor with dissemination limited to skin, bone marrow, and/or liver

differentiated NB (e-**Figs. 26.20** and **26.21**). GNB with intermixed features typically has a uniform grayish-tan mucoid cut surface, which is shared with some poorly differentiated NBs and GNs (e-**Fig. 26.22**). A neuroblastic tumor with one or more discrete nodules with variable dimensions in a background of grayish-tan, firm tissue is the gross appearance of nodular GNB (e-**Fig. 26.23**). Some neuroblastic tumors are entirely hemorrhagic and may have undergone near total cystic degeneration (with or without calcifications).

Though NB is often referred to one of the "small blue cell tumors", it is a neoplasm whose varied morphology can be a histopathologic challenge in some cases. Under the rubric of stromal-poor NB, there are three microscopic subtypes: poorly differentiated, differentiating, and undifferentiated NB. In addition to the typing, an assessment of the mitotic-karyorrhexis index (MKI) is determined by the number of tumor cells in mitosis or undergoing apoptosis with nuclear fragmentation in 5,000 cells (low <100; intermediate 100 to 200; high >200). The low and high MKI is readily apparent in most cases by the absence or presence of mitotic figures and karyorrhectic debris in most high power microscopic fields.

a. *Poorly differentiated stromal poor NB* is the most common subtype and in a well-preserved and prepared section, the tumor cells are arranged in lobules which are separated by a fibrovascular, nonschwannian stroma. An appreciation of the lobular architecture may be compromised in those cases with hemorrhage, necrosis, and/or fibrosis as either spontaneous or treatment-related changes (e-**Fig. 26.24**). Dystrophic calcifications may be extensive and are usually found in areas of necrosis. A background of eosinophilic fibrils (neuritic processes) may be confined to the center of Homer-Wright rosettes or be present as a more diffuse finding in the background of the small cells with little apparent cytoplasm and uniformly hyperchromatic nuclei (e-**Fig. 26.25**); these tumors in young children with low stage disease have a low MKI (e-**Fig. 26.25**). Finely dispersed chromatin may be present in preserved nuclei or in touch imprint preparations (e-**Fig. 26.26**). The tumor cells are typically immunoreactive for chromogranin and synaptophysin, but also for CD56 and neuronspecific enolase. Vimentin, CAM5.2, and CD99 are nonreactive.

b. *Differentiating stromal poor NB* is the second most common pattern and is characterized by an abundance of neurofibrillary processes when compared to the overall cellularity. Homer-Wright rosettes are often readily identified, as is evidence of larger neuroblastic cells with progression to ganglion cell differentiation with nuclear enlargement, a single small nucleolus, and amphophilic cytoplasm; the latter fully mature ganglion cells are only infrequently present (e-**Fig. 26.26**). The threshold for the interpretation of a differentiating NB is that 5% or greater of tumor cells are in some stage of dyssynchronous gangliocytic differentiation. If in doubt, the tumor should be designated as poorly differentiated NB.

c. *Undifferentiated stromal poor NB* is simply a primitive round cell neoplasm which requires immunohistochemistry to establish the phenotype of the neoplasm. Rosettes and neuropil are not present (e-**Fig. 26.27**). The tumor cells may have prominent nucleoli, which often indicates a *MYCN*-amplified NB (*Oncotarget* 2017;9:6416). Mitotic figures may be evident as well. These tumors are more likely to express vimentin, but are generally immunoreactive for chromogranin, synaptophysin, MAP2, and CD56 (e-**Fig. 26.27**).

d. *Stromal (schwannian) rich NBs* are represented by the two ganglioneuroblastic (GBN) subtypes, intermixed GBN and nodular GBN, and stromal predominant GN.

Intermixed GNB and GN have virtually identical gross features of a circumscribed, but nonencapsulated mass measuring up to 10 cm with a uniform, grayish-tan mucoid cut surface. In extra-adrenal sites, the periphery of the mass may blend into the formed, discrete capsule as in the case of a schwannoma but which is uncommon in GBNs and GN. Dystrophic calcifications are usually not apparent in the macroscopic examination, but may be noted in the microscopic findings. In order to fulfill the schwannian-rich designation, greater than 50% of the tumor should be composed of spindle cells whose features are those of a schwannoma (e-**Fig. 26.28**); these spindle cells are S-100 protein and collagen type IV immunoreactive. In both the case of an intermixed GNB and GN, the initial impression may be a schwannoma in the absence of the islands of dyssynchronous differentiation of neuroblasts to immature or dysplastic ganglion cells in the intermixed GNB, and differentiated ganglion cells in GN. Thorough sampling of these tumors is necessary to insure that the diffuse, stromal-rich neuroblastic tumor is fully characterized.

The second subtype of GNB is the nodular type which is recognized at gross examination as one or more nodules with hemorrhage and/or necrosis; these nodules are composed of poorly differentiated or differentiating NB which are surrounded by stromal dominant GN or stromal rich GNB (e-**Fig. 26.29**). The nodules should be assessed for their MKI.

e. *Stromal dominant neuroblastic tumor* or GN is an intermixed GNB without the islands of neuroblasts. These tumors are generally diagnosed in older children and into adulthood. In addition to the adrenal, GNs present in the retroperitoneum and posterior mediastinum. In the adrenal, GN measures 3 to 8 cm whereas in extra-adrenal sites, the tumors are larger at 8 to 20 cm. GN is a circumscribed, glistening, greyish to whitish-tan mass without any apparent capsule (e-**Fig. 26.30**). In the adrenal, GN is confined to the gland, but in extra-adrenal sites the tumor blends at least microscopically into the adjacent soft tissues, or on occasion enters into an intervertebral foramen like NBs. The ganglion cells are generally mature and are distributed irregularly in the schwannian stroma (e-**Fig. 26.31**). Scattered collections of lymphocytes and dystrophic calcifications may be seen.

f. *Molecular genetic abnormalities and prognosis* are correlative variables. Amplification *MYCN* is present in approximately 25% of NBs; it has been long appreciated that its presence is correlated with high-risk disease and an unfavorable prognosis. There is also the association of *MYCN* amplification with unfavorable histology which includes poorly differentiated stromal poor NB with high MKI with or without prominent nucleoli, undifferentiated NB with or without high MKI or nucleoli, and nodular GNB with high MKI nodules. Expression of CD44 correlates with nonamplified *MYCN* and low stage favorable outcome disease, whereas overexpression of ALK is associated with stromal poor differentiated NB and high stage NB. ALK-positive NBs may indicate the presence of heterozygous germline mutation in *ALK* as a susceptibility gene for familial NB; the other susceptibility gene is *PHOX 2B* (*Crit Rev Oncol/Hematol* 2016;107:163). There are numerous other favorable and unfavorable biomarkers and various chromosomal aberrations (+17q, −11q, −1p, −14q).

Risk assessment is a complex integrated process which takes into account the age at diagnosis (< or > 18 months), stage of the tumor, pathologic subtype, MKI (low or high) and *MYCN* nonamplified or amplified (Table 26.5). Undifferentiated NB and GNB, nodular with high MKI and amplified *MYCN,* are considered high risk tumors whereas GNB, intermixed and stromal dominant GN are regarded as low risk tumors.

The prognosis of a poorly differentiated NB is based on multiple factors: age, primary site, pathologic subtype, MKI, biologic markers, and stage of disease (localization and metastasis) (Table 26.5). Despite all of the pathologic and molecular refinements in the characterization of NBs, age (<1 year old) and pathologic stage remain the most significant determinants of outcome (*Pediatr Hematol Oncol* 2017;34:165; *Curr Pediatr Rev* 2018;14:73). Patients with extra-adrenal tumors tend to do better than those with adrenal-based NBs.

Neuroblastic tumors are categorized into favorable and unfavorable pathologic groups based on features that incorporate age at diagnosis, the MKI and *MYCN*. Tumors with favorable histopathology on the basis of histologic subtype and low

TABLE 26.5	International Neuroblastoma Pathology Committee Age-Linked Prognostic Classification	
Age Group	**Favorable Histology**	**Unfavorable Histology**
Any age	Ganglioneuroma Ganglioneuroblastoma, intermixed subtype, any MYCN	Neuroblastoma, undifferentiated subtype (any MKI), amplified (AMP)-MYCN
<18 months	Neuroblastoma, poorly differentiated with low or intermediate MKI, nonamplified (NA) MYCN Ganglioneuroblastoma, intermixed or nodular with low MKI, NA-MYCN	Neuroblastoma, poorly differentiated with high MKI, AMP-MYCN Neuroblastoma, differentiating with high MKI (>4% or 200/5,000 cells), AMP-MYCN Ganglioneuroblastoma, nodular, with undifferentiated or poorly differentiated nodules with high MKI
>18 months	Neuroblastoma, differentiating with low MKI, NA-MYCN Ganglioneuroblastoma, nodular, with differentiating nodule(s) with low MKI	Neuroblastoma, poorly differentiated (any MKI) Neuroblastoma, differentiating with intermediate or high MKI (>2% or >100/5,000 cells) Ganglioneuroblastoma, nodule, with undifferentiated or differentiating nodule(s) or nodule(s) with intermediate–high MKI
>5 years old		Neuroblastoma, any subtype ganglioneuroblastoma, nodular type

MKI have better outcomes. The molecular genetic markers associated with a poor prognosis are *MYCN* amplification and several chromosomal abnormalities (1p deletion, 14q deletion, 11q deletion, 17q gain) (*Cancer Genet* 2011;204:113).

g. *Posttreatment tumors* have features that can be seen in untreated neuroblastic tumors including necrosis of tumor cells with areas of hemorrhage, calcifications, and fibrosis. However, maturation of the neuroblastic component, with increased schwannian stroma and a shift along the spectrum from NB toward GN, are generally not seen in untreated tumors. The International Neuroblastoma Pathology Classification (INPC) does not apply to treated tumors so that a diagnosis of "neuroblastoma (or whatever the original classification) with treatment effect" should be rendered, and the histologic features enumerated; the treatment does not change the original favorable/unfavorable histology designation.

V. LESIONS OF THE EXTRA-ADRENAL PARAGANGLIOMA

A. Normal Anatomy and Histology. The extra-adrenal paraganglia are divided into two broad categories as they relate to the parasympathetic or sympathetic nervous system. The former are concentrated in the head and neck region with a close proximity to cranial nerves IX and XII and associated blood vessels, and are further divided into jugulotympanic, vagal, carotid body, laryngeal, and aorticopulmonary paraganglia. The aorticopulmonary paraganglia are distributed in parallel with the sympathetic nervous system along the paravertebral and para-aortic axis, and are further divided into cervical, intrathoracic, and intra-abdominal groups. Paraganglia are also found in the bladder, prostate, and gallbladder. All paraganglia have a similar composition of chief cells arranged in well-defined nests or Zellballen surrounded by peripheral sustentacular cells. Catecholamine concentrations tend to be higher in the sympathetic paraganglia (including the adrenal medulla). A greater proportion of sympathetic derived-PGLs are functional and noradrenergic (25% to 85% of cases) compared with those of parasympathetic origin (10% or less). Given the ubiquitous distribution of paraganglia, it is not surprising that these tumors present at diverse sites such as the cauda equina, skin, heart, and lung as some examples, and not a complete list. This group of tumors has either a germline or somatic mutation in one of 13 or more genes in 70% of cases (*Curr Opin Oncol* 2016;28:5).

B. **Extra-adrenal PGL** presents in a sporadic (70% to 75% of cases) or heredofamilial (25% to 30%) clinical setting, but in children it is almost always the latter with or without a PCC. Some of the various hereditary PGL syndromes are summarized in Table 26.4. In addition to PCC and PGLs in heredofamilial syndromes, they can be associated with RCC including the von Hippel-Lindau syndrome, SDHB-deficient syndrome, and several others (*Endocr Pract* 2017;28:253; *J Clin Endocrinol Metab* 2017;102:4013).

1. **Parasympathetic PGLs** have a predilection for the head and neck with an estimated incidence of 1:30,000 to 100,000. These tumors are found in association with cranial nerves IX and XII. Almost 60% of cases are carotid body tumors at the bifurcation of the internal and external carotid arteries. Other sites in the head and neck in approximate descending order of frequency are the glomus jugulare, glomus tympanicum (both of the latter in the middle ear), and the glomus vagale (which presents as a neck mass). The glomus jugulare arises in the adventitia of the jugular bulb (a dilated portion of the internal jugular vein at its origin at the jugular foramen) along the auricular branch of cranial nerve X (also known as Arnold's nerve) or the tympanic nerve (a branch of cranial nerve IX, also known as the nerve of Jacobson); the glomus tympanicum is contiguous with the tympanic nerve in the inferior temporal bone. Other less common sites in the head and neck include the larynx, paranasal sinus, salivary gland, orbit, and oral cavity. The thyroid and parathyroid rarely harbor PGLs.

   The carotid body tumor and glomus vagale are usually resected intact to reveal a firm to rubbery well-circumscribed mass with a fibrous pseudocapsule measuring 1 to 6 cm in greatest dimension. A greyish-tan to pale brownish surface is present on sectioning; focal hemorrhage may be seen. Groups of uniform pale staining tumor cells with finely granular nuclear chromatin are surrounded by a prominent and sometimes hemorrhagic fibrovascular network. Compressed spindle-shaped cells at the periphery of the cellular nests are S-100 protein positive sustentacular cells. There is typically more cellular pleomorphism, nuclear atypia, and hyperchromatism in PCC in contrast to PGLs, although individual case exceptions are acknowledged. Vascular invasion and infiltrative growth are unusual findings.

   There are some special problems associated with middle ear PGLs. These tumors are often submitted in a piecemeal fashion, and artifacts introduced during excision may yield an initial impression of a vascular tumor. Immunohistochemistry is helpful in establishing the diagnosis, and shows a phenotype of reactivity for chromogranin, synaptophysin, CD56, and focally for cyclin-D1 (*Otolaryngol Head Neck Surg* 2010; 143:531).

2. **Sympathetic (sympathoadrenal) PGLs** present in the abdomen-retroperitoneum in 80% or more of case, specifically the superior para-aortic region (45% of cases), region of the adrenal gland or renal hilum (10%), inferior para-aortic region (30%), and organ of Zuckerkandl or bladder (10%) (e-**Fig. 26.32**). The remaining 5% of cases are collectively reported in the gallbladder, kidney, urethra, prostate, spermatic cord, ovary, and vagina. Were the adrenal gland included in the discussion, it would be the most common site of "sympathetic PGL." Unlike the nonfunctional and infrequently metastasizing parasympathetic PGLs, sympathetic PGLs are more often malignant (25% to 65% of cases) with a metastatic potential in excess of that seen in PCCs (*J Clin Endocrinal Metab* 2011;96:717). In the absence of metastasis, many of the same problems exist in the reliable pathologic identification of a potentially malignant PGL as in the case of PCC (e-**Fig. 26.33**). Size (greater 100 g), confluent necrosis, mitotic and proliferative activity (Ki-67 index), absence of hyaline globules, and small cell morphology are some of the features that have been correlated with malignant behavior (*Histopathology* 2011;58:155).

3. **Gangliocytic PGL** usually arises in the periampullary portion of the duodenum, but is also rarely seen in the nasopharynx, lung, esophagus, mediastinum, pancreas, and

other intestinal sites (*Arch Pathol Lab Med* 2016;140:94). It occurs in patients over a wide age range as a solitary, polypoid mass that projects into the lumen from the ampulla of Vater and measures up to 7 cm in diameter. It is an infiltrative neoplasm with its epicenter in the submucosa, and is composed of three cell types in variable proportions, specifically spindle cells, epithelioid cells, and ganglion cells (**e-Fig. 26.34**). The spindle cells are elongated and have wavy nuclei resembling Schwannian cells, with S-100 and neurofilament immunopositivity; these cells can envelope the ganglion and epithelioid cells, analogous to sustentacular cells. The larger epithelioid cells are arranged in solid nests, ribbons, or pseudoglandular or papillary structures, and have neuroendocrine features including granular eosinophilic to amphophilic cytoplasm with uniform oval nuclei and finely stippled chromatin (**e-Fig. 26.35**); these cells express cytokeratin, chromogranin, and synaptophysin. The ganglion cells have atypical features, and there may be a morphologic continuum with the epithelioid cell population. In some cases, the ganglion cells may be inconspicuous. Recurrences are rare, but metastatic behavior is restricted to regional lymph nodes or liver.

VI. OTHER ADRENAL PARENCHYMAL LESIONS

A. **MYL** accounts for less than 5% of primary adrenal tumors and is commonly detected incidentally on imaging studies of the abdomen; however, these tumors are known to present in extra-adrenal sites (*Abdom Imaging* 2014;39:394). It is estimated that 10% of patients with CAH have a MYL (*Endocrine* 2018;59:7). These tumors can measure 20 cm or greater and weigh 2 kg, but the average size is 8 to 30 cm. A soft yellow to red-dish-brown cut surface is dependent on the volume of adipose tissue and hematopoietic elements. The usual microscopic appearance includes varying proportions of mature adipose tissue admixed with normal trilineage hematopoiesis (**e-Fig. 26.36**). Rarely, MYL contains a hematolymphoid neoplasm (*Am J Clin Pathol* 2018;150:406). Clonality has been demonstrated. Lipoma, AML, and liposarcoma are in the differential diagnosis.

B. **Adenomatoid Tumor,** like MYL, is usually detected as an incidentaloma. The tumor is well-circumscribed, solid or solid and cystic, and measures from 0.5 to 9 cm. Microscopically, the tumor is composed of tubules, cysts, papillary structures, and occasional solid sheets of low cuboidal cells (**e-Fig. 26.37**). The tumor cells may have cytoplasmic vacuoles with signet ring features (**e-Fig. 26.38**), but are mucicarmine negative for mucin. The tumor cells have the same immunophenotype as mesothelial cells with reactivity for vimentin, CK7, calretinin, and WT-1. The tumor is believed to arise from mesothelial inclusions within the adrenal gland. The main differential diagnoses include lymphangioma, metastatic carcinoma, and vascular tumors, especially epithelioid angiosarcoma.

C. **Mesenchymal Tumors** include lipoma, schwannoma, hemangioma, EBV-associated smooth muscle tumor, leiomyoma, leiomyosarcoma, angiosarcoma, perivascular epithelioid cell tumor, Ewing sarcoma-primitive neuroectodermal tumor, solitary fibrous tumor, and papillary endothelial hyperplasia.

D. **Lymphoma** is most commonly seen in previously diagnosed cases of non-Hodgkin lymphomas (NHL), and occurs in as many as 25% of cases at some point in the clinical course. Bilateral involvement is present in 75% to 80% of cases, and adrenal insufficiency is a known complication. Although primary adrenal lymphoma is uncommon, it is well-documented with diffuse large B-cell lymphoma as the most common pathologic type (*Ann Hematol* 2013;92:1583), although Burkitt lymphoma also occurs. Hodgkin lymphoma of the adrenal, even in case of secondary involvement, is rare.

E. **Sex Cord–Stromal Tumor** (SCST) of the adrenal and surrounding soft tissues is extremely rare and represents either adult-type granulosa cell tumor or LCT (*J Cytol* 2016;33:52; *Pathology* 2015;47:487). Considering the developmental relationship of the adrenal and gonad, the occurrence of a SCST in the adrenal is not entirely unexpected.

VII. ADRENAL CYSTS are relatively uncommon and are divided into four categories: parasitic cysts (7%), epithelial cysts (9%), pseudocysts (39%), and endothelial cysts (45%) (*Hum Pathol* 2013;44:1797).

A. **Pseudocysts** are discovered as another incidentaloma on CT imaging. The usual appearance is a well-defined cyst with water-like density and a median size of 6 to 10 cm in diameter. Pseudocysts are unilocular, are filled with yellow-brown to bloody amorphous semi-liquid material, and have a wall thickness of 1 to 5 mm. The densely hyalinized connective tissue of the wall may contain focal calcifications or even metaplastic bone formation, and entrapped cortical tissue may also be present. The smooth muscle in the wall of the cyst is continuous with the smooth muscle of the adrenal vein. An identifiable lining is absent. The differential diagnosis includes a cystic NB or PCC.

   B. Vascular Cysts are the most common type of adrenal cyst in some series (*Arch Pathol Lab Med* 2006;130:1722). Endothelial cysts are usually well circumscribed and multiloculated (**e-Fig. 26.39**). The endothelial cells are immunopositive for CD31, and if derived from lymphatic endothelium, then also positive for D2-40 (**e-Figs. 26.40**). Vascular malformations and lymphangiomas occur as other "vascular" lesions of the adrenal (*Hum Pathol* 2011;42:1013).

   C. Epithelial Cysts are divided into true glandular cysts and embryonal cysts (*World J Surg* 2006;30:1817), although in some classification schemes cystic adrenal tumors are also considered in the category of epithelial cysts. Mesothelial cysts also occur (*Endocr Pathol* 2008;19:203).

   D. Parasitic Cysts are a manifestation of echinococcal infection in the adrenal and retroperitoneum. The wall of the cyst is often calcified.

VIII. **METASTATIC NEOPLASMS** to the adrenal gland are second only to ACA as the most common adrenal tumor (*J Surg Oncol* 2014;109:31). Metastatic carcinoma is present in the adrenals in 25% to 30% of carcinoma-related deaths at autopsy. The lung is the most common primary site (adrenal metastases are found in 30% to 35% of cases) (**e-Fig. 26.41**) followed by the breast; other malignancies that frequently metastasize to the adrenals include adenocarcinomas of the kidney, stomach, and colon (**e-Fig. 26.42**); melanoma (10% to 15% or greater of cases) (**e-Fig. 26.43**); hepatocellular carcinoma; and urothelial carcinoma. RCC involves the adrenal by either direct extension from an upper pole tumor or metastasis in 5% to 10% of cases; metastatic RCC should always be differentiated from a primary adrenal cortical carcinoma. Other types of neoplasms arising in the retroperitoneum or as a metastasis to the adrenal can be differentiated in most cases by immunohistochemistry (Table 26.2).

Adrenal Gland Cytology

Cory Bernadt

I. **INTRODUCTION.** FNA is frequently used to evaluate adrenal gland mass lesions, and is performed under percutaneous CT and ultrasound guidance, or endoscopic ultrasound guidance for left adrenal lesions (*Diagn Cytopathol* 2005;33:26). FNA diagnosis of adrenal lesions has an accuracy of 98% and specificity of 100% (*Diagn Cytopathol* 1991;21:92). FNA biopsy of PCC is regarded as a relative contradiction due to possible induction of hypertensive crisis (*Radiology* 1986;159:733).

II. **SPECIFIC NEOPLASMS**

   A. MYL. The aspirate shows a mixture of mature adipose tissue and hematopoietic elements, including nucleated red blood cells, granulocytes and precursors, and megakaryocytes (*Acta Cytol* 1991;35:353).

   B. Adrenal Cortical Neoplasms. The distinction between adrenal cortical hyperplasia, ACA, adrenal cortical carcinoma, and normal adrenal cortical cells is not always possible in cytologic specimens. Radiologic correlation is essential.

   1. ACA yields moderately cellular smears that contain poorly cohesive sheets of epithelial cells with ill-defined and vacuolated cytoplasm, and abundant stripped small round uniform nuclei. Bubbly and vacuolated lipid background is prominent (**e-Fig. 26.44**). Scattered cells show nuclear atypia. Some cells may have cytoplasmic lipofuscin (*Diagn Cytopathol* 1999;21:92; *Acta Cytol* 1995;39:843; *Acta Cytol* 1998; 42:1352).

2. **Adrenal cortical carcinoma** yields richly cellular aspirates. It consists of more frequent single cells that have marked nuclear atypia, intact granular cytoplasm, eccentric nuclei, and necrosis (**e-Fig. 26.45**). The cytologic diagnosis of a well-differentiated adrenal cortical carcinoma is difficult (*Acta Cytol* 1997;41:385).

C. **PCC.** The cytomorphology shows similarity to that of other neuroendocrine tumors. The aspirate contains abundant isolated and loose clusters of malignant cells with intervening vasculature (**e-Fig. 26.46**). The isolated polygonal or spindle shaped cells exhibit poorly defined fragile cytoplasm and fine granular salt-and-pepper chromatin (**e-Fig. 26.47**). Red cytoplasmic granules can be seen on Romanowsky-type stains (*Acta Cytol* 1999;43:207).

D. **Metastatic Malignancy.** The most common malignancies metastatic to the adrenal are adenocarcinoma of the lung or breast (**e-Fig. 26.48**). The confirmation of metastasis is straightforward given a known malignant history. It is important to integrate clinical, laboratory, radiologic, cytologic, and immunocytochemical findings to differentiate primary neoplasms from metastasis (*Acta Cytol* 1995;39:843).

ACKNOWLEDGMENT

The author thanks Jing Zhai, an author of the previous edition of this chapter.

SUGGESTED READINGS

Brodeur GM, Hogarty MD, Bagatell R, Mosse YP, Marris JM. Neuroblastoma. In: Pizzo PA, Poplack DG, eds. *Principles and Practice of Pediatric Oncology*. 7th ed. Philadelphia, PA: Wolters Kluwer; 2016;30:772–797.

Hicks KJ, Cipriani N, Pytel P, Shimada H. The pineal, pituitary, parathyroid, thyroid and adrenal glands. In: Husain AN, Stocker JT, Dehner LP, eds. *Stocker & Dehner's Pediatric Pathology*, 4th ed. Philadelphia, PA: Wolter Kluwer; 2016:979–1011.

Lloyd RV, Osamura RY, Kloppel G, Rosai J, eds. *WHO Classification of Tumours of Endocrine Organs*. 4th ed. Lyon, France: IARC Press; 2017.

Lloyd RV, ed. *Endocrine Pathology: Differential Diagnosis and Molecular Advances*. 2nd ed. New York: Springer Publishing Company; 2010.

Nose V. *Diagnostic Pathology: Endocrine*. 2nd ed. Philadelphia, PA: Elsevier; 2019.

Rudzinski ER, Jarzembowski JA, Reyes-Mugica M, Sebire N, Shimada H. College of American Pathologists: protocol for the examination of specimens from patients with neuroblastoma. August 2016. https://cap.objects.frb.io/protocols/cp-pediatric-neuroblastoma-16protocol-3103.pdf.

27 Pituitary Gland
Richard J. Perrin

I. NORMAL ANATOMY AND HISTOLOGY. The pituitary gland (hypophysis, or "undergrowth") is located at the base of the brain, beneath the hypothalamus, within the sella turcica of the sphenoid bone. The smaller, posterior lobe of the pituitary contains the neurohypophysis (pars nervosa), which is connected to the hypothalamus via the pituitary stalk, or infundibulum ("little funnel"). Associated with the pituitary stalk is the infundibular portion (pars tuberalis) of the adenohypophysis. The other portions of the adenohypophysis form the anterior lobe (pars distalis) and vestigial intermediate lobe (pars intermedia); the latter contains remnants of Rathke's cleft (gland-like cystic spaces).

Histologically, on hematoxylin and eosin (H&E) stained sections, normal adenohypophysis (e-Fig. 27.1) is composed of three different cell types: acidophils (producing growth hormone [GH] or prolactin [PRL]), basophils (producing adrenocorticotrophic hormone [ACTH], thyroid stimulating hormone [TSH], luteinizing hormone [LH], and follicle stimulating hormone [FSH]), and chromophobes (hypogranulated acidophils and basophils); all are arranged in an acinar pattern. The acini are demarcated by a delicate fibrovascular stroma best visualized by histochemical reticulin stains. Although each acinus contains a mixed population of these cell types, the composition varies regionally. Acidophils dominate the lateral portions, basophils (ACTH and TSH) dominate the medial portions, and basophilic gonadotrophs (LH and FSH) are distributed uniformly. Occasionally with aging, basophils extend into the neurohypophysis; this phenomenon, termed "basophilic invasion," should not be misinterpreted as an infiltrating neoplasm. The posterior pituitary is composed of axons, axon terminals, and, sometimes, axonal swellings (spheroids) called Herring bodies, which contain vasopressin and oxytocin. Specialized glial cells (true "pituicytes") accompany the axons; these are generally considered to be the cells of origin for the related benign tumors pituicytoma and choristoma (granular cell tumor). Ectopic pituitary tissue can be found in the nasal cavity, sphenoid sinus, or rarely, within ovarian teratomas.

II. INTRAOPERATIVE EVALUATION AND TISSUE HANDLING. Intraoperative evaluations are frequently requested for pituitary neoplasms, most often to confirm the clinical diagnosis of pituitary adenoma. Although frozen sections usually provide adequate information to make an intraoperative diagnosis, a small (1 mm³) amount of tissue should be used for cytologic examination. Intraoperative cytologic smears or "touch preps" lack freezing artifacts that obscure nuclear details (e-Fig. 27.2); thus, they provide extremely valuable complementary information at the time of frozen section. Likewise, ample tissue should be reserved for paraffin embedding, free from freezing artifacts, to preserve antigenicity and morphologic features that might otherwise be compromised. This point is particularly important in the evaluation of a smaller microadenoma, which can easily be "lost" or exhausted through cavalier intraoperative processing. Finally, a small (1 mm³) amount of tissue should be reserved for ultrastructural examination; tissue fixed directly in 3% glutaraldehyde and embedded in plastic will retain fine structural features that cannot be recovered from formalin-fixed, paraffin-embedded tissue.

III. NONNEOPLASTIC LESIONS

    A. Pituitary Hyperplasia. Diffuse expansion of pituitary acini, best evaluated on reticulin-stained sections, is the histologic hallmark of pituitary hyperplasia. However, this diagnosis is often difficult to render with certainty. Nodular expansion of acini with one single hormonal cell type is noted in a variety of clinical scenarios, including pregnancy and estrogen therapy. It is also important to be cognizant of the naturally heterogeneous composition of the anterior pituitary, which favors acidophils laterally and basophils medially.

B. **Pituitary Apoplexy** (e-**Fig. 27.3.**). Spontaneous hemorrhage and infarction of the nonneoplastic pituitary or a pituitary neoplasm may represent a surgical emergency (in the setting of increased intracranial pressure, subarachnoid hemorrhage, or visual disturbance). For diagnosis of an underlying tumor in a partially necrotic specimen, a reticulin stain may prove more reliable than immunohistochemistry; immunohistochemistry should usually also be performed, but is often difficult to interpret in this setting.

C. **Lymphocytic Hypophysitis** is a rare autoimmune disorder of the adenohypophysis that progressively destroys the gland, resulting in panhypopituitarism. The posterior hypophysis may also be affected, resulting in diabetes insipidus. Lymphocytic hypophysitis occurs with greater frequency in pregnant or postpartum women. Subsets of patients also have other associated autoimmune disorders. Microscopically, the anterior pituitary demonstrates lymphoplasmacytic infiltrates *without* granuloma formation. The resulting glucocorticoid deficiency is often fatal if untreated.

D. **Granulomatous Hypophysitis.** This rare autoimmune disorder expands and selectively destroys the anterior pituitary with well-formed, noncaseating granulomas and a mild lymphocytic infiltrate. Radiologically, this condition may mimic adenoma, but it also often involves the thyroid, adrenals, and testes. Unlike lymphocytic hypophysitis, it shows no association with pregnancy.

E. **Rathke's Cleft Cyst** (e-**Fig. 27.4**) is a developmental abnormality that arises between the anterior and posterior lobes or in the infundibular stalk. Smaller examples are often detected incidentally. Lesions larger than 1 cm are usually symptomatic (e.g., cause hypopituitarism or visual disturbance related to compression of the optic chiasm). The cyst is lined by cuboidal to columnar epithelium that may or may not be ciliated, and may or may not contain goblet cells. Focally, the epithelium may show flattening and/or squamous metaplasia. The cyst contents are variably serous or mucoid. Xanthogranulomatous inflammation may be present in cysts that have undergone prior hemorrhage. Surgical resection is curative.

F. **Other.** Rarely, in the setting of hypopituitarism, only xanthogranulomatous inflammation is identified; such a finding may simply represent overwhelming reactive changes within a craniopharyngioma or Rathke's cleft cyst, but an entity "xanthogranuloma of the sellar region," generally restricted to the sella, has also been described. The pituitary may also become involved by systemic histiocytic disorders, such as Langerhans cell histiocytosis (LCH), Rosai–Dorfman disease, Erdheim–Chester disease, and xanthoma disseminatum. LCH, in particular, may involve the sellar/suprasellar region more often than is generally appreciated; diabetes insipidus is a common manifestation.

IV. **BENIGN NEOPLASMS**

A. **Pituitary Adenoma** is, by far, the most common sellar neoplasm. Tumors <1 cm are typically identified as microadenomas; those >1 cm, as macroadenomas; and those >4 cm, as giant adenomas. Microadenomas are most often functional (hormone producing), which explains why they draw clinical attention before reaching larger sizes. Nonfunctional tumors, which account for one-third of all adenomas, grow to a large size before drawing clinical attention. Often, large tumors produce so-called stalk effect, in which mild to moderate elevations of PRL hormone result from compression of the infundibular stalk, which blocks the transport of dopamine (formerly, PRL inhibitory factor) from the hypothalamus. Some macroadenomas may compress the normal pituitary tissue and cause panhypopituitarism. In many cases, macroadenomas are detected only after they compress the optic chiasm, producing bitemporal hemianopsia or other vision disturbance. Approximately half of nonfunctioning adenomas are referred to as **null cell adenomas**. These chromophobic (or less commonly, oncocytic) tumors have negative hormonal and transcription factor immunoprofiles despite showing reactivity for synaptophysin, and exhibit few, if any, secretory granules on ultrastructural analysis (oncocytic adenomas show abundant mitochondria). Although some null cell adenomas appear to express the alpha subunit of the glycoprotein hormones (LH, FSH, and TSH) and thus might be considered "silent" gonadotrophic or thyrotrophic adenomas, expression of the alpha subunit has also been documented in somatotroph adenomas (*Neurol Res* 1999;21:247), so this feature may have limited specificity.

Microscopically, adenomas lack the normal reticulin-rich acinar structure of the adenohypophysis. Instead, they may appear patternless, pseudorosette-rich, papillary, endocrine/organoid, or paraganglioma-like, and may focally form glands. In ambiguous cases, a reticulin stain may be useful for accentuating loss of acinar architecture. Adenoma tumor cells are typically larger than their nonneoplastic counterparts and have round-to-oval nuclei, delicate stippled ("salt and pepper") chromatin, and small or inconspicuous nucleoli. Occasionally, adenomas exhibit moderate to marked cytologic atypia, but this feature is not associated with aggressive behavior unless accompanied by elevated mitotic and/or proliferation indices (see below). Cytoplasmic quality varies within and among different adenoma (hormonal) sub-types, and may even vary among cells within an individual tumor, particularly in some (plurihormonal) tumors that secrete more than one hormone. Historically, a combination of cytologic, histochemical, and ultrastructural features have been and still can be used to subtype adenomas. However, immunohistochemical profiles of hormone expression and cell proliferation are now in widespread use for this purpose, and some centers are additionally using immunohistochemical transcription factor profiling (including PIT1, ER-alpha, GATA2, TPIT, and SF1) to classify adenomas. Nevertheless, familiarity with histomorphologic and histochemical features remains important.

For example, the presence of calcium and amyloid bodies, though rare, are clues for prolactinoma. In prolactinoma treated with dopamine agonists, fibrosis and smaller cells with high nuclear to cytoplasmic (N/C) ratios are common. Perivascular pseudorosettes usually indicate a gonadotrophic or null cell adenoma (e-**Fig. 27.5**). Deposits of Crooke's hyaline (ringlike cytoplasmic cytokeratin inclusions) are most commonly accumulated in nonneoplastic corticotropic cells in patients with hypercortisolism of any cause, but can also occur in a small subset of corticotroph adenomas (discussed below). Strong periodic acid–Schiff (PAS) staining suggests a corticotroph adenoma, whereas weak PAS positivity is seen in glycoprotein (FSH, LH, and TSH expressing) adenomas. Round, weakly eosinophilic, cytokeratin positive, paranuclear "fibrous bodies" in a relatively chromophobic tumor most often indicate a GH-producing adenoma (sparsely granulated subtype) (e-**Fig. 27.6**). In practice, of course, a combination of clinical, radiologic, and histologic features is used to subtype pituitary adenomas into useful categories.

B. Prolactinoma. Also called lactotroph adenoma, prolactinoma comes to clinical attention most commonly in women of reproductive age with amenorrhea and galactorrhea. Men with prolactinoma are usually asymptomatic or present with decreased libido, until the tumor grows to large size. Patients with prolactinoma are often treated medically with a dopamine agonist (e.g., bromocriptine) to impair adenoma cell growth and inhibit PRL production, but such agents are not cytotoxic. Tumors resected posttherapy usually show interstitial fibrosis, reduced cell size, and high N/C ratio, and may be reminiscent of small cell carcinoma (e-**Fig. 27.7**). However, they are usually positive for PIT1 and ER-alpha, at least focally positive for PRL, and display a low mitotic/proliferative index.

C. Corticotroph (ACTH-Producing) Adenoma. Corticotroph adenomas present most often as microadenomas, and account for 20% of all pituitary adenomas. These tumors, which may be as small as 1 or 2 mm, can be difficult to localize radiographically and intraoperatively. In such cases, a surgeon might employ inferior petrosal sinus sampling to evaluate lateralization and monitor the progress of resection. Even under these circumstances, exhaustive microscopic evaluation of the pathology specimen (examining multiple levels using reticulin and immunohistochemical stains) may yield no diagnostic findings. Fortunately, a postoperative drop in the patient's serum ACTH level may serve as evidence that the tumor was removed. Most ACTH adenomas are amphophilic-to-basophilic, deeply PAS positive, and arise in the central region of the gland where non-neoplastic corticotropic cells are concentrated. Crooke's hyaline, appearing as glassy eosinophilic cytoplasmic inclusions that ring the nucleus, results from hypercortisolism and represents an accumulation of cytokeratin filaments already present in corticotrophs (e-**Fig. 27.8**). Rare ACTH adenomas that exhibit Crooke's hyaline are called Crooke's adenoma. Other ACTH adenomas that show immunoreactivity for ACTH but do not secrete biologically significant amounts of the hormone and do not induce Cushing's syndrome are termed "silent corticotroph adenomas." Such tumors are more common in men, tend to be invasive, and do not come to clinical attention until they become large (macroadenomas). All these subtypes show nuclear immunoreactivity for TPIT.

D. **Somatotroph (GH Cell) Adenoma.** This subgroup of pituitary adenomas includes tumors with exclusive GH production (GH positive, PIT1 positive, ER-alpha negative, and PAS negative), tumors producing GH and PRL (mammosomatotroph adenomas with bifunctional cells, and mixed somatotroph and lactotroph adenomas with two cell types; both are immunopositive for PIT1 and ER-alpha), and plurihormonal adenomas (most positive for GH, PRL, TSH, PIT1, and other variable transcription factors). Somatotroph adenomas (e-**Fig. 27.9**) usually appear either intensely eosinophilic (densely granulated subtype, with abundant secretory granules visualized by electron microscopy) or chromophobic (sparsely granulated subtype), and show correspondingly strong or weak GH immunoreactivity. Aiding diagnosis, the chromophobic, sparsely granulated somatotroph adenoma (SGSA) cells often contain weakly eosinophilic, cytokeratin (CAM 5.2) reactive, paranuclear whorls known as fibrous bodies (e-**Fig. 27.6**). This distinction is important, as SGSAs have a relatively unfavorable clinical course and relative resistance to somatostatin (GH-inhibiting hormone) analogues such as octreotide. Particularly when resection is incomplete, treatment with GH receptor antagonists may be required; the systemic effects of somatotropic adenomas (acromegaly in adults, gigantism in adolescents) are mediated by insulin-like growth factor-1 (IGF-1), produced in the liver in response to GH. These tumors may appear in the setting of Carney's complex, McCune–Albright syndrome, familial isolated pituitary adenoma, and multiple endocrine neoplasia I (MEN I).

E. **Gonadotroph Adenomas** are more common in males and in the middle-aged and older. They are often nonfunctioning, and grow to a very large size before coming to clinical attention by compressing adjacent structures; invasion can occur, but is relatively less common in this subtype. Histologically, these tumors are usually chromophobic and often feature pseudorosettes, papillary architecture, or organoid features. Immunohistochemically, these tumors exhibit markedly variable reactivity for the beta subunits of LH and FSH, for their common α subunits, and for transcription factors SF1, GATA2, and ER-alpha.

F. **Thyrotroph Adenoma,** accounting for <2% of pituitary adenomas, may come to attention by causing hyperthyroidism. Examples without functional TSH production ("silent" thyrotroph adenomas) usually present at larger sizes, but invasion of adjacent structures is fairly common independent of hormone secretion. The cells of thyrotroph adenomas are usually chromophobic, and variably polygonal or somewhat spindled, with some nuclear pleomorphism. Thyrotroph adenomas are immunoreactive for PIT1 and GATA2, and a majority also silently co-expresses GH and PRL. In cases with incomplete resection, somatostatin analogues are often effective in reducing TSH secretion.

G. **Pituicytoma** ("infundibular astrocytoma"). This rare benign tumor is thought to arise from the specialized glial cells of the posterior pituitary. Radiographically, it shows strong postcontrast enhancement. Histologically, it exhibits a solid growth pattern and is formed by plump, spindled tumor cells arranged in short, interlacing fascicles. Rosenthal fibers and eosinophilic granular bodies are not present. Strong reactivity for Vimentin, S100, and TTF-1 (nuclear pattern), patchy reactivity for GFAP, and no reactivity for cytokeratins, synaptophysin, and neurofilament have been described (*J Neuropathol Exp Neurol* 2009;68:482). Mitotic figures are uncommon.

H. **Granular Cell Tumor of the Neurohypophysis** (GCT, choristoma). Like pituicytoma, this tumor is thought to derive from pituicytes; some consider these two tumors to be phenotypic variants. Although minute asymptomatic examples are quite common, larger symptomatic GCTs are relatively rare; the latter appear in the fifth or sixth decade with female predominance and commonly present as an enhancing sellar/suprasellar mass compressing the optic chiasm. Histologically, these tumors are formed by closely apposed polygonal cells with small nuclei and generous granular eosinophilic cytoplasm. Spindled/fascicular areas may also be present. Lymphocytic infiltrates are common and may be robust. Staining with PAS is resistant to diastase digestion. Immunoreactivity is strong for S100 and TTF-1, and variable for the lysosomal marker CD68; reactivity for pituitary hormones, synaptophysin, cytokeratins, neurofilament, and chromogranin A is not observed. Ultrastructurally, these cells show abundant phagolysosomes and no evidence of neurosecretory granules.

I. **Craniopharyngiomas** are discussed in detail in Chapter 39.

V. LOW-GRADE NEOPLASMS

A. **Aggressive ("Atypical") Pituitary Adenoma.** Beginning in 2004, the modifier "atypical" was applied to pituitary adenomas with nuclear immunoreactivity for proliferation marker Ki-67/MIB-1 in >3% of tumor cells and extensive nuclear immunoreactivity for p53; the term could also be applied to adenomas with Ki-67 labeling >10%, regardless of p53 status (*Neuroendocrinology* 2006;83:179). Relative to benign adenomas, these tumors were considered more likely to invade adjacent structures and to recur, but correlation of histology with clinical outcomes has been unsatisfactory. Currently, the WHO 2016 classification (Louis DN, Ohgaki H, Wiestler OD, Cavenee WK. *World Health Organization Histological Classification of Tumours of the Central Nervous System.* IARC Press. 2016) recommends that application of the word "atypical" be discontinued for tumors that meet the 2004 criteria. Instead, a descriptive phrase such as "**with aggressive features**" is favored, perhaps with a comment that adenomas with such features warrant close investigation and monitoring.

Of note, independent of mitotic/proliferative indices, the WHO 2016 classification system also emphasizes the relatively **aggressive clinical behavior of several pituitary adenoma subtypes**, specifically silent corticotroph adenoma, Crooke cell adenoma, SGSA, lactotroph adenoma (in men), and **plurihormonal PIT1-positive adenoma (silent subtype 3 adenoma).**

VI. HIGH-GRADE NEOPLASMS

A. **Pituitary Carcinoma** is a very rare neoplasm that cannot be diagnosed by its innate appearance or any known markers; instead, it is diagnosed by the presence of craniospinal or extracranial metastases. The Ki-67/MIB-1 and p53 labeling indices are typically high, but cytologic and histologic features are often benign. These tumors are usually functional, secreting PRL or ACTH. Its designation as a high-grade neoplasm may be inappropriate in the truest sense, but the term is applied to reflect its more aggressive clinical behavior.

ACKNOWLEDGMENT

The author thanks Sushama Patil and Arie Perry, authors of the previous edition of this chapter.

Reproductive Tract

Testis and Paratestis

Dengfeng Cao and Peter A. Humphrey

I. NORMAL ANATOMY. The normal adult testis is an ovoid paired organ, measuring 4.5 × 2.5 × 3 cm, and weighing approximately 20 g. The testes are suspended within scrotal sacs by spermatic cords. The testis is covered by a capsule composed of an outer tunica vaginalis lined by mesothelium, the collagenous tunica albuginea, and the inner tunica vasculosa. The tunica vaginalis forms a sac filled with serous fluid. The posterior portion of the testis not covered by a capsule is called the mediastinum and contains blood vessels, nerves, lymphatics, and the extratesticular rete testis.

The testicular parenchyma is subdivided into approximately 250 lobules containing seminiferous tubules separated by fibrous septae. The terminal portions of the seminiferous tubules drain into the tubuli recti that connect to the tubules of the rete testis at the mediastinum. The tubules of the rete testis anastomose with the ductuli efferentes, which form the head of the epididymis and empty into the vas deferens, which traverses the inguinal canal as a component of the spermatic cord. The testicular artery arises from the aorta and is the major source of vascular supply to the testes. The venous drainage occurs through numerous small veins that form a convoluted mass known as the pampiniform plexus that surrounds the testicular artery. These small veins anastomose to form the right testicular vein, which drains into the inferior vena cava, and two left testicular veins, which drain into the left renal vein.

Histologically, prepubertal and postpubertal seminiferous tubules are quite different. Prepubertal tubules are small, with few or no lumina, and contain mostly Sertoli cells with a few primordial germ cells (e-**Fig. 28.1**). Postpubertal seminiferous tubules are larger and harbor Sertoli cells and germ cells at varying stages of maturation ranging from spermatogonia, primary spermatocytes, secondary spermatocytes, spermatids, and spermatozoa (e-**Fig. 28.2**). Within the seminiferous tubules, the least mature germ cells—spermatogonia—are present along the basement membrane, while the most mature cells—elongate spermatids—are found at the luminal border. Primary and secondary spermatocytes are found in an adluminal position. The Sertoli cells abut the basement membrane and are aligned perpendicular to the membrane; their nuclei are round to oval with prominent nucleoli, and the cytoplasm has Charcot–Bottcher crystals which can occasionally be seen by light microscopy.

The interstitial tissue between the seminiferous tubules contains Leydig cells, vessels, and connective tissue. Leydig cells are arranged singly and in clusters (e-**Fig. 28.3**), and can be associated with nerves. They are large and irregularly spherical to polyhedral, with small spherical nuclei and abundant acidophilic cytoplasm. The cytoplasm can exhibit lipofuscin and rod-shaped Reinke crystals.

II. GROSS EXAMINATION, TISSUE SAMPLING, AND HISTOLOGIC SLIDE PREPARATION. Tissue samples of the testes received for surgical pathologic examination include testicular biopsies, and unilateral and bilateral orchiectomy specimens. Retroperitoneal lymph node dissection can be performed as part of a staging maneuver for testicular cancer.

A. Fine Needle Aspiration of the Testis in infertile patients (with sperm aspiration and cytopathologic examination) is occasionally performed. Cytologic touch imprints or wet preparations may be made at the time of open testicular biopsy in infertile patients to rapidly identify the presence of sperm. The role of cytology in the evaluation of testicular tumors is limited to diagnosis of lymph node metastases by fine needle aspiration. Although seminomas can usually be differentiated from nonseminomatous tumors, subtyping of nonseminomatous tumors cannot be reliably performed by cytology.

B. Testicular Biopsies, which can be open or percutaneous, are typically performed for evaluation of infertility. They are usually contraindicated in the evaluation of solid testicular masses, with the possible exception of epidermoid cysts which can be removed by excisional biopsy. Testicular biopsy specimens are usually received in Bouin's fixative. An accurate documentation of the number and size of the biopsy fragments and exact site(s) of the biopsy for each container should be made during gross dictation. The biopsy fragments should be inked with hematoxylin to facilitate identification during embedding, wrapped in lens paper, placed between sponges, and processed entirely. Three hematoxylin and eosin (H&E)-stained slides, each with three to four serial sections, should be prepared from each block.

C. Unilateral Simple Orchiectomy is performed in cases of testicular torsion. Gross examination of the testis similar to that for tumor cases should be performed. One section of the testicular parenchyma in relation to the capsule, and a section each of the epididymis and spermatic cord, should be submitted; description and sampling of focal lesions should also be performed.

D. Radical Orchiectomy is performed for testicular tumors. The specimen consists of the testis and paratesticular organs (surrounding tunica vaginalis, epididymis, soft tissue, and a segment of spermatic cord). In cases of tumor resection, the specimen should ideally be sent fresh and intact to the surgical pathology laboratory for immediate gross examination. Alternatively, when delay is anticipated, the specimen is placed in 10% buffered formalin and sent intact. In such cases, tumor morphology is often suboptimal due to poor fixation. The surgeon may occasionally bisect the specimen to aid fixation; this approach is not recommended as it prevents evaluation of involvement of the tunica by the tumor, as well as procurement of fresh tissue for ancillary studies.

The specimen is weighed, and measurements are recorded in three dimensions. The length and diameter of the resected segment of spermatic cord are noted separately. The external surfaces of the testis and spermatic cord are examined for involvement by tumor. The proximal shave resection margin of the spermatic cord is submitted in a separate cassette, and then the cord is then serially sectioned and inspected for tumor involvement; representative sections are submitted proximal to distal. The tunica vaginalis is opened anteriorly to show the tunica albuginea; presence of fluid, if any, within the sac is noted. The testis is then bisected anteroposteriorly through the epididymis, and serial sections are made parallel to this plane. Each slice is examined, and the tumor is described in relation to the epididymis and the tunica albuginea. The size, color, and consistency of the tumor should be noted. Foci of hemorrhage, necrosis, and variegation, as well as multifocality, if present, should be described. Photographs or digital images should be taken and tissue procured for tumor bank and ancillary studies such as flow cytometry and karyotyping, if necessary. The specimen should then be fixed overnight in an adequate amount of 10% buffered formalin before submission of one section per centimeter of tumor. Representative sections should include heterogeneous areas and sections of tumor in relation to uninvolved parenchyma, epididymis, and tunica albuginea. One section of grossly normal-appearing parenchyma should be included. If correlation of identified histologic tumor type with serum markers (alpha-fetoprotein [AFP] and human chorionic gonadotropin [hCG]) is not achieved, additional sections should be submitted (note that such correlation will not always be perfect because metastatic deposits may harbor different elements than the primary tumor).

E. **Retroperitoneal Lymph Node Dissection** is performed as a separate procedure. The specimen is received in 10% buffered formalin. During gross examination the tissue fragments should be measured in aggregate and carefully dissected to harvest as many lymph nodes as possible, and the size of the largest and the smallest putative nodes should be noted. Possible foci of tumor encountered during dissection should be measured and sampled. An effort should be made to sample any area(s) suspicious for viable tumor.

F. **Bilateral Orchiectomy Specimens** may be submitted as part of treatment of carcinoma of the prostate. Gross examination and sectioning are similar to that for unilateral simple orchiectomy. Prostate cancer is rarely encountered within these specimens.

III. DIAGNOSTIC FEATURES OF BENIGN DISEASES OF THE TESTIS

A. **Congenital Abnormalities**

1. **Cryptorchidism** is maldescent of the testis in which the testis is found, after 1 year of age, to be located high in the scrotum, within the inguinal canal, or in an intra-abdominal location. It is seen in 1% of males and it is unilateral in 80% of cases. Grossly, the prepubertal undescended testis differs little from normal, but after puberty the undescended testis is smaller. Histologically, there is a progressive loss of germ cells with age, along with decreased size of seminiferous tubules and increased thickness of tubular tunica propria. Sertoli cell nodules (e-**Fig. 28.4**), which are foci of tubules containing immature Sertoli cells and laminated calcific deposits, are often seen in cryptorchid testes. These are likely hyperplastic foci, although they have also been termed tubular adenoma of Pick. Rarely, Sertoli cell nodules can present as a mass (*Am J Surg Pathol* 2010;23:1874). Prominent Leydig cells are seen between seminiferous tubules and sometimes within the tubules. The major complications of cryptorchidism are infertility and germ cell neoplasia, ranging from germ cell neoplasia in situ (GCNIS) to invasive germ cell tumors, particularly seminoma, embryonal carcinoma (EC), and EC/teratoma. The risk of developing germ cell tumor is higher in the abdominal testis than inguinal testis. For patients >1 year of age, PLAP and CD117 immunostains can be useful in highlighting intratubular germ cell neoplastic cells.

2. **Anorchism and polyorchidism** are absence of testes and more than two testes, respectively. Testicular regression (vanishing testis) syndrome refers to a condition characterized by a rudimentary epididymis and spermatic cord with no identifiable testicular tissue.

3. **In testicular-splenic fusion**, encapsulated splenic tissue is found adjacent to the left testis, which can show germ cell aplasia in the seminiferous tubules.

4. **Adrenal cortical rests** are usually incidental, millimeter-sized nodules of adrenal cortical tissue that are detected along the pathway of descent of the testis, including along the spermatic cord and testis.

B. **Infertility.** The causes of infertility may be pretesticular, which include endocrine disorders involving the pituitary and adrenal glands; testicular, including genetic disorders; or posttesticular, which are mainly obstructive and include varicocele and cystic fibrosis. The evaluation of the patient includes a detailed clinical history, physical examination, semen analysis, tests of endocrine function, analysis of sperm function, and serology for antisperm antibody. Testicular biopsy (preferably open biopsy) is indicated in cases where an endocrine dysfunction has been ruled out. Biopsies from patients with azoospermia may show germ cell aplasia (Sertoli cell only) (e-**Fig. 28.5**), maturation arrest (e-**Fig. 28.6**), and/or normal spermatogenesis that points to an obstructive etiology (*Arch Pathol Lab Med* 2010;134:1197). Patients with oligospermia show a combination of one or more of the following: tubular hyalinization, fibrosis, hypospermatogenesis, normal or arrested spermatogenesis, and sloughing or disorganization. Although testicular biopsies are rarely performed in cases of endocrine dysfunction, the findings include small tubules with fibrosis and basement membrane thickening, and Leydig cell aplasia or hyperplasia. Synoptic-style reporting of testicular biopsies for infertility is described in Table 28.1.

TABLE 28.1	Reporting Infertility Biopsies

1. Method of obtaining sample
   a. Percutaneous testis sperm aspiration
   b. Incisional testis sperm extraction
   c. Orchiectomy/other
2. Presence/absence of testicular tissue
3. Seminiferous tubules
   a. Number
   b. Tunica propria: Normal/thickened
   c. Mean number of mature spermatids/tubule (count 20 tubules)
   d. Most advanced stage of spermatogenesis
   e. Sertoli cells: Present/absent
4. Interstitium
   a. Leydig cells: Present/absent/hyperplastic
   b. Amount of interstitial inflammation
   c. Presence of macrophages and mast cells
5. Extratesticular/Other comments
   a. Epididymis: Present/absent
   b. Vas deferens: Present/absent
   c. Immunohistochemical/special stains
6. Histologic diagnoses
   a. The most advanced histologic pattern is:
   b. The predominant histologic pattern is:

C. Inflammation and Infection

1. Epididymitis is typically more common and severe than orchitis, and is commonly related to urinary tract infection (from the urinary bladder, urethra, or prostate) by *Chlamydia, Neisseria, Escherichia coli,* or *Pseudomonas.* Tissue sampling is not needed for the diagnosis of orchitis and/or epididymitis.

2. Most cases of **orchitis** are due to infection that spreads from the vas deferens and epididymis. Infectious agents that can cause orchitis include bacteria, mycobacteria, fungi, viruses, or spirochetes.

   a. Tuberculous orchitis always emanates from another site and spreads into the testis from the epididymis or bloodstream. Both testes are usually involved. The testicular inflammatory infiltrate varies from nonspecific to caseating granulomas.

   b. Mumps orchitis is caused by a paramyxovirus. Microscopically, there is an initial interstitial lymphocytic inflammatory infiltrate, followed by a mixed infiltrate that can result in tubular atrophy and peritubular fibrosis.

   c. Syphilitic orchitis occurs prior to infection of the epididymis. Histologically, peritubular lymphocytes and plasma cells can be seen along with obliterative endarteritis and perivascular plasma cells. Gummas can form an intratesticular mass with central necrosis.

   d. Other types of orchitis include nonspecific granulomatous orchitis and malakoplakia. Before diagnosing nonspecific granulomatous orchitis, a specific infectious orchitis, sarcoidosis, lymphoma, and exuberant granulomatous inflammation associated with a germ cell neoplasm should be excluded.

D. Vascular Disorders

1. Systemic vasculitis can affect the testis, but isolated vasculitis involving only the testis is rare. Testicular vasculitis can cause infarction that clinically simulates a neoplasm. Most cases of testicular vasculitis are characterized by polyarteritis nodosa-like changes in small to medium-sized arteries, with transmural necrotizing inflammation (*Urology* 2011;77:1043).

2. Varicocele is an abnormal dilatation and tortuosity of veins of the pampiniform plexus of the spermatic cord.

3. Torsion and infarction generally occur in young men and in the setting of abnormal testicular descent. Initially there is congestion, edema, and hemorrhage, followed by hemorrhagic infarction (e-**Fig. 28.7**).

E. Atrophy can be caused by many factors including cryptorchidism, infection, chemoradiation, liver cirrhosis, exogenous gonadotropin releasing hormone analogue to treat prostate cancer, anabolic steroids, and environmental toxins. Nonetheless, the morphologic findings are similar. Grossly, the testis is small. Microscopically, the tubules are decreased in size and the tunica propria is thickened and hyalinized. End-stage atrophic tubules are completely hyalinized, without intraluminal cells (e-**Fig. 28.8**).

IV. GERM CELL TUMORS OF THE TESTIS. These are of germ cell origin in the vast majority of cases, with sex cord/gonadal stromal tumors occurring in 4% to 6% of cases. The highest incidence is found in Europe and parts of New Zealand. Populations in Africa and Asia show a much lower incidence. The 2016 World Health Organization classification of the neoplasms of the testis is given in Table 28.2. The major revision for the WHO classification of germ cell tumors in the testis is to divide them into two major categories: germ cell tumors derived from GCNIS, and germ cell tumors unrelated to GCNIS.

A. Germ Cell Tumors. Clinical diagnosis is usually made when the patient presents with a painless mass in the testis. Associated symptoms such as a dull ache in the scrotum or lower abdomen may be present. Less commonly, patients present with gynecomastia and thyrotoxicosis. In 10% of cases metastatic disease may produce presenting signs and symptoms. Patients with cryptorchidism are at an increased risk (about 3- to 5-fold) of developing germ cell neoplasia both in the cryptorchid as well as the normal contralateral testis. Patients with testicular microlithiasis, testicular atrophy, infertility, a family history of germ cell neoplasia, mixed gonadal dysgenesis (46,XY or 45,X/46,XY) mixed gonadal dysgenesis, testicular dysgenesis syndrome (TDS), or a previous history of GCNIS are also at an increased risk. The age of the patient as well as characteristic elevations in the levels of serum tumor markers in different subtypes of germ cell tumors can be very helpful in predicting tumor type. Prepubertal yolk sac tumor and prepubertal type teratoma are seen in infants and children, and only rarely is prepubertal type teratoma seen postpubertal patients (*Am J Surg Pathol* 2013;37:827); seminomas and nonseminomatous germ cell neoplasms (including EC, teratoma, yolk sac tumor, and choriocarcinoma) are found in adolescents and young adults; and spermatocytic tumor typically is found in patients older than 50 years (*Am J Surg Pathol* 2017; doi: 10.1097/PAS.0000000000001001). Serum AFP levels can be elevated in nonseminomatous germ cell tumors, especially those with a yolk sac tumor component, whereas serum beta-hCG levels are increased in choriocarcinoma and tumors with syncytiotrophoblasts, which include about 10% of seminomas. The levels of these tumor markers are monitored posttreatment and are indicators of residual disease.

Imaging studies such as ultrasound are extremely sensitive and inexpensive in evaluating testicular masses. Localization of the mass, including evaluation of extratesticular versus intratesticular sites of involvement, and presence of heterogeneity within the tumor can be accurately determined. Epididymal lesions cannot be characterized with a similar degree of sensitivity. Computed tomography and magnetic resonance imaging are not used as primary diagnostic tools but can be helpful in tumor staging.

B. Gross Examination. Diagnosis of Germ cell tumors is made by examination of H&E-stained sections (*J Clin Pathol* 2007;60:866), but gross examination can provide useful diagnostic clues as to tumor type. For instance, a white to gray, solid, homogenous, well-circumscribed appearance is characteristic of classic seminoma. Choriocarcinomas show extensive areas of hemorrhage and necrosis, whereas teratomas are multicystic and nodular, and may have grossly visible cartilage areas. ECs are smaller, soft, tan-white, and show hemorrhage and necrosis. Yolk sac tumors may show gelatinous, mucoid, and cystic areas. Lymphomas are fleshy and ill-defined, and often exhibit extratesticular extension. Scarring may represent a regressed germ cell tumor. Because many germ cell

TABLE 28.2 WHO Histologic Classification of Tumors of the Testis and Paratestis

Noninvasive germ cell neoplasia

Germ cell neoplasia in situ

Specific forms of intratubular germ cell neoplasia

Germ cell tumors derived from germ cell neoplasia in situ

Tumors of a single histologic type
  Seminoma
  Seminoma with syncytiotrophoblastic cells
  Embryonal carcinoma
  Yolk sac tumor
  Trophoblastic tumors
    Choriocarcinoma
  Trophoblastic neoplasms other than choriocarcinoma
    Placental site trophoblastic tumor
    Epithelioid trophoblastic tumor
    Cystic trophoblastic tumor
  Teratoma of postpubertal type
  Teratoma with somatic type malignancy

Tumors of more than one histologic type (mixed forms)

Germ cell tumors of unknown type: regressed germ cell tumors

Germ cell tumors unrelated to germ cell neoplasia in situ

Spermatocytic tumor

Teratoma, prepubertal type
  Dermoid cyst
  Epidermoid cyst
  Well-differentiated neuroendocrine tumor (monodermal teratoma)
Mixed teratoma and yolk sac tumor, prepubertal type

Yolk sac tumor, prepubertal type

Sex cord/gonadal stromal tumors

Pure forms

Leydig cell tumor
  Malignant Leydig cell tumor

Sertoli cell tumor
  Malignant Sertoli cell tumor
  Large cell–calcifying Sertoli cell tumor
  Intratubular large cell hyalinizing Sertoli cell neoplasia

Granulosa cell tumor
    Adult granulosa cell tumor
    Juvenile granulosa cell tumor

Tumors of the thecoma/fibroma group
    Thecoma
    Fibroma
    Fibrothecoma

Mixed and unclassified sex cord-stromal tumors
  Mixed sex cord-stromal tumors
  Unclassified sex cord-stromal tumors

Tumors containing both germ cell and sex cord/gonadal stromal elements
  Gonadoblastoma

TABLE 28.2	WHO Histologic Classification of Tumors of the Testis and Paratestis (*Continued*)

Miscellaneous tumors of the testis

Tumors of ovarian epithelial types
    Serous cystadenoma
    Serous borderline tumor
    Serous cystadenocarcinoma
    Mucinous cystadenoma
    Mucinous borderline tumor
    Mucinous cystadenocarcinoma
    Endometrioid adenocarcinoma
    Clear cell adenocarcinoma
    Brenner tumor

Juvenile xanthogranuloma

Hemangioma

Hematopoietic tumors

Tumors of collecting ducts and rete

Adenoma

Carcinoma

Tumors of paratesticular structures

Adenomatoid tumor

Malignant mesothelioma

Benign mesothelioma
    Well-differentiated papillary mesothelioma
    Cystic mesothelioma

Epididymal tumors
    Cystadenoma of the epididymis
    Papillary cystadenoma of the epididymis
    Adenocarcinoma of the epididymis

Squamous cell carcinoma

Melanotic neuroectodermal tumor

Nephroblastoma

Paraganglioma

Mesenchymal tumors of the spinal cord and testicular adnexae

Secondary tumors of the testes

From: Moch H, Humphrey PA, Ulbright TM, Reuter VE, eds. *WHO Classification of Tumours of the Urinary System and Male Genital System.* Lyon, France: IARC Press; 2017. Used with permission.

tumors are of mixed type, the importance of adequate sampling of heterogeneous areas cannot be overemphasized.

C. Noninvasive Germ Cell Neoplasia

1. **GCNIS,** a precursor of invasive germ cell tumor, and can be found in isolated form or adjacent to invasive germ cell tumors. Patients with infertility, cryptorchidism, intersex syndrome, gonadal dysgenesis, a history of invasive germ cell tumor in the contralateral testis, or a retroperitoneal germ cell tumor have an increased likelihood of development of GCNIS. The high sensitivity of testicular biopsy in detecting GCNIS makes it a useful screening tool in these subgroups of patients.

GCNIS is not recognizable grossly. Histologically, the seminiferous tubules show enlarged neoplastic cells with clear cytoplasm and prominent nucleoli, and often a thickened tunica propria (e-**Fig. 28.9**). Mitoses may be seen. Normal spermatogenesis is typically lacking. The surrounding stroma may show a prominent lymphocytic response. The presence of scattered neoplastic germ cells in the surrounding stroma qualifies as microinvasion (e-**Fig. 28.10**). Occasionally, the neoplastic cells spread along the tubules or the rete testis in a pagetoid fashion (e-**Fig. 28.11**). Periodic acid–Schiff histochemical stains highlight glycogen in the cytoplasm of GCNIS cells; immunohistochemically, positive stainings for PLAP, CD117 (c-kit), and OCT4 (e-**Fig. 28.12**) are observed (*Semin Diagn Pathol* 2005;22:33). In infants up to 1 year of age, and in patients with delayed germ cell maturation (cryptorchidism or gonadal dysgenesis), intratubular germ cells can resemble GCNIS morphologically and can be positive for PLAP and OCT4 (*Am J Surg Pathol* 2006;30:1427), so caution is advised in diagnosing GCNIS in these cases. SALL4 also stains GCNIS, with a stronger staining intensity than normal spermatogonia (*Am J Surg Pathol* 2009;33:1065). About 90% of pure GCNIS cases progress to invasive disease within 7 years.

2. Specific forms of intratubular germ cell neoplasia, may be seen in association with invasive seminoma (30%) and nonseminoma (15%, mostly EC; intratubular yolk sac tumor and intratubular teratoma are extremely rare). Spermatocytic tumor may also show intratubular growth; this form of noninvasive germ cell neoplasia is distinguished from GCNIS by distension and filling of tubules by the neoplastic germ cells.

D. Germ Cell Tumors Derived From GCNIS

1. Seminoma comprises almost 40% to 50% of all testicular germ cell tumors. Grossly, it has a homogeneous white to gray cut surface (e-**Fig. 28.13**). Necrosis may be seen, but hemorrhage and cystic change are uncommon. Histologically, the seminoma cells are relatively uniform with prominent nucleoli and a distinct cell membrane. The cytoplasm is typically clear but can be eosinophilic. The nuclei may have a squared appearance. Rarely signet ring-like (vacuolated) tumor cells can be seen in seminoma (*Am J Surg Pathol* 2008;32:1175). The cells grow as solid sheet or are separated into nests, clusters, or columns by delicate fibrous septae infiltrated by mature lymphocytes (e-**Fig. 28.14**). A parenchymal or intratubular granulomatous reaction may be present (e-**Fig. 28.15**). The granulomatous inflammation can be so extensive, both in the testis and draining lymph nodes, that it may obscure tumor cells resulting in a misdiagnosis of granulomatous orchitis. The tumor may entirely replace the normal testicular parenchyma, and may show an intratubular and less commonly an interstitial growth pattern. Other morphologic patterns include pseudoglandular (e-**Fig. 28.16**), tubular, cribriform, and occasionally microcystic appearances (*Am J Surg Pathol* 2005;29:500). Microcystic seminoma should be distinguished from yolk sac tumor and sex cord stromal tumors; this can be achieved with immunohistochemical markers including CD117 (e-**Fig. 28.17**), D2-40, AFP, glypican-3, OCT4, and inhibin (*Am J Surg Pathol* 2004;28:935; *Ann Diagn Pathol* 2010;14:331) (Table 28.3). Foci of scarring may indicate a regressed germ cell tumor, and areas of calcification should prompt a search for possible foci of gonadoblastoma. Although brisk mitotic activity (>6 mitoses per high-power field) is observed in some tumors, there is little evidence that this denotes a worse prognosis, although it has been hypothesized that this finding may indicate progression to EC. Marked cytologic atypia and mitoses have been used in the past to define "anaplastic seminoma," but this is not a currently recognized subtype of seminoma. Scattered multinucleated syncytiotrophoblasts are seen in up to 10% of seminomas (e-**Fig. 28.18**); this finding has no prognostic significance, but is important to diagnose such cases as seminoma with syncytiotrophoblastic cells because this may correlate with a mildly elevated serum HCG level. However, seminoma with syncytiotrophoblastic cells does need to be differentiated from choriocarcinoma; the lack of a mononucleated trophoblastic component is helpful in this regard. Other important entities in the differential diagnosis of seminoma include inflammatory conditions (especially in the presence of a prominent lymphocytic response), spermatocytic tumor, and sex cord stromal tumors (*Adv Anat Pathol* 2008;15:18).

TABLE 28.3 Immunophenotype of Testis Neoplasms

Tumor Type	LIN28	SALL4	PLAP	c-kit (CD117)	OCT4	CD30	AFP	AE1/AE3	CK7	EMA	Inhibin	CD45 (LCA)
Seminoma	+	+	+	+	+	–	–	v	v	–	–	–
Spermatocytic tumor	–/+	v	–	v	–	–	–	–	Nd	–	nd	–
Embryonal carcinoma	+	+	+	–	+	+	–	+	+		–	–
Yolk sac tumor	+	+	+	–/+	–	v	+	+	–	–	–	–
Sertoli/Leydig cell tumor	–	–	–/v	–	–	nd	nd	–/v	nd	v	v/+	–
Lymphoma	–	–	–	–	–/+	v	nd	–	nd	–	–	+

++: ≥80% of cases positive; v, variable staining (20% to 80% of cases); –: ≤20% of cases positive; nd = no data.
Modified from: *Semin Diagn Pathol* 2005;22:33, with additional data on LIN28 and SALL4.

2. EC occurs in young adults, most commonly as a component of a mixed germ cell tumor. Grossly, hemorrhage and necrosis are common (**e-Fig. 28.19**). The tumor cells are large and undifferentiated with an epithelial appearance, and are arranged in a solid, papillary, and/or glandular pattern (**e-Fig. 28.20**). Other uncommon growth patterns include nested (3%), micropapillary (2%), anastomosing glandular (1%), sieve-like glandular (<1%), pseudopapillary (<1%), and blastocyst-like (<1%) (*Am J Surg Pathol* 2014;38:689). Rare patterns include polyembryoma-like and diffuse embryoma-like. Nuclei are polygonal and vesicular with coarse chromatin, and they tend to overlap. Mitotic activity and necrosis are extensive. In two-thirds of cases, there is an applique appearance in which smudged and degenerating-appearing tumor cells appear applied to the periphery of tumor nests (*Am J Surg Pathol* 2014;38:689). In 11% of ECs, there is clear cytoplasm and a prominent cell membrane mimicking seminoma. Syncytiotrophoblastic cells are seen in nearly half of ECs (*Am J Surg Pathol* 2014;38:689). Intratubular spread can be seen in one quarter of cases, is typically present at the periphery, and frequently displays intratubular necrosis and microcalcifications. Dense lymphocytic infiltration and granulomatous inflammation can be seen in 7% and 3% ECs, respectively (*Am J Surg Pathol* 2014;38:689). Vascular invasion can be seen (**e-Fig. 28.21**) and should be differentiated from retraction artifact and artificial implantation during sampling. Pancytokeratin, SALL4, OCT4, and CD30 positivity is seen in tumor cells; PLAP and AFP are only focally positive in pure tumors. Epithelial membrane antigen (EMA) is negative, which is important in the differential diagnosis with somatic carcinomas (Table 28.3). Evaluation of H&E-stained slides is usually sufficient to establish the diagnosis; in occasional cases, immunohistochemistry is needed to help differentiate EC from yolk sac tumor, seminoma, large cell anaplastic lymphoma, and/or choriocarcinoma.

3. Yolk sac tumor (endodermal sinus tumor), postpubertal type, shows differentiation reminiscent of embryonic yolk sac, allantois, and extraembryonic mesenchyme. It is often found as a component in mixed germ cell tumors. YST is notorious for displaying multiple histologic patterns, including reticular (most common), microcystic, endodermal sinus-like (with Schiller–Duval bodies, characteristic but seen in only 1/3 cases), papillary, solid, glandular, alveolar, enteric, polyvesicular vitelline, and hepatoid patterns (**e-Fig. 28.22**). Rarely, a neoplastic spindle cell component has been observed in association with the myxomatous and reticular variants. The tumor cells are positive for AFP, glypican-3, SALL4, and LIN28 (**e-Fig. 28.23**). SALL4 and LIN28 stain far more tumor cells than AFP and glypican-3 (*Am J Surg Pathol* 2009;33:1065; *Hum Pathol* 2011;42:710). Yolk sac tumor in mixed germ cell tumors are often admixed with EC in a loose association pattern, so-called double-layered necklace pattern (**e-Fig. 28.24**), or polyembryoma-like pattern. EC nuclei are usually more pleomorphic, and immunostains can help in difficult cases (Table 28.3).

4. Trophoblastic tumors include choriocarcinoma, placental site trophoblastic tumor (PSTT), epithelioid trophoblastic tumor (ETT), and cystic trophoblastic tumor.

   a. Pure choriocarcinoma is extremely rare; instead, choriocarcinoma most commonly occurs as a component of mixed germ cell tumors. Grossly, necrotic and hemorrhagic nodules can be observed. Microscopically, the more viable peripheral areas show randomly admixed syncytiotrophoblasts, cytotrophoblasts, and intermediate trophoblasts, although one component may predominate giving rise to a monophasic tumor (**e-Fig. 28.25**). The tumor has a propensity for vascular invasion (**e-Fig. 28.25**). The differential diagnosis includes syncytiotrophoblast-rich seminoma, and isolated syncytiotrophoblasts found in nonseminomatous germ cell tumors.

   b. PSTT and ETT are rare and can be been within the testis or metastasis (*Am J Surg Pathol* 2015;39:1468). Morphologically, PSTT is composed of sheets of discohesive pleomorphic mononucleated cells that may invade blood vessels with associated fibrinoid change whereas ETT is composed of nodules and nests of squamoid trophoblastic cells with abundant eosinophilic cytoplasm with abundant extracellular fibrinoid material. Immunohistochemically, PSTT cells are p63- and human placental lactogen (HPL)+ whereas ETT cells are p63+ and HPL-. The tumor cells in both tumors are positive for GATA3.

   c. Cystic trophoblastic tumor is a minor component seen either in treated or untreated germ cell tumors and is associated with other types of germ cell components (teratoma, EC, yolk sac tumor, seminoma, and choriocarcinoma) *(Am J Surg Pathol* 2017;41:788). Microscopically, cystic trophoblastic tumor is cystic to partly solid with often intracystic fibrinoid material. The cysts are lined by mononucleated squamoid cells with eosinophilic to pale cytoplasm (frequently vacuolated), and pleomorphic nuclei with dense chromatin (often smudged) and inconspicuous mitotic activity. The tumor cells are positive for HCG, inhibin, and p63.

5. Teratoma, postpubertal type, is thought to arise from differentiation of other types of germ cell tumors, particularly GCNIS or seminoma. Pure teratomas are much less common than the finding of teratoma as an element of a mixed malignant germ cell tumor. Grossly, there are cystic and solid areas; cartilage (e-**Fig. 28.26**) and bone may be evident. Microscopically, teratomas may show well-differentiated elements derived from one (monodermal) or all three germ layers (ectoderm, mesoderm, and endoderm), or may be immature with fetal type tissue. Skin and its appendages, respiratory and intestinal-type epithelium, cartilage, and muscular tissue are common (e-**Fig. 28.27, A** and **B**); neural-type tissue is less frequent. Immature tissues can resemble renal blastema or embryonic neural tube (e-**Fig. 28.28**). Foci with the appearance of a primitive neuroectodermal tumor (PNET) have been classified as such if present in more than one low-power field. Prognostically, postpubertal type teratoma is a malignant germ cell tumor.

E. Germ Cell Tumors Unrelated to GCNIS

1. Spermatocytic tumor (previously known as spermatocytic seminoma) is rare and lacks the associations (i.e., cryptorchidism and GCNIS) commonly seen with classic seminoma *(Arch Pathol Lab Med* 2009;133:1985; *Am J Surg Pathol* 2019;43:1). This neoplasm is seen in older patients (mean age 52 years, range 19 to 81 years), and is more often than not unilateral. The mean tumor size is 5.7 cm (range 1.4 to 15 cm). Extratesticular extension is rare. Low-power view reveals either a predominantly multinodular or diffuse pattern. A small percentage of tumors may show fibrin at the periphery of tumor nodules. The tumor cells are of three types: small lymphocyte-like with dark nuclei and scant cytoplasm, intermediate with round nuclei and moderate eosinophilic cytoplasm, and large with single or multiple nuclei (e-**Fig. 28.29**). Uncommonly, the tumor is composed of predominantly intermediate sized cells, giving a monotonous appearance. Mitoses are frequent. The majority of tumors show intratubular spread. The presence of stromal edema may cause the tumor cells to appear to be nested or pseudoglandular. A lymphocytic or granulomatous response is seen in 8% and 1% tumors, respectively. Only four cases of metastatic pure spermatocytic seminoma have been reported, and so radical orchiectomy alone is curative for almost all patients with spermatocytic tumor. About 2% to 3% spermatocytic tumors undergo sarcomatous transformation, and the histologic types of sarcoma include spindle cell sarcoma, rhabdomyosarcoma, chondrosarcoma, and undifferentiated sarcoma. Spermatocytic tumor with sarcoma is an aggressive variant of spermatocytic tumor and no known etiology or familial predisposition has been reported, and most patients present with metastatic disease. The main differential diagnosis is with classic seminoma and lymphoma. Clinicohistomorphologic features and, if necessary, SALL4, PLAP, and OCT4 immunostains are useful in the distinction from classic seminomas (Table 28.3); lymphomas are more often bilateral and extratesticular, and have a more monomorphic cell population.

2. Yolk sac tumor, prepubertal type, mostly occurs in pure form and only rarely as a component admixed with teratoma. Only 6% patients are older than 5 years (*Am J Surg Pathol* 2015;39:1211). The serum AFP level is elevated in 90% patients. Morphologically it is similar to the postpubertal counterpart. Overall, prepubertal yolk sac tumors show a better prognosis than postpubertal yolk sac tumors, and even in advanced disease chemotherapy is still effective. The majority of prepubertal yolk sac tumors present with a stage I disease, significantly higher than postpubertal yolk sac tumors; among patients with stage I disease, the presence of two or more of the following features is associated with an adverse outcome: tumor size >4.5 cm, rete testis or epididymal invasion, and necrosis (*Am J Surg Pathol* 2015;39:1211). The major differential diagnosis for prepubertal type yolk sac tumor is juvenile granulosa cell tumor which shows overlapping morphologic features but can be reliably distinguished by immunohistochemical markers (juvenile granulosa cell tumor is inhibin+/ FOXL2+/WT1+/AFP-/glypican-3-/SALL4-/LIN28- whereas yolk sac tumor shows the opposite profile).

3. **Teratoma, prepubertal type,** including dermoid cysts and epidermoid cyst, are thought to arise through a different mechanism from postpubertal type teratoma. Dermoid cysts, which harbor keratinizing squamous epithelium and skin appendages, are very rare and are benign. Epidermoid cysts lack skin appendages and possibly represent monodermal teratomas; grossly, epidermoid cysts are distinctive with a ringlike "onion-skin" cut surface (e-**Figs. 28.30** and **28.31**). Compared with postpubertal type teratoma, prepubertal type teratomas have a more organized architecture and lack significant cytologic atypia (*Histopathology* 2017;70:335). Whether morphologically immature or mature, prepubertal type teratoma is biologically benign except for rare carcinoid tumors and other somatic-type malignancies arising from teratoma (see below). Prepubertal teratoma lacks an association with GCNIS and largely lacks 12p abnormalities (isochromosome or amplification). Most prepubertal teratomas are pure, but rarely they are mixed with prepubertal type yolk sac tumor.

Although the majority of prepubertal type teratomas occur in prepubertal patients, rarely they can be seen in postpubertal patients (*Am J Surg Pathol* 2013;37:827). They are not mixed with other germ cell components. Morphologically, they lack the cytologic atypia seen in postpubertal type teratoma or isochromosome 12p abnormalities. There is also no GCNIS, no tubular atrophy or scarring, no microlithiasis, and no impaired spermatogenesis. The teratoma components are frequently organoid and certain components are over-represented in these tumors, including ciliated respiratory epithelium and smooth muscle.

Well-differentiated neuroendocrine tumor (carcinoid tumor) is considered to be a pure form of monodermal prepubertal teratoma in the 2016 WHO classification. It may arise in association with dermoid cysts and epidermoid cysts (*Am J Surg Pathol* 2010;34:519). Rarely it is associated with carcinoid syndrome. It lacks an association with GCNIS. It typically grows in an organoid and trabecular pattern. Most cases lack mitotic activity. In the largest series, about 15% of tumors qualified as atypical carcinoid. Prognostically, typical carcinoids behave in an indolent fashion, however, most of the atypical carcinoids showed metastasis (*Am J Surg Pathol* 2010;34:519).

F. **Tumors of More Than One Histologic Type** (mixed forms), termed **mixed germ cell tumor**, are germ cell neoplasms composed of more than one type of tumor. They comprise approximately 30% of all germ cell tumors, and the most frequently encountered components include EC (in about half of cases), yolk sac tumor (about half), and teratoma (about 40%). About 40% of mixed malignant germ cell tumors also contain scattered syncytiotrophoblasts. A rare subtype of mixed germ cell tumor is polyembryoma with characteristic embryoid bodies with a central plate of EC (forming the dorsal amnion-like cavity) and a surrounding (ventral) yolk sac component. Mixed germ cell tumors with an embryonal component are predictive of a higher stage than tumors with a large seminomatous component, so for mixed tumors it is very important to quantitate, on a percentage basis, the amount of EC (as well as all other components). Tumors with a yolk sac or teratoma component show a lower incidence of metastatic disease.

G. **Somatic Type Malignancy Arising From Teratoma,** occurs in 3% to 6% germ cell tumors, mostly appearing in the metastatic sites after chemotherapy (*Am J Surg Pathol* 2014;38:1396). The types of malignancies reported include sarcomas (rhabdomyosarcoma > myxofibrosarcoma > spindle cell sarcoma NOS, undifferentiated pleomorphic sarcoma, leiomyosarcoma, osteosarcoma, gliosarcoma), carcinomas (adenocarcinoma NOS > mucinous, enteric type, endometrioid-like, papillary, pancreatobiliary type, signet ring), PNETs, glial and meningeal neoplasms, hematologic tumors, and nephroblastoma-like tumors. The diagnosis of somatic type malignancy arising from teratoma requires sarcoma overgrowth exceeding a 4× microscopic field, or carcinoma with invasive growth by the atypical epithelial cells or confluent growth exceeding a 4× microscopic field. Some sarcomatous tumors represent sarcomatoid yolk sac tumors as evidenced by positive staining for pancytokeratin, glypican-3, and SALL4 (*Am J Surg Pathol* 2014;l38:1396). Similarly, some adenocarcinomas may represent glandular yolk sac tumors.

H. **Regressed (So-Called Burnt-Out) Germ Cell Tumors** are germ cell tumors in which the primary tumor in the testis has undergone necrosis and fibrosis. This most commonly occurs with seminoma (*Am J Surg Pathol* 2006;30:858) and choriocarcinoma. The most specific histologic finding of a regressed germ cell tumor is a distinct scar (e-**Fig. 28.32**) in association with either GCNIS or coarse intratubular calcifications; however, many cases lack these latter two features (*Am J Surg Pathol* 2006;30:858). Some patients may present with metastatic disease, the only evidence of the testicular primary being a scar, with or without GCNIS.

I. **New Immunophenotypic Markers** that are transcription factors involved in the maintenance of stem cell pluripotency have been developed for germ cell tumors. These markers include SALL4, OCT4, NANOG, SOX2, and SOX17, and all demonstrate a nuclear pattern of expression. SALL4 labels all GCNISs, classic seminomas, ECs, and yolk sac tumors (*Am J Surg Pathol* 2009;33:1065). Choriocarcinoma, teratoma, and spermatocytic tumor are also variably positive for SALL4. Both OCT4 and NANOG label GCNIS, seminoma, and EC (*Am J Surg Pathol* 2004;28:935; *Histopathology* 2005;47:48). SOX2 only labels EC and teratoma (*Am J Surg Pathol* 2007;31:836; *J Pathol* 2008;215:21), and SOX17 labels GCNIS, seminoma, and yolk sac tumor (*Am J Clin Pathol* 2009;131:131; *J Pathol* 2008;215:21). Among these markers, SALL4 demonstrates the highest sensitivity and shows particular utility for yolk sac tumor diagnosis; for yolk sac tumors, SALL4 is much more sensitive than placental-like alkaline phosphatase (PLAP), AFP, and glypican-3 (*Am J Surg Pathol* 2009;33:1065). SALL4 is also particularly useful in differentiating metastatic germ cell tumors from metastatic carcinoma of nontesticular origin, a setting in which it has been found to be more sensitive than OCT3/4 (*Cancer* 2009;115:2640). However, SALL4 can be immunoreactive in some nongerm cell tumors, including a diffuse staining pattern, particularly gastric hepatoid carcinomas (*Am J Surg Pathol* 2010;34:533; *Pathol Res Pract* 2018;214:1707). Another marker that shows similar sensitivity to SALL4 but with a higher specificity is LIN28, an RNA-binding protein (*Hum Pathol* 2010;42:710). Recently, ZBTB16 has been found to be specific for yolk sac tumor with no expression in other types of germ cell tumors including seminoma, EC, choriocarcinoma, teratoma, and GCNIS; however, ZBTB16 is not as sensitive as SALL4 (*Mod Pathol* 2016;29:591). Both SALL4 and NBTB16 are also expressed in spermatogonia in both children and adults (*Am J Surg Pathol* 2009;33:1065; *Mod Pathol* 2016;29:591), a potential diagnostic pitfall that must be kept in mind (all new markers described above are also expressed in early fetal germ cells).

J. **Molecular Genetics** are not currently used in diagnosis. The only exception is detection of isochromosome 12p by fluorescence in situ hybridization to identify metastatic germ cell neoplasms, since gain of material in 12p is the most common structural chromosomal alteration in invasive germ cell tumors (*Mod Pathol* 2004;17:1309).

V. **NONGERM CELL TUMORS OF THE TESTIS AND PARATESTIS** include sex cord/gonadal stromal tumor, hematolymphoid tumors, tumors of collecting duct and rete testis, tumors of paratesticular structures, and mesenchymal tumors.

A. **Sex Cord/Gonadal Stromal Tumors** comprise 4% to 6% of all testicular tumors in adults and include Leydig cell tumor, Sertoli cell tumor (SCT), granulosa cell tumor, thecoma, and fibroma.

1. **Leydig cell tumors** are the most common and are known to occur in patients with gynecomastia, Klinefelter syndrome, and cryptorchidism. Grossly, the tumor cut surface is homogeneous, solid, and brown to yellow. The tumor cells are large and polygonal, and have abundant eosinophilic, lipid-laden cytoplasm (e-**Fig. 28.33**). The characteristic Reinke crystals are found in only 30% of cases. The tumor cells are positive for inhibin, calretinin, and Melan-A by immunohistochemistry. The main differential diagnoses are Leydig cell hyperplasia and syndromic adrenogenital tumors. Leydig cell tumors form a nodule without seminiferous tubules, whereas in Leydig cell hyperplasia the foci are bilateral and multifocal, and wrap around and extend between the tubules (e-**Fig. 28.34**); adrenogenital tumors are bilateral and dark brown, with pigmentation and fibrous stroma. About 90% of Leydig cell tumors are benign, but a constellation of features, including size >5 cm, cytologic atypia, increased mitotic activity, necrosis, and vascular invasion favors malignancy.

2. **SCTs** account for only 1% of all testicular tumors. Grossly, the mass is usually well-circumscribed with tan-yellow to white, sometimes hemorrhagic cut surfaces (e-**Fig. 28.35**). The known clinical associations are with Carney syndrome, Peutz–Jeghers syndrome (which can be associated with bilateral tumors), and androgen insensitivity syndrome. Large cell calcifying SCTs (e-**Fig. 28.36**) is considered to be a subtype of SCT. However, sclerosing SCT is no longer considered a specific subtype but rather part of the spectrum of SCT NOS (*Am J Surg Pathol* 2014;38:66; *Am J Surg Pathol* 2015;39:1390). Large cell calcifying SCTs do not show nuclear beta-catenin staining. SCTs should be distinguished from small incidental Sertoli cell nodules (benign and thought to be nonneoplastic) as can be seen in cryptorchid testes.

   Histologically, in the typical SCT the cytologically bland cells are arranged in tubules, potentially with retiform, tubular-glandular, and solid nodular areas. The tubules can be closed (solid) (e-**Fig. 28.37**) and are surrounded by a basement membrane. Intratubular growth can be present. The SCT cells are cytokeratin and sometimes inhibin and calretinin positive, but PLAP and OCT4 negative, by immunohistochemistry. Large cell calcifying SCT is seen sporadically and in the setting of Carney complex. Histologically, its tumor cells are characterized by abundant eosinophilic cytoplasm and calcifications; the stroma may be fibromyxoid and contain neutrophils. Malignant SCTs are rare (5%); features that are suggestive of malignant behavior include size >5 cm, local extratesticular spread, high-grade nuclear atypia, mitosis >5/10 hpfs, lymphovascular invasion, and necrosis (*Am J Surg Pathol* 1998;22:709).

3. **Intratubular large cell calcifying Sertoli cell neoplasia** is seen in patients with Peutz-Jeghers syndrome (*Am J Surg Pathol* 2007;31:827). All patients have gynecomastia. Morphologically, the expanded seminiferous tubules are filled with large Sertoli cells with eosinophilic to vacuolated cytoplasm admixed with eosinophilic basement membrane deposits. All reported tumors have behaved in a benign fashion.

4. **Adult granulosa cell tumors** are rare testicular tumors that occur in patients over a wide age range (from 14 to 87 years old) (*Am J Surg Pathol* 2014;38:1242). The mean tumor size is 2.8 cm (with a range from 0.5 to 6.0 cm). The predominant growth pattern is diffuse but other histologic patterns may also be seen including insular, spindled, microfollicular, trabecular, corded, watered-silk, palisading, and pseudopapillary. The tumor cells are similar to those in the ovarian counterparts with pale chromatin and frequent nuclear grooves. Mitotic activity is variable from 0 to 18/10 hpfs. Rarely the tumors may show necrosis and lymphovascular invasion. Most of these tumors behave in a benign fashion; however, rare cases with malignant behavior have been reported. The pathologic features that are associated with aggressive behavior include lymphovascular invasion, tumor size > 4 cm, and infiltrative border (*Am J Surg Pathol* 2014;38:1242).

5. **Juvenile granulosa cell tumor** occurs mainly in patients 6 months or younger (range 30 weeks gestational age to 10 years) (*Am J Surg Pathol* 2015;39:1159). It may occur in undescended testis and dysgenetic gonads. The tumor size ranges from 0.5

to 5 cm (mean 1.7 cm, median 1.5 cm) with a well circumscribed border in most cases. Grossly, a cystic component is seen in most cases. Microscopically, the tumor frequently shows a lobular pattern with variably sized follicles which contain basophilic and/or eosinophilic material. Rarely, follicles are not present within the tumor. The tumor cells typically grow diffusely within a fibrous or fibromyxoid stroma but they may have a corded or reticular appearance. The tumor cells have moderate to abundant cytoplasm with small to medium-sized nuclei and inconspicuous nucleoli, and only rare cases have nuclear grooves. There is abundant mitotic activity and apoptosis. The tumor cells are positive for WT1, FOXL2, SF1, inhibin, and SOX9. Juvenile granulosa cell tumor is biologically indolent (benign) after orchiectomy.

6. Fibrothecomas are very rare tumors in the testis. The mean size is 1.8 cm (0.5 to 7.0 cm). Most tumors are intratesticular but most abut the tunica albuginea; they may entrap seminiferous tubules. The tumor cells are ovoid or spindled without prominent nucleoli, and are arranged in storiform and fascicular patterns. Hypercellularity is seen in 50% tumors. No significant nuclear atypia is seen, and the mitotic activity is variable from 0 to 9 to 10/10 hpfs (*Am J Surg Pathol* 2013;37:1208). Testicular fibrothecomas are biologically benign tumors.

B. Mixed Germ Cell and Sex Cord/Gonadal Stromal Tumors include gonadoblastoma, most commonly seen in the setting of mixed gonadal dysgenesis, ambiguous genitalia, and 45X/46XY mosaicism. Microscopic examination shows two cell populations: a germ cell component resembling seminoma and a component resembling immature Sertoli cells (**e-Fig. 28.38**). Round deposits of basement membrane-like material and coarse calcification are common features. If left in place, gonadoblastoma will eventually develop into an invasive germ cell tumor (80% seminoma, 20% nonseminoma) and so patients are therefore treated with bilateral orchiectomy.

C. Miscellaneous Tumors of the testis include carcinoid tumors, tumors of ovarian epithelial types (serous cystadenoma, serous borderline tumor, serous carcinoma, mucinous cystadenomas, mucinous borderline tumor, mucinous cystadenocarcinomas, Brenner tumor, clear cell carcinoma, and endometrioid carcinoma), juvenile xanthogranuloma, nephroblastoma, and paraganglioma.

D. Hematolymphoid Neoplasms, of which the most common is malignant lymphoma, comprise 5% of all testicular malignancies. Lymphoma is the most common testicular tumor in men older than 50 years old (*J Clin Oncol* 2003;21:20), and is the most common bilateral tumor of the testis. The most common subtype is diffuse large B-cell lymphoma (80% to 90%). The growth pattern is typically intertubular (**e-Fig. 28.39**), and the main differential diagnosis is with seminoma and spermatocytic tumor. Immunostains can be helpful in establishing the diagnosis (Table 28.3); however, it should be pointed out that OCT4 can be immunoreactive in 20% testicular diffuse large B-cell lymphomas though the percentage of tumor cells is lower than that in seminoma (*Am J Surg Pathol* 2016;40:950). The prognosis is generally poor. Young age, low stage, and presence of sclerosis are indicators of a good prognosis. Isolated plasmacytoma of the testis is rare.

E. Tumors of the Collecting Ducts and Rete. Benign tumors of the rete include adenoma and adenofibroma. Adenoma can grow in several patterns including solid packed tubules, with a prominent cystic component (cystadenoma), papillary structures (papillary cystadenoma), and with a fibrous stromal component (adenofibroma).

One particular variant is Sertoliform cystadenoma (*Am J Surg Pathol* 2018;42:141); in this variant, besides the well-formed tubules, the other histologic patterns include individual tumor cells, festoons, branching tubules, solid sheets, and papillary structures (*Am J Surg Pathol* 2018;42:141). Occasionally the neoplasm may extend into adjacent seminiferous tubules. Sertoliform cystadenoma may show cytologic atypia and mitotic activity (up to 2/10 hpfs) but experience with these rare tumors is very limited (*Am J Surg Pathol* 2018;42:141). Immunohistochemically Sertoliform cystadenoma cells are typically positive for inhibin, WT1, and SF1.

Adenocarcinomas of the rete are very rare, and their diagnosis is subject to strict histologic criteria that include tumor centered on the testicular hilum, morphology distinct from any other testicular/paratesticular tumor, a solid growth pattern, transition between tumor and normal tissue, and absence of histologically similar extratesticular malignancy (especially lung and prostate). The main histologic patterns are tubuloglandular, retiform, Sertoliform, papillary, solid, solid with slit-like channels (Kaposiform), and sarcomatoid. The main differential diagnoses are extratesticular adenocarcinomas and mesothelioma. The tumor shows extensive regional spread and distant metastasis, and the overall prognosis is poor.

F. Tumors of the Paratesticular Organ

1. Benign

A. The most common benign neoplasm of the testicular adnexa is **adenomatoid tumor**, representing almost 60% of all cases. These are of mesothelial origin (*Semin Diagn Pathol* 2000;17:294) and arise in the upper or lower pole of the epididymis as solitary, round to oval nodules invariably <5 cm in size. Histologically, the tumor shows round to oval or slit-like tubules in a fibrous, hyalinized, and/or muscular stroma (e-**Figs. 28.40** and **28.41**). The lining cells are columnar or flat with vacuolated cytoplasm. Adenomatoid tumor may occasionally show necrosis or infarction (*Am J Surg Pathol* 2004;28:77) and infiltrate into adjacent testicular parenchyma. Adenomatoid tumors show immunoreactivity for cytokeratin, EMA, and mesothelial markers including calretinin, HBME1, D2-40, and WT-1 (*Mod Pathol* 2009;22:1228). The tumor should be differentiated from signet ring cell carcinoma and mesothelioma; tumors with a more diffuse growth pattern simulate Sertoli or Leydig cell tumors (inhibin positivity, lipofuscin pigment, and the presence of Reinke crystals favor Leydig cell tumor).

b. Another benign paratesticular tumor is **papillary cystadenoma of the epididymis** (e-**Fig. 28.42**). About two thirds of cases are seen in patients with von Hippel–Lindau disease, and in this setting the tumor tends to be bilateral.

c. A much rarer entity is **melanotic neuroectodermal tumor (retinal anlage tumor)**, which is composed of two cell populations: larger melanin-containing cells and smaller neuroblast-like cells.

2. Malignant

A. Malignant mesothelioma of the testicular adnexa has a microscopic appearance and immunophenotypic profile similar to mesothelioma of the pleura. The main differential diagnoses are with adenomatoid tumor, which is better circumscribed, and with carcinoma of the rete testis.

b. Primary adenocarcinoma of the epididymis is rare with fewer than 50 cases reported in the literature, and may histologically and cytologically simulate a cystadenoma due to the presence of columnar cells with clear cytoplasm containing glycogen. Rarely it can be mucinous (*Appl Immunohistochem Mol Morphol* 2015;23:308). Metastatic adenocarcinoma from other organs should also be excluded.

c. Desmoplastic small round cell tumor occurs in the epididymis of young adults. Molecular, genetic, histologic, and immunohistochemical features are similar to those of the tumor when it occurs at more conventional sites such as the peritoneum. The tumor should be differentiated from other small blue cell tumors such as malignant lymphoma and embryonal rhabdomyosarcoma.

d. Mesenchymal tumors of the scrotum, paratesticular organs, and spermatic cord include benign neoplasms such as lipoma, leiomyoma, neurofibroma, and granular cell tumor. Malignant mesenchymal tumors include liposarcoma, leiomyosarcoma (e-**Fig. 28.43**), malignant fibrous histiocytoma, and rhabdomyosarcoma (e-**Figs. 28.44** and **28.45**).

G. Secondary Malignancies include metastatic adenocarcinomas from the prostate (e-**Fig. 28.46**), lung, and colon, and melanoma.

VI. PATHOLOGIC STAGING by the most recent AJCC scheme applies only to postpubertal germ cell tumors and malignant sex cord-stromal tumors. (Amin MB et al., eds. *AJCC Cancer Staging Manual.* 8th ed. New York: Springer, 2017). Primary hematolymphoid tumors of the testis are staged according to the scheme for hematologic malignancies. There

is no AJCC staging system for spermatocytic tumor, prepubertal germ cell tumors, non-malignant sex cord/gonadal-stromal tumors, or paratesticular neoplasms. Clinical staging should be distinguished from pathologic staging.

VII. **REPORTING OF GERM CELL NEOPLASMS** should follow suggested guidelines (for example, College of American Pathologists Protocol for the Examination of Specimens From Patients With Malignant Germ Cell and Sex Cord-Stromal Tumors of the Testis; available at http://www.cap.org). When reporting mixed germ cell tumors, percentage of different subtypes/elements should be reported; it is particularly critical to assess for the presence and amount of EC. The basic elements that need to be included for the primary tumor are size, multifocality, and presence or absence of involvement of extratesticular tissues including the epididymis, tunica vaginalis (via penetration through the tunica albuginea), spermatic cord, and scrotum (if present). Involvement of rete testis and hilar soft tissue should be reported as well, but note that the rete testis is not considered to be an extratesticular structure. Pagetoid involvement of rete epithelium should be distinguished from stromal invasion as the latter is a worse prognostic factor. Tunica vaginalis invasion requires tumor cells to penetrate the visceral mesothelial layer (pT2). Spermatic cord involvement by germ cell tumor includes direct invasion (pT3) and lymphovascular invasion without stromal invasion (pT2). In all testicular germ cell tumors, lymphovascular should be documented as it indicates at least pT2 (there is no need to distinguish vascular from lymphatic invasion).

Prostate

Jennifer K. Sehn and Peter A. Humphrey

I. **NORMAL ANATOMY.** The normal weight of the prostate is 20 g for ages 20 to 50, and 30 g for ages 60 to 80. Anatomically, the prostate gland is composed of three zones: central zone, transition zone (where benign prostatic hyperplasia [BPH] occurs), and peripheral zone (where most carcinomas originate) (e-**Fig. 29.1**). Microscopically, the normal adult prostate is a branching duct-acinar glandular system embedded in a dense fibromuscular stroma (e-**Fig. 29.2**). The epithelium has two layers: a luminal or secretory cell layer and a basal cell layer. Normal central zone epithelium can have architectural patterns that include cribriform and Roman bridge-like structures (e-**Fig. 29.3**).

II. **GROSS EXAMINATION, TISSUE SAMPLING, AND HISTOLOGIC SLIDE PREPARATION.** The most common prostatic parenchymal tissue samples examined in surgical pathology laboratories in the United States are, in order, 18G needle cores, transurethral resection of prostate (TURP) chips, radical prostatectomy specimens, and fine needle aspirates.

A. **Needle Cores.** Needle core biopsy sample handling and processing begins in the room where the procedure is performed. The needle biopsy tissue should be immediately placed into a container with fixative, which is usually 10% neutral buffered formalin. Fixation in formalin should be for at least 6 hours. The number of cores received per container is highly variable, from 1 to >20. If the urologist and treating physician desire site-specific diagnosis, the core(s) should be placed in separate site-designated containers. Inking of cores to indicate site, with placement of cores marked with different colors into the same container, should not be performed because fragmentation renders site assignment impossible. Gross examination of prostate needle core tissue must include the size and number of tissue cores or fragments in each container. It is recommended that no more than two cores be submitted per cassette for processing and embedding to ensure that each core is adequately represented on the slides; some laboratories submit one core per cassette. Prostate cores can be marked with ink or hematoxylin, which facilitates identification during embedding and the ability to see the cores in the paraffin blocks. Regardless, the cores should be placed into a cassette after being put into a fine mesh envelope, wrapped in lens paper, sandwiched between sponge pads, or double-embedded in agar–paraffin wax. After processing, the cores should be embedded in the same plane, in the same direction, with even spacing. From each paraffin block, three hematoxylin and eosin (H&E)-stained slides should be prepared, with three to four serial sections on each slide. Some laboratories cut interval unstained sections on coated slides in case special studies such as immunohistochemistry are needed. Targeted biopsy of suspicious lesions identified on prostate magnetic resonance imaging (MRI) studies are sometimes performed. Clinical requests for frozen section diagnosis of prostate needle cores are rare and should be restricted to patients with clinical evidence of metastatic cancer who are to undergo immediate treatment (usually orchiectomy) for pain relief.

B. **TURP Chips.** The amount of prostate tissue resected in TURP procedures is variable, ranging from 5 to >75 g of tissue, with a mean of about 25 g. The gross description should include the aggregate weight of the chips. Recognizable gross features such as yellow coloration and induration can be recorded, but it has not been proven that chip color, size, or induration is linked to cancer presence, so gross selection of specific chips is not required. Although gross TURP chip sampling procedures are not standardized, one initial approach is to submit 12 g of chips or 6 to 8 blocks of tissue (with 1 to 2 g per cassette).

For specimens >12 g, the initial 12 g are submitted, with one cassette for every additional 5 g (*Arch Pathol Lab Med* 2009;133:1568). If the patient is younger than 60 years, all tissue should be submitted; all chip tissue should also be submitted if microscopic examination of partially submitted chips reveals carcinoma in <5% of tissue, or if high-grade prostatic intraepithelial neoplasia (PIN) or atypical glands (atypical small acinar proliferation) is found in sections of partially submitted chips. One H&E-stained slide, with one or two sections, is typically generated from each paraffin block of TURP chips.

C. **Open Suprapubic or Retropubic Simple Prostatectomy (Enucleation) Tissue.** The prostatic tissue from simple prostatectomies may be submitted to the pathology laboratory as a single mass or as pieces. The tissue should be weighed and sectioned at 3- to 5-mm intervals. The gross description should include size in three dimensions, weight, firmness, and coloration. Hard nodules should be sampled, and a total of eight cassettes or one cassette of tissue for each 5 g of tissue submitted. Additional tissue should be submitted if carcinoma is histologically detected in initial sections of partially submitted tissue, although no rules or recommendations exist on how many additional sections are required. One H&E-stained slide should be made per block.

D. **Radical Prostatectomy.** The entire prostate gland and seminal vesicles are excised in prostate cancer surgery using open retropubic or perineal approaches, or using laparoscopic (including robotic) approaches. The prostate gland and seminal vesicles are also resected in toto in radical cystoprostatectomy for bladder cancer.

1. **Pelvic lymph nodes.** Pelvic lymphadenectomy may be performed as a separate procedure, often laparoscopic, or during the radical prostatectomy operation. Sentinel lymph node sampling is not routinely performed.

   Frozen section analysis of the sampled lymph nodes may be requested for patients at risk for nodal metastasis, based on serum prostate-specific antigen (PSA) level, needle biopsy Gleason score, and clinical stage. All grossly recognizable lymph nodes should be examined by frozen section; cytologic touch imprints can be made at the same time. Frozen section diagnosis of metastatic carcinoma in lymph nodes is highly specific, but fairly insensitive. The low sensitivity rate of 58% to 73% is due to sampling error.

   Gross sampling of tissue after frozen section should entail submission of all grossly identifiable lymph node tissue and wide sampling of associated adipose tissue. The gross description of pelvic lymph nodes should include number, location, and size. One H&E-stained slide is made per paraffin block. Special studies to detect occult lymph node metastases, such as immunohistochemistry for cytokeratins or PSA, or reverse transcription–polymerase chain reaction (RT–PCR) for PSA RNA, are currently experimental and not performed in routine practice.

2. **Prostate gland and seminal vesicles.** The prostate gland and seminal vesicles from radical prostatectomy procedures may be received fresh or in fixative. All three dimensions and specimen weight should be recorded. Frozen section requests on fresh specimens are uncommon, and are usually made to evaluate margin status; this procedure has a high false-negative rate and is not standard practice. Fresh specimens are also used for tissue-banking protocols; after inking the entire outside of the specimen, tissue can be harvested from inside the gland while preserving the inked periphery. Alternatively, after inking, margin sampling, and seminal vesicle amputation (see below), the whole unfixed gland can be sectioned with a large sharp knife from apex to base at 4-mm intervals perpendicular to the prostatic urethra; areas suspicious for carcinoma, as judged by palpation or visual inspection, may be sampled by imprints, scrapes, core biopsy, or small wedge sections.

   Fixation of the inked radical prostatectomy specimens (sectioned or unsectioned) is accomplished by at least overnight (or 24- to-48 hour) room temperature immersion in 10% neutral buffered formalin at 10 times the volume of the specimen. For gross examination of unsectioned glands after inking, the seminal vesicles are amputated (including the soft tissue and prostatic tissue at the base of the seminal vesicles) and submitted separately as right and left seminal vesicles. The prostate weight without the seminal vesicles is recorded, and distal apical (urethral) and bladder neck margins are taken if not already submitted separately by the surgeon. The distal apical margin is evaluated by amputating the distal 5 to 10 mm of the gland, dividing it into the right and left sides, and submitting radial sections (as for a cervical cone biopsy). The bladder neck margin can be assessed by a thin 2-mm shave margin or by conization; the latter is recommended. Ink on tumor cells is indicative of a positive margin for cone sections and the peripheral margin, whereas tumor anywhere in shave margin tissue indicates a positive margin. Vasa deferentia stumps may be sampled using *en face* sections. The prostate gland is serially sectioned in a plane perpendicular to the urethra at 3- to 5-mm intervals using a long knife. The cut surfaces should be evaluated for gross evidence of BPH and carcinoma. Photographs or digital images can be used to document location and gross appearance of tissue in submitted cassettes. Diagrams (Fig. 29.1) or pictorial maps can also be used to indicate location of sections and any gross abnormalities. Correlation with prostate MRI findings, if available, can also be helpful in directing sampling of the gland.

Both complete embedding and partial embedding methods are acceptable (*Mod Pathol* 2011;24:6). Several protocols for partial submission have been published (*Scand J Urol Nephrol Suppl* 2005;216:34; *Mod Pathol* 2011;24:6). When there is grossly visible tumor, all lesions grossly suspicious for carcinoma should be submitted, along with distal apical and bladder neck margins and seminal vesicles. For cases with no grossly evident tumor, the posterior aspect of each transverse slice is submitted, as well as a mid-anterior block from each side, distal apical, and bladder neck margins, and the seminal vesicles. Sections should be submitted as quarters or halves of the prostate, depending on gland size. Whole-amount sections are rarely made and do not provide additional morphologic information. If no or minimal tumor is seen in initial sections of a partially submitted gland, all remaining tissue should be embedded (including any frozen tissue sent to a tissue bank). If still no tumor is

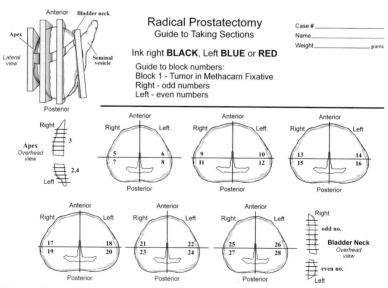

Figure 29.1 Diagram depicting guide to taking sections from a radical prostatectomy specimen. (Modified from True LD. Surgical pathology examination of the prostate gland. Practice survey by American Society of Clinical Pathologists. *Am J Clin Pathol* 1995;103:376.)

seen, basal cell and AMACR immunostains of atypical foci should be performed, and deeper sections should be obtained from block(s) from the region of the positive needle biopsy and areas of high-grade PIN (HG-PIN). If cancer remains undetected, the tissue blocks should be flipped, and histologic sections prepared from the new tissue faces (*Mod Pathol* 2011;24:6). Identity testing by short tandem repeat analysis can also confirm whether the radical prostatectomy specimen and prior prostate biopsy cores on which the diagnosis of carcinoma was originally rendered originated from the same patient, as there is a low but detectable rate of specimen provenance errors (usually that the prior biopsy was actually from a different patient) (*Am J Clin Pathol* 2013;139:93).

E. **Cystoprostatectomy.** The prostate gland in radical cystoprostatectomies performed for bladder cancer can be sampled by taking several sections of prostatic urethra and surrounding prostate tissue, any gross lesions, one block from the periphery of each side, and both seminal vesicles. The distal urethral shave margin is important in urothelial carcinoma cases. If prostate carcinoma is identified in the initial sections, additional sections should be submitted following the protocol for radical prostatectomy specimens (see above).

III. DIAGNOSTIC FEATURES OF COMMON DISEASES OF THE PROSTATE

A. **Inflammation and Infection.** Histopathologic identification of inflammatory cells in the prostate is common, but histologic identification of specific infectious agents is rare.

1. **Asymptomatic inflammatory prostatitis,** including acute neutrophilic inflammation and chronic lymphocytic, lymphoplasmacytic, or lymphohistiocytic inflammation, is common in all prostate tissue samples. Reporting this inflammation is optional; it may be useful to report if the inflammation is extensive or persistent in several needle core samples taken over time, because prostatic inflammation can raise the serum PSA. Inflammation can be associated with prostatic glandular atrophy and reactive nuclear changes including prominent nucleoli. Inflammation is more commonly associated with benign epithelial conditions, especially atrophy and BPH, compared with HG-PIN and carcinoma, where usually only a small percentage of foci (around 10%) are inflamed.

2. **Granulomatous prostatitis** can clinically elevate the serum PSA and/or present as a palpable abnormality. The most common type is nonspecific granulomatous prostatitis, which is thought to be a response to prostatic secretions released into the stroma by duct-acinar rupture. Microscopically, there is a lobulocentric noncaseating granulomatous inflammatory cell infiltrate with giant cells (e-**Fig. 29.4**). Variants include xanthogranulomatous prostatitis and so-called prostatic xanthoma. Other types of granulomatous prostatitis include infectious and postbiopsy/postresection cases. Infectious granulomatous prostatitis is most often Bacillus Calmette–Guérin (BCG) related in patients treated for bladder urothelial carcinoma (e-**Fig. 29.5**). Fungal prostatitis is rare and usually seen in immunosuppressed patients. Postbiopsy/resection granulomas are most often identified in TURP chip tissue, and are characterized by a fibrinoid central zone surrounded by palisading histiocytes.

B. **Atrophy** of prostatic glands is the benign condition most likely to be misdiagnosed as prostatic carcinoma by light microscopy. It is a common, age-related process that can be related to inflammation, hormones, obstruction, or ischemia. It can also be treatment-related, due to radiotherapy or hormonal therapy. Histologically, atrophy is defined as cytoplasmic volume loss. It is not necessary to subtype atrophy, but it is important to recognize the existence of different histomorphologic patterns including simple atrophy (with or without cystic change) (e-**Fig. 29.6**), sclerotic atrophy, partial atrophy (e-**Fig. 29.7**), and postatrophic hyperplasia (or hyperplastic atrophy) (e-**Figs. 29.8** and **29.9**). Atrophy can be confused with carcinoma because it is usually a small gland lesion that can show a pseudoinfiltrative pattern of growth, stromal sclerosis, nuclear atypia, and closely packed acini (in postatrophic hyperplasia). Atrophy can also be noted in cystically dilated peripheral zone glands (e-**Fig. 29.10**) and in cystic change in BPH nodules. Another diagnostic pitfall is that atrophic glands can show a fragmented basal cell layer and even loss of basal cells in a few glands by immunohisto-chemical stains (such as 34betaE12 and p63) (*Semin Diagn Pathol* 2005;22:88). Also, the selective but not specific marker for neoplastic epithelial cells alpha-methylacyl coenzyme A racemase (AMACR) can be immunopositive in atrophy, particularly partial atrophy.

C. **Metaplasia** or change in cell type in benign prostatic epithelium can be squamous, transitional cell (urothelial), mucinous, and eosinophilic. These metaplasias are usually secondary to inflammation, therapy, or injury. They are not preneoplastic.

1. **Squamous cell metaplasia** is most often an incidental finding associated with inflammation and infarction in BPH nodules. Microscopically, small solid nests or partially involved glands with a retained lumen are common (e-**Fig. 29.11**). Squa-moid cytoplasm and intercellular bridges may be evident, but keratin pearls are rare. Nuclear atypia, including prominent nuclei and mitoses, may be present in squamous metaplasia adjacent to infarcts. Squamous metaplasia after radiation or hormonal therapy can be more diffuse and is frequently immature with less cytoplasm and an absence of keratinization.

2. **Transitional cell or urothelial metaplasia** should be distinguished from urothelial cells that normally line the prostatic urethra and central ducts of the prostate. This is usually a focal, incidental finding with small solid nests or partial gland involvement by cytologically bland and uniform elongated cells, with some cells exhibiting nuclear grooves and cytoplasmic clearing (e-**Fig. 29.12**). It should be distinguished from urothelial carcinoma extending into prostatic ducts, a distinction readily made by morphologic evaluation.

3. **Mucinous metaplasia** is replacement of benign luminal epithelium by benign mucin-secretory cells. This is a focal, incidental microscopic finding in which the constituent cells have a granular blue cytoplasmic appearance (e-**Fig. 29.13**). Goblet cells and luminal secretion of the mucin are uncommon.

4. **Eosinophilic metaplasia** is the designation for benign epithelium with large supranuclear eosinophilic granules, which represent exocrine differentiation with lysosome-like granules. This uncommon and typically focal change is more often seen in prostatic ductal epithelium and is associated with variable degrees of chronic inflammation and atrophy. Paneth cell-like change, which is also characterized by large eosinophilic cytoplasmic granules, is usually seen in PIN and carcinoma and reflects neuroendocrine differentiation. Paneth cell-like alteration may be found in nonneoplastic prostatic epithelium after radiation.

D. **Hyperplasia.** BPH is a clinical diagnosis. Histologically, BPH can be diagnosed in TURP chips and simple and radical prostatectomy specimens, but it should not be diagnosed in needle biopsy tissue.

1. **Usual nodular epithelial and stromal hyperplasia** is the most common morpho-logic presentation of BPH. Grossly, the nodules, which characteristically arise in the transition zone and periurethral area, are multiple and vary from solid white to spongy with cystic change.

    a. **Pure stromal nodules (nodular stromal hyperplasia)** exist. Microscopically, the nodules can appear myxoid (e-**Fig. 29.14**), hyalinized, or leiomyomatous, with spindled, ovoid, or stellate cells. Prominent thick-walled blood vessels and lymphocytes may be noted.

    b. **Mixed epithelial and stromal hyperplasia** is most common, with variable admixtures of spindled stromal cells and complex benign glands with complex papillary and branching architecture (e-**Fig. 29.15**). Cystic change, inflammation, and basal cell hyperplasia are commonly detected in BPH nodules. Fibroadeno-matoid features (e-**Fig. 29.16**) can rarely be seen.

    c. **Epithelial predominant BPH nodules** (e-**Fig. 29.17**) are unusual.

    d. **Infarcts** can be identified in larger BPH nodules and can elevate serum PSA.

2. **Basal cell hyperplasia** is usually discovered in BPH nodules, but can also be found in peripheral zone needle biopsy tissue, often associated with inflammation.

Microscopically, there are two or more layers of basal cells arranged in acinar, cribriform, and solid growth patterns (e-**Fig. 29.18**). In usual basal cell hyperplasia, the basal cells are uniform and cytologically bland, whereas in so-called "atypical" basal cell hyperplasia prominent nucleoli are discerned. The term atypical should be avoided because no form of basal cell hyperplasia is a known risk factor for neoplasia.

3. **Cribriform hyperplasia** (e-**Fig. 29.19**), which is completely benign and not a risk factor for neoplasia, is an infrequently seen variant of BPH. The luminal lining cells are cytologically bland and there is a prominent rim of basal cells.

4. **Mesonephric remnant hyperplasia** is a very rare prostatic proliferation displaying a vaguely lobular or infiltrative pattern of small tubules with cuboidal epithelium and intraluminal, eosinophilic secretions (*Am J Surg Pathol* 2011;35:1054). Immunostains for high-molecular-weight cytokeratin (34betaE12) and/or p63 can be negative in some cases, and AMACR can be focally positive. These results may raise concern for prostatic adenocarcinoma, but helpful clues are negative prostate markers (PSA, PSAP, prostein, and/or NKX3.1) but positive PAX8 immunostains.

5. **Verumontanum gland hyperplasia** is a benign, small gland proliferation of the verumontanum and adjacent posterior urethra (e-**Fig. 29.20**). The closely packed glands can architecturally be confusing, but the lack of nuclear atypia and the presence of basal cells rules out carcinoma.

E. **Atypical Adenomatous Hyperplasia (Adenosis)** is a nodular proliferation of closely packed small acini (e-**Fig. 29.21**). It is invariably an incidental histologic finding, most often found in transition zone tissue in TURP chips or prostatectomy specimens. The densely packed small pale acini are sometimes intermingled with larger, more complex glands. Nuclear atypia is absent to minimal. The basal cell layer is fragmented, and, on average, 50% of glands completely lack basal cells. Of note, AMACR is diffusely positive in about 8% of cases. Adenosis can be mistaken for well-differentiated Gleason score 2 to 4 adenocarcinoma. It does not have known premalignant potential.

F. **PIN** is a proliferation of atypical epithelial cells in pre-existing ducts and acini (synonyms used in the past include atypical hyperplasia and dysplasia). Currently, PIN is graded as low-grade PIN and HG-PIN, although only HG-PIN has potential clinical significance and merits reporting. Isolated HG-PIN is diagnosed in about 5% to 10% of needle biopsies (*J Urol* 2006;175:820). It is found in the vast majority of radical prostatectomy specimens with prostatic carcinoma. Microscopically, there are four major structural patterns of HG-PIN growth: tufting, micropapillary, cribriform, and flat (*Mod Pathol* 2004;17:360) (Fig. 29.2; e-**Fig. 29.22**). These patterns are often admixed. At high power magnification, HG-PIN shows basal cells (which are typically reduced in number) and atypical luminal cells. Nuclear abnormalities that should be present to diagnose HG-PIN include increased nuclear size, increased chromatin clumping and content, and prominent nucleoli. The diagnosis can usually be made on H&E-stained sections. Immunostains for basal cells (34betaE12 and p63) and AMACR can be useful when the differential diagnosis is HG-PIN with outpouching versus HG-PIN with associated invasive adenocarcinoma (*Am J Surg Pathol* 2005;29:529). Routine immunostains are not helpful in differentiating HG-PIN versus intraductal carcinoma, which is largely a morphologic distinction; some labs utilize ERG and PTEN immunostains to facilitate classification in this setting (ERG more commonly positive in carcinoma, with loss of PTEN staining) (*Am J Surg Pathol* 2015;39:169; *Mod Pathol* 2018;31:S71). Occasionally, nuclear atypia and architectural features are intermediate between HG-PIN and intraductal carcinoma, in which case a diagnosis of "atypical intraductal proliferation" with a comment may be most appropriate (*Am J Surg Pathol* 2016;40:e67).

Isolated HG-PIN in needle biopsy and TURP chips has been considered a risk factor for subsequent detection of carcinoma on rebiopsy, although the level of risk has decreased with increased 10- to 12-core sampling of the prostate (*Urology* 2005;65:538; *Am J Surg Pathol* 2005;29:1201), such that not all patients necessarily need to undergo rebiopsy in the first year following diagnosis of isolated HG-PIN (*J Urol* 2006;175:820).

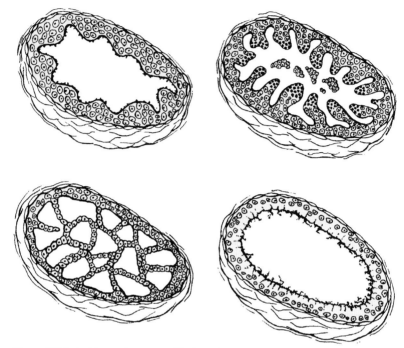

Figure 29.2 Architectural patterns of high-grade prostatic intraepithelial neoplasia (PIN). (From Humphrey PA. *Prostate Pathology.* Chicago: ASCP Press; 2003. Used with permission.)

However, patients with two or more cores with HG-PIN do appear to be at increased risk for subsequent detection of carcinoma and should be considered candidates for rebiopsy (*J Urol* 2009;182:485).

G. **Focal Glandular Atypia (Atypical Small Acinar Proliferation)** is a descriptive diagnosis for a gland or group of glands with architectural or cytologic atypia that does not allow for a definitive diagnosis of reactive atypia, atypical adenomatous hyperplasia, PIN, or carcinoma. If there is significant concern for malignancy, a diagnosis of focal glandular atypia, suspicious for carcinoma may be rendered. A diagnosis of atypia is applied in about 3% (range 1% to 9%) of needle biopsies (*J Urol* 2006;175:820). Distortion artifact, section thickness, and overstaining can contribute to difficulty in interpretation; immunostains for basal cells (34betaE12 and p63) and AMACR can be very useful in establishing a definitive diagnosis when atypia is the initial diagnosis in H&E-stained sections. Patients with a diagnosis of atypia or atypical small acinar proliferation (ASAP) in a needle biopsy should be clinically followed and rebiopsied, because about 43% of men are diagnosed with carcinoma on rebiopsy (*J Urol* 2006;175:820).

H. **Prostate Cancer,** which is acinar adenocarcinoma in the vast majority of cases, is a common malignancy in North America, Europe, and Australia, whereas it is less common in Asia.

1. **Risk factors.** Proven risk factors for adenocarcinoma include age, family history, and race. Prostatic adenocarcinoma is uncommonly diagnosed clinically before the age of 50, though a significant minority of men (around 31%) in their 30s and 40s have a small adenocarcinoma detectable at autopsy (*In Vivo* 1994;8:1459).

Hereditary prostatic adenocarcinoma accounts for about 10% of prostatic adenocarcinomas. Several candidate genes involved in hereditary transmission have been identified; genetic analysis is not routinely performed but may be useful in patients with metastatic, castrate-resistant prostate cancer for whom targeted therapies are being considered (*Cancer* 2018;124:3105). Probable risk factors include dietary fat and androgens; potential risk factors are cadmium, low vitamin D, low vitamin E, low selenium, herbicides, and sedentary lifestyle.

2. **Clinical diagnosis** of clinically localized prostate cancer is based on serum PSA and digital rectal examination (DRE). Serum PSA is widely used for early detection in the United States, although its use for screening is controversial. Serum PSA level is clearly related to risk for histologic diagnosis of carcinoma, but risk exists below the most often used 4.0 ng/mL prompt for biopsy (*N Engl J Med* 2013;347:215). The DRE is neither particularly sensitive nor specific for a diagnosis of prostatic carcinoma. Prostate MRI also is increasingly being adopted for evaluation of the prostate, with a lesion scoring system (PI-RADS) analogous to the one used in breast imaging (BI-RADS) (*Eur Urol* 2016;69:16). However, histopathologic tissue diagnosis remains the standard to establish a diagnosis of malignancy in the prostate.

Prostatic carcinoma generally does not cause symptoms until late in the course of the disease. Local growth into the urethra and bladder neck can cause increase in frequency and difficulty in urination. Metastatic spread to bone can produce pain in the lower back, chest, hip, legs, and shoulders. Response to treatment is followed by serum PSA determinations, and in some cases, radiologic studies.

3. **Histologic typing and diagnosis.** The 2016 World Health Organization (WHO) classification of neoplasms of the prostate is given in Table 29.1 (*Eur Urol* 2016;70:106).

4. **Acinar adenocarcinoma** of the prostate is by far the most common type of prostate cancer.

   a. **Gross diagnosis** of prostatic carcinoma is sometimes possible in radical prostatectomy tissues but not in needle biopsy or TURP chip tissues. Impalpable prostatic carcinomas detected due to an elevated serum PSA (clinical stage T1c) are difficult if not impossible to visualize on cut sections of radical prostatectomy specimens. When visible, the carcinoma can appear nodular and white to irregular and gray or white-yellow (e-**Fig. 29.23**).

   b. **Microscopic diagnosis** is based on a synthesis of a constellation of histologic attributes (Table 29.2) (*J Clin Pathol* 2007;60:35). Major criteria are architecture (pattern of growth), absence of basal cells, and nuclear atypia.

   The architectural patterns of cellular arrangement are well depicted in the Gleason grading diagram (Fig. 29.3). Well-differentiated prostatic adenocarcinoma of Gleason patterns 1 and 2 displays abnormal glandular arrangements in the form of well-circumscribed nodules of closely packed small acini (e-**Fig. 29.24**). Gleason pattern 3 usually presents as single, small, infiltrating glands (e-**Fig. 29.25**). Gleason pattern 4 is cribriform (e-**Fig. 29.26**), fused small acinar, or shows poorly formed glands. Gleason pattern 5 is composed of sheets, single cells, or comedocarcinoma (e-**Fig. 29.27**) (*Am J Surg Pathol* 2005;29:1228; *J Urol* 2010;183:433).

   Basal cell absence, the second major criterion, can sometimes be difficult to evaluate in H&E-stained sections, so in difficult cases and for small foci of adenocarcinoma (minimal or limited adenocarcinoma), immunohistochemical staining for basal cells using antibodies against high-molecular-weight cytokeratins (such as 34betaE12, also known as CK903) and p63 may be performed (e-**Fig. 29.28**). While a positive basal cell immunostain effectively rules out invasive adenocarcinoma, benign glands can focally lack a basal cell layer. In addition, intraductal carcinoma has a retained basal cell layer. Thus, basal cell immunostains must be interpreted in the context of the H&E histologic findings (*Semin Diagn Pathol* 2005;22:88).

TABLE 29.1   WHO Histologic Classification of Tumors of Prostate

Epithelial tumors

Glandular neoplasms

Adenocarcinoma (acinar)
 Atrophic
 Pseudohyperplastic
 Foamy gland
 Mucinous (colloid)
 Signet ring-like cell
 Pleomorphic giant cell
 Sarcomatoid

Prostatic intraepithelial neoplasia (PIN),
 high-grade

Intraductal carcinoma

Ductal adenocarcinoma
 Cribriform
 Papillary
 Solid

Urothelial carcinoma

Squamous tumors
 Adenosquamous carcinoma
 Squamous cell carcinoma

Basal cell carcinoma

Neuroendocrine tumors

Adenocarcinoma with neuroendocrine
 differentiation

Well-differentiated neuroendocrine tumor

Small cell neuroendocrine carcinoma

Large cell neuroendocrine carcinoma

Mesenchymal tumors

Stromal tumor of uncertain malignant
 potential

Stromal sarcoma

Leiomyosarcoma

Rhabdomyosarcoma

Leiomyoma

Angiosarcoma

Synovial sarcoma

Inflammatory myofibroblastic tumor

Osteosarcoma

Undifferentiated pleomorphic sarcoma

Solitary fibrous tumor

Solitary fibrous tumor, malignant

Hemangioma

Granular cell tumor

Hematolymphoid tumors

Diffuse large B-cell lymphoma

Chronic lymphocytic leukemia/small
 lymphocytic lymphoma

Follicular lymphoma

Mantle cell lymphoma

Acute myeloid leukemia

B lymphoblastic leukemia/lymphoma

Miscellaneous tumors

Cystadenoma

Nephroblastoma

Rhabdoid tumor

Germ cell tumors

Clear cell adenocarcinoma

Melanoma

Paraganglioma

Neuroblastoma

Metastatic tumors

Tumors of the seminal vesicles

Epithelial tumors

Adenocarcinoma

Squamous cell carcinoma

Mixed epithelial and stromal tumors

Cystadenoma

Mesenchymal tumors

Leiomyoma

Schwannoma

Mammary-type myofibroblastoma

Gastrointestinal stromal tumor

Leiomyosarcoma

Angiosarcoma

Liposarcoma

Solitary fibrous tumor

Hemangiopericytoma

Miscellaneous tumors

Choriocarcinoma

Seminoma

Well-differentiated neuroendocrine tumor

Lymphomas

Ewing sarcoma

Metastatic tumors

From: Moch H, Humphrey PA, Ulbright TM, Reuter VE, eds. *WHO Classification of Tumours of the Urinary System and Male Genital Organs.* Lyon, France: IARC Press; 2017. Used with permission.

TABLE 29.2 Criteria for Diagnosis of Prostatic Adenocarcinoma

Major criteria

Architectural: Infiltrative small glands or cribriform glands too large or irregular to represent high-grade prostatic intraepithelial neoplasia (PIN)

Single cell layer (absence of basal cells)

Nuclear atypia: Nuclear and nucleolar enlargement

Minor criteria

Intraluminal wispy blue mucin (blue-tinged or basophilic mucinous secretions)

Pink amorphous secretions

Mitotic figures

Intraluminal crystalloids

Adjacent high-grade PIN

Amphophilic cytoplasm

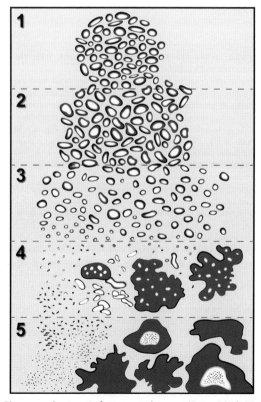

Figure 29.3 Gleason grades 1 to 5, from top to bottom. (From: Moch H, Humphrey PA, Ulbright TM, Reuter VE, eds. *WHO Classification of Tumours of the Urinary System and Male Genital Organs.* Lyon, France: IARC Press; 2017. Used with permission.)

TABLE 29.3 Immunophenotype of Prostatic Versus Urothelial (Transitional Cell) Carcinoma

Marker	Percentage of Cases Positive	
	Prostatic Carcinoma	Urothelial Carcinoma
PSA	94–100%	0%
PSAP	89–100%	0%
PSMA	92%	0%
NKX3.1	95%	0%
Prostein	100%	6%
GATA3	Rare, focal	86–>90%
p63	0–3%	81–96%
Thrombomodulin	0%	69–91%
Uroplakin III	0%	57%
High molecular weight cytokeratin[a]	0–10%[b]	65–100%

PSAP, prostate-specific acid phosphatase; PSMA, prostate specific membrane antigen.
[a]Detected by antibody 34betaE12.
[b]Mean = 3% prostatic carcinoma cases positive. Up to 20% of cases of metastatic prostatic carcinoma can be positive.

Nuclear atypia, the third of the major criteria, takes the form of nuclear enlargement and nucleolar enlargement.

The minor criteria (Table 29.2) tend to be found more often in adenocarcinoma, but are not specific for adenocarcinoma. Features considered specific for a diagnosis of prostatic adenocarcinoma include extraprostatic spread of prostatic glands, collagenous micronodules (also known as mucinous fibroplasia, e-Fig. 29.29), glomeruloid intraglandular projections (e-Fig. 29.30), and perineural invasion (e-Fig. 29.31). Of note, benign glands can abut intraprostatic nerves (*Am J Surg Pathol* 2005;29:1159).

c. **Immunohistochemical studies** are helpful in a minority of cases. The most commonly used immunostains are those for basal cells and for the neoplastic cell-selective marker (alpha-methylacyl coenzyme A racemase [AMACR or P504S]), and are usually used to assess a few atypical glands in a needle biopsy. AMACR is fairly sensitive for neoplastic prostatic epithelial cells (in both PIN and invasive carcinoma), staining 80% to 100% of adenocarcinomas, but is not specific as it can be found focally in benign glands (*Semin Diagn Pathol* 2005;22:88). Cocktails using p63 and AMACR or p63/34betaE12/AMACR antibodies are useful when a limited amount of tissue is available for staining (e-Fig. 29.28) (*Am J Surg Pathol* 2005;29:579; *Semin Diagn Pathol* 2005;22:88). PSA and GATA3 immunostains should be used for poorly differentiated carcinomas when the differential diagnosis is poorly differentiated prostatic adenocarcinoma versus poorly differentiated urothelial carcinoma (Table 29.3) (*Semin Diagn Pathol* 2005;22:88; *Am J Surg Pathol* 2014;38:e6). High-molecular-weight cytokeratin (34betaE12), p63, prostein (P501S), and NKX3.1 can be helpful if PSA and GATA3 are negative. PSA, PSAP, prostein, and/or NKX3.1 immunostains should always be performed when confronted with a metastatic adenocarcinoma of unknown primary origin in a man.

d. **Molecular studies** are not currently used to diagnose prostatic carcinoma, though commercially available gene expression assays may be used on archival prostate tissues from patients with low or favorable intermediate risk disease for prediction of prognosis/therapy response (including Prolaris, Decipher, Oncotype DX Prostate, and ProMark testing). Mismatch repair deficiency or microsatellite instability testing also may be considered in patients with regional or distant metastatic disease (National Comprehensive Cancer Network [NCCN] Guidelines Version 4.2018, 8/15/2018, https://www.nccn.org/professionals/physician_gls/PDF/prostate.pdf). Testing (including ConfirmMDx) also is available for evaluation of the likelihood that a patient does have unsampled prostate cancer when the prostate biopsies show no cancer.

5. **Variants of acinar adenocarcinoma** include atrophic, pseudohyperplastic, microcystic, foamy, mucinous (colloid), signet ring-like cell, pleomorphic giant cell, and sarcomatoid carcinoma (Table 29.1). Atrophic pattern adenocarcinoma displays decreased cytoplasm and can thereby mimic benign atrophy (e-**Fig. 29.32**). Such cytoplasmic volume loss can be seen with or without a history of hormonal or radiation therapy. Most cases are Gleason pattern 3. Pseudohyperplastic carcinoma is another malignancy that can resemble benign glands (*Am J Surg Pathol* 1998;22:1139). Here, the malignant glands simulate BPH glands (e-**Fig. 29.33**) in that they are complex with intraluminal papillary projections, undulating luminal surfaces, branching patterns, and/or cystic dilatation. Gleason grade assignment is pattern 3. Foamy gland carcinoma is characterized by xanthomatous cytoplasm and bland nuclei (e-**Fig. 29.34**); these carcinomas are usually Gleason score 6 or 7, but can be higher grade. Mucinous carcinoma of the prostate is defined as adenocarcinoma with at least 25% of the tumor composed of lakes of extracellular mucin (e-**Fig. 29.35**); this is a rare variant, with a Gleason grade pattern of 4 (usually) or 3. In the past this variant was thought to be more aggressive than usual acinar adenocarcinoma, but recent reports suggest otherwise. Signet-ring carcinoma of the prostate is also rare and clinically aggressive; the Gleason grade is 5. Sarcomatoid carcinoma of the prostate is rare (*Am J Surg Pathol* 2006;30:1316) and may be a homologous spindle cell malignancy or heterologous, with an osteosarcomatous (e-**Fig. 29.36**), chondrosarcomatous, or rhabdomyosarcomatous component. In one half of the men there is a history of prostatic adenocarcinoma treated by hormonal and/or radiation therapy; the outcome is poor. Microcystic adenocarcinoma (*Am J Surg Pathol* 2010;34:556) and pleomorphic giant cell carcinoma are rare. A variant morphologically resembling HG-PIN with dilated glands (PIN-like adenocarcinoma) also has been described but is rare (*Am J Surg Pathol* 2008;32:1060).

6. **Ductal adenocarcinoma** (not to be confused with *intraductal* adenocarcinoma, which is a pattern of growth rather than a distinct morphologic subtype) is the second most common subtype of prostatic adenocarcinoma (after acinar). Previously known as endometrioid adenocarcinoma, in pure form it accounts for about 1% of prostatic cancers and, when mixed with acinar adenocarcinoma, roughly 5% of prostatic cancers. Microscopically, these are usually papillary and/or cribriform adenocarcinomas (e-**Fig. 29.37**) that can arise centrally (causing urinary obstruction and hematuria) or peripherally. Cytologically, tall columnar neoplastic cells with cleared or amphophilic cytoplasm may be observed. Most patients present at a more advanced stage, and outcome is worse than that of acinar adenocarcinoma. Gleason grade is typically pattern 4. Serum PSA may be normal or only mildly elevated in patients with ductal adenocarcinoma.

7. **Intraductal carcinoma** is involvement of prostatic ducts by prostatic carcinoma (acinar subtype or otherwise), most commonly in the setting of high grade (Gleason score >7, mean Gleason score 8), high volume invasive carcinoma. By definition, the basal cell layer is retained, as can be demonstrated by immunostaining for basal cell markers (p63, 34betaE12). Tumor cells fill and often expand existing ducts and large acini with either solid or dense cribriform architecture (in which case the differential diagnosis includes invasive Gleason pattern 4 or 5 adenocarcinoma) or loose cribriform or micropapillary growth accompanied by marked nuclear atypia (exceeding the degree of atypia seen in HG-PIN) or comedonecrosis.

In rare cases where biopsies show purely intraductal carcinoma without detection of an invasive component, repeat biopsy or prostatectomy should be considered (*J Urol* 2010;184:1328).

Occasionally, an intraductal proliferation is encountered which shows architectural and cytologic features intermediate between HG-PIN and frank intraductal carcinoma, in which case a diagnosis of "atypical intraductal proliferation" is appropriate, accompanied by a comment about the association of intraductal carcinoma with invasive carcinomas (*Am J Surg Pathol* 2016;40:367).

8. **Rare types of prostatic carcinoma** include urothelial carcinoma (arising from central prostatic ducts), squamous and adenosquamous carcinoma (**e-Fig. 29.38**), basal cell carcinoma, and neuroendocrine carcinoma, including small cell and large cell neuroendocrine carcinoma (*Mod Pathol* 2004;17:316). It is important to exclude primary urethral and urinary bladder urothelial carcinoma before diagnosing primary prostatic urothelial carcinoma. An in situ component can be extensive in the prostate, with solid plugs of cytologically pleomorphic tumor cells, often with comedonecrosis and stromal inflammation; prostatic stromal invasion is typified by irregular solid nests and cords. Squamous cell and adenosquamous carcinomas of the prostate comprise less than 1% of all prostatic carcinomas, and in about two thirds of cases there is a history of hormonal and or radiation treatment (*Am J Surg Pathol* 2004;28:651). Average survival is 2 years. Basal cell carcinoma of the prostate includes malignant basaloid proliferations (basaloid or basal cell carcinomas) and also neoplasms that resemble, to a certain degree, adenoid cystic carcinomas of the salivary glands (*Am J Surg Pathol* 2003;27:1523). Basal cell carcinomas have several growth arrangements, including large basaloid nests with peripheral palisading and necrosis, a florid basal cell hyperplasia-like pattern, and an adenoid basal cell hyperplasia-like pattern (adenoid cystic carcinoma pattern). Small cell carcinoma of the prostate is quite rare and in one-half of cases is admixed with adenocarcinoma; the histologic appearance is similar to that of small cell carcinoma of the lung. In one-third of cases there is a history of prostatic adenocarcinoma followed by hormonal therapy (**e-Fig. 29.39**). A similar history is obtained in most cases of large cell neuroendocrine carcinoma of the prostate (*Am J Surg Pathol* 2006;30:684). Outcome is very poor for neuroendocrine carcinomas of the prostate.

9. **Mesenchymal neoplasms** are rare. The most common benign mesenchymal neoplasm is leiomyoma, and the most common malignant mesenchymal neoplasms are rhabdomyosarcoma in children and leiomyosarcoma in adults. Stromal tumors arising from specialized prostatic stroma include stromal tumors of uncertain malignant potential (STUMPs) (**e-Fig. 29.40**) and stromal sarcomas.

10. **Hematolymphoid neoplasms** may involve the prostate, including leukemia, lymphoma, Hodgkin disease, and multiple myeloma. Leukemic infiltrates almost always indicate secondary spread, usually of chronic lymphocytic leukemia. However, about one-third of prostatic lymphomas are primary, most commonly diffuse large B cell lymphoma.

11. **Miscellaneous neoplasms** rarely encountered in the prostate include cystadenoma, clear cell carcinoma of the utricle/prostate, paraganglioma, melanocytic neoplasms, and germ cell tumors.

12. **Secondary malignancy** in the prostate is overall uncommon, but can be seen in a substantial minority of patients with urothelial carcinoma of the bladder (**e-Fig. 29.41**), leukemia, and non-Hodgkin lymphoma.

13. **Treatment effects** can substantially alter the morphology of prostatic carcinoma, resulting in difficulty in diagnosis.

   a. **Hormonal androgen deprivation therapy** can cause a decrease in the number of glands, glandular atrophy, single tumor cells, nuclear pyknosis, and cytoplasmic vacuolization (**e-Fig. 29.42**). The carcinoma cells often resemble lymphocytes or histiocytes. PSA and pancytokeratin immunostains can be useful.

   b. **Radiation therapy** can induce striking nuclear atypia in benign glands. Positive basal cell and negative AMACR immunostains support a diagnosis of benign atypia. Adenocarcinoma postradiotherapy shows a decrease in number of neoplastic glands, poorly formed glands and single cells, cytoplasmic vacuolization, and nuclear pyknosis (e-**Fig. 29.43**). Immunostains for basal cells and AMACR can be useful in diagnosis in this setting (e-**Fig. 29.44**).

I. **Seminal Vesicles** are rarely the site of origin of primary disease, whether inflammatory or neoplastic. Amyloid can be identified in about 10% of seminal vesicles, as a function of aging; its presence does not indicate systemic amyloidosis unless there is also co-existing vascular amyloid deposition, which is rare. Seminal vesicles are usually examined for prostatic carcinoma as a part of pathologic staging.

J. **Prostatic Urethra** urothelium is subject to the same diseases as urothelium in the urinary bladder, namely inflammation, metaplasia (squamous metaplasia, urethritis cystica and glandularis, and nephrogenic metaplasia [adenoma]), hyperplasia, and neoplasms such as papilloma and carcinoma. However, primary isolated malignancies of the prostatic urethra are exceedingly rare, and malignancy in the prostatic urethra is most often due to secondary synchronous involvement by urothelial (transitional cell) carcinoma of the urinary bladder.

IV. **HISTOLOGIC GRADING OF PROSTATIC ADENOCARCINOMA.** Gleason grade is critical for patient prognosis. It is commonly used clinically, along with serum PSA level and clinical or pathologic stage, in tables (Partin tables) (http://urology.jhu.edu/Partin_tables/index.html) and nomograms (*J Urol* 2001;165:1562; *Cancer* 2009;15(Suppl):3107) to predict pathologic stage and response to treatment and outcome. Gleason score also is used to help generate risk groups that drive patient management (NCCN Guidelines Version 4.2018, 8/15/2018, https://www.nccn.org/professionals/physician_gls/PDF/prostate.pdf)

Grading should be performed using the Gleason system (Fig. 29.3). The so-called "grade group" (Table 29.4) (*Eur Urol* 2016;69:428), which is based on the Gleason score, should be reported in addition to the Gleason score. All adenocarcinomas of the prostate should be graded, except those that are posthormonal therapy or postradiotherapy (when radiation effect is evident). Grading is based solely on architecture and does not incorporate cytologic atypia or mitotic activity. At low magnification (40 to 100×), the most common pattern and the second most common pattern are summed to yield a score (on a scale of 2 to 10). Recent recommendations in application of the Gleason system include the following (*Am J Surg Pathol* 2005;29:1228; *J Urol* 2010;183:433; *Am J Surg Pathol* 2016;40:244; *Am J Surg Pathol* 2017;41:e1).

A. Do not (or rarely) assign a well-differentiated Gleason score 2 to 4 to carcinoma in a needle biopsy. This almost always represents undergrading.

B. When three grades are present in a needle biopsy, give most common grade and worst grade. Thus, if 3 + 4 + 5 are present, the Gleason grade is 3 + 5 = score of 8. In a radical prostatectomy, give the most common and second most common grades, but if there is a minor (<5%) tertiary high-grade 4 or 5 pattern, this should be noted.

C. If there is 95% high-grade pattern 4 or 5 and 5% or less of pattern 2 or 3, ignore the lower-grade component.

D. Any high-grade pattern (4 or 5) should be incorporated into a needle biopsy Gleason score. Thus, 98% pattern 3 and 2% pattern 4 in a needle biopsy is Gleason grade 3 + 4 = score of 7, with a comment indicating the percentage of pattern 4.

E. High-grade patterns also should be included in the radical prostatectomy Gleason grading. If only two Gleason patterns are present in a radical prostatectomy specimen

TABLE 29.4	Grade Group and Gleason Scores
Grade Group	**Gleason Score**
1	<= 6 (usually 3 + 3)
2	3 + 4 = 7
3	4 + 3 = 7
4	8 (4 + 4, 3 + 5, 5 + 3)
5	9 or 10 (4 + 5, 5 + 4, 5 + 5)

(e.g. 98% pattern 3 and 2% pattern 4), the minor high-grade component is included in the Gleason score as 3 + 4 = 7 (2% pattern 4)/grade group 2. If three Gleason patterns are present and the tumor consists mostly of low-grade adenocarcinoma, the minor high-grade component is included as a "minor pattern" (previously called "tertiary pattern"); for example, a tumor that is 80% pattern 3, 16% pattern 4, and 4% pattern 5 is Gleason score 3 + 4 = 7/grade group 2, with minor pattern 5 (4%).

F. Variants of prostatic adenocarcinoma can be graded (see above).

G. Cribriform adenocarcinomas are high-grade pattern 4.

H. For needle biopsies, provide grade by clinically submitted container, even if several cores are within the container. It may also be helpful to provide the Gleason grade for the core with highest Gleason score if different from the overall Gleason score for cores from that container.

I. Percentage of the tumor composed of Gleason patterns 4 and 5 should be reported; this is mandatory only for Gleason score 7 (3+4 or 4+3/grade groups 2 and 3) but may be helpful in any case where high-grade patterns are present.

V. PATHOLOGIC STAGING. Staging applies only to prostatic adenocarcinoma and follows the Tumor, Node, Metastasis (TNM) staging classification from the American Joint Committee on Cancer (AJCC) (Amin MB et al., eds. *AJCC Cancer Staging Manual.* 8th ed. New York: Springer, 2017). Clinical staging should be distinguished from pathologic staging.

A. Needle Biopsy. Pathologic staging is not performed. However, specific mention should be made of carcinoma seen in fat or in seminal vesicle tissue.

B. TURP Chips and Open Prostatectomy. Pathologic staging is not done, but for incidental carcinoma, the amount of carcinoma determined by light microscopic inspection of tissue involved will place the patient into clinical stage Tla or Tlb.

C. Radical prostatectomy and pelvic lymphadenectomy are used for pathologic staging.

1. pT2: Organ-confined prostatic carcinoma.

2. pT3: Extraprostatic extension (EPE) by carcinoma, diagnosed if carcinoma extends into posterolateral periprostatic adipose tissue (**e-Fig. 29.45**), beyond the outer boundary of normal prostatic glands at the anterior or apical prostate, or microscopically into the bladder neck. Note that carcinoma in skeletal muscle at apex does not always mean EPE. Site(s) and extent of EPE should be specified. EPE extent should be given as focal (only a few glands outside the prostate) or nonfocal. Capsular invasion is not part of the staging scheme. pT3b is seminal vesicle wall invasion (**e-Fig. 29.46**).

3. pT4: Gross involvement of adjacent structures (bladder, rectum, pelvic sidewall).

4. pN: If nodal metastases are present (pN1), the number of involved and total number of examined lymph nodes should be given.

5. pM: At time of radical prostatectomy, patients are clinical M0 (cM0). Distant metastases include nonregional lymph nodes (pM1a), bone (pM1b), and other sites (pM1c).

VI. REPORTING PROSTATE CANCER. Reporting should follow published guidelines (*Arch Pathol Lab Med* 2009;133:1568; *Mod Pathol* 2011;24:1). Templates for reporting are available (for example, see the College of American Pathologists Protocol for the Examination of Specimens From Patients With Carcinoma of the Prostate Gland, at http://www.cap.org).

For fine needle aspiration biopsy samples with carcinoma identified, grade should be given as well, moderately, or poorly differentiated.

For needle core biopsy samples, histologic type, Gleason grade, grade group, and amount of tumor should be provided. Amount of tumor should be quantitated as number of positive cores/total number of cores, percentage of tissue involved by carcinoma (by visual inspection), and linear millimeters of carcinoma per total millimeters of tissue. If present, periprostatic fat invasion, seminal vesicle invasion, perineural invasion, and lymphovascular space invasion should be reported.

For TURP and simple (enucleation) prostatectomy specimens, report the histologic type, Gleason grade, grade group, and amount of tumor. For Gleason grade, if three patterns are present, use the predominant and worst pattern of the remaining two. The percentage of tissue involved by tumor (by visual inspection) should be indicated; it is also recommended to report the number of positive chips per total number of chips. If present, periprostatic fat invasion, seminal vesicle invasion, perineural invasion, and lymphovascular space invasion should be reported.

For radical prostatectomy specimens, report histologic type, Gleason grade, grade group, amount of tumor, pathologic stage, and margin status. The amount of tumor should be reported as percentage of tissue involved by carcinoma (by visual inspection); greatest dimension of the dominant nodule (if present) may also be reported. For margins involved by carcinoma, the number and location of positive sites should be specified; the extent of margin positivity should be reported as limited (<3 mm) or nonlimited (>= 3 mm) (note: if a margin is positive for carcinoma without EPE, it is designated as pT2+). Evidence of prior treatment effect should be noted. Additional findings that may be reported include intraductal carcinoma, lymphovascular space invasion by carcinoma, inflammation, BPH, PIN, and adenosis.

Penis and Scrotum
Dengfeng Cao and Peter A. Humphrey

I. NORMAL ANATOMY. The penis is anatomically composed of three parts: posterior (root); central body or shaft; and anterior portion composed of glans, coronal sulcus, and foreskin (prepuce). In the shaft there are three cylinders of erectile tissues: a ventral corpus spongiosum surrounding the urethra and two corpora cavernosa. Histologically, the erectile tissues are characterized by numerous vascular spaces with surrounding smooth muscle fibers (**e-Fig. 30.1**). The tunica albuginea, a sheath of hyalinized collagen, encases the corpora cavernosa. All three corpora are surrounded by Buck's fascia, adipose tissue, dartos muscle, dermis, and a thin epidermis. Distally, the corpus spongiosum forms the conical glans, which is also composed of a stratified squamous epithelium, lamina propria, tunica albuginea, and corpora cavernosa. The coronal sulcus is a cul-de-sac just below the glans corona. The foreskin is a double membrane that has five layers: mucosal epithelium similar to glans epithelium, lamina propria, dartos smooth muscle, dermis, and epidermis.

The scrotum contains the testes and lower spermatic cords. It consists of skin that covers the dartos smooth muscle, fibers of the cremasteric muscle, and several layers of fascia. The skin is pigmented, hair-bearing, and loose, with numerous sebaceous and sweat glands. Lymphatic drainage is to the superficial inguinal lymph nodes.

II. GROSS EXAMINATION AND TISSUE SAMPLING. Tissue samples include mucosal or skin biopsies, penile urethral biopsies, foreskin resection specimens, and partial and total penectomy specimens.

A. Punch and Shave Biopsies of penile glans and skin should be handled as skin biopsies from other sites (see Chapter 38).

B. Foreskin Resection is indicated for primary carcinomas of this site. The entire periphery of the mucosal margin should be submitted as a shave resection margin (usually in three to four sections) or perpendicular margin depending on the distance between the carcinoma and the margin. The foreskin should then be pinned and fixed overnight in 10% formalin. Several full-thickness sections should be examined microscopically to permit evaluation of all five layers.

C. For **partial penectomy specimens,** the surgical margin of the penis is made 2 cm proximal to gross tumor extent. Three to four frozen sections are typically necessary to sample the cut surface of this margin. Permanent sections are taken as described below.

D. For **total penectomy specimens,** only proximal urethral and periurethral margin tissues should be submitted for frozen section, unless the mass is grossly close to or involves the skin, which should also then be sampled. For permanent sections of both partial and total penectomy specimens, the foreskin (when present) should be removed and handled as noted above. A thin 2-mm shave of all the structures of the shaft margin should be taken, if not already sampled by frozen section. One to three additional transverse sections should be taken from the glans. Any mass (es) should be sampled to demonstrate pattern of growth, depth of extension, and relationship to normal anatomic structures.

E. Lymph Nodes. There may be a clinical request for frozen section(s) of enlarged inguinal lymph nodes; if positive for carcinoma, a more extended ilioinguinal lymph node dissection may follow. Bilateral inguinal lymphadenectomy specimens may also be received after removal of the primary tumor and a course of antibiotics, or in patients with T2 tumors, high-grade tumors, or tumors with vascular invasion (*Critical Rev Oncol-Hematol* 2005;53:165).

A nomogram has been developed to predict nodal metastases using the presence of clinically palpable groin lymph nodes and histologic lymphovascular invasion in the primary tumor (*J Urol* 2006;175:1700). The utility of sentinel lymph node sampling is not yet settled. A prognostic index has also been generated to predict nodal metastasis (*Am J Surg Pathol* 2009;33:1049); this index incorporates histologic grade, deepest anatomic level involved by cancer, and the presence of perineural invasion by carcinoma.

III. DIAGNOSTIC FEATURES OF COMMON DISEASES OF THE PENIS AND SCROTUM

A. **Inflammation and Infection.** Three categories can be defined: inflammatory conditions specific to the penis and scrotum, systematic dermatoses (discussed in Chapter 38), and sexually transmitted diseases (*BJU Int* 2002;90:498).

1. **Phimosis,** the clinical condition in which the foreskin cannot be retracted behind the glans penis, is associated with fibrosis, inflammation, and edema of the prepuce. Histologically it is often characterized by lamina propria fibrosis with associated lymphoplasmacytic inflammation.

2. **Paraphimosis** is diagnosed clinically when the foreskin cannot be advanced back over the glans and becomes trapped between the coronal sulcus and the glands corona secondary to fibrosis and inflammation.

3. **Balanoposthitis** is inflammation of the glans penis and prepuce, usually in uncircumcised men with poor hygiene.

4. **Balanitis,** or inflammation of the glans, occurs in several forms.

   a. **Plasma cell balanitis (Zoon balanitis)** can clinically and grossly mimic carcinoma in situ, with presentation as brown or red patches or plaques. The histologic appearance can vary with time, and the inflammatory cell infiltrate can vary from patchy and lymphoplasmacytic (early) to dense and plasmacytic (later) (*Am J Dermatopathol* 2002;24:459).

   b. **Balanitis xerotica obliterans** (BXO) is lichen sclerosus of the glans and prepuce that macroscopically appears as a white patch or plaque. Histologically, the squamous epithelium is typically atrophic and hyperkeratotic, and shows basal layer vacuolization with a band of pale homogenous collagen in the upper dermis and an underlying lymphocytic infiltrate (e-**Fig. 30.2**). Complications include meatal stenosis (urethral stricture), and very uncommonly, squamous cell carcinoma.

   c. **Balanitis circinata** microscopically resembles pustular psoriasis and is seen in Reiter syndrome, which includes nongonococcal urethritis, conjunctivitis, and arthritis.

5. **Human papillomavirus (HPV) infection** can lead to condyloma acuminata. The growth is typically papillary or warty, and histologically papillomatosis, acanthosis, parakeratosis, and hyperkeratosis are found; intraepithelial neoplasia may also be present. Koilocytes with wrinkled nuclear membranes, nucleomegaly, cytoplasmic halos, and binucleation may be prominent or inconspicuous. Old lesions tend to show less prominent koilocytic changes. The causal HPV serotypes are usually 6 or 11, but it is not necessary to verify the presence of HPV. Bowenoid papulosis is also an HPV-related proliferation that presents with multiple 2 to 10 mm papules than can coalesce to form plaques; it is usually caused by serotypes 16, 18, and/or 35. Microscopically, although the appearance is similar to carcinoma in situ, the clinical course is typically self-limited and benign.

6. **Herpes simplex virus (HSV)** infection of the male genitalia is usually caused by subtype 2, which produces multiple vesicles. The diagnosis can be confirmed by scraping and performance of a Tzanck smear, which reveals multinucleated giant cells with intranuclear inclusions. Histologically the intraepithelial vesicles contain infected keratinocytes which show multinucleation, a nuclear ground-glass appearance, and molding.

7. **Scabies** is an infestation by a mite that burrows into the keratin layer of the epidermis with generation of erythematous papules and nodules. Detection of the mites may be accomplished via scrapes or biopsy. In tissue sections, the mite (400 μm long with an oval to round body), eggs, or egg walls, are diagnostic. A dermal lymphoid infiltrate with eosinophils and epidermal spongiosis are characteristic responses.

8. **Pediculosis pubis** is infection by *Pediculus pubis*, also known as the crab louse. Biopsy is not necessary; the lice may be seen by a magnifying lens.

9. **Syphilis** is caused by *Treponema pallidum*, a Gram-negative spirochete. The primary lesion, the chancre, is a single, round, crater-like painless ulcer with an indurated base (hard chancre) most often located on the glans or prepuce. Biopsy is not usually necessary, but if done (for example, when syphilis is not clinically suspected) shows a perivascular lymphoplasmacytic infiltrate. The spirochetes may be identified in the epidermis or in dermal perivascular regions by silver stains (Steiner, Dieterle, or Warthin–Starry) or immunohistochemical stains. The secondary and tertiary stages of syphilis are characterized by condyloma latum and gumma, respectively. Smears from the gray maculopapules of condyloma latum should be examined by dark-field microscopy for spirochetes since biopsy may yield nonspecific findings. The typical histologic features of condyloma latum include prominent epithelial hyperplasia and neutrophils in the epidermis, a dermal superficial lichenoid and deep perivascular plasma cell rich infiltrate, and endarteritis (superficial or deep). The gumma is a necrotic mass with surrounding granulomatous inflammation, with associated obliterative endarteritis with perivascular plasma cells. Special stains for *T. pallidum* are typically negative in these lesions.

10. **Gonorrhea** is caused by *Neisseria gonorrhoeae*, a Gram-negative diplococcus. Urethritis with urethral discharge may lead to urethral stricture. Biopsies are rarely performed.

11. **Lymphogranuloma venereum** is due to *Chlamydia trachomatis*. Vesicles, then ulcers, develop in the primary genital phase; biopsies are not useful for diagnosis of the primary phase. In the secondary stage, patients develop painful inguinal lymphadenopathy (bubo). Histologically, the lymph nodes initially demonstrate small suppurative foci followed by follicular hyperplasia and massive plasma cell infiltrates, which then coalesce to form large stellate abscesses surrounded by palisaded histiocytes and multinucleated giant cells, a nonspecific picture that can also be seen in cat scratch fever, tularemia, bubonic plague, and fungal and atypical mycobacterial infections. The organisms cannot be detected with special stains and the diagnosis requires culture.

12. **Granuloma inguinale (donovanosis)** is caused by *Calymmatobacterium granulomatis*, a Gram-negative intracellular bacillus. Infection results in ulcers. Smears or biopsy sections reveal large foamy histiocytes with inclusions (Donovan bodies), best visualized by Warthin–Starry or Giemsa stains. Long-standing disease may be associated with elephantiasis of the penis and scrotum.

13. **Chancroid or soft chancre** is caused by *Haemophilus ducreyi*, a Gram-negative rod, and is typified by painful nonindurated penile ulcers and lymphadenopathy. Histologically the lesions show a characteristic zonation phenomenon: upper layer with necrosis, fibrin, and neutrophils; middle layer with prominent granulation tissue and prominent blood vessels; and lower/deepest layer with an intense lymphoplasmacytic infiltrate. The organisms can be found in smears or histologic sections stained with Giemsa, Gram, or methylene blue stains.

14. **Molluscum contagiosum** is caused by a DNA pox virus and produces multiple small dome-shaped papules with a central umbilication. Biopsy sections show a crater with an acanthotic epidermis and the diagnostic intracytoplasmic viral eosinophilic inclusions (molluscum bodies or Henderson bodies).

15. **Penile infections in acquired immunodeficiency syndrome (AIDS)** include almost all sexually transmitted infections including gonorrhea, syphilis, herpes, candidiasis, chancroid, molluscum contagiosum, HPV, scabies, and Reiter syndrome.

16. **Sclerosing lipogranulomas** in the scrotum or penis are secondary to injections or topical application of oil-based chemicals. Sections show a foreign body, lymphoplasmacytic, and histiocytic reaction to lipid droplets that appear as cleared spaces.

17. **Hidradenitis suppurativa,** more typical of the sweat glands in the axilla, can also involve the scrotum. Acute and chronic inflammation, fibrosis, and even sinus tract formation can occur.

18. **Gangrene,** as a necroinflammatory process, can involve the scrotum due to a variety of insults. Fournier gangrene is an extreme fulminant infection of the genitals, perineum, or abdominal wall (*Int J Urol* 2006;13:960).

19. **Scrotal calcinosis** can occur due to calcification of dermal connective tissue (idiopathic) or in association with keratinous cysts. Multiple firm nodules are found, measuring several millimeters to several centimeters in greatest dimension, typically in the scrotum of younger men. Microscopically, calcific material is present with or without granulomatous inflammation and/or cyst wall remnants.

20. **Elephantiasis** or massive scrotal lymphedema is usually secondary to filariasis.

21. **Verruciform xanthoma** rarely occurs in the penis and scrotum (*J Urol* 1995;53:1625). Clinical and low-power microscopic examination may yield an impression of a wart; however, high-power microscopic examination reveals characteristic foamy to granular xanthomatous histiocytes within the dermal papillae.

B. **Miscellaneous Benign Nonneoplastic Conditions**

1. **Peyronie disease** presents with a painful bending of the erect penis. Histologically, there is fibrosis or fibromatosis of the tunica albuginea (e-Fig. 30.3). Rarely, calcification and ossification may occur in these fibrous plaques.

2. **Penile cysts**
   a. **Median raphe cyst** is most commonly located in the midline on the ventral aspect of the shaft. It is lined by pseudostratified, columnar, mucinous epithelial cells.
   b. **Mucoid cysts** are thought to arise from ectopic urethral mucosa, can be seen on the prepuce or glans, and are lined by stratified columnar epithelium with mucinous cells.
   c. **Epidermal inclusion cysts** are usually found on the penile shaft. They are also common in scrotal skin. They have the same appearance as elsewhere in the skin.

C. **Benign Epithelial Neoplasms** include squamous papilloma, common condyloma, and the very rare giant condyloma of Buschke–Lowenstein. Most reported giant condylomas likely represent warty or verrucous carcinomas. Grossly, giant condylomas are 5 cm in average diameter, and microscopically resemble a typical condyloma except for exuberant surface papillomatosis and pushing bulbous growth at the base. When carefully defined, they may be locally destructive but do not show malignant cytologic features or metastasize. Some of them may have associated invasive squamous cell carcinoma and therefore should be extensively sampled.

D. **Penile Intraepithelial Neoplasia (PeIN)** is the precursor to the invasive squamous cell carcinoma and can be divided into 2 main groups: HPV-related and non-HPV related (*Am J Surg Pathol* 2010;34:385). Histologically HPV-related PeINs are divided into basaloid, warty, and basaloid-warty subtypes whereas differentiated (simplex) PeIN is the non-HPV related subtype. Among the former, at least 18 types of high-risk HPV have been identified (*Am J Surg Pathol* 2017;41:820); HPV16 is the most common type associated with basaloid PeINs (at least six types identified, 71% HPV16) whereas warty PeINs harbor more marked heterogeneity in high-risk HPV subtypes (at least eight subtypes, 20% HPV 16). The majority of PeINs are multifocal with histologic heterogeneity (*Am J Surg Pathol* 2017;41:820). However, each lesion typically harbors one type of HPV.

Histologically basaloid PeIN is characterized by small to medium sized basaloid dysplastic squamous cells with a high nuclear/cytoplasmic ratio, whereas warty PeIN shows low papillary structures with acanthosis, cellular pleomorphism, and pleomorphic koilocytosis. Differentiated PeIN is characterized by hyperkeratosis, parakeratosis, hypergranulosis, acanthosis, elongated rete ridges, abnormal maturation, intraepithelial pearl formation, prominent intercellular bridges, and atypical basal or prickle layer cells.

Two specific variants of PeINs include erythroplasia of Queyrat (on the glans) and Bowen disease (on the penile shaft or prepuce). These are HPV-related (usually serotypes 16 or 18) intraepithelial proliferations. Grossly, erythroplasia of Queyrat appears as a sharply demarcated patch on the glans, whereas Bowen disease is a solitary, brownish-red plaque on the shaft or foreskin. Microscopically, the two lesions are similar and are composed of a full-thickness proliferation of pleomorphic basaloid cells that exhibit loss of polarity (e-**Fig. 30.4**). Traditionally, these two high-grade intraepithelial proliferations have been assigned grade III, while lower grade intraepithelial lesions have been graded as I or II.

E. Penile Cancer

1. **Risk factors for penile cancer** are phimosis, chronic inflammation, lichen sclerosus, smoking, ultraviolet (UV) radiation, radiotherapy, condyloma, HPV infection (usually type 16, less commonly type 18), and lack of circumcision (*J Am Acad Dermatol* 2006;54:364); the latter is an extremely strong risk factor.

2. **Clinical diagnosis.** Patients are typically 50 to 70 years of age and present with an exophytic or flat ulcerative mass of the glans, prepuce, or coronal sulcus. More than half of penile carcinomas occur in the glans (58%) followed by the foreskin (29%), whereas the penile shaft is much less commonly involved (7%); and more than one anatomic structure are involved in the remaining 6% cases (*Urology* 2012;79:804). Patients with advanced disease may present with pubic or scrotal skin nodules and inguinal lymph node metastasis. Magnetic resonance imaging of primary penile cancer can help define local tumor extent and any shaft involvement (*Radiographics* 2005; 25:1629).

3. **Histologic typing and grading.** The 2016 World Health Organization (WHO) classification of penile neoplasms is provided in Table 30.1. HPV-related penile squamous cell carcinomas include basaloid carcinoma and its papillary variant (papillary basaloid carcinoma), warty carcinoma and its variants (warty-basaloid carcinoma and clear cell carcinoma) and lymphoepithelioma-like carcinoma. Non-HPV related penile squamous cell carcinomas are divided into squamous cell carcinoma, usual type and its variants (pseudoglandular carcinoma and pseudohyperplastic carcinoma), verrucous carcinoma and its variant carcinoma cuniculatum, papillary carcinoma NOS, adenosquamous carcinoma, sarcomatoid squamous carcinoma, and mixed type of squamous cell carcinoma.

   A 3-tier grading system is recommended for penile squamous cell carcinoma. Grade 1 carcinomas include well-differentiated usual type squamous cell carcinoma, verrucous carcinoma, carcinoma cuniculatum, and pseudohyperplastic carcinoma. Warty carcinoma and moderately differentiated usual type squamous cell carcinoma are grade 2 tumors. Grade 3 carcinomas include poorly differentiated usual type squamous cell carcinoma, basaloid carcinoma, clear cell carcinoma, lymphoepithelioma-like carcinoma, and sarcomatoid squamous carcinoma (*Histopathology* 2018;72:893).

4. **Immunohistochemical studies** for penile squamous cell carcinomas are typically not needed. However, squamous cell markers (p63, p40, CK5/6, 34βE12) can be used to confirm the diagnosis in poorly differentiated squamous cell carcinoma and sarcomatoid carcinoma, and to distinguish these tumors from other malignant neoplasms including melanoma and sarcoma. Diffuse strong p16 staining is a reliable surrogate marker for high risk HPV infection in penile intraepithelial neoplasia and invasive squamous cell carcinoma (*Am J Surg Pathol* 2017;41:820).

5. **Molecular tests** for penile intraepithelial neoplasia and squamous cell carcinoma are not routinely performed. HPV typing is not usually necessary as p16 immunohistochemical staining is a more convenient and less expensive method. A recent study has shown that variable and multiple types of HPVs are present with multiple PeINs; however, unicentric PeIN is typically associated with a single genotype of HPV (*Am J Surg Pathol* 2017;41:820). There is a strong correspondence in the HPV genotypes between PeIN and an associated invasive carcinoma.

6. **Squamous cell carcinoma of usual type** accounts for 40% to 50% of penile cancers. Gross diagnosis is readily performed for penectomy specimens because most masses are several centimeters in diameter, and are usually solitary, firm, and ulcerated (e-**Fig. 30.5**). Multicentric tumors occur more frequently in the

TABLE 30.1	WHO Histologic Classification of Tumors of the Penis

Malignant epithelial tumors of the penis

Non-HPV–related squamous cell carcinoma

  Squamous cell carcinoma

    Usual carcinoma

    Pseudopapillary carcinoma

    Pseudoglandular carcinoma

  Verrucous carcinoma

    Pure verrucous carcinoma

    Carcinoma cuniculatum

  Papillary carcinoma, NOS

  Adenosquamous carcinoma

  Sarcomatoid squamous carcinoma

  Mixed squamous cell carcinoma

HPV-related squamous cell carcinoma

  Warty carcinoma

    Warty basaloid carcinoma

    Clear cell carcinoma

  Basaloid carcinoma

    Papillary basaloid carcinoma

  Lymphoepithelioma-like carcinoma

Precursor lesions

Penile intraepithelial neoplasia (PeIN)

  Low grade

  High grade

  Warty/Basaloid/Warty-basaloid PeIN

PeIN differentiated

Paget disease

Melanocytic lesions

Melanocytic nevus

Melanoma

Mesenchymal tumors

Lymphomas of penis

Secondary tumors

From: Moch H, Humphrey PA, Ulbright TM, Reuter VE, eds. *WHO Classification of Tumours of Urinary Tract and Male Genital Organs.* Lyon, France: IARC Press; 2017. Used with permission.

foreskin. Microscopic diagnosis is usually straightforward, but small superficial biopsies can be problematic in the differential distinction from pseudoepitheliomatous squamous cell hyperplasia. There are three major prognostically important growth patterns: superficial spreading, with horizontal growth and only superficial invasion; vertical growth, which is deeply invasive (**e-Fig. 30.6**); and multicentric. Histologically, they are graded as well, moderately and poorly differentiated using the WHO/ISUP 3-tier grading system (*Histopathology* 2018;72:893). Most usual squamous cell carcinomas are moderately differentiated with some keratinization (**e-Fig. 30.7**). Small nests, cords, and single neoplastic cells infiltrate into the lamina propria, corpus spongiosum, and uncommonly, the corpus cavernosum (**e-Fig. 30.8**). Poorly differentiated carcinoma may grow as sheets, with necrosis and a high mitotic rate. Local extension into several anatomic compartments may occur; for example, a carcinoma originating on the glans may spread to the foreskin, to skin of the shaft, and to the urethra. In very advanced cases, direct spread to inguinal, pubic, or scrotal skin can occur.

   a. Pseudohyperplastic carcinoma is an extremely well-differentiated variant of usual type squamous cell carcinoma and is commonly associated with lichen sclerosus (*Am J Surg Pathol* 2004;28:895). Microscopically, it is characterized by irregular downward growth of squamous nests with sharp borders and little stromal reaction. The tumor cells are well-differentiated with minimal to no atypia.

   b. Pseudoglandular carcinoma is another rare but aggressive variant of usual type squamous cell carcinoma (*Am J Surg Pathol* 2009;33:551). Microscopically, the squamous carcinoma cells show acantholytic or adenoid features characterized by solid nests with early necrosis or empty pseudoluminal spaces lined by one layer of squamous or cylindrical cells. Pseudoglandular squamous cell carcinoma is often deeply infiltrative and of high histologic grade.

7. **Verrucous carcinoma** is a very well-differentiated papillary neoplasm with hyperkeratosis, papillomatosis, and a broad pushing base (Fig. 30.1). The tumor cells are extremely well-differentiated with minimal deviation from normal squamous cells. Basal layer cells may show slight atypia. Carcinoma cuniculatum is a rare variant of verrucous carcinoma characterized by an endophytic deep penetrating and burrowing growth pattern (*Am J Surg Pathol* 2007;31:71).

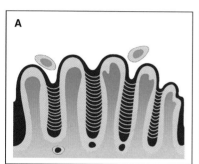
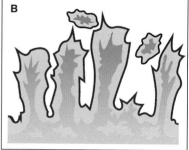
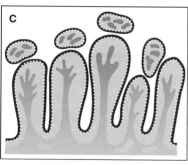
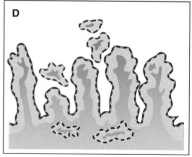

Figure 30.1 Verruciform tumors of the penis. **A:** Verrucous carcinoma with regular papillae, broad pushing base, and hyperkeratosis. **B:** Papillary carcinoma with irregular papillae and cores, and ragged infiltration at base. **C:** Giant condyloma, with branching cores and koilocytosis. **D:** Warty (condylomatous) carcinoma with irregular papillae and koilocytosis. (Modified from Young RH, Srigley JR, Amin MB, Ulbright TM, Cubilla AL, eds. *Tumors of the Prostate Gland, Seminal Vesicles, Male Urethra, and Penis*. Washington DC: Armed Forces Institute of Pathology; 2005:424.)

8. **Papillary carcinoma, NOS** is well-differentiated, hyperkeratotic, and has complex papillae and an irregular infiltrative base. It has a favorable prognosis (*Am J Surg Pathol* 2010;34:223).

9. **Adenosquamous carcinoma** is a rare non-HPV related penile carcinoma (*Am J Surg Pathol* 1996;20:156). Microscopically it is composed of mixed squamous and glandular components which can be separate or more often intermixed. The glandular component is typically a minority component. In one quarter of cases the carcinoma can be mixed, such as warty–basaloid, adenocarcinoma–basaloid, and squamous–neuroendocrine. Although it is generally considered as a non-HPV related tumor, high-risk HPV was reported in a recent case (*J Cutan Pathol* 2016;43:1226).

10. **Sarcomatoid (spindle cell) carcinoma** is an aggressive, high-grade, deeply invasive spindle cell malignancy with or without heterologous elements such as muscle, bone, and cartilage; coexisting carcinoma in situ or invasive carcinoma is usually evident (*Am J Surg Pathol* 2005;29:1152).

11. **Basaloid carcinoma** is the most common HPV-related penile squamous cell carcinoma. It has a nested growth pattern and comprises small, uniform, basaloid cells with high nuclear/cytoplasmic ratios and numerous mitoses (*Am J Surg Pathol* 1998:22;755) (e-**Fig. 30.9**). Papillary basaloid carcinoma is a rare variant of basaloid carcinoma and is characterized by exophytic papillary growth with tumor cells similar to basaloid carcinoma (*Am J Surg Pathol* 2012;36:869); it may contain an invasive carcinoma component which is similar to typical basaloid carcinoma. Basaloid carcinoma is an HPV-related carcinoma and immunohistochemically is diffusely positive for p16 (e-**Fig. 30.10**).

12. **Warty (condylomatous) carcinoma** is one of the verruciform carcinomas (the others being verrucous carcinoma and papillary carcinoma) (*Am J Surg Pathol* 2000;24:505). Microscopically, it is composed of condylomatous papillae lined by hyperkeratotic and clear cells of low to intermediate nuclear grade; koilocytic atypia may be prominent. Parakeratosis is also prominent. Warty-basaloid carcinoma is a variant composed of mixed warty and basaloid features. Clear cell carcinoma is a rare variant of warty carcinoma (*Am J Surg Pathol* 2016;40:917) and is characterized by solid growth with comedo-like or geographic necrosis and predominantly nonkeratinizing polyhedral to round clear cells.

13. **Lymphoepithelioma-like carcinoma** is another subtype of HPV-related penile squamous cell carcinoma (*Histopathology* 2014;64:312). Microscopically it is composed of poorly differentiated to undifferentiated cells with indistinct cell borders (syncytial growth) arranged in solid sheets, nests, trabeculae, or cords. Admixed is a dense lymphoplasmacytic and eosinophilic infiltrate.

14. Another rare subtype of penile squamous cell carcinoma that has not been included in the current WHO classification is **medullary carcinoma** (*Am J Surg Pathol* 2107;41:535). This is also an HPV-related poorly differentiated carcinoma with a moderate to dense tumor-associated inflammatory cell infiltrate composed of neutrophils, lymphocytes, plasma cells, and eosinophils.

15. **Rare types of primary penile carcinoma** include Merkel cell carcinoma, small cell carcinoma, sebaceous carcinoma, and invasive adenocarcinoma arising in association with extra-mammary Paget disease.

16. **Mesenchymal neoplasms** are rare and comprise only 5% of all penile tumors. The most common benign soft tissue tumors are vascular (hemangioma and lymphangioma), followed by neural, myxoid, and fibrous tumors. The most frequent malignant soft tissue tumors are Kaposi sarcoma and leiomyosarcoma (*Anal Quant Cytol Histol* 2005;28:193).

17. **Hematolymphoid neoplasms** include very rare primary penile lymphomas and secondary lymphomas. Penile lymphomas represent 2% of penile malignancies.

18. **Miscellaneous neoplasms** rarely encountered include melanoma (*J Urol* 2005; 173:1958).

19. Secondary malignancies are rare, with prostatic and urinary bladder carcinomas predominating (*Int J Surg Pathol* 2011;19:597; *Am J Surg Pathol* 2015;39:67). The corpus cavernosum is the most common site of metastasis, but the spongiosum, skin, and glans may also be involved.

F. Scrotal Cancer and Disease

1. Squamous cell carcinoma of the scrotum is usually detected as an invasive disease, but some examples of squamous cell carcinoma in situ have been reported. Its incidence is much lower than that of penile squamous cell carcinoma. Associations exist with exposure to soot (in chimney sweeps, described in 1775 by Sir Percival Pott), machine oil, psoriasis treated with coal tar, arsenic, psoralens/UV radiation, and HPV infection. Grossly, scrotal squamous cell carcinomas initially appear as a solitary nodule; later in their course they show ulceration and induration. Microscopically, most are well to moderately differentiated (**e-Fig. 30.11**). The tumor typically invades the scrotal wall, and larger cancers can involve the testis, spermatic cord, penis, and perineum. Initial metastatic spread is to ipsilateral inguinal lymph nodes. Outcome is related to tumor size and pathologic stage.

2. Basal cell carcinomas of scrotal skin are rare and have the same appearance as they do elsewhere in the skin.

3. Paget disease of the scrotum can be associated with underlying carcinoma of the urinary bladder, urethra, prostate, or eccrine sweat glands. The tumor cells in primary Paget disease are immunohistochemically positive for cytokeratin 7, GCDFP15, and GATA3 (*Diagn Pathol* 2017;12:51) (**e-Fig. 30.12**).

4. Sarcomas of the scrotal wall are rare and should be distinguished from paratesticular, intrascrotal sarcomas. By far the most common histologic type of scrotal wall sarcoma is leiomyosarcoma (**e-Fig. 30.13**), which likely arises from the dartos muscle.

IV. PATHOLOGIC STAGING OF PENILE CANCER.
The AJCC staging scheme for the penis only applies to squamous carcinoma and associated histologic subtypes (Amin MB et al., eds. *AJCC Cancer Staging Manual.* 8th ed. New York: Springer, 2017). The AJCC staging scheme for melanoma should be used for melanomas of the skin of the penis; the scheme for the urethra should be used for carcinomas arising in the penile urethra; and the scheme for soft tissue sarcomas (abdominal and thoracic visceral organs) for penile sarcomas. The AJCC staging scheme for cutaneous squamous cell carcinomas should be used for scrotal carcinomas.

V. REPORTING PENILE CARCINOMA.
Reporting should follow published guidelines (*Arch Pathol Lab Med* 2010;134:923; *Histopathology* 2018;72:893); templates are available to guide reporting (e.g., College of American Pathologists Protocol for the Examination of Specimens From Patients With Carcinoma of the Penis; available at http://www.cap.org). For circumcision and penectomy specimens, the following should be reported for the primary tumor: tumor size, histologic type, histologic grade (G1, G2, or G3), origin, depth of invasion (mm), anatomic level of invasion, structures involved, vascular and perineural invasion (if present), and status of the margins of resection. For regional lymph nodes, the report should include the number identified and their location, number involved by tumor, size of metastatic deposit (if present), and extracapsular extension (if present). Additional pathologic findings that can be noted (if present) are penile intraepithelial neoplasia and therapy-related changes.

31 The Ovary

Jennifer K. Sehn, Horacio M. Maluf, and
John D. Pfeifer

I. NORMAL GROSS AND MICROSCOPIC ANATOMY. The ovaries rest on both sides of the
uterus and are anchored by the broad ligament. Age and reproductive status greatly impact
the size and weight, which range from 3 to 5 cm and 5 to 8 g, respectively. The outer
surface of the ovary is white-tan and smooth during early reproductive years, but becomes
more bosselated with age due to repeated rupture of ovarian follicles. The cut surface is
organized into three ill-defined zones: an outer cortex, underlying medulla, and hilum.
The cortex and medulla contain cystic follicles, yellow or orange corpora lutea, and white
corpora albicantia.

Histologic sections of the ovary from a woman of reproductive age show a simple
cuboidal surface epithelial layer derived from the mesothelium. Within the ovarian cortex
and medulla, follicular structures composed of an inner layer of granulosa cells and an
outer layer of theca cells (e-Figs. 31.1 and 31.2), in varying phases of development, are
surrounded by a stroma comprised of closely packed s-shaped spindled cells and collagen
(e-Fig. 31.3). Centrally hemorrhagic corpora lutea composed of granulosa cells with
abundant eosinophilic cytoplasm and smaller theca cells (e-Figs. 31.4 and 31.5), as well
as white acellular corpora albicantia (e-Fig. 31.6), may also be seen. The hilum, where
the ovary connects to the broad ligament, is composed of abundant blood vessels, nerves,
and interspersed eosinophilic hilar cells that are histologically similar to the Leydig cells
of the testis (e-Fig. 31.7). The rete ovarii, the developmental analog of the rete testis that
is composed of slit-like spaces lined by nonciliated cuboidal epithelium, is also present in
the hilum (e-Fig. 31.8).

II. GROSS EXAMINATION AND TISSUE SAMPLING. The most common ovarian specimens
encountered in surgical pathology are from salpingo-oophorectomy (with or without
hysterectomy) or cystectomy (cyst excision) procedures. The weight and three-dimensional
measurements of the ovary and fallopian tube are recorded. The capsule should be inspected
for areas of rupture, adhesions, tumor involvement, or other abnormalities. If the capsule is
ruptured, an attempt should be made to determine whether it was ruptured preoperatively
or intraoperatively. The ovary is serially sectioned; solid, cystic, or papillary lesions are thoroughly sampled (one section per cm). If cysts are present, the color and consistency of the
cyst fluid are noted, and any areas of nodularity or papillary excrescences are sampled.

Prophylactic oophorectomy specimens, performed for a personal history of cancer or
family history of a hereditary cancer syndrome, are cut perpendicular to the long axis and
entirely submitted.

The surgical management of malignant primary ovarian tumors typically includes
a staging procedure, and so an ovary excised for a primary malignancy will usually be
accompanied by multiple peritoneal biopsies, the omentum, and occasionally by regional
lymph nodes. The small peritoneal biopsies are submitted entirely. The omentum must be
serially sectioned; if grossly visible tumor is present, it should be measured and only one
section need be submitted; when no tumor is identified, five to ten sections are submitted.
All identified lymph nodes from the lymph node dissections are submitted entirely; large
lymph nodes should be sectioned for optimal fixation and processing.

III. DIAGNOSTIC FEATURES OF COMMON BENIGN DISEASES OF THE OVARY

A. Inflammatory Diseases

    1. Infection of the ovary is almost always accompanied by infection of the fallopian
    tube (e-Fig. 31.9), systemic infection, or the development of a tubo-ovarian abscess

(e-Fig. 31.10). The most common cause of oophoritis is ascending pelvic inflammatory disease (PID), which typically causes intense pelvic pain and is usually polymicrobial. The ovary contains sheets of neutrophils and often shows paraovarian adhesions or adhesions to an inflamed fallopian tube. Severe PID may require hospitalization and treatment, while mild PID may resolve on its own. The subsequent fibrosis and scarring from PID is a leading cause of infertility (e-Fig. 31.11).

2. **Autoimmune oophoritis** typically presents with oligomenorrhea and infertility, and is often associated with other autoimmune disorders. The ovaries are normal in size but filled with a lymphoplasmacytic infiltrate in developing follicles and corpora lutea. Premature ovarian failure and premature menopause are the final sequelae of the disease.

3. **Noninfectious granulomas** may also be seen within the ovary. These may form secondary to systemic diseases such as sarcoidosis or represent a foreign body response following a pelvic or abdominal surgery, but the majority of cases is not related to a systemic disease. Unless they are accompanied by necrosis or other features of infectious granulomas, special stains are not necessary.

B. Cysts

1. **Follicular cysts** are commonly found in prepubescent and reproductive-aged women. Normal follicles measure up to about 1 cm in greatest dimension, while follicular cysts measure 3 to 10 cm in diameter and contain serosanguineous fluid. Most cysts are asymptomatic, but women may present with an abdominal mass or rupture. Follicular cysts are typically unilateral with a thin, smooth lining comprising an inner layer of granulosa cells and an outer layer of theca cells similar to normal follicles. Multiple follicular cysts may be associated with polycystic ovarian syndrome (PCOS) and McCune–Albright syndrome.

2. **Corpus luteum cysts** are also common in women of reproductive age. Like follicular cysts, they may present as a mass or with rupture. On gross examination, corpus luteum cysts are >3 cm, filled with thick hemorrhagic fluid, and rimmed by a yellow lining. Microscopically, the cyst has an undulating wall of luteinized granulosa cells (that have abundant, eosinophilic cytoplasm) with interspersed peripheral theca cells; the overall architecture is similar to that of a normal corpus luteum.

3. **Polycystic ovary syndrome (PCOS)** is an incompletely understood disease characterized by anovulation, infertility, hirsutism, and obesity. It is estimated that up to 10% of American women are affected by this syndrome, which typically presents between the ages of 20 and 30. In general, the ovaries are enlarged with a thickened, collagenized cortical surface; multiple, uniform follicles all in a similar phase of development (typically antral); and an absence of corpora lutea (indicating infrequent ovulation) (e-Fig. 31.12).

4. **Surface epithelial inclusion cysts** are common. They are thought to be formed by repeated invaginations of ovarian epithelium secondary to surface rupture with ovulation. By convention, inclusion cysts measure less than 1 cm in diameter; a cyst with similar morphology but greater than 1 cm is classified as a serous cystadenoma (see below). The cysts are lined by a single layer of bland flat, cuboidal, or ciliated columnar cells (e-Fig. 31.13). Psammoma bodies may be seen. It is hypothesized that benign, borderline, and low-grade serous epithelial neoplasms may arise from these inclusions.

5. **Paraovarian or paratubal cysts (rete ovary cysts)** are found in the hilar region of the ovary and arise from mesonephric (Wolffian) or paramesonephric (müllerian) duct remnants. Mesonephric cysts are lined by simple or stratified epithelium and have prominent muscular walls (e-Fig. 31.14). Paramesonephric cysts are lined by columnar epithelium with a mixture of ciliated and nonciliated cells similar to epithelial inclusion cysts (e-Fig. 31.13); hilus cells are often present in the wall.

6. **Endometriosis,** characterized by endometrial glands and stroma outside the uterus, is frequently seen in the ovary. Symptomatic patients typically present during the reproductive years with menstrual-associated pain and/or infertility. Grossly, the ovary shows a thickened cortex, surface adhesions, and one or multiple cyst(s) filled

with thick brown fluid resembling chocolate syrup, a constellation of findings often referred to as a chocolate cyst. Histologically, endometrial epithelium and stroma with associated hemosiderin-laden macrophages are diagnostic (e-Fig. 31.15). Endometriotic cysts frequently contain areas with reactive atypical cytologic features associated with acute inflammation, but areas of epithelial tufting, more complex architectural changes, or increased mitotic activity should raise suspicion for malignancy arising in endometriosis. Hyperplasias and neoplasms arising in endometriosis mirror those of the uterine endometrium (see Chapter 33). Although there is a classic association of clear cell carcinoma arising in endometriosis, the most common malignancy arising in endometriosis is endometrioid carcinoma. Serous carcinoma can also arise in endometriosis, albeit rarely.

C. Hyperplastic Changes

1. **Stromal hyperplasia**, defined as an increase in the cortex and medulla by nonluteinized ovarian stroma, and **hyperthecosis**, an increase by luteinized stromal cells in a background of stromal hyperplasia (e-Fig. 31.16), are changes most commonly seen in the sixth to seventh decades of life and in women with PCOS. The ovaries are enlarged bilaterally. While most women are asymptomatic, some present with estrogenic symptoms (including vaginal bleeding secondary to endometrial hyperplasia) or androgenic symptoms (including acne) due to hormone production by the luteinized cells.

2. **Hilus cell hyperplasia** is most common in postmenopausal women who also have stromal hyperplasia and hyperthecosis. The hilus cell proliferation rarely causes symptoms on its own. Microscopically, eosinophilic cells with hyperchromatic nuclei are arranged in nests or clusters found most often in the hilar region of the ovary. Elongated, eosinophilic intracytoplasmic inclusions, called Reinke crystals, may be seen (e-Fig. 31.17). Aggregates of hilus cells are often perineural.

D. Pregnancy Changes

1. **Solitary luteinized follicle cysts** are benign, unilocular, unilateral cysts that may grow up to 25 cm in diameter. They have the same lining as normal follicles, consisting of inner granulosa cells and outer theca cells. Lining cells can display significant cytologic atypia.

2. **Hyperreactio luteinalis** is characterized by symmetric, bilateral enlargement of the ovaries with multiple luteinized cysts. The condition is associated with high levels of human chorionic gonadotropin seen in multiple pregnancy, ovulation induction, and gestational trophoblastic disease. The cysts usually resolve in the months after completion of the pregnancy. Microscopically, the follicular cysts are lined by luteinized granulosa and theca cells with stromal edema.

3. **Pregnancy luteoma** is seen in the second half of pregnancy and is most common in multiparous African American women. The lesion consists of hyperplastic proliferations of luteinized cells, likely stromal and theca cells. Most pregnancy luteomas are incidental, but 25% of patients have symptoms of virilization. Grossly, the nodules are multiple (50%), bilateral (33%), yellow-brown, hemorrhagic, and soft. Microscopically, they are well-circumscribed collections of large eosinophilic cells that may have many mitotic figures (e-Fig. 31.18). The nodules usually regress after pregnancy.

E. Ovarian Torsion is frequently accompanied by torsion of the fallopian tube. Torsion is caused by twisting of the adnexa on its fibrovascular pedicle, impeding blood flow into and out of the adnexal structures, ultimately resulting in infarction. The ovary is often enlarged and hemorrhagic or dusky. Microscopically, there is extensive interstitial hemorrhage, edema, and necrosis of normal tissue. Not infrequently, there is an associated ovarian cyst or neoplasm. Pregnant women and women with adnexal masses are at increased risk, but torsion can occur in children, infants, and occasionally in utero. Patients typically present with acute abdominal pain, nausea, and vomiting; they also may have a palpable adnexal mass.

IV. OVARIAN NEOPLASMS. Table 31.1 shows the 2014 World Health Organization (WHO) histologic classification of tumors of the ovary.

TABLE 31.1	WHO 2014 Histologic Classification of Tumors of the Ovary

Epithelial tumors

Serous tumors
  Benign
    Serous cystadenoma, adenofibroma, surface papilloma
  Borderline
    Serous borderline tumor/atypical proliferative serous tumor
    Serous borderline tumor, micropapillary variant/noninvasive low-grade serous carcinoma
  Malignant
    Low-grade serous carcinoma
    High-grade serous carcinoma

Mucinous tumors
  Benign
    Mucinous cystadenoma, adenofibroma
  Borderline
    Mucinous borderline tumor/atypical proliferative mucinous tumor
  Malignant
    Mucinous carcinoma

Endometrioid tumors
  Benign
    Cystadenoma, adenofibroma, endometriotic cyst
  Borderline
    Endometrioid borderline tumor/atypical proliferative endometrioid tumor
  Malignant
    Endometrioid carcinoma

Clear cell tumors
  Benign
    Clear cell cystadenoma, adenofibroma
  Borderline
    Clear cell borderline tumor/atypical proliferative clear cell tumor
  Malignant
    Clear cell carcinoma

Brenner tumors
  Benign
    Brenner tumor
  Borderline
    Borderline Brenner tumor/atypical proliferative Brenner tumor
  Malignant
    Malignant Brenner

Seromucinous tumors
  Benign
    Seromucinous cystadenoma, adenofibroma
  Borderline
    Seromucinous borderline tumor/atypical proliferative seromucinous tumor
  Malignant
    Seromucinous carcinoma

Mesenchymal tumors
  Low-grade endometrioid stromal sarcoma
  High-grade endometrioid stromal sarcoma

Mixed epithelial and mesenchymal tumors
  Adenosarcoma
  Carcinosarcoma

TABLE 31.1 WHO 2014 Histologic Classification of Tumors of the Ovary (*Continued*)

Sex cord–stromal tumors
  Pure stromal tumors
    Fibroma
    Cellular fibroma
    Thecoma
    Luteinized thecoma associated with sclerosing peritonitis
    Fibrosarcoma
    Sclerosing stromal tumor
    Signet-ring stromal tumor
    Microcystic stromal tumor
    Leydig cell tumor
    Steroid cell tumor
    Steroid cell tumor, malignant
  Pure sex cord tumors
    Adult granulosa cell tumor
    Juvenile granulosa cell tumor
    Sertoli cell tumor
    Sex cord tumor with annular tubules
  Mixed sex cord–stromal tumors
    Sertoli–Leydig cell tumors (well differentiated, moderately differentiated, poorly
      differentiated, retiform, with or without heterologous elements)
    Sex cord–stromal tumors, NOS

Germ cell tumors
  Dysgerminoma
  Yolk sac tumor
  Embryonal carcinoma
  Nongestational choriocarcinoma
  Mature teratoma
  Immature teratoma
  Mixed germ cell tumor

Monodermal teratoma and somatic-type tumors arising from a dermoid cyst
  Struma ovarii (benign, malignant)
  Carcinoid (strumal carcinoid, mucinous carcinoid)
  Neuroectodermal-type tumors
  Sebaceous tumors (adenoma, carcinoma)
  Other rare monodermal teratomas
  Carcinomas (squamous cell carcinoma, others)

Germ cell–sex cord–stromal tumors
  Gonadoblastoma, including gonadoblastoma with malignant germ cell tumor
  Mixed germ cell–sex cord–stromal tumor, unclassified

Miscellaneous tumors
  Tumors of the rete ovarii (adenoma, adenocarcinoma)
  Wolffian tumor
  Small cell carcinoma, hypercalcemic type
  Small cell carcinoma, pulmonary type
  Wilms tumor
  Paraganglioma
  Solid pseudopapillary neoplasm

Mesothelial tumors
  Adenomatoid tumor
  Mesothelioma

(continued)

TABLE 31.1 WHO 2014 Histologic Classification of Tumors of the Ovary (*Continued*)

Soft tissue tumors
 Myxoma
 Others

Tumor-like lesions
 Follicle cyst
 Corpus luteum cyst
 Large solitary luteinized follicle cyst
 Hyperreactio luteinalis
 Pregnancy luteoma
 Stromal hyperplasia
 Stromal hyperthecosis
 Fibromatosis
 Massive edema
 Leydig cell hyperplasia
 Others

Lymphoid and myeloid tumors
 Lymphoma
 Plasmacytoma
 Myeloid neoplasms

Secondary tumors

From Kurman RJ, Carcangiu ML, Herrington CS, Young RH, eds. *WHO Classification of Tumours of Female Reproductive Organs.* Lyon, France: IARC Press; 2017. Used with permission.

A. Epithelial Tumors represent approximately two-thirds of all ovarian neoplasms. Ovarian surface epithelium may differentiate into any müllerian-type epithelium: serous (resembling fallopian tube), endometrioid (resembling endometrium), mucinous (resembling endocervix), clear cell, or Brenner. The standard of treatment for these tumors is surgery, with the goal of staging and optimally debulking the tumor, followed by chemotherapy for all but some categories of stage 1 tumors and borderline tumors.

1. Serous tumors are the most common subtype of ovarian epithelial tumors. The majority of serous tumors are benign (serous cystadenoma or adenofibroma) and occur in women of ages 30 to 40 years. About 15% are borderline (also known as atypical proliferative serous tumors). About 25% are malignant (low- or high-grade serous carcinoma). The neoplastic epithelium, particularly in benign and borderline tumors, resembles fallopian tube epithelium and contains ciliated and secretory cells.

 a. Serous cystadenoma/cystadenofibroma. These benign lesions make up over half of all serous tumors, and they are most commonly found in reproductive-aged women. Grossly, they are unilocular, smooth-walled cysts with varying amounts of fibrous stroma, usually ranging from 1 to 10 cm. Cystadenofibroma often has small, bulbous, cauliflower-like projections in the lining of the cyst; these should be distinguished from the friable papillary excrescences seen in serous borderline tumors (SBT) or serous carcinomas.

 Histologically, the cystadenoma lining is a single layer of columnar and usually ciliated epithelium (e-Fig. 31.19). Cystadenofibromas show broad, nonbranching stromal papillae lined by simple columnar ciliated epithelium (e-Fig. 31.20). The lining may be attenuated in longstanding lesions. Lesions without a cystic component are termed adenofibromas.

 b. Serous borderline tumors (SBT, also known atypical proliferative serous tumors) are predominantly cystic and generally present in perimenopausal women. As many as one-third are bilateral. These tumors have friable papillary excrescences with hierarchically branching stromal cores lined by mildly to moderately cytologically atypical epithelium that demonstrates mildly increased mitotic activity, epithelial stratification and tufting, and detached buds of epithelium (e-**Fig. 31.21**). Psammoma bodies are frequently seen. SBT may show areas of microinvasion, defined as clusters of cells with abundant eosinophilic cytoplasm in the stroma that span less than 5 mm in greatest extent (e-**Fig. 31.22**). Some have hypothesized that these strikingly eosinophilic cells are actually senescent, an interpretation supported by the fact that microinvasion does not alter the prognosis of SBT (*Am J Surg Pathol* 2014;38:743). Rarely, small foci of tumor cells lacking the "senescent" morphology are seen in the stroma; those cases must be extensively sampled to exclude low-grade serous carcinoma.

c. Although most SBT are confined to the ovary, extraovarian disease in the form of peritoneal "implants" may be present (e-**Figs. 31.23, 31.24**). Peritoneal implants are by definition noninvasive, but they may show desmoplastic changes (the so-called "noninvasive desmoplastic implant"). Desmoplastic implants have a "stuck-on" morphology, maintaining a clear interface between the surface implant and underlying tissue. Tumors with extraovarian lesions formerly classified as "invasive implants," which do show infiltration of the underlying tissue, in the current WHO classification are classified as low-grade serous carcinoma rather than SBT. Similarly, peritoneal tumor deposits with micropapillary (described below) or cribriform growth are considered to represent metastatic low-grade serous carcinoma rather than implants of SBT, regardless of whether the deposit is limited to the surface or appears infiltrative (*Am J Surg Pathol* 2001;25:419). Approximately 5% of tumors initially diagnosed as SBT evolve into low-grade serous carcinoma (*Am J Surg Pathol* 2005;29:707). Prognosis of SBT confined to the ovary is excellent.

SBT, micropapillary variant is considered to be a noninvasive low-grade serous carcinoma; the terms are synonymous in the current WHO classification. Cytologic atypia and mitotic activity is typically in line with that of a conventional low-grade serous carcinoma. Two morphologic patterns can be seen in these tumors: micropapillary or cribriform. In the micropapillary pattern, filiform micropapillae (five times as long as they are wide, with scant or absent stromal cores) project directly from larger papillae, without hierarchical branching (e-**Fig. 31.25**). The cribriform pattern is often associated with the micropapillary pattern and shows fusion of the tips of papillae with the formation of cribriform structures (e-**Fig. 31.26**). Micropapillary variant of SBT must have at least five linear millimeters (in any dimension) of confluent micropapillary/cribriform growth; otherwise, the tumor may be classified as SBT with focal micropapillary features. About half of micropapillary SBT/noninvasive low-grade serous carcinomas have metastatic disease (*Gynecol Oncol* 2014;134:267).

d. **Serous carcinoma** most commonly presents as bilateral masses with widespread peritoneal metastases. Grossly, the tumors are large and friable with multiloculated cysts and polypoid growths. Microscopically, the tumors may show a wide variety of architectural patterns including papillary, solid, and nested with slit-like spaces. Nuclear atypia is variable but often marked. By definition, serous carcinomas demonstrate destructive stromal invasion (e-**Fig. 31.27**). Psammoma bodies may be present. Exceptional cases present as purely cystic lesions and mimic a borderline tumor (e-**Fig. 31.28**).

Serous carcinomas are classified as high-grade or low-grade. Low-grade tumors (<12 mitoses/10 high-power fields and low-grade cytologic atypia) (e-**Fig. 31.29**) are frequently resistant to chemotherapy and are more appropriately treated surgically.

About half of low-grade serous carcinomas have *BRAF* and *KRAS* mutations. Virtually all high-grade serous carcinomas have mutations in *TP53*. As such, p53 immunohistochemical staining is occasionally helpful in substantiating a diagnosis of high-grade serous carcinoma; "mutant pattern" staining is either strong and diffuse or completely absent.

2. Mucinous tumors are the second most common type of surface epithelial tumor. The neoplastic epithelium resembles intestinal (goblet cells with intracytoplasmic mucin), gastric (foveolar), or endocervical (apical mucin with no cilia) epithelium. Eighty percent of these tumors are benign, 10% are borderline, and 10% are malignant. Because mucinous neoplasms are quite heterogeneous and a malignant component may be very focal, it is imperative that all mucinous neoplasms be well sampled (one to two sections per cm).

a. Mucinous cystadenomas are usually unilateral, multiloculated, and large (up to 50 cm). They have a smooth external surface and cyst lining. Microscopically, the cysts are lined by a single layer of tall columnar cells with bland basal nuclei, most often of intestinal type (**e-Fig. 31.30**). If there is a prominent stromal component, the lesion is termed a mucinous cystadenofibroma. Bilateral lesions should prompt consideration of metastatic well-differentiated adenocarcinoma. A classic association exists between mucinous cystadenoma and benign Brenner tumor; the two tumor types may be intermixed or occur adjacent to each other.

b. Mucinous borderline tumors (MBT)/atypical proliferative mucinous tumors also present as unilateral, multiloculated masses. They are most common in perimenopausal women. Grossly, these tumors have thick cyst walls, sometimes with papillary excrescences. Microscopically, MBTs have a stratified, tufted intestinal-type epithelial lining with mild-to-moderate nuclear atypia (**e-Fig. 31.31**).

By definition, borderline mucinous tumors do not demonstrate destructive stromal invasion. However, MBT can show areas of microinvasion, which consist of small foci of invasion either as small nests or individual cells (often with more eosinophilic cytoplasm), but foci should not exceed 5 mm in greatest linear extent (**e-Fig. 31.32**). MBT with intraepithelial carcinoma contain focal areas that demonstrate increased cytologic atypia with marked pleomorphism and prominent nucleoli (**e-Fig. 31.33**). No destructive stromal invasion is present, and the intraepithelial carcinoma does not appear to portend a worse prognosis (*Ann Surg Oncol* 2010;18:40). Extensive sampling (two sections per cm) should be performed to exclude invasive carcinoma in tumors that are >10 cm or have either microinvasion or intraepithelial carcinoma (*Int J Gynecol Pathol* 2004;31:524). Importantly, metastatic adenocarcinomas of gastrointestinal (particularly appendiceal) or pancreatobiliary primary can closely mimic MBT; unfortunately, immunohistochemical stains are not helpful in resolving that differential.

Borderline tumors with endocervical-type epithelium (15% of MBTs) have the hierarchical branching pattern of SBTs but the papillae are lined by mucinous epithelium; they are often associated with acute inflammation and frequently with endometriosis and bilaterality (**e-Fig. 31.34**). Some borderline tumors show a mixture of endocervical-type mucinous epithelium, serous epithelium, and even endometrioid epithelium; these tumors also have the hierarchical branching architecture of SBT and are also associated with endometriosis and bilaterality.

c. Mucinous carcinomas also present in perimenopausal women as unilateral, multiloculated cystic masses. Frank stromal invasion is present microscopically (**e-Fig. 31.35**), but mucinous carcinomas frequently demonstrate areas of benign and borderline-appearing mucinous epithelium as well. Two patterns of invasion are recognized. The expansile pattern shows crowded glands, little stroma, and sometimes a cribriform architecture. The destructive pattern shows infiltrative glands, frequently with a desmoplastic stromal response. Primary mucinous carcinoma of the ovary is very uncommon and usually occurs as a somatic-type malignancy arising in an ovarian teratoma; when stromal invasion is present, particularly of the destructive type, serious consideration must be given to metastatic involvement of the ovary by adenocarcinoma from a different site (including gastrointestinal or pancreatobiliary primary tumors). Similarly, dissecting pools of stromal mucin (pseudomyxoma ovarii, **e-Fig. 31.36**) should prompt evaluation of the appendix.

Features seen more commonly in metastatic disease include bilaterality, concomitant extraovarian disease, involvement of the external surface of the ovary, pseudomyxoma ovarii, and extensive lymphovascular space invasion. Metastatic adenocarcinoma from the colorectum will show abundant luminal karyorrhectic debris ("dirty necrosis"), a garland pattern of glands lining cystic spaces, an abrupt transition between viable and necrotic epithelium, and immunopositivity for CK20 and CEA but immunonegativity for CK7 and CA125 (e-**Fig. 31.37**). SATB2 is a recently described immunostain that has utility in establishing appendiceal or colorectal (hindgut) origin (*Am J Surg Pathol* 2016;40:419).

3. **Endometrioid tumors.** The majority of endometrioid tumors of the ovary are carcinomas. From 10% to 20% are associated with endometriosis, and about 15% have a concomitant endometrioid tumor of the endometrium. Squamous differentiation may be seen in all types of endometrioid tumors.

   a. **Benign endometrioid tumors** are adenofibromas/cystadenofibromas with organized endometrial glands arranged in a fibrous stroma. These are quite rare and can be distinguished from endometriosis by a lack of associated endometrial-type stroma and hemosiderin-laden macrophages.

   b. **Endometrioid borderline tumors/atypical proliferative endometrioid tumors** are very rare and frequently are associated with endometriosis, endometrioid adenofibroma, and/or endometrial hyperplasia. Grossly, these tumors may be solid or cystic. Their morphologic features are similar to those described for atypical hyperplasia of the endometrium, characterized crowded glands with nuclear stratification and mild-to-moderate cytologic atypia (e-**Fig. 31.38**). Intraepithelial carcinoma or microinvasion may occasionally be seen, but tumors demonstrating expansile gland proliferation spanning >5 mm or unequivocal stromal invasion should be classified as endometrioid carcinoma.

   c. **Endometrioid carcinomas** may be cystic or solid. Microscopically, they show villoglandular structures and/or tubular glands composed of a stratified layer of epithelial cells with smooth luminal borders (e-**Fig. 31.39**). Squamous metaplasia is common. By definition, destructive stromal invasion is present. These tumors are graded using the International Federation of Gynecology and Obstetrics (FIGO) grading scheme identical to that for endometrioid tumors, which is listed in Table 31.2. A variety of histologic variants can be seen, including secretory change (not to be confused with clear cell carcinoma), spindle cell morphology (not to be confused with carcinosarcoma or sex cord–stromal tumors), and sex cord–like (sertoliform) differentiation.

4. **Clear cell tumors.** The vast majority of clear cell tumors are frank adenocarcinomas; benign and borderline clear cell tumors are extremely rare. Clear cell carcinomas make up 5% of ovarian cancers and are often associated with endometriosis either in the ovary or elsewhere in the pelvis. They are also associated with age >50, nulliparity, and endometriosis. Grossly, clear cell adenocarcinomas are white-tan to yellow, solid and cystic masses. Histologically, the tumor grows in sheets, tubules, and/or papillae.

TABLE 31.2	FIGO Grading Scheme for Endometrioid Adenocarcinoma
Grade 1 or well-differentiated	Well-formed glands resembling villoglandular carcinoma of the uterine corpus[a] ≤5% solid tumor growth
Grade 2 or moderately differentiated	More complex glandular architecture Increased nuclear stratification 6–50% solid tumor growth
Grade 3 or poorly differentiated	Poorly formed glands, large sheets of cells >50% solid tumor growth

[a]Areas of squamous differentiation are not included when assessing the amount of solid tumor growth.

The large tumor cells have clear cytoplasm that may contain hyaline globules; the nuclei often jut into the lumen giving the cells a "hobnail" appearance. The stroma is densely hyalinized and eosinophilic (e-Fig. 31.40). These tumors are always high-grade and carry a poor prognosis.

5. Brenner tumors

a. Brenner tumors are usually unilateral and often an incidental finding. Grossly, they have a firm, white to tan, whorled cut surface but may show cystic spaces and calcification. Histologic sections show nests of oval epithelial cells with pale cytoplasm, uniform nuclei, and longitudinal nuclear grooves surrounded by abundant fibrous stroma, often with areas of calcification. Cystic spaces may contain eosinophilic material or be lined by mucinous epithelium (e-Fig. 31.41). Brenner tumors have an associated benign mucinous cystic component in 25% of cases.

b. Borderline Brenner tumors/atypical proliferative Brenner tumors are grossly cystic with papillary excrescences. Microscopically, the cysts and broad frond–like papillae are lined by a stratified epithelium resembling that of low-grade papillary urothelial carcinoma. Stromal invasion is absent (e-Fig. 31.42).

c. Malignant Brenner tumors may be solid or cystic. By definition, stromal invasion is present, and there is an identifiable borderline or benign Brenner component (e-Fig. 31.43). The invasive component may resemble low-grade or high-grade urothelial carcinoma, or even squamous cell carcinoma or adenocarcinoma.

6. Seromucinous tumors (cystadenoma/adenofibroma, borderline tumor, or carcinoma) are similar to the above-described tumor types but contain at least two types of müllerian epithelium (usually serous and endocervical mucinous types; each type must comprise at least 10% of the tumor cellularity).

7. Undifferentiated carcinoma in the ovary is uncommon and similar to undifferentiated carcinoma of the endometrium (see Chapter 33). Undifferentiated carcinoma is usually seen in association with low-grade endometrioid carcinoma. The prognosis is poor.

B. Mesenchymal Tumors in the ovary include low-grade and high-grade endometrioid stromal sarcomas, which are similar to endometrial stromal sarcoma of the uterus (see Chapter 33). These tumors are only rarely primary to the ovary; metastasis from the uterus should be excluded.

C. Mixed Epithelial and Mesenchymal Tumors of the ovary include adenosarcoma and carcinosarcoma (malignant mixed müllerian tumor), both of which are rare and analogous to tumors of the same names arising in the endometrium (see Chapter 33). Adenosarcoma consists of benign-appearing epithelial elements with a malignant stromal component; in carcinosarcoma, both the epithelial and mesenchymal elements are malignant (e-Fig. 31.44).

D. Sex Cord–Stromal Tumors. These tumors represent approximately 8% of ovarian tumors, and comprise the majority of the hormonally active ovarian neoplasms.

1. Fibroma–thecoma

a. Fibromas represent the most common of the sex cord–stromal tumors. They typically occur in perimenopausal women and are not hormonally active. Grossly, fibromas are unilateral, solid, and lobulated with a firm, white-gray cut surface. Cystic degeneration sometimes occurs. Histologically, they are characterized by interlacing bundles and storiform areas of spindle cells that show no atypia and few mitoses (e-Fig. 31.45). The tumor cells stain diffusely positive for vimentin and are usually negative for inhibin.

Fibromas may be associated with two syndromes: the Meigs syndrome (fibroma, ascites, and pleural effusion) and the Gorlin syndrome (basal cell nevus syndrome). In the Gorlin syndrome, fibromas occur in younger women or even children; are often multiple or bilateral; and are calcified.

b. Thecomas are unilateral solid tumors found most often in postmenopausal women. Hyperestrogenic symptoms are present in 50% to 80% of cases. Grossly, these tumors have a lobulated, yellow-tan cut surface. Histologically, thecomas comprise round-to-oval, lipid-laden theca cells in a fibromatous stroma with little atypia or mitotic activity (e-**Fig. 31.46**). These tumors are immunopositive for inhibin. Oil Red O fat stains (which require fresh–frozen tissue) highlight the intracellular lipid. When clusters of lutein cells (eosinophilic cells with large round nuclei) are present, the tumor is termed a luteinized thecoma (e-**Fig. 31.47**); this variant is more common in younger women and can be associated with sclerosing peritonitis.

2. Granulosa cell tumors

a. **Adult granulosa cell tumors** (AGCTs) are low-grade malignant neoplasms that occur most commonly in postmenopausal women but can occur at any age. AGCTs are the most common ovarian tumors with estrogenic manifestations (e.g., endometrial hyperplasia or carcinoma, and less commonly virilization). Hormonal manifestations may alert the clinician to the presence of a granulosa cell tumor, but patients more commonly present with an adnexal mass. In about 10% of cases patients present with hemoperitoneum from tumor rupture. The tumors are usually large (>10 cm) and unilateral. The cut surface is soft and yellow-tan with cysts and hemorrhage (e-**Fig. 31.48**).

These tumors exhibit a variety of histologic patterns including diffuse (e-**Fig. 31.49**), trabecular (e-**Fig. 31.50**), microfollicular, macrofollicular (e-**Fig. 31.51**), or gyriform (e-**Fig. 31.52**), and often more than one pattern is found within the same tumor. No matter the architecture, the cytology is usually bland with oval nuclei, longitudinal nuclear grooves, and a low mitotic rate (e-**Fig. 31.53**). The microfollicular and diffuse variants often contain characteristic Call–Exner bodies consisting of a small collection of eosinophilic material lined by palisaded granulosa cells (e-**Fig. 31.54**). AGCTs usually exhibit minimal cytologic atypia although areas of "bizarre" nuclei may occasionally be seen (e-**Fig. 31.55**).

AGCTs are usually confined to the ovary; spread outside the ovary is a poor prognostic factor. Tumors with high stage, large size, nuclear atypia, high mitotic activity, and a sarcomatoid pattern have a poorer prognosis, although tumors with none of these factors may recur. AGCTs are unusual in that they may recur decades after diagnosis.

b. **Juvenile granulosa cell tumors** (JGCTs) occur in children and young adults, typically under age 20 years. They usually present with a palpable mass and symptoms of hyperestrogenism such as breast development in children or menstrual irregularities in adolescents. The gross findings are similar to those of AGCTs with yellow-tan solid areas and interspersed blood-filled cysts.

Microscopically, JGCTs are characterized by solid sheets of cells mixed with small follicle-like spaces containing basophilic or eosinophilic secretions that are lined by more mature-appearing granulosa cells. Luteinization is prominent (e-**Fig. 31.56**). JGCTs exhibit more cytologic atypia and a higher mitotic rate than adult granulosa cells tumors. Nuclear grooves are not a feature (e-**Fig. 31.57**) of the cells.

JGCTs are usually confined to the ovary and high stage is a poor prognostic factor. Unlike their adult counterparts, patients with JGCT who recur usually do so within 2 years of diagnosis. Cytologic atypia is not a prognostic factor in JGCTs.

3. Sertoli and Sertoli–Leydig cell tumors

a. **Sertoli cell tumors** are rare, low-grade, nonfunctioning tumors that occur in women of child-bearing age. Grossly, they are yellow-tan, solid, lobulated tumors. Microscopically, they are composed of closely packed tubules separated by fibrous stroma. The tubules are lined by cuboidal to columnar cells with abundant pale eosinophilic cytoplasm with little atypia or mitotic activity.

b. **Sertoli–Leydig cell tumors** (SLCT) are rare, unilateral neoplasms that occur in young women and, in 30% of cases, secrete androgenic hormones. Grossly, these tumors average 10 cm in diameter, are yellow-orange to red-brown, and frequently have a nodular appearance with a central scar (e-**Fig. 31.58**). Well-differentiated

SLCTs contain tubules (similar to those seen in Sertoli cell tumors) and interspersed clusters of Leydig cells that have abundant eosinophilic cytoplasm (e-**Fig. 31.59**). SLCT of intermediate differentiation contain solid cords of Sertoli cells or may be very cellular (e-**Fig. 31.60**); Leydig cells may be difficult to find but are typically located at the periphery of cellular nodules, and the Leydig cells often show lipidization with foamy rather than eosinophilic cytoplasm (e-**Fig. 31.61**). Poorly differentiated SLCTs show densely packed atypical spindled cells resembling a sarcoma (e-**Fig. 31.62**).

Two morphologic variants of SLCT occur, usually in association with tumors of intermediate differentiation or poorly differentiated tumors. About 20% of SLCT harbor heterologous elements which take the form of intestinal-type mucinous glands (e-**Fig. 31.63**), carcinoid tumors, (which have a good prognosis), or rhabdomyoblastic or cartilaginous differentiation (which have a poor prognosis). About 15% of SLCTs contain in tubules and slit-like glandular structures, or micropapillary structures with dense fibrovascular cores (e-**Fig. 31.64**); these tumors are referred to as retiform variants. Retiform tumors are less likely to be androgen secreting and are more common in younger age groups (average age is 15 years). Distinction of this variant from yolk sac tumors may be difficult.

4. Steroid cell tumors are uncommon neoplasms composed of large cells with intracellular lipids that resemble Leydig cells or luteinized stromal cells.

    a. Stromal luteomas are benign, hormonally active steroid cell tumors that usually occur in postmenopausal women. Estrogenic manifestations are seen in 60% of cases; androgenic in 10% of cases. These well-circumscribed tumors grow within the ovarian parenchyma and have a yellow-brown cut surface. Microscopically, polygonal cells with eosinophilic cytoplasm grow in sheets, nests, and cords (e-**Fig. 31.65**). Degenerative changes may cause slit-like spaces within the tumor. Crystals of Reinke (slender, eosinophilic, rod-shaped crystals) are absent (e-**Fig. 31.17**). Stromal hyperplasia may occur in the ipsilateral or contralateral ovary.

    b. Leydig cell tumors are also benign steroid cell neoplasms found in postmenopausal women, although these tumors are more often androgenic or nonfunctioning. The majority of these tumors arise within the ovarian hilus (in which case the neoplasm can be referred to as a hilus cell tumor), although they also can occur in the ovarian stroma (in which case the neoplasm can be called a nonhilar Leydig cell tumor). The cut surface is yellow-brown with areas of hemorrhage. Microscopically, large polygonal cells with foamy or granular eosinophilic cytoplasm and round nuclei grow in cellular clusters separated by pink acellular areas (e-**Fig. 31.66**). In order to classify a tumor as a Leydig cell tumor, Reinke crystals must be identified.

    c. Steroid cell tumor, not otherwise specified (NOS) is a steroid cell tumor that does not meet the criteria for any of the types above. These are the most common of the steroid cell tumors, and may occur at any age. They are often hormonally active (50% androgenic, 10% estrogenic), and their gross morphology is similar to the other types of steroid cell tumor. Histologically, steroid cell tumor, NOS is composed of large cells with abundant granular cytoplasm separated by a vascular stroma. Reinke crystals are absent. A poorer prognosis is seen in tumors with necrosis, hemorrhage, an increased mitotic rate, or size greater than 7 cm.

5. Other sex cord–stromal tumors

    a. Sclerosing stromal tumors are rare benign neoplasms seen most often in girls and women less than 30 years of age. Grossly the tumor is firm to rubbery, white, and has areas of cystic degeneration. Histologically, cellular areas, consisting of both spindled cells and round cells with vacuolated cytoplasm, alternate with edematous and collagenized areas giving the tumor a pseudolobular appearance (e-**Fig. 31.67**).

    b. Sex cord tumors with annular tubules (SCTATs) occur in women of child-bearing age. In some women, the tumor occurs as a component of Peutz–Jeghers syndrome, in which case the SCTATs are small and incidental. Those unassociated with the Peutz–Jeghers syndrome form a large, solid, yellow mass. Histologically, the tumor is composed of well-circumscribed, ring-shaped tubules that contain central hyalinized material. The tubules are lined by cells with pale cytoplasm oriented toward the center of the tubule, with peripheral elongated nuclei (e-**Fig. 31.68**).

   c. Exceptionally rare purely stromal tumors of the ovary include signet-ring stromal tumor, microcystic stromal tumor, and fibrosarcoma.

E. Germ Cell Tumors

1. Teratomas

   a. Mature teratomas are the most common ovarian germ cell tumor. They occur most often in adult women of reproductive age, but may occur at any age. Grossly, they are usually cystic with a single solid nodule that may contain fat, teeth, bone, and many other tissue types. The cysts usually contain hair and soft yellow sebaceous debris. Microscopically, mature tissue from all three germ layers (ectoderm—skin or central nervous system elements; mesoderm—smooth muscle, teeth, bone; endoderm—respiratory epithelium, GI epithelium, thyroid) may be present (e-**Fig. 31.69**). The term dermoid cyst is commonly used to refer to mature cystic teratomas lined by squamous epithelium that contains skin appendages (e-**Fig. 31.70**). Mature cystic teratomas should be thoroughly sampled (one section per cm) in order to exclude an immature component, and to exclude malignant transformation of one of the mature components (a rare occurrence, more common in elderly women).

   b. Immature teratomas are rapidly growing malignant tumors that occur in children and young adults. They are unilateral and typically have solid and cystic components; the solid areas are generally more extensive than in a mature teratoma. Microscopically, they contain immature or primitive tissue (derived from any or all three germ cell layers) that is usually mixed with areas of mature tissue. The most common immature element is neuroectodermal and consists of rosettes, masses, or tubules of primitive neural cells (e-**Fig. 31.71**).

   Immature teratomas are graded based on the relative amount of immature tissue present (*Int J Gynecol Pathol* 1994;13:283). Tumors with more than one low-power field of immature neuroepithelium on any given slide are considered high-grade and require adjuvant chemotherapy.

   c. Monodermal teratomas are teratomas in which all the tissue is derived from one germ cell layer. **Struma ovarii** is the most common monodermal teratoma, and consists of mature thyroid tissue including follicles and colloid (e-**Fig. 31.72**). Secondary changes such as hyperplasia, adenoma, and even carcinoma may be seen.

2. Carcinoid tumors

of the ovary usually arise in a mature cystic teratoma. They most commonly have an insular or trabecular pattern identical to that seen in the gastrointestinal tract. The cells are small and uniform with round nuclei with stippled chromatin; goblet cell carcinoids are very uncommon. Metastasis from a primary carcinoid tumor outside the ovary must always be excluded; metastatic carcinoid tumors are more likely to be bilateral, larger, unassociated with a teratoma, and more commonly associated with carcinoid syndrome.

3. Dysgerminoma

is the most common malignant germ cell tumor. It occurs as pure dysgerminoma or as a component of mixed germ cell tumor. Dysgerminoma develops most commonly in adolescents and young women, and is frequent in patients with ovarian dysgenesis. Patients with dysgerminomas frequently have elevated LDH levels and occasionally mildly elevated hCG levels. Pure dysgerminomas have an excellent prognosis when treated by current therapeutic regimens.

   Grossly, dysgerminomas are large and solid with a smooth external surface and a lobulated gray-tan cut surface. The tumor should be thoroughly sampled (one section per cm) for microscopic examination to exclude other germ cell tumor types; special attention should be directed to hemorrhagic and cystic areas.

   Dysgerminomas are analogous to testicular seminomas and have an identical histologic appearance. They are composed of nests and sheets of uniform large round cells with abundant clear cytoplasm, large nuclei, and prominent nucleoli.

Tumor cells are separated by a lymphocyte-rich fibrous stroma (**e-Fig. 31.73**). Often a histiocytic or granulomatous infiltrate is present, and multinucleated syncytiotrophoblastic cells may also be identified (sometimes the former component can obscure the dysgerminoma cells). Dysgerminomas are immunopositive for placental alkaline phosphatase (PLAP), c-kit (CD117), OCT3/4, and SALL4.

4. Yolk sac tumors, also known as endodermal sinus tumors, occur in young women, usually with an associated elevated serum alpha fetoprotein (AFP) level. Yolk sac tumors grow rapidly and have often spread outside the ovary at the time of diagnosis. They are often a component of mixed germ cell tumors. Grossly, yolk sac tumors are unilateral and large, have a smooth external surface, and a solid and cystic yellow to tan cut surface. Hemorrhage and necrosis are often present.

Many different histologic patterns occur, including microcystic, endodermal sinus, macrocystic, solid, polyvesicular vitelline, papillary, hepatoid, and glandular. The microcystic pattern is the most common variant, and is composed of small cystic spaces lined by cuboidal to columnar cells with clear cytoplasm and large hyperchromatic nuclei (**e-Fig. 31.74**). The endodermal sinus pattern is the second most common pattern; this pattern features characteristic Schiller–Duval bodies (rounded fibrovascular papillae containing a single central vessel and lined by columnar tumor cells) (**e-Fig. 31.75**). The polyvesicular vitelline pattern is composed of abundant cystic structures lined by tumor cells that are embedded in a dense cellular stroma. Yolk sac tumors usually express keratins, alpha-1-antitrypsin, glypican 3, and AFP; immunostaining shows a lack of expression of EMA.

5. Embryonal carcinoma is rare in the ovary and is usually a component of mixed germ cell tumors. Half of cases occur in prepubertal girls, and half have elevated β-hCG levels. Grossly, these tumors are large (~17 cm) and solid with areas of hemorrhage and necrosis. Morphologically, the tumor is identical to embryonal carcinoma of the testis and is composed of large anaplastic cells with pale eosinophilic vacuolated cytoplasm that grow in sheets and nests. The nuclei are hyperchromatic with prominent nucleoli (**e-Fig. 31.76**). Atypical mitotic figures are common. Embryonal carcinomas express CD30, cytokeratin, PLAP, OCT 3/4, and SALL4.

6. Polyembryoma is a very rare, highly malignant neoplasm that usually is a component of a mixed germ cell tumor. Grossly, it presents as a unilateral solid mass with areas of hemorrhage and necrosis. Microscopically, the tumor is composed of embryoid bodies (embryonic disks lined by the endoderm on one side, the ectoderm on the opposite side, and the associated yolk sac and amniotic cavities).

7. Pure **choriocarcinoma** of the ovary is rare. It is most often seen as a component of a mixed germ cell tumor (i.e., nongestational), or as a metastasis from gestational trophoblastic disease.

Primary choriocarcinoma presents in children and adolescents; elevated β-hCG levels are invariably present. Grossly, the tumor mass is hemorrhagic, soft, and tan. Microscopically, both cytotrophoblast and syncytiotrophoblast are present. Cytotrophoblastic cells have centrally located hyperchromatic nuclei, prominent nucleoli, clear cytoplasm, and well-defined cytoplasmic borders; syncytiotrophoblastic cells are multinucleated and are immunopositive for hCG. While syncytiotrophoblast may be seen as a component of other germ cell tumors, cytotrophoblast is only seen in choriocarcinoma.

Nongestational choriocarcinoma (a germ cell tumor) should be distinguished from gestational choriocarcinoma (a form of gestational trophoblastic disease, see Chapter 37), a task which is readily accomplished by molecular testing with short tandem repeat (STR) analysis. Prognosis of nongestational choriocarcinoma is worse than that of choriocarcinoma arising in the setting of gestational trophoblastic disease.

8. Mixed germ cell tumors make up 10% of germ cell tumors. The most common combination is dysgerminoma and yolk sac tumor, although any combination can occur. The relative composition of the various histologic subtypes should be included in the final report, since it can impact therapy and prognosis.

F. **Germ Cell–Sex Cord–Stromal Tumors** include **gonadoblastoma,** a rare tumor that contains both germ cell and sex cord–stromal components. Most patients have gonadal dysgenesis, and over 90% have a Y chromosome. Approximately half of all cases harbor a malignant germ cell component, most often dysgerminoma. Gonadoblastoma is benign unless a malignant germ cell component is present. Grossly, the tumor is usually small with a yellow to gray cut surface and areas of calcification. Histologically, the tumor consists of admixed primitive germ cells and sex cord–stromal derivatives (that resemble immature granulosa cells and Sertoli cells) surrounded by abundant basement membrane-like material, often with calcification.

G. **Other Tumor Types**
1. **Small cell carcinoma of hypercalcemic type** is a highly malignant tumor with a poor prognosis that presents in young women (despite its name, this tumor is unrelated to small cell neuroendocrine carcinoma, the so-called "small cell carcinoma of pulmonary type", which rarely occurs in the ovary, but when it does is identical to small cell neuroendocrine carcinoma seen in other anatomic sites). Approximately two-thirds of patients manifest hypercalcemia. The tumor is generally large and unilateral with a soft, white-tan, lobulated cut surface that shows areas of hemorrhage and necrosis. Histologic examination demonstrates sheets of small cells with scant cytoplasm admixed with follicle-like spaces filled with eosinophilic fluid (e-Fig. 31.77). The tumor nuclei are round with coarse chromatin and prominent nucleoli (e-Fig. 31.78). Some tumor cells have globular hyaline inclusions producing a rhabdoid morphology. The tumor cells are usually positive for CK, EMA, WT-1, calretinin, CD10, and p53 and less commonly positive for vimentin, NSE, and chromogranin.
2. **Ovarian myxomas** are rare unilateral tumors composed of stellate and spindled cells in an abundant myxoid stroma. These tumors must be distinguished from pseudomyxoma ovarii, which is characterized by pools of mucin usually with associated strips of mucin-secreting epithelium.
3. Primary **hematopoietic malignancies** of the ovary are extremely rare; however, secondary ovarian involvement may be seen in up to one-half of all lymphomas. The tumors are generally bilateral with a fleshy cut surface. Microscopically, they resemble their nodal or marrow counterparts. The most common lymphoma with secondary involvement of the ovary is diffuse large B-cell lymphoma containing sheets of large noncohesive cells that have irregular nuclear contours and increased mitotic activity. Immunohistochemical stains such as CD45 (leukocyte common antigen), as well as B- and T-cell markers, can be used to demonstrate a hematopoietic origin in difficult cases.
4. **Other** tumors have also been rarely reported as primary in the ovary, including tumors of the rete ovarii and Wolffian remnants, Wilms tumor, paraganglioma, solid pseudopapillary neoplasm (identical to the same tumor type in the pancreas), mesothelial tumors (adenomatoid tumor, mesothelioma), and soft tissue tumors (identical to their counterparts in other sites).
5. **Metastases.** About 8% of ovarian tumors are metastases, of which most are derived from the gastrointestinal tract (especially the large intestine, stomach, and appendix), breast, uterine corpus, or cervix. In young girls, ovarian metastases may be from neuroblastoma, rhabdomyosarcoma, Ewing sarcoma/peripheral neuroectodermal tumor, and malignant rhabdoid tumor of kidney.

V. **STAGING OF OVARIAN MALIGNANCIES**
A. **Pathologic Staging.** Ovarian cancer is staged surgically. The staging procedure includes bilateral salpingo-oophorectomy, hysterectomy, and omentectomy; biopsies of multiple pelvic and abdominal peritoneal surfaces; and regional lymph node dissections. Cytologic examination of peritoneal washings is also performed. The most recent AJCC staging system is applied (Amin MB, Edge S, Greene F, et al., eds. *AJCC Cancer Staging Manual*, 8th ed. New York: Springer, 2017). In a simplification from the previous AJCC staging, a single staging scheme is used for malignant tumors originating in the ovary, fallopian tube, or peritoneum. Other notable changes include substaging of pT1

tumors (pT1c1, intraoperative capsule rupture; pT1c2, preoperative capsule rupture; pT1c3, malignant cells in ascites or peritoneal washings). In the absence of nodal (N0) or distant metastases (M0), the AJCC prognostic stage group is the same as the T stage (except reported with roman numerals, e.g., stage IC1 for pT1c1). Now, patients with nodal metastases also are substaged (N1a or N1b, corresponding to stage group IIIA1i or IIIA1ii, respectively) based on the size of the largest nodal deposit. Distant metastasis is defined as stage IV disease. Importantly, transmural involvement of the intestine (invasion from the serosa through the wall of the bowel and into the mucosa) is now defined as distant metastasis (stage IVB); specific examination of the bowel for transmural invasion must be performed during grossing, with histologic documentation of transmural involvement. Similarly, parenchymal involvement of the liver or spleen is also classified as stage IV, whether as an intraparenchymal metastatic nodule or via direct invasion from a capsular metastasis. FIGO stage, which mirrors AJCC prognostic stage grouping, may also be reported.

B. Items to Include in the Pathology Report. The final pathology report must include all required items listed in the College of American Pathologists (CAP) Protocol for the Examination of Specimens from Patients With Primary Tumors of the Ovary, Fallopian Tube, or Peritoneum (available at www.cap.org). These items include what procedures were performed, whether the ovarian and tubal surfaces were intact or ruptured (assessments best made upon initial receipt of the specimen, frequently in the frozen section area), anatomic origin of the tumor, size of the primary tumor(s), histologic type and grade, extent of involvement of other sites, ascitic/peritoneal fluid cytology findings, presence or absence of treatment response (if applicable), lymph node evaluation, and AJCC staging. Additional details may also be included in the report, as appropriate.

ACKNOWLEDGMENT

The authors thank Meredith Pittman and Phyllis Huettner, authors of previous editions of this chapter.

32

Fallopian Tube

John D. Pfeifer and Horacio M. Maluf

I. **NORMAL ANATOMY.** The fallopian tubes are formed from the Müllerian (paramesonephric duct) system and lie within the broad ligament between the ovary and the uterus. They conduct eggs from the surface of the ovary to the uterine cavity and are the usual sites of fertilization. Each fallopian tube is shaped like an elongated funnel and is divided into four parts from lateral to medial: infundibulum, ampulla, isthmus, interstitium; the infundibulum contains the fingerlike fimbriae distally.

The fallopian tube mucosa is branched and folded into plicae. The mucosa is lined by a nonstratified epithelium composed of three cell types: ciliated, secretory, and intercalated cells. The most common are the ciliated cells, followed by secretory cells, which together comprise over 90% of the cell population. The intercalated cells are seen as elongated nuclei sporadically present between the ciliated cells. The wall of the fallopian tube contains smooth muscle to aid in moving the fertilized egg into the uterus. The serosa contains abundant blood vessels and is continuous with the broad ligament.

II. **GROSS EXAMINATION, TISSUE SAMPLING, AND HISTOLOGIC SLIDE PREPARATION.** Fallopian tubes are usually received as a portion of a total abdominal hysterectomy–bilateral salpingo-oophorectomy specimen. Short cross-sections of fallopian tube are received after tubal ligation procedures. Ectopic pregnancy specimens also usually contain a portion of fallopian tube. Rarely, specimens are received for primary fallopian tube tumors.

At the grossing station, the length and diameter of the fallopian tube should be documented, as well as the presence or absence of a fimbriated end, or evidence of prior ligation. The serosal surface should also be assessed for the presence of adhesions, cysts, exudates, rupture, or metastatic tumor. The tube is then serially sectioned.

A. **Benign Specimens.** Three sections are submitted from a normal fallopian tube, specifically from the fimbriated end, ampulla, and isthmus end. Additional sections of any gross lesions are also submitted. Complete cross-sections must be identified from a tubal ligation specimen.

When examining an ectopic pregnancy specimen, an embryo and/or placental villi will often be grossly evident. Hemorrhagic areas, including blood clot, along with obvious villous or embryonic tissue, should be submitted for histologic examination. A section proximal to the site of the ectopic pregnancy should be obtained to identify potential causes (i.e., salpingitis isthmica nodosa)

B. **Neoplastic Specimens.** Primary tubal carcinoma specimens will show a dilated lumen filled with a papillary or solid tumor. An ovarian tumor secondarily involving the fallopian tube is more common than a primary fallopian tube tumor, and careful sectioning can help distinguish the two. Grossly papillary and solid areas should be sampled thoroughly (at least one section per centimeter of tumor), along with uninvolved areas. If possible, a section showing the tumor's relationship to the ovary should be submitted.

C. **Prophylactic Excision Specimens.** Fallopian tube specimens received as part of a prophylactic hysterectomy–oophorectomy from patients with hereditary cancer syndromes (for example, *BRCA1* syndrome) should be, together with the ovaries, entirely submitted for histologic examination. For the fallopian tube, the goal is to ensure sectioning and extensive examination of the fimbria (so-called SEE-FIM protocol), since the majority of early serous tumors occur in this area. The protocol (*Am J Surg Path* 2006;30:230) specifies that the entire tube is fixed for at least 4 hours to minimize loss of epithelium during manipulation, the distal 2 cm of the fimbriated end is transected, the fimbrial

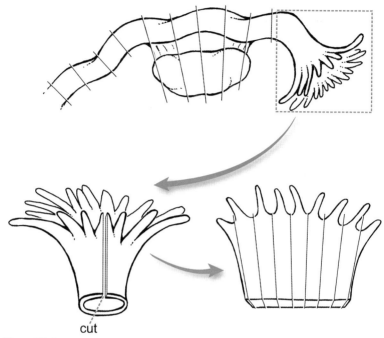

Figure 32.1 Approach to sectioning fallopian tube specimens received as part of a prophylactic hysterectomy–oophorectomy from patients with a hereditary cancer syndrome. Each tube and ovary should be entirely submitted for histologic examination; note that the fimbriated end of the tube should be transected, opened longitudinally, serially sectioned longitudinally, and then entirely submitted for microscopic examination.

mucosa is sectioned longitudinally into four pieces, the remainder of the tube is sectioned transversely every 2 to 3 mm, and that all the sections are submitted in toto (Fig. 32.1). This protocol has been incorporated into guidelines for the diagnosis of tubal, ovarian, and primary peritoneal carcinoma (*Mod Pathol* 2015;28;1101).

III. DIAGNOSTIC FEATURES OF COMMON DISEASES

A. Inflammatory and Nonneoplastic Lesions of the Fallopian Tube

1. **Cystic lesions.** Embryologic remnants may be found in the fallopian tube wall, usually as an incidental finding (e-**Fig. 32.1**). Paratubal cysts of Müllerian origin (ciliated lining) or Wolffian origin (columnar or stratified transitional lining) may be encountered; if the lining is atrophic secondary to compression, the two can be difficult to differentiate microscopically. A pedunculated paratubal cysts with a Müllerian epithelium present along the fimbriae is termed a Hydatid of Morgagni.

2. **Inflammatory lesions**

   a. **Acute salpingitis** usually presents in young to middle-aged women, is generally an ascending infection initiated by *Chlamydia trachomatis* or *Neisseria gonorrhoea,* and is often followed by polymicrobial infection (pelvic inflammatory disease [PID]). The damage to the tube that results from acute salpingitis may lead to infertility and/or ectopic pregnancy. Grossly, the tubal lumen may be distended by pus, blood, or secretions. Histologic sections show marked acute inflammation, with congestion and edema in the plicae and the tubal wall which often severely distorts the normal tubal architecture. The epithelial proliferation that accompanies the process can resemble an epithelial neoplasm (pseudocarcinomatous salpingitis) (e-**Fig. 32.2**).

  b. Chronic salpingitis is usually due to resolving acute salpingitis. Grossly, the tube is often enlarged, fibrotic, distorted, and adherent to the ovary or adjacent structures. Microscopically, a lymphoplasmacytic infiltrate is seen in the plicae. Fusion of the tubal plicae after resolution of acute salpingitis may lead to formation of follicle-like spaces, a histologic pattern known as salpingitis follicularis. Hydrosalpinx may be seen in end-stage chronic salpingitis, microscopically characterized by a dramatically thinned wall with few plicae and a lumen filled with clear fluid. Numerous adhesions are typically present on the serosal surface (e-**Fig. 32.3**).

  c. Granulomatous salpingitis may be caused by tuberculosis, fungal infection, Crohn disease, or sarcoidosis.

  d. Salpingitis isthmica nodosum typically presents in young women. It is associated with ectopic pregnancy and infertility, and has an unclear pathogenesis. Grossly, it presents as 1 to 2 cm diameter nodules in the wall of the fallopian tube isthmus. It is bilateral in 85% of cases. The lesions consist of outpouchings of tubal epithelium surrounded by a thickened wall of smooth muscle (e-**Fig. 32.4**).

  e. Pseudoxanthomatous salpingiosis and xanthogranulomatous salpingitis are characterized by accumulation of foamy histiocytes in the fallopian tube wall. The former is a manifestation of endometriosis, the latter, usually accompanied by other inflammatory cells, is seen in the context of PID. Changes similar to pseudoxanthomatous salpingiosis are seen in postablation tubal sterilization syndrome (PATSS).

3. Other nonneoplastic lesions of the fallopian tube

  a. The fallopian tube is a frequent site of involvement of **endometriosis**, primarily in women of reproductive age, which may be associated with infertility. Grossly, tubal endometriosis consists of dark brown serosal nodules. The microscopic findings include endometrial glands surrounded by a cuff of endometrial stroma with associated hemosiderin-laden macrophages and chronic inflammatory cells (e-**Fig. 32.5**).

  b. Ectopic pregnancy affects 1% to 2% of all conceptions, and the fallopian tube is the most common site; the most commonly involved region of the tube is the ampulla. Risk factors include prior ectopic pregnancy, salpingitis, congenital tubal anomalies, salpingitis isthmica nodosum, and endometriosis. Patients may present with tubal rupture and shock. Grossly, the fallopian tube is dilated and hemorrhagic with identifiable chorionic villi, with or without an identifiable embryo. Histologic sections should show chorionic villi or trophoblast in the tubal mucosa or wall (e-**Fig. 32.6**). Careful histologic examination is required to exclude a molar gestation. In problematic cases, immunohistochemistry for p63, interphase FISH, or DNA identity testing can be used for definitive diagnosis.

  Placental site nodules, which are thought to represent incomplete involution of a placental implantation site, have been described in the fallopian tube.

B. Neoplastic Lesions of the Fallopian Tube. The World Health Organization (WHO) histologic classification of tumors of the fallopian tube is presented in Table 32.1.

1. Benign tumors

  a. Adenomatoid tumor is the most common benign tumor of the fallopian tube. It is usually incidental, unilateral, and present grossly as a well-circumscribed, white-tan lesion in the tubal wall. It is derived from mesothelium, and the usual histologic pattern shows slit-like or glandular spaces lined by a single layer of flattened cuboidal cells (e-**Fig. 32.7**). The cells are immunopositive for cytokeratin, calretinin, and vimentin but negative for expression of factor VIII–related antigen and CD31, a profile that indicates a mesothelial rather than a vascular origin.

  b. Other benign tumors include adenomas, cystadenomas, adenofibromas, leiomyomas, and hemangiomas. Adenomas, cystadenomas, adenofibromas, and leiomyomas all resemble their ovarian and uterine counterparts.

TABLE 32.1 WHO Classification of Tumors of the Fallopian Tube

Epithelial tumors and cysts

Hydatid cyst

Benign epithelial tumors
  Papilloma
  Serous adenofibroma

Epithelial precursor lesion
  Serous tubal intraepithelial carcinoma

Epithelial borderline tumor
  Serous borderline tumor/atypical proliferative serous tumor

Malignant epithelial tumors
  Low-grade serous carcinoma
  High-grade serous carcinoma
  Endometrioid carcinoma
  Undifferentiated carcinoma

Others
  Mucinous carcinoma
  Transitional cell carcinoma
  Clear cell carcinoma

Tumor-like lesions
  Tubal hyperplasia
  Tubo-ovarian abscess
  Salpingitis isthmica nodosa
  Metaplastic papillary tumor
  Placenta site nodule
  Mucinous metaplasia
  Endometriosis
  Endosalpingiosis

Mixed epithelial–mesenchymal tumors
  Adenosarcoma
  Carcinosarcoma

Mesenchymal tumors
  Leiomyoma
  Leiomyosarcoma
  Others

Mesothelial tumors
  Adenomatoid tumor

Germ cell tumors

Teratoma
  Mature
  Immature

Lymphoid and myeloid tumors

Lymphomas

Myeloid neoplasms

From: Kurman RJ, Carcangiu ML, Herrington CS, Young RH, eds. *WHO Classification of Tumours of Female Reproductive Organs.* Lyon, France: IARC Press; 2017. Used with permission.

c. **Benign rests** can be incidentally found in the fallopian tube wall and include hilus cells, granulosa cells, and sex cord-like rests. Fibrous luminal nodules consist of a hyalinized core lined by a flattened epithelium within the lumen of the fallopian tube.

d. **Epithelial proliferations and metaplasias** are common in the fallopian tube.

   i. Mucinous and transitional cell metaplasia are the most frequent; the former can be associated with Peutz–Jeghers syndrome or rarely with mucinous neoplasms of the ovary, while the latter is an incidental finding.

   ii. Epithelial proliferations can have a papillary or nonpapillary appearance, and can exhibit a serous/secretory phenotype or rarely an endometrioid one. They lack the cytologic atypia and mitotic activity that characterizes STIC (see below).

   Detached papillary clusters with the morphologic features of borderline serous tumors and psammomatous calcifications are often seen in patients with advance stage borderline tumors/low-grade serous carcinoma. Whether these represent tumor precursors or entrapment of exfoliated cells remains undetermined, although the latter is more likely.

   Metaplastic papillary tumors are seen in pregnancy and postpartum and consist of a papillary lesion lined by eosinophilic nonstratified epithelium.

2. **Malignant tumors**

   a. **Primary fallopian tube carcinoma** is quite rare. Carcinomas typically occur in elderly women, and are usually widespread at the time of diagnosis with a correspondingly poor prognosis. Serum CA125 levels may be elevated. Grossly, the fallopian tube is distended by a papillary or solid tumor. Serous adenocarcinoma, which microscopically is identical to ovarian serous adenocarcinoma (e-**Fig. 32.8**), is the most common type of carcinoma.

   The etiology of primary fallopian tube carcinomas is unknown. However, the histologic and molecular demonstration that high-grade serous carcinomas may actually originate in the fallopian tube or fimbria (see below) suggests that the incidence of primary tubal carcinomas has been markedly underestimated.

   b. **Carcinoma in situ, also called serous tubal intraepithelial carcinoma (STIC),** is characterized by cellular stratification, loss of polarity, high-grade nuclear atypia, increased mitotic activity, and increased apoptosis, and is distinguished from carcinoma by the lack of stromal invasion (e-**Fig. 32.9**).

   Careful histopathologic examination of the fallopian tubes using the SEE-FIM protocol from cases of pelvic serous carcinoma has demonstrated that almost 50% of cases classified as arising in the ovary co-existed with a STIC, a finding that suggests many pelvic serous cancers originate from the tube/fimbria (*CM&R* 2007;5:35). Genetic analysis has provided further support for the concept that STIC represents a precursor of high-grade serous cancer (*Int J Gynecol Cancer* 2017;27:444). Consequently, a careful search for STIC is an important part of the pathologic examination of cases of pelvic serous carcinoma.

   A number of entities can mimic STIC (Table 32.2), including a range of benign hyperplasias, metaplasias, and reactive changes. And it has recently been demonstrated (by both histopathologic examination and molecular analysis) that many different types of primary non-gynecologic as well as gynecologic carcinomas can metastasize to the tubal mucosa and mimic STIC (*Arch Pathol Lab Med* 2017;141:1313). Immunohistochemistry can be useful in the setting of putative metastatic disease, with the caveats that p53 reactivity can be seen in many types of malignancies that may metastasize to the tube, and that p16 is likely to be expressed in STIC even in the absence of HPV infection.

   c. Other primary malignant tumors of the fallopian tube include endometrioid adenocarcinoma, clear cell adenocarcinoma, and **carcinosarcoma** (malignant mixed Müllerian tumor). The tumors microscopically resemble their ovarian and endometrial counterparts and are rare in the fallopian tube. Leiomyosarcoma can arise from the fallopian tube or adnexal soft tissue.

TABLE 32.2	Differential Diagnosis of Serous Tubal Intraepithelial Carcinomas (STIC)

Surgical (thermal) and other primary artifacts

Reactive hyperplasia/atypia of tubal epithelium

Arias-Stella phenomenon of tubal epithelium

Tubal metaplasia (papillary metaplastic tumor, transitional metaplasia, secretory metaplasia)

Tubal endometriosis

Metaplasia involving tubal endometriosis (papillary syncytial metaplasia)

Radiation-induced atypia

Metastasis from other gynecologic carcinoma (endometrium, cervix)

Metastasis from nongynecologic carcinoma (colon, upper GI track/pancreatobiliary, breast)

Compiled from *Arch Pathol Lab Med* 2013;137:126 and *Arch Pathol Lab Med* 2017;141:1313.

      d. Metastatic tumors are the most common category of malignancies involving the fallopian tube. Consequently, metastasis from a primary tumor at another site must always be excluded before making the diagnosis of a primary fallopian tube malignancy. Other primary tumors of the female reproductive tract, especially the ovary and endometrium, are the most frequent sources of metastases.

C. Reporting. The final report in any case of malignancy should include the histologic type and grade of the malignancy; the presence or absence of a precursor lesion (carcinoma in situ/STIC); tumor size, including depth and width; whether the malignancy is unifocal or multifocal; and the presence or absence of lymphovascular space invasion. Reporting should follow recommended guidelines (e.g., College of American Pathologists Protocol for the Examination of Specimens From Patients With Primary Tumors of the Ovary, Fallopian Tube, or Peritoneum, available at http://www.cap.org).

    The report should explicitly include all of the information required for assigning a stage, which by both FIGO and AJCC criteria is based on size, local extension, and lymph node metastasis (Amin MB et al., eds. *AJCC Cancer Staging Manual.* 8th ed. New York: Springer, 2017). Of note, the fallopian tube now shares the same staging system as the ovary and primary peritoneal tumors.

ACKNOWLEDGMENT

The authors thank Mitra Mehrad and Phyllis Huettner, authors of the previous editions of this chapter.

33 Uterine Corpus

Farhan A. Khan and Ian S. Hagemann

I. **NORMAL ANATOMY.** The uterus is a pear-shaped hollow organ with a normal weight of 40 to 80 g in adults. It is divided into the corpus, the lower uterine segment, and the cervix. The uterine cavity is triangular, measuring on average 6 cm in length. It is composed of an inner endometrial lining, a myometrium or muscular wall, and a serosal outer tunic continuous with the peritoneum. The peritoneal reflection is shorter anteriorly than posteriorly, because it reflects anteriorly over the bladder, and so can be used for orienting hysterectomy specimens.

II. **GROSS EXAMINATION, TISSUE SAMPLING, AND HISTOLOGIC SLIDE PREPARATION**

A. **Endometrial Biopsy and Curettage Specimens.** The most common endometrial tissue samples in surgical pathology are endometrial biopsy and curettage specimens. Endometrial biopsy samples are obtained from a relatively limited office sampling procedure in which no cervical dilation is required, while curettage is performed after cervical dilation in the operating room. The dimensions of the specimen (size range of the largest tissue fragments, or the dimensions of the tissue in aggregate) should be documented. The entire specimen should be submitted for microscopic examination, and three H&E-stained levels prepared for microscopic examination.

B. **Products of Conception are Usually Obtained by Curettage** (although the tissue is sometimes spontaneously passed). The dimensions of the specimen (size range of the largest tissue fragments, or the dimensions of the tissue in aggregate) should be documented. At least three cassettes should be submitted, focused on any villous tissue that is grossly present, both for confirmation of the presence of an intrauterine pregnancy and to rule out a molar gestation. If the initial three blocks do not contain villi, the remainder of the specimen should be submitted; if villi are still not identified, the possibility of an ectopic pregnancy exists, a result that should be immediately communicated to the clinician.

C. **Hysterectomy Specimens.** The type of hysterectomy (e.g., laparoscopic, abdominal, or vaginal, with or without salpingo-oophorectomy) should be determined, and the size, weight, and shape of the uterus recorded. (The processing of radical hysterectomy specimens, which differs substantially, is discussed in Chapter 34.) The uterine serosa should be carefully examined for any abnormalities, which should be sampled. The uterus is next bivalved in the coronal plane to show the endometrial cavity and endocervical canal, which are examined and measured. The maximum thickness of the endometrium and myometrium should also be noted. Both halves of the uterus then are serially sectioned. Taking sections parallel to the long axis of the uterus allows involvement of the lower uterine segment to be better evaluated.

1. For specimens excised for benign disease, sections of the anterior cervix, posterior cervix, anterior endomyometrium, and posterior endomyometrium are submitted. Additional sections of any identified lesions must also be submitted.

2. For specimens excised for malignancies, contiguous sections of both anterior and posterior endomyometrium, lower uterine segment, and cervix should be submitted. In addition, full-thickness sections of the anterior and posterior uterine wall should be taken to enable calculation of the depth of invasion. Representative sections from any other lesions must also be submitted.

III. ENDOMETRIUM

A. Dating

1. The endometrial mucosa is composed of glands and stroma. It is divided into the functional (luminal) layer and the basal (inner) layer. The basal cell layer acts as a reserve cell layer and is responsible for the regeneration of the endometrium after menses. The stroma is composed of endometrial stromal cells and blood vessels.

2. The menstrual cycle is divided into the menstrual phase, proliferative phase, and secretory phase. The onset of menstrual bleeding is defined as day 1 of the cycle. Menstrual endometrium, present for the first 4 days of the 28-day cycle, is characterized by glandular breakdown (karyorrhectic debris), stromal breakdown (dense balls of collapsed stroma with surrounding neutrophils and reactive epithelium), glandular secretory exhaustion, and background inflammation (e-**Figs. 33.1** and **33.2**)

Proliferative phase begins on day 4, and in an idealized 28-day cycle lasts until day 14, but this may greatly vary. During the early proliferative phase, the endometrium is thin and composed of straight, evenly spaced glands in a loose stroma (e-**Fig. 33.3**). By day 8 to 10, stromal edema due to estrogen causes increased endometrial thickening, and the glands become more coiled as the glands grow more rapidly than the stroma (e-**Fig. 33.4**). Throughout the proliferative phase, the epithelial lining in the glands show nuclear pseudostratification, and there is a high mitotic rate in both glands and stroma (e-**Fig. 33.5**).

The secretory phase begins with ovulation. In an idealized 28-day cycle, the secretory phase begins at day 14 and lasts 14 days, although it may range from 11 to 18 days. Following an interval phase from day 14 to day 15 (during which there are no dateable changes), the first dateable feature of early secretory phase is the appearance of subnuclear vacuoles on day 16, which appear as a clear zone between the basement membrane and the nucleus, pushing the nucleus toward the glandular lumen. On day 17, the epithelium exhibits uniform subnuclear vacuoles, giving the appearance of "piano keys" (e-**Fig. 33.6**). The vacuoles then move to the supranuclear position (day 18) and eventually are secreted into the glandular lumen (e-**Fig. 33.7**). Maximal stromal edema occurs during the mid-secretory phase, around day 22. At day 23, the stroma begins to condense, and the first signs of periarteriolar decidualization (where stromal cells acquire abundant, eosinophilic cytoplasm under the influence of progesterone) become apparent (e-**Fig. 33.8**). On day 25, this decidualization extends beneath the surface epithelium. Prominent glandular sawtoothing and maximal stromal decidualization occur on days 26 and 27 (e-**Fig. 33.9**). Numerous granular lymphocytes, marked stromal decidual change, and incipient glandular breakdown are the features of day 28 of the late secretory phase.

B. Pregnancy

1. The earliest gestation-related changes occur following the implantation of the blastocyst. These changes are characterized by decidualization of the stroma with edema; the glands exhibit distension with increased secretion and a serrated architecture (e-**Fig. 33.10**). By 4 to 8 weeks post implantation, the endometrial glands tend to become highly reduced and atrophic, and tissue samples will show markedly decidualized endometrial stroma. The epithelium that does remain may exhibit a physiologic response known as the "Arias-Stella reaction" characterized by glands that have a hypersecretory pattern and are lined by cells with enlarged, hyperchromatic nuclei that often jut into the gland lumens (e-**Fig. 33.11**). Having a history of pregnancy may protect the pathologist against interpreting these as neoplastic changes.

2. The placental implantation site, often seen in curettage specimens obtained because of a missed abortion, is characterized by decidualized stroma infiltrated by intermediate trophoblast. Intermediate trophoblasts have hyperchromatic angulated nuclei and amphophilic cytoplasm, and are often multinucleated (e-**Fig. 33.12**). Intermediate trophoblast also normally infiltrates maternal spiral arteries to replace the vascular smooth muscle, increasing the caliber of the vessels and increasing blood flow to the placenta (e-**Fig. 33.13**). Intermediate trophoblast also normally infiltrates myometrium which can occasionally be present in curettage specimens (e-**Fig. 33.14**).

3. **Placental site nodules** are incidental, usually microscopic findings that are characterized by small foci of hyalinized material with entrapped intermediate trophoblast cells, often with vacuolated cytoplasm (e-**Fig. 33.15**). They are thought to arise from the chorionic-type intermediate trophoblast of the fetal membranes which is also vacuolated. Placental site nodules are occasionally encountered in endometrial biopsies and curettage specimens but may also be seen in cervical specimens.

4. **Placenta accreta** is an abnormality of implantation that occurs when a layer of decidua is not present between the placental villi and the myometrium at the implantation site (e-**Fig. 33.16**); fibrin and intermediate trophoblast may be present between villi and myometrium in accreta. Cytokeratin, which will be positive in trophoblast and negative in decidua, can be used if the distinction is difficult on H&E. **Placenta increta** is present when villi invade into the myometrium, and transmural extension of villi with perforation is termed **placenta percreta**. Risk factors for placenta accreta include prior cesarean section, prior placenta previa, and prior instrumentation. All forms of implantation disorders may be associated with life-threatening hemorrhage and may require planned or emergent hysterectomy.

C. Exogenous Hormone Therapy

1. **Estrogen** causes proliferation of endometrial glands and stroma. Persistent exposure to estrogen (exogenous as well as endogenous estrogen as occurs with anovulatory cycles, obesity, or an estrogen-secreting tumor) causes endometrial proliferation, and without sufficient progesterone to stabilize the endometrium there will be glandular and stromal breakdown, often clinically interpreted as irregular menstrual bleeding. Microscopically, the findings include stromal condensation with formation of the so-called "exodus bodies" or "stromal blue balls," glandular degeneration and apoptosis of the glandular epithelial cells, and fibrin thrombi in stromal vessels (e-**Fig. 33.17**).

2. Prolonged exposure to **progestogens** results in endometrium with a characteristic pattern that includes underdeveloped, inactive glands in a background of a stroma that shows marked decidual change (e-**Fig. 33.18**).

3. **Tamoxifen** is primarily used for the treatment of breast cancer. In the endometrium, tamoxifen competitively binds to estrogen receptors (ERs) and acts as an agonist. Tamoxifen increases the risk of endometrial hyperplasia and adenocarcinoma (*Ann NY Acad Sci* 2001;949:237), and up to 20% of women on tamoxifen develop endometrial polyps (*Cancer* 92;2001;1151).

IV. COMMON BENIGN DISEASES OF THE ENDOMETRIUM

A. Endometritis

1. Acute endometritis is defined by the presence of acute (neutrophilic) inflammation in the stroma of nonmenstruating endometrium. In severe cases, neutrophils are present throughout the stroma, endometrial epithelium, and glandular lumens (e-**Fig. 33.19**). Acute inflammation present during the menstrual phase should not be interpreted as active infection. Acute endometritis is uncommon and is usually only seen in postpartum or postabortive scenarios.

2. Chronic endometritis is defined by the presence of plasma cells in the endometrial stroma. Associated features include glandular and stromal breakdown, and dyssynchronous glandular and stromal development (e-**Fig. 33.20**). The most common causes of chronic endometritis include *Chlamydia trachomatis*, *Ureaplasma urealyticum*, cytomegalovirus, and herpesvirus infection. Infection by *Actinomyces israelii* or *Neisseria gonorrheae* usually causes a mixed acute and chronic pattern of inflammation. Granulomatous inflammation is rare; common causes include *Mycobacterium tuberculosis* infection, fungal infection, sarcoidosis, and hysteroscopic ablation therapy.

B. Atrophy
is most commonly seen in postmenopausal women. Premenopausal causes include treatment with oral contraceptives or gonadotropin-releasing hormone analogs (leuprorelin, goserelin). Patients with premature menopause also show an atrophic pattern. Microscopically, the endometrium is composed of a thin layer of endometrial

glands lined by an attenuated layer of inactive epithelial cells surrounded by thin stroma. No mitotic activity is present (e-Fig. 33.21).

C. **Metaplasia** is the presence of any type of glandular epithelium other than the normal columnar type. Metaplasia is a common finding in perimenopausal and postmenopausal women, is often associated with abnormal uterine bleeding or recent use of exogenous hormonal therapy, and is a benign finding.

1. **Tubal metaplasia** consists of foci of normal tubal epithelium within the endometrial glands, including ciliated, nonciliated secretory, and intercalated cells. The ratio of the ciliated to nonciliated cells is cyclical and depends on hormonal influences.

2. **Ciliated cell metaplasia** is the most common form of metaplasia. It is composed of a layer of ciliated columnar cells with round to oval nuclei and abundant pale eosinophilic cytoplasm (e-Fig. 33.22). Ciliated cell metaplasia is a normal response of endometrial epithelium to various hormonal exposures. It is most commonly found in perimenopausal endometrium and is associated with endometrial polyps, anovulatory cycles, and exogenous hormonal therapy.

3. **Squamous metaplasia** (e-Fig. 33.23) is often caused by chronic irritation, and often takes the form of squamous morules or rounded, swirling nests of squamous cells. Squamous metaplasia must not be confused with endometrial hyperplasia or malignancy, although it can occur as a secondary change in both.

4. **Eosinophilic metaplasia** or eosinophilic change refers to glandular epithelium with abundant eosinophilic cytoplasm and a central round to oval nucleus (e-Fig. 33.24). It is often associated with a neutrophilic infiltrate, the formation of small epithelial papillae, and mild nuclear atypia. It is believed to be a degenerative change.

5. **Mucinous metaplasia** is rare. It is morphologically similar to endocervical mucinous epithelium in that it consists of columnar epithelium with basally located oval nuclei and abundant apical mucin (e-Fig. 33.25).

6. **Clear cell metaplasia** is also rare. It is characterized by columnar cells with round nuclei and clear cytoplasm.

D. **Endometrial Polyps** are local overgrowths of endometrial glands and stroma that protrude into the endometrial cavity. Polyps are present in about 20% to 25% of women and are frequently found in the peri- and postmenopausal periods. Grossly, polyps appear as broad-based to pedunculated lesions; some pedunculated polyps can extend into the endocervical canal, and even through the os. Microscopically, polyps are composed of endometrial glands within a spindled or fibrous stroma; the presence of thick-walled blood vessels within the fibrous stroma is the most common key to the diagnosis (e-Fig. 33.26). Frequently, the glands are variably shaped and irregularly distributed, and may run parallel to the polyp's surface.

Endometrial polyps may or may not cycle, and may show atrophy or metaplasia. Many polyps contain focal regions with architectural changes that resemble simple nonatypical hyperplasia; such findings are encompassed within the spectrum of endometrial polyp, and need not be separately diagnosed. In contrast, regions of complex or atypical hyperplasia should be diagnosed. Polyps may also harbor **serous endometrial intraepithelial carcinoma** (EIC) or frank serous carcinoma. Consequently, endometrial polyps should be entirely submitted for microscopic examination.

1. Foci of adenomyosis may become enlarged into polypoid projections, classified as **adenomyomatous polyps.** The endometrium in such polyps carries normal endometrial stroma and is invested with myometrium.

2. **Atypical polypoid adenomyoma** is characterized histologically by crowded, irregular endometrial glands with a complex architecture and cytologic atypia, in stroma that is predominantly composed of smooth muscle (e-Fig. 33.27). The lesion has a high rate of recurrence after incomplete surgical removal, and mainly occurs in premenopausal, nulliparous women. It is associated with a clinical history of infertility. If left untreated there is risk of progression to endometrioid adenocarcinoma.

E. **Disordered Proliferative Endometrium** is a category used to denote findings that fall short of simple hyperplasia. It exhibits a proliferative pattern with mild irregular branching and budding, with some cystic dilation. However, the gland-to-stroma ratio is not increased. The epithelium lining the glands is composed of stratified and columnar cells with no atypia. Mitotic activity is similar to that of normal proliferative endometrium (e-Fig. 33.28).

V. ENDOMETRIAL HYPERPLASIA AND SEROUS ENDOMETRIAL INTRAEPITHELIAL CARCINOMA

A. Endometrial Hyperplasia.
Endometrial hyperplasia results from unopposed estrogenic stimulation. Any disorder that causes an increase in endogenous or exogenous estrogenic stimulation such as polycystic ovarian disease, obesity, or some ovarian neoplasms (e.g., thecoma, granulosa cell tumor) can therefore predispose to endometrial hyperplasia. Abnormal bleeding is the major clinical symptom.

In the 2014 WHO classification (Table 33.1), hyperplasia is classified as nonatypical or with atypia. Numerous studies have demonstrated that the risk of progression to adenocarcinoma (specifically, endometrioid adenocarcinoma and its variants) is more highly correlated with the presence of cytologic atypia than the degree of architectural crowding (*Cancer* 1985;56:403).

1. **Hyperplasia without atypia** may be architecturally simple or complex. **Simple hyperplasia** shows a gland-to-stroma ratio that is slightly increased (more than 1:1) with prominent variability in the size of the glands, glandular budding, and cystic glandular dilation (e-Fig. 33.29). **Complex hyperplasia** is composed of crowded, architecturally complex glands with little intervening stroma. The gland-to-stroma ratio is elevated (at least 3:1) (e-Fig. 33.30). A diagnosis of hyperplasia should be made with extreme caution during the secretory phase of the endometrium because the glands are usually crowded in this phase; moreover, hyperplasia typically does not cycle.

2. **Atypical hyperplasia** is diagnosed based on the nuclear features of the endometrial glands. The most reliable indicators of cytologic atypia are an enlarged nucleus that is round rather than oval, that has coarse clumped chromatin, and that has a prominent nucleolus (e-Fig. 33.31). The presence of cytologic atypia must be distinguished from metaplasia and from the Arias-Stella reaction. Adjacent nonatypical nuclei may be an aid to diagnosis. Atypical hyperplasia is usually subcategorized as architecturally simple or complex.

B. Serous Endometrial Intraepithelial Carcinoma (EIC)
is the precursor to serous carcinoma. Microscopically, EIC is composed of glands lined by cells with the same cytologic abnormalities as serous carcinoma, but without evidence of stromal invasion (e-Fig. 33.32). A mutant pattern of p53 immunoreactivity (diffuse overexpression or complete loss) is typically present. The development of EIC is independent of prior unopposed estrogenic stimulation and typically arises in atrophic endometrium or in a polyp.

VI. EPITHELIAL MALIGNANCIES
are the most common gynecologic malignancy in women in developed countries.

A. Classification.
Endometrial cancer has classically been divided into two broad categories that differ in their clinical and pathologic features, as well as their underlying genetic abnormalities.

Type I tumors consist of endometrioid adenocarcinoma and its variants. They account for over 80% of endometrial tumors, and usually develop in postmenopausal women in their fifth or sixth decade with long-term estrogen stimulation. Type I tumors are strongly associated with diabetes and obesity and have a relatively good prognosis. The endometrial glands in type I tumors are strongly positive for estrogen and progesterone receptors. Genetically, they often show microsatellite instability and mutations in the *PTEN* tumor suppressor gene, *KRAS*, and *CTNNB1*, but assessment for these genetic abnormalities is not necessary for diagnosis.

Type II tumors, including serous carcinoma, clear cell carcinoma, and carcinosarcoma, usually occur in women in their sixth or seventh decade and are not associated with estrogen stimulation, and therefore do not occur in a background of atypical hyperplasia but rather in atrophic epithelium. They are more likely than type I tumors

TABLE 33.1   WHO Classification of Tumors of the Uterine Corpus and Gestational Trophoblastic Disease

UTERINE CORPUS

Epithelial tumors and precursors

Precursors
  Hyperplasia without atypia
  Atypical hyperplasia/endometrioid
    intraepithelial neoplasia

Endometrial carcinomas
  Endometrioid carcinoma
    With squamous differentiation
    Villoglandular
    Secretory
  Mucinous carcinoma
  Serous endometrial intraepithelial carcinoma
  Serous carcinoma
  Clear cell carcinoma
  Neuroendocrine tumors
    Low-grade neuroendocrine tumor
    Carcinoid tumor
    High-grade neuroendocrine carcinoma
    Small cell neuroendocrine carcinoma
    Large cell neuroendocrine carcinoma
    Mixed cell adenocarcinoma
    Undifferentiated carcinoma
    Dedifferentiated carcinoma

Tumor-like lesions
  Polyp
  Metaplasias
  Arias-Stella reaction
  Lymphoma-like lesion

Mesenchymal tumors

Leiomyoma
  Cellular leiomyoma
  Leiomyoma with bizarre nuclei
  Mitotically active leiomyoma
  Hydropic leiomyoma
  Apoplectic leiomyoma
  Lipomatous leiomyoma (lipoleiomyoma)
  Epithelioid leiomyoma
  Myxoid leiomyoma
  Dissecting (cotyledonoid) leiomyoma
  Diffuse leiomyomatosis
  Intravenous leiomyomatosis
  Metastasizing leiomyoma

Smooth muscle tumor of uncertain malignant potential

Leiomyosarcoma
  Epithelioid leiomyosarcoma
  Myxoid leiomyosarcoma

Endometrial stromal and related tumors
  Endometrial stromal nodule
  Low-grade endometrial stromal sarcoma
  High-grade endometrial stromal sarcoma
  Undifferentiated uterine sarcoma
  Uterine tumor resembling ovarian sex cord tumor

Miscellaneous mesenchymal tumors
  Rhabdomyosarcoma
  Perivascular epithelioid cell tumor
    Benign
    Malignant
  Others

Mixed epithelial and mesenchymal tumors
  Adenomyoma
  Atypical polypoid adenomyoma
  Adenofibroma
  Adenosarcoma
  Carcinosarcoma

Miscellaneous tumors
  Adenomatoid tumor
  Neuroectodermal tumors
  Germ cell tumors

Lymphoid and myeloid tumors
  Lymphomas
  Myeloid neoplasms

GESTATIONAL TROPHOBLASTIC DISEASE

Neoplasms
  Choriocarcinoma
  Placental site trophoblastic tumor
  Epithelioid trophoblastic tumor

Nonneoplastic lesions
  Exaggerated placental site
  Placental site nodule and plaque

Molar pregnancies
  Hydatidiform mole
  Complete
  Partial
  Invasive

Abnormal (nonmolar) villous lesions

to present at an advanced stage, and so have a relatively poor prognosis. *TP53* mutations are typical.

While the type I and type II taxonomy has been used as a conceptual framework for understanding endometrial cancer pathogenesis, it has long been recognized that there is substantial heterogeneity within, and overlap between, type I and II tumors; in addition, the type I and type II classification has never been part of formal staging schemes or risk stratification. Consequently, there has been an interest in whether molecular features can be used to better assess the biologic behavior of individual tumors to improve treatment decisions and outcomes, and the most comprehensive molecular study to date is that of The Cancer Genome Atlas (TCGA) project (*Gynecol Oncol Res Pract* 2016;3:14; *Nature* 2013;497:67). Molecular information was used to classify endometrioid and serous endometrial cancers into four groups that correlate with progression-free survival, specifically *POLE* ultra mutated (due to mutations that inactivate or suppress the proofreading of the POLE DNA polymerase), microsatellite instability hypermutated (due to post-replicative DNA mismatch repair deficiencies), copy-number low, and copy-number high. There is intense interest as to whether this type of molecular characterization can be used to improve patient outcomes more broadly.

1. **Endometrioid adenocarcinoma,** the prototype of type I tumors, usually arises in the uterine corpus and grossly usually consists of a raised to exophytic, pink-tan, hemorrhagic mass that projects into the endometrial cavity, but it may be grossly inconspicuous. Gross tumor dimensions are not particularly meaningful.

Microscopically, the tumor consists of irregular, confluent, complex glandular or villoglandular structures lined by stratified columnar cells with pleomorphic nuclei. The presence of areas with definitive cribriform architecture can be used to distinguish well-differentiated endometrioid adenocarcinoma from atypical hyperplasia. Foci of squamous differentiation, which should not be mistaken for a solid component of the tumor, are often encountered. Carcinoma may also have a maze-like pattern or show replacement of the stroma between glands by foamy macrophages.

Myometrial invasion is recognized by the presence of an irregular endometrial–myometrial border or by an associated desmoplastic and inflammatory stromal response (e-**Fig. 33.33**). Tumor involving adenomyosis (identified by the presence of adjacent normal glands or stroma) should not be interpreted as invasion. The depth of myometrial invasion compared with the full thickness of the myometrium, and the presence or absence of lymphovascular space invasion, should both be reported.

The FIGO grading system for endometrioid adenocarcinoma is based on the percentage of glandular and solid components (areas of squamous differentiation are not considered regions of solid growth). Tumors with 0% to 5% solid growth are grade 1, with 6% to 50% solid growth are grade 2, and with >50% solid growth are grade 3 (e-**Figs. 33.34–33.38**). Notable ("grade 3") nuclear pleomorphism inappropriate for the tumor architecture increases the tumor grade by one step.

a. Variants of endometrioid adenocarcinoma include villoglandular, secretory, mucinous, and squamous. The **villoglandular pattern** is diagnosed by the presence of a predominantly branching glandular architecture with central fibrovascular cores lined by stratified columnar cells containing elongated pleomorphic nuclei. The **secretory pattern** is characterized by glands composed of cells with supra- or subnuclear vacuoles resembling secretory endometrium. The **mucinous pattern** is defined by the presence of foci of endometrial glands lined by columnar cells with abundant intracytoplasmic mucin, often with a papillary architecture. **Squamous differentiation** (e-**Fig. 33.39**) is defined as the presence of sheets of squamous cells which are usually, but not always, nonkeratinizing.

b. The distinction between endocervical adenocarcinoma and endometrial adenocarcinoma is often difficult, especially on small biopsy specimens or when the tumor involves the lower uterine segment. The distinction has clinical significance, as endometrial adenocarcinomas are treated with simple hysterectomy and endocervical adenocarcinomas are treated with radical hysterectomy or radiation therapy. The clinical history can often be very helpful in the distinction. Women with endometrial cancer are typically obese and often diabetic; their uterus is often enlarged and they report menometrorrhagia or postmenopausal bleeding. Women with cervical cancer do not necessarily have a history of obesity, but are often smokers; they have a history of abnormal Pap tests or prior cervical intraepithelial neoplasia (CIN) or adenocarcinoma in situ (AIS), and are often symptomatic with postcoital spotting due to a friable mass. The presence of coexisting atypical endometrial hyperplasia, stromal foam cells, and benign morular squamous elements associated with carcinoma favor the diagnosis of endometrial adenocarcinoma, whereas adjacent cervical AIS or CIN favors endocervical adenocarcinoma. Immunohistochemistry can be useful when histologic features are ambiguous. The panel of ER, vimentin, carcinoembryonic antigen (CEA), and p16 can usually reliably distinguish between primary endometrial and endocervical adenocarcinoma, since ER and vimentin will be positive in endometrial and negative in endocervical adenocarcinoma, while CEA will only be positive in endocervical adenocarcinomas. Endocervical carcinomas are typically diffusely positive for p16 whereas endometrioid endometrial carcinomas show only patchy positivity. In situ hybridization with human papilloma virus (HPV) may also be helpful; endocervical adenocarcinomas should be positive and endometrial adenocarcinomas negative.

2. Serous carcinoma is characterized by cells with a high nuclear to cytoplasmic ratio and a high mitotic rate, that form a complex papillary architecture (e-Figs. 33.40 and 33.41). It is high-grade by definition. Deep myometrial and lymphovascular invasion are often present. The distinction between serous and grade 3 endometrioid tumors is often difficult and has high interobserver variability, but is clinically meaningful because the survival is significantly worse for serous carcinoma. Although not usually needed for distinguishing serous carcinoma from lower-grade endometrioid adenocarcinoma, p16 and p53 stains are sensitive and specific for serous carcinoma (in which p16 is positive and p53 shows a mutant pattern) when used to distinguish the tumor from grade 3 endometrioid adenocarcinoma.

3. Clear cell adenocarcinoma is a high-grade tumor composed of pleomorphic cells with hobnail cells (cells that protrude into the gland lumen), abundant clear or eosinophilic cytoplasm, and distinct cell borders, arranged in papillary, solid, and tubular structures, often admixed (e-Fig. 33.42). A characteristic feature is the presence of hyalinized stromal cores (e-Fig. 33.43). Clear cell adenocarcinoma is often at an advanced clinical stage at the time of presentation.

4. Mixed adenocarcinoma is defined as a tumor demonstrating a mixture of endometrioid adenocarcinoma (or its variants) together with serous, mucinous, or clear cell adenocarcinoma. By convention, the minor component must comprise at least 10% of the tumor.

5. Carcinosarcoma (malignant mixed müllerian tumor or MMMT) comprises approximately 10% of all uterine malignancies. The diagnostic criteria require the presence of both malignant epithelial and mesenchymal (sarcomatous) elements. Numerous genetic studies have demonstrated that both elements are derived from the same precursor, proving that the neoplasm does not represent a collision tumor. The tumor is now considered to represent a poorly differentiated endometrial carcinoma with metaplastic differentiation.

The tumor often presents as a mass prolapsing through the cervix. Grossly, carcinosarcomas are larger and fleshier than typical adenocarcinomas and are often described as polypoid. Microscopically, they consist of areas of adenocarcinoma (typically high-grade serous) intermixed with malignant mesenchymal elements of nearly any histology. The sarcomatoid elements are often rhabdomyosarcomatous, chondrosarcomatous, leiomyosarcomatous, or undifferentiated (e-Figs. 33.44 and 33.45). Extensive areas of necrosis are often present. Carcinosarcomas were formerly divided into homologous or heterologous type, with the former having only sarcomatous components thought to be native to the uterus, such as leiomyosarcoma, but this distinction is now recognized to have no clinical significance.

Carcinosarcoma generally has a poor prognosis. Specific adverse prognostic factors include the presence of a serous or clear cell epithelial component, deep myometrial invasion, cervical involvement, and lymphovascular space involvement. The grade of the tumor, type of mesenchymal element, and mitotic rate have no correlation with the outcome.

6. **Squamous cell carcinoma** of the endometrium is rare and usually occurs in postmenopausal women in association with pyometra and cervical stenosis. Microscopically, it is identical to squamous cell carcinoma of the cervix, and so must be distinguished from a cervical primary that has extended into the endometrium.

7. **Small cell neuroendocrine carcinoma** of the endometrium is extremely rare and comprises less than 1% of primary endometrial malignancies. The tumor has the same cytomorphology and immunophenotype as high-grade neuroendocrine tumors arising at other sites. Other neuroendocrine carcinomas are uncommon.

8. **Undifferentiated carcinomas** do not show differentiation toward any defined tumor pattern.

B. **Sentinel Lymph Node Processing.** Accurate staging is the most important determinant of therapy and prognosis in endometrial carcinoma, but the incidence of lymph node metastasis is low in patients with early-stage disease, and complete lymphadenectomy is associated with increased postoperative morbidity. Sentinel node biopsy has been validated as a means for accurate staging in endometrial cancer (*Lancet Oncol* 2017;18:384). While protocols vary, sentinel lymph nodes are typically evaluated by examining three H&E levels, with or without cytokeratin immunostaining.

In AJCC 8th edition staging, isolated tumor cells ≤0.2 mm in a lymph node are N0(i+), a micrometastasis ≤2 mm is N1mi, and a macrometastasis >2 mm is N1a. FIGO 2010 staging does not specifically comment upon isolated tumor cells.

C. **Screening for Lynch Syndrome.** Endometrial cancer is the most common presenting tumor in 50% of women with Lynch syndrome, and Lynch syndrome accounts for 2% to 4% of endometrial cancer overall (*Gynecol Oncol* 2012;125:414). Identification of Lynch syndrome–associated endometrial cancer allows screening for metachronous or synchronous colorectal and ovarian tumors, as well as cascade testing of family members. Professional guidelines recommend screening some or all endometrial cancer cases using either mismatch repair immunohistochemistry or microsatellite instability testing, followed by confirmatory germline testing of screen positives.

VII. **ENDOMETRIAL STROMAL TUMORS** are composed of small cells with scant cytoplasm that morphologically resemble stromal cells of proliferative endometrium. A subset of tumors exhibits variant morphologic patterns including smooth muscle differentiation, a fibromyxoid component, and sex cord–like/epithelioid patterns.

A. **Endometrial Stromal Nodules** are grossly tan to yellow, well-circumscribed lesions with a smooth border that range from 0.5 to 12 cm in greatest dimension. They are primarily located in the myometrium, and an obvious connection to the endometrium is not necessary for diagnosis. Histologically, these tumors are composed of sheets of small cells with scant cytoplasm and an accompanying vascular pattern reminiscent of the spiral arterioles present in the stroma of proliferative endometrium. These tumors stain strongly and diffusely positive for CD10 (although a minority of cases may show weak positivity) and negative for desmin. Since cellular leiomyomas and leiomyosarcomas are usually negative for CD10 but positive for desmin, immunohistochemistry can be helpful in difficult cases. Endometrial stromal nodules are benign and hysterectomy is curative. The t(7;17)(p15;q21) translocation, which produces a *JAZF1-SUZ12* fusion protein, is a recurring feature, but demonstration of its presence is not required for diagnosis.

B. **Low-Grade Endometrial Stromal Sarcoma** predominantly occurs in middle-aged women and does not share the same risk factors as endometrial carcinoma. On gross examination, endometrial stromal sarcomas exhibit a tan to yellow cut surface with an infiltrative border, often with foci of hemorrhage and necrosis. Microscopically, the tumor consists of cells with cytomorphology similar to those seen in endometrial stromal nodules, but with a higher rate of mitosis, greater nuclear pleomorphism, prominent stromal vascularity, and areas of collagenized stroma (e-**Fig. 33.46**). Finger-like protrusions into the myometrium and extensive lymphatic invasion are the hallmarks of this tumor. ER and CD10 immunostains are positive. The t(7;17) *JAZF1-SUZ12* is often present. The distinction from an endometrial stromal nodule must be made on histologic (not molecular) grounds.

C. **High-Grade Endometrial Stromal Sarcoma** is a destructive uterine mass composed of malignant round cells. Mitotic activity and necrosis are frequent. CD10 and ER immunostains are typically negative, and cyclin D1 is positive. There is sometimes a lower-grade spindle cell component that may be positive for CD10 and ER. HGESS is characterized by the translocation t(10;17)(q22;p13) that results in the *YWHAE-FAM22A/B* (*NUTM2A/B*) fusion. The prognosis of HGESS is worse than LGESS, but better than undifferentiated uterine sarcoma.

D. **Undifferentiated Uterine Sarcoma** is composed of sheets of pleomorphic undifferentiated cells with a moderate amount of cytoplasm and a high mitotic rate with frequent atypical forms. This tumor lacks the plexiform vasculature of LGESS, and is more pleomorphic than HGESS. Aberrant expression of CD10, cyclin D1, and smooth muscle markers (often focal) has been reported. These tumors have an aggressive course usually resulting in death within 3 years of diagnosis.

VIII. SMOOTH MUSCLE NEOPLASMS

A. **Leiomyoma** is the most common neoplasm of the uterus, and can occur as a submucosal, intramural, or subserosal lesion. Leiomyomas predominantly affect women of reproductive age; they can be found in 20% to 30% of women in their fourth decade, and more than 40% of women in their fifth decade. They tend to enlarge during pregnancy since they express estrogen and progesterone receptors. Grossly, leiomyomas are well-circumscribed lesions; they have a white-tan cut surface and are sharply demarcated from the adjacent myometrium. Microscopically, leiomyomas are composed of interlacing fascicles of closely packed cells with uniform elongated nuclei and eosinophilic cytoplasm (e-**Figs 33.47** and **33.48**). Degenerative changes including hyaline change, ischemic-type necrosis, and hydropic degeneration are often present.

1. **Cellular leiomyomas** have the same gross features as ordinary leiomyomas, but microscopically demonstrate increased cellularity with sheets of spindle cells with hyperchromatic elongated nuclei and a scant amount of eosinophilic cytoplasm (e-**Fig. 33.49**). There is no pleomorphism or increased mitotic activity. These lesions behave like classic leiomyomas. One important differential diagnosis for this lesion is endometrial stromal sarcoma. Endometrial stromal sarcomas lack a fascicular growth pattern, thick-walled vessels, and a cleft-like space between the lesion and adjacent myometrium; in addition, endometrial stromal sarcomas often have plaques of collagen and foamy cells which are not seen in leiomyomas. Endometrial stromal sarcomas are typically positive for CD10 and negative for H-caldesmon. Also, the presence of mast cells is a sensitive and specific finding favoring cellular leiomyoma, since these often have more than seven mast cells per high-power field.

2. **Epithelioid leiomyomas** are composed of predominantly epithelioid cells with eosinophilic to clear cytoplasm and fine nuclear chromatin. The cells are arranged in clusters and as single cells, with no pleomorphism. The mitotic rate is not elevated, and necrosis is absent. They behave the same way as classic leiomyomas.

3. **Symplastic leiomyoma** contains scattered enlarged, markedly atypical cells, often with multiple nuclei. However, the mitotic count is still less than 10 mitotic figures/10 hpf, and no necrosis is present. These lesions have the same benign behavior as classic leiomyoma.

4. **Mitotically active leiomyoma** contains up to 20 mitotic figures per 10 high-power fields (40× objective). This diagnosis is only appropriate when there is at most mild cytologic atypia and no tumor-type necrosis.

5. Lipoleiomyoma refers to a classic leiomyoma which contains islands of mature adipocytes. This variant has no clinical significance.

6. Myxoid leiomyoma consists of fascicles of uniform spindle cells surrounded by pools of myxoid edematous stroma. Large vessels are not uncommonly present.

B. **Benign Metastasizing Leiomyoma.** Many patients who have benign metastasizing leiomyoma have a prior history of hysteroscopy with dilation and curettage, or other procedures such as myomectomy or hysterectomy. Microscopically, benign metastasizing leiomyomas have the same histologic features as ordinary leiomyomas, although they may extend into adjacent vessels. The tumor cells can migrate to the lung, and lymph node involvement may be present. The differential diagnosis includes low-grade leiomyosarcoma, and a smooth muscle tumor of another site (such as GI or retroperitoneum) must be excluded. Some cases may respond to hormonal therapy.

C. **Intravascular Leiomyomatosis** refers to classic leiomyomas that grow into the lumen of the uterine or pelvic veins. The tumor may migrate or extend into the inferior vena cava, and even into the right heart. The tumor is composed of sheets of spindled to round cells with minimal atypia and rare mitoses, for which the differential diagnosis often includes low-grade endometrial stromal sarcoma. With local control, the tumor has an excellent long-term prognosis.

D. **Leiomyosarcoma** is the malignant counterpart of leiomyoma. It is the most common sarcoma of the uterus, with an incidence of 2 to 3 for every 1,000 women with leiomyomata. Leiomyosarcoma usually occurs in women over the age of 50 and has a higher rate of occurrence in African Americans. The clinical picture is often of a single or dominant, rapidly enlarging myomatous lesion. Some studies have suggested unopposed estrogen exposure as one of the underlying etiologies. The genetics of leiomyosarcomas have confirmed that they do not arise from leiomyomas.

Grossly, leiomyosarcoma consists of an irregular, soft, and fleshy mass with a pink-tan cut surface that has obvious foci of hemorrhage and necrosis. The tumor almost always demonstrates an ill-defined and infiltrating border. Microscopically, leiomyosarcoma is composed of sheets of pleomorphic spindle cells with elongated nuclei, high-grade cytologic atypia, and a high mitotic rate with frequent atypical mitotic figures (e-**Fig. 33.50**). A comprehensive study (*Am J Surg Pathol.* 1994;18:535) recommended that the diagnostic approach for leiomyosarcoma include evaluation of the degree of cytologic atypia (graded as mild, moderate, or severe), assessment of the presence or absence of coagulative tumor cell necrosis (CTCN, defined as an abrupt transition from viable cells to necrotic cells without a transition zone of hyalinized tissue or granulation tissue) (e-**Fig. 33.51**), and determination of the mitotic index (MI), as outlined in Table 33.2.

Leiomyosarcoma has a poor prognosis. The patient's age, tumor MI, and clinical stage of the disease at the time of presentation are among the important prognostic factors. Surgical intervention is the treatment of choice. Variants include epithelioid (clear cell) leiomyosarcoma and myxoid leiomyosarcoma; both are relatively rare.

E. **Smooth Muscle Tumor of Uncertain Malignant Potential (STUMP)** is the nomenclature used to designate problematic uterine smooth muscle neoplasms that fall between benign leiomyoma and leiomyosarcoma. Cases of STUMP represent tumors for which the classification by established criteria is uncertain.

IX. OTHER MYOMETRIAL DISEASES

A. **Adenomyosis** is defined as the presence of benign endometrial glands surrounded by endometrial stroma within the myometrium (conventionally at least 2.5 mm below the endomyometrial junction). Grossly, the adjacent myometrium can show a thick trabeculated pattern with punctate hemorrhage. Microscopically, the glands usually show an inactive pattern, or a pattern that is dyssynchronous with the endometrium (e-**Fig. 33.52**). The glands may be inconspicuous, particularly in postmenopausal women. Endometrial adenocarcinoma occasionally involves adenomyosis, but this occurrence is not considered myometrial invasion for staging purposes.

Prominent foci of adenomyosis may become elaborated into a mass-forming lesion, which is classified as an adenomyoma.

TABLE 33.2   Strategy for Diagnosis of Uterine Smooth Muscle Tumors

		CTCN Absent		CTCN Present
Mild atypia	MI <5	Leiomyoma	MI <10	STUMP
	MI ≥5	Mitotically active leiomyoma	MI ≥10	Leiomyosarcoma
Focal moderate–severe atypia	MI <5	Atypical leiomyoma	Any MI	Leiomyosarcoma
	MI ≥5	STUMP		
Diffuse moderate–severe atypia	MI <5	Atypical leiomyoma	Any MI	Leiomyosarcoma
	5 ≤ MI <10	STUMP		
	MI ≥10	Leiomyosarcoma		

CTCN, coagulative tumor cell necrosis; MI, mitotic index (mitotic rate per 10 high-power fields, 40× objective); STUMP, smooth muscle tumor of uncertain malignant potential.
Modified from Bell SW, Kempson RL, Hendrickson MR. Problematic uterine smooth muscle neoplasms. A clinicopathologic study of 213 cases. *Am J Surg Pathol* 1994;18:535–558; Ip PP, Cheung AN, Clement PB. Uterine smooth muscle tumors of uncertain malignant potential (STUMP): a clinicopathologic analysis of 16 cases. *Am J Surg Pathol* 2009;33:992–1005; and Zaloudek CJ, Hendrickson MR, Soslow RA, et al. In: *Blaustein's Pathology of the Female Genital Tract*, 6th ed. New York: Springer; 2011.

    B. Postoperative Spindle Cell Nodule is a benign lesion that usually occurs within a few weeks of endometrial instrumentation. It is grossly pink tan and friable. Microscopically, it consists of granulation tissue with surface ulceration, accompanied by a hypercellular proliferation of spindle cells with elongated nuclei, moderate amounts of pink cytoplasm, and a high mitotic rate arranged in fascicles. Numerous extravasated red blood cells are usually present. Post-operative spindle cell nodule must be distinguished from leiomyosarcoma; the former's distinct fascicular pattern of growth, lack of pleomorphism, and characteristic clinical presentation are clues to the correct diagnosis.

    C. Adenofibroma is a rare entity that usually occurs in postmenopausal women who present with abnormal bleeding. Microscopically, it is composed of a layer of epithelium with bland nuclear cytology that overlies a cellular fibrous stroma composed of fibroblasts and endometrial stromal cells. Adenofibroma is a benign entity and hysterectomy is curative.

    D. Adenosarcoma is characteristically a tumor of postmenopausal women. It is a rare neoplasm that arises most commonly from the endometrium and forms a large, polypoid, lobulated mass that may fill the entire endometrial cavity and prolapse through the cervical os. Microscopically, adenosarcomas are composed of benign glandular elements in a malignant stroma that shows increased cellularity, pleomorphism, and a mitotic rate of greater than 2 mitotic figures per 10 high-power fields (e-**Fig. 33.53**). The stroma is often condensed and hypercellular in periglandular areas and characteristically juts into gland lumens (e-**Fig. 33.54**).

    Adenosarcoma is best considered a tumor of low malignant potential, and has a better outcome than other uterine sarcomas. However, recurrence (which occurs in up to 25% of patients) is associated with very poor prognosis. Sarcomatous overgrowth is present when 25% of the tumor consists of pure sarcoma devoid of epithelial elements, and is also a poor prognostic factor.

X. GESTATIONAL TROPHOBLASTIC DISEASE. This group of diseases comprises abnormal trophoblastic proliferations that arise from the gestational trophoblast. In Western populations, about 0.1% of pregnancies are affected; patients are often at the extremes of reproductive age, and women with previous gestational trophoblastic disease are at higher risk.
    A. Hydatidiform Mole
        1. Complete molar pregnancies result from fertilization of an empty ovum. Complete moles are diploid, and may be either heterozygous (15% of cases, due to fertilization of an empty ovum by two sperm) or homozygous (85% of cases, due to fertilization of an empty ovum by a single sperm with subsequent endoreduplication). Complete moles classically present as a larger uterus than expected for the gestational age, with a so-called snowstorm pattern without fetal parts on the ultrasound; the patient's serum

hCG is usually elevated for the gestational age. Histopathologically, classic complete moles are composed of markedly enlarged villi with central villous cavitation (cisterns) and circumferential markedly atypical trophoblastic proliferation (e-**Fig. 33.55**). Due to paternal imprinting, a p57 immunostain is completely negative in the trophoblast of a complete mole. DNA short tandem repeat (STR) analysis shows only paternal alleles.

Early complete moles are usually associated with normal ultrasound and hCG levels, but with the advent of early ultrasound and better serum hCG screening, abnormal pregnancies are evacuated earlier which can complicate diagnosis. Microscopically, an early complete mole shows "claw-like" or "cauliflower-like" villous shapes, a blue mesenchymal-like stroma, labyrinthine stromal canaliculi, atypical implantation trophoblast, and circumferential trophoblastic hyperplasia at least focally (e-**Figs. 33.56–33.58**). Complete moles carry an increased risk of subsequent development of persistent gestational trophoblastic disease (up to 10% in Asian populations).

2. **Partial molar pregnancies** develop from fertilization of a normal ovum by two sperm, and so have a triploid karyotype. Patients may have a normal, elevated, or even low serum hCG for gestational age; fetal parts are sometimes present by ultrasound imaging. Histologically, partial moles are composed of two populations of villi; one population is essentially normal or small and fibrotic, and one population exhibits enlargement with at least focal cavitation, irregular claw-like villous outlines, trophoblastic inclusions, and subtle noncircumferential trophoblastic hyperplasia in the form of buds or lacy mounds (e-**Figs. 33.59** and **33.60**). p57 expression is retained in the trophoblast, and STR analysis shows biparental contributions and a triploid genotype. X/Y centromeric FISH may confirm an abnormal chromosomal complement, but may not be diagnostic since triploidy and sex chromosome trisomy will give similar results. Partial moles carry a small but increased risk of subsequent gestational trophoblastic disease.

3. **Invasive mole** is a sequela of molar pregnancy (either complete or partial) in which the villi and associated trophoblast invade the myometrium or blood vessels, or are deported to extrauterine sites (e-**Fig. 33.61**).

B. **Trophoblastic Neoplasms.** The clinical term "gestational trophoblastic disease" (or "neoplasia") is used to encompass a variety of pathologic entities including recurrent/invasive mole, choriocarcinoma, and other trophoblastic tumors.

1. **Choriocarcinoma.** Although molar pregnancies have a much-increased risk of subsequent development of gestational choriocarcinoma, this tumor can develop following any type of pregnancy, including normal gestations. Grossly, the tumor tends to be dark red due to its vascularity. Microscopically, choriocarcinoma is composed of sheets of highly atypical trophoblast with prominent hemorrhage and necrosis (e-**Fig. 33.62**). The trophoblast consists of alternating collections of syncytiotrophoblast and mononucleate trophoblast. Choriocarcinoma spreads hematogenously, and the most common metastatic sites are the lung, pelvis, vagina, liver, and brain. Choriocarcinoma is strongly positive for cytokeratin, hCG, human placental lactogen (hPL), and placental alkaline phosphatase by immunohistochemistry.

2. **Placental site trophoblastic tumor** is a tumor of implantation-site intermediate trophoblast. It typically presents as a mass which may be deeply invasive; serum hCG levels are usually only mildly elevated. Characteristic features include abundant eosinophilic fibrinoid deposition and dissection of individual smooth muscle cells by the neoplastic cells (e-**Figs. 33.63–33.65**). In this tumor, hCG staining is negative, p63 is negative, and the Ki-67 index is typically >1% (*Am J Surg Pathol* 2004; 28:1177). About 15% of cases exhibit malignant behavior. Unlike most forms of gestational trophoblastic disease, the tumor is not very responsive to chemotherapy.

3. **Epithelioid trophoblastic tumor** is composed of chorionic-type intermediate trophoblast. Morphologically, the tumor is composed of a uniform population of atypical mononucleate cells arranged in sheets and nests associated with eosinophilic material and surrounded by necrotic debris (e-**Fig. 33.66**). Immunostains for hCG are negative, but for p63 are positive; the Ki-67 index is >10%.

XI. SEROSAL DISEASES

A. **Endometriosis** affects 5% to 10% of women of childbearing age. Patients usually present with symptoms of pelvic pain, dyspareunia, secondary dysmenorrhea, and in some cases, infertility. Many cases remain asymptomatic. The three most common theories regarding its etiology are retrograde menstruation, serosal metaplasia, and a developmental abnormality. The most commonly involved sites include the ovary, uterine serosa, fallopian tube, peritoneum, and cul-de-sac. Oral contraceptives have been shown to have a protective role. Histologically, endometriosis is defined as the presence of endometrial glands surrounded by endometrial stroma; associated hemosiderin deposition and chronic inflammation are usually present. The diagnosis of "atypical endometriosis" is rendered when significant cytologic atypia (comparable to that seen in atypical endometrial hyperplasia) is present.

B. **Adenomatoid Tumor** is a benign peritoneal tumor that originates from the mesothelium. It most commonly involves the serosal surfaces of the uterus and fallopian tubes. Grossly, the tumor usually forms a tan 1 to 2 cm well-circumscribed nodule. Microscopically, the tumor is composed of tubular and slit-like spaces lined by a single layer of flattened cuboidal cells with bland cytology (**e-Fig. 33.67**). The cells are immunopositive for cytokeratin, D2-40, calretinin, and vimentin, but negative for factor VIII-related antigen and CD31, a profile that can be used to distinguish the tumor from metastatic carcinoma and vascular tumors. Adenomatoid tumor is clinically asymptomatic and usually found incidentally.

XII. OTHER MISCELLANEOUS NEOPLASMS

A. **Lymphoid Neoplasms** involving the uterine corpus (of which the most frequent is large B-cell lymphoma) most commonly represent a manifestation of disseminated disease. Primary disease of the uterus is extremely rare.

B. **Metastatic Tumors** only rarely involve the uterus. The most common primary tumors that spread to the uterus are those of breast, lung, stomach, gallbladder, thyroid, and melanoma. In most instances, uterine involvement by primary tumors of the ovary, cervix, bladder, and rectum/colon represents direct extension rather than hematogenous spread.

XIII. HISTOLOGIC GRADING, STAGING, AND REPORTING OF UTERINE CORPUS MALIGNANCIES.

The most recent staging system for carcinomas and carcinosarcomas of the uterine corpus is that of the 2017 Tumor, Node, Metastasis (TNM) American Joint Committee on Cancer staging classification (Amin MB, Edge S, Greene F, et al., eds. *AJCC Cancer Staging Manual*, 8th ed. New York: Springer, 2017). Sarcomas of the uterine corpus (e.g., leiomyosarcomas, endometrial stromal sarcomas, and adenosarcomas) have a separate AJCC staging classification, as do gestational trophoblastic neoplasms.

Reporting of uterine corpus tumors should follow recommended guidelines (e.g., Protocol for the Examination of Specimens From Patients With Carcinoma and Carcinosarcoma of the Endometrium; Protocol for the Examination of Specimens From Patients With Primary Sarcoma of the Uterus; and Protocol for the Examination of Specimens From Patients With Primary Gestational Trophoblastic Malignancy, all available at http://www.cap.org).

ACKNOWLEDGMENT

The authors thank Jena B. Hudson, John D. Pfeifer, and Phyllis C. Huettner, authors of the previous editions of this chapter.

SUGGESTED READINGS

Kurman JR, Carcangiu ML, Herrington CS, Young RH, Eds. *WHO Classification of Tumours of Female Reproductive Organs.* 4th ed. Lyon: International Agency for Research on Cancer; 2014.

Mazur MT, Kurman RJ. *Diagnosis of endometrial biopsies and curettings. A practical approach.* 2nd ed. Springer, 2005.

McCluggage WG. My approach to the interpretation of endometrial biopsies and curettings. *J Clin Pathol.* 2006;59:801–812.

34 Uterine Cervix

Ian S. Hagemann

I. NORMAL ANATOMY

A. **Gross.** The cervix is the tubular caudal portion of the uterus, divided into the ectocervix and endocervix. The ectocervix is smooth, covered by a reflection of the vaginal mucosa. The tan, rugous endocervix is a narrow canal that begins at the external os. The external os is round and small in the nulliparous state and becomes slit-like with parity. An internal os, or isthmus, marks the transition from the endocervix to the endometrium. The parametrial soft tissue, which attaches to the lateral aspects of the cervix, contains the uterine vessels and the ureters. The posterior cervix is the anterior wall of the pouch of Douglas, the space between the uterus and the rectum; the anterior cervix is immediately posterior and inferior to the bladder.

B. **Microscopic.** The ectocervix is generally covered by squamous epithelium in continuity with the vaginal epithelium, while the endocervix is lined by columnar mucinous epithelium. The transition from columnar to squamous epithelium through the process of squamous metaplasia occurs over a region of the cervical epithelium called the transformation zone. In low-estrogen states, the squamocolumnar junction is approximately at the external os. With higher levels of estrogen, the transition is observed on the portion of cervix visible in the vaginal vault. The transformation zone is important diagnostically because it is the site of most cervical epithelial tumors and their precursors (e-Fig. 34.1).

1. **Squamous epithelium.** The squamous epithelium is composed of a basal layer, intermediate layer, and superficial layer. The basal layer is one cell thick and has a relatively high nuclear/cytoplasmic (N/C) ratio. The N/C ratio decreases progressively from the basal layer to the superficial layer during normal maturation, and the superficial squamous cells tend to align with their longest axis parallel to the basement membrane. Directly sampled normal squamous epithelium in cytologic preparations shows individual and clustered superficial polygonal squamous cells with pyknotic nuclei, intermediate cells with somewhat larger nuclei, and more rounded parabasal cells with the highest N/C ratios. In the estrogenized state, superficial cells predominate.

2. **Columnar epithelium.** The mucinous columnar epithelium of the endocervix is one cell layer thick, with basal polarization of the cells' nuclei; little, if any, mitotic activity; and an N/C ratio of about 1:4. Mucinous columnar epithelium also lines the endocervical glands, which represent infoldings of the surface epithelium rather than true glands. Directly sampled endocervical columnar epithelium is seen in cytologic preparations as sheets of uniform round nuclei in a "honeycomb" arrangement or as single-layered strips of epithelium with basally oriented nuclei.

3. **Squamous metaplastic epithelium.** This is an expected finding in the transformation zone of cervical specimens. Histologically, in the immature form, the squamous epithelium underlies a layer of superficial residual columnar epithelium (e-Fig. 34.1); with full maturation it may appear very similar to native squamous epithelium. Metaplastic squamous cells in cytologic smears occur as either singly dispersed cells or as small sheets of cells, and they show cyanophilic cytoplasm and nuclear sizes and N/C ratios between those of normal intermediate and basal cells.

II. GROSS EXAMINATION, TISSUE SAMPLING, AND HISTOLOGIC SLIDE PREPARATION.
Cervical specimens for screening and diagnosis are obtained in several ways.

A. **Exfoliative Cytology (Pap Test).** See the section below on cytology of the uterine cervix for a discussion of the Pap test.

B. Biopsy. Colposcopic cervical biopsy specimens are small pieces of mucosa and superficial stroma that are taken, most often, from acetowhite areas identified visually. Documentation of the number and size of tissue fragments is important to ensure that the biopsy fragments are adequately represented on the slides. If a tissue fragment exceeds 4 mm in maximal dimension, it should be bisected prior to histologic processing. In general, the biopsy tissue should be wrapped in lens paper or placed between sponges to avoid loss during processing, and the tissue should be embedded such that the microscopic sections are perpendicular to the mucosal surface. Three hematoxylin and eosin (H&E)–stained levels are prepared for microscopic examination.

C. Curettage. Curettage specimens consist of numerous and often miniscule tissue fragments in mucus, so it is imperative to both filter the contents of the container and collect any tissue that may be adherent to the pad or paper submitted within the specimen container. It is necessary to wrap curettings in lens paper to avoid loss during processing. The specimens obtained from curettage procedures should be submitted in their entirety. Three H&E-stained levels are prepared for microscopic examination

D. Conization. Ideal cold knife cone excisional biopsy specimens consist of a single torus of ectocervix and cervical canal surrounded by stroma. Sutures placed by the surgeon enable the sections to be designated using clock-face positions, if desired. The endocervical margin must be inked differentially from the ectocervical margin; ink of indifferent color should also be placed on the stromal/radial margin. After fixation, the specimen should be radially sectioned, with each section encompassing the endocervical margin, the mucosal surface of the endocervical canal with the transformation zone, and the ectocervical margin, as shown in Figure 34.1.

E. Loop Electrosurgical Excision Procedure (LEEP). The key to correct processing of these specimens is identification of the endocervical margin; the ectocervix is smooth and tan-white, whereas the endocervix is tan and more rugous. The endocervical margin should be differentially inked from the ectocervical margin, and ink should also be placed on the stromal/radial margin. Radial sections should be taken perpendicular to the mucosa, encompassing the endocervical margin, transformation zone, and ectocervical margin in the same manner as for conization specimens (Fig. 34.1).

F. Radical Hysterectomy. Prior to opening the uterus, the parametrial soft tissue is inked, as it represents soft tissue margins of interest. The vaginal mucosal margins are also inked. The uterus is then bivalved. If no tumor is visible or the tumor does not appear to extend into the parametrial soft tissue, the parametrial soft tissue is removed, sectioned, and completely submitted. If the vagina appears free of tumor, shave margins are submitted. If tumor appears to extend into the parametrial soft tissue or vagina, radial sections are submitted to show the tumor's relationship to the margin. If a cervical mass is present, at least one section per centimeter of tumor, including the deepest extension

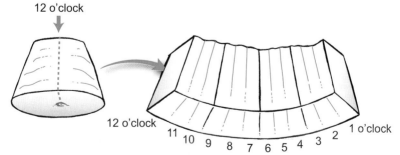

Figure 34.1 Sectioning of cervical excision specimens (cold knife cone biopsy or loop electrosurgical excision procedure).

into the cervical wall, is submitted. If no tumor is visible, the cervix is amputated and processed as a conization specimen.

III. DIAGNOSTIC FEATURES OF COMMON NONNEOPLASTIC DISEASES

A. Inflammation and Infection.
Acute cervicitis is a pattern of inflammation marked by a stromal and epithelial neutrophilic infiltrate, with associated stromal edema and reactive epithelial atypia. Reactive epithelium shows enlarged nuclei and prominent nucleoli in a pattern that may be confused with neoplasia. Acute cervicitis is usually a nonspecific diagnosis, as the inciting agent can be any of a wide variety of bacterial, fungal, or protozoan organisms. Chronic cervicitis consists of a lymphoplasmacytic infiltrate that is also nonspecific. Papillary endocervicitis is a term describing inflamed endocervical mucosa forming papillary structures, often containing numerous plasma cells.

1. **Noninfectious cervicitis.** Cervicitis can be due to irritation from chemical exposure, foreign materials (e.g., pessary, tampons), or surgical trauma. The cervix may also be a site of involvement in systemic inflammatory conditions such as collagen vascular disease. The type of inflammatory response may be neutrophilic, lymphoplasmacytic, or granulomatous.

2. **Infectious cervicitis**

    a. **Bacterial cervicitis.** *Neisseria gonorrhoeae* and *Chlamydia trachomatis* both produce a mucopurulent cervicitis that requires additional nonhistologic methods for specific diagnosis. With chronicity, *C. trachomatis* infection can result in follicular cervicitis, a pattern of intense lymphocytic infiltration that characteristically includes lymphoid aggregates with germinal centers (e-**Fig. 34.2**). Although often associated with *C. trachomatis*, follicular cervicitis is not specific for that infection.

    Actinomyces spp. infection is associated with intrauterine device (IUD) use and is often asymptomatic. The morphologic pattern is distinctive in that clusters of purple-red filamentous organisms are seen in curettings and smears, with associated "sulfur granules" consisting of clusters of neutrophils and organisms with a basophilic center.

    Bacterial vaginosis is characterized by "clue cells," squamous cells decorated with bacterial organisms. *Gardnerella vaginalis* and *Mobiluncus* spp. are both implicated in the disease.

    b. **Viral cervicitis.** Herpes simplex virus (HSV; primarily HSV type 2) infection is characterized by ulceration with enlarged nuclei, nuclear molding, multinucleation, and margination of the chromatin in virally infected epithelial cells at the edge of the ulcer (e-**Fig. 34.3**). Cytomegalovirus is distinctive for its nuclear and cytoplasmic inclusions within endothelial nuclei. Adenovirus is notable for its smudged epithelial nuclear inclusions. The poxvirus *Molluscum contagiosum* generates large round intensely eosinophilic cytoplasmic inclusions, as it does at cutaneous sites. Human papillomavirus (HPV) infection is closely tied to cervical neoplasia; its features are discussed in the sections below dealing with preinvasive and invasive squamous neoplasia.

    c. **Granulomatous cervicitis.** Infectious causes of granulomatous cervicitis include *Mycobacterium tuberculosis* and *Treponema pallidum*. As noted above, noninfectious etiologies are also in the differential diagnosis of granulomatous inflammation.

    d. **Fungal.** *Candida* spp. are commonly encountered in smears and are not necessarily pathogenic. They cannot be speciated reliably by morphology in either tissue sections or cervical smears.

    e. **Parasitic.** *Trichomonas vaginalis* is one of the most common sexually transmitted infections in women. Many infections are asymptomatic. In Papanicolaou-stained smears or liquid-based preparations, an ovoid organism with red cytoplasmic granules and an eccentric, pale nucleus is observed; in liquid-based preparations, squamous cells may be coated with the organism.

3. **Vasculitis.** Most cases of vasculitis involving the gynecologic tract are incidental, and the vasculitis is often confined to the cervix. However, some cases are associated with

known collagen vascular disease, and rare cases represent the first manifestation of a collagen vascular disorder (e-**Fig. 34.4**) (*Int J Gynecol Pathol* 2000;19:258).

B. Atrophy. Epithelial atrophy is seen in the postmenopausal state, when estrogen levels are decreased. As noted in the discussion of normal histology, high-estrogen states are associated with large numbers of superficial squamous cells; however, when the epithelium is thinned, the histologic picture is dominated by small cells with increased N/C ratios and nuclei at least as large or larger than those of normal intermediate cells. The overall appearance of a well-organized epithelial architecture and a lack of nuclear atypia distinguish atrophy from severe squamous dysplasia.

C. Metaplasia. Tubal metaplasia occurs most frequently in the upper endocervix. Transitional cell metaplasia is rare and recapitulates urothelium; it is not associated with a specific insult and must not be confused with neoplasia. Intestinal metaplasia is another uncommon metaplasia; it features columnar epithelium with goblet and Paneth cells.

D. Hyperplasia

1. Squamous hyperplasia consists of thickening of the epithelium with normal maturation. It occurs in situations of prolapse and chronic irritation.

2. Squamous papilloma is a benign squamous proliferation with fibrovascular cores. Squamous papilloma may be associated with HPV infection but it does not show classic koilocytic atypia.

3. Microglandular hyperplasia is an increase in glandular elements in the cervical stroma, with associated neutrophils. Seen in histologic sections, the exuberant proliferation sometimes has a cribriform architecture that can raise the question of neoplasia. However, microglandular hyperplasia shows no cytologic atypia, does not infiltrate the stroma, and is not associated with a desmoplastic reaction.

4. Lobular endocervical glandular hyperplasia is a benign proliferation of bland glands usually surrounding a central dilated gland and forming a well-circumscribed lobule. It is not HPV related. It must be distinguished from gastric-type endocervical adenocarcinoma (adenoma malignum), the latter of which is deeply invasive and shows features of malignancy.

5. Diffuse laminar endocervical glandular hyperplasia. In this entity, the proliferation is primarily in the very superficial aspects of the stroma and extends in a bandlike fashion with an intermingled lymphocytic infiltrate that may be dense.

E. Nabothian Cysts are pronounced dilatations of endocervical glands. They are extremely common (e-**Fig. 34.5**).

F. Endocervical Tunnel Clusters are superficial collections of endocervical gland ductal spaces.

G. Mesonephric Remnants and Mesonephric Hyperplasia are developmental remnants of the mesonephric (wolffian) duct that are occasionally identified in the deep stroma. Mesonephric remnants must not be confused with adenocarcinoma; helpful distinguishing features include the bland cytology of the lining epithelium, dense "bubble gum" luminal contents, and the absence of a desmoplastic stromal response (e-**Fig. 34.6**). Calretinin, androgen receptor, and GATA3 tend to be positive, and p16 only focally positive.

H. Postoperative Spindle Cell Nodule is a benign proliferation of fibroblasts that usually only occurs following surgical manipulation.

I. Endocervical Polyps are often identified colposcopically. They consist of an exophytic mass of benign glands and stroma usually with thick-walled vessels (e-**Fig. 34.7**). They must be carefully examined to exclude coexisting squamous dysplasia or a glandular neoplasm.

J. Inclusion Cysts are benign. Microscopically, they are filled with keratin debris and are related to surgical manipulation. Similar inclusions occur in the vagina following episiotomies.

K. Endometriosis can involve any layer of the cervical stroma, as well as the parametrial/paracervical soft tissue.

L. Decidual Change occurs in the cervical stroma during pregnancy. The nests of cells that show abundant amphophilic cytoplasm, a prominent cell border, and a single centrally placed nucleus are usually not visible grossly, but sometimes form polyps (e-**Fig. 34.8**).

M. The Arias-Stella Reaction, characterized by epithelial cells with nuclear enlargement and clear cytoplasm in response to progesterone, is most commonly seen in the uterine corpus in pregnancy, but may also occur in the cervix. The significance of the Arias-Stella reaction lies in the fact that it can easily be confused with a glandular neoplasm.

IV. CERVICAL NEOPLASIA. The World Health Organization (WHO) classification of cervical tumors is shown in Table 34.1.

TABLE 34.1 | WHO Classification of Tumors of the Uterine Cervix

Epithelial tumors

Squamous cell tumors and precursors
  Squamous intraepithelial lesions
    Low-grade squamous intraepithelial lesion
    High-grade squamous intraepithelial lesion
  Squamous cell carcinoma, NOS
    Keratinizing
    Nonkeratinizing
    Papillary
    Basaloid
    Warty
    Verrucous
    Squamotransitional
    Lymphoepithelioma-like
    Cervical intraepithelial neoplasia (CIN3) squamous cell carcinoma in situ
  Benign squamous cell lesions
    Squamous metaplasia
    Condyloma acuminatum
    Squamous papilloma
    Transitional metaplasia

Glandular tumors and precursors
  Adenocarcinoma in situ
  Adenocarcinoma
    Endocervical adenocarcinoma, usual type
    Mucinous carcinoma, NOS
      Gastric type
      Intestinal type
      Signet-ring cell type
    Villoglandular carcinoma
    Endometrioid carcinoma
    Clear cell carcinoma
    Serous carcinoma
    Mesonephric carcinoma
    Adenocarcinoma admixed with neuroendocrine carcinoma

Benign glandular tumors and tumor-like lesions
  Endocervical polyp
  Müllerian papilloma
  Nabothian cyst
  Tunnel clusters
  Microglandular hyperplasia
  Lobular endocervical glandular hyperplasia
  Diffuse laminar endocervical hyperplasia
  Mesonephric remnants and hyperplasia
  Arias-Stella reaction
  Endocervicosis
  Endometriosis
  Tuboendometrioid metaplasia
  Ectopic prostate tissue

(continued)

TABLE 34.1   WHO Classification of Tumors of the Uterine Cervix (*Continued*)

Other epithelial tumors
   Adenosquamous carcinoma
     Glassy cell carcinoma
   Adenoid basal carcinoma
   Adenoid cystic carcinoma
   Undifferentiated carcinoma

Neuroendocrine tumors
   Low-grade neuroendocrine tumor
     Carcinoid tumor
     Atypical carcinoid tumor
   High-grade neuroendocrine carcinoma
     Small cell neuroendocrine carcinoma
     Large cell neuroendocrine carcinoma

Mesenchymal tumors and tumor-like conditions

Benign
   Leiomyoma
   Rhabdomyoma
   Others

Malignant
   Leiomyosarcoma
   Rhabdomyosarcoma
   Alveolar soft-part sarcoma
   Angiosarcoma
   Malignant peripheral nerve sheath tumor
   Other sarcomas
     Liposarcoma
     Undifferentiated endocervical sarcoma
     Ewing sarcoma

Tumor-like lesions
   Postoperative spindle-cell nodule
   Lymphoma-like lesion

Mixed epithelial and mesenchymal tumors

Adenomyoma

Adenosarcoma

Carcinosarcoma

Melanocytic tumors

Blue nevus

Malignant melanoma

Germ cell tumors

Yolk sac tumor

Lymphoid and myeloid tumors

Lymphomas

Myeloid neoplasms

Secondary tumors

A. Benign

1. **Submucosal and stromal neoplasms.** Leiomyomas identical to those of the uterine corpus are also seen in the cervix.

2. **Blue nevus.** This benign melanocytic proliferation is common, noted clinically as a bluish discoloration of the cervical epithelium. Microscopic examination shows hyper-pigmented spindle cells infiltrating the stroma in a haphazard pattern (e-**Fig. 34.9**).

3. **Ectopic tissue.** While not neoplastic, several types of ectopic tissue may be seen in the cervix. The most common types of ectopic tissue are cutaneous adnexal structures and mature cartilage. Prostatic ectopia has also been noted to occur on occasion (e-**Fig. 34.10**) and is important to recognize to avoid overdiagnosis of a glandular malignancy.

B. Malignant and Premalignant Squamous Lesions.

Worldwide, cervical cancer is the third most common malignancy and the fifth most common cause of cancer mortality in women. Effective screening programs have dramatically reduced deaths due to cervical cancer in the developed world, but gains have been more modest elsewhere.

The major risk factor for cervical cancer is sexually transmitted HPV infection. Although there are more than 40 different HPV serotypes that infect the female genital tract, high-risk serotypes (including 16, 18, 35, 39, 45, 51, 56, and 58) are associated with a markedly increased risk of severe squamous dysplasia and subsequent cervical squamous cell carcinoma. Immunodeficiency may increase the likelihood of persistent infection and may increase the risk of subsequent epithelial malignant transformation. Host factors such as smoking, concomitant sexually transmitted diseases, high parity, and oral contraceptive use may also increase the risk of malignant transformation among already infected women. For example, among women with HPV infection, smoking doubles to quadruples the odds in favor of malignant transformation (*Cancer Causes Control* 2003;14:805; *J Natl Cancer Inst* 2002;94:1406).

1. **HPV infection.** The viral cytopathic effect that results from HPV infection is termed koilocytosis and consists of nuclear enlargement with irregular nuclear borders, condensed chromatin, occasional binucleation or multinucleation, and a perinuclear halo. Flat lesions that exhibit koilocytosis are usually associated with low-risk HPV types 6 and 11. High-risk HPV types such as HPV 16 and 18 encode proteins that have the capacity to immortalize keratinocytes through the ubiquitin-mediated degradation of the tumor suppressors p53 and pRb. Malignant transformation is not a committed endpoint of HPV infection, but its likelihood may be enhanced by environmental and host factors as discussed above.

2. **Low-grade squamous intraepithelial lesion (LSIL),** also known as mild dysplasia, and formerly known as cervical intraepithelial neoplasia grade 1 (CIN1), is defined by disordered maturation and cytologic abnormalities of the lower one-third of the squamous epithelium, often with koilocytic changes in the upper two-thirds of the epithelium (e-**Fig. 34.11**). Use of SIL terminology has been recommended throughout the lower anogenital tract (*Arch Pathol Lab Med* 2012;136:1266). Most cases of LSIL will regress (*Int J Gynecol Pathol* 1993;12:186). p16 is typically negative, but can be positive in some cases.

3. **High-grade squamous intraepithelial lesion (HSIL),** encompassing moderate or severe dysplasia and formerly known as cervical intraepithelial neoplasia grade 2 or 3 (CIN2 and CIN3), is defined by disordered maturation and cytologic abnormalities extending into the middle or top third of the epithelium, respectively (e-**Figs. 34.12** and **34.13**). Excision of HSIL is warranted because progression to invasive carcinoma occurs in a higher percentage of these lesions as compared with LSIL/CIN1 (*Int J Gynecol Pathol* 1993;12:186). The disease is caused by high-risk HPV, so p16 will be diffusely positive and Ki-67 will show proliferation in the middle or top third of the epithelium.

4. **Invasive squamous cell carcinoma** is recognized by penetration of the epithelial basement membrane by neoplastic squamous cells with an associated desmoplastic stromal response (e-**Fig. 34.14**). The invasive tumor cells often exhibit paradoxical maturation evidenced by abundant eosinophilic cytoplasm.

a. **Superficially invasive squamous cell carcinoma** is defined as a tumor that is not visible clinically, that invades ≤3 mm from the basement membrane of the adjacent surface epithelium or endocervical gland from which it arises, and that extends ≤7 mm in greatest lateral extent (International Federation of Gynecology and Obstetrics [FIGO] stage IA1). When no lymphatic or vascular involvement is present, when the entire lesion is excised, and when no dysplasia is present at the margins of excision, the potential for lymph node metastasis or recurrence is very low. Long-term follow-up studies have shown that the group of patients harboring residual invasive carcinoma in a hysterectomy specimen after conization for microinvasive squamous cell carcinoma with maximum invasion of ≤1 mm is 0%; when invasion is ≤3 mm the recurrence and lymph node metastasis rates are <1%. For lesions between 3 and 5 mm in depth, the recurrence and lymph node metastasis rates increase to 2% and 4%, respectively (*Pathol Ann* 1995;30:103). Most studies find 3 mm of invasion to be a cutoff beyond which recurrence and lymph node metastasis risk becomes significant.

b. **Squamous cell carcinoma variants**

   i. **Keratinizing tumors** contain keratin pearls and nests of tumor cells with central keratin; cytoplasmic keratinization and keratohyalin granules are also present. Intercellular bridges can be identified.

   ii. **Nonkeratinizing tumors** show cytoplasmic keratinization of individual cells and intercellular bridges, but keratin pearls and nests of tumor cells with central keratin are not present. The distinction between keratinizing and nonkeratinizing types has no clinical significance in current practice. Some tumors previously classified as nonkeratinizing type have subsequently been identified as small cell carcinomas, accounting for their supposedly poor prognosis.

   iii. **Basaloid carcinoma** features cells with scanty cytoplasm that resemble basal-type squamous cells. Only rare nests of tumor cells show central keratin. This variant has an aggressive behavior.

   iv. **Verrucous carcinoma** is a very well-differentiated squamous cell carcinoma that betrays its malignant character only in its invasion of the stroma along broad pushing borders. There is minimal cytologic atypia, and viral cytopathic effect is absent. Aggressive local invasion and recurrence after excision are common. Metastasis is uncommon.

   v. **Warty carcinoma** is a rare squamous malignancy that shows definitive stromal invasion but also prominent cytologic features of HPV infection. It may behave less aggressively than other well-differentiated squamous cell carcinomas.

   vi. **Papillary squamous cell carcinoma** is an exophytic tumor in which epithelium resembling HSIL covers fibrovascular cores. Koilocytosis is not characteristic. Although much of the tumor may have the appearance of a precursor lesion, definitive stromal invasion is present in the deep aspects of the lesion. Therefore, superficial biopsies of papillary lesions should be interpreted with caution.

   vii. **Lymphoepithelial-like carcinoma** resembles the nasopharyngeal tumor of the same name. The tumor consists of syncytial sheets and islands of undifferentiated epithelioid cells that have eosinophilic cytoplasm and large vesicular nuclei with prominent nucleoli in a background that contains an intense lymphocytic infiltrate.

C. **Glandular Neoplasms**

   1. **Adenocarcinoma in situ (AIS)** is an HPV-associated glandular lesion (most strongly associated with HPV serotypes 16 and 18) that is a precursor to invasive adenocarcinoma. Cytologically, AIS is characterized by loss of cytoplasmic mucin, cellular stratification, cellular crowding, nuclear enlargement, and atypia, and apically situated mitotic figures and epithelial apoptotic debris (e-**Fig. 34.15**). The various subtypes can mimic endocervical, endometrial, or intestinal epithelium, and can have a papillary or cribriform architectural pattern. AIS is often seen in conjunction with SIL.

A number of series show that a positive margin for AIS in a cone biopsy predicts the presence of either an invasive adenocarcinoma or the recurrence of AIS (*Gynecol Oncol* 2000;79:207), and AIS thus requires complete excision.

2. **Microinvasive adenocarcinoma.** The FIGO definition of microinvasive adenocarcinoma is the same as that of microinvasive squamous cell carcinoma. It is a difficult diagnosis; the subjectivity of histologic assessment and relative infrequency of in situ adenocarcinoma have presented challenges in elucidating the natural behavior of microinvasive adenocarcinoma. What is known is that it carries a good prognosis. When invasion is ≤2 mm, lymph node metastases essentially do not occur (*Obstet Gynecol* 1985;65:46; *Obstet Gynecol* 1997;89:88; *Int J Gynecol Pathol* 2000;19:29).

3. **Invasive adenocarcinoma.** Infiltrating glands with cribriform and papillary structures are the architectural characteristics of invasive adenocarcinoma. A desmoplastic stromal reaction helps to distinguish adenocarcinoma from both AIS and the hyperplastic entities described above (e-**Fig. 34.16**).

   a. **Mucinous (usual) adenocarcinoma.** Most primary mucinous adenocarcinomas have cytologic features resembling endocervical glands. The cells are cuboidal to columnar and show nuclear pleomorphism, nuclear atypia, and many mitoses. The relatively abundant cytoplasm stains positively with mucicarmine. Unlike benign endocervical glands, ER and PR are lost, and p16 is positive reflecting the role of HPV. Mucinous adenocarcinomas with goblet cells that have an overall morphology more similar to intestinal epithelium are termed intestinal variants.

   b. **Minimal deviation adenocarcinoma (adenoma malignum, gastric-type adenocarcinoma).** This rare entity comprises only 1% of primary adenocarcinomas of the cervix. The glandular epithelium has a gastric phenotype, and is so bland in appearance that these lesions may not be recognized as malignant on biopsy or curettage specimens; increased mitotic activity and cytologic atypia may be present focally but are not prominent. The diagnosis rests on the presence of deep infiltration, aggregation of glands around vessels or nerves, and a stromal reaction, features that are easiest to assess on cone biopsy or hysterectomy. The incidence of this lesion is increased in Peutz–Jeghers syndrome, but most cases are nonsyndromic. Hormone receptors are absent and p16 is negative, as this tumor is not caused by HPV.

   c. **Endometrioid adenocarcinoma.** Comprising 30% of cervical adenocarcinomas, endometrioid adenocarcinoma of the cervix is identical in appearance to its counterpart in the endometrium. When well differentiated, the lesion shows tall columnar cells without mucin. It may be very difficult to distinguish a cervical primary lesion from direct extension into the cervix of a tumor of the uterine corpus. Immunohistochemistry may be useful, as endocervical adenocarcinomas are generally expected to express monoclonal CEA and p16, while endometrial adenocarcinomas tend to be negative for these two markers and positive for vimentin and ER. Care should be taken when using immunohistochemistry, because neither of these profiles has 100% specificity.

   d. **Well-differentiated villoglandular adenocarcinoma** is considered to be a subtype of endometrioid adenocarcinoma. It shows an exophytic growth pattern with glandular and villous elements, little nuclear pleomorphism, and a low mitotic rate, all quite similar to an intestinal villous adenoma (e-**Fig. 34.17**). There is value in the recognition of the well-differentiated villoglandular variant as this is a tumor of young women and has a favorable prognosis (*Gynecol Oncol* 1997;64:147).

   e. **Clear cell adenocarcinoma.** This tumor's association with in utero diethylstilbestrol (DES) exposure has made it widely recognized. Although rare, the tumor can occur in patients without a DES exposure history as well. Clear cells with hobnail morphology are observed in solid, papillary, and tubular arrangements. The presence of this tumor in the cervix should prompt a search for a primary tumor of the ovary, endometrium, or vagina, which are sites where this entity is much more common.

    f. Serous adenocarcinoma rarely occurs as a cervical primary tumor.

    g. Mesonephric adenocarcinoma. This lesion differs from mesonephric remnants in its cytologic atypia, crowding, and increased mitotic activity. It arises in the deep lateral cervical walls, and a variety of architectural patterns is characteristic, including tubular, papillary, solid, and retiform. The behavior of this very rare tumor is generally indolent, if the tumor is low stage.

D. Other Carcinomas

    1. Adenosquamous carcinoma. Both squamous and glandular differentiation are observed in this lesion. To be diagnostic, invasive glandular and squamous components must be present; that is, adenocarcinoma with adjacent squamous dysplasia is not adenosquamous carcinoma. The epidemiologic profile is similar to that of squamous cell carcinoma and adenocarcinoma.

    2. Glassy cell carcinoma is considered a subtype of adenosquamous carcinoma that occurs in young women. It carries a poor prognosis because it is unresponsive to radiotherapy; progression is rapid and distant metastases are common. Microscopically, the tumor consists of sheets of pleomorphic cells with granular eosinophilic cytoplasm, nucleoli, and brisk mitotic activity. The tumor is usually infiltrated by eosinophils and plasma cells. An in situ precursor lesion is not typically found in association with this tumor.

    3. Adenoid cystic carcinoma is a rare cervical tumor found mostly in postmenopausal African-American women who present with abnormal bleeding and a pelvic mass. This tumor shows cystic spaces filled with eosinophilic hyaline material or basophilic mucin surrounded by palisades of epithelial cells. The tumor architecture may be tubular, cribriform, or solid. Adenoid cystic carcinoma of the cervix typically shows more cytologic atypia than its salivary gland counterpart, but displays the same tendency for perineural invasion and local aggressiveness. HPV is involved in the pathogenesis.

    4. Mucoepidermoid carcinoma (MEC) is not currently recognized as a distinct entity in the WHO classification of cervical tumors. Tumors with striking similarity to the analogous tumor of the salivary gland do occur in the cervix, however, with epidermoid, intermediate, and mucin producing cells. Interestingly, it has been shown that when strict histologic criteria are applied, cervical tumors with mucoepidermoid morphology harbor the same t(11;19)(q21;p13) as salivary gland MEC (*Am J Surg Pathol* 2009;33:835). This suggests that MEC may actually be an entity distinct from adenosquamous carcinoma in the cervix.

    5. Adenoid basal carcinoma. This tumor occurs in a population similar to that of adenoid cystic carcinoma. It also shows a nested cribriform architecture. The epithelium, however, is composed of more uniform, round to oval, basophilic cells, often with squamous differentiation, without significant atypia or increased mitotic activity. There is often associated CIN. Correct identification of this lesion is important because it is low grade and does not have aggressive behavior; in fact, some have suggested that the tumor is more appropriately termed adenoid basal epithelioma (*Am J Surg Pathol* 1998;22:965).

E. Neuroendocrine Neoplasms.
A variety of neuroendocrine neoplasms may rarely occur in the cervix. The classification of these tumors is similar to that of neuroendocrine tumors of the lung.

    1. Carcinoid. These tumors are organoid in their architecture and are composed of small, oval to spindle cells with granular cytoplasm. Mitoses are rare in typical carcinoid tumors. Immunoreactivity with neuroendocrine markers synaptophysin, chromogranin A, and neuron-specific enolase is the rule.

    2. Atypical carcinoid. Moderate cytologic atypia and the presence of 5 to 10 mitotic figures/10 high power fields are sufficient to classify a carcinoid as atypical; at least small foci of necrosis are often present (*Arch Pathol Lab Med* 1997;121:34). These tumors generally retain the organoid architecture of typical carcinoids. Their biologic behavior is difficult to assess systematically due to the subjectivity involved in separating atypical carcinoids from typical carcinoids and large cell neuroendocrine carcinomas.

3. Large cell neuroendocrine carcinoma. These tumors show frequent vascular invasion, have higher mitotic activity than atypical carcinoids (>10 mitotic figures/10 high power fields), and show loss of the organoid architecture seen in less aggressive neuroendocrine tumors. There may be focal adenocarcinoma-like areas with abundant cytoplasm and large nucleoli. Necrosis is frequent. The prognosis is poor, similar to that of small cell carcinoma.

4. Small cell carcinoma. Histologically identical to its counterpart in the lung, small cell carcinoma (also known as high-grade neuroendocrine carcinoma) is a tumor of variably sized, round to oval to spindle cells with scant cytoplasm, high mitotic activity, nuclear molding, and frequent crush artifact (e-**Fig. 34.18**). Necrosis may be extensive. Clinical series are small due to the rarity of the tumor, but the prognosis is uniformly poor. HPV is present, p16 is positive, and TTF-1 is also often positive and therefore is not useful in distinguishing primary from metastatic cases.

F. **Mesenchymal Neoplasms.** A wide variety of sarcomas may be primary to the cervix, including leiomyosarcoma, embryonal rhabdomyosarcoma, endometrioid stromal sarcoma, alveolar soft part sarcoma, and angiosarcoma (e-**Fig. 34.19**).

G. **Mixed Epithelial and Mesenchymal Neoplasms**

1. Adenosarcomas are polypoid lesions that microscopically consist of large papillae of malignant stroma covered with benign endocervical epithelium. The stroma can have many different appearances; it can consist of plump, mitotically active spindle cells or more undifferentiated round cells similar to those of small cell carcinoma. Heterologous sarcomatous elements may be present, with skeletal muscle, cartilage, adipose, or osseous differentiation. Prognosis after excision is apparently good, although only small numbers of cases have been reported.

2. Carcinosarcoma (malignant mixed müllerian tumor [MMMT]) also presents as a polypoid mass. In contrast to its more common counterpart in the uterine corpus, the malignant epithelial component is more often squamous or basaloid, as opposed to glandular. The sarcomatous component is usually homologous, with a spindle-cell morphology similar to that of fibrosarcoma. In limited series of MMMT of the cervix, it appears that the prognosis is better than that of MMMT of the uterine corpus.

H. **Hematolymphoid Neoplasms.** Lymphoma of the cervix is usually a part of systemic disease.

I. **Melanoma.** Primary melanoma of the cervix is rare. Vaginal bleeding with a cervical mass is a common presentation. The tumor is usually low stage at presentation, but the prognosis is dismal. Morphologically, the tumor is similar to melanomas of other sites, although cervical melanomas have been noted for a tendency toward a spindle-cell morphology. Melanin pigment is variable from tumor to tumor. It is important to identify a junctional component in this lesion if it is to be classified as primary to the cervix; otherwise, a thorough search for another primary site is indicated.

J. **Secondary Malignancies.** Most metastases to the cervix arise from tumors at other sites in the reproductive tract. Aside from the uterus and ovary, the gastrointestinal tract and breast are the most common origins of cervical metastases.

V. **PATHOLOGIC AND CLINICAL STAGING OF MALIGNANCIES**

A. **American Joint Committee on Cancer (AJCC) and FIGO.** The staging by both FIGO and AJCC criteria (Amin MB, Edge SB, Greene FL, et al., eds. *AJCC Cancer Staging Manual.* 8th ed. New York: Springer; 2017) is based on size, local extension, and lymph node metastasis.

B. **Additional Information.** The final report in any case of malignancy should explicitly include all of the information required for assigning a stage as well as other information of clinical interest not required for staging and follow recommended guidelines (College of American Pathologists Protocol for the Examination of Specimens from Patients with Primary Carcinoma of the Uterine Cervix, available at http://www.cap.org).

For the cervix, the report should include: (1) the histologic type and grade; (2) the presence or absence of precursor lesions (either CIN or AIS); (3) tumor size, including depth and width; (4) whether the malignancy is unifocal or multifocal; (5) presence or absence of lymphovascular space invasion; (6) presence or absence of vaginal, paracervical/parametrial, or uterine extension; (7) margin status; (8) presence or absence of lymph node or distant metastases.

Cytopathology of the Uterine Cervix

Cory Bernadt

I. SPECIMEN TYPES

A. Liquid-Based Preparations are the most widely used modality for cervical screening (Pap test). A brush is used to sample the cervix and the sample is placed in appropriate transport fluid for the proprietary system used in the laboratory, be it ThinPrep (Hologic, Inc., Marlborough, MA) or SurePath (BD Diagnostics-TriPath, Burlington, NC). Advantages of this modality include a cleaner background, a monolayer of cells, increased diagnostic sensitivity, and ease of performance of HPV assays.

B. Conventional Smears are made by using a spatula and/or brush to sample the cervix, smearing the endo- and ectocervical samples on a glass slide, and then immediately fixing the sample. Papanicolaou (Pap) staining is performed in the laboratory.

II. EXFOLIATIVE CYTOLOGY OF THE CERVIX

A. Squamous Cells. A spectrum of squamous cells, ranging from small parabasal and metaplastic cells with dense cytoplasm and relatively high N/C ratios (e-**Fig. 34.20**), to intermediate cells with medium-sized round nuclei with open chromatin and polygonal cytoplasmic outlines (e-**Fig. 34.21**), to superficial cells with polygonal shapes and small pyknotic nuclei (e-**Fig. 34.22**) is seen in normal cervical smears and liquid-based preparations.

B. Glandular Cells. The classic appearance of endocervical glandular cells is sheets of regularly spaced cells forming a so-called "honeycomb" pattern (e-**Fig. 34.23**); varying degrees of disruption of this architecture herald reactive and neoplastic change. Endometrial cells are smaller and form more three-dimensional aggregates in cytology preparations; they are also typically more degenerated than endocervical cells. Careful attention to nuclear details such as the chromatin pattern and nuclear contours is required to separate glandular neoplasia from reactive atypia.

III. THE BETHESDA SYSTEM

was developed in 1988 with the objective of standardizing terminology to promote better communication between the laboratory and clinicians. The third edition of the system was promulgated in 2015.

A. Adequacy. A statement of adequacy is required. Cellularity should be 5,000 cells for a liquid-based preparation, and this can be reproducibly and quickly estimated with experience and with the use of reference images. The 5,000-cell threshold should not be rigidly applied in vaginal and posttherapy (radiation or chemotherapy) specimens. Having 75% of squamous cells obscured by blood or inflammation renders a specimen unsatisfactory, as does improper labeling or slide breakage.

B. Negative for Intraepithelial Lesion or Malignancy

1. Microorganisms should be reported. Various causes of vaginitis can be detected cytologically.

    a. _Trichomonas vaginalis_ is seen as a pear-shaped structure, approximately 30 μm in diameter. It has a small pale nucleus and red cytoplasmic granules. The flagella are often difficult to appreciate (e-**Fig. 34.24**).

b. **Bacterial vaginosis** is marked by the presence of "clue cells," which are cocco-bacilli-coated squamous cells (e-**Fig. 34.25**). This is reported as "shift in flora suggestive of bacterial vaginosis."

c. **Actinomyces** shows filamentous organisms and the "sulfur granules" described above. This infection is associated with IUDs.

d. **Candida albicans** is responsible for most cases of vulvovaginal candidiasis. Although the fungus can be a commensal microorganism, when it is accompanied by acute inflammation the infection is usually symptomatic. Budding year and/or pseudohyphae are seen (e-**Fig. 34.26**).

e. **Herpes genitalis** is usually caused by HSV type 2. Nuclear enlargement, chromatin margination, multinucleation, nuclear inclusions, and nuclear molding are evident (e-**Fig. 34.27**).

2. **Other nonneoplastic findings**

a. **Reactive changes/repair** in squamous cells include nuclear enlargement with or without multinucleation, round and smooth nuclear contours, even chromatin distribution, and small nucleoli. In reparative change, there may be vacuolization of the cytoplasm and some of the cells may be elongated, clustering together in a streaming pattern. The relative abundance of cytoplasm and lack of true nuclear atypia differentiate this from neoplastic squamous proliferations (e-**Fig. 34.28**). Reactive endocervical cells may show even greater nuclear enlargement, multinucleation, mild hyperchromasia, and prominent nucleoli (e-**Fig. 34.29**).

b. **IUD.** The recognition of IUD-related changes is particularly important in cervical smears, as the singly dispersed cells with vacuolated cytoplasm and large nuclei seen in this reactive condition can mimic adenocarcinoma. Despite nuclear enlargement, truly atypical nuclei are not seen. Correlation with the history is key when IUD-type changes appear.

c. **Normal-appearing glandular cells status post hysterectomy** may represent metaplastic change, adenosis, or misplaced fallopian tube remnants. They are not considered an epithelial cell abnormality.

C. **Epithelial Cell Abnormality**

1. **Squamous**

a. **Atypical squamous cells of undetermined significance (ASC-US)** have nuclei 2.5 to 3 times the size of an intermediate cell nucleus. There is minimal nuclear hyperchromasia and a somewhat increased N/C ratio. Reflex HPV testing is preferred. While the predictive value of an ASC-US/HPV-positive sample varies with patient age, in general, the 5-year risk for histologic HSIL and cancer for an ASC-US/HPV-positive Pap test is 18% (*N Engl J Med* 2013;369:2324).

b. **ASC, cannot exclude HSIL** are approximately the size of squamous metaplastic cells, with associated nuclear enlargement resulting in an appearance approaching that of a HSIL. However, they usually lack the severe hyperchromasia and abnormal nuclear contours of HSIL. Colposcopy is recommended after this interpretation regardless of HPV result, since 30% of patients will have CIN2 or greater on follow-up (*Am J Obstet Gynecol* 2003;183:1383).

c. **LSIL** is a cytologic lesion with nuclei greater than three times the size of an intermediate nucleus. Despite the increased nuclear size, N/C ratios are relatively preserved. Nuclei are generally hyperchromatic and may have nuclear contour irregularities. Multinucleation and koilocytic halos are common, but not required (e-**Fig. 34.30**).

d. **HSIL** displays cells that are smaller and show less cytoplasmic maturity than LSIL. The nuclei are generally hyperchromatic with very irregular contours and frequently demonstrate prominent indentations or grooves. The dysplastic cells occur singly and in syncytial-like aggregates (e-**Fig. 34.31**).

e. **Squamous cell carcinoma** has nuclear abnormalities that are equal to or more severe than those of HSIL, with the addition of prominent nucleoli (e-**Fig. 34.32**). An inflammatory/proteinaceous background (the so-called "tumor diathesis") favors invasive squamous cell carcinoma, although the diathesis is seen less prominently in liquid-based preparations.

2. Glandular

a. Atypical glandular cells show nuclear enlargement, mild nuclear hyperchromasia, variable pleomorphism, and increased N/C ratios. Often in these cases, only incomplete features of adenocarcinoma are present. Although not always possible, every attempt should be made to state whether the abnormal cells are endometrial or endocervical in origin.

b. AIS of the endocervix shows glandular groups with nuclear stratification, crowding, and sometimes a characteristic "feathering." The nuclei are generally elongate and lack nucleoli (**e-Fig. 34.33**). Mitoses and apoptotic bodies may be present.

c. Adenocarcinoma of the endocervix can be detected by cervical cytology in approximately 80% of cases. However, only 22% of endometrial adenocarcinoma cases are evident in Pap tests (*Acta Cytol* 2007;51:47). The cells of endocervical carcinoma can be arranged singly or in three-dimensional clusters, and they show clearly malignant nuclear features including pleomorphism, hyperchromasia, irregular nuclear contours, and occasional large nucleoli. Cytoplasmic vacuoles are often present (**e-Fig. 34.34**). Cytologically, it can be difficult to distinguish endometrial and endocervical origins.

D. Other. The Bethesda System calls for the use of this category in cases showing endometrial cells in a woman ≥45 years of age. Clinical correlation is required to assess the significance of such cells. The absence of a squamous intraepithelial lesion must also be documented in the report when "other" is utilized.

IV. ANCILLARY TESTING

A. HPV Testing is recommended in most cases of ASC-US as a reflex test and as a cotest in women ≥30 years. It is performed on the unused portion of a liquid-based sample. There are several HPV tests that are FDA approved for performance in association with cervical cytology. These assays test for a number of high-risk HPV subtypes, and may provide genotyping for individual HPV types (e.g., HPV 16 and 18).

B. Immunohistochemical Assays such as p16, ProExC, and Ki67 have been incorporated into the practice of histopathology, but the data on their use for cytology specimens is not well developed.

C. Automated Screening of Cervical Cytology Specimens is now in wide use, with FDA approval. The system used depends upon the proprietary liquid-based Pap test used in the laboratory.

ACKNOWLEDGMENT

The authors thank Michael E. Hull, author of the previous edition of this chapter.

SUGGESTED READINGS

Massad LS, Einstein MH, Huh WK, et al. 2012 Updated consensus guidelines for the management of abnormal cervical cancer screening tests and cancer precursors. *J Low Genit Tract Dis* 2012;17:S1.

Schiffman M, Solomon D. Cervical-cancer screening with human papillomavirus and cytologic cotesting. *New Engl J Med* 2013;369:2324.

Vagina
Tiffany Y. Chen and Ian S. Hagemann

I. NORMAL ANATOMY. The vagina is derived from the müllerian ducts and is composed of three layers: mucosa, muscularis propria, and adventitia. The mucosa is composed of squamous epithelium overlying a lamina propria that contains a rich vascular and lymphatic network with scattered stromal cells that may show multinucleation. The anterior and posterior fornices are formed by the protrusion of the cervix into the vaginal vault. The posterior fornix is deeper than the anterior fornix.

II. BENIGN CONDITIONS

A. Infectious Diseases

1. **Vulvovaginal candidiasis** is a common condition that predominantly affects adult women in their second and third decades. Up to 70% of women will experience at least one episode in their lifetime. Common predisposing factors include antibiotic use, steroid use, oral contraceptive use, immunosuppression, and uncontrolled diabetes. Pruritus, erythema, and a thick white vaginal discharge are the most common symptoms. Histologically, squamous epithelial hyperplasia with hyperkeratosis and/or parakeratosis is seen. Foci of neutrophilic infiltration of the squamous epithelium are commonly present. *Candida* can be present in the form of budding yeasts as well as pseudohyphae, highlighted on GMS or other special stains.

2. **Bacterial vaginosis** is most commonly found among adult women. It is caused by *Gardnerella vaginalis*, a bacillus which usually grows when the vaginal flora shifts toward a more acidic environment. A watery, malodorous discharge without significant inflammation is a common symptom. Microscopically, the bacteria overgrow and cover the squamous cells producing so-called clue cells.

3. **Trichomoniasis,** a sexually transmitted disease, is caused by *Trichomonas vaginalis*, an oval protozoon with flagella. Microscopically, the organisms are identified by their blue-pink body, elongated nuclei, and flagella.

4. **Herpes simplex infection** is a sexually transmitted disease caused by herpes simplex virus (HSV). Grossly, the virus causes a mucosal ulceration within a few days to 2 weeks following the exposure. These lesions are highly infectious until crusting, with final scarring occurring within 2 to 3 weeks of initial symptoms. The majority of cases are caused by HSV-2, and recurrence is higher with infection by HSV-2 than by HSV-1.

   Microscopically, the ulcerated lesions are characterized by epithelial necrosis with associated degenerated cells containing viral inclusions, best identified at the periphery of the ulcer. The cells with viral inclusions have characteristic features including multinucleation and ground glass nuclei with a rim of chromatin condensation at the nuclear border surrounded by a cytoplasmic halo.

5. **Actinomyces** infection is most commonly seen in women with noncopper intrauterine contraceptive devices.

B. Inflammatory Diseases

1. **Atrophic vaginitis** occurs most commonly in postmenopausal women but can also occur during the postpartum period. Grossly, the primary finding is punctate hemorrhage of the vaginal mucosa. Microscopically, the squamous cells show decreased glycogen due to lower estrogen levels. Atrophy can be distinguished from vaginal intraepithelial neoplasia by the monotony of the cell population, uniform chromatin, the lack of cytologic atypia, and the low mitotic rate.

2. Crohn disease can result in rectovaginal fistula formation and is associated with fibrosis, chronic inflammation, and granulomas. The differential diagnosis includes vaginal fistulas of other etiologies including radiation therapy, perforated colonic diverticulum, or as a complication of hysterectomy.

3. Stenosis, ulceration, and necrosis are well-described sequelae of radiation therapy. Stenosis can also follow severe bullous erythema multiforme (Stevens–Johnson syndrome).

C. Cysts

1. Müllerian cysts are the most common type of vaginal cyst, and can be lined by endocervical, endometrial, or endosalpingeal type epithelium (e-**Fig. 35.1**).

2. Epithelial inclusion cysts are lined by keratinizing squamous epithelium and filled with white keratinous debris. They most commonly arise in areas of previous trauma such as episiotomy sites.

3. Mesonephric cyst. Also known as Gartner duct cysts, they are usually located along the anterolateral wall of the vagina (along the path of the mesonephric duct). This type of cyst is lined by low cuboidal, nonmucinous epithelium.

4. Bartholin gland cysts are thought to develop from obstruction of the ducts of Bartholin glands, which normally open to the vestibule. The cyst lining varies from squamous to transitional to mucin-secreting (e-**Fig. 35.2**).

D. Adenosis occurs in about 30% of women who were exposed to diethylstilbestrol (DES) in utero, and is associated with an increased risk of clear cell adenocarcinoma (see section on clear cell adenocarcinoma below). Adenosis usually involves the upper third of the vagina, but the middle third or lower third is affected in about 10% of cases. Grossly, adenosis presents as a red erythematous granular lesion. Microscopically, adenosis is defined by the presence of columnar epithelium of endometrial or endocervical type in the vaginal mucosa or underlying submucosa (e-**Fig. 35.3**).

E. Endometriosis of the vagina comprises less than 10% of cases of pelvic endometriosis. The diagnosis requires two of three components: Müllerian-type epithelium (most commonly endometrioid), endometrial-type stroma, and hemosiderin-laden macrophages. The presence of endometrial-type stroma can be used to distinguish endometriosis from adenosis (e-**Fig. 35.4**).

III. BENIGN NEOPLASMS. The WHO classification of vaginal tumors is given in Table 35.1.

A. Epithelial

1. Squamous papilloma is often asymptomatic and can occur at any age. Grossly, it usually presents as a cluster of papillary lesions. Microscopically, squamous papillomas have a fibrovascular core and are lined by benign squamous epithelium.

2. Fibroepithelial polyps most commonly occur in adult women during their reproductive years. They occur in the lower third of the vagina and grossly have a soft and papillary surface. Microscopically, they are composed of squamous epithelium with underlying hypocellular fibrovascular stroma. Atypical myofibroblasts are common in the stroma. Scattered multinucleated cells with bizarre atypical nuclei may also be seen (e-**Fig. 35.5**). However, rhabdomyoblasts and a cambium layer are not present and mitotic figures are rare; these features, together with patient age, distinguish fibroepithelial polyp from sarcoma botryoides.

3. Condyloma acuminatum is caused by human papilloma virus (HPV) serotypes 6 and 11. Microscopically, it is composed of papillary fibrovascular cores lined by squamous epithelium with acanthosis, hyperkeratosis, and parakeratosis. Viral cytopathic effect (koilocytosis) is also present characterized by nuclear enlargement and irregularity, chromatin clumping and hyperchromasia, occasional bi- or multinucleation, and perinuclear clearing.

B. Mesenchymal

1. Leiomyoma is the most common benign mesenchymal tumor of the vagina in adults, with a mean age at presentation of 40 years. Leiomyomas rarely affect children. The tumor most commonly develops in the submucosa. Grossly, it consists of a well-circumscribed, firm mass with a white-tan cut surface. Microscopically, the tumor is composed of fascicles of spindle cells with elongated uniform nuclei, fine chromatin,

| TABLE 35.1 | WHO Histologic Classification of Tumors of the Vagina |

Epithelial tumors

Squamous cell tumors and precursors
  Squamous intraepithelial lesions
    Low-grade squamous intraepithelial lesion
    High-grade squamous intraepithelial lesion
  Squamous cell carcinoma, NOS
    Keratinizing
    Nonkeratinizing
    Papillary
    Basaloid
    Warty
    Verrucous
  Benign squamous lesions
    Condyloma acuminatum
    Squamous papilloma
    Fibroepithelial polyp
    Tubulosquamous polyp
    Transitional cell metaplasia

Glandular tumors

Adenocarcinomas
  Endometrioid carcinoma
  Clear cell carcinoma
  Mucinous carcinoma
  Mesonephric carcinoma

Benign glandular lesions
  Tubulovillous adenoma
  Villous adenoma
  Müllerian papilloma
  Adenosis
  Endometriosis
  Endocervicosis
  Cysts

Other epithelial tumors

Mixed tumor

Adenosquamous carcinoma

Adenoid basal carcinoma

High-grade neuroendocrine carcinoma

Small-cell neuroendocrine carcinoma

Large-cell neuroendocrine carcinoma

Mesenchymal tumors

Leiomyoma

Rhabdomyoma

Leiomyosarcoma

Rhabdomyosarcoma, NOS
  Embryonal rhabdomyosarcoma

Undifferentiated sarcoma

Angiomyofibroblastoma

Aggressive angiomyxoma

Myofibroblastoma

Tumor-like lesions

Postoperative spindle cell nodule

Mixed epithelial and mesenchymal tumors

Adenosarcoma

Carcinosarcoma

Lymphoid and myeloid tumors

Lymphomas

Myeloid neoplasms

Melanocytic tumors

Nevi
  Melanocytic nevus
  Blue nevus

Malignant melanoma

Miscellaneous tumors

Germ cell tumors
  Mature teratoma
  Yolk sac tumor

Others
  Ewing sarcoma
  Paraganglioma

Secondary tumors

From Kurman RJ, Carcangiu ML, Herrington CS, Young RH, eds. *WHO Classification of Tumours of Female Reproductive Organs.* Lyon, France: IARC Press; 2017. Used with permission.

smooth nuclear membranes, and a moderate amount of eosinophilic cytoplasm. Mitotic figures are rare.

2. **Genital rhabdomyoma** is a rare tumor of the vagina that shows skeletal muscle differentiation. It affects middle-aged women, and patients usually present with vaginal bleeding or dyspareunia. Grossly, it is a solid, polypoid to nodular lesion that creates a bulging mass under the mucosa. Microscopically, rhabdomyoma is composed of loosely interweaving bundles of spindle cells with oval nuclei, abundant eosinophilic cytoplasm, and occasional cross-striations. Nuclear pleomorphism and mitotic activity are absent. Immunohistochemical stains for skeletal muscle markers such as

desmin, myogenin, and MyoD1 are positive. Rhabdomyoma can be distinguished from rhabdomyosarcoma based on the absence of a dense layer of atypical neoplastic cells beneath the epithelium, cytologic atypia, and mitotic activity.

3. **Angiomyofibroblastoma** is a benign tumor that occurs in the vagina and vulva. Grossly, it has a well-circumscribed outline with a white-tan cut surface, and can range from 0.5 to 14 cm in maximal dimension. Microscopically, it is composed of fascicles of spindle cells that have abundant eosinophilic cytoplasm, elongated nuclei, and minimal to no atypia, although scattered multinucleated cells may be present. Architecturally, the cells form alternating hyper- and hypocellular areas, with accentuation of the hypercellular areas around vessels. The absence of red blood cell extravasation and stromal mucin distinguishes this entity from aggressive angiomyxoma. Surgical excision is the treatment of choice.

4. **Myofibroblastoma** (also known as superficial cervicovaginal myofibroblastoma) is a well-circumscribed, polypoid-shaped benign tumor that occurs in the vagina and vulva of middle aged and elderly women. Histologically, it is characterized by a proliferation of bland stellate and spindled cells within a variably cellular stroma ranging from loose, myxomatous, and edematous, to dense nodular collagen arranged in a lace-like pattern (e-**Fig. 35.6**). Immunohistochemical stains are positive for desmin, smooth muscle actin (SMA), CD34, and estrogen and progesterone receptors.

5. **Aggressive angiomyxoma** predominantly affects the sacroiliac soft tissue and perineum of women in their fifth decade. Grossly, it presents as a large mass with a gelatinous, soft cut surface. Microscopically, it is composed of bland spindle cells with delicate eosinophilic cytoplasmic processes scattered throughout a hypocellular myxoid stroma. Medium to large thick-walled hyalinized vessels are commonly present; loose fibrillar arrangements of collagen fibers (so-called myoid bundles) are typically found around the thick-walled vessels (e-**Fig. 35.7**). The stromal cells are usually immunopositive for SMA and desmin. The tumor does not metastasize, but can show locally aggressive behavior, and is difficult to excise to negative margins.

6. **Postoperative spindle cell nodule** is a pseudosarcomatous lesion that most commonly appears at the site of an excision, a few weeks to months after the surgery. Grossly, it presents as a small friable reddish mass in the vaginal vault. Microscopically, it is composed of fascicles of spindle cells with stromal granulation tissue and extravasated red blood cells. Although atypical mitotic figures can be seen, atypical nuclear cytology is not present. The differential diagnosis of postoperative spindle cell nodule includes vaginal leiomyosarcoma. A clinical history of a recent surgery can aid diagnosis.

7. **Müllerian papilloma** is a benign papillary tumor of childhood. It typically occurs in the upper vaginal wall of children with a mean age of 5 years. Microscopically, it is composed of a complex branching fibrovascular core surrounded by hypocellular stroma covered by bland cuboidal to columnar epithelial cells that show no atypia. Mitotic figures are not seen.

IV. MALIGNANT NEOPLASMS

A. Epithelial

1. **Vaginal intraepithelial neoplasia** is a premalignant, HPV-associated lesion that primarily affects women 20 to 40 years old. The disease is sexually transmitted, with the same risk factors as cervical intraepithelial neoplasia (CIN), including low age at first intercourse and increased number of sexual partners. Vaginal intraepithelial neoplasia is divided into two tiers: low-grade squamous intraepithelial lesion (LSIL; formerly known as vaginal intraepithelial neoplasia grade 1 or VAIN 1) and high-grade squamous intraepithelial lesion (HSIL; formerly known as vaginal intraepithelial neoplasia grades 2 and 3, or VAIN 2 and 3) (*Arch Pathol Lab Med* 2012;10:1266). Both vaginal LSIL and HSIL are commonly associated with high-risk HPV, especially type 16 (*Obstet Gynecol.* 2018;132:261). The majority of low-grade lesions regress spontaneously, although about 5% of cases of LSIL progress to higher grades of dysplasia and invasive carcinoma. Progression to higher grade may take several years to a decade.

Grossly, squamous intraepithelial lesions appear as an exophytic to verrucopapillary lesion. Microscopically, the squamous epithelium shows nuclear atypia (nuclear enlargement, hyperchromasia, and irregular nuclear membranes) with koilocytosis and an increased number of mitotic figures above the parabasal layer. Grading is based on the extent to which the thickness of the squamous epithelium shows atypia; LSIL is defined as the loss of maturation of the lower third (e-**Fig. 35.8**), whereas HSIL is loss of maturation in the lower two thirds (e-**Fig. 35.9**) or full thickness (e-**Fig. 35.10**) of the squamous epithelium. LSIL is managed by observation, but the preferred treatment of HSIL is local excision or laser ablation.

2. **Squamous cell carcinoma** of the vagina accounts for 85% of vaginal carcinomas and occurs most commonly in women between the ages of 60 and 80 years. Squamous cell carcinoma is usually associated with HPV infection. Squamous cell carcinoma often metastasizes to the regional lymph nodes, and has a predilection for distant metastasis to lung and bone.

3. **Verrucous carcinoma** is a variant of squamous cell carcinoma. It is a slowly growing, well-differentiated tumor with a warty gross appearance. Microscopically, it demonstrates verruciform architecture with minimal nuclear epithelial atypia, and a pushing rather than infiltrative margin. Local excision is the treatment of choice. Local or distant metastasis is extremely rare.

4. **Clear cell adenocarcinoma** rarely occurs in women who do not have a history of DES exposure. The lifetime risk of developing clear cell carcinoma in women exposed to DES is about 0.1%, with a mean age of 20 years. In women who have not been exposed to DES, clear cell adenocarcinoma develops in the postmenopausal years around the age of 60. Patients typically present with bleeding or a grossly visible mass of the cervix or the vagina.

Histologically, clear cell carcinoma is composed of cells with pleomorphic and hyperchromatic nuclei with abundant clear cytoplasm; hobnailing is often a prominent feature. The malignant cells may form papillary or tubulocystic structures. The most common metastatic sites are the regional lymph nodes and lung.

5. **Other epithelial malignancies.** Primary adenocarcinoma of the vagina of non-clear cell type is rare; most nonclear cell adenocarcinomas represent metastasis from the endocervix or endometrium, or other sites such as the ovary, colon, or breast. The non-clear cell types of adenocarcinoma that most frequently involve the vagina include mucinous, serous, endometrioid, and adenosquamous (e-**Fig. 35.11**).

B. Mesenchymal

1. **Sarcoma botryoides** (a subtype of embryonal rhabdomyosarcoma) is the most common malignant vaginal tumor in children, usually affecting girls younger than 5 years. It is commonly located submucosally and grossly appears as grapelike clusters of tumor that fill (and in some cases protrude from) the vagina. Microscopically, the tumor is composed of cells with elongated small nuclei and a moderate amount of bright eosinophilic cytoplasm. For diagnosis, at least one microscopic field must show the malignant cells forming a condensed layer (a so-called cambium layer) beneath an intact epithelium (*Pediatr Dev Pathol* 1998;1:550). The tumor cells are immunopositive for skeletal muscle markers such as actin, desmin, MyoD1, and myogenin. Surgical excision with radiation and chemotherapy is the treatment of choice, and the prognosis is usually excellent.

2. **Leiomyosarcoma** is the most common malignant vaginal sarcoma of adults. Grossly, the tumor is typically a mass of 3 to 5 cm in maximal dimension. Microscopically, the tumor is identical to its counterparts at other sites in the female reproductive tract (e-**Fig. 35.12**) and stains positively for SMA.

The criteria for distinguishing leiomyosarcoma from smooth muscle tumors of uncertain biologic potential are not as well defined for vaginal tumors as for tumors of the myometrium. Current recommendations are that tumors larger than 3 cm in maximal dimension with an infiltrating margin, moderate to marked cytologic atypia, and ≥5 mitoses per 10 high-power fields be diagnosed as leiomyosarcoma (*Obstet Gynecol.* 1979;53:689).

C. Other Tumors

1. Malignant melanoma of the vagina is a rare tumor. It most commonly occurs in postmenopausal women in the lower third of the vagina. Grossly, it can present as a bulky mass with or without pigmentation. Microscopically, the cells have the same cytomorphology as the cells of cutaneous malignant melanoma. Immunohistochemical stains for S100, Sox10, HMB-45, Melan-A, and vimentin are positive in the malignant cells; immunostains for cytokeratin are negative. Vaginal melanomas are treated surgically; radiation and chemotherapy have not proven effective. The prognosis is very poor, and the recurrence rate is high.

2. Metastasis to the vagina from primary tumors of other sites is rare, except for vaginal recurrence of cervical or endometrial cancer which is a relatively common scenario. Other metastatic tumors to the vagina usually originate from the ovary, colon, or breast.

V. STAGING AND REPORTING OF VAGINAL CARCINOMAS. The staging of vaginal carcinomas, by both FIGO and AJCC criteria, is based on size, local extension, and lymph node metastasis. Of note, AJCC staging now recognizes lymph nodes with isolated tumor cells (Amin MB, Edge SB, Greene FL, et al., eds. *AJCC Cancer Staging Manual*. 8th ed. New York: Springer; 2017). There is no AJCC staging system for mucosal melanoma of the vagina.

Reporting of vaginal neoplasms should follow recommended guidelines (e.g., College of American Pathologists Protocol for the Examination of Specimens From Patients With Primary Carcinoma of the Vagina, available at http://www.cap.org).

ACKNOWLEDGMENT

The authors thank Rao Watson, John D. Pfeifer, and Phyllis C. Huettner, authors of the previous edition of this chapter.

36

Vulva

Tiffany Y. Chen and Ian S. Hagemann

I. **NORMAL ANATOMY.** The vulva or external female genital region encompasses the mons pubis, labia majora, labia minora, clitoris, and vestibule. The entire vulva except for the vestibule is covered by keratinized, stratified squamous epithelium. The epithelium of the vestibule is glycogenated squamous epithelium. The lateral aspects of the labia majora and the mons pubis contain hair follicles. Sebaceous glands are present in the labia majora and the perineum. The clitoris is lined by keratinizing stratified squamous epithelium overlying paired corpora cavernosa that contain vascular spaces surrounded by nerves.

The urethral meatus, major vestibular glands (Bartholin glands; e-**Fig. 36.1**), minor vestibular glands, paraurethral glands (Skene glands), and vagina all open onto the vulva. The Bartholin glands are paired glands that open posterolaterally on the hymenal ring; they are composed of acini lined by cuboidal mucus-secreting epithelium that drain into a duct that may be lined by mucus-secreting, transitional, or squamous epithelium depending on the location from deep to surface. Skene glands open on either side of the urethral meatus and are composed of acini lined by mucus-secreting epithelium that open into ducts lined by transitional epithelium.

II. **GROSS EXAMINATION, TISSUE SAMPLING, AND HISTOLOGIC SLIDE PREPARATION**

A. **Vulvar Biopsies** should be oriented as for skin biopsies (see Chapter 38) and three H&E-stained levels examined.

B. **Vulvar Resections.** It is helpful to ask the surgeon to orient the specimen with a diagram or labeled sutures so that orientation can be maintained during processing. The margins of resection should be inked and, depending on the location of the resection, the periurethral, vaginal, and perianal margins need to be noted. In cases with an obvious malignant neoplasm, one section per centimeter of tumor, including the areas closest to the deep margin, lateral margin, and/or other margins are recommended. In cases where no tumor is observed grossly, the entire specimen should be submitted. Because many gynecologic oncologists consider resection for squamous cancer in this area to be adequate only if tumor is greater than 8 mm from the margin (*Cancer* 2002;95:2331), radial rather than shave margins should be taken of all but the most obviously negative margins so that the distance from tumor to margin can be measured.

III. **DIAGNOSTIC FEATURES OF COMMON DISEASES OF THE VULVA.** Many inflammatory and neoplastic conditions that affect the skin will also affect the vulva. These are discussed in the skin chapters (Chapters 38 and 39). This section only covers those conditions for which the vulva is a common site of disease.

A. **Inflammation**

1. **Bartholin abscess** presents as a painful swelling in the area of the Bartholin gland. Microscopically, there is acute inflammation of the Bartholin duct, glands, and connective tissue, with purulent luminal contents. The etiology includes *Neisseria gonorrhea*, *Staphylococcus*, or other aerobic or anaerobic organisms. Treatment includes excision, drainage, and appropriate antibiotics.

2. **Hidradenitis suppurativa** presents as painful subcutaneous nodules in areas containing apocrine glands, particularly the vulva and axilla. Initial changes include acute and chronic inflammation around hair follicles, which progress to abscess formation, sinus tract formation, and dermal scarring (e-**Fig. 36.2**). Treatment may include laser ablation or total excision of the involved area.

3. **Crohn disease** may present as vulvar or perianal erythema, ulceration, abscesses, or fistulas between bowel and vulva, or between two different areas of vulva. Microscopically, there is acute and chronic inflammation of the deep dermis, often with associated noncaseating granulomas, fistulas, or sinus tracts (e-**Fig. 36.3**).

B. **Infection**

1. *Candida* **infection** is a chronic inflammatory condition of the vulva that is associated with diabetes, but is also seen in the general population. It often presents with pruritus and clinically shows areas of redness with thickened, edematous skin. Microscopically, there is acanthosis with acute and chronic inflammatory cells in the epithelium, and parakeratosis with neutrophils. Often fungal organisms are visible on H&E stain in the keratin layer; they are easily identified by silver stains.

2. **Syphilis** is a sexually transmitted disease caused by the spirochete *Treponema pallidum*. The primary lesion of syphilis, the chancre, develops in about half of women within 3 weeks of infection, and is characterized by one to sometimes multiple painless, clean-based ulcers. The ulcer heals in 2 to 6 weeks without a scar. Secondary syphilis develops within 6 weeks to 6 months and is characterized by the development of a rash on the palms, soles, and mucosal surfaces, as well as elevated plaques and papules (termed condylomata lata) on the vulva and mucosal surfaces.

On microscopic sections, the chancre shows epidermal ulceration, dermal acute and chronic inflammation with numerous plasma cells, and severe arteritis. Condylomata lata are characterized by marked epidermal acanthosis and hyperkeratosis, dermal inflammation with numerous plasma cells, and arteritis. The organisms may be detected by Warthin–Starry, Steiner, Dieterle, or immunostains; no organisms are seen in some cases of active infection.

3. **Human papillomavirus (HPV) infection.** Condyloma acuminatum, also referred to as a genital wart, is the result of sexually transmitted infection caused by human papilloma virus types 11 (75% of cases) or 6 (25% of cases). It presents as asymptomatic, usually multiple or confluent, papillary or papular lesions, and may occur anywhere on the vulva or perianal region.

Microscopically, condylomata of the vulva typically have a fibrovascular stalk. The epithelium exhibits acanthosis, papillomatosis, hyperkeratosis, dyskeratosis, and an accentuated granular cell layer (e-**Fig. 36.4**). Viral cytopathic effect, termed koilocytosis, takes the form of cytoplasmic clearing around enlarged nuclei with irregular nuclear outlines and clumped chromatin (e-**Fig. 36.5**). Vulvar condylomata usually follow a protracted course. They may grow rapidly during pregnancy and then regress after delivery. Small condylomas may be treated with topical agents while large ones are excised, or treated with laser ablation or cryotherapy.

4. **Herpes simplex virus (HSV).** Infection with HSV type 2, or less commonly type 1, is typically heralded by fever, dysuria, and severe pain. Painless vesicles then appear which progress to an intensely painful ulcer. The ulcer typically heals in about 2 weeks. Microscopically, epithelial ulceration is surrounded by virally infected keratinocytes that exhibit multinucleation, "ground glass" nuclear chromatin, or eosinophilic nuclear inclusions (e-**Fig. 36.6**).

5. **Molluscum contagiosum** in adults is a sexually transmitted disease caused by infection with the *Molluscum contagiosum* poxvirus. The lesions are 3- to 6-mm diameter papules with a characteristic central depression or umbilication, and are usually asymptomatic, although perianal lesions may be pruritic. Microscopic features (e-**Fig. 36.7**) include formation of a cup-shaped papule with marked epidermal acanthosis, and intracytoplasmic inclusions that are initially eosinophilic but become more basophilic as the lesion ages. Most lesions regress spontaneously.

C. **Noninfectious Squamous Lesions**

1. **Lichen sclerosus,** previously known as lichen sclerosus et atrophicus, presents as symmetric plaque-like areas of white, thinned epithelium that may be superficially ulcerated. In advanced cases there may be scarring of involved areas and stenosis of the introitus.

Microscopically, lichen sclerosus can be divided into three stages. In early stages, inflammation at the dermal–epidermal junction is only patchy. In the mid-stage, there is some epithelial atrophy, loss of rete ridges, and a band-like lymphocytic infiltrate in the upper dermis. The late stage shows a homogenous and watery superficial dermis (e-Fig. 36.8). Treatment involves high-dose corticosteroids. Postmenopausal women with lichen sclerosus have a small risk of developing differentiated VIN (see below) and squamous cell carcinoma.

2. Lichen simplex chronicus (formerly "squamous hyperplasia") typically occurs in adults and presents as a localized area of pruritus (*J Reprod Med* 2007;52:3). It is thought to be a nonspecific response triggered by a variety of irritants. Clinically, the area is white or red, with accentuated skin markings and sometimes areas of excoriation. The characteristic feature on microscopy is marked acanthosis without atypia, increased mitotic activity, inflammation, often with features that overlap other specific dermatoses (e-Fig. 36.9). Hyperkeratosis may be present. The dermis is normal. Treatment includes limiting exposure to irritants, topical corticosteroids, and antipruritic agents.

D. Cystic Lesions

1. Bartholin cyst. Obstruction of the Bartholin duct leads to the accumulation of secretions and the formation of a cystic dilatation of the duct. The epithelium lining these cysts may be squamous, transitional, or mucinous. Cysts can be treated by drainage, marsupialization, or excision of the gland.

2. Keratinous cysts (also known as epidermal inclusion cysts) occur at any age and typically affect the labia majora. They are small, measuring just a few millimeters in maximal dimension, and are filled with white cheesy material without hair. Microscopically, they are lined by stratified squamous or flattened epithelium. They can be excised if symptomatic.

3. Mucus cysts occur in the vestibule and are lined by mucinous epithelium with or without squamous metaplasia. They are probably the result of occlusion of minor vestibular glands.

IV. TUMORS. The WHO classification of tumors of the vulva is presented in Table 36.1.

A. Benign Tumors and Tumor-Like Lesions

1. Fibroepithelial polyps are also known as acrochordons or skin tags. They may be hyperpigmented, hypopigmented, or flesh-colored, and typically occur on hair-bearing skin. They usually have a papillomatous or pedunculated growth pattern and a soft cut surface. Microscopically, the epithelium may be thickened with hyperkeratosis, or may be flattened. The stroma contains loose bundles of collagen and may be edematous. Fibroepithelial polyps are clinically insignificant but can be excised if they are cosmetically unacceptable.

2. Papillary hidradenoma is a benign tumor that originates from apocrine sweat glands. It presents as a dome-shaped mass, usually less than 2 cm in diameter, arising between the labium majus and labium minus. The mass may ulcerate and bleed, but is usually asymptomatic. Microscopically, papillary hidradenoma forms tubules and acini lined by a luminal layer of epithelial cells and an outer layer of myoepithelial cells (e-Figs. 36.10 and 36.11). Cytologic atypia and mitotic activity are rare. These lesions exhibit a pseudocapsule, and caution should be exercised before interpreting compression of glandular epithelium at the periphery as invasion. Local excision is curative.

3. Granular cell tumors may be seen in many sites, but about 7% involve the vulva. They usually present as a painless, slowly growing subcutaneous mass involving the labia majora, clitoris, or mons pubis. On gross examination they are not encapsulated. Microscopically, they are composed of sheets of large cells with abundant, eosinophilic, granular cytoplasm and relatively small, uniform nuclei separated by hyalinized stroma (e-Fig. 36.12). It is important not to interpret this finding as squamous cell carcinoma on a superficial biopsy. The cytoplasm of the neoplastic cells is PAS positive and diastase resistant; immunohistochemically, the cytoplasm is positive for S-100 and myelin basic protein.

TABLE 36.1 WHO Histologic Classification of Tumors of the Vulva

Epithelial tumors

Squamous cell tumors and precursors
  Squamous intraepithelial lesions
    Low-grade squamous intraepithelial lesion
    High-grade squamous intraepithelial lesion
    Differentiated-type vulvar intraepithelial
      neoplasia
  Squamous cell carcinoma
    Keratinizing
    Nonkeratinizing
    Basaloid
    Warty
    Verrucous
  Basal cell carcinoma
  Benign squamous lesions
    Condyloma acuminatum
    Vestibular papilloma
    Seborrheic keratosis
    Keratoacanthoma

Glandular tumors
  Paget disease
  Tumors arising from Bartholin and other
    specialized anogenital glands
    Bartholin gland carcinomas
      Adenocarcinoma
      Squamous cell carcinoma
      Adenosquamous carcinoma
      Adenoid cystic carcinoma
      Transitional cell carcinoma
    Adenocarcinoma of mammary gland type
    Adenocarcinoma of Skene gland origin
    Phyllodes tumor, malignant
  Adenocarcinomas of other types
    Adenocarcinoma of sweat gland type
    Adenocarcinoma of intestinal type
  Benign tumors and cysts
    Papillary hidradenoma
    Mixed tumor
    Fibroadenoma
    Adenoma
    Adenomyoma
    Bartholin gland cyst
    Nodular Bartholin gland hyperplasia
    Other vestibular gland cysts
    Other cysts

Neuroendocrine tumors
  High-grade neuroendocrine carcinoma
    Small-cell neuroendocrine carcinoma
    Large-cell neuroendocrine carcinoma
  Merkel cell tumor

Neuroectodermal tumors

Ewing sarcoma

Soft tissue tumors

Benign tumors
  Lipoma
  Fibroepithelial stromal polyp
  Superficial angiomyxoma
  Superficial myofibroblastoma
  Cellular angiofibroma
  Angiomyofibroblastoma
  Aggressive angiomyxoma
  Leiomyoma
  Granular cell tumor
  Other benign tumors

Malignant tumors
  Rhabdomyosarcoma
    Embryonal
    Alveolar
  Leiomyosarcoma
  Epithelioid sarcoma
  Alveolar soft part sarcoma
  Other sarcomas
    Liposarcoma
    Malignant peripheral nerve sheath tumor
    Kaposi sarcoma
    Fibrosarcoma
    Dermatofibrosarcoma protuberans

Melanocytic tumors

Melanocytic nevi
  Congenital melanocytic nevus
  Acquired melanocytic nevus
  Blue nevus
  Atypical melanocytic nevus of genital type
  Dysplastic melanocytic nevus

Malignant melanoma

Germ cell tumors

Yolk sac tumor

Lymphoid and myeloid tumors

Lymphomas

Myeloid neoplasms

Secondary tumors

From Kurman RJ, Carcangiu ML, Herrington CS, Young RH, eds. *WHO Classification of Tumours of Female Reproductive Organs*. Lyon, France: IARC Press; 2017. Used with permission.

Granular cell tumor is treated with wide local excision; margins should be assessed carefully as the tumor may recur if not completely excised. Malignant granular cell tumors of the vulva are very rare and are best diagnosed in the presence of distant metastases.

4. **Leiomyomas** are the most common soft tissue tumor of the vulva. They present as painless masses. Like leiomyomata elsewhere, they are grossly well circumscribed with a firm, whorled cut surface. Microscopically, they are identical to leiomyomata in the uterus, composed of interlacing fascicles of smooth muscle cells with no atypia, necrosis, and only occasional mitotic figures. The criteria for distinguishing benign from malignant smooth muscle tumors in the vulva are not as well established as they are in the uterus. Excision is the treatment of choice.

B. Malignant Neoplasms and Their Precursors

1. **Vulvar intraepithelial neoplasia (VIN).** The usual type of VIN (u-VIN) is associated with HPV infection. A second type, differentiated VIN (d-VIN), is not caused by HPV (although HPV may sometimes be present incidentally). The salient features of these types are presented in Table 36.2 (*Crit Rev Oncol Hematol* 2008;68:131).

   a. **Usual type VIN** (u-VIN) is analogous to CIN in the cervix. It is almost always caused by high-risk HPV infection (HPV 16 most frequently). The gross appearance is variable; it usually forms discrete plaques, which may be flat, hyperkeratotic, or pigmented.

   Microscopically, u-VIN shows nuclear enlargement, irregularity, and hyperchromasia. Mitotic figures are common and are frequently atypical. The warty subtype has a growth pattern similar to a condyloma and microscopically exhibits acanthosis, hyperkeratosis, and parakeratosis; koilocytotic atypia and multinucleation are common. The basaloid subtype is usually flat without hyperkeratosis or parakeratosis; the cells are small and resemble the cells of the basal epithelium, and features of viral cytopathic effect are not prominent. Mixed types with both warty and basaloid features also occur.

   Microscopically, u-VIN can be graded according to the thickness of the dysplastic changes: VIN 1 with dysplasia limited to the lower third of the epithelium, and VIN 2 and VIN 3 with dysplasia extending into the middle and top third, respectively (e-**Figs. 36.13** and **36.14**). Based on the assumption that VIN 2 and 3 are due to high-risk HPV, p16 should be positive in these lesions and Ki-67 should show proliferation in the middle or top third of the epithelium, respectively (*Arch Pathol Lab Med* 2012;136:1266).

   b. **Differentiated VIN** (d-VIN) is much less commonly associated with high-risk HPV and is often seen in the setting of lichen sclerosus.

TABLE 36.2	Comparison of Vulvar Intraepithelial Neoplasia (VIN) Types	
	VIN, Usual Type (u-VIN)	**Differentiated VIN (d-VIN)**
Age	Younger, reproductive age	Postmenopausal
Etiology	HPV related	Not HPV related Associated with lichen sclerosus
Histology	• Easily identifiable nuclear atypia and abnormal mitoses • Viral cytopathic effect • Warty, basaloid, mixed subtypes	• More subtle nuclear atypia; abundant eosinophilic cytoplasm • No viral cytopathic effect
Grading	VIN 1, VIN 2, or VIN 3	Considered high grade
Diagnostic terms	Vulvar LSIL (for VIN 1) Vulvar HSIL (for VIN 2 or 3)	Differentiated VIN
Progression	Lower probability	Higher probability (keratinizing SCC)

Microscopically, d-VIN has subtler dysplastic changes than u-VIN. Characteristic findings include acanthosis, parakeratosis, and elongation of the rete ridges, often with keratinization at the tips of the rete. The cells do not show viral cytopathic effect, but rather have enlarged nuclei with prominent nucleoli and abundant eosinophilic cytoplasm (**e-Fig. 36.15**). Frequently there is edema between keratinocytes with prominence of the intercellular bridges. Marked atypia is characteristically seen in the basal layer, and these cells will show a mutant p53 expression pattern. d-VIN has a high risk of progression to squamous cell carcinoma. Excision is the treatment of choice.

  c. LAST/ISSVD terminology. The Lower Anogenital Squamous Terminology working group and International Society for the Study of Vulvovaginal Disease have recommended (Table 36.2) that usual VIN be diagnosed using the terms "low-grade squamous intraepithelial lesion" (LSIL; for lesions meeting VIN 1 criteria) and "high-grade squamous intraepithelial lesion" (HSIL; for lesions meeting VIN 2 or 3 criteria) (*Obstet Gynecol* 2016;127:264). The term "differentiated VIN" is recommended for that entity. Reporting vulvar LSIL as VIN is not recommended because of the potential for overtreatment.

2. Squamous cell carcinoma may be an incidental finding in a resection for VIN, may develop in the background of lichen sclerosus or an inflammatory dermatosis, or may develop in women with no history of VIN. Tumors may be exophytic, endophytic, or plaque-like and may be located anywhere on the vulva.

On microscopic examination, nests of invasive carcinoma will exhibit nuclear atypia, increased mitotic activity, and will be associated with a reactive and desmoplastic stroma. A characteristic feature is keratinization in nests deep in the stroma (**e-Fig. 36.16**). Tumors may show warty, keratinizing, verrucous, basaloid, or mixed features.

3. Melanoma, though rare, is the second most common malignancy of the vulva after squamous cell carcinoma. Common presenting symptoms include bleeding, a mass, and pain. Vulvar melanomas may be flat or polypoid, and are usually pigmented; they often have satellite lesions. Vulvar melanomas very uncommonly arise from a nevus.

The clinical and microscopic features of vulvar melanoma are the same as those of melanomas arising elsewhere (**e-Figs. 36.17** and **36.18**) and are covered in detail in Chapter 40. Important features to note are the thickness, presence or absence of ulceration, histologic pattern, degree of inflammation, presence of vascular or perineural invasion, and the presence of satellitosis. Most vulvar melanomas exhibit an acral-lentiginous pattern, but those arising on vulvar skin are more likely to be superficial spreading. Treatment is wide local excision aiming for 1 to 2 cm wide clear margins, which can be difficult to obtain in the vulva without compromising vital structures. The prognosis for vulvar melanoma is poorer than for melanoma of other skin sites.

4. Paget disease tends to affect elderly women and presents with patchy, erythematous, excoriated areas of vulvar skin and epithelium. Microscopically, the squamous epithelium is infiltrated by enlarged cells, either individually or in clusters, that hug the dermal–epidermal junction (**e-Fig. 36.19**). These cells have abundant mucinous cytoplasm, large nuclei with small nucleoli, and often form small glands within the epithelium. These Paget cells may also involve adnexal structures.

Immunohistochemistry is very helpful in distinguishing Paget disease from melanoma, which may appear morphologically similar. The neoplastic cells of Paget disease will be positive for cytokeratin (cytokeratin 7 is commonly used), but negative for HMB-45; melanoma has the opposite staining pattern.

Unlike in the breast, vulvar Paget disease does not necessarily indicate the presence of an underlying lesion. Cases of Paget disease associated with underlying carcinoma (usually vulvar adnexal adenocarcinoma, rectal adenocarcinoma, or bladder carcinoma) have a significantly worse prognosis, so careful gross and microscopic examination of excision specimens is warranted. In some cases, the Paget disease itself is the precursor lesion for an associated invasive process. Achieving and ascertaining negative margin status is a significant problem in Paget disease.

V. STAGING AND REPORTING OF VULVAR CARCINOMAS. The most recent AJCC staging of vulvar carcinomas (Amin MB, Edge SB, Greene FL, et al., eds. *AJCC Cancer Staging Manual.* 8th ed. New York: Springer; 2017) depends on size, stromal invasion, and extension beyond the vulva/perineum. Extension to adjacent structures including the lower one-third of the urethra or vagina upstages the carcinoma to T2; more distant extension is required in T3.

Important factors affecting lymph node staging include size of the metastasis, presence of extranodal extension, number of positive nodes, and ulceration of the overlying skin. The role of sentinel lymph node biopsy in the management of patients with vulvar squamous cell carcinoma continues to be evaluated (*Curr Opin Obstet Gynecol* 2004;16:65). The intensiveness of the histopathologic evaluation (including immunohistochemistry) determines the frequency at which metastases are identified, which is important since even small metastases/isolated tumor cells are associated with a small but increased risk for the presence of more extensive metastatic disease (*Curr Opin Oncol* 2010;22:481).

Melanoma of the vulva is staged according to the classification for melanoma of the skin.

Reporting of vulvar neoplasms should follow recommended guidelines (College of American Pathologists Protocol for the Examination of Specimens From Patients With Primary Carcinoma of the Vulva, available at http://www.cap.org).

ACKNOWLEDGMENT

The authors thank Danielle H. Carpenter, John D. Pfeifer, and Phyllis C. Huettner, authors of the previous edition of this chapter.

SUGGESTED READINGS

Kurman RJ, Carcangiu ML, Herrington CS, Young RH, eds. *Tumours of the Breast and Female Genital Organs.* 4th ed. Lyon, France: International Agency for Research on Cancer; 2014.
Pirog EC. Pathology of vulvar neoplasms. *Clinics Surg Pathol* 2011;4:87–111.

37

Placenta
Mai He

I. NORMAL ANATOMY. The placenta consists of three parts: fetal membranes, umbilical cord, and placental disk.

The fetal membranes insert at the edge of the disk and envelop the fetus and amniotic fluid. Microscopically, they are composed of a cuboidal amniotic epithelium with underlying connective tissue, a chorionic layer (composed of connective tissue, intermediate trophoblast, and degenerated villi), and sometimes a layer of decidua (gestational endometrium) (e-Fig. 37.1).

The umbilical cord is composed of two umbilical arteries (e-Fig. 37.2) and one umbilical vein (e-Fig. 37.3) surrounded by Wharton jelly, a paucicellular connective tissue matrix. Its outer surface is lined by a layer of cuboidal amniotic epithelium.

The placental disk is typically oval and microscopically composed of chorionic villi surrounded by maternal blood in the intervillous space. The chorionic villi contain vessels of the fetal circulatory tree embedded in mesenchymal stroma (e-Fig. 37.4). A layer of cytotrophoblast encompasses the villous stroma, and this is surrounded by a layer of syncytiotrophoblast that is in contact with the intervillous space. The maternal surface of the placental disk, which is adjacent to the uterine wall, contains variable amounts of fibrin, intermediate trophoblast, and decidua. The umbilical cord inserts near the center of the placental disk, and branches of the umbilical cord vessels arborize (with artery over vein) over the shiny fetal surface of the disk. Microscopically, the fetal surface of the disk is lined by amnion and chorion; its surface is lined by amniotic epithelium.

II. GROSS EXAMINATION, TISSUE SAMPLING, AND HISTOLOGIC SLIDE PREPARATION

A. Fetal Membranes. The fetal membranes should be assessed for completeness. The presence of green, blue, or brown staining indicating meconium or hemosiderin staining, should be noted. The membranes should be inspected for amniotic bands, nodules of amnion nodosum (see below) or squamous metaplasia, and hemorrhage. A strip of membranes should be cut from the rupture site to the disk insertion site (one end grasped by a forceps, the strip rolled around the forceps, and the roll then eased off the forceps into formalin). At least one cross-section of this membrane roll should be examined.

B. Umbilical Cord. The length of the cord should be measured, including any detached segments. The distance from the insertion to the disk edge should be measured as this gives a rough estimate of where in the uterus the placenta was implanted. Note should be made of marginal insertion (at the disk edge), or velamentous/membranous insertion (into the membranes). The coiling index of cord should be documented. Abnormalities of cord color (meconium staining) should be noted. Focal abnormalities such as stricture, hematoma, knots, nodules (e-Figs. 37.5 to 37.7), plaques, or amniotic bands should be noted and measured. Cross-sections should be made at regular intervals throughout the cord length, and the number of vessels and the presence of thrombi should be noted. At least two cross-sections of cord should be examined microscopically, avoiding the area just above the insertion site where the two umbilical arteries fuse.

C. Disk. The disk should be assessed for completeness and measured in three dimensions. After examining and removing the membranes and cord, the unfixed disk should be weighed. The fetal surface of the disk, which is covered by amnion and chorion, is examined for the same abnormalities as the membranes. The branches of the umbilical cord vessels are examined for lacerations, calcifications, and thrombi. The maternal surface of the disk is examined for retroplacental hematomas, indentations, or other focal abnormalities. The disk is then sliced at 1-cm intervals, and each slice is examined and palpated. The color, location (central vs. peripheral), size, texture (firm vs. spongy), demarcation (whether well-circumscribed or ill-defined), and a number of all focal lesions are recorded. An estimate of the percentage of the placental parenchyma involved by each type of process is noted. Any organized blood clot in the container is weighed. At least two full-thickness sections of central placenta that include fetal and maternal surfaces should be submitted, as well as sections of focal lesions.

Placental weight percentile. The percentile of the trimmed placental weight should be determined using a gestational age-specific weight chart. Small for gestational age (SGA) is defined by placental weight less than 10th percentile, appropriate for gestational age (AGA) when placental weight is between 10th and 90th percentile, and large for gestational age (LGA) when placental weight is more than 90th percentile.

D. Multiple Gestation. Placentas from twin gestations may have completely separate disks, a fused disk with two gestational sacs, or a fused disk and just one gestational sac (monoamniotic). If present, the dividing membranes should be inspected. The percentage of placental parenchyma associated with each twin should be determined. A roll of the dividing membranes should be made, as well as for the fetal membranes of each twin; at least one cross-section of the rolls should be examined microscopically to confirm the gross and ultrasound impression of chorionicity. The chorionic plate vessels should be inspected for anastomoses. In monochorionic or monoamniotic placentas, the type of anastomoses (artery to artery, artery to vein, vein to vein) should be investigated by air/ink injection and recorded, keeping in mind that arteries cross over veins. Note should be made of unpaired large vessels as these likely represent areas of physiologically important deep artery-to-vein anastomoses.

III. DIAGNOSTIC FEATURES OF COMMON DISORDERS OF THE PLACENTA

A. Fetal Membranes

1. Meconium. With recent meconium passage the fetal plate and membranes will be yellow-green and slimy. With longstanding meconium passage, the membranes, fetal plate, and even the umbilical cord will be dull brown. Microscopically, the reactive amniotic epithelium is stratified with pyknotic nuclei and cytoplasmic vacuoles. There is marked edema between the amnion and chorion. Macrophages in this area are filled with yellow-brown, waxy, meconium pigment (e-**Fig. 37.8**). Pigmented macrophages may also be seen in the chorion and decidua.

Meconium passage may be the result of neurologic maturity in the fetal intestines, but may also be associated with chronic in utero hypoxia, or stressors closer to delivery. Rarely meconium induces vascular wall necrosis in umbilical vessels.

2. Hemosiderin deposition may stain the fetal plate and membranes brown or green. Microscopically, the membranes do not show the epithelial stratification, tufting, and edema seen with meconium. Membrane macrophages contain refractile pigment that is positive with an iron stain. Sometimes a layer of hemosiderin is deposited in the basement membrane beneath the amniotic epithelium (e-**Fig. 37.9**). Diffuse chorioamniotic hemosiderosis is an indication of chronic peripheral separation (chronic abruption) or chronic bleeding, and is associated with oligohydramnios in the absence of membrane rupture, preterm delivery, and chronic lung disease.

3. Amnion nodosum forms small, gray-white, discrete nodules or plaques that may occur anywhere on the cord or fetal membranes but are most common on the fetal plate near the cord insertion. These nodules, which represent vernix caseosa, are easy to remove with a cotton swab. Microscopically they consist of fetal squamous cells, amniotic epithelial cells, and sometimes fetal hair (e-**Fig. 37.10**). Sometimes nodules of amnion nodosum become re-epithelialized by contiguous amniotic epithelium.

Amnion nodosum is the result of oligohydramnios. It therefore serves as a marker of conditions such as renal agenesis that may cause decreased fluid production, and can also alert to possible complications of oligohydramnios such as pulmonary hypoplasia and limb positioning abnormalities.

4. **Squamous metaplasia** is difficult to remove with a cotton swab. Microscopically, squamous metaplasia in the placenta is identical to that elsewhere in the body. Squamous metaplasia is not clinically significant.

5. **Amniotic bands** may appear as shredded amnion on the fetal surface of the placenta or as thin adhesion-like threads connecting one part of the fetal plate to another, connecting the fetal plate to the umbilical cord, or attached to the fetal digits or other fetal parts. Microscopically they are composed of fibrous tissue often with no attached amnion. Amniotic bands are associated with a wide variety of abnormalities in the fetus including digital amputations (**e-Fig. 37.11**), cleft lip and palate, and body-wall defects. Characteristically, the defects are asymmetric; no two cases are identical, and the spectrum of defects in any given case does not fit into a recognizable genetic syndrome. Amniotic band syndrome only extremely rarely recurs in a subsequent gestation.

6. **Fetus papyraceous.** Occasionally a mummified remnant of an embryo from much earlier in gestation will be compressed on the fetal membranes (**e-Fig. 37.12**), referred to as fetus papyraceous. It may represent an unrecognized twin gestation or may be the result of selective termination of a higher-order gestation.

B. Umbilical Cord

1. **Length abnormalities.** The normal umbilical cord is 55 to 60 cm long. Short cords (<35 to 40 cm) occur in about 5% of gestations; they are usually associated with conditions of decreased fetal movement such as amniotic bands, oligohydramnios, body-wall defects, fetal neuromuscular disorders, and arthrogryposis. Long cords (>80 cm) occur in about 5% of gestations; long cords are associated with an increased likelihood for encirclement around the fetal neck or other body part, knots, cord prolapse, and marked cord twisting.

2. **Single umbilical artery (SUA).** The incidence of SUA (**e-Fig. 37.13**) is about 1%, and SUA is about four times more common in twins. There is a strong association between SUA and congenital malformations, mortality, and low birth weight. In some cases of SUA, a small atrophic remnant of the second artery can be seen (**e-Fig. 37.14**).

3. **Abnormal cord insertion**

   a. **Marginal insertion.** In marginal insertion, the umbilical cord inserts at the edge of the disk (<1 cm from the nearest margin) (**e-Fig. 37.15**). This occurs in 6% to 18% of placentas.

   b. **Velamentous insertion.** In velamentous insertion, the umbilical cord inserts into the fetal membranes (**e-Fig. 37.16**). This insertion abnormality is seen in about 1% of placentas. In about 75% of these cases, the vessels branch within the membranes before the branches insert into the placental disk; in 25% of cases the cord vessels run through the membranes without branching. Because the branches of the umbilical cord are not protected by Wharton jelly, they are at risk for compression, thrombosis, and laceration.

4. **Umbilical cord knots.** About 1% of umbilical cords have a true knot (**e-Fig. 37.17**), which may be loose or tight. Differences in the diameter and color of the cord on either side of the knot should be noted. Cords with size differences, particularly with a dusky appearance between the knot and the fetus, are likely to be associated with an adverse outcome. The cord on either side of the knot should be examined microscopically for thrombi, a feature that suggests a clinically important knot. The knot should be untied in the fresh state to look for persistent grooving of Wharton jelly, a feature that suggests chronic tightening. The fetal mortality rate for umbilical cord knots is reported to be between 5% and 11%.

5. **Umbilical cord coiling.** The normal cord has a left-handed twist, a feature that is thought to increase turgor, preventing compression of cord vessels. A coiling index can be determined by counting the number of complete turns divided by the length of the cord (normal average 2 coils per 10 cm). Hypocoiled cords (<1 coil per 10 cm) and hypercoiled cords (>3 coils per 10 cm) have been associated with a variety of adverse outcomes.

6. Umbilical cord stricture is a focal area of cord that is markedly narrowed with a depletion of Wharton jelly, fibrosis, and often thrombosis of the umbilical cord vessels. The most common location for a stricture is the area adjacent to the umbilicus. There is a high association between cord stricture and stillbirth, especially early in gestation. Most cases also show excess twisting.

7. Umbilical cord hematomas occur once in every 5,500 deliveries, although small hematomas have been documented in 1.5% of cases following ultrasound-guided cord blood sampling. Hematomas nearly always occur in the portion of cord closest to the fetus and present as a fusiform swelling with a dark, hemorrhagic color. Large hematomas have a perinatal mortality rate of 50%, whereas small ones have very low fetal morbidity or mortality.

C. Circulatory Disorders. It is now recommended that the term **maternal vascular malperfusion (MVM)** be used instead of maternal vascular or uteroplacental underperfusion. It is also recommended that the term **fetal vascular malperfusion (FVM)** be used instead of fetal thrombotic vasculopathy (*Arch Pathol Lab Med* 2016;7:698).

1. Infarcts are firm and well circumscribed, with one edge usually abutting the maternal surface of the disk (e-**Fig. 37.18**). Early infarcts are red whereas older infarcts are white. Sometimes there is central hemorrhage. Microscopically, there is collapse of the intervillous space which crowds the villi together (e-**Fig. 37.19**). Depending on the age, the trophoblast may be pale and degenerative (recent) or show little staining with only ghost outlines of villi (longstanding).

Infarcts are common, occurring in 10% to 25% of term placentas from normal pregnancies, typically at the periphery. Extensive infarction, infarcts >3 cm, infarcts that occur in the central placenta, and infarcts in the first or second trimester of pregnancy are clinically significant and often indicate significant underlying maternal disease such as preeclampsia, collagen vascular disease, or a hereditary thrombophilic condition. Infarcts are caused by an interruption in the maternal blood supplied by a given spiral artery to an area of placental tissue.

Extensive infarction may cause fetal hypoxia, intrauterine growth restriction, periventricular leukomalacia in preterm infants, or fetal death.

2. Massive perivillous fibrin/fibrinoid deposition (MPFD). When large amounts of fibrin(oid) are deposited in the placenta, a firm, white or yellow, slightly gritty, ill-defined mass forms (e-**Fig. 37.20**). Often small pockets of red, villous tissue are interspersed within strands of white fibrin(oid). Microscopically, there is expansion of the intervillous space by eosinophilic fibrinoid material pushing the villi away from each other (e-**Fig. 37.21**); clusters of extravillous trophoblast proliferate in the fibrinoid material, and the villi entrapped in this fibrinoid material become ischemic. The amount of fibrin(oid) deposition needed for diagnosis of massive perivillous fibrin(oid) deposition or to be associated with an adverse outcome for the fetus is not well established. Some studies have found that entrapment of 20% of the central-basal terminal villi is associated with adverse outcomes (*Arch Pathol Lab Med* 1994;18:698); others have defined clinically significant fibrin deposition as fibrin extending from the fetal to maternal surface and entrapping 50% of villi on at least one slide (*Pediatr Dev Pathol* 2002;5:159). Massive perivillous fibrin(oid) is associated with intrauterine growth restriction, periventricular leukomalacia in preterm infants, and fetal death, and may recur in subsequent pregnancies.

The term maternal floor infarct is a misnomer in that it is a form of fibrin(oid) deposition, not infarction. It is defined as perivillous fibrin/fibrinoid deposition surrounding at least one-third of the villi adjacent to the basal plate, often with extension of fibrin(oid) into the underlying decidua. Maternal floor infarct is quite uncommon, seen in far fewer than 1% of placentas. It is associated with similar adverse outcomes as MPFD (Obstet Med 2018;1:17).

3. Decidual vasculopathy is abnormal or incomplete remodeling of the maternal spiral arteries. In the placentas of normal women, intermediate trophoblast remodels the intramyometrial segments of the spiral arteries late in the first trimester or early in the second trimester by replacing smooth muscle and elastic tissue with fibrinoid material, converting these vessels into flaccid tubes and thereby dramatically increasing the blood flow to the placenta; in pathologic conditions such as preeclampsia, the remodeling of these intramyometrial segments of spiral arteries does not occur. One form of decidual vasculopathy is absence of this physiologic transformation (e-Fig. 37.22); this condition can only be diagnosed in the decidual tissue adherent to the maternal surface of the placenta. A second form of decidual vasculopathy is acute atherosis; in this condition the spiral arteries exhibit fibrinoid necrosis, infiltration by lipid-laden macrophages, and often a chronic inflammatory infiltrate (e-Fig. 37.23). Vessels with acute atherosis, while already narrow, often have superimposed thrombi further reducing the blood flow through them. Acute atherosis can be diagnosed in the decidual tissue adherent to the maternal surface of the placenta but is most frequently seen in decidual spiral arteries in the membrane roll.

4. **Subchorionic fibrin deposition** is common and appears as firm, oval, tan-white, slightly raised plaques of the fetal surface of the placenta, beneath the amnion and chorion. On cut section, it is laminated and clearly beneath the membranes but above the villous tissue (e-Fig. 37.24). Microscopically, sections show layers of blood and fibrin beneath the chorion. Subchorionic fibrin plaques are not clinically significant.

5. **Retroplacental thrombohematomas** occur in about 4.5% of gestations. They are organized blood clots beneath the maternal surface of the placenta that indent the placental surface. Recent retroplacental hematomas are soft, red, easily dislodged, and are often seen in the specimen container rather than adherent to the placenta by the time the placenta arrives in the laboratory. Older hematomas are firm, brown, and densely adherent with definite placental indentation (e-Fig. 37.25). Microscopically, retroplacental hematomas consist of organized blood clot and fibrin, and the underlying placental parenchyma may be infarcted depending on how long the hematoma has been present (e-Fig. 37.26). Sometimes the villi immediately beneath the thrombohematoma exhibit villous stromal hemorrhage (intravillous hemorrhage) in which the vessels are disrupted and the stroma contains extensive red cells (e-Fig. 37.27).

   Retroplacental hematoma is an important cause of stillbirth. Although retroplacental hematoma and the clinical syndrome of placental abruption share many of the same risk factors, in only a third of cases with clinically identified abruption will a retroplacental hematoma be found on placental examination (likely associated with rapid delivery before clot can form), and in only a third of cases where retroplacental hematoma is identified on placental examination will there be a history of placental abruption (likely small and clinically insignificant).

6. **Intervillous thrombohematomas (thrombi)** are very common lesions, seen in up to 50% of normal placentas and 78% of placentas from complicated pregnancies. They are well-circumscribed, round to oval, very firm lesions with a laminated cut surface (e-Fig. 37.28). Recent intervillous thrombohematomas are red, whereas older ones are white. They are usually located midway between the fetal and maternal surfaces. Microscopically, they are composed of layers of red cells and fibrin devoid of villi. A thin rim of infarcted villous tissue may be present at their periphery.

   The blood in intervillous thrombohematomas is of both maternal and fetal origin, and so they serve as markers of fetomaternal hemorrhage. There is a very good correlation between the number of intervillous thrombohematomas in the placenta and the degree of fetomaternal hemorrhage as measured by the Kleihauer–Betke test on maternal blood. Fetomaternal hemorrhage may be associated with fetal anemia, fetal thrombocytopenia, fetal death, and maternal sensitization to fetal antigens that are not shared *(Pathol Res Pract* 2017;4:301).

7. **Subamniotic hematomas** are liquid collections of blood that pool between the amnion and chorion of the fetal plate (e-Fig. 37.29). Microscopically, they may be

difficult to demonstrate as the blood drains out once a cut is made. Subamniotic hematomas are not usually clinically significant.

8. **Marginal hematomas** occur in about 2% of placentas. They are wedge-shaped collections of blood at the margin of the placenta where the fetal membranes meet the placental disk (e-**Fig. 37.30**). Often there is blood clot beneath the free membranes in this area. Marginal hematomas are usually not clinically significant.

9. **Massive subchorial thrombosis** (Breus mole) is a very rare condition, occurring in fewer than 1 in 1,000 placentas. It is defined as a red thrombus measuring at least 1 cm in thickness immediately beneath the chorionic plate (e-**Fig. 37.31**). Microscopically, sections show an organizing blood clot. The pathogenesis of this rare condition is uncertain.

10. **Fetal thrombotic vasculopathy.** As noted above, it is now recommended to use the term **fetal vascular malperfusion (FVM)** instead of fetal thrombotic vasculopathy. Occlusion of vessels in the fetal circulatory system can involve the large umbilical cord vessels, the chorionic plate vessels, or the smaller fetal vessels within the chorionic villi. Because there is one continuous circulation between the fetus and the placenta during gestation, thrombotic lesions in the placenta, particularly when extensive, may serve as a marker for thrombotic or embolic lesions in the circulation of the fetus itself. Fetal vascular obstruction in the placenta is usually related to stasis, hypercoagulability, or vascular damage. Very often the vascular damage is associated with severe acute vasculitis of chorionic or umbilical cord fetal blood vessels. The prevalence of FVM is not known.

On gross examination, collections of avascular terminal villi appear as well-circumscribed pale areas of parenchyma of varying sizes that retain the same spongy consistency as the surrounding placental tissue (e-**Fig. 37.32**). Microscopically, these areas appear as villi with dense, eosinophilic, nearly acellular stroma with an absence of vessels (e-**Fig. 37.33**). The villi are normally spaced without collapse of the intervillous space as is seen in infarcts, a lesion with which avascular terminal villi may be confused grossly. A second pattern, formerly termed hemorrhagic endovasculitis but now referred to as villous stromal vascular karyorrhexis, is characterized by karyorrhexis of fetal cells such as endothelium, stroma, or blood cell elements (e-**Fig. 37.34**). In this pattern, the villi are more cellular than in avascular terminal villi and show degenerating fetal capillaries and fragmented red cells. Thrombosis of arterial or venous fetal blood vessels can also be seen.

Two patterns of FVM are recognized, and either may be low grade or high grade. The first is segmental FVM, indicating thrombotic occlusion of chorionic or stem villous vessels, or stem vessel obliteration. It is associated with complete obstruction to the villi downstream. The second is global FVM, indicating partially obstructed umbilical blood flow with venous ectasia, intramural fibrin deposition in large vessels, and/or small foci (five villi per focus) of avascular or karyorrhectic villi. It is associated with obstruction that is partial or intermittent even though the lesions can be distributed over much of the placenta.

11. **Chorangiomas** are placental hemangiomas. They are found in about 1% of placentas and are usually small. Typical chorangiomas are well circumscribed, red or gray, and have a firmer consistency than the surrounding parenchyma (e-**Fig. 37.35**). Sometimes fibrous septae form lobules within the chorangioma. Chorangiomas are frequently found under the chorionic plate and at the placental margins. Microscopically, chorangiomas are composed of small capillary-type vessels with a few intermixed larger vessels (e-**Fig. 37.36**). Chorangiomas do not undergo malignant transformation, and most are incidental findings with no clinical consequences. A similar villous capillary lesion is chorangiomatosis. Large or multiple chorangiomas may cause polyhydramnios, preterm delivery, antepartum bleeding, hydrops fetalis, fetal anemia or thrombocytopenia, fetal growth restriction, and cardiomegaly. Infants with placentas containing chorangiomas have a higher than expected incidence of hemangiomas elsewhere.

12. **Chorangiosis** is defined as the presence of ≥10 capillaries per terminal villus in 10 terminal villi in at least three different regions of the placenta (e-**Fig. 37.37**). Care should be taken to distinguish chorangiosis from congestion that makes the vessels appear more prominent. Chorangiosis is found in about 5% of placentas, typically at term. It is associated with congenital anomalies, maternal diabetes, maternal anemia, smoking, twin gestations, and delivery at high altitude.

D. Implantation Disorders

1. In **placenta accreta**, the placenta is abnormally adherent. On gross examination, the placenta is often severely disrupted or fragmented due to attempts to remove it manually. Sometimes thick areas of gray myometrial tissue will be visible on the maternal surface. Microscopically, the key feature is an absence of decidua between villi and myometrium (e-**Fig. 37.38**). The presence of fibrin and trophoblast between villi and myometrium is typical. Trophoblast is cytokeratin immunopositive, which is a feature that can be used to distinguish it from decidual cells of endometrial origin. Risk factors for placenta accreta include prior cesarean section with placenta previa overlying the uterine scar, and prior instrumentation.

   Placenta increta is present when villi invade into the myometrium, and transmural extension of villi with perforation is termed **placenta percreta**. All forms of implantation disorders may be associated with life-threatening hemorrhage and may require planned or emergent hysterectomy.

2. **Placenta extrachorialis.** Usually the fetal membranes insert at the edge of the disk. In placenta extrachorialis the membranes insert away from the disk edge, leaving a portion of the disk uncovered by fetal membranes. There are two types of extrachorialis, and they are best distinguished on gross examination. In circummarginate placentation, the junction between the membranes and the disk is relatively smooth and flat. In circumvallate placentation this junction forms a thick, rolled ridge (e-**Fig. 37.39**). A given placenta may exhibit partial or complete extrachorial placentation and may exhibit a combination of circummarginate and circumvallate placentation. The percentage of the disk circumference involved by each type should be recorded.

   Circummarginate placentation is not clinically significant. Complete circumvallate placentation is thought to be caused by chronic abruption or peripheral separation at the disk edge and is often associated with diffuse chorioamniotic hemosiderosis (see above).

3. **Shape abnormalities.** The placental disk is usually oval or round, but a variety of shape abnormalities may be seen, the most common or important of which follow.

   a. **Succenturiate (accessory) lobe.** In about 3% to 5% of placentas, a small portion of placenta (the succenturiate lobe) is completely separated from the main disk by membranes devoid of underlying villi. The umbilical cord almost always inserts into the main disk; the branches of the main vessels that supply the succenturiate lobe are at an increased risk of thrombotic events.

   b. **Bilobed placenta.** Occasionally the placenta will form two distinct lobes of approximately equal size, usually connected at one edge by villous tissue. The umbilical cord usually inserts between the lobes. The clinical significance of bilobed placenta, if any, has not been established.

E. Maternal Disease.

Many of the most common and clinically important maternal diseases affecting women during pregnancy have the shared feature of abnormal uteroplacental blood flow, which results in a characteristic set of changes in the placenta and significant impact on the growth of fetus.

1. **Preeclampsia** is the most common maternal disease to occur in pregnancy, complicating from 2% to 7% of all pregnancies. It is defined as the development of hypertension with proteinuria or generalized edema after 20 weeks of gestation. Eclampsia is diagnosed when seizures occur in the setting of preeclampsia. Preeclampsia is a leading cause of maternal and fetal morbidity and mortality.

   On gross examination, the placentas of preeclamptic women are often small. Decidual vasculopathy may be present (e-**Figs. 37.22** and **37.23**). The villi exhibit changes related to abnormal uteroplacental blood flow. They are small with an increased number of syncytial knots and accelerated villous maturity (hypermaturity) and exhibit a prominent cytotrophoblast layer, increased villous stroma, and a thickened trophoblastic membrane (e-**Fig. 37.40**). Placentas from preeclamptic women are more likely to have infarcts, and the infarcts are more likely to be larger and/or more numerous. There is also an increased incidence of retroplacental hematomas in the placentas of preeclamptic women.

2. **Diabetes.** The placental findings in diabetes are variable because the duration and severity of the disease are highly variable. Women with longstanding diabetes and significant vascular disease may show placental changes similar to those seen in preeclampsia. The placentas in the majority of cases, however, are larger and heavier than normal. The microscopic findings are not specific but are nonetheless characteristic. The villi are often edematous and immature for gestational age (delayed villous maturity/maturation). The cytotrophoblast is prominent. There is irregular thickening of the trophoblastic basement membrane. Chorangiosis, decidual vasculopathy, avascular terminal villi, and SUA are increased in frequency.

Women with diabetes are more likely to deliver stillborn infants or infants with malformations and/or macrosomia. There is no relationship between these adverse outcomes and the severity of the placental findings (*Placenta* 2014;12:1001).

3. **Maternal thrombophilic disorders.** There is increased interest in the relationship between hereditary thrombophilic disorders (such as protein C and S deficiency, factor V Leiden, and hyperhomocysteinemia) and pregnancy complications. Although controversial, it appears that various hereditary thrombophilic conditions, alone and in combination, are associated with an increased number and larger infarcts, acute atherosis, spiral artery thrombi, retroplacental hematomas, and fetal thrombotic vasculopathy.

4. **Sickle cell disease.** The placentas from women with sickle cell disease may be small and may have an increased number of infarcts. A characteristic finding is the presence of sickled maternal erythrocytes in the intervillous space (e-**Fig. 37.41**). Sickled maternal red cells may also be seen in the placentas of women with sickle cell trait.

F. **Multiple Gestations**
1. **Types of placentation**
   a. **Diamniotic dichorionic.** In this type of placentation, the placental disks may be completely separate or fused. Each fetus is enveloped by its own gestational sac composed of amnion and chorion. The dividing membranes are thick. Sections show amniotic epithelium from each twin with fused chorion from both twins (e-**Fig. 37.42**).

      Dizygous (fraternal) twins exhibit diamniotic dichorionic placentation, but about 25% of monozygous (identical) twins also exhibit this type of placentation if the blastocyst splits within the first 3 days postfertilization. Because diamniotic dichorionic twins do not share vascular anastomoses, these twins are the least likely to have complications such as fetal loss, preterm delivery, and twin–twin transfusion syndrome (TTTS).

   b. **Diamniotic monochorionic placentation.** In this type of placentation, the placental disks are typically fused. Each fetus is enveloped by its own gestational sac lined by amnion. A single chorionic layer surrounds both sacs so that the dividing membranes are composed of only fused amnion from each sac with no intervening chorion (e-**Fig. 37.43**).

      Twins with monochorionic placentation are monozygous. This type of placentation is seen in about 75% of monozygous twins and results when the blastocyst splits between 4 and 7 days after fertilization. Twins with monochorionic placentation usually share vascular anastomoses and are therefore at risk for complications such as fetal loss, preterm delivery, and TTTS.

   c. **Monoamniotic placentation.** In monoamniotic placentation, the twins share a gestational sac, and therefore there are no dividing membranes (e-**Fig. 37.44**).

Twins with monoamniotic placentation are monozygous, but only 1% of twins are monoamniotic. This type of placentation results when the blastocyst splits between 8 and 13 days after fertilization. Monoamniotic twins have a very high rate of complications, with only 50% surviving to term. They share vascular anastomoses, so are at risk for the associated complications noted above for monochorionic twins. In addition, because they share the same gestational sac, these twins have a high rate of umbilical cord accidents.

2. **TTTS** complicates about 15% of monochorionic twin gestations. It is the result of a chronic imbalance of blood flow across the two placental circulations. The vascular anastomoses normally seen in monochorionic placentas may be artery-to-artery, vein-to-vein, or artery-to-vein. The artery-to-vein anastomoses are usually at the capillary level and are not visible on gross examination, but are the most important physiologically as they allow blood to flow in only one direction and therefore can result in a chronic blood flow imbalance. Twins with artery-to-artery anastomoses are much less likely to develop TTTS because these anastomoses tend to cancel any circulatory imbalances that occur. Hemodynamic imbalance may also be affected by the type of cord insertion (especially a velamentous cord in the donor twin) and extensive infarction or other abnormalities of the placenta in one twin (with resultant increased placental resistance).

Often the twins are discrepant in size. The donor twin supplies blood for both twins and is hypovolemic, oliguric, and oligohydramnic. The donor twin may be anemic and hypoglycemic, with small and pale organs. The placental territory of this twin is usually large, bulky, and pale with edematous villi and increased nucleated red cells in fetal vessels. The recipient twin experiences circulatory overload resulting in polyuria, polyhydramnios, and eventually hydrops fetalis; this twin develops heart failure, hemolytic jaundice, and kernicterus, with heavy and congested organs. The placental territory of this twin is small, firm, and congested (*Pediatr Dev Pathol* 2013;4:237).

G. Infection. Intrauterine infections can have important consequences for the fetus including abortion, stillbirth, active infection after birth, and long-term sequelae such as cerebral palsy, blindness, deafness, and learning disabilities. There are two patterns of placental infection: ascending and transplacental. Ascending infections are the most common and are typically caused by bacteria. They result in inflammation of the fetal membranes (chorioamnionitis) and inflammation of the umbilical cord (funisitis). Transplacental infections are much less common and may be caused by viruses, protozoa, and some bacteria. The placenta usually shows chronic and sometimes acute inflammation within the villi (villitis). Most cases of villitis, however, do not have an infectious etiology but instead represent villitis of unknown etiology (VUE).

1. **Ascending infections** are caused by aerobic or anaerobic organisms that travel through the cervix or uterine soft tissues to the amniotic cavity. Ascending infections complicate about 4% of term deliveries but a much higher percentage of preterm deliveries. Both the mother and the fetus (after about 20 weeks) respond to the infection. Maternal neutrophils emigrate from vessels in the decidua through the chorion and eventually into the amnion (e-**Fig. 37.45**). They also marginate from the intervillous space to the subchorionic fibrin under the fetal plate of the placenta, and eventually emigrate through the chorion and amnion of the fetal plate. Fetal neutrophils emigrate from chorionic plate vessels toward the amnion. They also emigrate from the umbilical cord vessels to stroma, a process termed funisitis (e-**Fig. 37.46**). A staging and grading system has been developed to assess the extent and severity of both the maternal and fetal inflammatory response (*Pediatr Dev Pathol* 2003;6:435).

In term gestations there is a relationship between the time elapsed since membrane rupture and the likelihood of developing chorioamnionitis; in preterm gestations it is thought that the chorioamnionitis precedes and contributes to the development of membrane rupture. There is also a relationship between acute chorioamnionitis, funisitis, and adverse fetal outcome such as neonatal sepsis, neonatal pneumonia, cerebral palsy, chronic lung disease, and necrotizing enterocolitis. Some of these complications may be directly related to infection and others to the effect of prematurity, but the fetal response to infection that includes release of cytokines and other molecules (termed the Fetal Inflammatory Response Syndrome) also likely plays a role in pathogenesis. Adverse outcomes are more tightly linked to funisitis, and are greater for arteritis than phlebitis; funisitis associated with vascular thrombi has the highest complication rate of all. These associations have provided the rationale for staging and grading the inflammatory response in the fetal membranes and umbilical cord as referenced above.

2. **Transplacental infections** reach the placenta by hematogenous spread from the mother. They are usually caused by viruses or protozoa such as those of TORCH infections (*Toxoplasma gondii*, rubella, cytomegalovirus [CMV], and herpes simplex virus [HSV]), but some bacteria, most notably *Treponema pallidum* and *Listeria monocytogenes*, may also be spread transplacentally.

   The tissue response pattern to infections spread transplacentally is villitis. In cases of villitis there are usually no findings on gross examination, although occasionally small yellow nodules may be seen. Microscopically, the villi contain an inflammatory infiltrate, usually composed of only lymphocytes and histiocytes but occasionally containing plasma cells and neutrophils (e-**Fig. 37.47**). Sometimes multinucleated giant cells are seen. Villitis may be necrotizing or nonnecrotizing; necrotizing villitis, in which there is destruction of the trophoblastic membranes with fibrin deposition causing affected villi to agglutinate, is most common. This abnormal agglutination, rather than the inflammation, is the feature that is most easily recognized on low-power examination. Usually villitis is randomly distributed throughout the placenta, but sometimes villitis only involves the basal villi. There are subtle features that suggest a specific etiology in some cases; some of the most common of these are detailed below.

   a. **CMV.** On gross examination, the placenta may be small, normal, or enlarged and pale. The characteristic microscopic features are necrotizing lymphoplasmacytic villitis, villous plasma cells, stromal hemosiderin, necrotizing vasculitis, and areas of villous vessel sclerosis. Cases often show areas of active villitis as well as areas of scarred villi. In about 20% of cases, viral inclusions are seen involving the fetal capillaries, villous stromal cells, or trophoblast (e-**Fig. 37.48**). Immunohistochemistry, in situ hybridization, and polymerase chain reaction (PCR) may all be used to confirm a diagnosis of CMV in cases with a clinical suspicion or suggestive microscopic features.

      CMV infections are usually acquired in utero and are more commonly the result of a primary infection rather than reactivation of latent viral infection. Infected women are usually asymptomatic.

   b. **HSV** infections are typically acquired during delivery through an infected birth canal and therefore usually do not cause abnormalities in the placenta. Occasionally, however, the virus may be transmitted as an ascending infection, causing acute necrotizing lymphoplasmacytic chorioamnionitis with viral inclusions in the amniotic epithelium, or acute funisitis. The virus may also be transmitted hematogenously, giving rise to necrotizing or nonnecrotizing villitis. Immunohistochemistry and in situ hybridization may be helpful in confirming infection. Disseminated HSV infection may cause severe disease or death of a newborn.

   c. **Parvovirus B19.** On gross examination, the placenta is often large for gestational age and pale, as would be expected in any condition causing fetal anemia. Microscopically, the villi are edematous and there are numerous nucleated fetal red cells in the villous vessels. Many of the red cell precursors contain eosinophilic intranuclear glassy inclusions with peripheral margination of the chromatin (e-**Fig. 37.49**). Immunohistochemistry or in situ hybridization may be useful in confirming the diagnosis.

      Parvovirus causes a mild disease with a rash in children and is usually asymptomatic in adults. Pregnant women are more severely affected with a flulike syndrome and polyarthralgia; most fetuses are unaffected by maternal infection. Because red cell precursors, endothelial cells, and cardiac myocytes are specific targets for parvovirus, fetal anemia and eventual hydrops fetalis can cause fetal death.

d. Human immunodeficiency virus (HIV) is usually transmitted from mother to child at delivery or through breastfeeding in the postnatal period. Transplacental transmission is the least common method of spread. The role of the placenta in promoting or preventing the spread of HIV is unclear. There are typically no gross abnormalities. The microscopic features are not specific and are controversial.

e. Syphilis is caused by the spirochete *T. pallidum*. Placentas from cases of syphilis may be normal but are often markedly enlarged, bulky, and edematous. Microscopically, many cases show a classic triad of large, hypercellular, immature villi; villous vascular proliferation with perivascular fibroblastic proliferation and medial hypertrophy; and villitis that is usually chronic but may be acute, plasmacytic, or granulomatous. However, this triad is seen in only 43% of cases, although two of the three features is seen in another 47% of cases. In addition to the triad, some cases show necrotizing funisitis or lymphoplasmacytic deciduitis. Special stains for spirochetes may identify organisms although often the number of organisms is very low (e.g., one per slide). PCR identifies cases even when staining is negative.

f. Toxoplasmosis is caused by the protozoal organism *Toxoplasma gondii*, and the placental findings in congenital toxoplasmosis are highly variable. The placenta may be normal but is often very large and edematous. Microscopically, the villitis is subtle and nonnecrotizing or results in fibrotic villi. The inflammatory infiltrate is lymphohistiocytic. Occasionally, true granulomas are present in the inflammatory infiltrate. In addition to villitis, some cases show a plasmacytic infiltrate in the decidua, chronic chorioamnionitis and funisitis, and thrombosis and calcification of the large vessels of the chorionic plate. The encysted organism may be present in the cord, membranes, decidua, or villi but it is not associated with inflammation and is very difficult to identify. Tachyzoites released from the cysts cause marked inflammation and necrosis. Immunohistochemistry, immunofluorescence, and PCR may all aid in the diagnosis.

g. *Listeria monocytogenes.* The pathologic features of listerial infections differ in several respects from those of other transplacental infections. The placenta is typically normal on gross examination but occasional small, yellow-white microabscesses can be seen. Microabscesses, which feature an abundance of neutrophils between the villous stroma (intervillous abscess) and the trophoblast as well as extensive necrosis, are present microscopically (**e-Fig. 37.50**). Occasionally, palisaded histiocytes and multinucleated giant cells will be seen. Usually acute chorioamnionitis is also present. The organism is a small rod-shaped or curved gram-positive coccus that can be found in amniotic epithelial cells, and immunohistochemistry may be more sensitive than routine special stains for its identification.

Listeriosis can have devastating consequences for the fetus. It may cause spontaneous abortion, prematurity, neonatal sepsis, meningitis, and death. Infections at birth are typically associated with sepsis and death.

3. VUE. In most cases of villitis, an infectious etiology is not identified; these cases are referred to as **villitis of unknown etiology** or simply VUE. Serologic studies of both the infant and mother can be used to exclude many infectious causes if clinically indicated. Most cases of VUE are seen in the third trimester, and the placenta is normal on gross examination. Microscopically, about 85% of cases are very mild or mild; most are necrotizing and have a lymphohistiocytic inflammatory infiltrate. Sometimes there is vasculitis of the stem villus vessels with associated downstream avascular terminal villi (so called VUE with obliterative vasculopathy). The inflammatory cells in VUE are of maternal origin.

There are two theories about the pathogenesis of VUE. One theory proposes that VUE is a response to an unrecognized infectious agent, although many cases have been studied with increasingly sophisticated techniques and no agent has been identified. The other theory proposes that VUE is an immunologic phenomenon, specifically a host-versus-graft reaction; the maternal origin of the inflammatory cells, the tendency of VUE to recur, and the increased incidence of autoimmune diseases in the mother all support this theory.

In most cases of VUE, the fetus is unaffected. Adverse fetal outcomes in the form of intrauterine growth restriction, long-term neurologic deficits, oligohydramnios, abnormal nonstress tests, abnormal pulsed flow Doppler studies, abnormal biophysical profiles, and perinatal mortality are related to the severity of the villitis.

4. **Chronic histiocytic intervillositis.** Chronic intervillositis can be associated with adverse pregnancy outcomes and can be recurrent. Microscopically, at low power, the intervillous space has higher cellularity, which in higher power demonstrates intervillous infiltrates of histiocytes (**e-Fig. 37.51**). The diagnosis can be confirmed by CD68 immunohistochemistry (**e-Fig. 37.52**).

5. **Eosinophilic/T-cell vasculitis** may occur in a chorionic plate vessel and it consists of T lymphocytes and eosinophils (**e-Fig. 37.53**).

6. **Chronic chorioamnionitis** is the most common lesion in late spontaneous preterm birth and is characterized by the infiltration of maternal CD8+ T cells into the chorioamniotic membranes. The lesion is frequently accompanied by VUE, evidence of maternal antifetal antibodies, and deposition of complement in the umbilical vein.

7. **Chronic deciduitis** consists of the presence of severe, extensive lymphocytic infiltration with abundant plasma cells of the basal plate of the placenta. This lesion is more common in pregnancies resulting from egg donation and has been reported in a subset of patients with premature labor (**e-Fig. 37.54**).

ACKNOWLEDGMENT

The author thanks Phyllis C. Heuttner, the author of the previous edition of this chapter.

SUGGESTED READINGS

Benirschke K, Burton GJ, Baergen RN. *Pathology of the Human Placenta*. 6th ed. New York: Springer; 2012.

Khong TY, Mooney EE, Ariel I, et al. Sampling and definitions of placental lesions: Amsterdam placental workshop group consensus statement. *Arch Pathol Lab Med* 2016;7:698–713.

Skin: Nonneoplastic Dermatopathology

Margareth Pierre-Louis and Ilana S. Rosman

I. **NORMAL MICROANATOMY.** Microscopically, the skin is composed of three compartments: the epidermis (keratinizing epithelium), dermis (connective tissue matrix), and subcutis (layer of adipose tissue).

The epidermis, a stratified squamous epithelium, rests on a normally conspicuous basement membrane. The keratinocytes of the basal layer (stratum basale) have a generative function and are anchored to the basement membrane by hemidesmosomes. Immediately above the basal layer is the spinous layer (stratum spinosum), within which desmosomes—eosinophilic processes that connect adjacent keratinocytes—are visible by light microscopy. Above the spinous layer is the granular layer (stratum granulosum), which features intracytoplasmic basophilic keratohyalin granules. The granular cell layer is one to three cells thick and forms a water-tight barrier. The most mature and outermost cell layer of the epidermis, the cornified layer (stratum corneum), is composed of flat keratinocytes without nuclei. Keratinocyte transit time through all layers of the epidermis is approximately 28 days.

Cells other than keratinocytes are also present in the epidermis. Melanocytes originate in the neural crest and are normally located in the basal layer slightly beneath the basal keratinocytes. A melanocyte is histologically distinct with a rounded, hyperchromatic nucleus as compared with the more elongated nucleus of the basal keratinocyte. Melanocytes sometimes show pericytoplasmic clearing as an artifact of fixation, attributable to their lack of desmosomes. The melanocyte to basal keratinocyte ratio varies from 1:10 on the truncal skin to 1:3 on the facial skin; the ratio is affected by sun exposure. Melanocytes produce melanin, which has an ultraviolet light–protective function. Melanin is packaged in melanosomes that are exported to adjacent keratinocytes via slender, elongated dendritic processes.

Langerhans cells are suprabasal dendritic cells that function as antigen presenting cells. Langerhans cells are visible only via special stains, or in aggregates in inflammatory disorders and in Langerhans cell histiocytosis; when visible, they have characteristic reniform or coffee bean–shaped nuclei. Merkel cells, located along the stratum basale, are also histologically apparent. They have recently been determined to be derived from progenitor keratinocytes and are presumed to serve in tactile perception.

Small, slender, regularly spaced downward extensions of the epidermis (rete) divide the superficial dermis into papillae. The papillary dermis, located immediately beneath the basement membrane, is composed of fine collagen and elastic tissue fibers and contains the capillary loops of the vascular plexus. The reticular dermis, with haphazardly arranged thick collagen bundles, is separated from the papillary dermis by the superficial vascular plexus. Elastic fibers, a component of both the papillary and reticular dermis, are usually visible only with special stains.

The dermis contains adnexal structures, arrector pili muscles, nerves, and blood vessels. Adnexal structures in the skin include hair follicles, and eccrine, apocrine, and sebaceous glands. Eccrine glands develop as downgrowths of the epidermis. They are present as secretory coils in the deep dermis and have a vertically oriented duct that communicates directly through the epidermis by way of a pore (acrosyringium). Apocrine glands develop from the follicular unit and communicate to the surface via the follicular infundibulum. Like eccrine glands, apocrine glands have deep coils and vertically oriented ducts, although apocrine coils have larger central spaces and display decapitation secretions, with eosinophilic cytoplasmic apical blebs. Like apocrine glands, sebaceous glands are outgrowths of the follicular infundibula. They form lobules that connect to the follicle via a small duct and are composed of peripheral basaloid germinative cells and central mature sebocytes with vacuolated cytoplasm.

Hair follicles have varied features depending on the type of hair produced and on the phase within the hair cycle: active growth (anagen), involution (catagen), or resting (telogen). The infundibular portion of the follicle, which extends from the epidermal surface (follicular ostia) to the sebaceous duct, is histologically identical to the epidermis. The isthmus has trichilemmal keratinization and extends from the sebaceous duct to the insertion point of the arrector pili muscle (the bulge). The lower segment of the follicle extends from the bulge to the bulb.

Terminal anagen hair follicles extend into the subcutis, while the bulbs of vellus hairs sit within the reticular dermis. Miniaturized hairs appear similar to vellus hairs with a thin hair shaft, but also leave a fibrous streamer (stela) within the deep dermis and subcutis. On horizontal sections, telogen follicles have basophilic stellate epithelium while catagen follicles have an eosinophilic corrugated center with numerous apoptotic cells in the outer root sheath (e-**Fig. 38.1A,B**). Both telogen and catagen hairs leave stelae as they involute. In a 4-mm punch biopsy of normal scalp sectioned horizontally, there are approximately 35 follicles in Caucasians, 20 follicles in African Americans, and 15 follicles in Asians. The normal telogen count (telogen and catagen follicles divided by total hair count) is approximately 10% to 15%.

The subcutis is composed of mature adipose tissue separated into lobules by fibrous septa. A fully lipidized adipocyte has a crescentic, barely visible nucleus that is displaced to the periphery of the cell by the accumulated lipid. The deep vascular plexus separates the subcutis from the reticular dermis.

II. COMMON DESCRIPTIVE TERMS

A. Acantholysis—Loss of attachment(s) between keratinocytes (e-**Fig. 38.2**).

B. Acanthosis—Thickening of the epidermis or epidermal hyperplasia (e-**Fig. 38.3**).

C. Bulla—Fluid-containing space in the epidermis, greater than 1 cm in size.

D. Dyskeratosis—Abnormal keratinization that results in altered eosinophilic cytoplasm (e-**Fig. 38.4**).

E. Epidermotropism—Migration of malignant cells into the epidermis (e-**Fig. 38.5**).

F. Exocytosis—Migration of benign inflammatory cells into the epidermis, commonly seen in association with spongiosis (e-**Fig. 38.6**).

G. Hypergranulosis—Thickening of the granular layer (e-**Fig. 38.7**).

H. Hyperkeratosis—Thickening of the stratum corneum.

I. Orthokeratosis—Mature stratum corneum composed of superficial keratinocytes without nuclei. Basket-weave pattern on nonacral skin; densely compact on acral skin (e-**Fig. 38.8**).

J. Parakeratosis—Abnormally retained keratinocyte nuclei in the stratum corneum (e-**Fig. 38.9**).

K. Spongiosis—Fluid/edema-creating space between adjacent keratinocytes in the stratum spinosum (e-**Fig. 38.10**).

L. Vacuolar alteration—Clearing of basal keratinocyte cytoplasm secondary to inflammation, leaving a "bubbly" appearance at the dermoepidermal junction (e-**Fig. 38.11**).

Punch biopsy

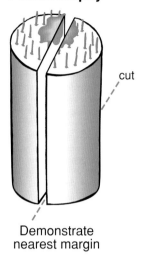

cut

Demonstrate
nearest margin

Figure 38.1 Gross processing of a punch biopsy.

III. GROSS EXAMINATION AND TISSUE SAMPLING. The skin biopsy/excision is generally received in the laboratory in a fixative such as 10% formalin. Specimens for direct immunofluorescence (DIF) should be submitted in Michel's medium. The gross description should include the tissue size in centimeters (length × width × thickness), presence or absence of epidermis, color, presence or absence of hairs, and alterations to the epidermal surface (including dimensions, color, and distance to the nearest margin for discrete lesions). All surfaces, except the epidermis, must be inked prior to sectioning; two or more colors is required if orientation for specific margin identification is provided.

Shave or punch biopsies with a greatest epidermal dimension of less than 0.3 cm are submitted for processing without sectioning. Specimens with a greatest epidermal measurement of at least 0.4 cm are sectioned vertically through the epidermis resulting in pieces of relatively uniform thickness (approximately 0.2- to 0.3-cm thick) (Figs. 38.1 and 38.2). Most punch biopsies received in dermatopathology are 4 mm in diameter and should be bisected vertically. As seen in Figure 38.1, if an epidermal lesion is present, sectioning that will best represent the lesion and its relationship to the nearest margin is optimal. Biopsy

Shave biopsy

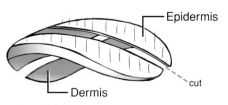

Epidermis

cut

Dermis

Figure 38.2 Gross processing of a shave biopsy.

Punch biopsy
for alopecia

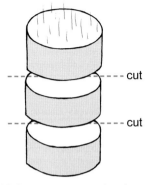

- - - - - cut

- - - - - cut

Figure 38.3 Gross processing of an alopecia biopsy.

tissue is otherwise sectioned along the longest epidermal axis. Sponges can help prevent distortion of the tissue during processing.

Punch biopsies of the scalp for the evaluation of alopecia are sectioned horizontally to permit evaluation of follicular density and architecture at various tissue levels (Fig. 38.3). The 4-mm punch biopsy is considered standard for evaluating alopecia. The specimen is bisected horizontally at the level of the dermis–subcutis junction and the two pieces of tissue are placed cut-side down in the tissue cassette and subsequently embedded with this orientation. If embedded and sectioned appropriately, the superficial sections include a peripheral rim of epidermis. Ten levels should be cut with a PAS stain performed on the last section. Additional sectioning can be performed if all elements of the follicular architecture are not visualized. If two biopsies of the scalp are received for the same condition, one may be processed as a typical punch biopsy (vertically bisected).

For elliptical excisions, if the ellipse is oriented by a suture or any other means, inks of different colors are applied to the two long margins to allow specific margin identification. Sections of an ellipse should be taken at regular intervals of 2 to 3 mm to allow a reasonable assessment of the true margin. Laboratories vary in their handling of the tip ends of ellipses; the recommended method is illustrated in Figure 38.4.

Frozen sections may be helpful in evaluating margins of cutaneous carcinomas; however, frozen sections are never indicated for melanocytic neoplasms as they may compromise diagnosis based on subsequent permanent sections.

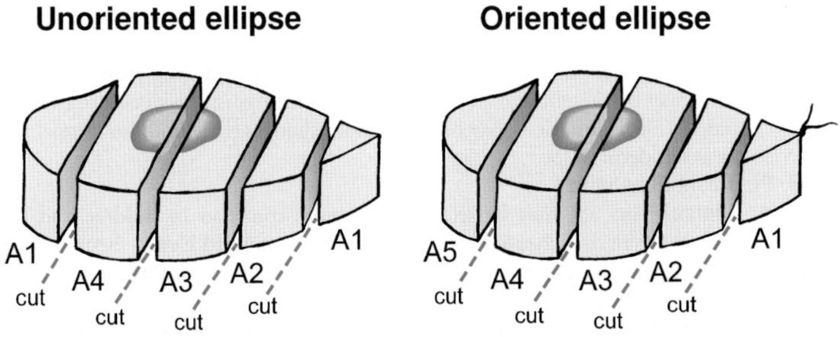

Unoriented ellipse

A1
cut
A4
cut
A3
cut
A2
cut
A1

Oriented ellipse

A5
cut
A4
cut
A3
cut
A2
cut
A1

Figure 38.4 Gross processing of an elliptical excision specimen.

IV. INFLAMMATORY DERMATOSES

A. **Lichenoid/Interface:** Characterized by basal keratinocyte damage with vacuolar alteration, dyskeratosis, and pigment incontinence (interface) or an additional band of lymphocytes in the upper dermis that obscures the dermoepidermal junction (lichenoid).

1. **Lichen planus**
   a. **Clinical:** Violaceous, flat-topped, pruritic papules, and plaques. Most common in adults; can involve the skin, hair, nails, and mucous membranes.
   b. **Microscopic:** Compact orthohyperkeratosis, irregular acanthosis, alternating wedge-shaped hypergranulosis and hypogranulosis, obscuring band of lymphocytes at the dermoepidermal junction, dyskeratotic keratinocytes in and under the epidermis, rete with a "saw-tooth" pattern, melanophages in the superficial dermis (e-Fig. 38.12).

2. **Erythema multiforme (EM)/Stevens–Johnson syndrome (SJS)/toxic epidermal necrolysis (TEN)**
   a. **Clinical:** EM—symmetric, targetoid lesions on palms and soles and sometimes mucosa; associated with multiple triggers (recurrent herpes simplex virus [HSV], mycoplasma infection). SJS and TEN—cutaneous erythematous lesions associated with mucosal ulcerations and cutaneous sloughing, typically triggered by medications. SJS involves <10% of the body surface area (BSA); TEN >30% BSA.
   b. **Microscopic:** Vacuolar alteration, aggregates of dyskeratotic keratinocytes throughout the epidermis, possible subepidermal bulla with full-thickness epidermal necrosis, variable perivascular lymphocytic inflammation with or without eosinophils (e-Fig. 38.13).

3. **Lupus erythematosus**
   a. **Clinical:** May involve the skin only and/or multiple other organ systems; clinical lesions vary based on the type of cutaneous lupus. Acute—associated with systemic lupus; erythematous "butterfly" rash on the central face. Subacute—annular, erythematous lesions with scale on sun-exposed skin. Discoid (chronic)—hyperpigmented, atrophic plaques with scarring on face, ears, and scalp (with associated alopecia).
   b. **Microscopic:** Features vary based on the type of cutaneous lupus, but most have interface dermatitis, often also with superficial lymphoplasmacytic inflammation, deep perivascular and periadnexal lymphoplasmacytic inflammation, and increased dermal mucin (e-Fig. 38.14). Additional studies may be helpful: PAS for basement membrane thickening, colloidal iron for mucin, CD123 to highlight sheets of plasmacytoid dendritic cells within the infiltrate. DIF of well-established lesions shows granular IgG, IgM, and/or C3 deposition at the basement membrane.

4. **Graft versus host disease (GVHD)**
   a. **Clinical:** Acute—morbilliform eruption with sudden onset that favors acral sites and often occurs before gastrointestinal/hepatic manifestations. Chronic—may resemble lichen planus (lichenoid GVHD) or morphea (sclerodermoid GVHD).
   b. **Microscopic:** Acute—interface dermatitis associated with sparse lymphocytes (satellite cell necrosis) (e-Fig. 38.15). Findings are often subtle and may be indistinguishable from changes seen in response to marrow engraftment (cutaneous eruption of lymphocyte recovery), viral exanthema, and drug eruptions. Eosinophils may be present and do not necessarily distinguish between drug eruptions and GVHD. Chronic—may have lichenoid changes (lichenoid) or dermal sclerosis (sclerodermoid).

5. **Pityriasis lichenoides**
   a. **Clinical:** Any age may be affected, but more common in children and young adults. Pityriasis lichenoides et varioliformis acuta (PLEVA)—hemorrhagic or crusted papules, rarely associated with systemic symptoms. Pityriasis lichenoides chronica (PLC)—small, scaly, red-brown thin papules.
   b. **Microscopic:** Mild spongiosis with variable vacuolar alteration and inflammation. PLEVA—wedge-shaped lymphocytic infiltrate, extravasated erythrocytes,

dyskeratoses within the upper epidermis (**e-Fig. 38.16A**). PLC—parakeratosis, sparse perivascular lymphocytic infiltrate; features subtler than in PLEVA (**e-Fig. 38.16B**).

B. **Psoriasiform:** Characterized by regular elongation of the rete.

1. **Psoriasis**

   a. **Clinical:** Vulgaris—most common presentation with symmetric, erythematous plaques with thick, white, or silvery scale on the extensor surfaces (knees, elbows); may have scalp involvement with well-demarcated scaly plaques; nails may demonstrate oil spots, pitting, and ridging. Guttate—acute with multiple drop-like, mildly scaly, erythematous papules. Pustular—erythematous plaques studded with pustules.

   b. **Microscopic:** Vulgaris—confluent parakeratosis, absent granular cell layer, regular elongation of the rete, neutrophils in the stratum corneum (Munro microabscess) and stratum spinosum (spongiform pustule of Kogoj), widely dilated papillary dermal vessels, thinning of the suprapapillary plates, increased suprabasal keratinocyte mitoses, and sparse superficial lymphocytic infiltrate (**e-Fig. 38.17A,B**). Guttate—mounds of parakeratosis with neutrophils; often with spongiosis and without fully developed psoriasiform hyperplasia. Pustular—subcorneal and spongiform collections of neutrophils with mild epidermal hyperplasia; may have rare eosinophils. Pre-treatment biopsy often associated with altered features.

2. **Lichen simplex chronicus (LSC)**

   a. **Clinical:** Thick, hyperkeratotic plaques caused by chronic rubbing or scratching.

   b. **Microscopic:** Compact hyperorthokeratosis, hypergranulosis, thick and elongated rete with dermal fibrosis (**e-Fig. 38.18**). Apparent acral-type epidermis with the presence of hair follicles suggestive of LSC ("hairy palm" sign).

3. **Other:** Psoriasiform hyperplasia may be seen in chronic spongiotic dermatitis, dermatophytosis, pityriasis rubra pilaris, prurigo nodularis and mycosis fungoides.

C. **Spongiotic**

1. **Eczema/atopic dermatitis/allergic or irritant contact dermatitis**

   a. **Clinical:** Erythematous, scaly patches or plaques; age/gender and distribution vary with inciting agent. Atopic dermatitis in children classically periflexural.

   b. **Microscopic:** May have acute, subacute, or chronic spongiotic changes. Acute—intraepidermal spongiotic vesicles, minimal parakeratosis, often with numerous eosinophils within dermis (**e-Fig. 38.19A**). Subacute—parakeratosis, irregular epidermal hyperplasia (**e-Fig. 38.19B**). Chronic—mild spongiosis, psoriasiform hyperplasia, compact ortho- and parakeratosis. PAS should be performed to exclude dermatophytosis in any spongiotic dermatitis.

2. **Pityriasis rosea**

   a. **Clinical:** Scaly erythematous plaques in "Christmas tree–like" pattern on the trunk; self-limited eruption lasting approximately 8 weeks.

   b. **Microscopic:** Mounds of parakeratosis, irregular acanthosis, spongiosis, and mild superficial perivascular lymphocytic infiltrate with extravasated erythrocytes (**e-Fig. 38.20**). May have prominent lymphocyte exocytosis.

3. **Eosinophilic spongiosis**

   a. **Clinical:** Varied, depending on the etiology. Etiologies include allergic contact dermatitis, arthropod-bite reactions, early pemphigus or pemphigoid, and the first stage of incontinentia pigmenti.

   b. **Microscopic:** Variable spongiosis with exocytosis of eosinophils (**e-Fig. 38.21**).

4. **Other:** Spongiosis may be seen in scabies, drug eruptions, early and partially treated psoriasis, and mycosis fungoides.

D. **Vesiculobullous:** Characterized by a vesicle or bulla.

1. **Bullous pemphigoid**

   a. **Clinical:** Tense blisters on an erythematous base more common in elderly; often pruritic. A variant, pemphigoid gestationis, occurs in pregnancy and postpartum period. Cicatricial pemphigoid is a closely related disease with mucosal involvement and scarring (*Autoimmun Rev* 2017;16:445).

b. Microscopic: Subepidermal bulla with eosinophils in the blister cavity and/or in the dermis (**e-Fig. 38.22**). A variant without significant inflammation also occurs. DIF shows diffuse linear deposition of C3 and IgG (C3>IgG) at the basement membrane zone. ELISA studies for autoantibodies to bullous pemphigoid antigens (BP180, BP230) have largely supplanted indirect immunofluorescence (IIF) for diagnosis and to follow treatment response.

2. Superficial pemphigus (foliaceus, vulgaris)

a. Clinical: Flaccid bullae that extend easily with lateral pressure. Cutaneous erosions only in pemphigus foliaceus; oral erosions additionally present in pemphigus vulgaris (*Nat Rev Dis Primers* 2017;11;3:17026; *Clin Rev Allergy Immunol* 2018;54:36).

b. Microscopic: Subcorneal (foliaceus) or suprabasal (vulgaris) vesiculation with acantholysis and variable inflammation, typically neutrophils and/or eosinophils (**e-Fig. 38.23A,B**). DIF shows intercellular IgG and C3. ELISA studies for autoantibodies to desmoglein 1 (foliaceus) or 3 (vulgaris) have largely supplanted IIF for diagnosis and to follow treatment response.

3. Porphyria cutanea tarda

a. Clinical: Blistering of sun-exposed skin, especially dorsal hands with scarring and milia (small subepidermal cysts).

b. Microscopic: Pauci-inflammatory subepidermal bulla on acral skin. Dermal papillae extend into the blister floor (festooning) (**e-Fig. 38.24**). DIF may show deposition of C3, immunoglobulins, and/or fibrin at the basement membrane zone and within superficial dermal blood vessel walls. Pseudoporphyria has identical histologic and immunofluorescent findings (*F1000Res* 2017;6:1906).

4. Dermatitis herpetiformis

a. Clinical: Highly pruritic vesicles and excoriations on symmetric extensor surfaces (elbows, knees, and buttocks) associated with gluten-sensitive enteropathy.

b. Microscopic: Neutrophils in the dermal papillae with small subepidermal clefts (papillary dermal microabscesses) (**e-Fig. 38.25**). DIF shows granular IgA at the dermal papillae (*Clin Dermatol* 2012;30:56).

E. Granulomatous: Characterized by a variable number and arrangement of histiocytes with or without lymphocytes (*Semin Diagn Pathol* 2017;34:301; *Clin Rev Allergy Immunol* 2018;54:131).

1. Granuloma annulare

a. Clinical: Localized or generalized, annular and erythematous papules, plaques or patches, or subcutaneous nodules.

b. Microscopic: Histiocytes palisading around altered eosinophilic or basophilic dermal collagen with increased interstitial mucin; often with associated perivascular lymphocytic infiltrate (**e-Fig. 38.26A,B**).

2. Necrobiosis lipoidica

a. Clinical: Chronic plaque with depressed yellow/orange center and raised erythematous or hyperpigmented border; usually pretibial. May be associated with diabetes.

b. Microscopic: Horizontal layers of fibrotic dermal collagen alternating with zones of histiocytes and admixed plasma cells. Infiltrate may extend into the subcutis (**e-Fig. 38.27**).

3. Sarcoidosis

a. Clinical: Highly variable; annular lesions, areas of hypopigmentation, ichthyosis-like changes, alopecia, subcutaneous nodules, and/or nonspecific reactions such as erythema nodosum. Predilection for areas of cutaneous injury, such as scars and tattoos. Up to one-third of patients with systemic sarcoidosis have skin lesions. Also seen with oncologic immune modulators (*Curr Opin Pulm Med* 2017;23:492).

b. Microscopic: Noncaseating granulomas with tight aggregates of histiocytes without significant inflammation (**e-Fig. 38.28**). Presence of polarizable foreign material does not reliably distinguish between sarcoidosis and foreign-body reaction. Special stains should be performed to exclude infection.

F. Vascular Disease: Characterized by damaged/incompetent endothelial cells.

1. Leukocytoclastic vasculitis

    a. Clinical: Palpable purpura, generally on the extremities. Clinical variants include Henoch–Schönlein purpura, acute hemorrhagic edema of childhood, urticarial vasculitis, and mixed cryoglobulinemia (*Curr Opin Rheumatol* 2017;29:39).

    b. Microscopic: Involves the vessels at the interface of the papillary and reticular dermis (superficial vascular plexus) with perivascular neutrophils, nuclear debris (leukocytoclasia or karyorrhexis), fibrinoid necrosis of the vessel walls, and extravasation of erythrocytes (e-**Fig. 38.29**). DIF may be positive for immunoglobulins and C3 within vessel walls. In Henoch–Schönlein purpura (IgA vasculitis) there is deposition of IgA within vessel walls (*Am J Dermatopathol* 2018;40:661).

2. Occlusive vasculopathy

    a. Clinical: Varied presentations include purpura, livedo reticularis, and ulcers.

    b. Microscopic: Occlusion of any of the vessels in the cutaneous vasculature with fibrin thrombi (coumadin necrosis, heparin necrosis, disseminated intravascular coagulation, thrombotic thrombocytopenic purpura, heritable disorders of coagulation) or amorphous eosinophilic material (essential cryoglobulinemia). Cholesterol emboli may be seen after instrumentation. Vascular calcification can lead to vascular occlusion if extreme (calciphylaxis).

3. Neutrophilic dermatoses

    a. Clinical: Includes several entities often reactive to underlying systemic disease (often malignancy or autoimmune disorder). Sweet syndrome—abrupt onset of erythematous to dusky nodules and plaques with fever and leukocytosis; up to 20% associated with underlying malignancy, typically hematogenous. Pyoderma gangrenosum—clean-based ulcers with violaceous undermined borders; associated with pathergy (spread of lesion or new lesion occurring after trauma, instrumentation, or debridement); more than half of affected patients have underlying systemic disease including inflammatory bowel disease and hematologic disorders (*J Am Acad Dermatol* 2018;79:987; *ibid* 2018;79:1009).

    b. Microscopic: Diffuse dermal infiltrate of neutrophils. Sweet syndrome—infiltrate in superficial dermis associated with marked subepidermal edema, neutrophilic debris (leukocytoclasia), and sometimes secondary vasculitis (e-**Fig. 38.30**). Pyoderma gangrenosum—ulcerated epidermis; infiltrate may extend deeper into dermis and/or subcutis; may have granulomatous features; special stains should be performed to exclude infection.

4. Urticaria

    a. Clinical: Pruritic wheals (edematous papulonodules) that last less than 24 hours. Persistence for more than 24 hours, burning rather than itching, and resolution of lesions with purpuric macules suggestive of urticarial vasculitis.

    b. Microscopic: May appear histologically normal at low power. Sparse perivascular and interstitial infiltrate; predominant cell type is neutrophil and/or eosinophil (e-**Fig. 38.31**). No associated necrosis or vasculitis. Dermal edema may be noted, and there may be neutrophils in the vascular lumina (*Immunol Allergy Clin North Am* 2014;34:1).

5. Pigmented purpuric dermatosis (capillaritis)

    a. Clinical: Multiple clinical variants, most common: Schamberg disease—numerous pinpoint red-brown macules ("cayenne pepper") sprinkled on lower extremities, usually self-limited and asymptomatic; lichen aureus—solitary or multiple golden-brown patches on the trunk or extremities.

    b. Microscopic: Lymphocytes surrounding superficial dermal capillaries; scattered extravasated erythrocytes and siderophages, which can be highlighted by Perls iron stain (e-**Fig. 38.32**). Some vacuolar alteration may be present.

G. Panniculitis: Characterized by inflammatory changes to the septae or lobules of the subcutaneous adipose tissue.

1. **Erythema nodosum (septal)**
   a. **Clinical:** Single or multiple painful erythematous nodules on shins, although other sites can be involved; predilection for young adults. Associated with multiple systemic diseases and medications, including inflammatory bowel disease, sarcoidosis, leukemia/lymphoma, antibiotics, salicylates, and oral contraceptives.
   b. **Microscopic:** Inflammation and fibrosis of the septae with relative sparing of lobules; neutrophils and edema in early lesions with variable lymphocytes, multinucleate giant cells, histiocytes, and eosinophils with associated fibrosis in later lesions (e-**Fig. 38.33**) (*J Clin Pathol* 2015;68:954; *Dermatol Online J* 2014;16:22376).

2. **Erythema induratum/nodular vasculitis (lobular)**
   a. **Clinical:** Single or multiple erythematous nodules on the posterior lower leg/calf; any age/gender can be affected.
   b. **Microscopic:** Lobular infiltrate of histiocytes in well- to poorly formed granulomas; lymphocytes, neutrophils, and plasma cells may also be present. Vasculitis variably present with mixed inflammation and necrotizing changes (e-**Fig. 38.34A,B**).

3. **Calcifying panniculitis/calciphylaxis (lobular)**
   a. **Clinical:** Depends on underlying systemic pathology including disorders of coagulation, peripheral vascular disease, localized trauma/inflammation, and calciphylaxis of renal failure. Typically subcutaneous firm nodules on the buttocks and thighs that ulcerate (*J Cutan Med Surg* 2017;21:425; *Am J Dermatopathol* 2017;39:795).
   b. **Microscopic:** Stippled basophilic calcium deposits in and around small vessels within the adipose tissue, with lipophages; variable inflammation.

4. **Lipodermatosclerosis (lobular)**
   a. **Clinical:** Indurated erythematous or hyperpigmented plaques on the inferior lower extremities.
   b. **Microscopic:** Variably sized cysts within the fat lobules that have a complex eosinophilic cuticle with frond-like excrescences (arabesque or membranous lipodystrophy); minimal/no inflammatory response; septal fibrosis and thickening (e-**Fig. 38.35**).

V. COMMON CUTANEOUS INFECTIONS
A. Viral

1. **Molluscum contagiosum**
   a. **Clinical:** Single to multiple, 1 to 2 mm, dome-shaped, umbilicated papules, most common in healthy children and young adults. Atypical clinical presentations in immunosuppressed patients.
   b. **Microscopic:** Exo/endophytic, acanthotic, and papillomatous epidermis, with classic homogeneous eosinophilic cytoplasmic inclusions (Henderson–Patterson bodies) that displace and compress keratinocyte nuclei into peripheral crescents; keratinocyte cytoplasm has violaceous hue (e-**Fig. 38.36**).

2. **Verruca**
   a. **Clinical:** Single to multiple, hyperkeratotic (verrucous) lesions. Vulgaris—common in school-aged children and immunosuppressed patients; often on digits. Plana—flat-topped papules. May spread to adjacent skin by trauma such as scratching or shaving (*Acta Dermatoven APA* 2011;20:145).
   b. **Microscopic:** Vulgaris—compact hyperorthokeratosis with parakeratosis at the peaks of a papillomatous epidermis; hypergranulosis due to increased number and size of irregular keratohyalin granules (viral keratohyalin); keratinocytes with large irregular hyperchromatic nuclei with conspicuous perinuclear halo (koilocytes); elongated rete that bow inward toward the center of the lesion (e-**Fig. 38.37A,B**). Multiple large irregular eosinophilic cytoplasmic inclusions in some forms of palmoplantar verrucae (myrmecial) (e-**Fig. 38.38A,B**). Plana—mild hyperorthokeratosis (basket weave), hypergranulosis/viral keratohyalin, scattered koilocytes, epidermal acanthosis with a flat surface and base (e-**Fig. 38.39**).

3. Condyloma acuminatum
  a. **Clinical:** Single or multiple, skin-colored, verrucous papules/plaques on external genitalia, perineum, and/or near the anus (*Best Pract Res Clin Obstet Gynecol* 2014;28:1063).
  b. **Microscopic:** Variable parakeratosis with compact orthokeratosis, acanthosis with mild papillomatosis, viral keratohyalin, and koilocytes in varying amounts (often less conspicuous than in verruca) (e-**Fig. 38.40**). If there is keratinocyte dysplasia/dysmaturation, testing for high risk human papillomavirus (HPV) serotypes (16 and 18) can be performed. Striking cytologic atypia can also be incited by topical treatment with agents such as podophyllin.

4. Herpes (herpes simplex virus [HSV]/varicella zoster virus [VZV])
  a. **Clinical:** Primary herpes simplex—painful, grouped vesicles on an erythematous base that ulcerate. Primary varicella—vesicles on an erythematous base following a 1- to 2-day prodrome. Lesions appear in crops, crust in less than 24 hours. Most common in children. Recurrent varicella (zoster)—grouped vesicles on an erythematous base in a dermatomal distribution (may be generalized in immuno-suppressed patients); typically preceded by pain or tingling.
  b. **Microscopic:** Intraepidermal vesicle with ballooning and reticular degeneration and acantholysis; variable inflammation with lichenoid changes, neutrophils and/or eosinophils; viral cytopathic change of affected keratinocytes with multinucleation, margination of chromatin, and molding of nuclei (e-**Fig. 38.41A,B**). Changes may be restricted to the follicular epithelium. In older lesions, "ghosts" of multinucleated keratinocytes are present within an inflammatory scale crust. Immunohistochemical stains are available to distinguish between HSVI, HSVII, and VZV.

B. **Fungal:** The most common fungal organism present on the surface of the skin is the yeast form of *Malassezia* sp. (*Pityrosporum*). These small ovoid forms in the stratum corneum are typically incidental and usually not reported. If they are present deep to follicular infundibulum and associated with inflammation and/or follicular rupture, consider *Pityrosporum* folliculitis.

1. Dermatophytosis (tinea)
  a. **Clinical:** Annular scaly erythematous plaques on the body (corporis), face (faciei), feet (pedis), or associated with alopecia on the scalp (capitis) or beard (barbae). Thickened and/or discolored nails (onychomycosis).
  b. **Microscopic:** Fungal hyphae within the stratum corneum and/or follicular epithelium/infundibulum, sometimes visible without the use of special stains such as Gomori methenamine silver (GMS)/PAS. All other changes highly variable, including parakeratosis, intracorneal neutrophils, and dermal inflammation (e-**Fig. 38.42A,B**). Clippings of nails for evaluation of fungus are processed after softening in a phenol solution (such as a depilatory) and should always be stained for organisms since hyphae are usually invisible without special stains.

2. Angioinvasive fungus
  a. **Clinical:** Necrotic papules/plaques in severely immunosuppressed patients; frequently with systemic symptoms. Common causative organisms include *Aspergillus*, *Fusarium*, and *Zygomycetes*; culture needed to definitively speciate.
  b. **Microscopic:** Ischemic necrosis of the epidermis and/or dermis; extravasation of erythrocytes; fungal hyphae present in mid to deep dermal blood vessels of all sizes with extension through the vascular wall; inflammation type and amount variable and may be absent (e-**Fig. 38.43**).

3. Traumatically implanted fungus/dematiaceous fungus
  a. **Clinical:** Variable, from scaly and erythematous, to nodular and verrucous; often at sites of trauma or implantation of vegetable matter, may see foreign material such as a wood splinter. Verrucous lesions are common in chromomycosis; draining sinuses in mycetoma.
  b. **Microscopic:** Pseudocarcinomatous epidermal hyperplasia and/or ulceration; mixed acute, chronic, and granulomatous inflammation (e-**Fig. 38.44A**); brown/

golden hyphae and spore forms (Medlar bodies or "copper pennies") can be seen depending on the organism (e-**Fig. 38.44B**).

4. Other fungal: Many fungal organisms can cause skin infections with variable presentations in immunocompetent and immunocompromised patients. Granulomatous inflammation, pseudoepitheliomatous hyperplasia, and/or parasitized macrophages are histologic clues to deep fungal infection; GMS should be performed in these settings. Blastomycosis presents with budding yeasts; histoplasmosis with small yeasts, often with a clear halo, within parasitized macrophages.

C. Bacterial

1. Impetigo

a. Clinical: Honey-colored crusted papules and plaques, often around the nose and mouth in children. Bullous form mimics other blistering disorders with flaccid bullae and erosions usually caused by *Staphylococcus aureus* or *Streptococcus pyogenes.*

b. Microscopic: Gram-positive cocci and numerous neutrophils within the stratum corneum and superficial epidermis or within subcorneal vesicles in bullous impetigo.

2. Staphylococcal scalded skin syndrome

a. Clinical: Flaccid bullae and erosions, painful erythema often in perioral, genital, and intertriginous areas with crusting, fissuring, and desquamation. No involvement of mucous membranes. Typically in children under 6 years old, but also in patients with renal failure and caused by epidermolytic toxins released by *S. aureus.*

b. Microscopic: Subcorneal bulla formed by acantholysis with minimal inflammation and no organisms (e-**Fig. 38.45**).

3. Syphilis

a. Clinical: Oral or genital ulcers in primary syphilis (chancre); reddish-brown scaly thin papules in secondary syphilis, often with involvement of the palms. Caused by *Treponema pallidum* and spread through sexual contact.

b. Microscopic: Numerous presentations, but in secondary syphilis classic findings include mixed pattern dermatitis with psoriasiform and lichenoid changes with numerous plasma cells (e-**Fig. 38.46A,B**). *T. pallidum* immunohistochemical stain confirms diagnosis by highlighting spirochetes within the epidermis.

4. Other bacterial: Deep bacterial infections can occur within the dermis (cellulitis), subcutis (ecthyma) and/or follicles (furunculosis). Abscess formation or suppurative dermatitis with or without involvement of the subcutis should trigger Gram stain; findings must be correlated with tissue cultures.

D. Mycobacterial

1. Atypical mycobacteria

a. Clinical: Variable. Nodules, ulcers, and/or plaques. *Mycobacterium marinum* is a common causative organism in healthy individuals with history of exposure to fresh or salt water.

b. Microscopic: Noncaseating granulomas with or without suppurative changes. Pseudoepitheliomatous changes are common (e-**Fig. 38.47A**). Ziehl–Neelsen and Fite stains may highlight acid-fast bacilli (e-**Fig. 38.47B**), often within vacuoles surrounded by neutrophils. Tissue cultures important for confirming diagnosis.

VI. NONLYMPHOID INFILTRATES

A. Eosinophil Infiltrates

1. Dermal hypersensitivity reaction

a. Clinical: Varied depending on the etiology. Edematous erythematous papulonodule in arthropod bites; morbilliform (erythematous macules and fine papules) in drug eruptions (*Clin Rev Allergy Immunol* 2014;50:189).

b. Microscopic: Superficial and deep perivascular lymphocytic infiltrate with eosinophils; may have associated dermal edema and spongiosis, particularly in arthropod bites (e-**Fig. 38.48A,B**). Deep infiltrate more common in arthropod bites. Clues to a drug eruption include associated purpura, slightly increased dermal mucin, and dyskeratotic keratinocytes.

B. Mast Cell Infiltrates
1. Cutaneous mastocytosis
- **a. Clinical:** Solitary mastocytoma—red-brown papulonodule that spontaneously involutes; seen in children. Urticaria pigmentosa (UP)—generalized, red-brown macules or papules. Positive Darier sign (development of a wheal after rubbing) in both solitary mastocytoma and UP. Telangiectasia macularis eruptiva perstans (TMEP)—multiple, telangiectatic, and slightly pigmented macules.
- **b. Microscopic:** Variable number of mast cells within the superficial dermis; admixed eosinophils, associated edema, and basal hyperpigmentation (e-Fig. 38.49). TMEP—subtle; slightly increased number of mast cells surrounding superficial dilated blood vessels; CD117 or tryptase IHC preferred for visualization of mast cells (*Annu Rev Pathol* 2017;12:487).

C. Histiocytic Infiltrates
1. Juvenile xanthogranuloma
- **a. Clinical:** Solitary or multiple red-brown papulonodules, often in children and young adults. Spontaneous involution in children.
- **b. Microscopic:** Nodular dermal infiltrate of mononuclear cells with admixed inflammatory cells, particularly eosinophils and neutrophils; Touton giant cells (multinucleated cells with peripheral wreath of nuclei surrounded by abundant foamy cytoplasm) characteristic but may be seen in other entities (e-Fig. 38.50).

2. Xanthomas
- **a. Clinical:** Varied including multiple red-yellow papules (eruptive xanthomas) and periocular yellow plaques (xanthelasma).
- **b. Microscopic:** Collections of foamy histiocytes in the superficial and mid dermis. Extracellular lipid in eruptive xanthomas.

3. Langerhans cell histiocytosis
- **a. Clinical:** When skin is involved, yellow-brown scaly or crusted papules in a seborrheic distribution (scalp, face, groin, buttocks). Self-limited form in neonates (congenital self-healing histiocytosis) regresses by 3 months.
- **b. Microscopic:** Papillary dermal edema with clusters and sheets of mononuclear cells with abundant eosinophilic or amphophilic cytoplasm and reniform nuclei (e-Fig. 38.51). Often admixed inflammatory cells, particularly eosinophils. Histiocytes stain with S-100, CD1a, and langerin (CD207). BRAF VE1 immunohistochemistry (IHC) to detect the *BRAF* V600E mutation can be helpful for treatment purposes (*Arch Pathol Lab Med* 2015;139:1211; *J Am Acad Dermatol* 2018;78:579).

VII. DERMAL DEPOSITS
A. Myxoma
1. **Clinical:** Usually solitary skin-colored papule or nodule; most common in adults with no site predilection. May be sporadic or syndromic (Carney complex).
2. **Microscopic:** Dermal lesion composed of wispy blue material with delicate spindle cells; usually moderately well circumscribed but not encapsulated (e-Fig. 38.52). Stains such as colloidal iron or alcian blue at low pH can be used to confirm the presence of interstitial mucin, but are not typically necessary.

B. Digital Mucous Cyst
1. **Clinical:** Solitary, dome-shaped, cystic nodule on the distal finger/toe near a joint or nail.
2. **Microscopic:** Compact hyperorthokeratosis; acellular, wispy blue material in the papillary dermis. Technically is a pseudocyst.

C. Calcinosis Cutis
1. **Clinical:** Ranges from small firm papules, to plaques, to nodules.
2. **Microscopic:** Basophilic deposits within the dermis or subcutis (e-Fig.38.53).

D. Osteoma Cutis
1. **Clinical:** Ranges from firm papules on the face at sites of acne scars, to incidental changes in cysts, and benign or malignant cutaneous neoplasms.
2. **Microscopic:** Trabecular bone with fatty replacement of the marrow cavity and/or hematopoiesis; osteoblasts in Haversian canals; sometimes osteoclasts (e-Fig. 38.54).

E. Gout
1. **Clinical:** Nodules/dermal deposits; ear or periarticular sites.
2. **Microscopic:** Dermal or subcutaneous nodular amorphous pink deposits with variable surrounding foreign-body giant cell reaction. After routine tissue processing, birefringent needles are not detectable (e-**Fig. 38.55A,B**).

F. Amyloidosis
1. **Primary cutaneous**
   a. **Clinical:** Macular and lichen—pebbled/pigmented areas on the upper back and shins, respectively. Nodular—solitary or multiple nodules.
   b. **Microscopic:** Amorphous deposits of pink-orange or slightly basophilic material with clefting ("cracked earth"). Macular—histologically normal at low power with subtle amyloid deposits within dermal papillae. Lichen—similar to macular amyloidosis with hyperkeratosis and acanthosis. Nodular—dermal aggregates of amyloid with or without plasma cells (e-**Fig. 38.56**). Congo red or crystal violet stains can be used to confirm the presence of amyloid.

2. **Systemic**
   a. **Clinical:** Papular or nodular lesions; periorbital ecchymoses ("pinch purpura").
   b. **Microscopic:** Hyaline deposits in the dermis or amyloid rings around blood vessels and adipocytes.

VIII. KERATINOUS CYSTS. Keratinous cysts are epithelial-lined cystic structures in the dermis and/or subcutis. They vary in the manner of keratinization and/or cyst contents.

A. Infundibular Type (Follicular)
1. **Clinical:** Solitary, slow-growing, mobile nodule with small opening to the skin (punctum).
2. **Microscopic:** Lined by stratified squamous epithelium with orthokeratotic (basket weave) keratin and an intact granular layer, but devoid of rete; contains laminated orthokeratin (e-**Fig. 38.57**). Mixed inflammation and foreign body reaction occur with rupture.

B. Trichilemmal Type (Pilar)
1. **Clinical:** Solitary or multiple, smooth, firm nodule(s); most common on the scalp.
2. **Microscopic:** Lined by stratified squamous epithelium with an abrupt transition to compact orthokeratotic keratin; the granular layer is absent. Keratinocytes become larger and cuboidal with pale abundant cytoplasms toward the lumen. Contains compact eosinophilic keratin which may be focally calcified (e-**Fig. 38.58**).

C. Steatocystoma
1. **Clinical:** Solitary (simplex) or multiple (multiplex), firm, yellow or skin-colored cystic nodules.
2. **Microscopic:** Undulating cyst lined by a thin stratified squamous epithelium that is covered with a homogeneous eosinophilic cuticle; sebaceous glands communicate with the cyst cavity which is usually devoid of contents (e-**Fig. 38.59**).

D. Vellus Hair Cyst
1. **Clinical:** Multiple small skin-colored papules; most common on the chest and axillae.
2. **Microscopic:** Small cyst lined by stratified squamous epithelium showing either epidermal or trichilemmal keratinization with multiple small vellus hairs intermixed with keratin (e-**Fig. 38.60**).

IX. DISORDERS OF COLLAGEN AND ELASTIN
A. Morphea/Localized Scleroderma
1. **Clinical:** Indurated plaques; slightly erythematous to violaceous during the inflammatory stage; ivory white or hyperpigmented with chronicity. Most common on the trunk or extremities in children or young adults (*Curr Rheumatol Rev* 2017;13:86).
2. **Microscopic:** Thick hypocellular collagen bundles replace normal collagen within the dermis; decreased adipose tissue around eccrine coils; loss of adnexal structures with retention of arrector pili muscles; flattened dermal–subcutaneous interface (e-**Fig. 38.61A,B**). In early stages, variable perivascular and periadnexal inflammation with lymphocytes and plasma cells. Some cases show overlapping features of morphea and lichen sclerosus.

B. **Lichen Sclerosus**
1. **Clinical:** Slightly depressed, ivory white patches/plaques with tissue paper–like surface. Preferentially involves female genitalia; more common past middle age, but also occurs in premenarche. Extragenital lesions most common on hair-bearing skin. Called *balanitis xerotica obliterans* when glans penis/prepuce affected. Increased risk of squamous cell carcinoma in long-standing genital lesions.
2. **Microscopic:** Compact hyperorthokeratosis, epidermal atrophy, and characteristic homogenization of collagen within the papillary dermis; variable lichenoid inflammation with early lesions mimicking lichen planus; dilated vessels and edema may be prominent within papillary dermis (e-**Fig. 38.62**) (*Mod Pathol* 1998;11:844).

X. **DISORDERS OF EPIDERMAL MATURATION AND KERATINIZATION**
A. **Acantholytic Dyskeratosis**
1. **Clinical:** Varied, including malodorous, erythematous lesions in seborrheic areas (Darier disease) or intertriginous areas (Hailey–Hailey disease), solitary pruritic lesions on the trunk (Grover disease), solitary warty lesions (warty dyskeratoma).
2. **Microscopic:** Suprabasal clefting with variable acantholysis and dyskeratosis (e-**Fig. 38.63**). Darier disease—also has distinctive granular keratinocytes that are perfectly round (corps ronds), or parakeratotic and acantholytic (corps grains). Hailey–Hailey disease—full-thickness acantholysis with less prominent dyskeratosis. Warty dyskeratoma—cup-shaped or cystic architecture with acantholytic dyskeratosis. Any of these changes may be seen in Grover disease (*J Cutan Pathol* 2019;46:6).
B. **Porokeratosis**
1. **Clinical:** Single or multiple, erythematous, thin papules with a thread-like scale at their border; usually on sun-damaged skin (*Eur J Dermatol* 2014;24:533).
2. **Microscopic:** One or more cornoid lamella consisting of a diagonal column of parakeratotic keratin overlying a focus of epidermis with hypogranulosis and scattered dyskeratotic keratinocytes (e-**Fig. 38.64**). Often with atrophic epidermis between the cornoid lamellae and patchy superficial chronic inflammation.

XI. **ALOPECIA**
A. **Nonscarring Alopecia:** Characterized by retention of sebaceous lobules and follicular units, typically with normal total hair count. Telogen count and degree of miniaturization particularly important in nonscarring alopecia. Most nonscarring alopecias have minimal inflammation, with the exception of alopecia areata (*J Cutan Pathol* 2017;44:53).
1. **Alopecia areata**
   a. **Clinical:** Well-circumscribed, round, smooth patches of hair loss on the scalp; may involve beard area or eyebrows. Occurs at any age. Varied clinical course ranging from sporadic hair loss with complete resolution to progressive hair loss involving the entire scalp and body. Tapered shedding telogen hairs ("exclamation point" hairs) may be present (*Clin Rev Allergy Immunol* 2018;54:68).
   b. **Microscopic:** Acute to subacute—peribulbar lymphocytic infiltrate with or without scattered eosinophils (e-**Fig. 38.65A**); subacute to chronic—markedly increased catagen/telogen count (may be near 100%) with prominent miniaturization with or without subtle inflammation (e-**Fig. 38.65B**).
2. **Androgenetic alopecia**
   a. **Clinical:** Decreased hair density over frontotemporal areas, crown and vertex in men, and over frontal/parietal scalp in women with retention of the frontal hairline. May be subtle in women with widening of the central part.
   b. **Microscopic:** Prominent miniaturization of hair follicles with scant perifollicular chronic inflammation; may have slightly increased telogen count (20% to 25%) (e-**Fig. 38.66**).
3. **Telogen effluvium**
   a. **Clinical:** Disturbance in the hair cycle resulting in increased shedding of hair. Mild, diffuse thinning of hair; sometimes not clinically appreciable. Precipitating event typically 3 months prior to the onset of hair loss. Causes include childbirth, major surgery, severe illness, and medications.
   b. **Microscopic:** Increased telogen count (typically 20% to 50%) without miniaturization.

4. Trichotillomania

a. **Clinical:** Well-demarcated areas of alopecia with unusual shape (angulated, linear, curved) and broken hairs of varied lengths. Seen in children and young adults. Caused by repeated manipulation (twirling, plucking, pulling) of hairs.

b. **Microscopic:** Increased catagen/telogen hairs, trichomalacia (distorted follicular architecture), and pigment casts (clumps of pigment within follicular infundibula or ostia) (e-**Fig. 38.67A,B**) (*Actas Dermosifiliogr* 2015;106:158).

B. Scarring Alopecia:
Characterized by inflammation, dermal and perifollicular fibrosis, loss of sebaceous lobules, and decreased hair count secondary to destruction of hair follicles. Inflammatory scarring alopecias eventually progress to end-stage alopecia (Brocq alopecia, pseudopelade) with extensive dermal fibrosis and markedly decreased hair count with the absence of follicular units leaving residual fibrotic tracts/stelae (*J Clin Pathol* 2001;28:333; *Acta Dermosifiliogr* 2015;106:260).

1. Discoid lupus erythematosus

a. **Clinical:** Indurated erythematous or violaceous plaques that progress to alopecia with atrophy, scarring, depigmentation, and scale.

b. **Microscopic:** Variably dense lymphoplasmacytic infiltrate surrounding superficial portions of hair follicles and eccrine coils in the deep dermis. Epidermal changes include atrophy, interface dermatitis, thickened basement membrane zone (best appreciated with PAS stain), and plugging of follicular ostia (e-**Fig. 38.68A,B**).

2. Lichen planopilaris

a. **Clinical:** Hair loss with perifollicular erythema and scaling. Frontal fibrosing alopecia—variant with hair loss in eyebrows and frontotemporal scalp in a band-like distribution. More common in women, particularly postmenopausal.

b. **Microscopic:** Perifollicular fibrosis and lichenoid inflammation surrounding superficial portions of hair follicles leading to destruction of affected follicles and loss of sebaceous glands (e-**Fig. 38.69**). Variable epidermal changes ranging from normal, to lichenoid or interface change.

3. Central centrifugal cicatricial alopecia

a. **Clinical:** Progressive permanent hair loss over the central crown or vertex. Occiput typically spared. More common in African American women.

b. **Microscopic:** Selective destruction of hair follicles with loss of sebaceous glands, leaving fibrotic tracts and hair shaft fragments surrounded by granulomatous inflammation. Remaining follicles have varying degrees of perifollicular fibrosis. Patchy chronic inflammation in early stages. Premature desquamation of the inner root sheath (keratinization occurring below the level of the isthmus) and eccentric epithelial atrophy are common findings but not pathognomonic (e-**Fig. 38.70**).

ACKNOWLEDGMENT

The authors thank Samuel J. Pruden II, Kimberley G. Crone, and Anne C. Lind, authors of the previous editions of this chapter.

Skin: Nonmelanocytic Tumors

Tiffany Y. Chen, Matthew Hedberg, and Leigh Compton

The WHO classification of tumors of the skin is presented in Table 38.1.

I. BENIGN TUMORS OF THE EPIDERMIS

A. Seborrheic Keratosis

1. **Clinical:** Single or multiple discrete papules or plaques, typically measuring 0.5 to 1.0 cm; variably pigmented and with a waxy, "stuck-on" appearance; wide anatomic distribution excluding hands and palms; most commonly found in people >30 years of age.

TABLE 38.1	WHO Classification of Skin Tumors

Keratinocytic/epidermal tumors

Carcinomas
  Basal cell carcinoma NOS
    Nodular basal cell carcinoma
    Superficial basal cell carcinoma
    Micronodular basal cell carcinoma
    Infiltrating basal cell carcinoma
    Sclerosing/morphoeic basal cell carcinoma
    Basosquamous carcinoma
    Pigmented basal cell carcinoma
    Basal cell carcinoma with sarcomatoid differentiation
    Basal cell carcinoma with adnexal differentiation
    Fibroepithelial basal cell carcinoma
  Squamous cell carcinoma NOS
    Keratoacanthoma
    Acantholytic squamous cell carcinoma
    Spindle cell squamous cell carcinoma
    Verrucous squamous cell carcinoma
    Adenosquamous carcinoma
    Clear cell squamous cell carcinoma
    Other (uncommon) variants
      Squamous cell carcinoma with sarcomatoid differentiation
      Lymphoepithelioma-like carcinoma
      Pseudovascular squamous cell carcinoma
      Squamous cell carcinoma with osteoclast-like giant cells
  Squamous cell carcinoma in situ (Bowen disease)
  Merkel cell carcinoma

Carcinoma precursors and benign simulants
  Premalignant keratoses
    Actinic keratosis
    Arsenical keratosis
    PUVA keratosis
  Verrucae
    Verruca vulgaris
    Verruca plantaris
    Verruca plana
  Benign acanthomas/keratoses
    Seborrhoeic keratosis
    Solar lentigo
    Lichen planus-like keratosis
    Clear cell acanthoma
    Large cell acanthoma
    Warty dyskeratoma
    Other benign keratoses

Melanocytic tumors

Melanocytic tumors in intermittently sun-exposed skin
  Low-CSD melanoma (superficial spreading melanoma)
  Simple lentigo and lentiginous melanocytic nevus
  Junctional nevus
  Compound nevus

(continued)

TABLE 38.1   WHO Classification of Skin Tumors (*Continued*)

Dermal nevus
Dysplastic nevus
Nevus spilus
Special-site nevi (of the breast, axilla, scalp, and ear)
Halo nevus
Meyerson nevus
Recurrent nevus
Deep penetrating nevus
Pigmented epithelioid melanocytoma
Combined nevus, including combined BAP1-inactivated nevus/melanocytoma

Melanocytic tumors in chronically sun-exposed skin
Lentigo maligna melanoma
Desmoplastic melanoma

Spitz tumors
Malignant Spitz tumor (Spitz melanoma)
Spitz nevus
Pigmented spindle cell nevus (Reed nevus)

Melanocytic tumors in acral skin
Acral melanoma
Acral nevus

Genital and mucosal melanocytic tumors
Mucosal melanomas (genital, oral, sinonasal)
Mucosal lentiginous melanoma
Mucosal nodular melanoma
Genital nevus

Melanocytic tumors arising in blue nevus
Melanoma arising in blue nevus
Blue nevus NOS
Cellular blue nevus
Mongolian spot
Nevus of Ito
Nevus of Ota

Melanocytic tumors arising in congenital nevi
Melanoma arising in giant congenital nevus
Congenital melanocytic nevus
Proliferative nodules in congenital melanocytic nevus

Appendageal tumors

Malignant tumors with apocrine and eccrine differentiation
Adnexal adenocarcinoma NOS
Microcystic adnexal carcinoma
Porocarcinoma
Porocarcinoma in situ
Malignant neoplasms arising from spiradenoma, cylindroma, or spiradenocylindroma
Malignant mixed tumor
Hidradenocarcinoma
Mucinous carcinoma
Endocrine mucin-producing sweat gland carcinoma
Digital papillary adenocarcinoma
Adenoid cystic carcinoma
Apocrine carcinoma

TABLE 38.1   WHO Classification of Skin Tumors (*Continued*)

Squamoid eccrine ductal carcinoma
Syringocystadenocarcinoma papilliferum
Secretory carcinoma
Cribriform carcinoma
Signet-ring cell/histiocytoid carcinoma

Benign tumors with apocrine and eccrine differentiation
Hidrocystoma/cystadenoma
Syringoma
Poroma
Syringofibroadenoma
Hidradenoma
Spiradenoma
Cylindroma
Tubular adenoma
Syringocystadenoma papilliferum
Mixed tumor
Myoepithelioma

Malignant tumors with follicular differentiation
Pilomatrical carcinoma
Proliferating trichilemmal tumor
Trichoblastic carcinoma/carcinosarcoma
Trichilemmal carcinoma

Benign tumors with follicular differentiation
Trichoblastoma
Pilomatricoma
Trichilemmoma
Trichofolliculoma
Pilar sheath acanthoma
Tumor of the follicular infundibulum
Melanocytic matricoma
Spindle cell–predominant trichodiscoma

Tumors with sebaceous differentiation
Sebaceous carcinoma
Sebaceous adenoma
Sebaceoma

Site-specific tumors
Mammary Paget disease
Extramammary Paget disease
Adenocarcinoma of anogenital mammary-like glands
Hidradenoma papilliferum
Fibroadenoma of anogenital mammary-like glands
Phyllodes tumor of anogenital mammary-like glands

Tumors of hematopoietic and lymphoid origin

Mycosis fungoides
Folliculotropic mycosis fungoides
Granulomatous slack skin
Pagetoid reticulosis
Sezary syndrome

(*continued*)

TABLE 38.1 **WHO Classification of Skin Tumors (*Continued*)**

Primary cutaneous CD30+ T-cell lymphoproliferative disorders
  Lymphomatoid papulosis
  Primary cutaneous anaplastic large cell lymphoma
Cutaneous adult T-cell leukemia/lymphoma
Subcutaneous panniculitis-like T-cell lymphoma

Cutaneous manifestations of chronic active EBV infection
  Hydroa vacciniforme-like lymphoproliferative disorder
Extranodal NK/T-cell lymphoma, nasal type

Primary cutaneous peripheral T-cell lymphomas, rare subtypes
  Primary cutaneous gamma-delta T-cell lymphoma
  Primary cutaneous CD8+ aggressive epidermotropic cytotoxic T-cell lymphoma
  Primary cutaneous acral CD8+ T-cell lymphoma
  Primary cutaneous CD4+ small/medium T-cell lymphoproliferative disorder

Secondary cutaneous involvement in T-cell lymphomas and leukemias
  Systemic anaplastic large cell lymphoma, ALK positive
  Systemic anaplastic large cell lymphoma, ALK negative
  Angioimmunoblastic T-cell lymphoma
  T-cell prolymphocytic leukemia
Primary cutaneous marginal zone (MALT) lymphoma
Primary cutaneous follicle center lymphoma
Primary cutaneous diffuse large B-cell lymphoma, leg type
Intravascular large B-cell lymphoma
EBV-positive mucocutaneous ulcer
Lymphomatoid granulomatosis

Cutaneous involvement in primarily extracutaneous B-cell lymphomas and leukemias
  Mantle cell lymphoma
  Burkitt lymphoma
  Chronic lymphocytic leukemia/small lymphocytic lymphoma

T-lymphoblastic and B-lymphoblastic leukemia/lymphoma
  T-lymphoblastic leukemia/lymphoma
  B-lymphoblastic leukemia/lymphoma
Blastic plasmacytoid dendritic cell neoplasm
Cutaneous involvement in myeloid leukemia
Cutaneous mastocytosis
  Mast cell sarcoma
  Indolent systemic mastocytosis
  Aggressive systemic mastocytosis
  Systemic mastocytosis with an associated hematologic neoplasm
  Mast cell leukemia

Histiocytic and dendritic cell neoplasms
  Langerhans cell histiocytosis
  Indeterminate cell histiocytosis/indeterminate dendritic cell tumor
  Rosai–Dorfman disease
  Juvenile xanthogranuloma
  Erdheim–Chester disease
  Reticulohistiocytosis

Soft tissue and neural tumors

Adipocytic tumors
  Atypical lipomatous tumor
  Dedifferentiated liposarcoma

TABLE 38.1 WHO Classification of Skin Tumors (*Continued*)

Lipoma
Spindle cell/pleomorphic lipoma
Angiolipoma
Nevus lipomatosus superficialis

Fibroblastic, myofibroblastic, and fibrohistiocytic tumor
Myxoinflammatory fibroblastic sarcoma
Dermatofibrosarcoma protuberans
Giant cell fibroblastoma
Bednar tumor
Fibrosarcomatous dermatofibrosarcoma protuberans
Plexiform fibrohistiocytic tumor
Superficial fibromatosis
Dermatofibroma (fibrous histiocytoma)
Epithelioid fibrous histiocytoma
Fibromas
  Fibroma of tendon sheath
  Calcifying aponeurotic fibroma
  Sclerotic fibroma
  Nuchal-type fibroma
  Gardner fibroma
  Pleomorphic fibroma
  Elastofibroma
  Collagenous fibroma
Superficial acral fibromyxoma
Cutaneous myxoma
Dermatomyofibroma
Myofibroma
Myofibromatosis
Plaque-like CD34+ dermal fibroma
Nodular fasciitis

Smooth muscle tumors
Cutaneous leiomyoma
Cutaneous leiomyosarcoma (atypical smooth muscle tumor)

(Myo)pericytic tumors
Glomus tumor
  Glomuvenous malformation (glomangiomyoma)
  Glomus tumor of uncertain malignant potential
  Malignant glomus tumor
Myopericytoma
Angioleiomyoma

Vascular tumors
Cutaneous angiosarcoma
  Hemangioendotheliomas
  Composite hemangioendothelioma
  Kaposiform hemangioendothelioma
  Pseudomyogenic hemangioendothelioma
  Retiform hemangioendothelioma
  Epithelioid hemangioendothelioma
Kaposi sarcoma
Atypical vascular lesion
Cutaneous epithelioid angiomatous nodule

(*continued*)

TABLE 38.1	WHO Classification of Skin Tumors (*Continued*)

Hemangiomas
  Cherry hemangioma
  Sinusoidal hemangioma
  Microvenular hemangioma
  Hobnail hemangioma
  Glomeruloid hemangioma
  Spindle cell hemangioma
  Epithelioid hemangioma
  Tufted hemangioma
  Angiokeratoma hemangioma
  Infantile hemangioma
  Rapidly involuting congenital hemangioma
  Non-involving congenital hemangioma
  Lobular capillary hemangioma
  Verrucous venous malformation
  Arteriovenous malformation
Lymphangioma (superficial lymphatic malformation)

Neural tumors
  Neurofibroma
  Solitary circumscribed neuroma
  Dermal nerve sheath myxoma
  Perineurioma
  Malignant perineurioma
  Granular cell tumor
  Malignant granular cell tumor
  Schwannoma
  Malignant peripheral nerve sheath tumor
  Epithelioid malignant peripheral nerve sheath tumor
  Malignant triton tumor

Tumors of uncertain differentiation
  Atypical fibroxanthoma
  Pleomorphic dermal sarcoma
  Myxofibrosarcoma
  Epithelioid sarcoma
  Dermal clear cell sarcoma
  Ewing sarcoma
  Primitive nonneural granular cell tumor
  Cellular neurothekeoma

CSD, chronic skin damage.
From Elder DE, Massi D, Scolyer RA, Willemze R, eds. *WHO Classification of Skin Tumours*. Lyon, France: IARC Press; 2017. Used with permission.

    2. Microscopic: Exophytic or endophytic lesion sharply demarcated from adjacent epidermis, composed of basaloid and often homogeneous cells with variable degrees of squamoid differentiation; intraepidermal pseudocysts filled with loose orthokeratotic keratin are common. There are many microscopic patterns, the most common being hyperkeratotic, acanthotic, reticulated, and clonal. Features of irritation are commonly seen (**e-Fig. 38.71**), including squamous eddies. While irritated seborrheic keratosis (ISK) can be confused for squamous cell carcinoma in situ, it lacks overt cytologic atypia.

  B. Clear Cell Acanthoma

    1. Clinical: Uncommon; slowly growing, pink to brown, dome-shaped nodule or small plaque, most frequently on the extremity of middle-aged and elderly individuals.

2. **Microscopic:** Sharply demarcated proliferation of keratinocytes with pale/clear cytoplasm, agranulosis, parakeratosis, and an intralesional neutrophilic infiltrate. PAS stain highlights cytoplasmic glycogen (e-**Fig. 38.72**).

II. PREMALIGNANT AND MALIGNANT TUMORS OF THE EPIDERMIS

A. Actinic Keratosis

1. **Clinical:** Scaly, erythematous papules or nodules on sun-exposed skin particularly on the head and neck, upper and lower extremities; more common in fair-skinned individuals.

2. **Microscopic:** Irregular buds of atypical keratinocytes emanate from the basal epidermis; patchy parakeratosis and agranulosis that spare adnexal ostia; dyskeratotic cells and solar elastosis may be present. Dysplasia does not involve the full thickness of the epidermis. Atypical epithelium may extend down adnexal structures (e-**Fig. 38.73**). Hypertrophic variant shows an acanthotic epidermis, and a thickened alternating hyperkeratotic and parakeratotic scale.

3. **Genetics:** Displays a high rate of chromosomal aneuploidy, including frequent loss of heterozygosity of 17p, 17q, 9p, 9q, and 3p. *TP53* mutations and overexpression of cyclin D1 are common.

B. Squamous Cell Carcinoma in Situ (Bowen Disease)

1. **Clinical:** Sharply demarcated, scaly to hyperkeratotic macule, papule, or plaque; most common in sun-exposed areas (particularly the face and legs); more common in fair-skinned, older individuals.

2. **Microscopic:** Keratinocytes with enlarged, hyperchromatic nuclei and variable amounts of cytoplasm occupy the full thickness of the epidermis; variable acanthosis, hyperparakeratosis, agranulosis, dyskeratosis, multinucleate cells, mitoses above the basal layer, and loss of maturation; the neoplastic cells populate adnexal structures. May show pagetoid growth as single cells and small nests within a thickened epidermis (e-**Fig. 38.74**).

3. **Genetics:** Increased expression and mutation of *TP53* have been observed. Allelic deletion of one or more chromosome 9q markers has also been detected in occasional lesions. HPV is frequently detected at periungual and anogenital sites but may be found within tumors across any anatomic distribution.

C. Invasive Squamous Cell Carcinoma (*J Clin Pathol* 2006;33:191; *IBID* 2006;33:261)

1. **Clinical:** Early lesions are firm, skin-colored, or erythematous nodules; later lesions are shallow ulcers with peripheral elevation, induration, and scale crust; most common in fair-skinned, older individuals on sun-exposed areas and in immunocompromised patients. Important stratifiers in the most recent AJCC staging scheme (Amin MB, Edge S, Greene F, eds. *AJCC Cancer Staging Manual*, 8th ed. New York: Springer, 2017) of head and neck cutaneous tumors include size (cutoffs of 2 cm and 4 cm), presence of high-risk features (depth of invasion >6 mm, perineural invasion, nodal metastases with extranodal extension, poor differentiation, location on the ear, temple, cheek, and lip), and invasion of bone.

2. **Microscopic:** Acanthosis, invasion of the dermis by individual or nested keratinocytes with variable amounts of cytoplasm and nuclear pleomorphism, dyskeratosis, and swirls of parakeratotic keratin (keratin pearls). There may be dermal desmoplasia and variable inflammation. Tumors are graded on the degree of differentiation: well-differentiated tumors show abundant keratinization, obvious intracellular bridges (e-**Fig. 38.75**); moderately differentiated tumors have less obvious keratinization with increased nuclear to cytoplasmic ratios and a greater degree of disorganization; poorly differentiated tumors lack keratinization, and may show anaplastic or sarcomatoid features and marked nuclear pleomorphism (*Dermatol Surg* 200;26:521).

D. Basal Cell Carcinoma

1. **Clinical:** Variable presentation; most commonly a slowly growing, dome-shaped, firm papule with a pearly, telangiectatic surface; primarily arise on the head, neck, and trunk. The most common skin cancer in Caucasians; rarely metastasizes unless neglected (*Front Oncol* 2015;11:3011; *IBID* 2015;11:3023).

2. **Microscopic:** Variable histology with common features including basaloid cells with hyperchromatic nuclei and scant cytoplasm. Basaloid islands show peripheral palisading, mitoses, and apoptosis; mucin is often seen within and surrounding tumor nodules and causes a histologic retraction artifact separating the basaloid cells from the surrounding stroma (e-Fig. 38.76). Of the many subtypes described two have particular clinical significance: Superficial BCC, which is entirely connected to the epidermis, may be treated conservatively with topical agents or by electrodessication and curettage. Infiltrative BCC, which is composed of small angulated and infiltrative nests of basaloid cells, may follow a more aggressive clinical course and is more likely to display perineural invasion.

3. **Genetics:** Mutations of genes *PTCH1* on chromosome 9q22.3 and *SMD* on chromosome 7q31–32 involved in activating the hedgehog signaling pathway have been identified in both sporadic basal cell carcinomas and basal cell nevus syndrome (also known as the Gorlin syndrome, a rare autosomal dominant (AD) disorder characterized by numerous basal cell carcinomas, odontogenic keratocysts, fibromas, various bone abnormalities, and central nervous system malignancies).

III. **TUMORS OF THE CUTANEOUS APPENDAGES.** Tumors of the cutaneous appendages or adnexa have a complex, multi-tiered nomenclature. A traditional system organizes the tumors based on their origin from one of the normal cutaneous appendages: hair follicle, sebaceous gland, eccrine gland, or apocrine gland. However, complex adnexal tumors also occur that show multiple lines of differentiation; therefore, a tumor's precise histogenesis is not always clear (*J Clin Pathol* 2012;65:819).

A. **Benign Appendage Tumors** (*J Clin Pathol* 2007;60:129; *J Dermatol* 2017;44:259)

1. **Hair follicle tumors**

   a. **Trichofolliculoma**

      i. **Clinical:** Rare; solitary, small (<1 cm), skin-colored nodule on the face, especially the nose and earlobe. There is often a central umbilication filled with keratin and sometimes a protruding tuft of fine hairs.

      ii. **Microscopic:** One or more cystically dilated hair follicles with radiating follicles that project into a relatively cellular stroma; secondary follicles may be vellus or large terminal hairs in any stage of the hair cycle, are sometimes misshapen, and may give rise to tertiary hair follicles (e-Fig. 38.77).

   b. **Trichoepithelioma**

      i. **Clinical:** Usually solitary, skin-colored papule, most commonly on the central face; if multiple, associated with AD inheritance. The desmoplastic variant is a solitary, firm annular lesion with a raised border and central depression that occurs exclusively on the face.

      ii. **Microscopic:** Relatively well-circumscribed dermal tumor composed of islands of basaloid cells with pilar differentiation in a cellular eosinophilic stroma; papillary mesenchymal bodies are characteristic; small keratinous cysts and foci of calcification are often present. The tumor epithelium may mimic basal cell carcinoma, but there is no retraction artifact or mucinous stroma (e-Fig. 38.78). The desmoplastic variant shows a well-circumscribed lesion in the upper and mid-dermis composed of cords or small nests of basaloid cells in a sclerotic stroma (e-Fig. 38.79). It may be confused with a syringoma, the surface of a microcystic adnexal carcinoma, or morpheaform basal cell carcinoma (*Arch Pathol Lab Med* 2017;141:1490).

   c. **Trichoadenoma (of Nikolowski)**

      i. **Clinical:** Rare; solitary skin-colored or grey nodule on the face or buttocks.

      ii. **Microscopic:** Well-demarcated dermal tumor composed of multiple cyst-like structures that are frequently interconnected by multilayered keratinizing pilar-type squamous epithelium. There is an associated paucicellular, fibrotic stroma. The cysts contain keratinous debris but no hair shafts (e-Fig. 38.80).

   d. **Dilated pore of Winer**

      i. **Clinical:** Common; comedo-like lesion on the head and neck, or trunk.

      ii. **Microscopic:** Cystically dilated hair follicle filled with loose keratin and lined by acanthotic, stratified squamous epithelium with irregular budding (e-Fig. 38.81).

e. Trichilemmoma

- **i. Clinical:** Solitary, wart-like or dome-shaped, skin-colored papule on the face and neck; multiple lesions are associated with the Cowden syndrome.
- **ii. Microscopic:** Well-circumscribed, endo-exophytic tumor composed of clear squamoid cells with glycogenated cytoplasms; tumor extends from the epidermis with a lobular configuration; thin peripheral rim of palisading columnar cells lined by a thick, eosinophilic basement membrane (e-**Fig. 38.82**). The desmoplastic variant shows variable amounts of small nests and single cells within a sclerotic desmoplastic stroma, imparting an infiltrative appearance and is not associated with the Cowden syndrome.
- **iii. Genetics:** The Cowden syndrome has an AD inheritance pattern and is associated with *PTEN* tumor suppressor gene mutation in 70% to 80% of patients. Other clinical manifestations aside from multiple trichilemmomas include sclerotic fibromas, hamartomatous gastrointestinal polyps, and increased risks of breast, thyroid, and endometrial cancers.

f. Pilomatrixoma (pilomatricoma, calcifying epithelioma of Malherbe)

- **i. Clinical:** Firm, deep-seated nodule; most common on the head and neck region and upper extremities; onset frequently in childhood.
- **ii. Microscopic:** Sharply demarcated tumor in the lower dermis and subcutis; composed of large, irregularly shaped tumor islands and intervening stroma; individual islands have basophilic matrical cells at the periphery that transition into larger, paler supramatrical cells and finally give rise to centrally located cornified shadow cells. In addition, features commonly observed include dystrophic calcifications, a mixed inflammatory infiltrate, hemosiderin, melanin, bone, and foreign-body giant cells (e-**Fig. 38.83**).

2. Eccrine tumors (*J Clin Pathol* 2007;60:145)

a. Syringoma

- **i. Clinical:** Usually multiple, skin-colored, small, firm papules on the lower eyelids and cheeks; more common in women; onset often at puberty.
- **ii. Microscopic:** Multiple small ducts in a dense fibrous stroma in the upper dermis; ducts are lined by two layers of cuboidal epithelium, and sometimes are "tadpole" or "comma-like"; solid nests and strands of tumor cells can be present (e-**Fig. 38.84**).

b. Eccrine (or apocrine) mixed tumor (chondroid syringoma)

- **i. Clinical:** Solitary, firm, dermal, or subcutaneous nodule on the head and neck or extremities of adults.
- **ii. Microscopic:** Well-circumscribed dermal tumor of small epithelial cells arranged as solid nests, small clusters, and ducts within a prominent myxoid, cartilaginous, and/or fibrous stroma (e-**Fig. 38.85**).

c. Cylindroma, spiradenoma, and spiradenocylindroma.
Although cylindroma and spiradenoma have distinct histopathologic features, they lie along a spectrum and some experts classify lesions with overlapping features as spiradenocylindroma. Collectively, these tumors may occur sporadically or as part of the Brooke–Spiegler syndrome.

- **i. Clinical:** Sporadic lesions present as solitary nodules on the head and neck or, less commonly, extremities of adults. Multiple lesions are associated with AD inheritance as part of the Brooke–Spiegler syndrome.
- **ii. Microscopic:**
  - **(a) Cylindroma**—poorly circumscribed dermal tumor composed of irregularly shaped nests of basaloid cells surrounded by a thick eosinophilic basement membrane; cells at the periphery show palisading and have hyperchromatic nuclei. The cellular nests fit together in a "jigsaw" pattern (e-**Fig. 38.86**).
  - **(b) Spiradenoma**—one or more sharply demarcated dermal nodule(s) of small basaloid cells mixed with paler cells and lymphocytes that display trabecular to solid architecture (e-**Fig. 38.87**).

(c) Spiradenocylindromas—hybrid features of cylindroma and spiradenoma with at least 10% of the tumor being represented by each.

iii. Genetics: The Brooke–Spiegler syndrome has an AD inheritance pattern and is associated with *CYLD* tumor suppressor gene mutation. In addition to multiple cylindromas, spiradenomas, and spiradenocylindromas, patients may develop trichoepitheliomas. Rarely, malignant neoplasms arise in association with a pre-existing benign tumor (*Head Neck Pathol* 2016;10:125).

d. Poroma group (including eccrine poroma, dermal duct tumor, hidroacanthoma simplex, and poroid hidradenoma)

i. Clinical:

(a) Eccrine poroma—solitary, sessile, or slightly pedunculated pink nodule; often on the plantar or palmar skin, or at other locations with sweat glands.

(b) Dermal duct tumor—a solitary, firm nodule on the head, neck, and extremities.

(c) Hidroacanthoma simplex—a solitary plaque or nodule on the extremities and trunk; clinically resembles SK or basal cell carcinoma.

(d) Poroid hidradenoma—similar to dermal duct tumor; a solitary, firm nodule on the head, neck, or extremities.

ii. Microscopic: All four entities are composed predominantly of monomorphous, round basophilic cells (poroid cells) and fewer large, eosinophilic squamoid cells (cuticular cells); ductules and intracytoplasmic vacuoles representing rudimentary ductules may be seen on histology and highlighted by epithelial membrane antigen (EMA) or carcinoembryonic antigen (CEA) immunostains. Necrosis en masse is often a feature. The neoplasms differ in their low-power architecture and lesions with combined patterns are common.

(a) Eccrine poroma—interconnected aggregates of tumor emanate from the undersurface of the epidermis with an intervening fibrotic stroma; has a well-circumscribed, smooth outer silhouette (e-**Fig. 38.88**).

(b) Dermal duct tumor—small aggregates of tumor present entirely within the reticular dermis without connection to the overlying epidermis; has a variably myxoid and hyaline stroma.

(c) Hidroacanthoma simplex—small aggregates of tumor are confined to the epidermis; has a broad, horizontal orientation.

(d) Poroid hidradenoma—large; solid, and cystic nodules of tumor confined to the reticular dermis with a variably myxoid and hyaline stroma.

e. Hidradenoma (acrospiroma, nodular hidradenoma, solid-cystic hidradenoma, apocrine/eccrine hidradenoma, and clear cell hidradenoma)

i. Clinical: Solitary nodule, 0.5 to 2.0 cm or more in diameter; no site predilection; disputed histogenesis.

ii. Microscopic: Variable histologic appearance as reflected by the nosology; usually a circumscribed, nonencapsulated, multilobular, dermal tumor with variable proportions of cystic and solid areas; tumor cells have variable clear or eosinophilic cytoplasm and are round, fusiform, or polygonal. Duct-like structures are typically present, have a squamous appearance, and may be highlighted by immunostains for EMA or CEA. The stroma varies from rather fine, fibrous tissue to dense hyalinized collagen (e-**Fig. 38.89**).

3. Sebaceous hyperplasia and tumors

a. Sebaceous hyperplasia

i. Clinical: Yellow to whitish papules with central umbilication; typically occur on the face of older individuals. It may mimic a basal cell carcinoma.

ii. Microscopic: Multiple large, but otherwise normal, sebaceous lobules centered on a sometimes dilated hair follicle (e-**Fig. 38.90**).

b. Sebaceous adenoma and sebaceous epithelioma (sebaceoma)

i. Clinical: Rare; solitary or multiple, pink or flesh-colored nodules on the face or scalp of adults; usually <1 cm in dimension; may present as part of the Muir–Torre syndrome.

ii. **Microscopic:** Multiple circumscribed sebaceous lobules usually centered in the superficial to mid-dermis. Sebaceous adenoma is composed of peripheral basaloid germinative cells, a predominance of central mature sebaceous cells (50% or greater), and a variable zone of transitional forms (e-**Fig. 38.91**). In sebaceous epithelioma, by contrast, germinative basaloid cells predominate (50% or greater) (*Pathology* 2017;49:688; *Surg Pathol Clin* 2017;10:367).

iii. **Genetics:** The Muir–Torre syndrome has an AD pattern of inheritance and is associated with mutations in DNA mismatch repair genes (*MSH2, MSH6, MLH1,* and *PMS2*), with mutation in *MSH2* being the most common. These mutations correlate with the loss of MMR protein expression as may be demonstrated by immunohistochemical studies, and with microsatellite instability as demonstrated by molecular testing. In addition to developing sebaceous tumors, affected families also develop a variety of visceral carcinomas as seen in the Lynch syndrome (particularly colorectal and endometrial carcinomas).

c. **Fibrofolliculoma/trichodiscoma.** Once considered follicular neoplasms, these entities are now favored to be derived from the immature sebaceous gland epithelium known as the mantle.

i. **Clinical:** Solitary or multiple skin-colored papules; most commonly occur on the face; multiple lesions are seen in the Birt–Hogg–Dubé syndrome.

ii. **Microscopic:** A spectrum of changes with fibrofolliculoma at one end and trichodiscoma at the other. Fibrofolliculoma is composed of thin, anastamosing strands of basaloid epithelium extending from centrally located, dilated hair follicle infundibulum; there is a distinct and dense fibrous and collagenous stroma that forms a nodule around the epithelium. Trichodiscoma is composed of a variably fibrous and myxoid stroma surrounded by lobules of mature sebaceous glands with a configuration likened to "baseball mitts" (e-**Fig. 38.92**).

iii. **Genetics:** The Birt–Hogg–Dubé syndrome has an AD pattern of inheritance associated with mutations in the *FLCN* gene encoding folliculin. Other clinical manifestations include pulmonary cysts and renal cell carcinoma (*Am J Clin Dermatol* 2018;19:87).

4. **Apocrine tumors**

a. **Apocrine hidrocystoma**

i. **Clinical:** Solitary, translucent to bluish nodule; predominantly occurs on the face.

ii. **Microscopic:** Cyst composed of an outer myoepithelial layer and an inner layer of cuboidal to columnar cells with apocrine decapitation secretion; pseudopapillary projections may be present (e-**Fig. 38.93**).

b. **Syringocystadenoma papilliferum**

i. **Clinical:** Varied; most commonly a raised, warty plaque on the scalp; associated with nevus sebaceous in approximately one-third of cases (*J Dermatol* 2016;43:175).

ii. **Microscopic:** Characteristic sharp transition from the keratinized follicular epithelium at the surface to the endophytic glandular epithelium composed of luminal columnar to cuboidal cells and outer myoepithelial cells; dermal glandular component shows ductal and papillary architecture and is surrounded by a chronic inflammatory infiltrate that almost invariably includes plasma cells (e-**Fig. 38.94**).

iii. **Genetics:** Allelic deletions of the *PTCH1* gene on chromosome 9q22 and loss of heterozygosity at chromosome 9p21 have been reported in syringocystadenoma papilliferum.

5. **Complex adnexal tumors: Nevus sebaceous of Jadassohn (organoid nevus)**

a. **Clinical:** Yellow or waxy, patch or plaque with alopecia on the scalp (most common), face, neck, or trunk; present at birth or first noticed in early childhood.

b. **Microscopic:** Complex hamartoma involving the epidermis, pilosebaceous unit, and ducts/glands; variable epidermal acanthosis, papillomatosis, and abnormally formed/abortive hair follicles with bulbs that do not extend into the subcutis; increased numbers of large sebaceous glands are present around and after puberty;

dilated apocrine glands are found in up to 50% of cases (e-**Fig. 38.95**). Secondary tumors may develop, such as syringocystadenoma papilliferum.

B. Malignant Tumors of the Cutaneous Appendages are rare and far less common than their benign counterparts. As with the benign tumors discussed above, a malignant neoplasm can arise from any of the normal skin appendages and more than one lineage may be present within a single tumor (*Surg Pathol* 2017;10:383).

1. Extramammary Paget disease

a. Clinical: A red scaly plaque, typically in areas rich in apocrine glands such as the anogenital region and, less commonly, the axilla; usually pruritic and slowly spreading. An underlying adnexal carcinoma is present in approximately 20% to 25% of cases; visceral carcinoma (rectal, prostate, bladder, cervix, or urethra) is present in 10% to 15% of cases.

b. Microscopic: Similar to the mammary Paget disease, there are large, epithelioid tumor cells with pleomorphic nuclei and abundant pale cytoplasm arranged predominantly as single cells and as small nests within the epidermis. The tumor cells are concentrated in the lower epidermis and randomly dispersed throughout the epidermis. Special stains may be needed to distinguish the extramammary Paget disease from melanoma in situ (MIS) and squamous cell carcinoma in situ with pagetoid features; the tumor cells are positive by mucicarmine and periodic acid–Schiff (PAS) stains; CEA, EMA, and low–molecular-weight keratin immunostains are positive; Melan-A/Mart-1 and S-100 immunostains are negative (e-**Fig. 38.96**).

2. Microcystic adnexal carcinoma (MAC)

a. Clinical: Plaque-like lesion; most commonly occurs on the upper lip or other sites on the face (*Dermatol Surg* 2017;43:1012).

b. Microscopic: Deeply infiltrative, poorly circumscribed nests and cords of basaloid cells and keratinocytes with ductal differentiation, often with a characteristic "paisley tide tadpole" shape and embedded within a sclerotic stroma. Differential diagnosis includes desmoplastic trichoepithelioma, morpheaform basal cell carcinoma, and syringoma.

3. Sebaceous carcinoma

a. Clinical: Most commonly presents as a firm, tan-yellow nodule on the eyelid of elderly patients; poor clinical course with high rates of metastasis.

b. Microscopic: Nodules and sheets of basophilic cells with variable amount of cytoplasmic lipid; mitotic figures, nuclear atypia, necrosis, and lymphovascular invasion are common; immunoreactive to EMA, androgen receptor, high–molecular-weight cytokeratin, and p63.

c. Genetics: Patients with multiple sebaceous neoplasms including sebaceous carcinoma are associated with the Muir–Torre syndrome (see above).

IV. BENIGN AND MALIGNANT TUMORS OF MESENCHYMAL ORIGIN. Classification of mesenchymal neoplasms is based on the mature, nonneoplastic tissue from which they are believed to be derived: blood vessel, nerve, smooth muscle, skeletal muscle, bone, cartilage, fibrous tissue, neuroendocrine tissue, or hematopoietic elements. These tumors are discussed in more detail in the chapters on hematolymphoid and soft tissue malignancies; only the most common entities will be discussed here (*Pediatr Dev Pathol* 2018;21:150).

A. Vascular Tumors

1. Lobular capillary hemangioma (pyogenic granuloma)

a. Clinical: Common; rapidly developing polypoid or pedunculated, red, eroded papules or nodules that bleed easily; occur on mucous membranes and skin.

b. Microscopic: Exophytic, frequently ulcerated proliferation of capillaries divided into lobules by fibrous tissue septae; variably cellular, often surrounded by a collarette of epidermis (e-**Fig. 38.97**).

2. Arteriovenous hemangioma (acral arteriovenous tumor)

a. Clinical: Solitary, usually asymptomatic, red or purple, enlarging or bleeding papule averaging 4 mm in diameter; most common on the lips, perioral skin, nose, and eyelids of middle-aged to elderly men.

   b. **Microscopic:** Well-circumscribed, nonencapsulated vascular tumor in the upper to mid-dermis; composed of closely packed, large-caliber, thick-walled, and thin-walled vessels (e-**Fig. 38.98**).
3. **"Cherry" angioma (senile angioma, Campbell de Morgan spot)**
   a. **Clinical:** Solitary or multiple, tiny, bright red papules, predominantly on the trunk and proximal extremities; common in adults, almost universal in the elderly.
   b. **Microscopic:** Early lesions with one or more dilated interconnecting thin-walled vessels in the papillary dermis. Established lesions are polypoid with an epidermal collarette and are composed of dilated and congested vascular channels in the papillary dermis (e-**Fig. 38.99**).
4. **Angiokeratoma**
   a. **Clinical:** Single or multiple, red to black papule(s) or plaque(s) that may be warty or hyperkeratotic; multiple variants exist with characteristic clinical presentations and carrying various eponyms.
   b. **Microscopic:** Markedly dilated and congested papillary dermal vessels form cavernous channels that have an intimate association with the epidermis, associated with irregular acanthosis and variable hyperkeratosis (e-**Fig. 38.100**). Angiokeratomas are often thrombosed.
5. **Lymphangioma (cystic lymphatic malformation)**
   a. **Superficial lymphangioma (lymphangioma circumscriptum)**
      i. **Clinical:** Multiple, localized, scattered, or grouped translucent vesicles or papulovesicles; may be red or purple due to intralesional hemorrhage and thrombus formation; usually congenital, sometimes presents later in childhood and is rare in adults. There may be a deeper component.
      ii. **Microscopic:** Multiple dilated, thin-walled lymphatic channels in the papillary and upper reticular dermis; epidermis is sometimes acanthotic and forms a collarette (e-**Fig. 38.101**).
   b. **Deep lymphangioma (including cavernous lymphangioma and cystic hygroma)**
      i. **Clinical:** Usually solitary, rubbery, skin-colored nodules that may result in swelling of the soft tissue; most common on the face, trunk, and extremities; varies from spongy to a large cystic tumor. Most are present at birth or the first few years of life.
      ii. **Microscopic:** Variable; in general, there are irregularly dilated vascular channels of variable size in the dermis, subcutis, and deeper tissue. The vessels are thin or thick walled and contain luminal proteinaceous fluid or lymphocytes. There is no endothelial atypia or mitotic activity. The intervening stroma is unremarkable or fibrotic (e-**Fig. 38.102**).
6. **Glomus tumor and glomangioma**
   a. **Clinical:** Painful, solitary or multiple, red to purple subungual macule(s); may be a nodule at other sites. Glomangioma is less painful.
   b. **Microscopic:** Well-circumscribed or encapsulated dermal tumor composed of sheets of glomus cells surrounding blood vessels. The glomus cells are homogeneous with eosinophilic cytoplasm and dense, round nuclei. The tumor stroma is fibrous and often pale staining (e-**Fig. 38.103**). A glomangioma is predominantly vascular and has fewer glomus cells (e-**Fig. 38.104**). The glomus cells are immunopositive for smooth muscle actin and negative for endothelial markers such as CD31.
7. **Kaposi sarcoma**
   a. **Clinical:** Early lesions are ecchymotic macules or patches; later lesions are bluish or purple papules, nodules, plaques, and tumors; all are palpable. There are four clinical subtypes with similar cutaneous findings: Classic, African (endemic), epidemic (human immunodeficiency virus [HIV]-associated), and iatrogenic (immunosuppressive therapy related). Regardless of the type, currently classified as a tumor of intermediate biologic potential by the WHO. The etiologic agent is human herpes virus type 8 (HHV-8) in all types.

b. Microscopic: Early lesions show a dermal proliferation of irregular slit-like vascular channels with extravasated erythrocytes, hemosiderin, and plasma cells; the endothelial cells are plump or inconspicuous and without significant cytologic atypia. The vascular channels infiltrate between collagen bundles and surround existing blood vessels and appendages (promontory sign) in the patch stage (e-**Fig. 38.105**). With the plaque stage there are increased spindle cells between the poorly defined slit-like vessels. In the tumor stage, spindled cells form short fascicles, mitoses become more prominent, and intracytoplasmic eosinophilic hyaline globules (PAS positive) can be identified within tumor cells (e-**Fig. 38.106**).

8. Epithelioid hemangioendothelioma

a. Clinical: Firm, tan-pink subcutaneous nodules and plaques, uncommonly involving the dermis, measuring several centimeters in maximal diameter; common sites are the trunk and extremities. Occurs primarily in adults and has a slight female predilection. Now classified as a low-grade sarcoma, cutaneous lesions that are fully excised carry an excellent prognosis.

b. Microscopic: Sheets and cords of large polyhedral tumor cells in the subcutis/dermis. The tumor cells have amphophilic cytoplasm, prominent cytoplasmic vacuoles, and round nuclei often with small nucleoli; the cells have a tendency to grow around pre-existing large vessels. The stroma is variably fibrous or myxoid. Mitotic figures and necrosis may be seen and predict worse clinical behavior. The tumor cells are immunoreactive for endothelial cell markers CD31, CD34, and ERG and, in up to 50% of cases, keratin (e-**Fig. 38.107**).

9. Angiosarcoma

a. Clinical: Single or multifocal, purpuric or black plaque(s) on the head and neck of elderly patients, or purplish-red papules or polypoid tumors in the chronically edematous skin associated with lymphedema and/or prior radiation.

b. Microscopic: Poorly circumscribed and often multifocal proliferation of anastomosing, infiltrative vascular channels in the dermis and subcutis with prominent extravasation of erythrocytes and hemosiderin. The vascular channels are lined by crowded, variably plump, and atypical endothelial cells; papillary processes sometimes extend into the lumens of the vessels. Poorly differentiated tumors with an epithelioid cellular morphology may resemble carcinoma or melanoma. The tumor cells are immunoreactive for endothelial cell markers such as CD31, CD34, and ERG (e-**Fig. 38.108**).

B. Neural and Neuroendocrine Tumors

1. Traumatic neuroma

a. Clinical: Usually a firm, pea-sized nodule in the subcutis and deep soft tissue at sites of previous injury; may be painful.

b. Microscopic: Irregularly arranged nerve fascicles embedded in fibrous scar tissue; there are scattered mast cells (e-**Fig. 38.109**).

2. Solitary circumscribed neuroma (palisaded and encapsulated neuroma)

a. Clinical: Not uncommon; usually solitary, skin-colored or pink papule, most common on the face of middle-aged adults; slowly growing, painless, and <6 mm in diameter.

b. Microscopic: Well-circumscribed and partially encapsulated dermal nodule composed of short fascicles of bland spindle cells with amphophilic cytoplasm and serpiginous nuclei that appear parallel to each other within a single fascicle. No intervening fibrous tissue is present (e-**Fig. 38.110**). Spindle cells are diffusely immunoreactive for S-100 and Sox-10, and the partial capsule may be highlighted by an EMA immunostain.

3. Neurofibroma

a. Clinical: Soft, skin-colored, pedunculated papules or nodules. Multiple lesions in a segmental or widespread distribution are related to neurofibromatosis. The plexiform type is associated with NF1.

b. **Microscopic:** A nonencapsulated dermal or subcutaneous tumor characterized by loosely arranged, wavy spindle cells in a pale-staining stroma; the stroma contains small-caliber vessels and mast cells. The spindle cells tend to surround adnexal structures rather than displace them (**e-Fig. 38.111**). The plexiform type shows tumor cells of similar cytomorphology replacing large nerves, imparting a "bag of worms" appearance at low power. Tumor cells are immunoreactive for S-100 and Sox10.

4. **Cutaneous schwannoma (neurilemmoma)**
   a. **Clinical:** Uncommon, slowly growing, usually solitary tumor/nodule with a predilection for the limbs of adults. The neoplasm can be either sporadic or associated with neurofibromatosis 2 (NF-2). Schwannomas are more commonly seen in the deep soft tissue, intracranially, or intraspinally.
   b. **Microscopic:** Similar to their soft tissue counterpart; form a circumscribed and encapsulated subcutaneous/dermal nodule. The tumor cells are spindled Schwann cells with indistinct cytoplasmic borders arranged in interlacing fascicles. There are hypercellular areas (Antoni A) containing rows or palisades of nuclei aligned around eosinophilic cellular processes (Verocay bodies) and hypocellular (Antoni B), often myxoid areas. No axons are present. Tumor cells are immunoreactive for S-100 and Sox10 while the capsule stains positive for EMA (**e-Fig. 38.112**).

5. **Merkel cell carcinoma**
   a. **Clinical:** Rapidly growing, often ulcerated, red nodule or plaque usually arising on the sun-exposed skin of the elderly, particularly on the head, neck, and extremities; majority of cases are associated with Merkel cell polyoma virus (MCPyV). Current AJCC staging strongly depends on the tumor size and the presence of bone, muscle, fascia, or cartilage invasion (*J Am Acad Dermatol* 2018;78:433).
   b. **Microscopic:** Trabeculae, nests, and sheets of small cells with scant cytoplasm, indistinct cytoplasmic borders, vesicular nuclei with nuclear molding, and multiple small nucleoli that infiltrate the entire dermis and sometimes the subcutis; apoptotic forms and mitoses are frequent; local intralymphatic spread is commonly observed. The tumor cells are positive for neuron-specific enolase, chromogranin, and synaptophysin and have a characteristic "paranuclear dot-like" staining pattern for low–molecular-weight keratin such as CK20. The tumor cells are immunonegative for CD45, S-100, and TTF-1, allowing distinction from hematopoietic and melanocytic neoplasms, as well as metastatic small cell carcinoma of the lung (**e-Fig. 38.113**) (*Clin Lab Med* 2017;37:485).
   c. **Genetics:** Deletion of chromosome 1p36 is commonly seen; numerous other chromosomal abnormalities have been described, of which trisomy 6 is the most common (*Nat Rev Dis Primers* 2017;26;3:17077).

6. **Granular cell tumor**
   a. **Clinical:** Asymptomatic, solitary, skin-colored nodule <3 cm in diameter; multiple lesions in about 10% of cases; most common in adults and women; malignant counterpart is exceedingly rare.
   b. **Microscopic:** Nonencapsulated, dermal-based tumor composed exclusively of large polyhedral cells with abundant fine to coarsely granular eosinophilic cytoplasm, and small, oval, centrally located nuclei. The granular cells infiltrate between collagen bundles and surround adnexal structures. The epidermis may be markedly acanthotic as in pseudocarcinomatous hyperplasia (**e-Fig. 38.114**). Tumor cells are immunoreactive for S-100 and Sox-10.

C. **Fibrous and Fibrohistiocytic Tumors**
   1. **Keloid**
      a. **Clinical:** Firm, pink to purple, mildly tender, bosselated tumors that usually develop at sites of previous injury; most common on the upper back, shoulders, presternal area, and ear lobes of dark-skinned individuals.
      b. **Microscopic:** A nodule of haphazardly arranged, broad, homogeneous, brightly eosinophilic collagen bundles outlined by large, pale-staining fibroblasts in the superficial dermis (**e-Fig. 38.115**).

2. Fibrous histiocytoma (dermatofibroma) and variants

a. Clinical: Most common cutaneous mesenchymal neoplasm; wide range of ages and anatomic sites; reddish-brown hyperpigmented papule or nodule. Cellular variant is typically larger and arises on the extremities or head and neck of young men; reexcision is advised due to recurrence and rare reports of metastasis.

b. Microscopic: Dermal tumor composed of bland spindled cells with variable amounts of pale cytoplasm; arranged in short fascicles or a storiform configuration; characteristic collagen entrapment seen at the edge of the lesion. Inductive changes including epidermal hyperplasia and, less commonly sebaceous hyperplasia, may be present (e-**Fig. 38.116**). Cellular variant composed of more elongate spindle cells; a fascicular architecture predominates; commonly extends into the subcutis. Numerous histologic variants described including aneurysmal and atypical.

c. Genetics: Recurrent mutations involving *PKC* across a variety of histologic subtypes confirm FH as a true neoplasm.

3. Dermatofibrosarcoma protuberans

a. Clinical: Solitary or multiple polypoid nodules arising in an indurated plaque on the trunk or extremities of young adults; slowly growing locally aggressive tumor; rarely metastasizes but risk increases when there is fibrosarcomatous transformation.

b. Microscopic: Cellular dermal tumor composed of homogeneous spindle cells arranged in a storiform or cartwheel pattern; tumor cells infiltrate between the adnexa and there is characteristic extension into the subcutis with fat trapping; occasional mitotic figures can be found, and atypia is mild. The epidermis is normal, atrophic, or ulcerated (e-**Fig. 38.117**). DFSP may undergo fibrosarcomatous transformation characterized by increased cellularity, cytologic atypia, frequent mitoses, and characteristic herringbone architecture. DFSP is strongly and diffusely immunoreactive for CD34 but the expression may be weaker or absent in areas of fibrosarcomatous change.

c. Genetics: The tumor characteristically exhibits the translocation t(17;22) (q22;q13) which results in the production of a COLIA1-PDGFB fusion protein.

4. Angiofibroma

a. Clinical (major types)

i. Fibrous papule of the face: A solitary, firm, dome-shaped, often flesh-colored lesion on the nose or central face.

ii. Pearly penile papules: Tiny white papules, 1 to 3 mm in diameter, arranged in groups or rows on the coronal margin of the penis.

iii. Adenoma sebaceum (tuberous sclerosis): Multiple papules or nodules with a predilection for the butterfly area of the face.

b. Microscopic: Dermal fibrosis with dilated small vessels having plump endothelial cells and variably enlarged, angulated, or stellate fibroblasts. Concentric fibrosis around the blood vessels is more prominent in the adenoma sebaceum than in the fibrous papule of the face (e-**Fig. 38.118**).

c. Genetics: Mutations of two genes, *TSC1* on chromosome 9 and *TSC2* on chromosome 16, are identified in patients with tuberous sclerosis.

5. Acquired digital fibrokeratoma (acral fibrokeratoma)

a. Clinical: A solitary, thin, keratotic nodule on a digit or acral surface.

b. Microscopic: Hyperkeratosis, epidermal acanthosis, and a dense fibrocollagenous dermal nodule with variable number of vessels and fibroblasts (e-**Fig. 38.119**). Differential diagnosis includes the accessory digit, which may have the similar features but also increased and disorganized neural tissue.

6. Acrochordon (skin tag, soft fibroma, fibroepithelial polyp)

a. Clinical: Flesh-colored, pedunculated papules or nodules with irregular or smooth surfaces; most common at the site of friction, especially on the axilla, neck, groin, and eyelids; incidence increases with age; more common in obese women.

b. Microscopic: Polypoid lesion with variable epidermal changes and well-vascularized, loose dermal connective tissue. A variable amount of fat can be seen in the dermis of larger lesions (soft fibroma). No appendages are present (e-**Fig. 38.120**).

D. Fatty and Muscular Tumors

1. Lipoma
   a. Clinical: Common, asymptomatic, soft, subcutaneous nodule.
   b. Microscopic: Unremarkable mature adipocytes are surrounded by a thin fibrous capsule; unlike normal subcutaneous tissue there is a paucity of fibrous septae.

2. Angiolipoma
   a. Clinical: Often multiple/sequential, painful, subcutaneous nodules of the extremities or trunk; usually appears after puberty.
   b. Microscopic: Varying proportions of mature adipose tissue and small-caliber blood vessels with fibrin thrombi, surrounded by a thin fibrous capsule, and arranged vaguely into lobules by fine incomplete fibrous septae (e-**Fig. 38.121**).

3. Dermal pleomorphic lipoma/spindle cell lipoma
   a. Clinical: Soft, painless slow-growing nodules; compared with their subcutaneous counterparts, intradermal lesions have a broad anatomic distribution and a predilection for females.
   b. Microscopic: Spindle cell lipomas are composed of bland spindle cells, mature adipocytes, and ropey collagen with a myxoid background. While subcutaneous tumors are well demarcated, dermal lesions show an infiltrative border. In addition to the aforementioned histologic features, pleomorphic lipomas also display multinucleated "floret-like" giant cells and rare lipoblasts. Both entities are immunoreactive for CD34 and show abnormal loss of RB protein expression.
   c. Genetics: Associated with *RB1* deletion, which is also found in mammary-type myofibroblastoma, cellular angiofibroma and superficial acral fibromyxoma (*Mod Pathol* 2018;31:1862).

4. Leiomyoma
   a. Clinical: Solitary or multiple red nodules; often painful.
   b. Microscopic: Pilar leiomyoma is a circumscribed, nonencapsulated tumor composed of interlacing smooth muscle bundles (e-**Fig. 38.122**). **Scrotal leiomyomas** are similar but often have ill-defined or focally infiltrative margins. **Angioleiomyoma** is a deep dermal/subcutaneous, well-circumscribed nodule of interlacing smooth muscle bundles with multiple thick-walled vessels (e-**Fig. 38.123**).

5. Atypical intradermal smooth muscle neoplasm (AISMN) and leiomyosarcoma.
   Tumors that are confined to the dermis should be classified as AISMN given the demonstrated lack of risk for metastasis; the designation cutaneous leiomyosarcoma should be reserved for those lesions that invade the subcutaneous tissue, which carry a low risk for metastasis (*Appl Immunohistochem Mol Morphol* 2013;21:132).
   a. Clinical: Slowly growing nodule; most commonly occurs on the trunk and lower limbs of elderly men.
   b. Microscopic: Intersecting fascicles of spindle cells with cigar-shaped nuclei and abundant brightly eosinophilic cytoplasm; differentiated from leiomyoma by the presence of nuclear atypia and mitoses; necrosis is uncommon. Tumor cells are immunoreactive for SMA, desmin, and h-caldesmon. Up to 50% of tumors may show focal positivity for keratins.
   c. Genetics: Loss of PTEN staining by IHC has recently been reported in AISMN; *PTEN* mutations and chromosomal losses have also been reported in deep soft tissue and uterine leiomyosarcomas. Importantly, PTEN staining by IHC does not reliably differentiate malignant uterine leiomyosarcoma from benign uterine leiomyoma, and so the role of immunohistochemical staining for PTEN in AISMN is unclear at this time.

V. CUTANEOUS LYMPHOID INFILTRATES.
These infiltrates are highly varied and encompass reactive lymphoid infiltrates, primary cutaneous lymphoma, and cutaneous involvement by systemic/nodal lymphoma. With the exception of mycosis fungoides, determination of whether the skin is the primary or a secondary site of a lymphoma requires a complete clinical examination for appearance and distribution of cutaneous lesions, the presence or absence of lymphadenopathy and/or organomegaly, systemic symptoms, and peripheral

blood smear abnormalities. In contrast to nodal lymphomas (of which B-cell lymphomas comprise the vast majority), approximately 70% of cutaneous lymphomas are of T-cell origin, of which mycosis fungoides is the most common (accounting for about 50% of all cutaneous lymphomas). The updated World Health Organization–European Organization for Research and Treatment of Cancer (WHO-EORTC) consensus classification (Swerdlow SH, Campo E, Harris NL, et al. WHO classification of tumours of haematopoietic and lymphoid tissue. 4th ed. Lyon: IARC Press) is the most current classifications of cutaneous lymphomas, and is uniformly accepted by pathologists, dermatopathologists, dermatologists, and oncologists (*Semin Cutan Med Surg* 2018;37:61).

A. Cutaneous Lymphoid Hyperplasia (Pseudolymphoma, Reactive Lymphoid Hyperplasia, Lymphocytoma Cutis)

1. Clinical: Single or multiple erythematous papules, nodules, or plaques; wide anatomic distribution; occur secondary to any number of insults such as arthropod bites, infection, vaccinations, foreign material, and as a form of drug eruption.

2. Microscopic: Dense dermal infiltrate of lymphocytes, histiocytes, plasma cells, and eosinophils that may extend to the subcutis. Germinal centers may be present. Infiltrate may be B- or T-cell predominant but immunohistochemical and in situ hybridization studies reveal a reactive pattern: normal CD4 to CD8 ratio, CD43 expression limited to T-cells, and polytypic expression of kappa and lambda light chains.

The differential diagnosis includes the following cutaneous B-cell lymphomas: marginal zone, follicular center cell and small lymphocytic types (*Clin Lab Med* 2017;37:547).

B. Mycosis Fungoides

1. Clinical: Patches, plaques, and/or tumors with a wide anatomic distribution; most common in middle-aged to elderly persons, but may occur in children. Usually pruritic, may present with or develop erythroderma; clinical course is usually indolent. Mycosis fungoides (MF) is, as a rule, limited to the skin, with widespread distribution and a protracted disease course. Extracutaneous spread may occur in advanced stages, mainly to lymph nodes, liver, spleen, lungs, and blood. Malignant cells of mycosis fungoides involving the blood in advanced stages are cerebriform in appearance and called Sézary cells. Disease progression involving peripheral blood must be distinguished from the primary Sézary syndrome, a rare T-cell lymphoma that presents as a triad of erythroderma, generalized lymphadenopathy, and malignant T-cells (Sézary cells) in the peripheral blood.

The TNMB staging scheme for MF and Sézary syndrome according to the International Society for Cutaneous Lymphomas (ISCL) and the EORTC depends on the degree of skin, node, visceral, and blood involvement (*Blood* 2007;110:1713). The T-stage (tumor stage) depends on the skin surface area involvement and number of tumors. The N-stage (node stage) depends on the clonality, presence of cerebriform nuclei, and degree of lymph node architecture effacement. The M-stage depends on the level of visceral involvement. In addition to clonality, the B-stage (blood stage) of peripheral blood involvement also depends on blood tumor burden. The current AJCC staging scheme also follows the ISCL-EORTC scheme.

2. Microscopic: Histologic features vary with clinical presentation; epidermal changes range from atrophic to psoriasiform; spongiosis may be disproportionate to the intraepidermal lymphocytes. Immunohistochemical studies reveal the infiltrate to be most commonly composed of CD3- and CD4-positive T-cells that display partial to complete loss of CD2, CD5, and/or CD7. Reactive CD8-positive T-cells are usually present in the dermis. Rarely, tumor cells are CD8 positive and CD4 negative.

a. Patch-stage/early mycosis fungoides is histologically subtle. A patchy, paucicellular band of lymphocytes is present in a fibrotic papillary dermis; lymphocytes extend into the epidermis (epidermotropism); intraepidermal lymphocytes are larger than the dermal lymphocytes and have hyperchromatic, cerebriform nuclei; lymphocytes are separated from keratinocytes by a halo and file along the basal layer of the epidermis (the so-called "string of beads" pattern). Aggregates of atypical intraepidermal lymphocytes (Pautrier microabscesses) are rare. Dermal lymphocytes align along fibrotic papillary dermal collagen bundles (**e-Fig. 38.124**).

b. Plaque stage has easily identifiable Pautrier microabscesses in the epidermis and a more prominent band of lymphocytes in the upper dermis (e-**Fig. 38.125**).

c. Tumor stage shows a dense nodular or diffuse infiltrate filling the dermis and extending into the subcutis; epidermotropism may be lost; eosinophils may be conspicuous. There may be transformation to a large cell phenotype that is often positive for CD30 by IHC (*J Am Acad Dermatol* 2014;70:205).

3. Genetics: Some human leukocyte antigen (HLA) class II alleles (specifically HLA-B8, Aw31, and Aw32) are more prevalent among patients with mycosis fungoides. There is also an increased rate of aberrations involving multiple chromosomes, including chromosomes 1, 6, 11, 8, 17, 13, 15, and 9, in advanced-stage disease.

C. Primary Cutaneous CD30+ Lymphoproliferative Disorders are the second most common form of cutaneous T-cell lymphoproliferative disorders and represent a spectrum of diseases including primary cutaneous anaplastic large cell lymphoma (cALCL), lymphomatoid papulosis (LyP), and borderline cases. Primary cutaneous ALCL and LyP show considerable histologic overlap and are best distinguished on the basis of clinical presentation and course. Further, based on histologic grounds alone, it can be impossible to differentiate cutaneous involvement by systemic ALCL from these entities.

1. Primary cutaneous anaplastic large cell lymphoma (cALCL)

  a. Clinical: Solitary or localized, large (>2 cm), often ulcerated, red/brown tumors; mostly in adults. Partial regression is common; complete spontaneous regression is rare; extracutaneous involvement is possible.

  b. Microscopic: Nodular or diffuse dermal infiltrate composed of sheets of cohesive CD30+ atypical cells, frequently involving the superficial subcutis. The atypical cells have large rounded or irregular vesicular nuclei; prominent, centrally placed nucleoli; and ample clear to amphophilic cytoplasm. A nonneoplastic mixed inflammatory infiltrate is present (e-**Fig. 38.126**). The large lymphocytes in cutaneous ALCL stain positive for CD4, show variable loss of pan T-cell markers (CD2, CD3, etc.), and stain negative for anaplastic lymphoma kinase-1 (ALK-1) which is frequently positive in systemic ALCL.

  c. Genetics: Clonal rearrangement of TCR genes is detected in >90% of cases of primary cutaneous ALCL. However, the translocation t(2;5)(p23;q35) characteristic of systemic ALCL is rarely, if ever, found in primary cutaneous ALCL.

2. Lymphomatoid papulosis (LyP)

  a. Clinical: Recurrent crops of papules, nodules, and plaques at different stages of evolution, mainly on the trunk and extremities of young adults. Spontaneous regression occurs within a few weeks or months; the course may last for decades. Correlation with clinical lesion size, behavior, and distribution is required for diagnosis. Patients with LyP should have lifelong monitoring since 5–25% of patients develop a lymphoma, such as Hodgkin lymphoma or anaplastic large cell lymphoma.

  b. Microscopic: Five histologic subtypes have been described; the three most are:

   i. Type A: Wedge-shaped, mixed cellular infiltrate of small lymphocytes, eosinophils, neutrophils, and histiocytes, mixed with variable numbers of large atypical lymphocytes that may have hyperchromatic nuclei or resemble the neoplastic cells of ALCL (e-**Fig. 38.127**).

   ii. Type B: Histology similar to plaque-stage mycosis fungoides.

   iii. Type C: Histology similar to ALCL.

       The characteristic immunophenotype of the tumor cells is CD30+/CD3+/CD4+, and CD8/EMA negative. CD30-positive cells in Type B may be rare.

  c. Genetics: Clonal rearrangement of TCR gene can be found in at least 40% of LyP lesions. Chromosome deletions and rearrangements of chromosomes 1, 7, 9, and 10 have also been demonstrated.

D. Primary Cutaneous Diffuse Large B-cell Lymphoma (DLBCL), also known as DLBCL-leg type, is a rare B-cell lymphoma in the skin with no evidence of extracutaneous involvement.

1. Clinical: Predominantly affects the elderly, especially women; solitary or clustered reddish brown tumors, often on a distal leg (*Am J Hematol* 2016;91:1052).

2. **Microscopic:** Dense, diffuse dermal infiltrate of large, atypical cells with round to ovoid nuclei, vesicular chromatin, prominent nucleoli, and moderate amounts of pale to basophilic cytoplasm; mitoses are readily identifiable. Infiltrate stains positive for B-cell markers (CD20, CD79a, Pax-5) and is usually positive for bcl-2 and bcl-6. Most cases stain positive for MUM-1 and FOXP1.

3. **Genetics:** Unlike systemic DLBCL, primary cutaneous lesions do not harbor the translocation t(14;18)(q32;q21) but have frequent translocations involving *c-MYC*, *BCL*, and *IGH* (*J Invest Dermatol* 2017;137:1831).

VI. **CUTANEOUS METASTASIS.** The skin is an uncommon site for metastasis from visceral malignancies. Carcinoma may reach the skin by direct extension from an underlying tumor, by lymphatic and/or hematogenous spread as part of systemic involvement, or by accidental implantation during a diagnostic or surgical procedure. Metastases tend to occur on the skin near the primary malignancy; metastasis to sites distant from the primary tumor is more common in tumors that demonstrate angioinvasion.

A. **Clinical:** Common anatomic locations for cutaneous metastases include the head and neck, chest, and abdomen. Lesions appear as nonspecific painless papules or nodules. Most commonly, they represent the spread from primary tumors of the lung, breast, or kidneys (i.e., renal cell carcinoma).

B. **Microscopic:** Cutaneous metastases are generally histologically similar to their primary malignant counterpart.

ACKNOWLEDGMENT

The authors thank Nathan C. Walk, Yumei Chen, Anne C. Lind, Friederike Kreisel, and Dongsi Lu, authors of the previous editions of this chapter.

Skin: Melanocytic Lesions

Louis P. Dehner

I. **INTRODUCTION.** Cutaneous melanocytic lesions are among the most commonly biopsied or excised skin specimens in those areas of the world inhabited in part by light-skinned individuals. Even though a particular lesion is pigmented, not all such lesions are melanocytic; SK, pigmented actinic keratosis, and pigmented basal cell carcinoma are some of the more common nonmelanocytic but pigmented lesions encountered among skin biopsies (e-**Figs. 38.128, 38.129**). The latter three lesions do not exhaust the list which also includes pigmented dermatofibroma, pigmented dermatofibrosarcoma protuberans (Bednar tumor), postinflammatory pigmentation, and scars (e-**Figs. 38.130, 38.131**) (*Clin Dermatol* 2002;20:212). In turn, there are those other lesions without a suspicion for melanoma that are melanomas on microscopic examination (*Clin Dermatol* 2014;32:324). Even a small number of clinically suspected pigmented SKs are malignant melanomas (MMs) on pathologic examination.

Melanocytic proliferative lesions of the skin are categorized into acquired and congenital types which reflect differences not only in clinical presentation, but also pathogenesis. The overwhelming majority of melanocytic lesions of the skin are acquired and the process begins in infancy and continues into later childhood and beyond (*J Am Acad Dermatol* 2016;75:813). It is generally acknowledged in numerous studies that there is a correlation between the number of melanocytic nevi and the risk for cutaneous MM (*J Clin Oncol* 2006;24:3540; *Cancer Epidemiol Biomarkers Prev* 2015;24:817). It is proposed that two pathways exist for the development of cutaneous MM: the chronic sun injury and head and neck pathway as lentigo maligna (lentiginous MM), and the route of precursor nevi (intermittent sun exposure) arising on the trunk and extremities as superficial spreading MM (SSMM). It is the combination of environmental factors, in particular ultraviolet radiation (UVR), and genetic factors such as skin coloration, susceptibility genes, and activation of mitogenic-activated protein kinase (MAPK) pathway that create the biologic stage for the clinical appearance of cutaneous MM (*N Engl J Med* 2015;373:1926). The various melanocytic lesions and their MAPK and other genetic aberrations are summarized in Table 38.2.

There are seemingly countless challenges which are offered by melanocytic lesions in general that reflect their heterogeneous morphology. For that reason, it takes a great deal of experience to acquire a sense of familiarity with these lesions, and not surprisingly, there is a high degree of discordant interpretations even among expert pathologists (*Hum Pathol* 1996;27:528; *J Am Acad Dermatol* 2010 62:751; *BMJ* 2017;357:2813). It is also not surprising that the misdiagnosis of MM is second only to breast cancer as a source of medical liability claims against the pathologist (*Mod Pathol* 2006;19:5148; *Dermatol Clin* 2012;30:593).

II. **ACQUIRED MELANOCYTIC PROLIFERATIONS.** Within this category of lesions there exists benign, malignant, and acknowledged borderline lesions. The patterns of proliferation of neoplastic melanocytes are the following: (1) those restricted to the basal epidermis as single cells in a confluent or nonconfluent lentiginous pattern (note: repopulation of melanocytes along with reconstituted basal epidermis after a skin resection can produce nonconfluent lentiginous-like features); (2) regularly distributed junctional nevomelanocytes are accompanied by dermal nests in the papillary and/or reticular dermis in **compound nevus** (e-**Fig. 38.132**). When there is loss of the dermal nesting pattern within the depths of the dermis, especially around hair follicles, as individual nevus cells whose overall cell size and nuclear size are reduced, the phenomenon is known as maturation or more appropriately senescence with depth. The single-cell pattern of nevus cells at or below the hair follicle is a feature associated with **congenital nevus**. If the nevus cells with depth appear the same size as those at or near the junction, retain their nucleoli, and have scattered individual or grouped mitotic figures, the lesion may represent a nevoid melanoma (e-**Fig. 38.133**) (*Surg Pathol Clin* 2009;2:531). (3) Dermal nests or individual nevus cells are the features of a **dermal nevus** (e-**Fig. 38.134**). The dermal nevus can have a papillomatous configuration in the epidermis with a resemblance to SK, or the contoured epidermis of a fibroepithelial polyp or skin tag. Abundant eosinophilic stroma within the background of a nevus can produce a resemblance to a neurofibroma, the so-called neurotization, or tactile-like bodies. The dermis may have a sclerotic appearance. Metastatic MM in the skin typically features circumscribed but nonnested tumor cells, either at the dermoepidermal junction or within the reticular dermis, and can have an innocuous nevoid appearance.

Other dermal-based melanocytic nevi include the blue nevus (BN) family of lesions (including BN and cellular blue nevus [BN]). Pigmented epithelioid melanocytoma and neurocristic hamartoma are uncommon types of dermal-based lesions.

A. **Simple Lentigo, Solar Lentigo, Lentiginous or Atypical Melanocytic Hyperplasia (LAMH), Lentiginous Dysplastic Nevus (LDN), and Lentigo Maligna (Lentiginous MM in Situ).** These pigmented lesions have in common an increase in the density of melanocytes, nevomelanocytes, or melanoma cells in the basal layer of the epidermis. All of these lesions except for the LAMH present as a pigmented macule (*Clin Dermatol* 2014;32:88).

   1. **Simple lentigo** is ubiquitous in its distribution and has a sharply delineated focus of pigmented linear hyperplasia of melanocytes with some elongation of rete ridges and absence of solar elastosis (e-**Fig. 38.135**).

   2. **Solar lentigo** (SoL) is characterized by hyperplasia of rete ridges with intense pigmentation of the rete tips, all in a background solar elastosis (*J Am Acad Dermatol* 1997;36:444) (e-**Fig. 38.136**). The hyperplastic melanocytes generally lack atypia, but the differential diagnosis is lentiginous melanoma in situ (LMIS) so that Melan A or HMB-45 is useful in the delineation of the melanocytic proliferation beyond the apparent focus of hyperpigmentation, or expansion of atypical melanocytes into the

TABLE 38.2 Mutational Landscape of Melanocytic Lesions

Gene	Congenital Melanocytic Nevus (%)	Common Acquired Nevus (%)	Blue Nevus (%)	Spitz Nevus (%)	Atypical Spitz Tumor (%)	Spitz-like (Spitzoid Melanoma) (%)	Common MM (%)
BRAF	5–15	~80	—	5–6	5–6	30–40	40–70
NRAS	70–90	2–3	—	2–3	2–3	Rare	15–20
HRAS	N/A	N/A	—	10–20	15–16	Rare	Rare, if at all
ROS, ALK, NTRK1, RET, ROS1, MET	N/A	N/A	—	50–55	55–60	35–40	—
GNAQ/GNA11	—	—	70–80[a]	—	—	—	—
CDKN2A	—	—	—	—	—	±	12–15
KIT	—	—	—	—	—	—	3–4
KRAS	—	—	—	—	—	—	3–5

[a]GNAQ/GNA11 mutations in 80% uveal melanoma (*N Engl J Med* 2010;363:2191).

upper layers of the epidermis or into and around hair follicles. Of note, some concern has been expressed whether Melan A immunostaining tends to overestimate the number of actual atypical melanocytes in this context (*J Cutan Pathol* 2016;35:931; *J Cutan Pathol* 2011;38:775). MiTF or Sox-10 staining is an alternative approach. SoL may not have club-like elongations of the rete ridges but only basal melanosis on a base of dermal elastosis; SoL may also reside adjacent to LMIS which is potentially problematic when the more serious pathology has not been sampled.

3. **Lentiginous dysplastic nevus** (LDN) has very similar histologic features to SoL except for the presence of melanocytic nests at the tips and along the side of the rete ridges.

4. **Lentiginous melanoma in situ** (LMIS), like SoL, is seen in chronic sun-damaged skin of the head and neck and upper posterior trunk. The differential diagnosis between LDN and LMIS is not always sharp, and may be arbitrated with immunohistochemical staining. A dense population of atypical melanocytes concentrated in the basilar region, possibly an occasional nest with nevoid features in some cases, extension down the hair follicle, and some pagetoid spread are the basic histologic features of LMIS. In some cases, the involved epidermis has a true or artifactual cleft lifting it from the dermis. The atypical melanocytes trail along the basal layer generally without an abrupt transition to uninvolved skin as in most, but not all, LDNs. The atypical melanocytes may be interrupted by an apparent focus without atypical cells (the so-called skip focus). Approximately 10% to 15% of LMIS have an invasive MM in the skin excision so that thorough sampling is required (*J Am Acad Dermatol* 2015;73:193). Ascertainment of tumor-free margins is difficult since an edge of a resection may demonstrate scattered or individual melanocytes. Both mucous membrane and acral MM have similar lentiginous features to the chronic sun-damaged LMIS.

5. **Atypical melanocytic hyperplasia or proliferation** is a poorly defined but convenient designation for a lentiginous proliferation overlying an otherwise unremarkable dermal nevus and lichenoid keratosis. Nests of melanocytes can occur in the midst of lichenoid inflammation producing a diagnostic dilemma of junction nevus versus pseudonevus (*J Cutan Pathol* 2011;38:797).

B. Common Acquired Melanocytic Nevi

1. **Junctional melanocytic nevus** is first appreciated in children and less often in adults, especially in those beyond the age of 50 years. The nests of nevomelanocytes are regularly distributed at the tips of rete ridges, typically in the absence of any obvious single-cell or lentiginous component (e-**Fig. 38.137**).

2. **Compound melanocytic nevus** is defined by a combined junctional and dermal nevomelanocytic pattern. The junctional nests are variably prominent to the extent that they may be overlooked on initial review especially in those lesions with a substantial dermal component (e-**Fig. 38.132**). The nests in the suprapapillary dermis are pressed against the basal epidermis so that it is difficult to be certain whether the nests are junctional or not. The dermis is occupied to a greater or lesser degree by relatively uniform, discrete, but often crowded nests of nevomelanocytes which tend to become smaller in size from the superficial to the deeper dermis. Like the junctional nests, the overall configuration of the entire nevus is one of architectural symmetry. If the dermal nests are tending to fuse, the growth becomes confluent, and the presumed nevomelanocytes retain their size and nucleoli similar to the superficial dermal population, the possibility of a **nevoid** or **small cell MM** must be considered, a lesion that shows the minimal so-called maturation with depth with retention of nucleoli and deep mitotic figures (e-**Fig. 38.133**) (*Surg Pathol Clin* 2009;2:521).

3. **Compound melanocytic nevus with architectural disorder (dysplastic nevus)** and its junctional counterpart are characterized by the following histopathologic features (e-**Fig. 38.138**): (1) basilar nevomelanocytic proliferation with nested and nonconfluent lentiginous (single cells) features; in the compound lesion, junctional nests are three rete ridges beyond the dermal nests (the so-called shouldering); (2) mild to moderate atypia; (3) lamellar fibroplasia; (4) fusion of rete; and (5) mild inflammation and vascular reaction in superficial dermis (*J Am Acad Dermatol* 2012;67:e1;

Dermatol Clin 2012;30:389). By definition, there is nevomelanocytic atypia of a mild to moderate degree in these lesions, but it may be more worrisome in some cases to the point of recommended reexcision. It has been reported that the architecturally disordered nevus is less likely to have BRAF V600E expression (*J Am Acad Dermatol* 2018;79:221).

C. **Acquired Melanocytic Nevi With Unique Clinical and/or Pathologic Features.** These various lesions include the halo, Meyerson, special site, ancient, persistent, and combined nevi.

1. **Halo (Sutton) nevus** is clinically recognized as a sharp zone of hypopigmentation around various types of nevi from the common acquired, to Spitz, to congenital nevi (*Int J Dermatol* 2015;54:e433). The dense lymphocytic infiltrate, rich in CD8+ T-lymphocytes, may partially or focally obscure the nevomelanocytic process (**e-Fig. 38.139**). Histologic features of a halo nevus can be present without the clinical halo.

2. **Meyerson nevus** is another example of a localized inflammatory reaction in the superficial dermis and epidermal spongiosis in the presence of an acquired or congenital nevus. Lymphocytes with some eosinophils are present.

3. **Special site nevi** or those with site-related atypia include the following sites: breast, axilla, ear, scalp, genitalia (vulva and penis), and acral location (*Am J Dermatopathol* 2016;38:867). The histologic features in many respects overlap with those of the architecturally disordered or dysplastic nevus. Those nevi on the breast and vulva are especially problematic.

4. **"Ancient" nevus** is predominantly dermal and is otherwise unremarkable except for the presence of large pleomorphic cells scattered among otherwise small nevomelanocytes. Foci of perivenular sclerosis and pseudoangiomatous changes are often present.

5. **Persistent (recurrent) nevus** usually makes its reappearance within 12 months after a shave biopsy. Recurrent pigmentation may simply represent a hyperpigmented scar or irregularly distributed junctional nests with or without dermal nests in the midst of a dermal scar (**e-Fig. 38.140**).

6. **Combined nevus** is defined as a nevus with two or more distinctive populations or patterns of nevomelanocytes (*Am J Surg Pathol* 2011;35:1540). Most commonly, an acquired or architecturally disordered nevus is accompanied by a BN, DPN, or Spitz nevus. The Spitz nevus and DPN are prone to have atypical features.

D. **Deeply Pigmented Nevomelanocytic Lesions.** This group of lesions has overlapping histopathologic features of exclusive spindle or epithelioid cells, or some combination of these two cytomorphologies (*J Clin Pathol* 2015;68:963). These lesions in aggregate constitute a minority of nevomelanocytic proliferations.

1. **Deep penetrating nevus** (DPN), also known as plexiform spindle cell nevus, has a distinctive architecture of a sharply demarcated, wedge-shaped, spindle cell, and/or epithelioid proliferation whose base is toward the epidermis and tip is toward the reticular dermis or subcutis (**e-Fig. 38.141**). There is often a junctional or compound nevus in association with the DPN, but distinct from it, so that the DPN represents a type of combined nevus.

   DPN is a solitary, deeply pigmented lesion that presents on the upper half of the body in individuals less than 30 years. The differential diagnosis includes CBN and psammomatous pigmented schwannoma. Another nevomelanocytic lesion with DPN-like features is the **clonal nevus** with its focal nests of atypical epithelioid nevus cells, also known as an inverted type A nevus, or nevus with focal atypical epithelioid components (NFAEC). A junctional nevus component is more common in the NFAEC than the DPN.

2. **Pigmented spindle cell nevus of Reed**, because of the presence of Kamino bodies, has led some experts to favor Spitz nevus (SN). In this lesion, the symmetrically pigmented spindle nevomelanocytic proliferation is localized to the epidermal–dermal junction, or includes contiguous nests also in the papillary dermis (**e-Fig. 38.142**). Pagetoid melanocytosis is seen, as well as patchy atypia, which can cause some concern about pigmented spindle cell MM.

3. **Blue (BN) and cellular blue (CBN) nevi** are dermal-based lesions usually accompanied by intense pigmentation in most but not all cases. BN is composed of a circumscribed focus of spindled and dendritic nevomelanocytes in the superficial dermis where the cells interdigitate between bundles of collagen (e-**Fig. 38.143**). An epithelioid variant of BN appears on occasion; sclerosis in the background is another feature. CBN, unlike BN, is a nodular lesion with a predilection for the scalp and gluteal region. In the superficial dermis, this lesion resembles a BN, but the well-circumscribed nodular portion may bulge into the subcutis (e-**Fig. 38.144**). The nodule is variably cellular with small to somewhat larger epithelioid and/or smaller spindle cells, with a peripheral population of pigmented spindle cells and melanophages.

4. **Pigmented epithelioid melanocytoma (PEM, epithelioid blue nevus)** is a heavily pigmented, dermal-based nodule which may occupy the full thickness of the dermis by spindle and epithelioid cells as single cells, nests, and fascicles. The polygonal or epithelioid nevomelanocytes may display worrisome atypia. PEM may be accompanied by another type of nevus (SN, deep penetrating nevus). Lymph node metastasis is reported, but in most cases that is the full extent of the disease (*Br J Dermatol* 2016;174:1115). PEM occurs sporadically or as a manifestation of the Carney complex (*Eur J Endocrinol* 2015;173:M85).

5. **Dermal melanocytosis** presents clinically as a nevus of Ota, or Ito, or mongolian spot. It is generally unnecessary to biopsy these lesions since the clinical presentation is diagnostic. However, there is a resemblance to BN, but without the lentil shape and a more dispersed pattern of spindle and dendritic melanocytes within various layers of the dermis (e-**Fig. 38.145**).

E. **Spitz Nevus (SN) and Other Spitzoid Tumors.** This group of lesions presents as a morphologic spectrum of similar appearing nevomelanocytic neoplasms which are composed of spindle and/or epithelioid cells.

1. **Spitz nevus** and variants occur throughout life, but 10% to 20% of cases are diagnosed in the first three decades and at least 40% at or before age 15 years. There are also rare congenital examples. Approximately 10% of nevomelanocytic lesions in children are SN; children 10 years or younger constitute 65% of pediatric SN (*Pediatr Dev Pathol* 2018;21:252).

   SN is a solitary dome-shaped, flesh-colored papulonodule measuring 1 cm or less that has a predilection for the head and neck and upper extremity in 60% of cases. The overwhelming majority of cases have the following histologic features in some combination (e-**Fig. 38.146**): (1) symmetrical nodule; (2) epidermal hyperplasia; (3) superficial vascular ectasias (which accounts for the clinical impression of pyogenic granuloma in some cases); (4) vertically oriented junctional spindle and/or epithelioid nevomelanocytes with intercellular clefts; (5) Kamino (eosinophilic) bodies; (6) a nested or confluent spindle and/or epithelioid dermal pattern (pure epithelioid SN may be BAP-1 deficient) (*J Am Acad Dermatol* 2018;79:525); (7) reduction in the cell size and prominence of nuclei with depth in dermis; and (8) typical mitotic figures in junctional and superficial nevoid cells if present at all. The growth into the dermis may have a wedge-shaped pattern similar to DPN which is typically densely pigmented.

2. **Atypical spitzoid tumor and spitzoid melanoma** are generally characterized by asymmetrical growth, enlarged hyperchromatic and pleomorphic nuclei within the deeper aspects of the lesion, and mitotic figures also within the depths of lesion (e-**Figs. 38.147, 38.148**). The lesions remain problematic in terms of diagnosis even among experts (*Pediatr Dev Pathol* 2018;21:252).

III. **CONGENITAL MELANOCYTIC NEVUS.** By definition, congenital melanocytic nevus (CMN) is one that is recognized at or soon after birth and is present in up to 2% of neonates, though some may not be identified until later childhood as a so-called tardive CMN (*Clin Dermatol* 2015;33:368). CMNs are classified on the basis of size (as projected on their adult size): small, <1.5 cm; medium, 1.5 to 2.0 cm; large, 20 to 40 cm; and giant, >40 cm). Giant CMN occurs in 1:20,000 to 50,000 live births, is accompanied by neurocutaneous melanosis in 10% of cases, and is complicated by MM in 2% to 6% of cases (*Pediatr Dev Pathol* 2018;21:252).

Like common acquired melanocytic nevus, the histologic patterns are junctional, compound, and dermal; however, the diagnostic features of CMN are encountered at or below the level of the hair follicles where the nevomelanocytes are present as individual small cells trailing through the reticular dermis and into the subcutis along the fibrous septa or into the adipose tissue (e-**Fig. 38.149**). Nevomelanocytes also track along and around adnexa, nerves, and vessels. In those cases where the nevomelanocytes surround adnexa, but do not extend into the depths of the reticular dermis, the lesion may be qualified as having "congenital features" rather than "congenital melanocytic nevus." Of these two patterns, a lesion confined to the dermis has been designated CMN type I and a deeply infiltrative lesion as type II (*Am J Dermatopathol* 2015;37:31).

Proliferative nodule(s) (PN) presents as one or more nodular and/or hyperpigmented foci within a large or giant CMN. It is a distinctive focus of larger atypical cells in the midst of the smaller nevomelanocytes. Mitotic figures are generally few in number with some exceptions. Before the appreciation of the PN as benign, this nodule(s) was commonly interpreted as MM.

IV. MALIGNANT MELANOMA. MM of the skin accounts for 90% or more of all cases of melanoma, but there are several other primary sites for melanoma including the eye, mucous membranes in the head and neck, vulva, vagina, urethra, and anus. In the United States, the incidence has increased from 6.8 to 20.1 per 100,000 from 1973 to 2007 with an increase in incidence of 3% per year during this period (*J Natl Cancer Inst* 2016;doi:10.1093). It is a disease of fair-skinned individuals; the trunk and lower extremities in females, and the trunk, upper extremities, and head and neck in males, are the sites of predilection. Though cutaneous MM constitutes 5% or less of all primary cutaneous malignancies, it accounts for 50% or more of tumor-related deaths. Approximately 15% of those with MM on presentation have metastasis in a lymph node, viscera, or nonprimary cutaneous site, and 5% have a metastatic MM without a known primary site. UVR exposure is regarded as the pathogenetic factor and there are two postulated pathways (*Cancer Epidermiol* 2017;48:147): (1) early development of multiple melanocytic nevi in children followed by intermittent UVR exposure with MMs arising from extremities and trunk as SSMM; or (2) chronic UVR exposure of the skin of the head and neck, dorsal hand, and upper back through successive stages from LMIS to invasive MM. Specific mutations in the MAPK pathway (*BRAF* or *NRAS*) are the initial genetic events in melanomagenesis (*N Engl J Med* 2015;373:1926).

A. Pathologic Types of Melanoma. Three basic histopathologic types of cutaneous MM are recognized, although there are also several variants: SS; lentigo maligna, and nodular types (*Hematol Oncol Clin N Am* 2009;23:501). Some of the other variants include acral lentiginous, desmoplastic, nevoid, spitzoid, signet-ring, and rhabdoid MM.

1. **Melanoma in situ** (MIS) has been discussed above in the section on lentiginous nevomelanocytic proliferations. In addition to lentigo maligna, which is the most common pattern of MIS, SSMM often has an in situ component; however, exclusive MIS, SS type is uncommon (e-**Figs. 38.135, 38.150**). The head and neck is the most common site of MIS; most of these lesions are lentigo maligna or lentiginous MIS (*J Am Acad Dermatol* 2015;73:181).

2. **Superficial spreading MM (SSMM)** is the most common pattern among the three basic types. It presents on the trunk in males and lower extremity in females as a generalization, since it is seen on any body site. The BRAF V600E pathway that is associated with the number of nevi and intermittent sun exposure is correlated with this pattern. Junctional nests and infiltration of the epidermis by individual, often epithelioid cells, with a confluent pattern are the epidermal features of SSMM. The nests of cells, containing abundant eosinophilic or pigmented atypical cells, have an irregular distribution along the epidermal–dermal junction where invasion is identified as a patchy or confluent process. Any superficial nest formation often gives way to the formation of sheets of tumor cells, individual cells, or small irregular clusters (e-**Fig. 38.151**). Pigment incontinence and a variably intense lymphocytic infiltrate

are other features. Prominent nucleoli are maintained in tumor cells in all levels of dermal invasion. The number of mitotic figures tends to vary.

3. **Lentigo maligna melanoma** (LMM) is characterized by its lentiginous pattern of atypical cells along the junction, together with occasional nests and pagetoid spread in some cases. The pattern of dermal invasion may be a solitary, or as more than one focus along the length of the MIS (e-**Fig. 38.152**). Individual atypical cells in the papillary dermis are always problematic; these cells are likely macrophages in many instances. Individual nests of highly atypical tumor cells, or spindle cells in a desmoplastic stroma (desmoplastic melanoma [DM]), are the features of LMM. In the latter setting, neurotrophic involvement can be seen.

4. **Desmoplastic melanoma** (DM) is regarded as a variant of LMM with its predilection for the head and neck, where lentiginous MIS and marked solar elastosis are indicative of chronic solar injury. Because DM is predominantly dermal based, an overlying junctional lentiginous proliferation may not be apparent in the biopsy. The spindle cells often have enlarged, hyperchromatic nuclei, but some cases may have less impressive nuclear abnormalities and may even be bland appearing. A myxoid, desmoplastic stroma serves as the background with separation of the cells (e-**Fig. 38.153**). Neurotropic growth as either perineural or intraneural involvement is a feature of DM. Most DMs, but not all DMs, are S-100 positive and virtually all are SOX10 positive.

5. **Nodular melanoma** (NM) accounts for 15% of cutaneous MM, compared with 15% to 20% for SSMM and 10% to 12% for LMM (*Arch Dermatol* 2012;148:30). NM pursues a vertical rather than a radial growth phase, unlike SSMM and LMM, which accounts for its disproportionate fatality rate of 35% to 40%. NM presents as a polypoid or nodular mass, often with ulceration and without site preference. If present, the junctional component does not extend beyond the nodule as in the case of SSMM with a nodule. Microscopically, the lesion is composed of a monotonous population of high-grade, rounded tumor cells with abundant mitotic figures (e-**Fig. 38.154**). The Breslow thickness is significantly greater in NM than either SSMM or LMM, except in the case of DM.

B. **Immunohistochemistry.** IHC in nevomelanocytic lesion and MM largely relies on antibodies to S-100 protein, Melan-A/MART1, HMB-45, SOX10, p16, and MITF (*J Cutan Pathol* 2008;35:433; *Hum Pathol* 2014;45:191). These markers are especially helpful in the following settings.

1. Poorly differentiated epithelioid and spindle cell neoplasms with MM in the differential diagnosis which present as a primary or metastatic tumor. S-100 remains the most sensitive marker for MM, but SOX10 should be used in conjunction with S-100 since MM infrequently can lose its immunophenotype especially in the presence of a spindle cell pattern.

2. Lentiginous nevomelanocytic lesions that have the differential diagnosis of LDN versus lentigo maligna (lentiginous MIS). Melan-A/MART1 is useful in the demonstration of the pattern of a continuous, confluent proliferation of atypical melanocytes which helps to support an interpretation of lentigo maligna, with a more limited radial pattern in LDN.

3. The combination of p16, HMB-45, and Ki-67 may be helpful to differentiate an atypical appearing compound melanocytic nevus from nevoid melanoma. Loss of p16, loss of HMB-45 gradient, and Ki-67 positive nuclei are supportive of nevoid melanoma.

4. Sentinel lymph node biopsies are routinely stained for S-100 protein, HMB-45, Melan-A, and/or Ki-67. These stains do not distinguish nevus cells from MM. Although most nevus cells are found in the capsule, this is not always the case. However, p16 (retained in nevus cells) may be helpful as well as nestin and SOX2 (*Arch Pathol Lab Med* 2018;142:815; *Mod Pathol* 2013;26:44).

5. Desmoplastic melanoma (DM), scar, malignant peripheral nerve sheath (MPNST) and other spindle cell neoplasms that have overlapping histologic features. Sox10 positivity serves to identify DM and MPNST from the others (*Histopathology* 2018; doi:10.1111). Only 40% to 50% of MPNST are S-100 protein positive in a patchy

distribution whereas most, but not all, DMs have a diffuse pattern of staining. Lentiginous MIS in the presence of a high-grade spindle cell or even bland spindle cell component establishes the diagnosis of DM.

C. Fluorescence in Situ Hybridization (FISH). This ancillary technique has its application in the assessment of a particularly troublesome melanocytic lesion. The standard 4 FISH probes, RREB1 (6p25), MYB (6q23), CCND1 (4q13), and centromere 6 (CEP 6), have been augmented in some studies by the addition of CDKN2A (9q21), centromere 9 (CEP 9), and MYC (8q24) (*Pathology* 2017;49:740; *Mod Pathol* 2018; doi: 10.1038). Another group of melanocytic lesions which has drawn attention in the utilization of FISH is the spitz/spitzoid lesion (*Pathology* 2016;48:113). The interpretation of the results should always be integrated with the clinicopathologic context since the diagnostic accuracy of the FISH technique is far from being absolute (*Am J Dermatopathol* 2016;38:253).

D. Pathologic Staging of MM. Staging of cutaneous MM has undergone several modifications in the last several years, but the basic principles remain tumor thickness (Breslow thickness now rounded out to 0.1 rather than 0.01 mm), the presence or absence of ulceration, and spread to regional lymph nodes as detected by sentinel lymph node biopsy (SLNB) (clinically occult) or clinically detected disease, and spread to distant sites (lung, liver) (*Am Surg Oncol* 2018;25:2105). Modifications have been made in the T1 category which includes T1a (<0.8 mm without ulceration) and T1b (0.8 to 1.0 mm with or without ulceration, and <0.8 mm with ulceration). There is a well-established correlation between Breslow thickness and survival; although mitotic activity in MM is still regarded as important in the outcome of the patient, problems are acknowledged in the reproducibility of findings so that mitotic figures have been eliminated in the assessment of T1a and T1b. The recent AJCC staging scheme also contains some alterations in the N-category of lymph node metastasis and presence or absence of in transit, satellite, or microsatellite metastases; definition of distant metastasis (M) has been refined to many more subgroups and also includes normal or elevated serum lactic dehydrogenase (Amin MB, Edge S, Greene F, et al., eds. *AJCC Cancer Staging Manual*, 8th ed. New York: Springer, 2017). Reporting should follow suggested guidelines (e.g., see the College of American Pathologists Protocol for the Examination of Specimens From Patients With Melanoma of the Skin, at http://www.cap.org).

V. MELANONYCHIA. Brownish to black pigmentation of a nail(s) has melanocytic and non-melanocytic causes (*Dermatol Clin* 2015;33:185). Longitudinal melanonychia is a band or strip from the base to the edge of the nail caused by melanin excess as a reaction with the overproduction of melanin in otherwise normal-appearing melanocytes (lentigo), to an acral junctional nevus, or to the rare subungual MM (*Br J Dermatol* 2017;27:275).

ACKNOWLEDGMENT

The author thanks Anne C. Lind, Nils Becker, and Emily A. Bantle, authors of the previous editions of this chapter.

SUGGESTED READINGS

Abbas O, Miller DD, Bhawan J. Cutaneous malignant melanoma: update on diagnostic and prognostic biomarkers. *Am J Dermatopathol* 2014;36(5):363–379.

Elder DE, Massi D, Scolyer R, Willemze R. *WHO Classifications of Skin Tumours*. 4th ed. Lyon, France: IARC Press; 2017.

Gershenwald JE, Hess KR, Ross MI, et al. Melanoma of the skin. *AJCC Cancer Staging Manual*, 8th ed. 2017; 47:563–585.

Pimiento JM, Larkin EM, Smalley KSM, et al. Melanoma genotypes and phenotypes get personal. *Lab Invest* 2013;93(8):858–867.

Yaman B, Akalin T, Kandilo lu G. Clinicopathological characteristics and mutation profiling in primary cutaneous melanoma. *Am J Dermatopathol* 2015;37(5):389–397.

Nervous System

39

Central Nervous System: Brain, Spinal Cord, and Meninges

Richard J. Perrin and Sonika M. Dahiya

I. **INTRODUCTION.** This chapter provides a baseline approach to common neuropathologic entities that are encountered in the daily practice of surgical pathology.

II. **ANATOMY AND HISTOLOGY.** The central nervous system (CNS) consists of cerebrum, cerebellum, brain stem, spinal cord, meninges, 12 paired cranial nerves, and the blood vessels supplying these structures. The brain and spinal cord are enclosed within the skeletal confines of the cranium and vertebral column. The mature (adult) brain weighs around 1,200 to 1,400 grams. The meninges covering the brain and spinal cord are of two principle types: (1) the dense fibrous dura mater and (2) the more delicate leptomeninges (pia and arachnoid mater). The cerebrum is divided into right and left hemispheres by a thick dural fold: the falx cerebri. A second dural fold between the cerebrum and cerebellum (tentorium cerebelli) divides the brain into supra- and infratentorial compartments. Infratentorially, the midbrain, pons, and medulla oblongata (cranial to caudal) form the brain stem, which is connected to the cerebellum by three (superior, middle, and inferior) cerebellar peduncles. The supratentorial compartment contains cerebral cortex (frontal, temporal, parietal, and occipital lobes), white matter, and deep gray nuclei, such as basal ganglia, thalamus, and hypothalamus. The term "neuraxis" is sometimes used to refer to brain and spinal cord; thus, lesions that involve brain parenchyma are said to be "intra-axial" (e.g., astrocytoma, central neurocytoma, ependymoma), and those located outside of the parenchyma are referred to as "extra-axial" (e.g., meningioma, hemangiopericytoma [HPC]/solitary fibrous tumor [SFT], and schwannoma of cranial nerve VIII). Similarly, in the spine, the terms "intramedullary" and "extramedullary" are used to denote lesions within or adjacent to the spinal cord parenchyma, respectively.

The CNS is composed of gray and white matter. Neuronal cell bodies and dendrites reside mostly in the gray matter (cortex and deep gray nuclei), and axons create the framework of the white matter. Glial cells (astrocytes, oligodendroglial cells, and microglia) are also present in different proportions in these two tissues. Oligodendrocytes are more populous in the white matter; their processes form the sheaths of myelin that insulate CNS axons. The eosinophilic, finely granular to fibrillary material between cell bodies, often referred to as "neuropil," is formed by the processes of neurons (axons and dendrites) and glial cells. Neuronal morphology varies significantly, with cell body size ranging from <15 μm (e.g., small neocortical granular stellate neurons) to 100 μm (Betz cells of the primary motor cortex). For descriptive purposes, neocortical pyramidal neurons are often considered the morphologic prototype. These cells contain abundant amphophilic cytoplasm,

583

clumpy basophilic Nissl substance, a large round central nucleus, a prominent nucleolus, coarse proximal cytoplasmic processes, and a prominent apical dendrite oriented perpendicular to the cortical surface. Ependymal glial cells form a ciliated cuboidal epithelium that lines the ventricles and central canal and focally transitions with the epithelium of the choroid plexus. The choroid plexus, which produces cerebrospinal fluid (CSF) within the ventricles, has papillary architecture; its branching fibrovascular cores are lined by a specialized cuboidal epithelium with a hobnailed apical surface.

III. INTRAOPERATIVE EVALUATION, GROSS EXAMINATION, AND TISSUE SAMPLING. Evaluation of a surgical neuropathology specimen often begins with an intraoperative consultation, which may be requested by the surgeon: (1) to confirm the presence of lesional tissue; (2) to provide a preliminary diagnosis that will guide surgical management (e.g., aggressive surgery for a well-circumscribed tumor like ependymoma, limited biopsy for lymphoma, culture sample to microbiology for abscess or granulomatous inflammation); and (3) to sample fresh or frozen tissue for ancillary studies (e.g., Western blot for Creutzfeldt–Jakob disease [CJD], molecular pathology, tumor banking, karyotyping). For optimal evaluation, specimens should ideally be submitted on Telfa nonstick gauze pads saturated with normal saline. Tissue that has been soaked in saline is certainly acceptable, but is more likely to fragment during transport and may demonstrate more severe freezing artifacts. Fresh brain tissue, especially small biopsy specimens, should never be placed on dry gauze or tissue paper because subsequent tissue retrieval from these materials is almost impossible. Water content may be reduced through very gentle blotting on a clean dry plastic surface, but fresh brain tissue is very fragile, and improper handling can introduce cellular touch and crush artifacts.

For intraoperative diagnosis, small portions of the fresh specimen should be chosen for freezing, for cytologic smear or touch preparations, and for possible ultrastructural examination. When multiple pieces of tissue are received, sampling more than one piece for each of these preparations may yield a more accurate intraoperative diagnosis. However, freezing or otherwise exhausting the entire specimen for intraoperative diagnosis should be avoided, for several reasons. First, the techniques available during intraoperative examination seldom yield sufficient information for a definitive final diagnosis; most diagnoses require the fine histologic detail afforded by paraffin sections and information from immunohistochemical stains and other ancillary molecular tests. Second, freezing introduces artifacts (e.g., ice crystals, clumping of nuclear chromatin). These artifacts persist when the residual tissue is processed for permanent sections, can easily compromise the accuracy of the final diagnosis (for example, permanent sections of previously frozen oligodendroglioma tissue often show artificially irregular, hyperchromatic nuclear features reminiscent of neoplastic astrocytes), and can impair the performance and interpretation of some ancillary studies that are increasingly performed for diagnosis and prognosis. Third, on some occasions, surgical attempts to obtain additional diagnostic material from the patient cause bleeding or other complications that prevent further tissue acquisition.

The manner in which intraoperative specimens are processed for diagnosis is just as important as tissue selection. For optimal results, frozen sections of CNS tissue require techniques that differ somewhat from those commonly used in surgical pathology. Before any tissue is frozen, a block of embedding compound (OCT, poured into an empty tissue well within the cryostat) should be frozen fast to a cryostat chuck. After freezing, the chuck and OCT block are removed sharply and inverted. The tissue to be frozen should be placed centrally on the flat surface of the frozen OCT block, immediately covered with a minimal amount of liquid OCT, and frozen from above by a flat, prechilled metallic weight (e-**Fig. 39.1**). Once the tissue is frozen, multiple 5-μm thick sections are cut, affixed to slides, immersed briefly in 95% alcohol, and stained with hematoxylin and eosin (H&E) for intraoperative diagnosis. This process maximizes rate of freezing and minimizes (but does not eliminate) ice crystal formation. Cytologic evaluation by smear preparation is extremely helpful because it lacks freezing artifacts and preserves nuclear details. Smears can be prepared by gently compressing a very small amount of representative tissue between two glass slides, gently sliding them apart, and immediately fixing both smeared slides in

95% alcohol (e-Fig. 39.2). Lastly, a small tissue fragment (1 mm³) should also be fixed in glutaraldehyde and stored for potential electron microscopic studies, particularly if the intraoperative diagnosis is unclear.

In contrast, gross examination and tissue sampling for permanent sections is less complicated for neuropathologic specimens than for most other surgical pathology specimens. Most neuropathologic specimens are small and/or fragmented, limiting full appreciation of meaningful gross features. Even when large resection specimens are submitted intact, gross abnormalities are often absent or subtle. In fact, radiologic imaging is commonly considered the "gross pathology" for CNS biopsies. In either case, specimens are usually entirely submitted for histologic analysis after adequate formalin fixation (a few hours for smaller specimens; overnight for large specimens). This practice is particularly important because most neuropathologic processes are heterogeneous. Even when the diagnosis seems clear, if a resection specimen is too large for complete processing, it should still be extensively sampled. For similar reasons, resected tissue that appears morcellated by Cavitronic UltraSound Aspiration (CUSA) or similar processes should not be dismissed as worthless; such material may show histologic artifacts (e.g., variable autolysis that must be carefully distinguished from true necrosis) that are absent from mechanically resected tissue, but, occasionally, it provides essential clues to the final diagnosis.

A. CNS Biopsy for Special Circumstances. Brain and sometimes meningeal biopsies for nonneoplastic indications are occasionally performed (e.g., nonresolving chronic meningitis, neurosarcoidosis). Similarly, a "blind" frontal lobe biopsy is sometimes obtained for neurodegenerative disorders that do not have a clearly defined etiology, particularly in younger patients. When a prion protein disease like CJD is suspected, a neuropathologist should be given advance notice, and should be involved from the outset. One piece of cortex from the biopsy should be snap frozen for Western blot analysis by a reference laboratory such as the National Prion Disease Pathology Surveillance Center (NPDPSC) (special shipping containers must be used, and specific procedures must be followed; see http://www.cjdsurveillance.com/). The remaining tissue should be fixed in 10% neutral buffered formalin for 24 hours, followed by immersion in 88% to 98% formic acid (undiluted stock solution) for 1 hour, prior to routine processing. If initial histologic examination reveals pathologic features consistent with CJD or fails to suggest an alternative diagnosis to explain clinical findings, paraffin-embedded material (blocks or unstained slides) must accompany the frozen specimen to the reference laboratory to allow immunohistochemistry to be performed; histomorphologic CJD pathology can be patchy within the brain (even when the abnormal protein is widespread), and rare cases of CJD are caused by a protease-sensitive prion, requiring immunohistochemical rather than immunoblot analysis for definitive diagnosis (*Ann Neurol* 2010;68:162). Lab equipment (gloves, instruments, etc.) are decontaminated with 1N sodium hydroxide solution for a minimum of 1 hour or, alternatively, in 10% or 20% bleach solution for 1 hour, followed by autoclaving; many disinfection protocols that may be more or less appropriate for particular circumstances have been reported (*Infect Control Hosp Epidemiol* 2010;31:107). Frozen tissue diagnosis *should not* be attempted on tissues suspected of prion protein diseases.

B. Ancillary Studies
1. **Electron microscopy (EM).** The utilization of EM for diagnosis of CNS lesions has declined over the last several decades. It is labor intensive, time consuming, and expensive, and it is mainly used by neuropathologists to evaluate nerve and muscle biopsies. However, ultrastructural evaluation remains invaluable for many other neuropathologic diagnoses, including CADASIL, neuronal ceroid lipofuscinoses, and for distinguishing ambiguous brain tumor cases (e.g., anaplastic or otherwise unusual meningiomas and ependymomas).
2. **Immunohistochemistry** as an ancillary diagnostic test is now routinely used in evaluation of complex surgical neuropathology cases, especially in the area of tumor neuropathology. Frequently utilized antibodies and their immunoreactivity for common tumor types are summarized in Table 39.1.

TABLE 39.1 Typical Immunostains and Molecular Test Results for Common CNS Neoplasms

Tumor	Positive (+)	Positive or Negative (±)	Negative (−)
Pilocytic astrocytoma	GFAP	BRAF p.V600E, BRAF fusion (FISH), NF (few entrapped axons)	IDH-1, YKL-40
Glioblastoma, IDH wildtype (primary)	GFAP, YKL-40, NF (axons), S-100, CK	ATRX, p53	IDH-1,[a] CAM 5.2
Diffuse astrocytoma, IDH wildtype	S-100, GFAP, gain Chr 7 (FISH)	ATRX, p53	IDH-1,[a] 1p19q codeletion (FISH), CK,[b] LCA, SYN, HMB-45
Glioblastoma, IDH-mutant	S-100, GFAP, IDH-1,[a] ATRX, p53		CK,[b] LCA, SYN, HMB-45
Diffuse astrocytoma, IDH mutant	S-100, GFAP, IDH-1,[a] ATRX, p53		CK,[b] LCA, ATRX, p53
Oligodendroglioma, IDH mutant, 1p19q Codeleted	S-100, GFAP,[c] IDH-1, 1p19q loss (FISH)	SYN (dot-like)	
Diffuse midline glioma, H3 K27M-mutant	H3 K27M (nuclear), S-100, Olig2	GFAP, p53 (50%)	H3 K27me3 (nuclear)
Ependymoma	S-100, GFAP, D2-40, and CD99 (lumens)	EMA (luminal), CK	LCA, SYN, IDH-1
Ependymoma, RELA fusion positive	C11orf95-RELA fusion (FISH); L1CAM (correlates with FISH, but nonspecific), S-100, GFAP, D2-40 and CD99 (lumens)	EMA (luminal), CK	LCA, SYN, IDH-1
Choroid plexus tumors	S-100, CK, VIM, transthyretin[d]	GFAP	EMA, CEA
Metastatic carcinoma	EMA and CK, CK7 (lung), CK20 (colon), TTF1 (lung), CAM 5.2	CEA, S-100, SYN	GFAP, LCA, HMB-45, IDH-1
Melanoma	S-100, HMB-45, Melan-A (MART-1)	BRAF p.V600E	GFAP, CK, LCA, IDH-1
Lymphoma	LCA, CD20 (L26), CD79a	EMA[e]	CK, GFAP, HMB-45, SYN, CD3
Meningioma	EMA, VIM, PR,[f] INI1/BAF47 (retained) SSTR2A	S-100, CD34, CK[g]	GFAP, HMB-45, SOX10
Hemangiopericytoma/Solitary fibrous tumor	Stat6 (nuclear), VIM, CD99, bcl-2, Factor XIIIa[h]	CD34	EMA, CK, GFAP, S-100
Medulloblastoma (see text for subtypes)	SYN, INI1/BAF47(retained)	S-100, GFAP, NeuN, β-cat, GAB1, YAP1, p53, reticulin, iso17q (FISH), MYCN/MYC amp (FISH)	CK, LCA, EMA, LIN28A

Embryonal tumor with multilayered rosettes, C19MC-altered	C19MC amplification/fusion (FISH), LIN28A (cytoplasmic, cell clusters), SYN, VIM, INI-1/BAF47 (retained)	CK, EMA, CD99	GFAP
Atypical teratoid/rhabdoid tumor	VIM, EMA, CK, actin	SYN, GFAP, desmin, AFP	PLAP, β-hCG, LCA, INI-1/BAF47[l]
Ganglioglioma	SYN, NF, CG, GFAP	BRAF p.V600E, CD34, Neu-N	CK, EMA, PLAP
Central neurocytoma	SYN, Neu-N	GFAP, S-100, Olig2	IDH-1, NF, CG, CK, LCA
Schwannoma	S-100,[j] CD34, Coll IV,[i] SOX10	GFAP, HMB-45[k]	EMA, NF, CK, SSTR2A
Paraganglioma	SYN, CG, S-100[i]	NF	GFAP, CK, HMB-45
Hemangioblastoma	S-100, NSE, inhibin	GFAP	CK, EMA
Germinoma	OCT4, D2-40,[n] c-kit (CD117),[m] PLAP	β-hCG,[n] CK	AFP, EMA, HMB-45, LCA
Yolk sac tumor	AFP, CK	PLAP, c-kit[m]	β-hCG, GFAP, OCT4, EMA
Choriocarcinoma	β-hCG, CK, EMA	PLAP	AFP, OCT4, GFAP, HMB-45
Embryonal carcinoma	CK, OCT4, PLAP, CD30	c-kit,[m] AFP, EMA, D2-40[m]	β-hCG, LCA, HMB-45
Teratoma	CK, EMA	AFP, PLAP	β-hCG, c-kit

IDH-1 (p.R132H) stains the majority of IDH-mutant diffuse gliomas; IDH1 and IDH2 gene sequencing is necessary for examples with uncommon mutations.

[a] CAM 5.2 recommended, because CK (AE1/AE3) AE1/AE3 stains reactive astrocytes and frequently stains gliomas.

[b] Strongly positive in minigemistocytes and gliofibrillary oligodendrocytes.

[c] Not specific for choroid plexus.

[d] Positive in myeloma.

[e] Nuclear PR reactivity is strong in most WHO I meningiomas, weaker or absent in WHO grades II and III.

[f] Positive in secretory variant.

[g] Characteristic pattern of scattered, individual immunoreactive cells.

[h] Loss of INI-1/BAF-47 immunoreactivity from nuclei is observed in the vast majority of ATRT; reactivity is retained in most other pathologies.

[i] Diffuse, strong expression.

[j] Positive in melanotic schwannomas.

[k] Positive in sustentacular cells.

[l] Membranous pattern in germinoma, cytoplasmic in embryonal carcinoma/yolk sac tumor.

[m] Positive in syncytiotrophoblasts, present in a minority of cases.

AFP, α-fetoprotein; BAF47, also called SNF5 and INI1; β-hCG, β-human chorionic gonadotropin; CAM5.2, cytokeratin negative in glial cells; CEA, carcinoembryonic antigen; CG, chromogranin; CK, cytokeratin; Coll IV, collagen type IV; D2-40, podoplanin; EMA, epithelial membrane antigen; GFAP, glial fibrillary acid protein; IDH-1, isocitrate dehydrogenase 1; LCA, leukocyte common antigen; NF, neurofilament; NSE, neuron-specific enolase; PLAP, placental alkaline phosphatase; PR, progesterone receptor; SYN, synaptophysin; TTF1, thyroid transcription factor 1; VIM, vimentin; YKL-40, chitinase-3-like 1.

a. **Glial markers.** The most commonly used glial marker in neuropathology practice is glial fibrillary acid protein (GFAP). This intermediate filament protein is fairly (but not completely) specific for glial lineage. However, it does not reliably distinguish astrocytic, oligodendroglial, and ependymal tumors from one another, and may also be encountered in other tumors with glial differentiation, such as choroid plexus tumors, medulloblastomas, other embryonal neoplasms, and gangliogliomas (GGs). GFAP can even be detected to some extent in nonglial neoplasms, such as nerve sheath and cartilaginous tumors.

b. **Neuronal markers.** Some of the most commonly used neuronal markers include neurofilament (NF) protein, synaptophysin (SYN), chromogranin, and Neu-N.

SYN, a protein associated with presynaptic vesicles, is one of the more sensitive markers of neuronal differentiation in common use. It is typically found even in the most primitive neuronal tumors (e.g., CNS embryonal neoplasms) and is very useful for highlighting dysplastic or neoplastic ganglion cells, pituitary adenomas and carcinomas, carcinoid tumors, neurocytomas, paragangliomas, and metastatic neoplasms with neuroendocrine differentiation. One major disadvantage of SYN is that it fails to differentiate native (entrapped) neuropil from tumor neuropil. It should also be noted that SYN is faintly expressed by a reasonable proportion of tumors (e.g., pilocytic astrocytomas [PAs]) that are generally not considered to have neuronal differentiation. In some cases, this feature is actually somewhat useful; for example, classic oligodendrogliomas show dot-like paranuclear reactivity for SYN.

NF is a heteropolymer composed of three subunits that are unique to neurons and axons. Cortical dysplasias and tumors with mature albeit dysmorphic neuronal elements, such as GGs, often stain for NF; however, more primitive neuronal tumors such as medulloblastomas are often negative. In addition, NF also stains normal axons, a property that is of great utility for distinguishing solid versus infiltrative growth patterns by highlighting entrapped axons in the latter (e-**Fig. 39.3**).

Neu-N is a marker of advanced neuronal differentiation; it has the advantage of clearly staining neuronal nuclei and cell bodies rather than surrounding neuropil. As a result, it is particularly useful for identifying architectural abnormalities in cortical dysplasia, and for highlighting neuronal loss (e.g., in mesial temporal sclerosis) and neurons entrapped within infiltrative tumors. Most neoplastic ganglion cells in GGs are negative for Neu-N; this feature can be useful because entrapped cortical neurons are virtually always strongly positive.

c. **Epithelial markers.** The commonly used epithelial markers in surgical neuropathology include pan-cytokeratin (CK; AE1/AE3), epithelial membrane antigen (EMA), and CAM 5.2. CKs are used predominantly in the diagnosis of metastatic carcinomas, but are also used to identify craniopharyngiomas, chordomas, and choroid plexus tumors. Due to cross-reactivity with GFAP, gliomas (and reactive astrocytes) may show CK reactivity, a major pitfall in the differential between glioblastoma (GBM) and metastatic carcinoma. In such instances, cytokeratin CAM 5.2 is recommended, because gliomas (and reactive astrocytes) are usually negative—except when they are harboring adenoid and/or epithelioid features. EMA is frequently used in the identification of meningiomas, which, unlike true epithelial tumors, usually display minimal to no CK expression (secretory meningioma is an exception). EMA is also useful in the diagnosis of ependymomas, along with CD99 and D2-40 antibody (podoplanin).

d. **S-100 protein** is a marker of neuroectodermal cells, including melanocytes, glia, Schwann cells, chondrocytes, and the sustentacular cells in tumors such as paraganglioma, pheochromocytoma, and olfactory neuroblastoma. In conjunction with collagen IV, which stains basement membranes, S-100 is particularly helpful for demonstrating Schwannian differentiation in benign and malignant peripheral nerve sheath tumors.

e. **Proliferation markers** are used in conjunction with mitotic counts in brain tumors to guide determination of tumor grade and prognosis. Most widely used is murine monoclonal antibody MIB-1, raised against protein Ki-67, which labels nuclei that are not in the G_0 resting phase of the cell cycle.

f. **Molecular markers.** Recently, several antibodies have been developed that may be used in lieu of more complicated molecular tests for diagnosis and prognosis of various neoplasms.

   i. ***INI1/BAF47* deletions** are detected in ~70% of atypical teratoid/rhabdoid tumors (AT/RT); however, loss of the corresponding INI1 protein is even more common than the genetic alteration. Loss of this protein can be demonstrated by a lack of nuclear immunoreactivity in tumor cells, amidst retained nuclear reactivity in associated nonneoplastic cells.

   ii. **Isocitrate dehydrogenase (*IDH1/IDH2*) mutations** are present in most diffuse gliomas, with the notable exceptions of primary (de novo) GBM and diffuse midline glioma, H3 K27M-mutant; IDH mutations appear to play a fundamental and early role in oncogenesis (*N Eng J Med* 2009;360:765). The most common mutation is in the *IDH1* gene (p.R132H); this mutation introduces a neoepitope that is recognized by monoclonal antibody IDH-1. Diagnostically, this immunohistochemical stain shows greatest promise for its potential to distinguish low-grade diffuse glioma from gliosis (*Am J Surg Pathol* 2010;34:1199; *Acta Neuropathol* 2010;119:509). Prognostically, the presence of this mutation is favorable.

   iii. **H3 K27M mutation** helps to define diffuse midline glioma, H3 K27M-mutant (WHO grade IV), but it is not restricted to that entity, which must also be defined by its adjectives diffuse and midline. This mutation can appear in any one of three histone genes (*H3F3A, HIST1H3B, HIST1H3C*), but all three can be detected by IHC (nuclear stain) using the same antibody. By reducing PRC2 activity, this mutation leads to decreased H3 K27 trimethylation in histones, allowing a companion IHC test for loss of nuclear H3 K27me3 to confirm the H3 K27M IHC result.

   iv. **LIN28A cytoplasmic reactivity**, though not specific, is strong and diffuse in most examples of embryonal tumor with multilayered rosettes (ETMR), and has been proposed as a surrogate for C19MC amplification, to support that diagnosis (*Acta Neuropathol* 2012;124:875).

3. **Molecular diagnostics** involves the measurement of diagnostically or prognostically relevant pathologic features at the DNA (epigenetic, genomic [nuclear or mitochondrial]), messenger RNA (mRNA), or protein levels. Molecular diagnostics has taken on an important role in the evaluation of CNS tumors because these analyses often provide theragnostic and prognostic information that is of great value to oncologists. Not infrequently, molecular diagnostics are also essential for establishing a definitive diagnosis—particularly after the paradigm shift of molecularly defining neoplasms introduced by the 2016 WHO Classification System (Louis DN, et al. *WHO Classification of Tumours of the Central Nervous System.* Lyon, France: IARC; 2016).

   Abundant tumor-related mRNAs (e.g., kappa and lambda light chain restriction in plasma cell neoplasms) can be measured in formalin-fixed, paraffin-embedded (FFPE) tissue sections using in situ hybridization (ISH). However, detection of less abundant gene products is often limited by the degradation and cross-linking of RNA in FFPE tissue. Consequently, such markers are generally measured by RT-PCR and quantitative RT-PCR.

   The most common and practical approaches to detect larger changes in DNA (deletions of chromosomal regions, amplifications of oncogenes, or loss of specific tumor suppressor genes) include fluorescence ISH (FISH) and quantitative PCR techniques. FISH has the advantages of simplicity, morphologic preservation, and minimal tissue and purity requirements. However, FISH is insensitive to very small deletions/amplifications, whole arm losses/gains, substitution mutations, or epigenetic modification (e.g., methylation).

Perhaps the most notable use of FISH in surgical neuropathology is to detect co-deletion of chromosomal arms 1p and 19q as a diagnostic hallmark of adult oligodendroglioma (*Acta Neuropathol* 2016;131:803). Other clinical applications of FISH include detection of: gain of chromosome 7 to distinguish diffuse astrocytoma (DA) from gliosis; *EGFR* amplification and/or 10q/*PTEN* deletions in undersampled GBM; 22q11.2 deletion (*INI1* locus) to distinguish AT/RT from variants of medulloblastoma (*Hum Pathol* 2001;32:156) (see also antibody BAF47/INI-1 discussed above); 17q gain as a surrogate for isochromosome 17q (i17q) and *NMYC* or *MYC* amplifications to diagnose, stratify, and predict outcome for medulloblastomas; C19MC amplification to diagnose ETMR (see also antibody for LIN28A); meningioma-associated deletions (*NF2*, *DAL1*, 1p, 14q) to distinguish anaplastic meningiomas from other malignancies or benign meningiomas from foci of meningothelial hyperplasia; and (9p21) to provide prognostic information about higher-grade meningiomas and gliomas.

One of the most common uses of PCR-based techniques in neuropathology is to detect O6-methylguanine-DNA methyltransferase (*MGMT*) gene methylation, which blocks *MGMT* transcription. As the *MGMT* gene product plays an important role in DNA repair, GBMs with this epigenetic modification show greater sensitivity to alkylating agents (like temozolomide) and radiation therapy (*N Eng J Med* 2005;352:987).

IV. BASIC ELEMENTS OF CNS PATHOLOGY. The cells and tissues of the CNS are capable of displaying diverse histologic abnormalities. A few of these are pathognomonic for a given disease, but most diseases require a constellation of findings to suggest a diagnosis.

A. Neurons

1. **Axonal injury.** When an axon is damaged and the associated neuron survives, the axon itself may form a swelling, or axonal spheroid, at the site of injury. If the axon is severed, in most cases the distal portion will disintegrate in an active cellular process called Wallerian degeneration. In some cases, the axotomized neuron will undergo "chromatolysis", in which the cell body appears mildly swollen and achromatic; this change reflects a loss of Nissl substance that occurs as the cell alters its metabolism to allow repair of its damaged axon.

2. **Apoptosis.** If neuronal injury is severe enough to cause "cell death", neurons may undergo apoptosis (as occurs in the basis pontis and subiculum from hypoxic ischemic injury late in gestation, a pattern labeled with the misnomer "pontosubicular necrosis"); in this process, the nucleus becomes fragmented and specific enzyme cascades destroy the rest of the cell. Alternatively, neurons may undergo necrosis.

3. **Necrosis.** The classic histologic appearance of acute neuronal necrosis includes: (1) variably intense cytoplasmic eosinophilia (accounting for the name "red neurons") and (2) shrunken pyknotic nuclei (e-**Fig. 39.4**). Red neurons require 12 to 24 hours to develop *within a living brain*; individuals who die within minutes or a few hours of an ischemic stroke do not show red neurons in affected region(s). Although red neurons are commonly caused by ischemia, many insults (e.g., hypoxia, hypoglycemia, epilepsy, herpes simplex virus [HSV] infection) can also cause neuronal necrosis. It is important to note that a common artifact caused by overmanipulation of fresh brain tissue can cause normal healthy neurons to (superficially) resemble red neurons. Fortunately, neurons affected by this so-called "dark cell change" usually show more basophilia than red neurons, a nucleus that is less distinct within the cell body, and an apical dendrite that resembles a spiral or corkscrew (e-**Fig. 39.5**).

4. **Ferrugination**. Occasionally, damaged neurons around the edge of a remote infarct or traumatic injury become encrusted with basophilic iron and calcium salts. This condition is often referred to as mineralization or ferrugination.

5. **Binucleation** of neurons, rare in normal brains, is infrequently noted in dysplastic/malformative processes (e.g., tuberous sclerosis [TS]), in certain neoplasms (e.g., GG), and in Alzheimer disease (AD) (*Neuropathol Appl Neurobiol* 2008;34:457) (e-**Fig. 39.6**).

6. **Intraneuronal inclusion bodies** form within neurons under many different circumstances. Some are pathognomonic, some are associated with one or more diseases; others appear to have no pathologic significance.

   a. **Pick bodies** are round, tau-positive intracytoplasmic neuronal inclusions. In Pick disease (a form of frontotemporal dementia), these are argyrophilic by Bielschowsky and Bodian (but not Gallyas) silver stains and are abundant in neurons of the cortex, hippocampus, and dentate gyrus. A similar (but less abundant, Gallyas positive) inclusion is seen in corticobasal degeneration.

   b. **Lewy bodies (LBs).** Classic LBs, which occur within pigmented neurons of the brainstem (e.g., substantia nigra pars compacta, locus coeruleus, Raphe nuclei), are spherical cytoplasmic inclusions with an eosinophilic core and a pale halo [e-**Fig. 39.7**]). By contrast, cortical LBs appear as subtle spheres of homogeneous eosinophilia. Making detection even more difficult, cortical LBs are not argyrophilic. Fortunately, LBs all show immunoreactivity for ubiquitin and α-synuclein (e-**Fig. 39.8**). These lesions (along with similar inclusions [Lewy neurites] that appear within cell processes) are seen in LB disorders (e.g., Parkinson disease [PD], and dementia with Lewy bodies [DLB]).

   c. **Marinesco bodies** are small, eosinophilic, strongly ubiquitin-positive intranuclear inclusions located chiefly in pigmented brain stem neurons (e-**Fig. 39.9**). These have no clinically significant pathologic association.

   d. **Neurofibrillary tangles (NFT)** (e-**Fig. 39.10**) are argyrophilic intracytoplasmic filamentous aggregates of hyperphosphorylated tau protein. Characteristic of AD and many other neurodegenerative "tauopathies," they may be seen in rare GGs and some epilepsy resection cases.

   e. **Hirano bodies** are brightly eosinophilic rod-shaped or elliptical cytoplasmic inclusions that occur within the proximal dendrites of neurons, particularly in the hippocampus. Though not specific for AD, they are particularly numerous in brains with AD pathology (e-**Fig. 39.11**).

   f. **Granulovacuolar degeneration (GVD)** is common in hippocampal pyramidal neurons in AD, and less common in older brains without AD. GVD resembles many small bubbles, each with a small basophilic granule.

   g. **TDP-43 neuronal cytoplasmic inclusions (NCIs),** as the name suggests, are immunoreactive for TDP-43. Though characteristic of a subset of frontotemporal dementias, NCI are also common in hippocampal sclerosis (HS) of aging (*Arch Pathol Lab Med* 2017;141:1113), and in the temporal lobes of individuals with advanced AD (*Acta Neuropathol* 2016;131:571).

   h. **Bunina bodies** are eosinophilic, ubiquitin- and TDP-43-immunoreactive, intracytoplasmic inclusions that form in motor neurons in sporadic and many cases of familial amyotrophic lateral sclerosis (ALS).

B. Astrocytes

1. **Reactive astrocytosis.** Normally, astrocytes are evenly dispersed (albeit with regional variation), mitotically silent, and GFAP positive. In most forms of brain injury, astrocytes become hypertrophic, increase their GFAP content, and may proliferate. Reactive astrocytes have prominent stellate processes and, often, abundant eccentrically distributed glassy cytoplasm that inspires the moniker "gemistocyte". Nevertheless, reactive astrocytes generally maintain an even distribution, and do not exhibit nuclear atypia (though there are exceptions [e.g., radiation exposure] to this latter observation). Grossly, tissues affected by chronic astrocytosis are usually firm; thus, some use the term gliotic to describe brain tissues that appear unusually firm or rubbery.

2. **Bergmann gliosis** refers to an accumulation of astrocytic nuclei (usually in association with neuron loss) within the Purkinje cell layer of the cerebellum.

3. **Alzheimer type II astrocytes,** with swollen pale nuclei and minimal visible cytoplasm, appear in hyperammonemic states (e.g., liver failure, Wilson disease). In the cortex and striatum, these nuclei are round with a prominent nucleolus (e-**Fig. 39.12**); in the pallidum, dentate nucleus, and brainstem they may be irregular and lobated.

4. **Corpora amylacea** are basophilic, round, concentrically lamellated aggregates of polyglucosan (polyglucosan bodies) that develop within astrocytic processes. Common in normal brains, particularly near ventricular and pial surfaces, these become more numerous with age. Similar structures (Lafora bodies) form in far greater numbers in astrocytes and neurons (and in eccrine sweat glands) in Lafora body disease.

5. **Rosenthal fibers (RFs)** are brightly eosinophilic, somewhat refractile, irregular/beaded structures that range from ~10 to 40 μm in diameter. EM reveals them as swollen astrocytic processes filled with electron-dense amorphous granular material and glial filaments. RFs are commonly observed in PA, but are also commonly seen in nonneoplastic tissues adjacent to slowly growing neoplasms (e.g., craniopharyngioma, ependymoma) and chronic lesions (e.g., cysts, syrinx, vascular malformations); such RF-abundant tissue reaction is called "piloid gliosis" (e-Fig. 39.13).

6. **Eosinophilic granular bodies (EGBs),** though not present in nonneoplastic astrocytes, are found in slowly growing astrocytic and glioneuronal tumors (PA, GG, and pleomorphic xanthoastrocytoma [PXA]). EGBs appear on H&E sections (or cytologic smear preparations) as refractile clusters of small, round hyaline droplets, and are PAS positive (e-Fig. 39.14).

C. **Microglia,** normal immune cell residents of the brain, are of monocytic lineage (and are consequently immunoreactive for leukocyte common antigen [LCA/CD45] as well as CD68 and CD163). Even in a "resting" state, they play a vital role in monitoring the parenchyma for abnormalities (e.g., antigens, complement, interleukins, cytokines). In response to various signals, these cells undergo "activation" whereupon they change their morphology (appearing as irregular elongated so-called "rod cells"), become motile, and intensify their communication with other cells via secreted factors (e.g., cytokines and interleukins). They may also participate in limited phagocytosis. Small clusters of activated microglial cells (microglial nodules) are characteristic of viral encephalitis and may be seen decorating dying neurons, in a process called "neuronophagia". Capacity for phagocytosis increases in the setting of injury, infection, or demyelinating disease when microglia differentiate into macrophages. Monocytes and macrophages may also be recruited into the CNS from the systemic circulation. Occasionally, brisk mitotic activity among macrophages in these settings (particularly in tumefactive multiple sclerosis (MS), which radiographically resembles GBM) can cause diagnostic confusion with gliomas. Gliomas themselves often contain large numbers of microglial cells, which appear to play a role in tumorigenesis (*Cancer Res* 2008;68:10358).

D. **Cerebral Edema** is an increase in brain volume due to increased water content. Depending on its pathogenesis, cerebral edema can be classified as vasogenic, cytotoxic, osmotic, or interstitial (resulting from obstructive hydrocephalus). However, combinations of different edema types often coexist. In vasogenic edema (more common type), the fluid collection is predominantly extracellular and results from breakdown of the blood–brain barrier. In cytotoxic edema, the fluid accumulation is intracellular, the result of impaired Na/K-ATPase function in glial cells, caused by toxins, ischemia, or various other conditions. Osmotic edema results when osmolality of the brain interstitial fluid exceeds that of the plasma. Interstitial edema results from transependymal flow from the ventricles in the setting of obstructive hydrocephalus.

E. **Hydrocephalus,** an abnormal increase in the intracranial volume of CSF associated with dilatation of all or part of the ventricular system, may be classified as communicating, noncommunicating (obstructive), normal pressure, or *ex vacuo*.

1. **Noncommunicating** hydrocephalus results from physical blockage of CSF flow, usually by tumor compressing a narrow channel, such as the foramen of Monro or cerebral aqueduct.

2. **Communicating** hydrocephalus results from impaired resorption of CSF, as may occur in the setting of subarachnoid hemorrhage or meningitis; less commonly, it may result from increased CSF production (e.g., by a choroid plexus papilloma).

3. **Normal pressure hydrocephalus (NPH),** characterized classically by the clinical triad of dementia, ataxia, and incontinence, is poorly understood. NPH may represent a

circumstance in which production and resorption of CSF reach a new equilibrium after a prolonged period of impaired resorption.

4. Hydrocephalus *ex vacuo* describes a state of ventricle expansion due to loss of adjacent parenchyma or generalized cerebral atrophy (as occurs in AD).

F. Intracranial Pressure (ICP) and Brain Herniation. Normally, the cranial cavity contents (blood, brain, and CSF) are maintained in volumetric balance within the rigid skull and dura. ICP increases when this balance is strained, as may result from diffuse brain edema, increased cerebral blood flow and blood volume, or development of space-occupying lesions (e.g., tumor, abscess, hematoma, or large edematous infarct). Elevated ICP, if not treated, can cause herniation, wherein portions of expanded brain are compressed by rigid dural reflections or bony structures. Herniation syndromes include subfalcine (cingulate gyrus), transtentorial (uncal), and cerebellar tonsillar/brainstem herniations. Tonsillar/brainstem herniation is often fatal and results in death due to compression of cardiorespiratory centers in the medulla. In contrast, uncal herniation causes compression of vessels and nerves adjacent to the tentorium, leading to posterior cerebral artery infarcts and so-called "blown" pupils from involvement of sympathetic fibers at the periphery of cranial nerve III.

G. Duret (Secondary Brain Stem) Hemorrhage occurs when penetrating pontine arteries (which arise perpendicularly from the basilar artery) become kinked in association with brainstem herniation; the resulting acute hemorrhagic infarction of the pons is often fatal.

V. NEOPLASMS OF THE CNS. For most CNS tumors, incidence varies greatly with age and gender. Among adults, metastases, GBM, and meningioma are the most common CNS neoplasms; among children, PA, medulloblastoma, and ependymoma are far more common. Likewise, tumors often differ in their radiographic features and propensity for certain anatomic sites. For this reason, microscopic evaluation of a CNS biopsy specimen is incomplete without considering the neuroradiologic findings that describe the targeted lesion in situ. Indeed, neuroradiologic assessment can be considered to be the neuropathologist's surrogate for gross examination. Imaging studies are particularly helpful when evaluating small biopsy samples. For example, a ring-enhancing GBM that has been undersampled in a biopsy procedure may show only features of low-grade DA on histologic slides. Thus, considering the radiologic findings in conjunction with histologic features can help with assessments of biopsy adequacy and, in turn, reduce the risk of misdiagnosis.

Thus, patient age and gender, tumor location, and radiographic features are all extremely important for narrowing the differential diagnosis for a CNS biopsy. The WHO currently lists more than 100 types of CNS tumors and their variants (Table 39.2); of note, the recent AJCC staging scheme for CNS tumors reflects the WHO approach to classification (Amin MB et al., eds. *AJCC Cancer Staging Manual.* 8th ed. New York: Springer, 2017). Table 39.3 organizes the common CNS tumor diagnoses based on location, patient age, and imaging characteristics. Because a final diagnosis may not be obvious from an initial histomorphologic examination, it is worthwhile to begin with a broad differential based on a specimen's general histopathologic pattern; Table 39.4 lists eight major histopathologic patterns that may be encountered, along with their most commonly associated diagnostic entities.

In 2016, the WHO Classification System for CNS tumors was changed in a fundamental way. Now, many neoplasms are ultimately defined by molecular characteristics, often one or more genetic alterations considered to be specific for that diagnosis. To represent this new system succinctly in pathology reports, an integrated diagnosis is rendered that often includes a tumor name based on histomorphologic features, followed by the defining molecular characteristic(s); reporting should follow suggested guidelines (for example, see the College of American Pathologists Protocol for the Examination of Specimens From Patients With Tumors of the Central Nervous System, at http://www.cap.org). When the required tests fail, or are not available, or are electively not performed to confirm a histomorphologic diagnosis, the acronym NOS (short for not otherwise specified) can be applied. The rationale and application of this approach has been explained (*Brain Pathol* 2014;24:429). More recently, a new term NEC (not elsewhere classified) has been introduced to reflect diagnoses where molecular results are available but do not allow

TABLE 39.2 WHO Classification and Grading of Central Nervous System (CNS) Tumors

	I	II	III	IV
Tumors of neuroepithelial tissue				
Diffuse astrocytic and oligodendroglial tumors				
Diffuse astrocytoma, IDH-mutant, IDH-wildtype or NOS		*		
Gemistocytic astrocytoma, IDH-mutant				
Anaplastic astrocytoma, IDH-mutant, IDH-wildtype or NOS			*	
Glioblastoma, IDH-mutant, IDH-wildtype or NOS				*
Giant cell glioblastoma, IDH-wildtype				*
Gliosarcoma, IDH-wildtype				*
Epithelioid glioblastoma, IDH-wildtype				*
Diffuse midline glioma, H3 K27M mutant				*
Oligodendroglioma, IDH-mutant and 1p/19q co-deleted or NOS		*		
Anaplastic oligodendroglioma, IDH-mutant and 1p/19q codeleted or NOS			*	
Oligoastrocytoma, NOS		*		
Anaplastic oligoastrocytoma, NOS			*	
Other Astrocytic Tumors				
Pilocytic astrocytoma	*			
Pilomyxoid astrocytoma	not assigned			
Subependymal giant cell astrocytoma	*			
Pleomorphic xanthoastrocytoma		*		
Anaplastic pleomorphic xanthoastrocytoma			*	
Ependymal tumors				
Subependymoma	*			
Myxopapillary ependymoma	*			
Ependymoma		*		
Papillary		*		
Clear cell		*		
Tanycytic		*		
Ependymoma, RELA fusion-positive				
Anaplastic ependymoma			*	
Other gliomas				
Astroblastoma				
Chordoid gliomas of the 3rd ventricle		*		
Angiocentric glioma	*			
Choroid plexus tumors				
Choroid plexus papilloma	*			
Atypical choroid plexus papilloma		*		
Choroid plexus carcinoma			*	
Neuronal and mixed neuronal-glial tumors				
Dysplastic gangliocytoma of cerebellum (Lhermitte–Duclos)	*			
Desmoplastic infantile astrocytoma/ganglioglioma	*			
Dysembryoplastic neuroepithelial tumor	*			
Gangliocytoma	*			
Ganglioglioma	*			
Anaplastic ganglioglioma			*	
Central neurocytoma		*		
Extraventricular neurocytoma		*		
Cerebellar liponeurocytoma		*		
Papillary glioneuronal tumor	*			
Rosette-forming glioneuronal tumor of the 4th ventricle	*			
Paraganglioma	*			

TABLE 39.2 WHO Classification and Grading of Central Nervous System (CNS) Tumors (*Continued*)

	I	II	III	IV
Tumors of the pineal region				
Pineocytoma	*			
Pineal parenchymal tumor of intermediate differentiation		*	*	
Pineoblastoma				*
Papillary tumor of the pineal region		*	*	
Embryonal tumors				
Medulloblastoma				*
Desmoplastic/nodular medulloblastoma				*
Medulloblastoma with extensive nodularity				*
Anaplastic medulloblastoma				*
Large cell medulloblastoma				*
Embryonal tumor with multilayered rosettes, C19MC-altered				*
Embryonal tumor with multilayered rosettes, NOS				*
Medulloepithelioma				*
CNS neuroblastoma				*
CNS ganglioneuroblastoma				*
CNS embryonal tumor, NOS				*
Atypical teratoid/rhabdoid tumor				*
CNS embryonal tumor with rhabdoid features				*
Tumors of cranial and paraspinal nerves				
Schwannoma (neurilemoma, neurinomas)	*			
Cellular	*			
Plexiform	*			
Melanotic	*			
Neurofibroma	*			
Atypical				
Plexiform				
Perineurioma, NOS	*	*	*	
Perineurioma, (Intraneural)	*			
Malignant perineurioma			*	
Malignant peripheral nerve sheath tumor (MPNST)		*	*	*
Epithelioid MPNST		*	*	*
MPNST with divergent differentiation		*	*	*
Melanotic MPNST		*	*	*
MPNST with perineurial differentiation		*	*	*
Meningioma				
Meningothelial	*			
Fibrous (fibroblastic)	*			
Transitional (mixed)	*			
Psammomatous	*			
Angiomatous	*			
Microcystic	*			
Secretory	*			
Lymphoplasmacyte rich	*			
Metaplastic	*			
Chordoid		*		
Clear cell		*		
Atypical		*		
Papillary			*	
Rhabdoid			*	
Anaplastic (malignant)			*	

(*continued*)

TABLE 39.2	WHO Classification and Grading of Central Nervous System (CNS) Tumors (*Continued*)			

	I	II	III	IV
Mesenchymal, nonmeningothelial tumors				
Lipoma				
Angiolipoma				
Hibernoma				
Liposarcoma				
Desmoid-type fibromatosis				
Benign fibrous histiocytoma				
Myofibroblastoma				
Inflammatory myofibroblastic tumor				
Fibrosarcoma				
Malignant fibrous histiocytoma				
Leiomyoma				
Leiomyosarcoma				
Rhabdomyoma				
Rhabdomyosarcoma				
Chondroma				
Chondrosarcoma				
Osteoma				
Osteosarcoma				
Osteochondroma				
Hemangioma				
Hemangioblastoma	*			
Epithelioid hemangioendothelioma				
Hemangiopericytoma/Solitary fibrous tumor	*	*		
Anaplastic hemangiopericytoma			*	
Angiosarcoma				
Kaposi sarcoma				
Ewing sarcoma–peripheral PNET				
Melanocytic lesions				
Meningeal melanocytosis				
Meningeal melanocytoma				
Meningeal malignant melanoma				
Meningeal melanomatosis				
Tumors of the hematopoietic system				
Malignant lymphomas/primary CNS lymphomas				
B-cell lymphoma				
Diffuse large B-cell lymphoma				
Immunodeficiency-associated CNS lymphomas				
AIDS-related				
EBV-positive				
Lymphomatoid granulomatosis				
Low-grade B-cell lymphoma				
Marginal zone B-cell (MALT) lymphoma of the dura				
Plasmacytoma				
Intravascular large B-cell lymphoma				
T-cell lymphoma				
Anaplastic large-cell lymphoma, ALK-positive, ALK neg				
NK/T-cell lymphoma				
Histiocytic tumors				
Langerhans cell histiocytosis				
Rosai–Dorfman disease				
Erdheim–Chester disease				
Juvenile xanthogranuloma				
Histiocytic sarcoma				

TABLE 39.2	WHO Classification and Grading of Central Nervous System (CNS) Tumors (*Continued*)	I	II	III	IV
Germ cell tumors					
Germinoma					
Embryonal carcinoma					
Yolk sac tumor					
Choriocarcinoma					
Teratoma					
Mature					
Immature					
Teratoma with malignant transformation					
Mixed germ cell tumor					
Tumors of the sellar region					
Craniopharyngioma		*			
Adamantinomatous		*			
Papillary		*			
Granular cell tumor of the neurohypophysis		*			
Pituicytoma		*			
Spindle cell oncocytoma of the adenohypophysis		*			

Modified from Louis DN, Ohgaki H, Wiestler OD, Cavenee WK. *WHO Classification of Tumours of the Central Nervous System.* Lyon, France: IARC Press; 2017.

TABLE 39.3	Common CNS Tumor Diagnosis by Location, Age, and Imaging Characteristics

Location	Child/Young Adult	Older Adult
Cerebral/supratentorial	Ganglioglioma (TL, cyst-MEN) DNT (TL, intracortical nodules) Embryonal tumor (solid, E) AT/RT (infant) Pleomorphic xanthoastrocytoma (cyst-MEN)	Grade II–III glioma (NE) GBM (ring E, butterfly) Mets (gray–white junctions, E) Lymphoma (periventricular, E)
Cerebellar/infratentorial	Pilocytic astrocytoma (cyst-MEN) Medulloblastoma (vermis, E) Ependymoma (4th v., E) Choroid plexus papilloma (4th v.) AT/RT (infant)	Mets (multiple, E) Hemangioblastoma (cyst-MEN) Choroid plexus papilloma (4th v.)
Brain stem	Diffuse midline glioma with H3 K27M mutation/"brain stem glioma" (pons) Pilocytic astrocytoma (dorsal brain stem)	Diffuse midline glioma with H3 K27M mutation (multifocal) RGNT (4th ventricle, aqueduct)
Spinal cord (intra-axial)	Ependymoma Pilocytic astrocytoma (cystic)	Ependymoma Diffuse astrocytoma (ill-defined) Paraganglioma (filum terminale) Myxopapillary ependymoma (filum terminale)

(*continued*)

TABLE 39.3	Common CNS Tumor Diagnosis by Location, Age, and Imaging Characteristics (*Continued*)	
Location	**Child/Young Adult**	**Older Adult**
Extra-axial/dural	Secondary lymphoma/leukemia	Meningioma Metastases Hemangiopericytoma/solitary fibrous tumor Secondary lymphoma/leukemia
Intrasellar	Pituitary adenoma Craniopharyngioma Rathke cleft cyst	Pituitary adenoma Rathke cleft cyst
Suprasellar/hypothalamic/ optic pathway/3rd v.	Germinoma/germ cell tumor Craniopharyngioma Pilocytic astrocytoma Pilomyxoid astrocytoma	Colloid cyst (3rd v.)
Pineal	Germinoma/germ cell tumor Pineocytoma Pineoblastoma Pineal cyst	Pineocytoma Pineal cyst
Thalamus	Pilocytic astrocytoma AA/GBM	AA/GBM Lymphoma
Cerebellopontine angle	Vestibular schwannoma (NF2)	Vestibular schwannoma Meningioma
Lateral ventricle	Central neurocytoma SEGA (tuberous sclerosis) Choroid plexus papilloma Choroid plexus carcinoma (infant)	Central neurocytoma SEGA (tuberous sclerosis) Choroid plexus papilloma Subependymoma
Nerve root/paraspinal	Neurofibroma (NF1) MPNST (NF1)	Schwannoma Meningioma Secondary lymphoma Neurofibroma (NF1) MPNST

AA, anaplastic astrocytoma; AT/RT, atypical teratoid rhabdoid tumor; CNS, central nervous system; DNT, dysembryoplastic neuroepithelial tumor; E, enhancing; GBM, glioblastoma; MEN, mural enhancing nodule; MPNST, malignant peripheral nerve sheath tumor; NE, nonenhancing; NF, neurofilament; PNET, primitive neuroectodermal tumor; SEGA, subependymal giant cell astrocytoma; TL, temporal lobe; v., ventricle.

for a specific designation according to revised WHO 2016 guidelines (*Acta Neuropathol* 2018;135:481). The two classes of tumors that have been most dramatically affected by this change of approach are the CNS embryonal neoplasms of children and the diffuse gliomas of adults.

A. **Diffuse Gliomas.** Previously classified largely by the cytomorphology and graded according to histologic features (principally atypia, mitotic density, microvascular proliferation (MVP)/endothelial hyperplasia (EH), and necrosis), the diffuse gliomas are now classified according to the presence/absence of several genetic changes that are thought to drive neoplastic transformation and progression. The most important changes at present include mutations in *IDH1/2*, *ATRX*, and *TP53* genes, and co-deletion of chromosomal arms 1p and 19q, gain of chromosome 7, monosomy chromosome 10, loss of

TABLE 39.4 Major Histopathologic Patterns in Surgical Neuropathology

I. Parenchymal Infiltrate with Hypercellularity
- Diffuse glioma
- Central nervous system lymphoma
- Infections
- Inflammatory demyelinating disease
- Organizing infarct
- Reactive gliosis

II. Discrete Mass (Pure)
- Metastasis
- Ependymoma
- Subependymoma
- Subependymal giant cell astrocytoma (SEGA)
- Central neurocytoma
- Pineocytoma
- Primitive/embryonal tumor (e.g., atypical teratoid rhabdoid tumor)
- Choroid plexus papilloma
- Cerebral cavernous malformation/cavernous angioma/cavernoma
- Hemangioblastoma

III. Solid and Infiltrative Process
- Pilocytic astrocytoma
- Pleomorphic xanthoastrocytoma
- Glioblastoma/gliosarcoma
- Ganglioglioma
- Dysembryoplastic neuroepithelial tumor
- Primitive/embryonal tumor (e.g., medulloblastoma/primitive neuroectodermal tumors)
- Choroid plexus carcinoma
- Germ cell tumors
- Craniopharyngioma
- Central nervous system lymphoma
- Sarcoma
- Abscess and other forms of infection

IV. Vasculocentric Process
- Central nervous system lymphoma
- Lymphomatoid granulomatosis
- Intravascular lymphoma
- Vasculitis
- Meningioangiomatosis
- Acute demyelinating encephalomyelitis (ADEM)
- Amyloid angiopathy and lobar hemorrhage
- Amyloid beta related angiitis (ABRA)
- Arteriolosclerosis
- Cerebral autosomal dominant arteriopathy with subcortical infarcts and leukoencephalopathy (CADASIL)
- Vascular malformation
- Infection (e.g., aspergillus)
- Neurosarcoidosis
- Thromboembolic disease

(continued)

TABLE 39.4 Major Histopathologic Patterns in Surgical Neuropathology (*Continued*)

V. Extra-axial Mass
- Meningioma
- Hemangiopericytoma
- Solitary fibrous tumor
- Sarcomas
- Schwannoma
- Metastasis
- Melanoma/melanocytoma
- Secondary lymphoma/leukemia/plasmacytoma
- Paraganglioma
- Sarcoidosis/granulomatous diseases
- Inflammatory pseudotumors
- Calcifying pseudotumor of neuraxis
- Histiocytosis (e.g., Rosai–Dorfman disease)

VI. Meningeal Infiltrate
- Meningeal carcinomatosis (or lymphomatosis, gliomatosis, melanomatosis, meningiomatosis, etc.)
- Diffuse leptomeningeal glioneuronal tumor
- Meningitis
- Sarcoidosis/granulomatous diseases
- Collagen vascular disease
- Inflammatory disorder (e.g., Castleman disease, IgG4-related pachymeningitis)

VII. Destructive/Necrotic Process
- Cerebral infarct
- Tumor with treatment effect
- Infection
- Vasculitis
- Severe demyelinating disease

VIII. Subtle Pathology or Near Normal Biopsy
- Hypothalamic hamartoma
- Low-grade glioma
- Cortical dysplasia/tuber
- Mesial temporal sclerosis
- Heterotopia
- Ischemic disease
- Neurodegenerative disease
- Benign cysts
- Reactive gliosis
- Hepatic encephalopathy
- Cerebral edema
- Viral encephalitis

chromosome 10q/*PTEN*, *EGFR* amplification, and H3 K27M mutations. However, this field is still evolving, with emphasis on further stratification.

1. Diffuse (infiltrating) astrocytoma (DA), IDH-mutant, WHO grade II. Diffuse gliomas are the most frequent primary CNS neoplasms in adults. Because they are diffusely infiltrative, complete resection is nearly impossible. On MRI, DAs are nonenhancing, T1 hypointense, T2/FLAIR hyperintense, ill-defined intra-axial masses that can occur throughout the neuraxis, but commonly involve the cerebral hemispheres. Patients generally present with new-onset seizures (the most common symptom, due to cortical involvement), headaches, or functional neurologic deficits, or when neuroimaging performed for another purpose detects a lesion. Grossly, these lesions may be subtle, or appear gray-tan to gelatinous and obscure the native gray–white junction. Microscopically, tumor cells invade adjacent cortex along white matter tracts. They aggregate around neurons and blood vessels and beneath pial and ependymal surfaces to produce the so-called secondary structures of Scherer. The cytologic features of astrocytic tumor cells can vary widely from being uniform and minimally atypical to highly pleomorphic in terms of both the cytoplasmic and nuclear features (e-**Fig. 39.15**). Cells with elongate, irregular, hyperchromatic nuclei with minimal cytoplasm are seen in fibrillary astrocytomas, whereas cells with eccentrically located nuclei and abundant eosinophilic cytoplasm characterize the gemistocytic variant. Tumor cells are often, but not invariably, immunoreactive to GFAP. For a DA to qualify for WHO grade II, it must exhibit no (or very low) mitotic activity, no MVP, and no necrosis. Most tumors with these radiographic and histomorphologic features carry mutations in *IDH1* (or *IDH2*), *ATRX*, and *P53*, and show the following immunohistochemical pattern: positive for IDH-1 p.R132H (cytoplasmic); negative for ATRX (loss of nuclear reactivity); positive for p53 (in a majority or strong minority of tumor cell nuclei). Such tumors receive the integrated diagnosis DA, IDH-mutant, WHO grade II.

2. **Diffuse (infiltrating) astrocytoma (DA), IDH-wildtype, WHO grade II.** A much smaller group of DAs (with the same radiographic and histomorphologic characteristics described just above) does not harbor *IDH1* or *IDH2* mutations; these cases require *IDH1/2* sequencing to rule out IDH mutation and may require additional testing to support the diagnosis. This entity is somewhat heterogeneous with molecular low-grade and high-grade groups (*NeuroOncol* 2017;19:1327). Cases in either group may show *MYB* amplification and/or *BRAF* p.V600E mutation, but "molecular high-grade" cases frequently also harbor *TERT* promoter mutation, and/or *EGFR* amplification, and/or *H3F3A* mutation, and/or combined chromosome 7 gain and 10 loss (*Acta Neuropathologica* 2018;136:805). Thus, IHC for BRAF p.V600E, FISH studies (for the *EGFR* locus on chromosome 7 and for the *PTEN* locus on chromosome 10q), and next-generation sequencing targeting these genes of interest may be applied to provide positive evidence to support the diagnosis. IHC for p53 and Ki-67 can also be helpful when they preferentially highlight a suspiciously large number of atypical nuclei. These IDH-wildtype low-grade DAs are rarely diagnosed because most are clinically and radiologically subtle, and may exhibit radiologic and histomorphologic low-grade features for only a short time before developing the classic appearance of IDH-wildtype GBM.

3. **Anaplastic astrocytoma (AA), WHO grade III** is a diffusely infiltrating glioma with a mean age of presentation in the fifth decade. AA may appear de novo, or through progression of a pre-existing IDH-mutant or IDH-wildtype DA. Like DA, AA preferentially involves the cerebral hemispheres. On MRI, AA is similar to DA, but may show faint, focal enhancement. Histologically, AA is distinguished by increased cellularity, pleomorphism, mitoses, and increased proliferative index. The defining feature that distinguishes AA from DA is mitotic activity, which should be evaluated in the context of sample size. In a limited (needle/core) biopsy, a single mitosis is sufficient to designate a glioma as anaplastic. However, in large resections there should be at least a few mitoses before the tumor is considered anaplastic. By definition, AAs do not have MVP or necrosis. It is worth noting, however, that many AAs harbor genetic features of IDH-wildtype GBM (see below) and have clinical outcomes similar to those of IDH-wildtype GBMs (defined by classic histologic features). For this reason, it is important to evaluate IDH-wildtype AAs for genetic features of GBM. **Gliomatosis cerebri** is no longer considered a WHO diagnosis, but remains a useful term to describe the growth pattern of an extensively infiltrative glioma that involves three or more lobes of the cerebrum and may extend into brain stem, cerebellum, and even spinal cord.

4. GBM **(ex multiforme; GBM), WHO grade IV** is the most malignant form of astrocytoma and also the most common diffuse glioma subtype. GBMs occur mostly

in adults but peak age of onset differs considerably between IDH-mutant and IDH-wildtype tumors. IDH-mutant tumors usually arise earlier in life, with a peak in the fourth and fifth decades (mean age = 45); IDH-wildtype GBMs, in the sixth to seventh decades (median age = 64). On imaging, GBMs show heterogeneous or ring enhancement, and are differentiated from AA histologically by EH, MVP, and/ or necrosis. EH is defined by the presence of multilayered vessel walls with enlarged, often cytologically atypical and mitotically active endothelial (and smooth muscle/ pericytic) cells. MVP describes abnormally frequent, unusual, reactive-appearing blood vessels, sometimes forming glomeruloid structures with multiple lumina (e-**Fig. 39.16**). These vascular changes often occur together and the terms are often used interchangeably. Necrosis may be characterized as palisading (hypercellular tumor cells arranged radially around a zone of central necrosis—formerly described as pseudopalisading) or geographic (nonpalisading, often caused by infarction). Interestingly, geographic necrosis may be more common in IDH-wildtype tumors, in which intravascular thrombosis is common; in contrast, IDH-mutant GBM actively inhibits clot formation. The genetic features of IDH-wildtype GBM are complex, involving considerable intertumor and intratumoral heterogeneity. The more common alterations include *TERT* promoter (*TERTp*) mutation (most common), *EGFR* amplification, *PTEN*/10q loss, *CDKN2A/2B* loss, *PDFGRA* amplification and/or variants in *TP53*, *PTEN*, *NF1*, *PIK3CA*, *PIK3R1*, *RB1*, *MDM2*, and *BRAF*; and others. Epigenetics can also differ across GBMs; *MGMT* promoter methylation is a very important favorable predictor of response to therapy. Beyond the fundamental diagnostic histologic features and genetic changes of GBM, several morphologic variants of GBM are recognized.

a. Small cell GBM (scGBM) usually presents de novo rather than progressing from a lower-grade astrocytoma. The term "small cell" is not intended to draw a morphologic comparison to the neuroendocrine carcinoma of the lung with the same name; instead, it may be considered a foil of the previously named giant cell GBM. scGBM has some features that resemble high-grade oligodendroglioma, and other features that provide genuine diagnostic clues. At low magnification, the hypercellular sheets of scGBM appear bland. At higher power, scGBM shows slightly oval or elongate (rather than round) nuclei with mild hyperchromasia and delicate chromatin, perinuclear halos, microcalcifications, and so-called chicken wire-like branching capillaries. However, unlike most oligodendrogliomas, its mitotic density is remarkably high (e-**Fig. 39.17**). This dissonance (bland histology and abundant mitotic figures) is often the first clue to the diagnosis (*Cancer* 2004;101:2318). Other helpful clues include radiographic ring-enhancement and, when present, focal EH and pseudopalisading necrosis. However, a subset of anaplastic oligodendrogliomas can show these features, and one-third of scGBMs do not (yet still behave clinically like other GBMs).

Fortunately, scGBM and oligodendrogliomas have immunohistochemical and molecular characteristics that distinguish them. The tumor cells in scGBM often contain thin, GFAP-positive cytoplasmic processes; GFAP reactivity in oligodendrogliomas is usually restricted to minigemistocytes, gliofibrillary oligodendrocytes, and entrapped reactive astrocytes. The MIB-1 (Ki-67) labeling index is typically much higher in scGBM than in most anaplastic oligodendrogliomas, though the ranges of these indices overlap. More importantly, reactivity with antibody IDH-1 is uniformly absent in scGBM (a primary GBM) and present in the majority of oligodendrogliomas. In addition, FISH studies have shown *EGFR* amplifications in ~70% and deletions of chromosome 10q in >90% of scGBMs (e-**Fig. 39.18**); these are rare in oligodendroglioma. In contrast, codeletion of chromosomal arms 1p and 19q (involving whole arms), now essential for a diagnosis of oligodendroglioma, is not observed in scGBM (though false positives can occur, depending on the 1p19q assay; e.g., with FISH assays in which only a small locus is tested, because of the genomic instability in GBMs).

b. **Epithelioid GBM (eGBM), WHO grade IV** is another rare variant of IDH-wildtype GBM, which, as the name implies, prominently features epithelioid (and some rhabdoid) cytology. It preferentially affects young adults and children, and has a very poor prognosis even among GBMs. Importantly, 50% of these tumors harbor a *BRAF* p. V600E mutation (and show reactivity for antibody VE1), which may make this tumor type sensitive to BRAF-inhibitor targeted therapy.

c. **Gliosarcoma (GS) WHO grade IV,** a variant of GBM, is often superficially located and, radiographically, deceptively circumscribed. GS exhibits astrocytic and sarcomatous elements, the latter usually resembling fibrosarcoma, leiomyosarcoma, or undifferentiated sarcoma. However, GS may also exhibit bone, cartilage, muscle, and even epithelial lines of differentiation; when the latter is present, the tumor may be called adenoid GBM. Molecular studies have demonstrated similar genetic abnormalities within all histologic elements within a tumor, suggesting a common cell of origin. The sarcomatous elements in GS are reticulin rich, typically negative for GFAP, and positive for vimentin, smooth muscle actin, muscle-specific actin (MSA), and so forth based on the sarcomatous differentiation pattern. In contrast, the glial regions are reticulin poor and GFAP positive. Although true sarcomas can arise in the CNS from the meninges, they are very rare; when confronted with a neoplasm in the brain that appears to be completely sarcomatous, exhaustive sampling for elements of glioma is prudent.

5. **Diffuse midline glioma, H3 K27M mutant, WHO grade IV.** This diagnosis represents a major step forward in the understanding of this class of gliomas. As the name suggests, these almost always involve midline structures, favoring the brainstem, thalamus, and spinal cord; in the brain stem, they were formerly known as "brainstem glioma" or "diffuse intrinsic pontine glioma". They are more common in children, but also appear in adults. Though they generally resemble DAs or AAs histomorphologically, the prognosis is worse, with 2-year survival reported to be <10%. The molecular and immunohistochemical features of this neoplasm are discussed above. A few important points worth mention include that a pair of specific antibodies can recognize the protein product of the underlying mutation and the histone methylation change that it causes; these tumors may have ATRX mutations (15%) and/or p53 mutations (50%), but are unlikely to harbor an IDH mutation; this mutation can sometimes occur in other tumor types (e.g., well-circumscribed tumors such as GG and ependymoma), but its presence should not be regarded as synonymous with a WHO grade IV diagnosis and outcome unless the tumor in question is both diffuse and midline.

6. **Oligodendroglioma, IDH-mutant, 1p/19q-codeleted, WHO grade II** comprises 10% to 25% of all adult gliomas, behaves less aggressively than astrocytoma, and shows slower progression and longer patient survival. Although molecular data (IDH mutation status and 1p/19q codeletion status) are mandatory for rendering a final integrated diagnosis, and molecularly defined DA and oligodendroglioma can show considerable overlap of histologic features, histomorphologic assessment remains important for establishing a tumor's diffusely infiltrative nature, for assigning an appropriate WHO grade, and for providing a favored diagnosis when ancillary testing fails or is unavailable. One of the more useful histologic features for distinguishing classic oligodendroglial neoplasms from astrocytic tumors is nuclear morphology; oligodendroglioma nuclei are nearly spherical, with delicate chromatin, crisp envelopes, and inconspicuous nucleoli (e-**Fig. 39.19**). Other helpful features include: artifactual clear perinuclear haloes that often appear after routine histologic processing; a delicate hexagonal array of capillaries that resembles "chicken wire"; mucin-rich microcystic spaces; microcalcifications; predominantly cortical involvement; and perineuronal satellitosis. Immunohistochemically, classic oligodendroglioma cells show diffuse reactivity for OLIG2 and no reactivity for GFAP. However, oligodendrogliomas often contain three cell types that do show reactivity for GFAP: minigemistocytes, gliofibrillary oligodendrocytes, and reactive astrocytes.

The mini-gemistocyte, named for its superficial resemblance to the larger astrocytic gemistocyte, has a belly of glassy eosinophilic cytoplasm and an eccentrically placed oligodendroglial nucleus. Gliofibrillary oligodendrocytes are indistinguishable from classic oligodendroglial tumor cells on H&E stained sections, but show a GFAP-positive rim of cytoplasm and a tadpole-like tail. Entrapped, nonneoplastic astrocytes generally retain their characteristic stellate morphology.

In addition to oligodendrogliomas, several other tumors exhibit the so-called "fried egg" appearance with rounded nuclei and clear perinuclear haloes; most notably DNT, PA, central neurocytoma, and clear cell ependymoma. Nevertheless, this differential diagnosis can usually be resolved using clinical information, other histologic clues (e.g., RFs, EGBs, atypical astrocytic nuclei), immunohistochemical stains (e.g., IDH-1, GFAP, Neu-N, SYN, NF, EMA, CD99, D2-40, MIB-1), and FISH studies (see below).

Molecular profiling of oligodendrogliomas is now routinely performed because this tumor type is fundamentally defined by IDH mutation and 1p/19q codeletion (e-**Fig. 39.20**). Most of these tumors (~96%) also harbor *TERTp* mutations, which enhance telomerase activity. All three changes (*IDH* mutation, 1p19q codeletion, *TERTp* mutation) are thought to be early events in tumorigenesis. Other genetic alterations fairly frequent in oligodendrogliomas are inactivating mutations in tumor suppressor genes *CIC* (located on 19q) and *FUBP1* (located on 1p). Compared with IDH-mutant astrocytomas, oligodendrogliomas lack *ATRX* alterations, behave less aggressively, are more sensitive to chemotherapy and radiation, and are thus considered "genetically favorable". Unfortunately, pediatric oligodendrogliomas generally do not show codeletion; those that do harbor the codeletion frequently occur in teenagers and older children and likely represent the "adult type" oligodendroglioma (*J Neuropathol Exp Neurol* 2003;62:53).

7. Anaplastic oligodendroglioma, IDH-mutant, 1p/19q-codeleted, WHO grade III.

Based on the criteria defined by the WHO, anaplastic oligodendroglioma must have "brisk" mitotic activity, and/or "conspicuous microvascular proliferation" along with increased cellularity and marked atypia. High-grade oligodendrogliomas additionally often show greater cytologic pleomorphism, epithelioid morphology, prominent nucleoli, and sharper cell borders. Necrosis, when present, is more often geographic rather than palisading. The exact density of mitoses has not been universally accepted, but a mitotic index of 6 or more per 10 high-power fields (40×) is often used to assign anaplastic grade III (based on *J Neuropathol Exp Neurol* 2001;60:248) in the absence of EH or necrosis. Anaplastic transformation can be focal or widespread. Some oligodendrogliomas appear otherwise low-grade, but contain hypercellular nodules with increased mitotic activity; such cases may be designated "oligodendroglioma with focal anaplasia", WHO grade III. Neuroimaging studies of anaplastic oligodendroglioma often, but not invariably, show patchy or homogeneous contrast enhancement. Ring enhancement, however, is uncommon.

8. Mixed oligoastrocytoma (MOA).

This diagnosis is included primarily for historical reasons; at many centers, this diagnosis was not uncommon until 2016, when the WHO adopted molecular features as the defining characteristics of oligodendroglioma and astrocytoma. Frequently now, as patients with this diagnosis return for follow-up care, their existing molecular findings are re-interpreted according to the 2016 WHO criteria, or the definitive molecular tests that are newly performed to render the most appropriate contemporary diagnosis. Most cases with a prior diagnosis of MOA can now be clearly reclassified as molecular astrocytoma or oligodendroglioma; only rarely examples with ambiguous patterns of molecular alteration encountered in routine clinical practice.

9. Pediatric diffuse gliomas.

Unlike their histologically similar counterparts that appear in older adults, pediatric diffuse gliomas are driven by very different molecular changes. **Pediatric oligodendrogliomas** and **pediatric DAs** do not harbor *IDH1/2* mutations, 1p/19q codeletion, or *ATRX* mutations; instead, >50% have alterations of

FGFR1, *BRAF*, or *MYB*, or *MYBL1*. Many **pediatric high-grade diffuse astrocytic tumors** may be categorized as either a diffuse midline glioma, H3 K27M mutant, WHO grade IV (described above) or a hemispheric high-grade DA of childhood. Both of these are driven by mutations that alter histones; the latter is usually H3.3 G34R (or G34V). **Hemispheric GBM of childhood** is driven by *NTRK* fusions in ~40% of cases; other genes altered include *TP53*, *ATRX*, *SETD2*, *CDKN2A* (deletion), and *PDGFRA*; adult alterations (e.g., those to *IDH1/2*, *TERTp*, *EGFR*) are rare. Diffuse gliomas presenting in adolescence and young adulthood appear to have molecular features that conform either to pediatric or to adult diffuse gliomas.

B. Circumscribed Astrocytomas

1. **Pilocytic astrocytoma (PA), WHO grade I** (e-Fig. 39.21) is a slowly growing, rather circumscribed neoplasm frequently occurring in children and young adults, with a predilection for the cerebellum. It also occurs in the optic pathway (engendering the term "optic pathway glioma", commonly associated with neurofibromatosis 1), hypothalamus, dorsal brain stem, spinal cord, and rarely, cerebral hemispheres. Classically, these tumors appear in imaging studies as cystic lesions with an enhancing mural nodule. In the brain stem, they may occur as exophytic lesions. Histologically, these tumors often exhibit a biphasic pattern in which compact pilocytic areas are interspersed with microcystic loose and/or spongy areas. PA is variably cellular and populated by bipolar cells with long hair-like (piloid) processes. RFs and EGBs commonly occur within the compact (dense) regions, and, though not specific for PA, provide very helpful diagnostic clues. Mitotic activity is low. The blood vessels within PAs are commonly hyalinized, and often exhibit linear "glomeruloid" tufts of EH. This feature, particularly when coupled with the marked nuclear atypia that commonly occurs in PA, can lead to confusion with high-grade glioma. However, the EH and nuclear atypia of PA have no negative prognostic significance; PAs usually follow a benign clinical course. In some cases, PA may focally resemble oligodendroglioma. Genetics: Most PAs are driven by genetic changes that affect the MAPK pathway. In cerebellar PAs, the most common alteration is *BRAF* fusion, with the regulatory domain replaced by that of another gene (usually *KIAA1549*); *BRAF* fusions can be detected by FISH or other molecular techniques. Most remaining PAs harbor *BRAF* pV600E (more common in supratentorial cases), *NF1* loss, or *FGFR1* alterations. Although extent of surgical resection is the strongest prognostic variable, *BRAF* fusion confers better prognosis in cases with incomplete resection; such patients may also benefit from MEK/mTOR inhibitor therapy.

2. **Pilomyxoid astrocytoma (PMA), WHO grade unassigned** is now considered a variant of PA (with similar genetic underpinnings) that presents in infants at a median age of 10 months, and favors the hypothalamus and optic chiasm. On MRI, PMA appears circumscribed and solid (not cystic), hypointense on T1 and hyperintense on T2, and shows homogenous contrast enhancement. The histologic hallmark of PMA is the presence of monomorphous bipolar cells in a markedly mucoid matrix, with a prominent angiocentric arrangement that resembles the perivascular pseudorosettes of ependymoma (e-Fig. 39.22). As defined, PMA does not show RFs or EGBs. Nuclear atypia is uncommon. Mitoses can be present. Vascular proliferation resembling that in PA is characteristic. Although not common, necrosis may be seen. The tumor cells show strong and diffuse immunoreactivity for GFAP, S-100, and vimentin. A subset of tumor cells is also positive for SYN. Clinically, PMAs are associated with adverse clinical outcomes relative to PAs, with frequent local recurrences and, often, CSF seeding at the time of diagnosis. It remains unclear whether these outcomes reflect inherent aggressiveness or the tendency for PMA to appear in surgically unfavorable anatomic locations. Given this ambiguity, the revised 2016 WHO classification scheme has withdrawn the previous assignment of WHO grade II to PMA.

3. **Pleomorphic xanthoastrocytoma, WHO grade II** is an epileptogenic neoplasm commonly located in the superficial cortical regions of the temporal lobe, often with meningeal attachment. Histologically, this tumor is composed of large

pleomorphic, variably GFAP-positive astrocytes, intermingled with less conspicuous spindled cells (e-Fig. 39.23). Some of the tumor cells have bizarre nuclei and nuclear pseudoinclusions, and multinucleated giant cells are common. EGBs are almost always evident. Xanthomatous tumor cells, though helpful, only occur in 25% of cases. Other features include perivascular plasmalymphocytic cuffing and scant mitoses. Reticulin silver stain highlights a network of basal laminae that surround individual tumor cells. Neuronal differentiation is often evidenced by reactivity for SYN and NF protein. Reactivity for CD34 is frequently observed. Grade II PXAs have a relatively favorable prognosis (81% 5-year survival). **Anaplastic (WHO grade III)** transformation, characterized by less pleomorphism, increased proliferative activity, necrosis, and/or MVP, occurs in 15% of PXAs; reticulin staining is often diminished in these examples. Genetically, ~60% of WHO grade II PXAs harbor *BRAF* pV600E mutation, though IHC for antibody VE1 often stains only a subset of cells; this mutation is less common in anaplastic PXA.

4. Subependymal giant cell astrocytoma (SEGA), WHO grade I is almost exclusively found in children and young adults with tuberous sclerosis. These well-circumscribed, intraventricular tumors usually occur near the foramen of Monro and cause symptoms associated with obstructive hydrocephalus. Imaging studies reveal contrast enhancement and calcification. Histologically the tumor cells may be spindled, epithelioid, or gemistocyte-like, and may appear in sweeping fascicles, large clusters, or perivascular pseudorosettes. The gemistocyte-like cells have abundant glassy eosinophilic cytoplasm and nuclei resembling those of ganglion cells, with fine granular chromatin and prominent nucleoli (e-Fig. 39.24); despite their name, they are more aptly considered large rather than giant. The hybrid astrocytic and neuronal features of SEGAs are also reflected in their immunohistochemical profile, with focal reactivity for both GFAP and one or more neuronal markers (e.g., SYN), as well as neural stem cell marker SOX2 (but not CD34). Mitoses are usually rare. MVP and necrosis are typically absent.

C. Ependymal Tumors

1. Ependymoma, WHO grade II (e-Fig. 39.25). Ependymomas occur as discrete enhancing masses. In children, they favor the posterior fossa; in young adults, the spinal cord. However, these associations are not absolute, and supratentorial tumors, often unassociated with the ventricles, can present in either age group. CSF dissemination occurs in <5% of the cases. Calcification in ependymoma is common when the lesion is located intracranially, whereas cyst formation is common in supratentorial cases. Smear preparations of ependymoma show relatively cohesive cells with uniform round to oval nuclei, fine chromatin, and fibrillary to epithelioid morphology; histologically, these tumor cells form perivascular pseudorosettes and, in 5% to 10% of cases, true ependymal rosettes. True rosettes (or ependymal canals) have central lumens reminiscent of the young central canal of the spinal cord (the central canal is often distorted in the adult spinal cord), whereas perivascular pseudorosettes have vessels at the center surrounded by a nucleus-free zone of radially oriented tumor cell processes. Ependymal canals, elongate versions of true rosettes, are typically seen in only the most differentiated examples. Immunohistochemically, most ependymomas exhibit reactivity for GFAP. Many cases also show reactivity for EMA, CD99, and/or podoplanin (antibody D2–40) along the luminal surface of true rosettes/ependymal canals or within paranuclear intracytoplasmic dot-like structures, thought to represent intracytoplasmic lumina. In difficult cases, EM studies can confirm ependymal differentiation by demonstrating long zipper-like intercellular junctions, microvilli, cilia, and/or intracytoplasmic lumina. Histomorphologic variants of ependymoma include the clear cell (mimics oligodendroglioma), cellular (mimics medulloblastoma or other embryonal tumors), tanycytic (mimics schwannoma or PA), and papillary (mimics choroid plexus tumors) subtypes. Rarely, ependymomas may contain cells with melanin pigment, or xanthomatous, signet ring, giant cell, or neuronal features. Ependymomas are usually treated with surgery alone, though some cases also receive adjuvant radiation. Extent of resection is the most reliable predictor of progression-free and overall survival. Other (poor) prognostic indicators include age <3 years, posterior fossa location, and anaplastic tumor grade. Grade II ependymomas have a 5-year progression-free survival rate of 60% to 80% as compared with 25% to 50% in anaplastic ependymomas. From a molecular perspective, recent findings suggest that ependymomas might be classified into nine groups: three within each anatomic region (i.e., supratentorial, posterior fossa, and spinal). Importantly, two of these groups have particularly unfavorable prognoses. One of these two groups, representing ~70% of pediatric supratentorial ependymomas and defined by the presence of a *RELA* fusion gene, is now considered to be a separate diagnostic entity by the 2016 WHO classification system (see Ependymoma, RELA fusion-positive, below). The other variant, ependymoma group A, usually appears in the lateral posterior fossa of infants, is often invasive, and has a balanced genome with a CpG island methylator phenotype ("CIMP"); evidence of global reduction of H3 K27me3 in these tumors (*Sci Transl Med* 2016;8:366) suggests that IHC for H3 K27me3 might serve as a surrogate diagnostic marker.

2. **Ependymoma, *RELA* fusion-positive, WHO grades II–III.** This entity is morphologically essentially indistinguishable from other ependymomas. Fortunately, FISH testing (e.g., using break-apart probes for the *RELA* locus) is diagnostic. *C11orf95-RELA* fusion causes constitutive activation of the NF-kB pathway, a potential therapeutic target. Immunoreactivity for L1CAM may serve as a surrogate marker for *RELA* fusion in supratentorial ependymomas.

3. **Anaplastic ependymoma, WHO grade III.** Several grading systems have been proposed for ependymomas, but no consensus has been achieved because correlations of grade with survival and clinical outcomes are lacking; thus, histologic grade is seldom used to guide treatment strategies. According to the WHO 2016 criteria, anaplastic ependymomas are characterized by increased cellularity, brisk mitotic activity, necrosis, and widespread MVP. Necrosis by itself does not warrant the diagnosis of anaplasia because lower-grade ependymomas also can show degenerative changes.

4. **Myxopapillary ependymoma, WHO grade I** is a slowly growing tumor of young adults that occurs almost exclusively in the cauda equina region where it arises from the filum terminale. Grossly, these tumors are encapsulated, intradural, sausage-shaped masses with a gelatinous interior. Histologically, the tumors show variable amounts of two patterns: ependymal and papillary. In papillary areas, the tumor cells form irregularly ovoid rings of cuboidal-to-columnar epithelium, each ring formed around a hyalinized central vessel, some fibrous stroma, and a rim of pale basophilic mucin. Pale, basophilic, often bubbly mucinous (myxoid) material also separates the papillae. In ependymal areas, the tumor cells are spindled and slender, and are arranged in loose fascicles and rather extravagant perivascular pseudorosettes (e-Fig. 39.26). The tumor cells are immunoreactive for GFAP, S-100 protein, and vimentin, with variable staining for EMA, CD99, and podoplanin (antibody D2-40). These tumors have a favorable prognosis following complete resection. If untreated or incompletely resected, rare cases can progress, develop anaplastic features, and invade surrounding tissues. Occasional ependymal tumors in this location show a mixture of myxopapillary and "typical" ependymoma features; the clinical behavior of such tumors is incompletely understood.

5. **Subependymoma, WHO grade I** is a benign, slowly growing, solid tumor related to ependymoma. The tumor is often asymptomatic, discovered incidentally on CT and MRI studies performed for other reasons. Occasionally, the tumor undergoes intratumoral hemorrhage and becomes life threatening by exerting mass effect. The prognosis is excellent following resection. Grossly, it appears as a sessile or pedunculated mass within one of the ventricles (lateral >4th >3rd). Histologically, it is lobulated and well demarcated. The tumor nuclei resemble those of ependymoma and (classically) appear in irregular clusters within a dense fibrillar background formed by tumor cell processes (e-Fig. 39.27). Mitotic figures are rare. Occasional pseudorosettes are not unusual. Secondary degenerative changes include microcyst formation, hemosiderin deposition, vascular hyalinization, myxoid change, and calcification.

Nuclear pleomorphism and MVP are occasionally seen; these do not warrant a higher-grade diagnosis. It is worth noting that subependymoma may appear as part of a compound ependymal tumor; in such cases, tumor grading should be assigned according to the ependymal component.

D. Choroid Plexus Tumors

1. **Choroid plexus papilloma, WHO grade I** (e-Fig. 39.28) is a benign lesion commonly located in the lateral ventricles in children, and in the 4th ventricle in adults. It typically presents with symptoms associated with obstructive hydrocephalus. Histologically, choroid plexus papilloma resembles normal choroid plexus. However, its fibrovascular cores are lined by a cuboidal-to-columnar epithelium that lacks the superficial intercellular spaces that impart a "cobblestone" appearance to normal choroid plexus. Mitotic activity is low. Clear cytoplasmic vacuoles are noted in some cases. Architectural complexity is limited. Occasionally, infarct-like necrosis may be present, but has no prognostic significance. Dystrophic calcifications are common and focal ependymal differentiation may be seen. Tumor cells show immunoreactivity for S-100, CAM 5.2, transthyretin (TTR), and GFAP (focally) but not for EMA and carcinoembryonic antigen (CEA). Reactivity for CK20 is uncommon.

2. **Atypical choroid plexus papilloma, WHO grade II** differs from typical choroid plexus papilloma by its defining feature of 2 or more mitotic figures per 10 randomly selected high-power fields; it also shows some preference for lateral ventricles and an increased tendency to metastasize (~17% of presenting cases). It may also show increased cellularity, nuclear pleomorphism, regional loss of papillary architecture, and necrosis, but these features are not required. Relative loss of reactivity for S100 and/or for TTR (lost in >50% of cells) may be prognostically unfavorable.

3. **Choroid plexus carcinoma (CPC), WHO grade III** (e-Fig. 39.29), usually presents in children under 3 years of age as an enhancing, intraventricular mass. These tumors are highly aggressive, often metastasize via the CSF, and are nearly uniformly fatal. Histologically, the tumors are more solid and complex than papillomas. High-grade cytology and frequent mitoses (usually >5 per 10 high-power fields) are the rule. Foci of necrosis are characteristic, and MVP may be seen. Focal small cell features may mimic embryonal tumors (ETs). Immunoreactivity for S-100, CAM 5.2, and TTR is characteristic, but S-100 and TTR may be lost. GFAP is variable; EMA and CEA are typically not observed. The differential diagnosis includes anaplastic ependymoma (GFAP+, CAM 5.2−, EMA+/−), GBM (GFAP+, CAM 5.2−), medulloblastoma/ET (SYN+, CAM 5.2−), and metastatic carcinoma (in older patients, EMA+, CEA+/−, S-100 +/−, CAM 5.2+). As CPC is frequently associated with Li-Fraumeni syndrome, germline testing for *TP53* may be warranted.

E. Other Glial Neoplasms

1. **Angiocentric glioma (AG), WHO grade I** (e-Fig. 39.30). First reported in 2005, AG is a rare supratentorial tumor associated with epilepsy in children and young adults. Radiographically, AG appears as a T2/FLAIR hyperintense, nonenhancing mass that expands the cortex with minimal mass effect. In some cases, a projection of the tumor extends to the ventricle. Histologically, AG shows uniform, slender spindled glial cells, often arranged either radially from or parallel to vessels, and, occasionally, perpendicular to the pia. AG shows some ependymal features, including dot-like immunoreactivity for EMA, and microvilli and zipper like junctions by electron microscopy, but shows an infiltrative growth pattern. The proliferation index is low. A defining genetic feature (*MYB-QKI* rearrangement) has been identified and its mechanisms of action described (*Nat Genet* 2016;48:273).

2. **Astroblastoma (AB), not yet graded** (e-Fig. 39.31). As with AG, AB is associated with epilepsy in children and young adults, but AB is also associated with headaches and vomiting, and shows a female predominance. On MRI, AB is usually large, lobulated, well-demarcated solid with an occasional cystic component, T2-isointense with gray matter, and enhancing. Histologically, AB bears some resemblance to ependymoma, but has stout (rather than fibrillar) cell processes that form the defining

astroblastic pseudorosettes. Vascular hyalinization is usually robust. In some tumors this architectural pattern assumes a papillary appearance. Like ependymoma and AG, AB shows dot-like immunoreactivity for EMA; reactivity for GFAP highlights the abbreviated cell processes within pseudorosettes. ABs showing >5 mitoses per ten 40× fields, anaplastic nuclear features, increased cellularity, MVP, and palisading necrosis are considered anaplastic/malignant, but may still be resectable due to this tumor's noninfiltrating growth pattern. *BRAF* p.V600E mutation has been reported in ~38% of ABs (*NeuroOncol* 2017;12:31).

3. **Chordoid glioma (CG) of the third ventricle, WHO grade II** is a rare tumor of adults that occurs almost exclusively in the vicinity of the anterior third ventricle and hypothalamus. Radiographically, CG is solid, well-demarcated, T2 intense, and strongly contrast enhancing. Histologically, as its name suggests, CG focally resembles chordoma, showing cords and clusters of eosinophilic epithelioid cells within a bubbly basophilic mucinous matrix; where mucin is lacking, these cells appear in sheets. Lymphoplasmacytic infiltrates are typically seen. Although CG shows modest immunoreactivity for EMA, its reactivity for GFAP, TTF-1, and CD34 (and absence of whorls, psammoma bodies, and physaliferous cells) helps to distinguish it from chordoid meningioma and chordoma. CGs lack genetic alterations typical of diffuse gliomas, and have recently been shown to harbor a recurrent kinase domain mutation in *PRKCA* with consequent activation of MAPK pathway (*Nat Commun* 2018;9:810).

F. Neuronal and Glioneuronal Neoplasms

1. **Ganglion cell tumor (GG and gangliocytoma), WHO grade I.** Ganglion cell tumors are epileptogenic and appear most often in the temporal lobes. On imaging, they commonly enhance and appear solid, cystic, or both. A cyst with an enhancing mural nodule is a common (but not specific) pattern. Microscopically, they are usually cortically based, microcystic, variably fibrotic, and calcified, and they often show perivascular lymphocytic cuffing (e-**Fig. 39.32**). Dysmorphic neurons (that may exhibit cytomegaly, vacuolated cytoplasm, coarse Nissl substance, irregular multipolar processes, and/or nuclear abnormalities including binucleation) are the defining feature. Architecturally, the ganglion cells are clumped or haphazardly arranged in comparison to the laminar well-ordered arrangement of the normal cortex. GGs have a variable glial component, typically astrocytic. Glial predominant GG may resemble DA, PA, or, infrequently, oligodendroglioma. Other features commonly noted include EGBs and Rosenthal fibers (though the latter is more common at the tumor periphery, and may result from piloid gliosis). Cortical dysplasia may be seen adjacent to GG. High-grade glial transformation is exceedingly rare and difficult to define precisely, but anaplastic GGs often show GBM-like features, including dense cellularity, atypia, high mitotic index, MVP, and necrosis. The glial component is immunoreactive for GFAP; the neuronal component is variably immunoreactive for SYN (highest sensitivity), NF, and chromogranin, but is usually negative or minimally positive for Neu-N. Often, a subset of cells both within and adjacent to the tumor shows immunoreactivity for CD34. These CD34+ cells are "spider-like", characterized by long, stellate, ramified processes, and are thought to represent progenitor cells. About 20% to 60% of GGs are positive for *BRAF* p.V600E, with immunoreactivity usually favoring ganglion cells. GGs generally have a favorable prognosis after surgical resection.

2. **Desmoplastic infantile astrocytoma (DIA) and desmoplastic infantile ganglioglioma (DIG), WHO grade I** (e-**Fig. 39.33**) typically occur in children younger than 2 years and are located superficially within the frontoparietal region. Radiologically, these are very large, attached to the dura, brightly enhancing, and are associated with a very large, occasionally multiloculated cyst. Histologically, they are biphasic. In areas that are rich in collagen IV and reticulin, the tumor cells are arranged in a storiform or fascicular pattern. The astrocytic cells, spindled and gemistocytic, are often inconspicuous within the desmoplastic background, but can be identified by GFAP immunostaining. The neuronal component (present in DIG, absent in DIA) is also

subtle because the polygonal neuronal tumor cells are often considerably smaller than those of conventional GG. The other phase of the tumor resembles embryonal neoplasms, with abundant small cells and many mitotic figures, and lacks reticulin and collagen. EH and necrosis may be observed but are not associated with an unfavorable prognosis. *BRAF* p.V600E mutation has been reported in small subsets (~10%) of DIA/DIGs.

3. **Dysplastic cerebellar gangliocytoma (DCG) (Lhermitte–Duclos disease), WHO grade I.** This unique cerebellar tumor is often associated with Cowden syndrome (*PTEN/MMAC-1* mutation). Patients with DCG often present with cerebellar dysfunction and/or obstructive hydrocephalus. DCG, which is T1 hypointense and T2 hyperintense on MRI, has a characteristic striped appearance with both modalities. Microscopically, DCG presents as a unilateral expansion of cerebellar folia wherein the internal granular layer is replaced by dysmorphic ganglion cells; there is no glial component. Abnormal vascular proliferation is sometimes noted, and white matter is occasionally vacuolated. Evaluation for other features of Cowden syndrome is warranted in patients with DCG.

4. **Central neurocytoma, WHO grade II** (e-Fig. 39.34) occurs in the lateral ventricles near the foramen of Monro in young or middle-aged patients, and often presents with signs and symptoms of obstructive hydrocephalus. On imaging studies, these masses are large, globular, enhancing, and often calcified. Histologically, the tumor cells have a uniform appearance with round nuclei, finely granular chromatin, inconspicuous nucleoli, sparse eosinophilic or clear cytoplasm, and delicate fibrillar cell processes (in contrast to the coarse processes of glial tumors). These cells often appear in solid monotonous sheets that may also exhibit prominent chicken-wire vasculature, and/or neurocytic (Homer Wright) rosettes, and/or perivascular pseudorosettes, and/or calcifications. Thus, the differential diagnosis often includes oligodendroglioma and (clear cell) ependymoma. In most cases, the brain/tumor interface of central neurocytoma is solid/pushing rather than infiltrative. Immunohistochemistry shows diffuse and strong immunoreactivity with SYN, variable reactivity for Neu-N and NF, and focal reactivity for GFAP. This neoplasm lacks *IDH* mutations, and codeletion of chromosomes 1p and 19q has been reported only rarely (in hindsight, reflecting 2016 criteria, such reports may actually represent unrecognized oligodendroglioma).

Occasionally, neurocytoma occurs within the parenchyma of the cerebral hemispheres, cerebellum, or spinal cord; diagnosed as **extraventricular neurocytoma WHO grade II**, this tumor often exhibits more pronounced ganglion cell and astrocytic differentiation. A small subset of "atypical" neurocytomas (central and extraventricular) with MVP, necrosis, and elevated mitotic and proliferative indices (three mitoses per 10 hpf and MIB-1 index of 2% or more) show more rapid recurrence, but are still considered WHO grade II. A rare cerebellar neoplasm resembling neurocytoma but with adipocytic differentiation, *TP53* mutation, and focal GFAP expression, **cerebellar liponeurocytoma, WHO grade II**, is a distinct entity.

5. **Dysembryoplastic neuroepithelial tumor (DNT), WHO grade I** is a benign, slowly growing tumor of adolescents and young adults with history of longstanding, drug-resistant partial seizures. On imaging, DNT appears in an area of expanded cerebral cortex, with a predilection for the medial temporal lobe. DNT is T1 hypointense, T2/FLAIR hyperintense, and nodular; some "complex" varieties show enhancement (see below). Microscopically, "simple" DNT demonstrates only the "specific glioneuronal element"; patterned intracortical mucin-rich nodules each exhibit a network of bundled axons and delicate capillaries that divide the mucin into microcystic pools. This network is decorated by oligodendroglioma-like cells and occasional stellate astrocytes, and some of the microcytic pools show morphologically normal "floating" neurons (e-Fig. 39.35). Mitotic figures are rare to absent. Oligodendroglioma-like cells show reactivity for OLIG2, and no reactivity for GFAP. Reactivity for CD34 and BRAF p.V600E (~30%) in DNT is variable. Complex DNT consists of the specific glioneuronal element with an additional component referred to as "glial nodules" which are

histologically identical to PA, GG, diffuse glioma, or another glial neoplasm. Cortical dysplasia may be seen adjacent to DNTs. Simple DNTs are commonly misdiagnosed as oligodendrogliomas, but can be distinguished from adult oligodendroglioma by the lack of *IDH* mutation; in children, *FGFR1* alteration is common to pediatric oligodendroglioma-like tumors and DNT so cannot be used to distinguish these two entities. If sampling is incomplete, complex DNTs may be misdiagnosed according to the glial nodule subtype that is present. Therefore, review of clinical history and radiographic imaging is essential in evaluating specimens from temporal lobe epilepsy surgical resections. DNT has a benign course and postsurgical seizure resolution is common.

6. **Papillary glioneuronal tumor (PGNT), WHO grade I.** This is a contrast-enhancing, well-circumscribed, solid or cystic lesion that appears most commonly in the periventricular white matter, usually in the temporal lobe. Patients, most commonly young adults, present with seizures, headaches, and vision disturbance. Histologically, as the name suggests, these tumors have glial and neuronal elements, and a papillary appearance. The glial element (GFAP-positive) forms a loose layer of spindled-to-cuboidal cells closely apposed to the surfaces of hyalinized fibrovascular cores; between these pseudopapillary structures are the neuronal tumor cells (SYN positive), which can range morphologically from neurocytic to ganglion cell-like. Mitotic activity, atypia, vascular proliferation, and necrosis are rare to absent in most cases (e-**Fig. 39.36**). Rare cases with Ki-67 proliferation indices >5% may have increased risk of progression or recurrence.

7. **Rosette-forming glioneuronal tumor (RGNT), WHO grade I** is most common in young adults, always involves the ventricular system of the posterior fossa, and in unusual cases may extend upward into the proximal supratentorial ventricles. Consequently, RGNT usually presents with sequelae of obstructive hydrocephalus (e.g., headache, ataxia). MRI shows RGNT to be circumscribed and solid, T2 hyperintense, T1 hypointense, and in some cases, heterogeneously enhancing. Histologically (e-**Fig. 39.37**), RGNT is biphasic, characterized by a uniform population of small neurocytic cells and a second glial element that resembles pilocytic astrocytoma. The neurocytic cells have hyperchromatic round nuclei and a small amount of cleared cytoplasm; classically, they form single or clustered rosettes and pseudorosettes within a relatively hypocellular eosinophilic matrix of astrocytic tumor cell processes. The centers of these rosettes and pseudorosettes are more intensely eosinophilic and contain fine, SYN-immunoreactive cell processes. The surrounding matrix shows immunoreactivity for GFAP, and may exhibit EGBs and RFs. Mutations in *PIK3CA* and *FGFR1* have been reported, but mutations in *IDH1/2*, *BRAF* p.V600E, and *BRAF* fusions are lacking. Surgical resection is curative.

8. **Diffuse leptomeningeal glioneuronal tumor (DLGT), no WHO grade assigned**. Usually appearing in childhood (male:female = 1.7:1), this very rare neoplasm is characterized by oligodendroglial cytology and widespread nodular leptomeningeal growth (T2 hyperintense on MRI) favoring spine and posterior fossa. Histologically it is usually low grade, but some tumors have mitotic activity or MVP and show decreased survival. The *KIAA1549-BRAF* fusion has been reported in ~75% of tested cases, with frequent concurrence of 1p deletion. More recently, by methylation array, DLGT have been divided into two subgroups with distinct clinical and molecular features (*Acta Neuropathol* 2018;136:239).

9. **Paraganglioma, WHO grade I** usually affects the cauda equina/filum terminale and jugulotympanic regions.

G. Pineal Parenchymal Tumors (PPT)

1. **Pineocytoma, WHO grade I** is more common in adults. On MRI, pineocytoma appears as a T1 hypo- or isointense, T2 hyperintense, uniformly enhancing, often calcified, discrete mass in the region of the pineal gland. Through mass effect, pineocytoma often causes increased ICP and upward gaze palsy (Parinaud syndrome). Histologically, pineocytoma tumor cells (SYN+, Neu-N+), with round-to-oval nuclei, salt and pepper chromatin, inconspicuous nucleoli, and poorly demarcated cell

borders, often form pineocytic rosettes (large, exaggerated Homer Wright rosettes) (e-**Fig. 39.38**). Mitotic activity is very low. Pineocytomas may be difficult to distinguish from normal pineal tissue in a small biopsy, although a lobular pattern with gliovascular septae favors the latter. A rare pleomorphic variant of pineocytoma with large ganglion cells, bizarre multinucleated giant cells, degenerative atypia, and low mitotic activity has no known prognostic significance.

2. **Pineoblastoma, WHO grade IV** is a rapidly growing malignant tumor that predominantly occurs in children and very young adults. Occasionally, pineoblastomas occur in association with bilateral retinoblastoma ("trilateral retinoblastoma"). On MRI, pineoblastomas are inconsistent: hypo- to isointense on T1, hypo- to hyperintense on T2, with homogeneous or heterogeneous enhancement. Their borders appear more infiltrative than those of pineocytoma, and leptomeningeal metastasis (through CSF dissemination) is common at presentation. Grossly, they are soft, friable, and poorly demarcated. Hemorrhage and necrosis may be present. Calcification is rare. Histologically, they resemble other "small blue cell tumors" (e.g., ETs), as described below. The primitive-appearing cells, with little cytoplasm and hyperchromatic, molded nuclei, are densely packed in sheets, occasionally interrupted by Homer Wright rosettes, Flexner–Wintersteiner rosettes (which have a central lumen), and zones of necrosis. Mitotic activity is generally high. Invasion of the adjacent pineal gland and leptomeninges is common. Immunoreactivity for neuronal markers (e.g., NF, SYN, chromogranin, and neuron-specific enolase) is weak and focal relative to that seen in pineocytoma. Occasionally, these tumor cells may additionally express antigens related to photoreceptor or pineal differentiation, including retinal S-antigen, rhodopsin, and melatonin.

3. **Pineal parenchymal tumor of intermediate differentiation (PPTID), WHO grades II—III,** appears at any age but is more common in adults, and accounts for almost half of PPTs. Radiographically, PPTIDs show heterogeneous distributions of T1 hypointensity, T2 hyperintensity, and marked enhancement. Histologically, PPTID is rather cellular, lacks pineocytic rosettes, and has slightly more pronounced cytologic atypia and higher mitotic/proliferative activity than pineocytoma (MIB-1 indices range from 10% to 16% for PPTID, versus 1% to 2% for pineocytoma). PPTID appears in two main patterns: *diffuse*, with mildly irregular round-to-oval nuclei arranged in a sheet-like pattern, and *pseudolobulated*, wherein tumor cells are divided into lobules delineated by vessels. Although not official WHO criteria, higher-grade (III) is assigned to PPTID when the mitotic index exceeds six mitoses per ten 40× fields or when immunoreactivity for NF protein is nearly absent (*Brain Pathol* 2000;10:49). For this reason, definitive grading is best reserved for resection (rather than limited biopsy) specimens. For low-grade and high-grade PPTID, recurrence (~22% vs. 56%, respectively), craniospinal spread (15% vs. 28%), and 5-year survival rates (74% vs. 39%) are intermediate between those of pineoblastoma and pineocytoma.

4. **Papillary tumor of the pineal region (PTPR), WHO grade II or III,** has been reported in children and adults, with a peak in the third decade. MRI shows a large, well-circumscribed, T2-intense, enhancing (occasionally cystic) mass in the vicinity of the pineal gland. Histologically, as the name implies, PTPR does exhibit papillary features; large, pale-to-eosinophilic tumor cells form columnar epithelia around hyalinized vessels (e-**Fig. 39.39**). In other, more solid areas, tumor cells with round-to-oval nuclei and rather clear or vacuolated cytoplasm may form true ependymal rosettes. Mitotic activity is variable (0-to-10 per 10 high-power objective fields), and necrosis may be seen; EH is usually not observed. PTPR does not infiltrate the pineal gland.

This histologic appearance resembles that of ependymoma. Further, both tumors can show focal membranous and dot-like reactivity for EMA (PTPR is thought to arise from the specialized ependymal cells of the subcommissural organ). The key features that distinguish PTPR are minimal reactivity for GFAP and strong reactivity for CK18. Importantly, PTPR is also immunoreactive for TTR, so this marker does not distinguish choroid plexus neoplasms from PTPR. Official grading criteria have not yet been defined; however, a mitotic index of 3 or more per ten 40× fields has been associated with poorer prognosis.

H. CNS Embryonal tumors (ET), most common in children, are so-named because their histology (primitive appearing "small blue cells") is reminiscent of elements of the embryonic nervous system. These tumors are bulky, grow rapidly, and seed the CSF pathways. All ETs are inherently malignant (WHO grade IV); however, the prognoses for these tumors vary widely, as some respond very well to current treatments and others do not. Having undergone re-classification in the 2016 WHO system, ETs now include: medulloblastoma; AT/RT; ETMR, C19MC altered; and "other CNS ETs". This last category, encompassing tumors that would previously have been called "CNS primitive neuroectodermal tumors (PNET)", now includes cerebral neuroblastoma, ganglioneuroblastoma, medulloepithelioma (without C19MC alteration), and any other embryonal neoplasm that does not belong in the other categories. Though the term PNET is no longer recognized in the 2016 WHO brain tumor classification system, it remains in the medical literature and in existing pathology reports that are reviewed for ongoing patient care.

1. Medulloblastoma, WHO grade IV, the most common embryonal CNS tumor, is thought to originate either from remnants of the external granular layer or from the fourth ventricular germinal matrix. On imaging, the tumor is often a T1 hypointense, T2 hyperintense, noncalcified, and homogeneously contrast-enhancing cerebellar mass with restricted diffusion. In approximately one-third of classic cases, the tumor has already seeded the CSF pathways focally (with "drop metastases" in the lumbosacral spinal cord) or diffusely ("icing" the subarachnoid space) at the time of presentation. Distant metastases, most often involving bone and lymph nodes, are rare. Medulloblastomas are routinely classified in two different ways that show incomplete correspondence; by histomorphology and by biologic/genetic underpinning.

Histologic subtypes of medulloblastoma include classic/undifferentiated, desmoplastic/nodular, with extensive nodularity, large cell, and anaplastic.

Classic/undifferentiated medulloblastoma (e-**Fig. 39.40**), the most common subtype, usually arises from the cerebellar midline and appears as a patternless sheet of abundant small tumor cells with hyperchromatic nuclei and minimal apparent cytoplasm. The nuclei show a degree of molding and are often described as round-to-oval or "carrot-shaped". Nucleoli are inconspicuous. Mitotic figures and apoptotic bodies are often abundant. MVP and necrosis may be present, but are not prominent. Forty percent of cases exhibit Homer Wright rosettes (tumor cells surrounding small islands of delicate fibrillary tumor neuropil). In addition to seeding the CSF, this tumor often re-invades the cerebellar parenchyma from the subarachnoid space via Virchow–Robin spaces.

The desmoplastic/nodular variant (e-**Fig. 39.41**), accounting for ~30% of cases, usually arises laterally, and has a characteristic low power appearance of rounded, pale islands separated by dark internodular tissue. The pale islands (reticulin free) contain cells with a relatively neurocytic phenotype that have round to oval nuclei, open chromatin, moderate cytoplasm, cell processes that form a neuropil-like stroma, and little mitotic activity. The internodular tissue (reticulin-rich) is formed by densely packed, primitive-appearing cells with hyperchromatic, malleable nuclei, smudged chromatin, little cytoplasm, and high proliferative activity. This variant is genetically distinct and has a slightly more favorable prognosis than other subtypes (*Acta Neuropathol* 2006;112:5).

Another prognostically favorable variant is "medulloblastoma with extensive nodularity". This rare tumor, found almost exclusively in infants, radiographically may resemble a cluster of grapes (T1 imaging, postcontrast). Histologically, it resembles the desmoplastic variant, but is dominated by pale, reticulin-free nodules with neuronal differentiation; primitive areas are diminished. After treatment, this tumor has been reported to undergo complete gangliocytic differentiation.

In contrast, the rare large cell variant of medulloblastoma behaves relatively aggressively and is less responsive to therapy. As its name suggests, the cells of large cell medulloblastoma have relatively more cytoplasm than those of classic medulloblastoma, as well as larger nuclei, vesicular chromatin, and prominent nucleoli. It is worth noting, however, that this large cell histologic pattern may not be uniform within a tumor, and intermixed anaplastic tissue, described below, is often associated.

Anaplastic features in medulloblastomas include cellular pleomorphism, cytomegaly, hyperchromasia, markedly elevated mitotic index, atypical mitoses, abundant apoptotic bodies, apoptotic lakes, and cell wrapping (**e-Fig. 39.42**). Although the common co-occurrence of large-cell and anaplastic features has led some to advocate a monolithic large-cell/anaplastic medulloblastoma category, anaplasia can be observed in classic medulloblastomas that lack large cell features.

Biologic/genetic subtypes of medulloblastoma include: WNT-activated (Group 1), 10% of cases; *SHH*-activated (Group 2), 30% of cases, further sub-divided into *TP53* mutant and *TP53*-wildtype groups; non-WNT/non-SHH (Groups 3 and 4), 20% and 40% of cases, respectively.

Most WNT-activated (Group 1) medulloblastomas appear in the cerebellar midline of children and young adults (not infants), have classic histomorphology, and may exhibit relatively invasive growth. Most (~85%) also show monosomy 6 and/or mutation of *CTNNB1* (beta-catenin gene), leading to WNT pathway activation. Group 1 medulloblastomas have a very favorable prognosis, with excellent response to surgery and adjuvant therapy. *P53* mutations do not confer worse prognosis in this subtype.

SHH-activated (Group 2) medulloblastomas are a heterogeneous group. Those with *TP53* wildtype status (about one-third of Group 2 cases) generally correspond to the desmoplastic/nodular and extensively nodular histologic variants, and show an excellent response to therapy. In contrast, cases with TP53 mutation usually exhibit classic or large cell/anaplastic histomorphology, and prognosis is poor; germline testing for *TP53* alterations is generally warranted in such cases.

Non-WNT/non-SHH (Group 3 and Group 4) medulloblastomas can be divided into either group 3 or group 4 by gene expression profiling, but with considerable overlap and limited clinical utility. Group 3 tumors affect infants and children equally, can show classic or large cell/anaplastic morphology, usually harbor isochromosome 17q, often show *MYC* gene amplification or *MYC* gene fusion (and/or MYC protein overexpression), and have a poor prognosis. Group 4 tumors preferentially affect children rather than infants, show classic morphology, and have an intermediate prognosis, but are not as well characterized as groups 1, 2, and 3.

Although gene sequencing remains the gold standard for classification of genetic subtypes of medulloblastoma, such analyses can take considerable time, and rare cases show no clear genetic underpinning to account for otherwise clear evidence of pathway activation (e.g., for SHH pathway activation). Fortunately, four immunohistochemical markers (Beta-catenin, GAB1, YAP1, and p53) and cytogenetic tests for isochromosome 17q and *MYC* amplification can serve as excellent surrogate markers to categorize most medulloblastomas and provide prognostic information.

Immunohistochemistry for beta-catenin, showing reactivity within tumor cell nuclei (indicating translocation from the cytoplasm) serves as a surrogate marker for WNT pathway activation (Group 1); however, this immunostain is often difficult to interpret, and some mutated tumors show only patchy or focal nuclear staining. Fortunately, Group 1 (WNT) tumors are also YAP1 positive and GAB1 negative. In contrast, Group 2 (SHH) tumors show only cytoplasmic reactivity for beta-catenin, and are positive for both YAP1 and GAB1; to subdivide Group 2, strong p53 immunoreactivity in a majority of tumor nuclei can serve as a rapid, temporary surrogate for *TP53* mutation analysis. Finally, Groups 3 and 4 are negative for YAP1 and GAB1, show only cytoplasmic reactivity for beta-catenin, and may show evidence of isochromosome 17q. Importantly, further prognostic information can be derived from assessments for *MYC* amplification and anaplastic/large cell histology; both of these features are independent predictors of poor prognosis.

Otherwise, medulloblastomas are generally positive for SYN and variably positive for GFAP, and have high MIB-1 (Ki-67) labeling indices. They also retain nuclear immunoreactivity for INI1; this feature should be tested routinely in all embryonal neoplasms of the posterior fossa to rule out AT/RT, which shows "loss" of nuclear expression.

The 5-year survival rate for medulloblastoma overall is 60%, following current treatment protocols (gross total resection, craniospinal radiation therapy, and adjuvant chemotherapy). Patients with WNT-activated tumors or the extensively nodular variant of SHH-activated tumors fare relatively better; other patients, particularly when younger than 3 years and/or with limited surgical resections and/or with CSF dissemination, have relatively unfavorable prognoses. Although the standard treatment of cytotoxic therapy and craniospinal radiation is often life-saving, it can also introduce significant neurologic impairment in young patients, particularly those younger than 3 years.

2. **Embryonal tumor with multilayere drosettes (ETMR), C19MC-altered, WHO grade IV.** This entity, defined by a combination of multilayered, mitotically active rosettes and amplification/fusion of the *C19MC* locus at 19q13.42, appears supratentorially (~70%) or in the posterior fossa of children <4 years of age as a large contrast-enhancing mass, potentially with cysts and/or calcifications. Allowing some histologic variability, it includes ETs previously called ependymoblastoma, showing "multilayered" true rosettes (with central lumens) that blend into a surrounding sheet of dense tumor cells (e-Fig. 39.43), ET with abundant neuropil and true rosettes (ETANTR) (e-Fig. 39.44), and a subset of medulloepitheliomas defined by arrangements of neoplastic neuroepithelium reminiscent of the developing neural tube. Immunohistochemistry for CAM5.2, EMA, and CD99 may highlight rosettes; SYN will highlight better-differentiated neuropil-like areas. Reactivity for LIN28A, a negative regulator of let-7 tumor suppressor microRNAs, is strong in the rosettes and poorly differentiated areas of ETMR, but is not specific. A definitive diagnosis requires molecular (e.g., FISH) testing for genetic alterations that drive increased expression of the cluster of microRNAs at the *C19MC* locus. Prognosis is usually very poor, even with combination therapies.

3. **Other CNS ETs (all WHO grade IV).** Under the revised 2016 WHO classification of CNS tumors, many ETs (e.g., medulloblastoma, ETMR, AT/RT) can be defined by specific morphologic and/or molecular features; however, several ETs currently lack specific molecular traits and must be categorized on the basis of morphology and by exclusion.

   a. **Medulloepithelioma** is characterized by primitive embryonal cells forming a multilayered to pseudostratified neuroepithelium that is arranged into tubular structures resembling the embryonic neural tube. Some tumors with these histomorphologic features harbor *C19MC* alterations (and express LIN28A) and are, therefore, considered ETMRs. Other examples also express LIN28A, but lack *C19MC* alteration; these await identification of an expected diagnostic genetic signature.

   b. **CNS neuroblastoma** is formed by sheets of primitive neuroepithelial cells and interspersed areas of neurocytic differentiation that feature Homer Wright rosettes. Necrosis and calcifications are common.

   c. **CNS ganglioneuroblastoma** appears morphologically similar to CNS neuroblastoma, but additionally features scattered dysmorphic neuronal/ganglionic forms.

   d. **CNS ET, NOS** includes cases in which poorly differentiated neuroepithelial cells show variable capacity for neuronal, astrocytic, myogenic, or melanocytic differentiation.

4. **AT/RT, WHO grade IV** (e-Fig. 39.45) is a densely cellular tumor of infants and young children (most <3 years old, male predominance) that can occur anywhere in the neuraxis. Radiographically, AT/RT is usually large, cystic, hemorrhagic, focally necrotic, and heterogeneously enhancing; not uncommonly, nodular leptomeningeal spread is found at presentation. Histologically, AT/RT is defined by rhabdoid cells with eccentrically placed vesicular nuclei, prominent nucleoli, and large eosinophilic paranuclear whorls of intermediate filaments. Unfortunately, rhabdoid cells may appear only focally, or perhaps not at all, in a biopsy specimen; tissue heterogeneity

is common in AT/RT. A small blue cell component is seen in 65% of cases and may predominate. For this reason, AT/RT can easily be confused with medulloblastoma (particularly the large cell/anaplastic variant) or other ETs. Other areas of AT/RT may show glial, mesenchymal, epithelial or papillary features, potentially conjuring an even broader differential diagnosis. Complicating histologic evaluation further, AT/RT typically shows immunoreactivity for vimentin, EMA, CK, and smooth muscle actin, and often, for SYN and GFAP. Because AT/RT can mimic other entities and is relatively common among infantile CNS tumors, a very low threshold should be maintained to rule out this diagnosis when confronted with a tumor in a child under 3 years of age. Fortunately, a highly sensitive and specific immunohistochemical stain for INI1 can distinguish almost all AT/RTs from other ETs. INI1, the protein product of the *INI1/BAF47/hSNF5* tumor suppressor gene on chromosome 22q11, is a component of the SWI/SNF complex, which functions to alter chromatin structure. Most AT/RTs result from biallelic inactivation of this gene, and hence virtually all AT/RTs show loss of intranuclear reactivity for INI1 (intratumoral endothelial cells often provide a convenient internal positive control). Of note, only ~70% of cases show deletion or mutation of this locus, despite showing loss of the protein. A small subgroup of AT/RTs that do not show loss of INI1 may, instead, harbor mutation/inactivation *of SMARCA4*, another gene in the SWI/SNF complex, with consequent loss of BRG1 protein expression. AT/RTs are highly aggressive tumors; mean survival is 17 months.

I. Tumors of the Meninges

1. Meningiomas, which bear cytologic resemblance to the arachnoidal cells that normally inhabit the inner surface of the dura, are most often intracranial and extra-axial, appearing over the cerebral convexities, parasagittally along the falx cerebri, along the skull base or tentorium, or in the optic nerve sheath. Less commonly, meningiomas appear within the spine, wherein thoracic segments are favored. Rarely, meningiomas occur within a ventricle, presumably arising from the tela choroidea, a leptomeningeal invagination at the base of the choroid plexus. Most meningiomas occur in adults between 20 and 60 years of age, with a peak incidence around 45 years and a slight female preponderance (female:male = 3:2). Spinal meningiomas are particularly more common in women (female:male = 9:1). Radiation-induced meningiomas (which can appear two or more decades after radiotherapy for other brain tumors [or, historically, for tinea capitis]) are well recognized but represent a minority of cases. Many benign meningiomas (WHO grade I) grow slowly and come to clinical attention incidentally or only after they have grown to very large size and have begun to cause headaches, seizures, or focal neurologic deficits by compressing adjacent structures. In contrast, atypical (WHO grade II) and anaplastic (WHO grade III) forms can be aggressive, showing more rapid growth, a greater propensity to recur following resection, and, in some cases, invasion of the CNS parenchyma. It is important to note, however, that even a benign meningioma can show invasion of soft tissue and bone, and may come to clinical attention after invading (for example) the orbits or sinuses; invasion of soft tissue and bone is not considered a criterion for WHO grading. On imaging, most meningiomas are extra-axial, homogeneously enhancing lesions; heterogeneous enhancement and/or evidence of necrosis are suggestive of a higher grade. Trailing of the enhancement into adjacent dura is a useful radiologic sign (the so-called "dural tail") but can also be observed in other dura-based tumors. Hyperostosis of the adjacent skull is a suggestive radiographic finding that is somewhat more specific, and is often associated with bone invasion.

Grossly, meningiomas are spherical to lobulated, firm or rubbery, usually well-circumscribed, and firmly attached to the inner surface of the dura. Meningiomas that occur along the sphenoid wing may grow en plaque as flat, carpet-like masses. Most invade the underlying dura or dural sinuses but do not involve the pia or the underlying CNS.

The microscopic features of meningioma are highly variable; 13 histologic variants (discussed below) are recognized by the WHO classification system (**e-Fig. 39.46**).

However, the patterns that characterize these variants often appear together within a single tumor. Consequently, some features appear at least focally in most meningiomas and provide relatively reliable diagnostic clues. Although cytologic smear preparations of meningioma occasionally fail due to excessive collagen deposition within the tumor parenchyma, those that succeed usually show three-dimensional clusters (sometimes exhibiting whorls) of epithelioid to spindled cells reflecting their rather cohesive nature. Tumor cell nuclei are generally round to oval and often contain intranuclear pseudoinclusions (cytoplasmic invaginations) and nuclear clearings. These latter features are characteristic, but not specific. Likewise, concentric microcalcifications (psammoma bodies) provide some diagnostic reassurance. Histologically, the most common cytoarchitectural patterns in meningioma are fibrous (fascicles of spindled cells) and meningothelial (dominated by whorls and fascicles); identification of these patterns—even focally—may provide the strongest initial clue to diagnosis, particularly when an uncommon histologic pattern dominates. In problematic cases, immunohistochemistry is indispensable for confirming the diagnosis. Some of the common differential diagnoses for meningioma subtypes are provided in Table 39.5. Most meningiomas display strong reactivity for SSTR2A, patchy or weak membranous reactivity for EMA, and reactivity within nuclei for progesterone receptor (though reactivity for PR is less common among atypical and anaplastic tumors). Relevant for the often-encountered differential diagnosis of schwannoma versus meningioma for a spindled CNS neoplasm, reactivity for collagen IV and SOX10 are not observed in meningioma, and S100 reactivity is typically patchy rather than diffuse. In unusual

TABLE 39.5 | **Common Differential Diagnosis for Meningioma Subtypes**

Variant	Differential Diagnoses
Meningothelial/transitional	Metastatic carcinoma Meningothelial hyperplasia
Fibrous/Fibroblastic	Schwannoma
Psammomatous	Reactive process
Angiomatous (vascular)	Hemangioblastoma Atypical meningioma (degenerative atypia)
Microcystic	Diffuse or pilocytic astrocytoma Clear-cell meningioma
Secretory	Metastatic adenocarcinoma (e.g., thyroid)
Lymphoplasmacyte rich	Inflammatory process
Metaplastic (bone, cartilage, xanthomatous, myxoid, fat, etc.)	Soft tissue tumors
Clear cell (WHO grade II)	Metastatic renal cell carcinoma Microcystic meningioma Hemangioblastoma
Chordoid (WHO grade II)	Chordoma Chordoid glioma of third ventricle Epithelioid hemangioendothelioma
Papillary (WHO grade III)	Papillary ependymoma Astroblastoma Hemangiopericytoma Metastatic malignancy
Rhabdoid (WHO grade III)	Metastatic malignancy Atypical teratoid rhabdoid tumor (AT/RT) GBM/gliosarcoma

circumstances, when immunohistochemistry fails to provide diagnostic clarity, EM may be helpful; meningioma cells have interdigitating cell processes with scattered desmosomes, and do not secrete a basement membrane. FISH for common genetic changes (discussed below) may also be useful for guiding diagnosis.

a. Histologic variants, grading, and prognosis. Roughly 80% of meningiomas are considered histologically benign (WHO grade I) and have a low risk of recurrence after gross total resection (~5% at 5 years, ~20% at 20 years). Atypical (WHO grade II) meningiomas constitute 15% to 20% of cases and have a higher risk of recurrence (~30% or more at 5 years). Anaplastic (WHO grade III) meningiomas account for 1% to 2% of cases, are associated with even higher recurrence rates, and often prove fatal (median survival <2 years). After histologic grade, the most influential prognostic factor for recurrence is extent of surgical resection; subtotally resected benign meningiomas have a recurrence rate of ~30% to 40% at 5 years. Other prognostic factors include male gender and young age; each is unfavorable. Genetic characteristics of a meningioma also influence prognosis.

One determinant of WHO grade is histologic pattern. Meningothelial, fibrous, transitional, psammomatous, angiomatous, microcystic, secretory, lymphoplasmacyte-rich, and metaplastic variants are considered WHO grade I unless they have additional superimposed features (discussed below) that independently reach criteria for assignment of a higher grade. Tumors dominated by chordoid or clear cell histology show greater propensity to recur and are classified as WHO grade II. Tumors with abundant papillary and rhabdoid histology show an aggressive clinical course and warrant a diagnosis of WHO grade III. Often, a tumor will exhibit more than one pattern; in this circumstance, the dominant histologic subtype dictates which grade is assigned. Nevertheless, when a histologic pattern characteristic of a higher grade is observed even focally, it should be mentioned in the resulting pathology report. It is worth mentioning that, in addition to the 13 histologic variants currently recognized by the WHO classification system, a few other histologic patterns have been described but have not been designated as variants; these include Rosette-formation, and meningioma with oncocytic, mucinous, sclerosing, whorling-sclerosing, GFAP-expressing, and granulofilamentous inclusion-bearing features.

b. Atypical meningioma, WHO grade II (e-Fig. 39.47). In addition to meningiomas with a dominant clear cell or chordoid pattern, atypical meningiomas include those with increased mitotic activity (4 or more mitotic figures per 10 contiguous high power [40× objective] fields) or three or more of the following histologic features: (1) generally increased cellularity; (2) "small cell change", in which focal areas show small dense nuclei and diminished cytoplasm, reminiscent of clusters of lymphocytes; (3) prominent ("macro") nucleoli; (4) uninterrupted patternless or sheet-like growth (loss of architecture); and (5) foci of spontaneous or geographic necrosis not induced by embolization or radiation (*Am J Surg Pathol* 1997;21:1455). Consistent with increased mitotic activity, atypical meningiomas also generally exhibit moderately elevated Ki-67 (MIB-1 antibody) labeling indices. Because measurements of Ki-67 labeling index can show interinstitutional variability, this feature is not officially considered in the WHO grading system. However, it does represent a reasonable surrogate for mitotic activity when cytologic preservation is poor or when a specimen is particularly small. As mentioned above, invasion of dura, bone, and soft tissue is not considered in assignment of histologic grade; however, invasion of the CNS does warrant a WHO grade II diagnosis (see below).

c. Brain invasion. Brain invasion by meningioma is characterized by entrapped islands of brain parenchyma at the periphery of the tumor and/or irregular, tongue-like protrusions of tumor tissue into attached (usually gliotic) brain parenchyma. Perhaps surprisingly, on H&E sections, this phenomenon can be quite subtle, so immunohistochemistry for GFAP is often warranted for confirmation (**e-Fig. 39.48**). Brain invasion may occur in tumors that are otherwise histologically benign, atypical, or anaplastic. Though brain invasion has historically been assumed to be a "malignant" feature, clinicopathologic correlation studies have revealed statistical outcomes more consistent with atypical meningiomas. Therefore, brain-invasive meningiomas are considered WHO grade II even when their histologic patterns are otherwise benign.

d. **Anaplastic (malignant) meningioma, WHO grade III.** Anaplastic meningiomas that are not overtly papillary or rhabdoid must exhibit a markedly elevated mitotic density, reaching 20 or more mitotic figures per ten 40× fields, or show histologic features of frank malignancy reminiscent of carcinoma, melanoma, and high-grade sarcoma (*Cancer* 1999;85:2046) (**e-Fig. 39.49**). Consequently, the differential diagnosis for these anaplastic meningiomas often includes one or more of these malignant tumors. Complicating this situation somewhat is the tendency for meningioma to receive and harbor metastatic carcinoma from outside the CNS (most commonly breast and lung). In such cases, when immunohistochemical data are insufficient to support a diagnosis with confidence, ultrastructural and FISH studies probing for genetic changes common to meningioma may be useful. FISH studies may additionally provide prognostic information (discussed below).

e. **Genetic changes in meningioma.** Most meningiomas of all grades show loss of chromosome 22 or 22q, site of the *NF2* gene, thought to be important for tumor development; neurofibromatosis type II is associated with multiple meningiomas, and ~60% of sporadic meningiomas (mostly fibroblastic and transitional) harbor *NF2* mutations. Some other variants show some association with other genes (e.g., meningothelial with *AKT1*; secretory with *TRAF7* and *KLF4*; clear cell with *SMARCE1*; rhabdoid with *BAP1*). Also of note are location-associated signatures (e.g., *NF2* mutation and loss of 22q in convexity meningiomas; *AKT/SMO/TRAF7* mutation in skull base meningiomas). Genetic alterations with prognostic implications that occur later in meningioma progression include loss of the *CDKN2A/p16* region on 9p21. Present in the majority of anaplastic meningiomas, loss of 9p21 is associated with decreased survival; tumors that lack this alteration show survival patterns more consistent with atypical rather than anaplastic grade. *TERTp* mutations, present in ~6% of atypical and ~20% of anaplastic meningiomas, also have prognostic significance, dramatically shortening median progression-free survival from many years to ~10 months.

2. **Hemangiopericytoma (HPC)/Solitary Fibrous Tumor (SFT), WHO grades I–III** (**e-Fig. 39.50**). These two uncommon tumors are now considered to represent a single neoplastic entity, defined by the common characteristic of aberrant intranuclear STAT6 immunoreactivity/*NAB2-STAT6* gene fusion (*Acta Neuropathol* 2013;125:651). In the CNS, a three-tier classification system is now applied to these tumors: benign SFT (WHO grade I), HPC (WHO grade II), and anaplastic HPC (WHO grade III).

Radiologically, they resemble meningioma; they are dura-associated, solid, uniformly enhancing, and appear in a similar anatomical distribution. However, unlike meningioma, HPC does not show intratumoral calcification, and can be associated with bone lysis rather than hyperostosis. In addition, HPC appears hypervascular by angiography, and may receive a dual blood supply from the meninges and brain. Microscopically, this hypervascularity is contributed by slit-like vascular channels that are lined with flattened endothelial cells and by frequent ectatic, thin-walled, branched "staghorn vessels". Although such vessels are not specific, they provide a very helpful diagnostic clue. The parenchyma of these tumors is usually biphasic. Cellular areas of HPC contain oval-to-epithelioid cells with round nuclei and scant cytoplasm that are densely arranged in a random or vaguely nested pattern with little intervening stroma; collagen is not prominent. Within this dense background, paucicellular areas of HPC appear as pale islands.

Hypocellular areas of SFT are strongly collagenous and hyalinized. Cellular areas of SFT are composed of a patternless or mildly fascicular arrangement of elongated spindled-to-oval cells that are intermixed with brightly eosinophilic, interlaced collagen bundles. Mitotic figures are generally sparse (when present, mitoses must not exceed a density of 4 per ten 40× fields), and other anaplastic features are not observed. When the cellular areas of SFT become particularly dense, they may resemble HPC.

A diagnosis of anaplasia for HPC requires ≥5 mitotic figures per ten 40× fields; such tumors often also exhibit necrosis, hypercellularity, moderate to severe nuclear atypia, and/or hemorrhage. In ambiguous cases, special stains can guide diagnosis. The most definitive diagnostic tests are STAT6 immunohistochemistry (which will show nuclear localization of normally cytoplasmic STAT6) or cytogenetic/molecular testing for *NAB2/STAT6* gene fusion. However, other stains can also support the diagnosis. HPC shows, at best, only focal immunoreactivity for CD34, but has abundant stromal reticulin fibers that surround cells individually and in small groups; SFT stains strongly for CD34 and is reticulin-poor. Assessment of mitotic index and/or staining with MIB-1 antibody may also be helpful. Relevant for distinguishing these from other tumors (e.g., meningioma), both show reactivity for vimentin, bcl-2, and CD99, and no reactivity for S-100, CD31, EMA, and progesterone receptor. FISH studies can also be helpful for this purpose, as loss of chromosome 22q is usually not observed in HPC. It is worth noting, however, that loss of 9p21, a poor prognostic marker in high-grade meningiomas, has been reported in about 25% of HPCs.

J. Hemangioblastoma (HB), WHO Grade I. Sporadic cases of this benign, slowly growing, highly vascular neoplasm occur most often in the posterior fossa of adults, favoring the cerebellum. HBs located elsewhere (e.g., brain stem, spinal cord, retina, cerebrum), particularly when multiple and/or occurring in younger patients, are more commonly associated with von Hippel–Lindau disease (VHL); therefore, discovery of an HB with any of these unusual characteristics warrants thorough screening for other manifestations of VHL (e.g., endolymphatic sac tumor, pheochromocytoma, pancreatic cyst or islet tumor, renal cyst or clear cell carcinoma, and papillary cystadenoma of the epididymis) and genetic testing and counseling. On imaging studies, the classic HB is well-circumscribed, intra-axial, and cystic, with an enhancing mural nodule that is hypervascular on angiography. Microscopically, HBs have two main components: stromal and vascular. Stromal cells show variable morphology, but typically are large and polygonal with vacuolated (lipid laden) cytoplasm (e-Fig. 39.51). Karyomegaly and nuclear ("degenerative") atypia among these stromal cells are common and without significance. The vascular component is characterized by thin-walled channels lined by flattened endothelial cells. Based on the relative prominence of these two components, two histologic variants (cellular and reticular) have been described; the less common stroma-rich cellular variant may show greater Ki-67 labeling index and has a propensity to recur. Mast cells are common within HBs and foci of extramedullary erythropoiesis are present in a minority of cases, induced by stromal cell production of erythropoietin. Occasionally, these tumors produce brisk piloid gliosis in the adjacent brain parenchyma. Based on radiographic and histologic patterns, the differential diagnosis often includes PA and metastatic renal cell carcinoma (RCC), requiring immunohistochemical stains such as D2-40/podoplanin or inhibin (positive in stromal cells), as well as EMA, CD10, PAX8, and RCC (all variably positive in RCC) and GFAP (positive in PA and most often negative in stromal cells).

K. Tumors of the Sella and/or Suprasellar Region (Other Than Pituitary Adenomas)

1. Craniopharyngiomas, WHO grade I, due to their location, may present clinically with hormonal abnormalities, vision disturbance, and obstructive hydrocephalus. These partly cystic, histologically benign epithelial tumors are thought to originate from Rathke's pouch epithelium. On MRI, these tumors often show T1 bright cyst contents and postcontrast enhancement of solid areas and any cyst capsule(s). Two morphologically distinct subtypes have been described, adamantinomatous and papillary; the former shows heterogeneous calcifications on CT, whereas the less common papillary variant does not.

a. **Adamantinomatous craniopharyngiomas** occur more commonly in children aged 5 to 15, but show a second peak in the 5th and 6th decades. Grossly, any cyst contents have the appearance of dark green-brown "machine oil". Calcifications are frequently noted. Microscopically, this variant resembles adamantinoma of the bone (tibia) and ameloblastoma of the jaw. The adamantinomatous variant is formed by a complex squamous epithelium that shows: "basal palisading" (a columnar orientation of the most peripheral layer of nuclei); an overlying zone of moderate cellularity in which focal areas resemble a network of processes over a cleared background ("stellate reticulum"); and central keratinization which produces nodules of pale, anucleate, cohesive cell remnants ("wet keratin") (e-**Fig. 39.52**). Areas of xanthogranulomatous inflammation and abundant cholesterol clefts are common. The border of this tumor is usually irregular and adherent to surrounding structures, and the adjacent parenchyma typically shows robust piloid gliosis. Though histologically benign, its adherent, somewhat invasive nature leads to frequent recurrence, even after gross total resection. Consequently, adamantinous craniopharyngioma can cause considerable morbidity, particularly given its close association with the optic chiasm and pituitary. About 95% of cases harbor *CTNNB1* (beta-catenin) mutations, leading to activation of the WNT pathway.

b. **Papillary craniopharyngioma** (e-**Fig. 39.53**) is less common than the adamantinomatous variant, is not typically seen in children, and most commonly occurs in the third ventricle or suprasellar region rather than in the sella itself. Grossly, it is seldom cystic; any cysts observed contain clear fluid rather than "machine oil." Calcifications are absent, and the interface with the brain is smoother and less adherent. Histologically, the papillary variant is formed by a well-differentiated, nonkeratinizing squamous epithelium that overlies broad, loose fibrovascular cores. The basal layer shows increased density, but without strong palisading. Beyond the apical surface, the tissue degrades (undergoes dehiscence), effectively leaving crude pseudopapillae of viable tissue around stromal cores. Occasionally, the epithelium may show focal cilia or goblet cells. In spite of clearer demarcation from the adjacent brain tissue in the papillary variant, most groups comparing the two forms have reported similarly high rates of recurrence. *BRAF* p.V600E mutations have been found in up to 95% of cases.

2. **Langerhans Cell Histiocytosis (LCH)** is mentioned here only to underscore its predilection for this region within the CNS; it is discussed further below.

L. **Germ Cell Tumors (GCT).** Included in this category are germinoma (homologous to testicular seminoma and ovarian dysgerminoma), teratoma, yolk sac tumor, embryonal carcinoma, and choriocarcinoma. Typically, these brain tumors occur in children or young adults. A pineal location, classically associated with increased ICP and Parinaud syndrome, is more common in males; a suprasellar location, classically associated with diabetes insipidus, vision changes, and hypopituitarism, is slightly more common in females. In some cases, both areas are involved. Less common sites include the basal ganglia and thalamus. On MRI, most GCT are heterogeneously T2 hyperintense and show heterogeneous enhancement. Calcification and complexity are common in teratomas, and hemorrhage is strongly associated with choriocarcinoma. Histologically, these tumors are homologous to their gonadal and mediastinal counterparts. Occasionally, the marked lymphocytic infiltrate and/or granulomatous response seen in germinomas can mask the underlying large, clear cells with central round nuclei and large nucleoli that define the neoplasm. In such cases, immunostaining for CD117 (membranous pattern), OCT4 (nuclear pattern), and PLAP (cytoplasmic and membranous pattern), may be applied to aid diagnosis (Table 39.1, e-**Fig. 39.54**). Rare germinomas contain syncytiotrophoblastic elements and should not be confused with choriocarcinoma; such tumors can also have associated increased CSF and serum levels of beta-HCG. Pure germinomas are exquisitely radiosensitive and have an excellent prognosis; those with syncytiotrophoblastic cells show a greater tendency to recur, and modestly less favorable survival. Mature teratomas follow a benign clinical course and may be cured by gross total resection. Yolk sac tumors, embryonal carcinoma, and choriocarcinoma (and mixed tumors composed of more than one of these elements) confer less favorable prognoses.

M. Lymphomas and Histiocytic Tumors

1. Primary CNS lymphomas (PCNSLs) are malignant lymphomas that occur in the absence of systemic lymphoma. PCNSL is more common among, but not exclusive to, elderly or immunosuppressed patients. On imaging, PCNSLs occur as single or multiple homogeneously enhancing lesions; some appear well-circumscribed (resembling, for example, a metastasis or tumefactive MS) and others appear somewhat diffuse (resembling a diffuse glioma). A periventricular location is common. These lesions often respond dramatically to steroid therapy, at least initially, reflecting the direct cytotoxic effect of steroids on B-lymphocytes. Although this radiographic response may provide a diagnostic clue, steroid treatment is usually withheld when possible until a tissue diagnosis is secured.

Microscopically, most PCNSLs appear as parenchymal and angiocentric infiltrates of highly atypical lymphocytes (e-**Fig. 39.55**) accompanied by nonneoplastic CD3+ T-cells. The neoplastic cells usually have centroblast-like or immunoblast-like morphology and are immunoreactive for B-lymphocyte markers (e.g., CD20, CD79a); most PCNSLs are considered diffuse large B-cell lymphomas (DLBCL). PCNSLs with DLBCL features can be stratified into germinal center (CD10+, BCL+/−, MUM1−) or nongerminal cell (CD10−, BCL+/−, MUM1+) types, analogous to their systemic counterparts. Although the prognostic relevance of this sub-categorization is questionable in the CNS, identification of the germinal center pattern (unusual in PCNSL) should heighten suspicion for possible systemic DLBCL that has metastasized to the CNS. Affected vessels show mural expansion by this mixed population, a feature that can be highlighted by reticulin stain. In some cases, nonneoplastic foamy histiocytes and reactive astrocytes may also be abundant in the parenchyma. Necrosis and evidence of Epstein–Barr virus (EBV) (by immunostain or ISH for EBER) are features associated with acquired immunodeficiency syndrome (AIDS) or immunosuppression-associated PCNSL.

Uncommon variants of lymphoma that affect the CNS include *lymphomatoid granulomatosis*, an angiodestructive, EBV-driven, high-grade B-cell lymphoma that affects the brain in 25% of cases (more commonly, the lung and skin), features fibrinoid angionecrosis and poorly formed granulomas (lymphohistiocytic nodules), and leads to vascular occlusion and infarcts; *intravascular B-cell lymphoma*, a high-grade extranodal B-cell lymphoma characterized by its restriction to vessel lumina and similar tendency to cause vascular occlusion and infarcts; *anaplastic large cell* (positive for CD30 and EMA, and sub-categorized by *ALK* translocation/expression); and *T-cell lymphomas*, which are encountered only rarely as PCNSLs. When lymphoma metastasizes to the CNS (secondary CNS lymphoma) it typically appears in epidural, dural, or leptomeningeal locations and is accompanied by systemic disease. The converse also holds; lymphoma appearing in epidural, dural, or leptomeningeal locations is likely to represent metastasis from the periphery. Notable exceptions to this rule are *extranodal MALT lymphoma of the dura*, which is histologically similar to MALT lymphomas (positive for CD20; negative for CD5 and CD10) and often mimics meningioma clinically and radiographically; and *myeloid sarcoma*, which occupies the meninges, exhibits necrosis and marked atypia, and shows variable reactivity for myeloperoxidase, CD68, CD163, CD117, CD34, and CD99 (though myeloid sarcoma may occur in the setting of AML).

2. Histiocytic disorders

a. Langerhans cell histiocytosis (LCH) is a term officially endorsed by the Histiocyte Society to replace previous terms (e.g., Hand–Schuller–Christian disease [HSCD], eosinophilic granuloma, histiocytosis X). LCH, the most common of the histiocytic tumors, primarily affects children with a median age of 12 years. The most common manifestation seen by neuropathologists involves an isolated osteolytic lesion of the skull ("eosinophilic granuloma") that may also involve the underlying meninges and cortex. When multiple, such lesions may be accompanied by hypothalamic involvement (consistent with HSCD). Although it is rare to encounter isolated involvement of the hypothalamus, pituitary, and optic chiasm (e-**Fig. 39.56**), this region shows radiographic changes in approximately 50% of cases with disseminated LCH, and 25% of children with multifocal disease present with diabetes insipidus. Histologically (e-**Fig. 39.57**), LCH is characterized by Langerhans cells accompanied by variable amounts of nonneoplastic reactive elements that may include eosinophils, neutrophils, macrophages, lymphocytes, plasma cells, and multinucleated giant cells. Langerhans cells are recognizable morphologically by their grooved so-called "coffee bean" nuclei; immunohistochemically by reactivity for S100, CD1a, and langerin (CD207); and ultrastructurally by the presence of Birbeck granules. Of note, approximately 50% of LCH cases harbor a *BRAF* p.V600E mutation; lesser numbers are driven by other mutations affecting the same cell-signaling pathway (e.g., MAP2K1 >> MAP3K1 or ARAF). In addition, reactivity for CD1a (MTB-1 monoclonal antibody) is observed not just in LCH, but also in anterior pituitary cells (Am J Surg Pathol 2016;40:812).

b. **Non-LC Histiocytic disorders** are far less common in the CNS. Intracranial **Rosai–Dorfman disease** (e-**Fig. 39.58**) affects children and adults and can mimic meningioma; it most often affects the meninges as a contrast-enhancing mass, and may induce a nonneoplastic hyperplastic response in the associated arachnoidal cells. However, the other constituents of the tumor include plasma cells, lymphocytes, and, most importantly, scattered large pale histiocytes (S-100+, CD68+, CD1a–) with prominent nucleoli. In a majority of cases, these large histiocytes exhibit the diagnostic feature of emperipolesis (engulfment of lymphocytes or plasma cells). No genetic alterations common to Rosai–Dorfman disease have been detected. **Erdheim–Chester disease** affects adults and may involve any part of the CNS or its coverings. Meningeal and perivascular lesions feature foamy histiocytes (S100 variable, CD68+, CD1a–, factor XIIIa+) but cells in the parenchyma may resemble activated microglia or neoplastic astrocytes. Sparse lymphocytes, plasma cells, eosinophils, and multinucleated histiocytes may also be seen. Definitive diagnosis usually requires correlation with clinical and radiologic evidence of systemic involvement, particularly bone pain and sclerosis of the long bones. About 50% of Erdheim–Chester disease cases have the *BRAF* p.V600E mutation. **Juvenile xanthogranuloma (JXG)** (e-**Fig. 39.59**) usually appears as an isolated cutaneous nodule in children, but can also occur as an isolated lesion in the brain or meninges. The histiocytes of JXG are S-100–, CD68+, CD1a–, Factor XIIIa+, CD11c+ and lysozyme–, a phenotype similar to that of plasmacytoid monocytes. Scattered touton giant cells, lymphocytes, and eosinophils are commonly seen. JXG is benign, but may cause seizures. **Histiocytic sarcoma** is a very rare tumor that shows cytologic atypia, necrosis, and a high proliferative index; stains reliably only with macrophage markers CD68 and CD163; is negative for CD23 and CD35 (follicular dendritic cell sarcoma antigens); and is associated with poor prognosis.

N. **Metastatic Tumors to the CNS** are the most common CNS neoplasms, which occur in up to 30% of adult and 6% to 10% of pediatric cancer patients. Common sources in adults include carcinomas of lung, breast, kidney, and colon, as well as melanomas. In children, leukemia, lymphoma, osteogenic sarcoma, rhabdomyosarcoma, and Ewing sarcoma are the most common primaries. Prostate, breast, lung, and kidney carcinomas are the most common sources of metastases to the spinal cord. Radiologically, the majority of CNS metastases implant in the cerebral hemispheres at the junction of cortex and white matter, appear well-circumscribed, and show ring-like or diffuse contrast enhancement. Histologically and immunophenotypically, metastases usually resemble their primary tumors (if only focally); because primary tumors may be idiosyncratic and heterogeneous, it is always worthwhile to review slides from a putative primary tumor, whenever possible.

VI. INFLAMMATORY AND INFECTIOUS DISORDERS

A. Inflammatory demyelinating disorders are characterized by myelin loss with relative preservation of axons; this finding is often accompanied by abundant foamy macrophages and perivascular lymphocytes. Classic radiographic examples of myelin disorders are not generally biopsied, but when clinical and/or radiologic data are unusual or ambiguous, neurosurgery may be consulted to obtain a tissue sample. Some of the commonly encountered demyelinating disorders include MS, acute disseminated encephalomyelitis (ADEM)/perivenous encephalomyelitis, neuromyelitis optica (NMO), and demyelinating viral infections such as progressive multifocal leukoencephalopathy (PML).

1. **Multiple sclerosis (MS)** is an idiopathic demyelinating disorder with genetic, environmental, and infectious influences. Historically, several sub-types have been described, including (but not limited to) relapsing-remitting, secondary progressive, primary progressive, acute monophasic (Marburg disease), and acute tumefactive. The relapsing-remitting form (RRMS), characterized by intermittent attacks and partial recovery from neurologic deficits during periods of remission, is more common in young adults (women > men; 2:1) and is the most common form in the United States (~80% of cases). Less common forms involve rapid, unremitting clinical deterioration—either de novo (primary progressive MS [PPMS]) or in the setting of RRMS (secondary progressive MS [SPMS]). Demyelinative MS plaques in these subtypes most often involve white matter periventricularly, and the optic pathway, brain stem, and/or spinal cord. Radiographically, chronic inactive plaques are hypointense on T1 and diffusion-weighted images; plaques with active inflammation are hyperintense on T2 and show postcontrast enhancement. This latter feature can be responsible for some radiologic diagnostic uncertainty in cases of Marburg disease or acute tumefactive MS. In acute tumefactive MS, a large isolated plaque appears as a T2-hyperintense, peripherally enhancing lesion that resembles a high-grade glioma or lymphoma. Although the rim of enhancement around the demyelinative lesion may be incomplete (forming a horseshoe-shaped profile that would be highly unusual in a neoplasm), this feature is not specific enough for conclusive diagnosis. Consequently, such lesions, though uncommon, are often biopsied. At frozen section, tumefactive MS can represent a great diagnostic challenge; in such cases, examination of a cytologic smear preparation is often very helpful as it preserves important cellular details (such as those of lipid-laden macrophages) that can be obscured by freezing artifact. Microscopically, an active demyelinative MS plaque shows (1) loss of myelin, (2) relative preservation of axons, (3) perivascular nonneoplastic lymphocytic infiltrates, (4) numerous foamy macrophages, (5) reactive astrocytosis, and (6) cerebral edema. Mitotic activity among astrocytes and macrophages may be brisk, but nuclear atypia should be minimal. Granular mitoses and Creutzfeldt cells (which contain multiple micronuclei), though not specific for MS lesions, are characteristic. Myelin loss with axonal sparing (which distinguishes this lesion from an axon-destroying infarct) is best visualized by comparing Luxol fast blue (LFB)–periodic acid Schiff (PAS) stained sections to others stained with Bielschowsky silver or NF protein immunohistochemistry (e-**Fig. 39.60**). On LFB–PAS sections, the border of demyelination is usually abrupt, and blue-green debris (partially metabolized myelin) is visible within macrophages. In rare cases that cannot be satisfactorily diagnosed with special stains, molecular and/or FISH studies can be applied to evaluate for lymphoma- or glioma-associated genetic changes.

2. **Acute disseminated encephalomyelitis (ADEM)/perivenous encephalomyelitis** represents an unusual autoimmune response among children and young adults induced by recent infection (days to weeks; most commonly measles, but also mumps, varicella, influenza, rubella, *Campylobacter jejuni*, and *Mycoplasma pneumoniae*) or vaccination (first described with smallpox and later with rabies). Symptoms include headache, fever, and vomiting followed by weakness, ataxia, and visual and sensory loss, with progression to stupor and seizures. Radiologically, ADEM usually appears as many small T2-weighted and FLAIR hyperintensities in subcortical and periventricular white matter and the spinal cord; the deep gray matter and cortex may also

be affected. This clinico-radiographic pattern is characteristic enough that biopsy is not always performed. Nevertheless, when obtained, biopsy material of this disease process shows perivenous demyelination with axonal sparing, mononuclear infiltrates, macrophages, activated microglia, and occasional petechial hemorrhages. This pattern resembles that of the acute monophasic form of experimental allergic encephalomyelitis (EAE) produced in rodents by immunization with myelin components, providing support for the notion that ADEM results from a myelin-directed, cross-reactive immune response to a foreign antigen.

3. **"NMO"** (formerly known as Devic disease) is a demyelinating disorder that classically involves optic nerves and large segments of the spinal cord simultaneously, but may also involve other sites (NMO spectrum disorders). NMO is caused by auto-antibodies to anti-aquaporin 4, an astrocyte water channel, enriched in processes at the glia limitans, and present at high levels in spinal cord, diencephalon, and periventricular areas. Histologically, NMO can mimic MS very closely, but is frequently more destructive, showing less axonal preservation and resembling infarction. Granulocytes and eosinophils, which may mediate the damage to oligodendrocytes, can also provide a clue to diagnosis. Loss of GFAP (and AQP4) immunoreactivity within lesions (preserved or increased in MS) provides stronger diagnostic evidence; some cases will also exhibit swelling of astrocytic cell bodies and processes (clasmatodendrosis) at the periphery of a lesion. Fortunately, most cases can be diagnosed clinically by serology for circulating NMO-IgG (directed at AQP4).

4. **Demyelinating viral infections.** Viral infections that commonly cause CNS demyelination include human immunodeficiency virus (HIV leukoencephalopathy and vacuolar myelopathy [HIVL, HIVVM]), human T-cell lymphotropic virus-1 (HTLV-associated myelopathy/tropical spastic paraparesis [HAM/TSP]), JC virus (PML), and measles virus (subacute sclerosing panencephalitis [SSPE]).

    a. White matter damage by **HIV** is thought to be mediated by virally infected macrophages and giant cells; oligodendrocytes are not directly infected. HIVL is often associated with HIV-associated encephalitis (HAVE), but begins earlier, often introducing cognitive impairment (up to 50% of AIDS patients develop dementia ascribed to HIVL and HIVE). Histologically, HIVL may show subtle white matter pallor, with variable numbers of microglial nodules, macrophages, and multinucleated giant cells. HIVVM targets the spinal cord in ~25% of AIDS cases, producing vacuolar myelopathy in the dorsal and lateral columns that resembles subacute combined degeneration (vitamin B12 deficiency).

    b. **HAM/TSP,** characterized by paraparesis, spasticity, and hyperreflexia of the lower extremities and positive Babinski sign, affects 1% to 5% of individuals seropositive for HTLV-1. As clinical presentation suggests, HAM/TSP preferentially affects the lateral columns (corticospinal tracts), most severely in the thoracic spinal cord; corresponding changes (T2 hyperintensity, thoracic spinal cord atrophy) are visible radiologically. Though biopsy is uncommonly undertaken, histology of the cord shows leptomeningeal and perivascular lymphocytic infiltrates, foamy macrophages, widespread myelin loss, and axonal dystrophy of the lateral columns.

    c. **PML** is caused by reactivation of a latent JC papovavirus (much of the general population is seropositive) in the setting of immunosuppression (e.g., lymphoproliferative disorders, AIDS, monoclonal antibody treatments for autoimmune diseases). Patients experience 3 to 6 months of progressive neurologic symptoms that reflect the anatomic distribution of the lesions, which favor the subcortical and deep cerebral white matter, cerebellum, and brainstem, and rarely involve the spinal cord. Personality changes are often prominent, followed by dementia and death. In some cases, restoration of immunocompetence may halt the disease; in other cases, the restored inflammatory response hastens clinical decline (immune reconstitution inflammatory syndrome [IRIS]). On MRI, the lesions of PML are T2-hyperintense, T1-hypointense, and nonenhancing; enhancement is common, however, in the setting of IRIS. Histologically, PML shows foci with myelin loss, a variably modest lymphocytic infiltrate (more pronounced in IRIS), and, within the center of larger lesions, few oligodendrocytes. Some oligodendrocytes show the hallmark lesion of PML, a large nucleus with marginated chromatin and a glassy inclusion that appears plum-colored on H&E sections (**e-Fig. 39.61**). Ultrastructurally, the papovavirus particles exhibit a so-called "stick and ball" or "spaghetti and meatballs" pattern. Also noted within and around these lesions are "pseudoneoplastic" astrocytes with atypical nuclei; these do not appear to produce or contain virus particles, and should not be mistaken for astrocytoma. Immunohistochemistry for JC virus proteins, EM, and ISH studies may be used to confirm the presence of the virus.

  d. SSPE (e-Fig. 39.62) is a rare sequela of measles in which a defective paramyxovirus targets oligodendrocytes and neurons, resulting in a slowly progressive encephalitis that results in coma and death. SSPE may present as many as 3 to 10 years after initial infection. Early in the course, radiographic findings are minimal; periventricular T2- and FLAIR hyperintensities appear late. Antimeasles IgG titers in CSF may be elevated. Histologically, SSPE shows large areas of myelin loss and neuron loss, leptomeningeal and perivascular lymphocytic infiltrates, and, most importantly, eosinophilic viral inclusions in the nuclei of oligodendrocytes and neurons. Diagnosis may be confirmed through immunohistochemistry for measles-virus-associated proteins.

B. CNS Infections may be broadly classified into meningitides, encephalitides, and abscesses.

  1. Infectious meningitis may be caused by bacteria, mycobacteria, viruses, fungi, and parasites. Although CSF analysis is often sufficient for diagnosis, biopsy is occasionally necessary.

   a. Bacterial meningitis is characterized in its acute stage by abundant neutrophils within the subarachnoid space and sub-pial reactive gliosis. Organisms are usually difficult to identify. In the chronic stage, neutrophils are supplanted by mononuclear cells, and granulation tissue and fibrosis may appear.

   b. Tuberculous meningitis can mimic bacterial meningitis, but more commonly exhibits a patchy granulomatous infiltrate of epithelioid histiocytes, multinucleated giant cells, and mononuclear cells. As with bacterial meningitis, organisms are difficult to identify even with acid fast stains; ancillary testing (PCR, culture) may aid diagnosis.

   c. Viral meningitis often shows meningeal and perivascular lymphocytic infiltrates that may extend into Virchow–Robin spaces. Because these infiltrates can be minimal and patchy, absence of inflammation on biopsy does not rule out the diagnosis. Identification of microglial nodules in the parenchyma supports an additional diagnosis of viral encephalitis.

   d. Fungal meningitis provokes a mononuclear/granulomatous inflammatory response similar to that of tuberculous meningitis, but the organisms are usually easily identified by histochemical stains (e.g., H&E, PAS, mucicarmine, GMS). Nevertheless, culture is required for definitive speciation. In contrast to yeast forms (*Histoplasma, Blastomyces, Cryptococcus),* pseudohyphal and hyphal organisms *(Candida, Aspergillus, Zygomycetes, Fusarium, Coccidioides)* can be angioinvasive and compromise blood supply, leading to infarction.

  2. Encephalitis is most often caused by viruses; less commonly, by parasites.

   a. Viral encephalitis is recognized histologically by the presence of meningeal and perivascular lymphocytes, accompanied by parenchymal microglial nodules. Occasionally, a microglial nodule may be observed around a dying neuron (a finding termed neuronophagia). Hundreds of viruses can cause encephalitis, and most do so without forming distinctive inclusions, so serologic/laboratory tests and clinical observations are usually required for diagnosis. Nevertheless, a small subset of pathogens is responsible for most clinically significant cases; a few of these entities are discussed here.

     i. West Nile virus (WNV) has become the leading cause of *epidemic* viral encephalitis in the United States within the last two decades, and now spans the continent. This arbovirus (arthropod-borne virus) has a peak in the summer or early autumn. In the acute phase, WNV can induce a neutrophil response that is visible in the meninges and CSF. In the chronic phase, microglial nodules are most abundant in the spinal cord, thalamus, and substantia nigra pars compacta. Unlike many others, WNV encephalitis is best diagnosed by detection of specific IgM in the CSF rather than by PCR.

ii. **Herpes encephalitis (HSV-1 > HSV2)** is the most common cause of *sporadic* viral encephalitis is the United States. Asymmetric, bilateral involvement of the temporal lobes is characteristic and, when severe, involves hemorrhage and necrosis. Clinically, involvement of the temporal lobes may cause hallucinations, agitation, personality changes, and psychosis. PCR testing of CSF for HSV shows high sensitivity and specificity, but sensitivity might be lower early in the course of infection. Histologically, in addition to perivascular lymphocytes and microglial nodules, biopsy material may show areas of necrosis with foamy macrophages and hemorrhage. Intranuclear Cowdry A ("owl's eye") and Cowdry B (eosinophilic translucent) inclusions may also be visible in some cases. Immunohistochemistry or ISH for HSV-1 and HSV-2 may be applied to confirm diagnosis.

iii. **Varicella zoster virus (VZV) encephalitis** is more common with immunosuppression, and targets several structures leading to different injuries. By infecting and damaging large and medium-sized vessels, VZV causes bland and hemorrhagic infarcts. By damaging small vessels, VZV causes small, deep, ovoid ischemic lesions, then infects the newly exposed oligodendrocytes, creating areas of demyelination; intranuclear Cowdry A inclusions (e-**Fig. 39.63**) are often visible within glial cells at the edges. Less commonly, VZV infects ependymal cells, causing ventriculitis.

iv. **HIV encephalitis** (microglial nodule encephalitis), in conjunction with HIV leukoencephalopathy, is associated with the dementia commonly associated with AIDS. The pathology features widespread, robust microglial nodules with associated lymphocytes, reactive astrocytes, and occasional multinucleated giant cells that harbor the virus. Neurotoxic cytokines and other damaging chemical agents (e.g., reactive oxygen species) may also play a role in this poorly understood dementia, which is also associated with cortical and subcortical atrophy.

v. **Rocky Mountain spotted fever** is caused by rickettsia, but can mimic viral encephalitis and is therefore mentioned here. This organism targets vascular endothelium and smooth muscle cells, and thus produces vasculitis, thrombosis, microinfarcts, and petechial hemorrhage without fibrinoid necrosis. Microglial nodules and mononuclear infiltrates with a leptomeningeal and perivascular distribution are commonly seen.

b. **Parasitic encephalitis**

i. **Neurocysticercosis** (e-**Fig. 39.64**), caused by the pork tapeworm *Taenia solium*, is the most common CNS parasitic infection worldwide, and a common cause of seizures. The larvae form thin-walled cysts in muscle, brain, eyes, liver, and lung; each cyst contains a scolex, the pathognomonic radiographic and histologic feature of the lesion. Microscopically, the cyst wall has three layers: an eosinophilic 3μ cuticle, a thin cellular layer, and an inner hypodense reticular layer. Death of the organism triggers a brisk mixed (neutrophils, lymphocytes, eosinophils) and granulomatous inflammatory response. Over months to years, inflammation subsides and the cyst becomes fibrotic and, eventually, a small calcified nodule.

ii. **Cerebral malaria** affects fewer than 10% of infected individuals, favoring those without immunity (<4 years of age, foreign visitors). Presenting symptoms include fever, headache, backache, photophobia, vomiting, variable neurologic deficits, and seizures. The event that defines this disorder is the deposition/lodging of parasitized erythrocytes within the microvasculature of the brain. This process is accompanied by petechial hemorrhages in the white matter around necrotic vessels. Over time, as these ring hemorrhages are resorbed by microglia, macrophages and astrocytes, they are called Dürck granulomas. Prompt treatment with corticosteroids and antimalarial drugs reduces mortality, which remains common.

iii. **Amebic encephalitis (AE)** is caused by several organisms, including *Naegleria fowleri*, *Balamuthia mandrillaris,* and *Acanthamoeba* species; *Entamoeba histolytica* tends to form abscesses. *N. fowleri,* usually encountered during fresh water swimming, enters the CNS through the cribriform plate; the others enter hematogenously from other infected organs. Clinically, AE with *N. fowleri* presents in previously healthy children and young adults as acute meningitis, and progresses to coma and death in 2 to 3 days. Histologically, mononuclear inflammation of the meninges is scanty, but the adjacent brain shows extensive hemorrhagic necrosis. Organisms are visible in the subarachnoid space and around vessels. These trophozoites bear a striking resemblance to (rather small) foamy macrophages but have a prominent central nucleolus. AE with *B. mandrillaris* and *Acanthamoeba* has a similar dismal prognosis, but a more chronic course.

iv. **Toxoplasmosis** is seen in neonates as a congenital infection (one of the TORCH infections: toxoplasma, other, rubella, cytomegalovirus, herpes) that leads to microcephaly with dystrophic calcifications. Infection later in life may cause fever, a maculopapular rash, and malaise or may be asymptomatic. In the setting of subsequent immunosuppression (particularly AIDS) a dormant infection can undergo reactivation and present with multiple deep-seated and/or cortical enhancing lesions. Grossly, when present, the focal lesions of cerebral toxoplasmosis are multiple, discrete, and necrotic; less commonly, toxoplasmosis may appear as a more diffuse encephalitis. Histologically (e-Fig. 39.65), the necrotic lesions show peripheral mixed inflammatory infiltrates, neovascularization, and gliosis. Perivascular inflammation and fibrinoid necrosis of vessels may also be seen. Though H&E stains are usually adequate for identifying *Toxoplasma gondii* organisms (encysted bradyzoites, free and intracellular tachyzoites [2 to 8 μ]), immunostains for the protozoan offer greater sensitivity and specificity. In unusual cases when cerebral toxoplasmosis manifests diffusely without necrotic foci, histologic changes include microglial nodules and reactive astrocytosis.

3. Brain abscess may be caused by bacteria, protozoa, or fungi. Most cases result from direct spread from the paranasal sinuses, middle ear, or dental root; others travel hematogenously from another site. In children, congenital heart defects may allow septic emboli to bypass the filter of the pulmonary circulation; in adults, lung infections and endocarditis are the most common sources of hematogenous inoculation. Damaged brain tissue and immunosuppression contribute in some cases. Abscesses mature over a 2-week period. Days 1 and 2 involve endothelial swelling and neutrophil invasion; over days 3 and 4, necrosis and macrophages are prominent and lymphocytes and plasma cells join the infiltrate; over days 5 to 7, granulation tissue (fibrosis, MVP, mixed inflammation, and macrophages) forms around the necrotic center; over days 8 to 14, the capsule becomes strengthened by collagen and fibrosis, traversed by radially oriented capillaries, and surrounded by gliosis.

C. Granulomatous Inflammation

1. Sarcoidosis. The CNS is affected in 5% of cases; most often, the basal meninges, cranial nerves, optic tracts, and/or hypothalamus are involved. Facial nerve palsy is the most common presenting symptom, but other focal deficits also occur, reflecting loss of function of affected structures. CNS-only sarcoidosis is quite rare, but cases of systemic sarcoidosis that also affect the CNS often receive neurosurgical/neuropathologic attention because the neurologic symptoms are so worrisome. Radiographically, the involved structures show postcontrast enhancement. Grossly, the meninges and cranial nerves may appear nodular and thickened. Microscopically, affected structures show epithelioid granulomas with giant cells (e-**Fig. 39.66**). Necrosis, though it may be seen focally, is not a usual feature of neurosarcoidosis, and should encourage consideration of other diagnoses. Because sarcoidosis is a diagnosis of exclusion, all reasonable efforts to exclude other etiologies for granulomatous inflammation (e.g., fungal, tuberculous, and rheumatologic) must be made. Ultimately, a pathologic diagnosis no more specific than "granulomatous inflammation" (accompanied by an appropriate written comment) is usually warranted, leaving the clinical diagnosis of sarcoidosis to the clinician.

VII. SEIZURE DISORDERS. Surgically curable seizure disorders are broadly classified into neoplastic and nonneoplastic lesions. Distinct neoplastic entities that generate chronic seizures include DNT, GGs, and PXAs, and are discussed above. Common nonneoplastic entities are discussed below.

A. Hippocampal (Mesial Temporal) Sclerosis (HS) is a disorder characterized by neuronal loss and gliosis of the hippocampus and, in some cases, adjacent mesial temporal structures such as the amygdala and entorhinal cortex. Clinically, HS is associated with longstanding complex partial seizures, most often beginning near the turn of the first decade. Radiographically, the hippocampus is small, and affected structures show T2 and FLAIR hyperintensity and evidence of hypometabolism. Surgical treatment often involves amygdalohippocampectomy. Histologically, the hippocampus shows variable neuronal loss and gliosis, most pronounced in areas CA1 (Sommer's sector) and CA4 (the endofolium of Ammon's horn) (e-**Fig. 39.67**). In more advanced cases, area CA3 and the subiculum may be similarly affected. Neurons within the dentate gyrus are often reduced in number and, in some cases, may appear dispersed or split into two layers. Because this diagnosis requires accurate identification of neuronal populations defined only by anatomic landmarks, the hippocampal specimen must be carefully oriented when it is sectioned for histology; ideally, it is resected in one piece that can (in most cases) be sectioned perpendicular to its long axis to reveal the desired classic "seahorse" architecture. Not uncommonly, HS resection specimens demonstrate a second pathology (a minute tumor or a malformation of cortical development [MCD] [see below]) that could otherwise independently account for seizures; such findings mirror the clinicopathologic experience that seizure activity can both engender and arise from HS. After resection, most patients experience a significant reduction in seizure frequency or are cured altogether. (The term HS is also used to describe entities with similar gross and histologic [H&E] findings that result from other unrelated causes, such as hypoxic-ischemic injury or an incompletely understood neurodegenerative process that preferentially affects the very elderly and usually involves NCIs of phosphorylated TDP-43 protein [see above].)

B. Malformation of cortical development (MCD) is a general term applied to a wide range of developmental abnormalities that affect the cortex. These abnormalities come to attention most often as epileptogenic foci, and are thought to account for up to 25% of cases of intractable epilepsy.

Grossly and radiographically, MCD may appear as (1) ectopic bands or nodules of cortical tissue in the white matter (heterotopias); (2) a firm, focal cortical expansion (cortical tuber); (3) an area of smooth, unfolded cortical ribbon (agyria/lissencephaly); (4) an area of cortical ribbon with few, broad gyri (pachygyria); (5) an area of cortex with many small irregular gyri and fused sulci (polymicrogyria); (6) an area with a blurred gray-white junction (some focal cortical dysplasias, FCD); or (7) ostensibly normal tissue (other FCDs).

Histologically, MCD shows similar variability. Heterotopias contain gray matter neuropil and abnormally arranged neuronal elements. Cortical tubers are formed by aggregates of large so-called "balloon cells" with abundant glassy eosinophilic cytoplasm and an eccentrically placed neuron-like nucleus (e-**Fig. 39.68**). Tubers may occur sporadically in isolation or in greater numbers in the setting of TS; the lesion itself is histologically identical in the two settings. Consequently, a tuber is best diagnosed as a form of FCD (called "type IIB" by the most recent International League Against Epilepsy [ILAE] classification system [*Epilepsia* 2011;52:158], and called "Taylor type" by a previously reported classification system [*J Neurol Neurosurg Psych* 1971,34:369]); this approach is particularly prudent when a clinical history of TS has not been provided. Agyria and pachygyria appear most commonly as a four-layered (rather than six-layered) cortical ribbon. Polymicrogyria has been described as having two-layered and/or four-layered areas within the cortex, but the most consistent feature is a fusion of two adjacent molecular layers through what would otherwise be a sulcus.

The term 'focal cortical dysplasia' describes a collection of entities for which the neuropathologic classification system has evolved over the last five decades. The most recent consensus classification system is that of the ILAE, which incorporated and expanded upon the pre-existing nomenclature of the Palmini system (*Neurology* 2004;62(Suppl3):52). The most striking and easily recognized form of FCD within the Palmini system is type IIB or Taylor type as discussed above; some other forms are more subtle, featuring enlarged dysmorphic neurons (type IIA), hypertrophic pyramidal neurons within layers 2 and 3 with mild lamination abnormalities (type IB), or isolated abnormalities in cortical lamination, including neuronal clumping, loss of columnar organization, absent layers, and so forth (type IA). In the Palmini system, inappropriately migrating neurons (appearing within the molecular layer, or in increased numbers within the white matter) are considered mild malformations of cortical development (mMCD, types I and II, respectively). Particularly in subtle cases, immunohistochemistry for NeuN (to accentuate neuronal cytoarchitecture), NF protein (to stain the somata of enlarged, atypical neurons), GFAP, and CD34 (to reveal poorly defined, highly branched cells associated with MCDs) (*Acta Neuropathologica* 1999;97:481) may facilitate diagnosis.

Although the ILAE system does not modify the Palmini definitions of type IIa or IIb, it does reconfigure type I. ILAE Ia describes lesions with radial dyslamination of cortical neurons; ILAE Ib, lesions with tangential dyslamination; ILAE Ic, with both radial and tangential dyslamination. The ILAE system also adds a third tier of classification when FCDs occur in the context of other lesions; ILAE IIIa describes FCD in the setting of HS; and ILAE IIIb describes FCDs with co-existing epilepsy-associated neoplasms; ILAE IIIc describes FCDs associated with vascular malformations. Although some neuropathologists question the practical utility of finely subclassifying FCDs (particularly the more subtle forms) at a time when etiologies and clinical significance is lacking, advocates would argue that large case series, accurately classified and studied by molecular techniques, might yield new insights. In turn, any such insights and downstream discoveries would be more likely to help patients who have been accurately subclassified.

C. Other Seizure-Associated Disorders encountered less often are hemimegalencephaly, Rasmussen encephalitis, hypothalamic hamartoma, and Sturge–Weber angiomatosis.

VIII. VASCULAR DISORDERS

A. Vascular Malformations are classified into four groups: arteriovenous malformation (AVM), cerebral cavernous malformation (CCM)/cavernoma, capillary telangiectasia (CT), and venous angioma (VA). CT and VA are asymptomatic and seldom encountered in surgical pathology, so will not be discussed further.

1. Arteriovenous malformations (AVMs) are usually supratentorial and are thought to be congenital; 50% come to clinical attention in the third, fourth, or fifth decades due to hemorrhage. Other AVMs induce seizures or, less often, slowly grow and cause a constellation of progressively worsening headaches and focal neurologic deficits. Angiography and MRI provide a diagnosis, reveal abnormal flow characteristics, and identify the supplying and draining vessels of these lesions to facilitate intervention planning. Some AVMs are embolized or coiled by interventional radiology in lieu of or prior to resection. Grossly, superficially located AVMs typically show dilated, thick-walled draining veins on the cortical surface; cut sections show a disorganized mass of blood vessels of varying mural thickness and diameter, with associated atrophic, relatively firm (gliotic) brain parenchyma. Histologically, AVMs are characterized by an array of abnormal blood vessels that show evidence of remodeling and degenerative changes (arteries with medial hyperplasia, collagen deposition, and complex restructuring of the internal elastic lamina; veins with thick collagenous walls). In some vessels, mixed arterial and venous features may be identified. Among the abnormal blood vessels, the intervening parenchyma shows atrophy, astrocytosis (sometimes piloid gliosis), and, often, hemosiderin deposits. Masson trichrome stain and an elastin stain (VVG) can be used to reveal features of the vascular pathology that are subtle on routine sections. If embolization has been performed prior to resection, intravascular foreign material may be identified; if sufficient time has elapsed, a foreign body giant cell reaction may be visible.

2. **CCM** (also called cavernous angioma, cavernous hemangioma, and cavernoma) is a vascular malformation characterized by large, thin-walled ectatic vessels or sinusoids that are closely packed with minimal intervening brain parenchyma (**e-Fig. 39.69**). CCMs are usually supratentorial but may occur anywhere in the CNS or leptomeninges. Autopsy studies have estimated the prevalence of sporadic CCMs to be approximately 1 in 200 individuals. As many as 50% of patients with these lesions develop seizures and/or recurrent headaches. In addition, these lesions exhibit an annual 1% chance of hemorrhage. Because such hemorrhages are not at high pressure they are usually not fatal; however, they may cause focal neurologic deficits, and do increase risk of seizures and subsequent hemorrhage several-fold. Brainstem lesions are associated with worse prognosis. Radiographically, T2-weighted images show a heterogeneous center with a surrounding rim of hypodensity that corresponds to deposits of hemosiderin; gradient-echo MRI shows greater sensitivity for this "ferruginous penumbra" and therefore can detect smaller lesions. Grossly, CCMs appear spongy and dark red with golden brown hues (hemosiderin deposition) and, occasionally, calcifications. Microscopically, the vascular component described above shows only a single layer of endothelium and lacks a muscular layer and an internal elastic lamina; the peripheral rim of resected tissue contains hemosiderin-laden macrophages and gliotic parenchyma with axonal spheroids. Areas of fibrosis, xanthomatous degeneration, and calcification are common. Although most cases are sporadic, some are familial and inherited in autosomal dominant fashion. Affected individuals often have multiple CCMs. The genes in question have been named *CCM1, CCM2,* and *CCM3*, and encode KRIT1, MGC4607/malcaverin, and PDCD10.

B. **Primary Angiitis of the CNS (PACNS).** Inflammation of the CNS vasculature may occur as part of a systemic vasculitis (e.g., giant cell arteritis, polyarteritis nodosa) or may be CNS-specific (PACNS). PACNS more commonly afflicts males in late middle age. Symptoms are highly variable, but are generally multifocal, intermittent, progressive, and, by definition, strictly neurologic. On MRI, PACNS may show nothing more than multiple ischemic microinfarcts; the angiographic finding of alternating luminal stenosis and dilatation (beads on a string), while characteristic, is neither sensitive nor specific for the disorder. CSF cytology may show mild lymphocytic pleocytosis, another nonspecific finding. To establish the diagnosis, meningeal/brain biopsy is performed. Histologically, the key feature of PACNS is segmental granulomatous inflammation of small and medium-sized arteries, featuring transmural lymphocytic infiltrates and expansion of the intima by histiocytes and multinucleated giant cells. Fibrinoid necrosis is characteristic, but not required. Associated parenchyma often shows changes associated with ischemic injury. As is the case for sarcoidosis, other potential causes of granulomatous vasculitis (including acid-fast bacilli, fungus, and intravascular amyloid [see CAA and ABRA, below]) must be excluded, and the most appropriate pathologic diagnosis is often, simply, "granulomatous vasculitis". Although prognosis is poor without treatment, immunosuppression (prednisone, with or without cyclophosphamide) has been effective in some cases.

C. **Congophilic (or Cerebral) Amyloid Angiopathy (CAA),** as the name suggests, is characterized by deposits of amyloid in leptomeningeal and superficial cortical vessels. By far, the most common substrate of this disease is amyloid-beta 1–40; approximately 80% of neuropathologically confirmed AD cases show CAA at least focally. Not surprisingly, therefore, CAA commonly affects the elderly. These deposits can disrupt physiologic autoregulation of blood flow, and may contribute to cognitive dysfunction. Most often, however, CAA comes to clinical attention only when it becomes severe enough to compromise vessel integrity. The superficial lobar hemorrhage that can result from CAA can cause mass effect and may resemble intratumoral hemorrhage; consequently, surgical evacuation is often performed for decompression, occasionally with some degree of parenchymal resection to determine the cause. This circumstance illustrates why CNS hematoma evacuation specimens must be examined very thoroughly for even the smallest fragments of brain tissue. Microscopically, involved vessels show amyloid deposits that can be appreciated on routine and special (Congo red and thioflavin S) stains (e-Fig. 39.70). Immunohistochemistry can be used to identify the amyloidogenic peptide involved; cases that do not show reactivity for amyloid-beta may be tested for rarer forms (not associated with AD) caused by deposition of cystatin C (Icelandic type), integral membrane protein 2B (ITM2B, British type or Danish type), gelsolin (Finnish type), or TTR (meningovascular amyloidosis). Although inflammation is usually absent, specimens must be evaluated for **amyloid beta related angiitis (ABRA)**, a form of granulomatous vasculitis (e-Fig. 39.71) that may respond to immunosuppressive therapy.

D. Cerebral Autosomal Dominant Arteriopathy With Subcortical Infarcts and Leukoencephalopathy (CADASIL) (e-Fig. 39.72) is caused by missense mutations of the *Notch3* gene. The abnormal protein accumulates in granules (PAS-positive, osmiophilic) within the walls of small arteries, the smooth muscle layer degenerates, and the vessel walls become thickened and fibrotic; this process gradually diminishes capacity for and regulation of perfusion. CADASIL usually presents in the fifth or sixth decade of life with classic migraine, multiple subcortical ischemic strokes, psychiatric disturbance and, later, dementia. In this context, T2 hyperintensities in anterior temporal lobes and external capsules on MRI are strongly suggestive. Although the symptoms of CADASIL arise from the brain, the disease also affects peripheral tissues, including the skin. Histologic and ultrastructural examination of arterioles in the skin (or brain) provides the diagnosis. Worthy of note, however, a rare, otherwise identical clinical/radiologic syndrome with an autosomal recessive inheritance pattern (appropriately named CARASIL, linked to the *HTRA1* gene) lacks these granular osmiophilic inclusions. This circumstance provides an example in which molecular (genetic) testing should play a greater role in the future to establish diagnosis.

E. Cerebral Infarcts. Most often, biopsies of infarcts are performed when glioma is in the differential diagnosis, particularly in young patients. Gross and microscopic features of a cerebral infarct change over time. In the acute stage (1 to 3 days), red necrotic neurons, vacuolated neuropil, and variable neutrophilic infiltrates are present. Subacute infarcts (days to weeks) demonstrate capillary proliferation with prominent endothelial cells, numerous foamy macrophages, and reactive astrocytes that are typically more common at the periphery. Because such reparative lesions may exhibit mitotic figures, necrosis, and MVP (consistent with GBM), care must be taken to recognize their reactive and histiocytic components, particularly during an intraoperative microscopic evaluation. Large infarcts eventually evolve into cystic lesions with a weblike network of delicate blood vessels, sparse gliotic parenchymal remnants, and a few residual macrophages. Infarcts disrupt and destroy axons, a feature often helpful in distinguishing infarcts from demyelinative processes such as MS in which the axons are relatively spared. Once an infarct is diagnosed, identifying its cause is the next step; when the specimen at hand provides no insight, clinical correlation is required.

IX. NEURODEGENERATIVE DISORDERS. Although some of these affect children and adolescents, most come to clinical attention after the fifth or sixth decades. An increasing number of neurodegenerative diseases can be diagnosed by identifying changes in DNA, biologic fluids, peripheral biopsy material, or radiographic images. Nevertheless, few treatments are currently available in clinic for neurodegenerative disorders, and most of them remain idiopathic, progressive, and fatal. Consequently, CNS biopsy performed explicitly to diagnose a neurodegenerative disease is rare. These disorders usually appear in a surgical pathology specimen incidentally (e.g., when some brain is removed to evacuate a life-threatening hematoma) or when unusual clinical/radiologic data suggest that securing a definitive tissue diagnosis warrants the risk of brain biopsy. In the future, as treatments for these disorders pass through clinical trials and into the clinic, it is likely that diagnosis will increasingly rest on genetic, radiologic, and fluid (CSF or serum/plasma) biomarker studies and microscopic examination of peripheral tissues (e.g., leukocytes in the setting of neuronal ceroid lipofuscinoses) rather than a more invasive brain biopsy. Nevertheless, recognizing these disorders in surgical specimens remains important and may become even more critical as treatments become available.

A. **Alzheimer disease (AD),** the most common neurodegenerative disorder, is characterized histologically by neuron loss, gliosis, and the presence of extracellular beta-amyloid peptide deposits (diffuse, cored, and neuritic plaques) and NFT (intraneuronal aggregates of hyperphosphorylated tau protein) in the neocortex and hippocampus (e-**Fig. 39.73**). Plaque deposition begins 10 to 15 years before the onset of very mild dementia of the Alzheimer type (a term for the clinical manifestations of AD). Degree of cognitive impairment appears to correlate with the severity and extent of NFT pathology, which appears early in the mesial temporal lobes and, subsequently, spreads outward to involve the parietal and frontal lobes; in most cases, the occipital lobe is relatively spared. Neuroimaging techniques (to assess atrophy, metabolism, and amyloid burden within the brain), and CSF biomarker measurements (e.g., of amyloid beta peptide and tau protein, among others) now allow reasonable antemortem confirmation of AD pathology, but techniques for antemortem staging of AD (e.g., using PET imaging with tracers that bind NFTs) and for the detection of coincident pathologies (e.g., LB disease) are not yet ready for practical application. For these and other reasons, recognition of the histologic changes of AD remains important. Currently, there are four leading sets of criteria for the neuropathologic diagnosis of AD: Khachaturian, CERAD, NIA/Reagan, and NIA-AA. Technically, the Khachaturian system, which evaluates only the presence of amyloid plaques within any portion of neocortex, is the only one that can be applied faithfully to a limited brain biopsy; officially, CERAD requires sampling of numerous cortical areas (possible only at autopsy) for a semiquantitative assessment of neuritic plaques; NIA/Reagan additionally requires assessment of the anatomical distribution of NFT pathology within the brain; and NIA-AA incorporates information from both CERAD and NIA-Reagan. Nevertheless, since NFT pathology correlates most reliably with degree of cognitive impairment and the frontal lobe is generally affected later in the disease process, the presence of plaques and NFTs in a biopsy specimen from the frontal lobe should suggest that AD pathology may be responsible for or may be contributing to a patient's cognitive symptoms. The deposits of AD are best visualized by modified Bielschowsky silver staining, thioflavin S or T (using fluorescence microscopy), or by immunohistochemistry for amyloid beta peptide and for phosphorylated tau protein. As discussed above, CAA often accompanies AD pathology.

B. **Lewy Body Disease (LBD).** This generic term is intended to unify several clinicopathologic diagnoses that feature this intraneuronal inclusion (described above) and the related Lewy neurite (e-**Fig. 39.8**). Advanced LB pathology, either alone or in conjunction with AD, is associated with ~10% to 15% of dementia cases. LB pathology has been proposed (in the setting of clinical PD) to begin within the gut, spreading from the enteric nervous system through the vagus nerve to the medulla, and to spread rostrally, reaching the dopaminergic neurons of the substantia nigra in middle stages, and the neocortex in later stages. In parallel, many patients with PD develop dementia ~10 years after motor symptoms. Therefore, identification of these lesions in a frontal lobe biopsy specimen at sufficient density provides reasonable evidence that a patient may be suffering from dementia related to LB disease (*Neurology* 2005;65:1863). Because these lesions can be subtle on H&E sections of the neocortex, and because they are not argyrophilic on Bielschowsky stained sections, immunohistochemistry for (ideally, phosphorylated) alpha-synuclein is required for definitive identification; this stain should therefore be applied routinely, particularly when symptomatology is suggestive of PD or DLB, or when other relevant pathologies (e.g., AD, CJD) are not detected,

C. **Creutzfeldt–Jakob Disease (CJD)** (e-**Fig. 39.74**). The desire to diagnose or rule out CJD as a cause of rapidly progressive dementia (developing in approximately two years or less) has been one of the leading clinical scenarios prompting brain biopsy. However, with improving radiologic and CSF laboratory tests (e.g., RT-QuIC) to diagnose CJD, brain biopsy for this purpose may be waning. CJD is a transmissible spongiform encephalopathy (TSE; others include Gerstmann–Strauss–Scheinker (GSS) syndrome, fatal insomnia, and kuru) that is classically characterized by a clinical triad of myoclonus, periodic shortwave EEG activity, and rapidly progressive dementia. Diffusion weighted (DWI) and FLAIR MRI commonly show restricted diffusion within the striatum and cerebral cortex. Though the condition is, technically, transmissible, most cases are sporadic, affecting one person per million individuals per year with a peak age of onset of 60; 10% of cases are familial, attributable to mutations in the prion gene *PRNP*. Only rare examples are actually the result of apparent transmission, resulting from inoculation with tissues or instruments inadvertently contaminated by misfolded pathogenic prion protein from another individual with CJD. Microscopically, CJD cases show neuronal loss, gliosis, and spongiform change (small, sharply defined, punched out vacuoles). These histologic changes appear in an anatomic pattern suggested by radiographic changes, but evaluation is typically limited to a right frontal cortex biopsy specimen. Within the cortex, the spongiform change of CJD should span the entire thickness of the cortical ribbon; other dementing conditions may show vacuolation that appears similar and is limited to superficial layers. It is worth noting, however, that the histologic changes in CJD may be anatomically patchy and, therefore, very subtle or invisible in a limited biopsy specimen. It is also worth noting that biopsies of individuals with CJD may also show pre-existing histologic changes associated with other dementing illnesses, so identification of abundant amyloid plaques, NFTs, or LBs does not rule out the possibility of CJD. For this reason in particular, immunoblotting and immunohistochemical analysis for the abnormally folded (usually protease-resistant) proteins are essential for definitive diagnosis. Cerebellar amyloid plaques are noted in only about 5% of cases.

D. **New Variant CJD (nvCJD)** is a rare form of TSE linked to bovine spongiform encephalopathy (BSE). Unlike CJD, nvCJD affects a younger demographic (adults younger than 40), typically has a longer clinical course characterized by behavioral changes more often than dementia, and shows an additional thalamic (pulvinar) abnormality on DWI, T2, and FLAIR MRI. Microscopically, the most characteristic feature is the presence of numerous amyloid plaques (florid plaques; 4 PRP positive, amyloid beta negative) in the cerebral and cerebellar cortices. The few hundred cases reported since 1996 are clustered in the United Kingdom and France, and are thought to stem from an outbreak of BSE that affected the UK cattle industry in 1986. Perhaps reflecting the incubation period and changes in cattle industry practices, the incidence of nvCJD in the United Kingdom has dwindled, so the diagnosis is now quite rare.

ACKNOWLEDGMENTS

The authors thank Sushama Patil and Arie Perry, authors of the previous edition of this chapter.

Cytology of the Central Nervous System

Jessica Petrone and Souzan Sanati

I. **SPECIMEN TYPES.** The most common specimen type obtained for cytologic evaluation of pathologic conditions of the CNS is CSF. Rarely, stereotactic fine needle aspiration (FNA) of cysts or masses of the CNS is used to provide specimens for cytologic diagnosis.

A. **Cerebrospinal fluid (CSF).** Several methods have been developed for concentration of samples obtained via lumbar puncture, including cytocentrifugation and membrane filtration. Slides prepared via the cytocentrifugation technique are usually DiffQuik stained since leukemic involvement of the CSF is the most common malignant diagnosis and its features are best visualized on DiffQuik stained slides; the limited amount of material obtained (0.5 to 1.0 mL) usually precludes allocating material for Papanicolaou and other stains. Although the precise proportions vary by practice setting, most CSF specimens obtained for headaches and mental status changes show reactive (e-Fig. 39.75) or nonspecific features, and usually contain benign lymphocytes and monocytes (e-Fig. 39.76). Other normal cells which can be found in CSF specimens include ependymal and choroidal cells (e-Fig. 39.77). These cells usually present in small numbers as small clusters or isolated cells with round, central nuclei and moderate amounts of cytoplasm. Microscopic brain fragments have a fibrillary texture and are usually seen in samples taken directly from the ventricles. Germinal matrix cells can be seen in CSF samples from neonates. Contamination with chondrocytes or bone marrow elements can be seen if the needle was placed too far anteriorly while obtaining the specimen.

1. **Traumatic tap.** CSF samples that consist predominantly of peripheral blood are diagnosed as "negative for malignant cells" with the caveat that the sample may represent a traumatic tap (which occurs in about one quarter of cases). When a CSF sample shows leukemic involvement in the presence of peripheral blood, the possibility of CSF sample contamination by peripheral blood blasts should be raised. In this situation the specimen is best classified as "noncontributory" and a repeat sample should be obtained.

2. **Infectious processes.** Peripheral blood contamination can result in presence of variable numbers of polymorphonuclear neutrophils in a CSF sample; however, abundant neutrophils in the absence of blood contamination should raise the possibility of acute meningitis. Prompt diagnosis is crucial, since it can be fatal if not treated promptly (e-Fig. 39.78). Aseptic meningitis gives a picture of an increased number of mature appearing lymphocytes and monocytes with a small proportion of atypical lymphocytes (e-Fig. 39.79). Suspicion of an infectious process should prompt additional work-up including microbiologic cultures and molecular techniques to identify the source of infection. With the advent of highly active antiretroviral therapy (HAART), AIDS-related CSF lesions have become rare in recent years (*J Neurovirol* 2005;11(Suppl 3):72).

3. **Lymphoma and leukemia.** A primary diagnosis of lymphoma or leukemia should not be made in the absence of flow cytometric analysis of the cells to demonstrate a clonal process. A diagnosis of involvement by lymphoma or leukemia may be rendered if malignant appearing lymphoid cells or cells consistent with blasts are present (e-Figs. 39.80 to 39.85) in a patient with a previously proven history of lymphoma or leukemia. The diagnosis is straightforward when the specimen is hypercellular, but in hypocellular samples the diagnosis can be challenging. Blasts can have variable cytomorphologies, but in general, most blasts show enlarged nuclei, fine chromatin, and prominent nucleoli.

4. **Metastasis.** Cytologic examination of CSF can be used to document CNS involvement in patients who have a known history of malignancy; for example metastatic carcinoma (e-Fig. 39.86), melanoma (e-Fig. 39.87), and leukemia and lymphoma (e-Fig. 39.88). In cases of metastasis, the diagnosis should be confirmed by immunocytochemical stains or by comparison of the cytologic material with the patient's primary malignancy. The diagnostic approach to the rare metastatic tumors of unknown origin that present in the CSF is the same as for tumors of unknown origin presenting at other sites (*Semin Oncol* 1993;20:206).

B. **Stereotactic Brain FNA** is an uncommon procedure, and the choice of the preparatory method is dependent upon the type of tissue aspirated. Involvement by a known primary lesion should be confirmed by comparison of the cytologic specimen with the prior diagnostic material. Fluid or purulent fine needle aspirates should be cultured as well as submitted for cytologic evaluation.

C. Diagnostic Categories

1. **Negative for malignancy.** This diagnosis is rendered for CSF specimens in which only benign cellular elements, and primarily mature appearing lymphocytes and/or monocytes are present.

2. **Atypical cytology.** This diagnosis is rendered when there are rare atypical cells but for which there is inadequate material for ancillary studies. This diagnosis should prompt the collection of additional material for either flow cytometric or immunocytochemical evaluation.

3. **Suspicious for malignancy**. This diagnosis is rendered when there are rare cells highly concerning for involvement by a malignant process, but when the findings are nonetheless insufficient for definitive diagnosis.

4. **Positive for malignancy.** This diagnosis is rendered when there is both quantitative and qualitative evidence of a malignant neoplasm. Ancillary tests can be used to provide a definitive diagnosis as to the type of neoplasm.

D. Special Techniques. Special techniques, such as confirmatory FISH, can be performed on CSF samples (**e-Fig. 39.89**).

ACKNOWLEDGMENT

The authors thank Lourdes R. Ylagan, an author of the previous edition of this section.

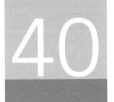

40 Nerve Biopsies

Robert E. Schmidt

Successful use of nerve biopsy requires a discussion between the clinician and neuropathologist since the clinical differential diagnosis may dictate an unusual sampling scheme, for example, vasculitis in which multiple cross-sections may be required for diagnosis.

I. NORMAL PERIPHERAL NERVE AND METHODS OF ANALYSIS. The sural nerve, a cutaneous sensory nerve to the lateral foot, is typically biopsied without stretching or use of intraneural anesthetic. The nerve is divided into a portion for fixation in formalin for paraffin embedding, and a portion for fixation in glutaraldehyde for plastic sections and possible electron microscopy. The entire nerve is typically used rather than dissected into individual fascicles. The portion (~1 cm) of the nerve fixed in formalin should be cut into 3-mm segments and examined in cross-section with paraffin-embedded H&E sections, thioflavin-S histochemistry, and possible immunohistochemistry.

An **H&E stained cross-section** of the sural nerve (e-Fig. 40.1) contains 6 to 12 fascicles, each surrounded by flattened perineurial cells. Outside the perineurium is the epineurium, containing connective tissue and an anastomotic vascular network. Often individual myelinated axons can be seen in H&E stained material (e-Fig. 40.2). The endoneurium (the space inside the perineurial cell layer and outside the axon/Schwann cell units) contains fluid, collagen, capillaries, venules, fibroblasts, macrophages/monocytes, and scattered mast cells. Immunohistologic localization is useful for the demonstration of neurofilaments (a rough measure of axon number, e-Fig. 40.3), amyloid, immunoglobulins, subtypes of inflammatory cells, and growth factors and their receptors.

One-μm thick **plastic embedded sections** (e-Fig. 40.4) provide a wealth of information. Myelinated axons range in diameter from 2 to 18 μm, and are coarsely separated into small (mean of 4 μm) and large (average 12 μm) myelinated axon populations (e-Figs. 40.5 and 40.6) with myelin thickness related directly to axonal diameter. The patterns of nerve damage visible in plastic sections may be characteristic (although rarely pathognomonic) of certain disease entities or pathogenetic processes. Qualitative information is provided on the degree of myelinated axon loss, distribution of axon loss, presence of active axonal degeneration or demyelination, identification of regenerative clusters of axons, swollen axons, onion bulb formation, the nature of cellular infiltrates, or amyloid deposition. Groups of unmyelinated axon populations are detectable in plastic sections (e-Fig. 40.6).

Ultrastructure provides additional detail and is the only definitive method to evaluate unmyelinated axons (e-Fig. 40.7), which are 3 to 4 fold more numerous than myelinated axons in the sural nerve and typically are less than 2 μm in diameter.

If necessary, lengths of individual lightly fixed, osmicated myelinated axons can be dissected or "teased" out of a fascicle with pins. Each myelin internode, maintained by a single Schwann cell, ranges from 0.2 to 1.8 mm in length, increasing linearly with axon diameter. Ongoing activity or residua of past episodes of demyelination or axonal degeneration are readily identified.

Morphometry provides quantitative data concerning axon number and axon size-frequency distribution. Large axons are lost in uremia, abetalipoproteinemia, thallium, arsenic, acute intermittent porphyria, cisplatin, vincristine, and Friedreich ataxia. Small axons are selectively damaged (Fig. 40.1) in amyloidosis, some forms of diabetic neuropathy, acute pandysautonomia, Fabry disease, and hereditary sensory and autonomic neuropathies (HSANs).

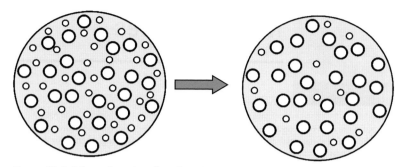

Figure 40.1 Selective loss of small myelinated axons. Normal fascicle is on the **left**.

II. THREE BASIC PATHOLOGIC MECHANISMS CHARACTERIZE NEUROPATHIES

A. Axonal Degeneration is the most common pattern in biopsies, resulting in degeneration of the axon and its myelin sheath (**e-Figs. 40.8** and **40.9**). Often the distal portions of the longest axons are preferentially involved (i.e., distal axonopathy or dying-back neuropathy). Myelin destruction and its early catabolism occurs in the Schwann cell, producing the myelin "ovoid" of teased fibers, and is subsequently continued in hematogenously and endogenously derived macrophages which engulf the debris. Early regenerative events begin immediately with the proliferation of Schwann cells and their processes which accumulate within the original basal lamina of the axon/Schwann cell unit as "bands of Büngner" which are conduits for regenerating axonal sprouts. Schwann cells increase their synthesis of growth factors as trophic and tropic stimuli. Maturing axons form regenerative clusters (**e-Fig. 40.10**) of thinly myelinated axons within the original Schwann cell's basal lamina and, with time, one axon emerges and begins to function and the others regress. Such a regenerated axon characteristically has a myelin sheath relatively thin for its axon's caliber. Teased fiber preparations of a regenerated axon show a distinctive and uniform internodal length regardless of axon diameter. The end stage of a chronic neuropathy may consist of rare preserved axons, scattered fibroblasts, and Schwann cells and may provide little information concerning the process which preceded it.

Axonal degeneration shares mechanisms with wallerian degeneration (WD) which is the reaction of axons and myelin distal to a crush injury. In WD, many axons show simultaneous involvement and are often at the same histologic stage; in axonal degeneration it is typical to find degenerating, regenerating, and normal axons together, some of which may have a distinctive pathologic signature (Fig. 40.2).

B. Segmental Demyelination represents preferential damage to one or several internodes of the myelin sheath, directly to myelin or to its Schwann cell, with relative axonal sparing as seen in this teased fiber preparation (**e-Fig. 40.11**). Schwann cell proliferation results in the replacement of each lost myelin internode by several shorter internodes resulting in variation in internodal length along individual teased fibers.

C. Secondary Demyelination preferentially, nonrandomly involves selected axons, which may be atrophic or damaged, while entirely sparing others. It may reflect an abnormal axon–Schwann cell interaction resulting in secondary myelin loss. Uremic neuropathy is the prototype.

III. TOXIN-INDUCED NEUROPATHIES.
A huge number of toxins and drugs (Table 40.1), including many whose neuropathic toxicity limits their clinical usefulness, produce neuropathy, likely with different mechanisms. One group of axonal degenerations targets axonal transport, others selectively affect neurofilaments or microtubules. Acrylamide can result in distinctive neurofilament and tubulovesicular aggregates involving distal portions of axons. Zinc pyridinethione and bromophenylacetylurea preferentially target reversal of the polarity of axonal transport resulting in terminal swellings. Lead, diphtheria toxin,

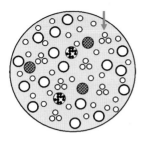 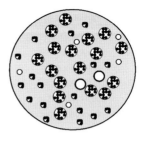

**Axonal
Degeneration**

**Wallerian
Degeneration**

Figure 40.2 Axonal degeneration versus wallerian degeneration. Axonal degeneration is typically characterized by simultaneous axonal degeneration, regenerative clusters (*arrow*), and axons with pathologic signatures (crosshatched) compared with synchronous and uniform degeneration of most axons in a fascicle in wallerian degeneration.

perhexiline, lysolecithin, and hexachlorophene are prominent toxins preferentially directed at the Schwann cell/myelin sheath, resulting in demyelination. Many therapeutic agents may induce peripheral nerve disease. Heavy metals (e.g., arsenic, mercury, thallium, gold) are well known for their toxic effects on peripheral nerves. Neuropathic industrial and environmental agents have resulted in epidemics of toxic neuropathy.

IV. **ISCHEMIC NEUROPATHIES.** The nerve vascular supply (i.e., vasa nervorum) is rich and anastomotic, requiring a substantial decrease in nerve blood flow to interrupt function. Vasculitis (i.e., vasculopathy with angionecrosis) is frequently patchy, resulting in asymmetric nerve involvement (mononeuritis multiplex), emphasizing the need for thorough sampling of the nerve biopsy. Polyarteritis nodosa, the vasculitic prototype, is characterized by epineurial arteries damaged by polymorphonuclear leukocytes, macrophages, monocytes, fibrin (e-**Figs. 40.12** and **40.13**), and a range of axonopathy rarely culminating in infarction. There may be inter- or intrafascicular variability in axon loss (Fig. 40.3, e-**Figs. 40.14** and **40.15**). Fibrotic recanalized vessels mark previous sites of vasculitic damage.

Patients with collagen vascular diseases may clinically present with mononeuritis multiplex histologically comparable to that of polyarteritis nodosa or a minimal epineurial perivascular mononuclear cell infiltrate (i.e., microvasculitis) lacking angionecrosis. Epineurial perivascular collections of a few mononuclear cells are common, and some authors consider them, in isolation, to be of little pathologic importance in the absence of loss of vascular continuity or vasculopathy. Alternatively, they may represent an early or mild vascular injury, or represent an area adjacent to more substantial vasculopathy. Immunoglobulin and complement deposition within the vascular wall in collagen vascular diseases may reflect the deposition of circulating immune complexes not specific for nerve.

V. **METABOLIC NEUROPATHIES** constitute a pathogenetically heterogeneous group.

A. **Diabetes.** There is a complex spectrum of neuropathies in diabetes which may have different pathogenetic mechanisms:

1. **Symmetrical sensori(motor) polyneuropathy** is the most well-known variety of diabetic neuropathy, presenting with distal, largely sensory problems which may culminate in stocking-glove anesthesia. Patients may develop neuropathy after years of recognized diabetes or present de novo with neuropathic symptoms. Typically, distal axon loss is accompanied by vasculopathy (e-**Fig. 40.16**). Schwann cells, perineurial cells, and endothelial cells are enveloped by thickened basement membranes, thought to reflect resistance to degradation because of the formation of advanced glycation end products. Some patients with painful dysesthesias and a normal

TABLE 40.1	Partial List of Agents Causing Toxic Neuropathies	
Metals	**Toxins**	**Drugs**
Aluminum	Acrylamide	Almitrine
Arsenic	Allyl chloride	Amiodarone
Cadmium	Buckthorn	Bortezomib
Gold	Carbon disulfide	Chloroquine
Lead	Dimethylaminopropionitrile	Cisplatin
Lithium	Dioxin	Clioquinol
Mercury	Ethanol	Colchicine
Tellurium	Ethylene oxide	Cyanide
Thallium	Hexacarbons and solvents	Dapsone
	Latrotoxin	Dichloroacetate
	Organophosphorus esters	Disulfiram
	Perchloroethylene	Doxorubicin
	Styrene	Ethambutol
	Toluene	Etoposide
	Toxic oil syndrome	Glutethimide
	Trichloroethylene	Hydralazine
	Vacor	Isoniazid
	Vinyl chloride	Metronidazole
	Xylene	Misonidazole
		Nitrofurantoin
		Nitrous Oxide
		Nucleosides
		Perhexiline
		Phenytoin
		Podophyllin
		Polychlorinated biphenyls
		Procainamide
		Pyridoxine (vitamin B6)
		Sodium cyanate
		Statins
		Suramin
		Tacrolimus (FK506)
		Taxanes (paclitaxel [Taxol], docetaxel)
		Thalidomide
		Vinca Alkaloids (Vincristine, Vinblastine)
		Zinc Pyridinethione

electrophysiologic examination show loss of intraepidermal axons in skin biopsies, a procedure becoming routine practice in some institutions. Multiple ischemic insults may summate to produce a symmetrical and uniform axon loss distally but this mechanism has not been universally accepted. Diabetes-induced oxidative stress may reflect deranged metabolism and/or mitochondriopathy.

2. **Asymmetric neuropathies** include radiculoplexus neuropathy (diabetic amyotrophy), truncal radiculopathy, upper limb mononeuropathy, and cranial nerve (chiefly III) palsies characterized by an inflammatory microvasculitis and/or perineuritis, possible immune complex and complement deposition, and a mild to marked axonopathy.

3. **Diabetic autonomic neuropathy** produces a large range of symptoms contributed by the sympathetic and parasympathetic nervous systems (also enteric and visceral sensory). Autonomic axons may be involved in symmetrical sensorimotor polyneuropathy or as more restricted involvement of autonomic fibers in the gut, bladder,

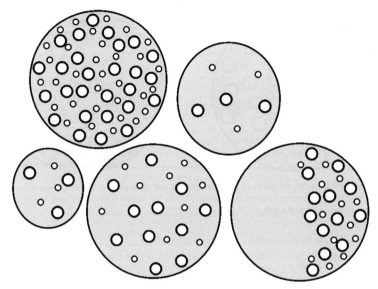

Figure 40.3 Ischemic pattern of axon loss. Intra- and interfascicular variability of axon loss is typical but not pathognomonic of a vasculitic/ischemic pathogenesis.

penis, and other organs. Studies of human diabetics and rodents show markedly swollen dystrophic axons in prevertebral sympathetic ganglia.

B. Uremia results in demyelination of relatively atrophic axons (i.e., secondary demyelination).

C. Others. Deficiencies of pyridoxine, thiamine, vitamin E (found in abetalipoproteinemia, cystic fibrosis, and biliary atresia), niacin, cobalamin, and multiple nutritional deficiencies (apparently resulting in an epidemic in Cuba) are associated with several forms of neuropathy. Hypothyroidism, acute intermittent porphyria, galactosemia, hepatic failure, acromegaly, chronic respiratory insufficiency, and critical illness may also be associated with neuropathy.

VI. NEUROPATHIES WITH AN IMMUNE-MEDIATED MECHANISM

A. Guillain–Barré Syndrome (GBS)

1. **Acute inflammatory demyelinating polyneuropathy (AIDP)** results in patchy myelin loss with residual debris and the appearance of naked demyelinated axons (**e-Figs. 40.17** and **40.18**). A perivascular epineurial and endoneurial T-cell rich infiltrate is coupled with macrophage infiltration (**e-Fig. 40.19**) and results in distinctive macrophage-mediated stripping of layers of otherwise normal appearing myelin (Fig. 40.4, **e-Figs. 40.20** to **40.22**). Circulating antibodies against endoneurial targets may secondarily gain access through a damaged blood–nerve barrier or be locally synthesized. Plasmapheresis and intravenous immunoglobulins may be useful treatment modalities. Eventually, Schwann cells proliferate and remyelinate the denuded internode (**e-Fig. 40.23**). Axonopathy and axon loss is seen, probably because of a noxious endoneurial environment containing cytokines and oxidative mediators.

2. **Acute motor axonal neuropathy (AMAN) and acute motor and sensory axonal neuropathy (AMSAN).** In these axonal forms of GBS the axon rather than myelin is the primary target and may produce acute motor (AMAN) or motor and sensory (AMSAN) dysfunction. Macrophages may be found adjacent to nodes of Ranvier or entering the periaxonal space, possibly targeting axons with a variable degree of axonal degeneration. Antibody may target a constituent of the node of Ranvier to which it

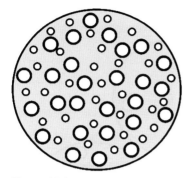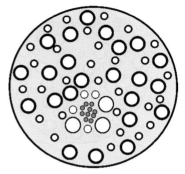

Figure 40.4 Acute inflammatory demyelinating polyneuropathy (AIDP). Patchy loss of myelin in large and small axons is accompanied by an inflammatory infiltrate (*solid dots*). Normal fascicle is on the **left**.

binds, fixes complement forming a membrane attack complex, recruits macrophages, and results eventually in axonal degeneration. Axonal GBS may be associated with a more aggressive course with poorer outcome, electrophysiologic and pathologic evidence of prominent axonopathy, relatively increased incidence of enteric *Campylobacter jejuni* infection, and a role for antibody directed against GM1 ganglioside. Different patterns of nerve injury seen in GBS may reflect the strain of infecting organism or host HLA alleles.

3. Miller Fisher Variant of GBS is distinguished from AIDP/AMAN by a distinctive presentation of ataxia, areflexia and ophthalmoplegia, and antibodies against the ganglioside GQ_{1b} which is concentrated at the nodes of Ranvier, particularly those of the oculomotor nerves.

B. Chronic Inflammatory Demyelinating Polyradiculoneuropathy (CIDP) is characterized by a symmetric progressive or relapsing/remitting, sensory and motor polyradiculoneuropathy, particularly involving proximal nerves. Perineurial inflammation and onion bulbs reflect its chronicity, but do not occur in all cases. CIDP may be a chronic form of GBS in which there is failure of regulatory T cells to suppress the typically monophasic attack of GBS. Its autoimmune pathogenesis involves $CD4^+$ and $CD8^+$ T cells, and possibly also anti-myelin antibodies. HLA subtype frequencies (e.g., HLA-DR2) differ between GBS and CIDP.

C. Anti–Myelin-Associated Glycoprotein (MAG) Neuropathy is a slowly progressive demyelinating neuropathy with an associated IgM monoclonal gammopathy (monoclonal gammopathy of unknown significance, MGUS) in which the antibody is directed against MAG, a molecule which supports myelin integrity. Anti-MAG antibodies deposited on portions of the myelin sheaths of peripheral nerve axons result in altered myelin periodicity, demyelination, and axonal degeneration. Immunosuppression and plasmapheresis have resulted in transient improvement. Rituximab, a mouse–human chimeric antibody against the B cell surface marker CD20, is reported to have clinical benefit.

D. Anti-Glycolipid, -Sulfatide, and -Ganglioside Neuropathies have been associated with a wide range of clinically identifiable acute and chronic neuropathy syndromes.

E. Anti-Hu Antibody Neuropathy is associated with paraneoplastic sensory neuropathy and likely reflects development of antibodies against shared antigens of small cell lung carcinoma and dorsal root ganglion neurons. Infiltration of $CD8^+$ T cells is also present.

F. Autoimmune Autonomic Neuropathy resulting in autonomic failure following a viral illness may be mediated by circulating antibodies against ganglionic nicotine acetylcholine receptor.

VII. GENETIC NEUROPATHIES

A. **Hypertrophic (Onion Bulb) Neuropathies.** The concentric proliferation of Schwann cells in response to multiple episodes of demyelination and subsequent remyelination results in onion bulbs, the defining pathologic hallmark of a group of neuropathies. Onion bulbs are visible in H&E stained nerves (e-**Fig. 40.24**), a pattern accentuated with immunolabeling for Collagen type IV (e-**Fig. 40.25**). Onion bulbs are best illustrated in plastic embedded nerve (e-**Fig. 40.26**) and with electron microscopy (e-**Fig. 40.27**). Nerves may be palpably enlarged and conduction velocities markedly decreased. Genetic analysis has identified mutations in myelin constituents (Po, PMP-22, myelin basic protein), including those localized to noncompact myelin near the paranode (MAG, connexin 32, neurofascin 155) and axonal proteins (Caspr, contactin, kinesin). A more complete catalogue can be found at several websites (e.g., http://www.molgen. ua.ac.be/CMTMutations/).

1. **Hypertrophic Charcot–Marie–Tooth disease (CMT1)** is inherited as an autosomal dominant condition resulting from a duplication or point mutation in the PMP-22 gene or a point mutation in P_o myelin protein (both needed for myelin compaction), a defect in the early growth response 2 gene (EGR2), or mutations of periaxin (a Schwann cell protein regulating its shape and axonal communication). Animal models have established a role for macrophage and lymphocytic infiltration in disease pathogenesis. X-linked CMT demonstrates a defect in the gene for connexin-32.

2. **Other types** (Table 40.2). Dejerine–Sottas syndrome (DSS, includes HMSN-III+) begins in early life, some cases of which have a demonstrable genetic defect in PMP-22, periaxin, GDAP1, EGR2, or myelin protein P_o. Refsum disease, caused by phytanic acid oxidase deficiency, also results in an onion bulb neuropathy.

B. **Hereditary Neuropathy With Pressure Palsies (HNPP).** Teased fiber preparations of this dominantly inherited neuropathy demonstrate marked focal hypermyelination (called tomaculi or sausages) characterized by redundant myelin folds, demyelination, and remyelination. Evidence suggests monosomy of the PMP-22 gene due to loss of a portion of chromosome 17.

C. **Hereditary Giant Axonal Neuropathy** results in axons distended by aggregates of neurofilaments and thinned myelin sheaths, a variety of CNS symptoms, and so-called kinky hair. Schwann cells and endothelial cells may also have aggregates of intermediate filaments. This neuropathy results from the disruption of the gene coding for the synthesis of gigaxonin which interferes with the microtubule network and its dynein motor.

D. **Hereditary Sensory and Autonomic Neuropathies (HSANs).** Included in this group are neuropathies with autonomic and sensory dysfunction, dominant and recessive forms of acral sensory neuropathy, familial dysautonomia, and congenital sensory neuropathy with anhidrosis, all of which are characterized by neuron loss in sensory and various sympathetic and parasympathetic ganglia.

VIII. AMYLOID AND RELATED NEUROPATHIES.

Amyloid represents an extracellular deposit of proteins arranged in a beta pleated sheet conformation forming 10- to 20-nm unbranched filaments which stain with thioflavin-S fluorescence and Congo Red (the latter polarizes light resulting in an apple green color). Amyloid neuropathy occurs in (1) primary (nonhereditary) amyloidosis (also composed of immunoglobulin derived amyloid); (2) amyloidosis associated with dysglobulinemia; and (3) hereditary amyloidosis (e.g., Andrade disease) in which the deposited amyloid is derived from transthyretin or other materials. Amyloid may be deposited within the endoneurium, in the endoneurial and epineurial vasculature (e-**Figs. 40.28** and **40.29**), or within epineurial connective tissue. Axon loss, particularly small axons, is typical. Immunostains may identify the amyloid source (e.g., kappa light chains in a myeloma patient).

IX. INFECTIOUS NEUROPATHIES

A. **Herpes Zoster (Shingles)** presents as a painful cutaneous vesicular rash corresponding to a dermatome in which DRG varicella virus has emerged from latency, initially established at the time of childhood chickenpox infection. In response to immunologic cues or other stimuli, virus activates, travels distally within axons forming a cutaneous

TABLE 40.2 Forms of Hereditary Neuropathy With Onion Bulbs and Tomaculi

Designation	Inheritance	Gene Defect	Pathology
CMT1A	AD	PMP-22	Onion bulbs (OB)
CMT1B	AD	Po	OB
CMT1C	AD	EGR2	OB
		LITAF/SIMPLE	OB
CMT1X	XD	Connexin 32	Axonal/OB
CMT2A	AD	Kinesin family member 1B (KIF1B)	Axonal/±OB
CMT2B	AD	RAB-7	Axonal/±OB
CMT2D	AD	Glycyl tRNA synthetase	Axonal
CMT2E	AD	Neurofilament-L	Axonal
		PMP-22, Po, Connexin 32	Axonal
CMT3 (DSS)	AD or AR	PMP-22, Po, EGR2,	OB
	(or de novo)	Periaxin, GDAP1	
CMT4A	AR	GDAP1	OB
CMT4B.1	AR	Myotubularin-related protein 2	Demyel + folds
CMT4B.2	AR	Set binding factor 2	OB + focal thickening
CMT4C	AR	SH3 & tetratricopeptide repeat domain 2	OB + focal thickening
CMT4D	AR	N-myc downstream	OB
(HMSN-LOM)		Regulated gene 1 (NDRG1)	
CMT4E	AR/AD	EGR2, Po	Severe myelin loss
CMT4F	AR/AD	Periaxin, PMP-22, Po, EGR2	OB (+ tomaculi)
HNPP	AD	PMP-22	Demyel + tomaculi

eruption (rarely myelitis), and produces hemorrhagic ganglioradiculitis (e-**Fig. 40.30**) infecting satellite and Schwann cells and neurons in trigeminal ganglia and DRG.

B. **Leprosy** is caused by *Mycobacterium leprae* infection, and results in loss of cutaneous sensation and motor function as the result of direct infection (lepromatous form) or as a result of a granulomatous response to the organism (tuberculoid form). The tuberculoid form involves the skin and adjacent nerves, in which few organisms are found (complicating distinction from sarcoid neuropathy). In patients with a compromised immune response to the organism, endoneurial fibrosis is accompanied by numerous organisms which can be demonstrated within Schwann cells (particularly those of unmyelinated axons) and endoneurial macrophages (lepra cells). The organism is particularly fond of Schwann cells, binding to laminin-α_2 (*Science* 2002;296:927).

C. **AIDS.** Several different types of neuropathy may develop in patients infected with HIV (Table 40.3) including GBS, CIDP, and necrotizing vasculitis (*Muscle Nerve* 2003;28:542). Distal sensory polyneuropath (DSP) shows prominent HIV-infected macrophage activation and lymphocytic (CD8$^+$>CD4$^+$) infiltration with local release of proinflammatory cytokines (IFN-γ, TNF-α, and IL-6) in the vicinity of degenerating axons and DRG neurons. The viral product gp120 results in neuronal apoptosis and direct local toxicity to axons and may increase vulnerability to dideoxynucleoside-induced neurotoxicity. Antiretroviral treatment may produce a clinical picture closely resembling DSP possibly due to direct mitochondrial toxicity. Skin biopsy is a sensitive and early monitor of the development of DSP, demonstrating loss of epidermal axons and axonal swellings, often in the absence of neuropathic changes in the sural nerve.

TABLE 40.3 Subtypes of HIV-Associated Neuropathy

Subtype of Neuropathy (NP)	Clinical Stage	Mechanism
1. Distal sensory NP	Advanced HIV	Macrophage mediated axonopathy
2. Toxic antiretroviral drug NP	Advanced HIV	Mitochondrial DNA synthesis
3. Mononeuritis multiplex		
Vasculitic form	Moderately advanced	Immune complex deposition
CMV multiple monoNP	Advanced HIV	CMV infection: Schwann cells, vessels
4. Inflammatory demyelinating NP		
GBS (demyelinating or axonal)	Early HIV	Immune dysfunction
CIDP	Early HIV	Immune dysfunction
5. Opportunistic infectious NP		
CMV polyradiculopathy	Advanced HIV	CMV necrotizing NP
Herpes zoster radiculopathy	Advanced HIV	VZV: Schwann cells and endothelium
6. Neoplastic (lymphoma)	Advanced HIV	Endoneurial infiltration
7. Autonomic neuropathy	Advanced HIV	
8. Diffuse infiltrative lymphocytosis	Moderately advanced	CD8 lymphocytosis/vasculopathy

   D. Lyme Disease. Cranial and peripheral nerves show an epineurial or perineurial perivascular lymphocytic/plasmacytic infiltrate (perivasculitis) and axonal degeneration. Organisms are not typically seen in involved nerves.

X. TRAUMATIC NEUROPATHY exists in many forms. Chronic nerve compression and entrapment is characterized by focal loss of myelin. More severe trauma with loss of nerve continuity may produce a traumatic neuroma, that is, a combination of degenerative and regenerative responses resulting in a disorganized aggregate of collagen and axonal "mini-fascicles" (e-**Figs. 40.31** and **40.32**). The distinctive appearance of mini-fascicles can be seen with immunohistochemistry for neurofilaments (which stains axons, e-**Fig. 40.33**) or epithelial membrane antigen (EMA, which stains the perineurium, e-**Fig. 40.34**), and in plastic sections (e-**Fig. 40.35**).

SUGGESTED READINGS

Bilbao JM, Schmidt RE. *Biopsy Diagnosis of Peripheral Neuropathy.* Switzerland: Springer International Publishing; 2015.

Kennedy WR. Opportunities afforded by the study of unmyelinated nerves in skin and other organs. *Muscle & Nerve* 2004;29:756–767.

Pestronk. *Neuromuscular Division Website.* Washington University School of Medicine. https://neuromuscular.wustl.edu/.

Spencer PS, Schaumburg HH, Ludolph AC. *Experimental and Clinical Neurotoxicology.* New York: Oxford University Press; 2000.

Zochodne DW. Diabetes mellitus and the peripheral nervous system: Manifestations and mechanisms. *Muscle Nerve* 2007;36:144–166.

SECTION X

Hematopoietic System

41 Lymph Nodes

Chen Yang, Friederike Kreisel, and Anjum Hassan

I. NORMAL ANATOMY. Lymph nodes are the most widely distributed collections of lymphoid tissue within the lymphoreticular system, which also includes the thymus, tonsils, adenoids, spleen, and Peyer patches. Due to their easy accessibility, lymph nodes are the most frequently examined lymphoid tissue for a lymphoreticular disorder. Microscopically, the lymph node shows four general components, namely, the primary and secondary follicles which are usually found near the capsule, the paracortex which surrounds the follicles and extends deeper into the node, the medullary region, and the sinuses (e-Fig. 41.1).

II. GROSS EXAMINATION, TISSUE SAMPLING, AND HISTOLOGIC SLIDE PREPARATION. Fresh lymphoid tissue should be examined by gross inspection, touch preparation to assess for:

A. Adequate sampling, and

B. Allocation for various ancillary studies

The fresh lymph node should be cut perpendicularly to the long axis, and materials for ancillary studies procured as follows:

1. Wet touch preparations fixed in 95% alcohol or formalin, for Papanicolaou or hematoxylin and eosin (H&E) staining

2. Air-dried touch preparations for Giemsa or Wright–Giemsa staining, cytochemistry (myeloperoxidase, nonspecific esterase, etc.), or cytogenetics (i.e., fluorescence in situ hybridization [FISH])

3. Fresh tissue (in RPMI 1640 medium or saline) for flow cytometry

4. Sterile fresh tissue for microbial cultures or cytogenetic analysis (karyotyping or FISH), if clinically requested

5. Paraffin-embedded tissue after fixation for routine H&E staining, immunohistochemistry, and special stains (e.g., Giemsa, periodic acid–Schiff [PAS], elastin, trichrome, Leder, etc.)

Procuring tissue for histology takes priority over other studies. The most commonly used fixative for permanent sections is 10% neutral buffered formalin. In some laboratories, B5 fixative is used in addition to 10% neutral buffered formalin because of the sharp nuclear detail it produces; however, this mercuric chloride–based fixative is very expensive and poses an environmental hazard. Furthermore, molecular studies cannot be carried out on B5-fixed paraffin-embedded tissue because it will generally yield poor polymerase chain reaction (PCR) amplification results.

III. DIAGNOSTIC FEATURES OF COMMON BENIGN DISEASES OF LYMPH NODES. In reactive lymphadenopathy there are five different architectural patterns to be recognized. It should be mentioned that in most cases of benign reactive lymphadenopathy, a combination of more than one architectural pattern may be present.

A. **Follicular Hyperplasia** (e-Fig. 41.2) is characterized by an increase in the number and size of B-cell germinal centers and is common in lymph node–draining sites of chronic inflammation. This pattern is also present in syphilitic lymphadenitis where, in addition to the marked lymphoid hyperplasia, thickening of the capsule by chronic inflammation, fibrosis, and neovascularization with arteritis and phlebitis, and a marked plasma cell infiltrate in the medullary region predominate. Rheumatoid lymphadenopathy and acute human immunodeficiency virus (HIV) lymphadenitis are other examples of marked follicular hyperplasia.

B. **Diffuse (Paracortical) Hyperplasia** shows expansion of the T-cell paracortical areas. This pattern is commonly seen in viral lymphadenitis (Epstein–Barr virus [EBV], cytomegalovirus [CMV], herpes) and vaccinia lymphadenitis revealing an expansion of the paracortex with increased immunoblasts, imparting a mottled appearance. Follicular hyperplasia and sinus dilation are often concurrent findings in this entity resulting in a mixed pattern of lymphoid hyperplasia. Phenytoin lymphadenopathy represents a relatively pure diffuse hyperplasia showing an expanded paracortical T-zone with numerous large immunoblasts, eosinophils, plasma cells, and neutrophils.

C. **Sinus Hyperplasia** describes increased cellularity within the medullary sinuses of lymph nodes. Sinus histiocytosis is seen in numerous nonspecific responses to chronic inflammation, as well as in lymph nodes draining solid tumors. Sinus histiocytosis with massive lymphadenopathy (Rosai–Dorfman disease) is characterized by markedly dilated sinuses filled with CD68+, S100+ histiocytes showing emperipolesis. Lipophagic reactions causing sinus histiocytosis with accumulation of phagocytosed fat include mineral oil ingestion, Whipple disease, and lymphangiography procedures. Prominent vacuoles in the histiocytes can generate signet-ring cell histiocytosis, a pattern that should not be confused with signet-ring cell carcinoma. Finally, vascular transformation of lymph node sinuses (e-Fig. 41.3) shows a sinus pattern, and it is important to distinguish this entity from the Kaposi sarcoma (e-Fig. 41.4). The latter can be distinguished from the former by the proliferation of spindle-shaped Kaposi sarcoma cells forming cleft-like vascular spaces that contain erythrocytes, many of which are extravasated.

D. **Granulomatous Lymphadenopathy** describes the formation of epithelioid granulomas in lymph nodes. Caseating granulomas are epithelioid granulomas that form central necrosis and caseation, and are typically seen in *Mycobacterium tuberculosis* lymphadenitis. Special stains for mycobacteria in paraffin-embedded tissue (Ziehl–Neelson, Fite–Faraco) will detect the bacilli as bright red, slender, beaded microorganisms (e-Figs. 41.5 and 41.6). *Mycobacterium leprae* lymphadenitis and histoplasma lymphadenitis are other examples of caseating granulomatous inflammation. Necrotizing, noncaseating granulomas are present in cat-scratch disease (e-Fig. 41.7) caused by *Bartonella henselae*, in which suppurative granulomas with stellate microabscesses surrounded by palisading histiocytes predominate. Kikuchi–Fujimoto lymphadenopathy is characterized by necrotizing granulomas containing karyorrhectic debris, but lacking neutrophils; this form of necrotizing lymphadenitis characteristically occurs in young Asian women. Nonnecrotizing, noncaseating granulomas are characteristic of sarcoidosis lymphadenopathy (e-Fig. 41.8), composed primarily of epithelioid histiocytes with scattered multinucleated giant cells, lymphocytes, and plasma cells. This type of epithelioid granuloma can also be seen in draining lymph nodes of the Crohn disease.

E. **Acute Lymphadenitis** is an acute inflammation in lymph nodes draining an infected focus. Acute lymphadenitis is almost exclusively bacterial in nature, and morphologic features range from focal infiltration by neutrophils to necrosis and suppuration with abscess formation.

IV. **INCIDENCE AND EPIDEMIOLOGY OF NON-HODGKIN LYMPHOMAS**
  A. **B-Cell Lymphomas** (see Table 41.3). B-cell lymphomas constitute the vast majority of lymphomas in North America and Europe, accounting for nearly 90% of all

lymphomas. Diffuse large B-cell lymphoma (DLBCL; ~31%) (e-Fig. 41.9) and follicular lymphoma (~22%) (e-Fig. 41.10) are the most common types. Immunosuppression, specifically due to HIV infection and immunosuppressive therapy to prevent graft versus host disease (GVHD), is associated with a markedly increased incidence of mature B-cell lymphomas, particularly DLBCL and Burkitt lymphoma (BL) (e-Fig. 41.11).

Low-grade B-cell lymphomas include follicular lymphoma grades 1, 2, and 3A, chronic lymphocytic leukemia/small lymphocytic lymphoma (CLL/SLL) (e-Fig. 41.12), nodal and extranodal marginal zone B-cell lymphoma (e-Fig. 41.13), and lymphoplasmacytic lymphoma, which are generally indolent and may present in a disseminated stage with bone marrow involvement. Mantle cell lymphoma (e-Figs. 41.14 and 41.15) and DLBCL represent clinically "intermediate-grade" B-cell lymphomas that generally show a more aggressive clinical behavior, but are potentially curable. The same applies to "clinically" aggressive B-cell lymphomas, which include BL, and precursor B-lymphoblastic leukemia/lymphoma. High-grade B-cell lymphoma (HGBL) is considered a new category in the WHO classification (Swerdlow SH, Campo E, Harris NL, et al., eds. *WHO Classification of Tumours of Haematopoietic and Lymphoid Tissues.* Lyon, France: IARC Press; 2017) where two types of HGBL are defined (see Table 41.1). The first category has *MYC* and *BCL-2* and/or *BCL-6* rearrangements, that is, the so-called double hit and triple hit lymphomas. The second category, which is not otherwise specified (NOS), encompasses cases that either have features intermediate between DLBCL and BCL or apparent blastoid morphology but by definition do not harbor a genetic double hit as defined above.

B. Monoclonal B-Cell Lymphocytosis (MBL) is defined by a monoclonal B-cell count of $<5 \times 10^9$/L in the peripheral blood in absence of lymphadenopathy, organomegaly, and extramedullary involvement or any other features of a B-cell lymphoproliferative disorder. It is classified into three categories: (1) CLL type (most common); (2) atypical CLL type; and (3) non-CLL type. It is reported that all CLL is preceded by MBL; however, not all MBL progresses to CLL. Due to clinical significance, MBL should be further classified into high count ($\geq 0.5 \times 10^9$/L) versus low count ($<0.5 \times 10^9$/L).

C. T-Cell Lymphomas. Mature T- and natural killer (NK)-cell malignancies are rare, accounting for only 10% to 12% of all non-Hodgkin lymphoma, and usually are more aggressive than B-cell lymphomas. The most common subtypes are peripheral T-cell lymphoma, NOS (~4% of all adult non-Hodgkin lymphomas and ~30% of peripheral T-cell lymphomas) (e-Fig. 41.16) and anaplastic large cell lymphoma (~3% of all adult non-Hodgkin lymphomas) (e-Fig. 41.17). In general, T- and NK-cell malignancies are much more common in Asia and are linked to viral infection with EBV (NK-cell lymphomas) (e-Fig. 41.18) and human T-cell leukemia virus (HTLV-1) (adult T-cell leukemia/lymphoma) (e-Fig. 41.19).

V. PATHOPHYSIOLOGY OF NON-HODGKIN LYMPHOMAS

A. B-Cell Lymphomas. Mature B-cell malignancies mimic stages of normal B-cell differentiation; therefore, classification is generally based on their morphologic and immunophenotypic resemblance to the normal B-cell counterpart (Fig. 41.1) (*Best Pract Res Clin Haematol* 2005;18:11). Normal B-cell development begins in the bone marrow where precursor B-lymphoblasts undergo immunoglobulin VDJ gene rearrangement and develop into IgM+, IgD+ naïve B-cells with surface immunoglobulin light chain and CD5 expression. These resting B-cells circulate in the blood and occupy primary follicles and mantle zones of secondary follicles. Malignant counterparts of CD5+ naïve B-cells are believed to be CLL and mantle cell lymphoma. Upon antigen stimulation, naïve B-cells undergo blastic transformation, migrate into the center of the primary follicle, and form the germinal center. These centroblasts are large lymphoid cells with vesicular chromatin and several eccentrically located nucleoli. They express BCL-6 and CD10 but switch off BCL-2 protein expression, therefore becoming susceptible to death through apoptosis. Centroblasts undergo intense proliferation that is accompanied by somatic hypermutation of their rearranged variable-region genes, giving rise to cells carrying receptors with high affinity for the stimulating antigen. This leads to a large pool of

TABLE 41.1 2016 WHO Classification of Lymphoid Neoplasms

Mature B-cell neoplasms
Chronic lymphocytic leukemia (CLL)/small lymphocytic lymphoma
Monoclonal B-cell lymphocytosis (MBL), CLL type
MBL, non-CLL type
B-cell prolymphocytic leukemia
Splenic marginal zone lymphoma
Hairy cell leukemia
Splenic B-cell lymphoma/leukemia, unclassifiable
Splenic diffuse red pulp small B-cell lymphoma
Hairy cell leukemia variant
Lymphoplasmacytic lymphoma
Waldenström macroglobulinemia
IgM monoclonal gammopathy of undetermined significance (MGUS)
Heavy chain diseases
μ heavy chain disease
γ heavy chain disease
α heavy chain disease
Plasma cell neoplasms
Non-IgM MGUS
Plasma cell myeloma
Solitary plasmacytoma of bone
Extraosseous plasmacytoma
Monoclonal immunoglobulin deposition diseases
Primary amyloidosis
Light chain and heavy chain deposition diseases
Extranodal marginal zone lymphoma of mucosa-associated lymphoid tissue (MALT lymphoma)
Nodal marginal zone lymphoma
Pediatric nodal marginal zone lymphoma
Follicular lymphoma
In situ follicular neoplasia
Duodenal-type follicular lymphoma
Testicular follicular lymphoma
Pediatric-type follicular lymphoma
Large B-cell lymphoma with *IRF4* rearrangement
Primary cutaneous follicle center lymphoma
Mantle cell lymphoma
In situ mantle cell neoplasia
Diffuse large B-cell lymphoma (DLBCL), NOS
Germinal center B-cell subtype
Activated B-cell subtype
T-cell/histiocyte-rich large B-cell lymphoma
Primary DLBCL of the CNS
Primary cutaneous DLBCL, leg type
EBV-positive DLBCL, NOS
EBV-positive mucocutaneous ulcer
DLBCL associated with chronic inflammation
Fibrin-associated DLBCL
Lymphomatoid granulomatosis, grade 1, 2
Lymphomatoid granulomatosis, grade 3
Primary mediastinal (thymic) large B-cell lymphoma
Intravascular large B-cell lymphoma
ALK-positive large B-cell lymphoma
Plasmablastic lymphoma

(*continued*)

TABLE 41.1   2016 WHO Classification of Lymphoid Neoplasms (*Continued*)

Primary effusion lymphoma
Multicentric Castleman disease
HHV8-positive DLBCL, NOS
HHV8-positive germinotropic lymphoproliferative disorder
Burkitt lymphoma
Burkitt-like lymphoma with 11q aberration
High-grade B-cell lymphoma (HGBL)
HGBL with *MYC* and *BCL2* and/or *BCL6* rearrangements
HGBL, NOS
B-cell lymphoma, unclassifiable, with features intermediate between DLBCL and classic Hodgkin
    lymphoma (CHL)

Mature T- and natural killer (NK)-cell neoplasms
T-cell prolymphocytic leukemia
T-cell large granular lymphocytic leukemia
Chronic lymphoproliferative disorder of NK-cells
Aggressive NK-cell leukemia
Systemic EBV-positive T-cell lymphoma of childhood
Chronic active EBV infection of T- and NK-cell type, systemic form
Hydroa vacciniforme–like lymphoproliferative disorder
Severe mosquito bite allergy
Adult T-cell leukemia/lymphoma
Extranodal NK/T-cell lymphoma, nasal type
Enteropathy-associated T-cell lymphoma
Monomorphic epitheliotropic intestinal T-cell lymphoma
Intestinal T-cell lymphoma, NOS
Indolent T-cell lymphoproliferative disorder of the gastrointestinal tract
Hepatosplenic T-cell lymphoma
Subcutaneous panniculitis-like T-cell lymphoma
Mycosis fungoides
Sézary syndrome
Primary cutaneous CD30-positive T-cell lymphoproliferative disorders
Lymphomatoid papulosis
Primary cutaneous anaplastic large cell lymphoma
Primary cutaneous γδ T-cell lymphoma
Primary cutaneous CD8-positive aggressive epidermotropic cytotoxic T-cell lymphoma
Primary cutaneous acral CD8-positive T-cell lymphoma
Primary cutaneous CD4-positive small/medium T-cell lymphoproliferative disorder
Peripheral T-cell lymphoma, NOS
Angioimmunoblastic T-cell lymphoma
Follicular T-cell lymphoma
Nodal peripheral T-cell lymphoma with T-follicular helper phenotype
Anaplastic large cell lymphoma, ALK positive
Anaplastic large cell lymphoma, ALK negative
Breast-implant–associated anaplastic large cell lymphoma

Hodgkin lymphomas
Nodular lymphocytic-predominant Hodgkin lymphoma
CHL
Nodular sclerosis CHL
Lymphocyte-rich CHL
Mixed cellularity CHL
Lymphocyte-depleted CHL

From Swerdlow SH, Campo E, Harris NL, et al., eds. *WHO Classification of Tumours of Haematopoietic and Lymphoid Tissues.* Lyon, France: IARC Press; 2017. Used with permission.

Normal and abnormal counterparts of B-cell progeny[a]

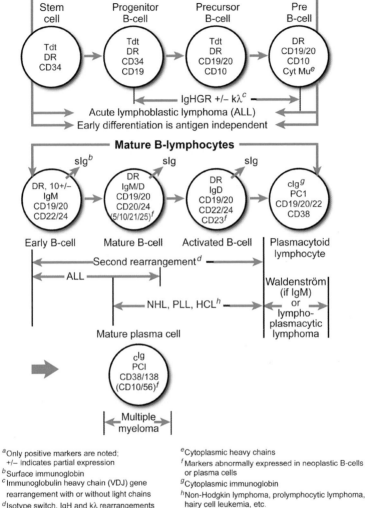

Figure 41.1 Brief overview of normal B-cell progeny and malignant counterparts.

B-lymphoid cells with intraclonal diversity. Centroblasts then mature into centrocytes, representing intermediate-sized lymphoid cells with irregular, cleaved nuclei and inconspicuous nucleoli. Centrocytes with mutations resulting in decreased affinity for antigen die by apoptosis, whereas centrocytes with high affinity for antigen are rescued from apoptosis by re-expressing BCL-2. Malignant counterparts of germinal center–derived B-cells are follicular lymphoma, a subset of DLBCL and BL. Via interactions with follicular dendritic cells through CD23 and with T-lymphocytes through CD40 ligand (CD40L), centrocytes switch off BCL-6 expression and differentiate into either memory cells or plasma cells. Memory cells are found in the marginal zone of follicles; they typically express immunoglobulin M (IgM) and lack expression of IgD, CD5, CD10, or CD23. Plasma cells home to the bone marrow; they lack surface immunoglobulin and pan-B-cell expression, but express CD79a, CD138, and cytoplasmic IgG or IgA. Neither memory cells nor plasma cells undergo further somatic hypermutation. Marginal zone B-cell lymphoma corresponds to post-germinal center cells, possibly memory cells of marginal zone type. Plasma cell myeloma is the malignant counterpart of bone marrow–homing Igg- or IgA-producing plasma cells.

B. T-Lymphocytes. Two major classes of T-lymphocytes exist based on the structure of the T-cell receptor (TCR). Approximately 95% of all T-cells are αβ T-lymphocytes that can be subdivided into CD4+ helper T-cells or CD8+ cytotoxic T-cells. Only 5% of T-cells are γδ cells, which are primarily found in the splenic pulp and intestinal epithelium and are not MHC restricted in their function because they do not express CD4 or CD8. The TCR is composed of either the αβ or γδ chains, each consisting of an external variable (V) and constant (C) domain. The TCR is complexed with CD3 that contains γ, δ, and ε chains. NK-cells do not have a complete TCR, but usually express the ε chain of the CD3 in the cytoplasm; therefore, NK-cells will stain positively with a polyclonal antibody to CD3. The malignant counterparts of γδ T-cells are believed to be hepatosplenic T-cell lymphoma (**e-Fig. 41.20**) and enteropathy-type T-cell lymphoma (**e-Fig. 41.21**). NK-cells share some immunophenotypic markers and functions with cytotoxic CD8+ T-cells; these include expression of CD2, CD7, CD8, CD56, CD57, granzyme B, perforin, and T-cell intracellular antigen (TIA-1).

Due to their broad cytologic spectrum, the absence of immunophenotypic markers of monoclonality, and general lack of specific genetic abnormalities, clinical presentation plays a major role in the subclassification of T- and NK-cell malignancies (Fig. 41.2). For example, hypercalcemia is associated with adult T-cell leukemia; hemophagocytic syndrome occurs more frequently in cytotoxic T-cell or NK-cell malignancies; persistent severe neutropenia is a relatively common clinical feature in T-cell granular lymphocyte leukemia (**e-Fig. 41.22**); and systemic symptoms of edema, pleural effusion, ascites, arthritis combined with anemia, and polyclonal hypergammaglobulinemia are relatively specific for angioimmunoblastic T-cell lymphoma (**e-Fig. 41.23**).

VI. A RATIONAL APPROACH TO GENERAL LYMPHOMA WORKUP. The classification of lymphomas may appear difficult; however, a systematic approach can be used to efficiently narrow the differential diagnosis for most cases. Needless to say, knowledge of clinical history and a basic complete blood count are required to guide the initial steps of the evaluation (e.g., to direct the immunophenotypic workup of the sample by flow cytometry), because tissue sections are often not available until the next day. The general algorithm (see Table 41.2) starts with the low-power appearance of the tissue section. Is the architecture nodular, follicular, diffuse, or mixed? What is the cell size; small (close to a normal lymphocyte), medium, or large (about three times the size of a normal lymphocyte)? What is the nuclear shape (cleaved nuclei of follicular lymphoma or round nuclear contours of chronic lymphocytic lymphoma)? Is the process high-grade (necrosis, starry-sky appearance, high mitotic rate)? The workup continues with a determination of the lineage and stage of maturation. As mentioned above, flow cytometry is usually extremely helpful in delineating the lineage, provided care is taken to save fresh tissue in RPMI medium and order appropriate markers; alternatively, immunohistochemistry can be performed on formalin-fixed, paraffin-embedded tissue. The workup concludes with evaluation of disease-specific markers such as cyclin D1 and anaplastic large cell lymphoma kinase (ALK-1), which can only be evaluated by immunohistochemistry in tissue sections.

Antigen markers useful in delineating and subclassifying lymphoid malignancies are the following:

A. Leukocyte Marker. CD45 (also known as leukocyte common antigen [LCA]) is expressed on all leukocytes.

Normal T-cell progeny[e]

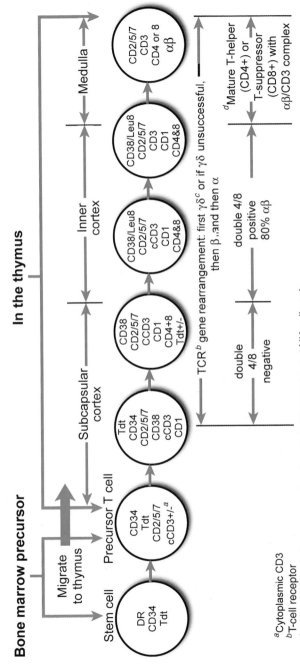

Figure 41.2 Brief overview of normal T-cell progeny.

[a]Cytoplasmic CD3
[b]T-cell receptor
[c]Gamma-delta chains expressed on immature thymocytes and NK-cells only
[d]Mature T-cells can circulate in peripheral blood and tissues
[e]Only positive markers are noted. Markers partially expressed or about to lose expression are noted by a "+/−".

TABLE 41.2 An Algorithm for the Workup of Lymphomas

Cell type: Are the cells lymphoid?

In a tissue section, what is the low-power architecture?

Cell size

Are the majority of cells small (same as a normal lymphocyte)? Or large (~3 times as big as a lymphocyte, or even bigger)?

Is there an even mixture of small and large cells? Are they anaplastic?

Nuclear shape

Do the cells have round nuclei with a smooth contour (noncleaved)? Or a round shape with a bumpy or notched contour (irregular)? Or a variable shape with deeply folded or grooved nuclei (cleaved)?

Histologic grade

Is necrosis present? Is there a "starry-sky" appearance? Are mitoses easy to find?

Lineage (by flow cytometry or immunohistochemistry)

Are the cells of B-lineage (generally CD19 and 20+) or T-lineage (generally CD3+)?

Maturation

Are the cells at a precursor (TdT+) or a mature (TdT−) stage of maturation?

If mature and of B-lineage, are they prefollicular, follicular, postfollicular, or effector cell stage?

If mature and of T-lineage, are they at a thymic or postthymic/effector cell stage?

Disease-specific markers

Do the cells express cyclin D1, BCL6, ALK-1, and so on?

Cytogenetic and molecular studies

   B. **Markers of Immaturity**
   1. TdT (terminal deoxynucleotidyl transferase, a specialized DNA polymerase; nuclear expression present only in pre-B and pre-T lymphoblasts)
   2. CD34 (present on pluripotent hematopoietic stem cells and progenitor cells of many lineages)
   3. CD10 (CALLA [common acute lymphoblastic leukemia antigen]; expressed on marrow pre-B-cells and mature follicular center B-cells)
   4. CD22 (present on pre-B-cells)
   5. cμ (cytoplasmic μ heavy chain)
   C. **Primarily B-Cell–Associated Markers**
   1. CD19 (present on marrow pre-B-cells, mature B-cells, but not on plasma cells)
   2. CD20 (present on marrow pre-B-cells and mature B-cells, but not on normal plasma cells)
   3. CD79a (present on mature and pre-B-cells, as well as on plasma cells)
   4. CD22 (transmembrane molecule, present on mature B-cells [cCD22] and pre-B-cells [cCD22])
   5. PAX-5 (also known as B-cell–specific activator protein [BSAP]; in normal hematopoiesis PAX-5 is expressed only by B-cells and is downregulated in plasma cells; this marker can be used in combination with other universal B-cell markers especially in the setting of anti-CD20 therapy effect)
   D. **Markers Helpful in Subclassifying Mature B-Cell Lymphomas**
   1. CD5 (expressed on all T-cells and small subset of B-cells, expressed on neoplastic CLL and mantle cell lymphoma cells)
   2. CD10
   3. CD11c (expressed in high levels on monocytes, macrophages, and NK-cells, as well in moderate levels on granulocytes; expressed on subsets of T- and B-cells)
   4. CD23 (present on activated mature B-cells)

5. CD38 (primarily expressed on mature B-cells and plasma cells)
6. CD43 (leukosialin, expressed on the surface of all leukocytes except resting B-cells; CD43 expression in B-cell lymphomas is highly correlated with CD5 and is therefore an indicator of aberrant B-cell populations)
7. BCL-6 (expressed normally in germinal center lymphocytes in the normal lymph node; it is distributed in a pattern reciprocal to that of BCL-2)
8. BCL-2 (present on T-cells and normal mantle B-cells; aberrantly expressed in a majority of B-cell lymphomas)
9. Cyclin D1 (cell cycle regulatory protein rearranged through the t(11;14) of mantle cell lymphoma; also expressed weakly in hairy cell leukemia and plasma cell dyscrasias; nuclear protein detectable in paraffin-embedded sections)
10. CD138 (Syndecan-1, expressed on most cases of myeloma, but also present in carcinomas)

E. **Markers of Clonality:** κ and λ immunoglobulin light chains

F. **Primarily T- and NK-Cell–Associated Markers:**

1. CD1 (expressed on cortical thymocytes and Langerhans cell histiocytes)
2. CD2 (present on all T-cells [thymic and peripheral T-cells] and NK-cells)
3. CD3 (lineage-specific marker for T-cells; cytoplasmic form also expressed in NK-cells)
4. CD5 (expressed on all T-cells and a small subset of B-cells)
5. CD7 (expressed on all T-cells and a small subset of myeloid precursor cells)
6. CD8 (present on cytotoxic subset of peripheral T-cells and on a subset of thymocytes and NK-cells)
7. CD16 (present on NK-cells and granulocytes)
8. CD56 (present on NK-cells and a subset of T-lymphocytes; also present on myeloma cells)
9. TIA-1 (cytotoxic granule–associated RNA-binding protein), granzyme B, and perforin (proteins released by cytotoxic T-cells, inducing apoptosis) are expressed in cytotoxic T- and NK-cells

G. **Flow Cytometry** can easily detect clonality in B-cell malignancies (normal κ to λ light chain ratio ranges between 1:1 and 4:1). Clonality for T-cell malignancies can only be detected by molecular or cytogenetic studies.

H. **Polymerase Chain Reaction (PCR).** PCR amplification methods to detect clonal *IgH* and *TCR* gene rearrangements can be utilized specifically in the setting of atypical lymphocytic proliferations, when histopathologic features fall short for a specific diagnosis of a non-Hodgkin lymphoma.

The 200 variable segments of the *IgH* gene contain three highly variable and mutation-prone regions termed complementary determining regions (CDR1, 2, and 3) that are interspersed between four conserved framework regions (FR1, 2, 3, and 4) that provide reliable targets for consensus primers. About 70% of B-cell malignancies harbor clonal rearrangements that are detectable with framework 3 primers, and about 15% to 20% of additional clonal rearrangements can be detected when framework 2 primers are used. Therefore, most laboratories use primers targeting frameworks 2 and 3 to detect at least 80% of all B-cell lymphomas.

The rearranged *TCRγ* gene is most suitable for clonal detection by PCR amplification in T-cell malignancies, because most T-lymphocytes harbor rearrangements in 1 of the 11 γ segments. Because many of these segments are homologous to one another, they can be targeted by a single consensus primer set. *TCRδ* and *TCRα* cannot be targeted because *TCRδ* is deleted during *TCRα* gene rearrangement, and because the diversity of possible *TCRα* rearrangements makes analysis difficult by current PCR technology.

I. **Cytogenetic Analysis** is a morphologic study of chromosomes to assess changes in their number and structure.

1. **Conventional karyotyping** requires viable cells, and analysis of chromosomes is performed according to their size and banding pattern after chromosome staining.

Although this study has become critical in the diagnosis and classification of acute leukemias, it is not frequently used as part of a routine diagnostic workup for lymph node biopsies.

2. **Fluorescence in situ hybridization (FISH)** uses one or more labeled probes directed toward specific portions of chromosomes. It is helpful in locating specific translocations, deletions, and amplifications of chromosomal regions. The advantage of FISH (see Chapter 57) is that it can be performed on nondividing nuclei (interphase nuclei), eliminating the need for cell culture. Furthermore, interphase FISH can be performed on a wide range of specimen types, such as peripheral blood smears, cytospin preparations, and paraffin-embedded tissue. Many of the classic chromosomal translocations that characterize specific lymphomas can be identified with interphase FISH techniques. Tables 41.3 and 41.4 summarize the characteristic morphologic, immunophenotypic, and genetic features of B-cell and T/NK-cell malignancies, respectively.

VII. **PLASMA CELL NEOPLASMS.** Plasma cells represent terminally differentiated B-cells. Their neoplasms are characterized by the secretion of a single homogenous immunoglobulin product known as the monoclonal or "M" component, which can be detected by serum and urine protein electrophoresis. The International Myeloma Working Group categorizes plasma cell neoplasms into plasma cell myeloma, monoclonal gammopathy of undetermined significance (MGUS), plasmacytomas, osteosclerotic myeloma (POEMS syndrome), and systemic immunoglobulin light-chain amyloidosis.

A. **Plasma Cell Myeloma** usually is characterized by multifocal bone marrow plasmacytosis causing osteolytic lesions, pathologic fractures, bone pain, hypercalcemia, and anemia (e-**Figs. 41.24** and **41.25**). The diagnostic criteria for plasma cell myeloma are outlined in Table 41.5. These criteria must be manifest in a symptomatic patient with progressive disease to diagnose symptomatic plasma cell myeloma. Clinical variants include asymptomatic (smoldering) myeloma when patients are asymptomatic and have no lytic bone lesions (Table 41.5); nonsecretory myeloma where serum M-protein may be absent but cytoplasmic M-protein can be demonstrated by immunohistochemistry (in the majority of patients) and abnormalities in serum light chains can be demonstrable (*Br J Hematol* 2003;121:749); and primary plasma cell leukemia (pPCL) characterized by the presence of >2 × 10^9/L peripheral blood plasma cells or plasmacytosis accounting for >20% of the differential white cell count, without a preexisting plasma cell myeloma. The circulating plasma cells may resemble plasmacytoid lymphocytes morphologically. Therefore immunophenotypic studies are extremely helpful in this setting. Unlike other myelomas, pPCL usually lacks aberrant expression of CD56 and is more likely to be associated with abnormal or unfavorable cytogenetics (Table 41.6).

B. **Patients With MGUS** are asymptomatic with no evidence of lytic bone lesions, but reveal a clonal plasma cell population in the bone marrow of <10% and an associated M component of <30 g/L. No lytic lesions or myeloma-related organ damage is present and a B-cell lymphoma with plasmacytic differentiation should be excluded.

C. **Plasmacytomas** manifest as a localized osseous or extraosseous lesion with no radiographic or morphologic evidence of bone marrow involvement (e-**Figs. 41.26–41.29**). The most common osseous location is the vertebral body, and the most common extraosseous location is the upper respiratory tract (Table 41.7).

D. **POEMS** syndrome represents an osteosclerotic myeloma with associated clinical features including polyneuropathy, organomegaly, endocrinology, monoclonal gammopathy, and skin changes. Lymph node biopsies in these patients may demonstrate Castleman-like features, specifically the plasma cell variant (*Blood* 2003;101:2496). The bone marrow shows plasmacytosis only in the vicinity of sclerotic lesions with less than 5% plasma cells elsewhere (*Blood Rev* 1996;10:75).

E. **Systemic Immunoglobulin Light-Chain Amyloidosis** is diagnosed by positive amyloid staining by Congo red in any tissue (fat aspirate, bone marrow, or organ biopsy); establishment of amyloid being light-chain related by direct examination using mass spectrometry-based proteomic analysis or immunoelectron microscopy; and evidence

TABLE 41.3	Characteristic Features of Different B-Cell Malignancies			
Disease	**Clinical Presentation**	**Morphology**	**Immunophenotype**	**Genetics**
CLL/SLL	Mostly asymptomatic, may present with fatigue, autoimmune hemolytic anemia, hepatosplenomegaly, lymphadenopathy; peripheral absolute lymphocytosis	**PB:** Small cells with coarsely clumped chromatin and inconspicuous nucleoli **LN:** Proliferation centers (PC) composed of "paraimmunoblasts" and prolymphocytes; large/confluent or highly proliferative PCs are adverse prognostic indicators	CD20 (weak), CD19, IgM, IgD, CD22 (weak), CD5, CD23, CD79a, CD43 ZAP-70-positive (IgVH unmutated) CLL with aggressive clinical course vs. ZAP-70-negative (IgVH mutated) CLL with indolent course	Trisomy 12, deletions at 13q14, deletions at 11q22–23 50–60% have somatic hypermutations, IgH clonally rearranged *TP53, NOTCH1, SF3B1, ATM,* and *BIRC3* mutations may have potential clinical relevance
Prolymphocytic leukemia	Marked splenomegaly without lymphadenopathy, rapidly rising lymphocyte count (>100 × 10⁹/L)	**PB:** Medium-sized cells with round nucleus, moderately condensed chromatin, and prominent central nucleolus	CD20 (bright), CD19, IgM, CD22, CD79a, FMC7, CD23 typically absent, CD5 present in 1/3 of cases	Complex karyotypes are common, abnormalities of *TP53* in ~50%, IgH clonally rearranged
Hairy cell leukemia	Predominantly middle-aged men, splenomegaly, pancytopenia with monocytopenia	**PB:** Small- to medium-sized cells with circumferential hairy projections **Spleen:** Red pulp infiltration (macroscopy: "bloody lakes")	CD19, CD20, CD22 (bright), CD79a, CD11c (bright), CD25 (bright), CD103, TRAP, DBA-44 in tissue sections	*BRAF* V600E mutations in vast majority of cases; *MAP-2K1/IGHV4-34* mutations in cases that lack *BRAF* mutation
Lymphoplasmacytic lymphoma/Waldenström macroglobulinemia	Monoclonal IgM serum paraprotein with associated hyperviscosity symptoms	Mixture of small lymphocytes, plasmacytoid lymphocytes, and plasma cells, Dutcher bodies	CD19, CD20, CD22, CD79a, CD38, surface and cytoplasmic IgM, no expression of CD5, CD23, or CD10	*MYD88* L265P mutation in most cases
Splenic marginal zone B-cell lymphoma	Splenomegaly, sometimes associated with autoimmune thrombocytopenia or anemia, peripheral lymphadenopathy uncommon	**PB:** Small- to medium-sized cells with polar villi (villous lymphocytes) **Spleen:** Both white pulp and red pulp infiltration	CD19, CD20, CD79a, IgM, and IgD, no expression of CD5, CD23, CD10, or CD43	Allelic loss of chromosome 7q21–32 in 40% of cases, trisomy 3 in rare cases, *IgH* clonally rearranged

(continued)

TABLE 41.3 Characteristic Features of Different B-Cell Malignancies (*Continued*)

Disease	Clinical Presentation	Morphology	Immunophenotype	Genetics
Extranodal marginal zone B-cell lymphoma (MALT lymphoma)	History of chronic inflammatory or autoimmune disorders (*Helicobacter pylori* gastritis, Hashimoto thyroiditis, Sjögren syndrome), GI tract most common site of involvement	Polymorphous infiltrate of centrocyte-like cells, monocytoid cells, small lymphocytes, scattered immunoblasts, and lymphoid cells with plasmacytic differentiation, "overrun follicles," lymphoepithelial lesions	CD19, CD20, CD79a, IgM, and no expression of CD5, CD23, CD10	t(11;18)(q21;q21) in ~25% to 50% of cases, t(14;18)(q32;q21) [*IgH/MALT1*], *IgH* clonally rearranged
Nodal marginal zone B-cell lymphoma	Localized or generalized lymphadenopathy	Marginal zone and interfollicular areas infiltrated by centrocyte-like B-cells, monocytoid B-cells, or small lymphocytes; plasma cell differentiation may be present	CD19, CD20, CD79a, IgM, no expression of CD5, CD23, CD10	The translocations associated with extranodal MZL are not detected; *IgH* clonally rearranged
Follicular lymphoma	Widespread peripheral and central lymphadenopathy, bone marrow involved in 40% of cases	Grade 1-2: 0-15 centroblasts per 40× HPF Grade 3A: >15 centroblasts per 40× HPF (centrocytes present, clinically = grade 1-2) Grade 3B: >15 centroblasts per 40× HPF (centrocytes absent, clinically = DLBCL)	CD19, CD20, CD22, CD79a, BCL-6, BCL-2, CD10	t(14;18)(q32;q21) rearrangement of the *BCL-2* gene leading to overexpression of the BCL-2 protein and survival advantage of malignant cells; *IgH* clonally rearranged
Mantle cell lymphoma	Lymphadenopathy, most common extranodal site is the GI tract (multiple lymphomatous polyposis)	May show vaguely nodular, diffuse, or mantle zone pattern, medium-sized lymphoid cells with irregular nuclear contours, may be blastoid in appearance	CD19, CD20, CD5, FMC-7, CD43, cyclin-D1, SOX11 in cyclin-D1 negative cases, lack of expression of CD23, CD10, BCL-6	t(11;14)(q13;q32), translocation between *IgH* and *BCL-1* genes; *IgH* clonally rearranged; two subtypes: one unmutated/minimally mutated *IGHV* and SOX11 positive; the other *IGHV* mutated and SOX11 negative (indolent)

Entity	Clinical	Morphology	Immunophenotype	Genetics
Diffuse large B-cell lymphoma, NOS	Rapidly enlarging, often symptomatic mass, often disseminated disease	Sheets of large cells with nuclear size equal or exceeding normal macrophage nucleus. Morphologic variants: Centroblastic, immunoblastic, T-cell/histiocyte-rich, anaplastic	CD19, CD20, CD22, CD79a. CD10+, BCL-6+, MUM1: germinal center B-cell-like (better overall survival than activated B-type). Coexpression of MYC and BCL-2 considered poor prognostic marker	IgH clonally rearranged, ~30% with abnormalities of 3q27 region involving BCL6
Mediastinal (thymic) large B-cell lymphoma	Mostly women in their third to fifth decades, large anterior mediastinal mass, sometimes with impending superior vena cava syndrome	Large cells with associated delicate interstitial fibrosis causing compartmentalization, possible thymic remnants, biopsy samples often small and obscured by profuse sclerosis and crush artifact	CD19, CD20, CD30 (weak), Ig, and HLA class I and II expression is often absent	IgH clonally rearranged; hyperdiploid karyotype, gains in chromosome 9p
Burkitt lymphoma	Highly aggressive lymphoma often presenting at extranodal sites or as acute leukemia, risk for central nervous system involvement, "endemic" Burkitt lymphoma with involvement of jaws and other facial structures, "sporadic" Burkitt lymphoma with abdominal masses	Medium-sized cells with basophilic vacuolated cytoplasm and regular nuclei with several small nucleoli, tingible body macrophages imparting "starry-sky" appearance	CD19, CD20, CD22, CD10, CD79a, BCL-6, no expression of TdT, BCL-2, Ki-67 index of nearly 100%	IgH clonally rearranged; t(8;14) in most cases; t(2;8) and t(8;22) rare. TCF3 or ID3 mutations in ~70% of cases

CLL, chronic lymphocytic leukemia; DLBCL, diffuse large B-cell lymphoma; GI, gastrointestinal; HLA, human leukocyte antigen; HPF, high-power field; Ig, immunoglobulin; LN, lymph node; MALT, mucosa-associated lymphoid tissue; MZL, marginal zone lymphoma; PB, peripheral blood; SLL, small lymphocytic lymphoma; TdT, terminal deoxynucleotidyl transferase; TRAP, tartrate-resistant acid phosphatase.

TABLE 41.4 Characteristic Features of Different T- and NK-Cell Malignancies

Disease	Clinical Presentation	Morphology	Immunophenotype	Genetics
T-cell prolympho-cytic leukemia	Aggressive disease with hepatosplenomeg-aly and generalized lymphadenopathy; marked lymphocytosis, usually >100 × 10^9/L, anemia and thrombocytopenia	**PB:** Medium-sized cells with nongranular cytoplasm, visible nucleolus, and cytoplasmic protrusions or blebs	CD3, CD2, CD7, CD4+/CD8- in 60%, CD4+/CD8+ in 25%, CD4-/CD8+ in 15%	inv(14)(q11;q32) in 80%, t(14;14) (q11;q32) in 10% involving *TCR-α/β* and *TCL-1*, clonally rear-ranged *TCR*
T-cell large granular lymphocyte leu-kemia	Indolent clinical course, severe neutropenia with/without anemia, mild to moderate lymphocytosis, moderate splenomegaly, rheumatoid arthritis, circulating immune complexes, hypergammaglobulinemia	**PB:** Large granular lymphocytes with abundant cytoplasm and fine or coarse azurophilic granules; **BM:** Interstitial infiltrate	CD3, TCR-α/β, CD8 in 80%, coexpression of TIA-1, CD57, perfo-rin, granzyme B, FasL (CD95), and FasL	Clonally rearranged *TCR*; *STAT3*, and *STAT5B* mutations in a subset of cases (the latter are more aggressive)
Aggressive NK-cell leukemia	More prevalent among Asians; fever, leuke-mic blood picture, constitutional symp-toms, cytopenias, hepatosplenomegaly, multiorgan failure due to increased serum soluble FasL level	**PB:** Lymphoid cells larger than normal LGL with slightly basophilic cytoplasm-containing granules, hyperchromatic nucleus	CD2, cCD3ε, CD56, TIA-1, granzyme B, perfo-rin, EB; no expression of surface CD3 or CD57	*TCR* not clonally rear-ranged, EBV present in clonal episomal form
Adult T-cell leukemia	Endemic in Japan, the Caribbean basin, parts of Central Africa; linked to HTLV-1, hypercalcemia; hepatosplenomegaly, increased LDH, associated T-cell immuno-deficiency with opportunistic infections	**PB:** Medium- to large-sized cells with polylobated nucleus ("flower cells")	CD2, CD3, CD5, CD4, CD25; lack CD7 expres-sion	Clonally integrated HTLV-1, clonally rearranged *TCR*
Extranodal NK/T-cell lymphoma, nasal type	More prevalent in Asia, Mexico, Central and South America; extensive midfacial destructive lesions, other extranodal sites include skin, soft tissue, testis, GI tract	Extensive ulceration and necrosis, angiocentric and angiodestruc-tive growth pattern, hyper-chromatic nucleus, intermixed inflammatory cells	CD2, CD56, cCD3ε, granzyme B, TIA-1, perforin, surface CD3 not expressed	*TCR* not clonally rear-ranged, EBV present in clonal episomal form

Enteropathy-type T-cell lymphoma	Associated with celiac disease and ulcerative jejunitis	Ulcerating mucosal mass in jejunum or ileum, broad cytologic spectrum, intermixed inflammatory cells	CD3, CD8+/−, CD103, TIA-1, granzyme, perforin	Clonally rearranged *TCR*, HLA DQA1*0501, DQB1*0201 genotype of celiac disease
Hepatosplenic T-cell lymphoma	Peak incidence in adolescents and young adults, marked hepatosplenomegaly with lymphadenopathy, more common in patients with immunosuppression	Sinusoidal infiltration of liver, spleen, and bone marrow by monotonous small- to medium-sized cells	CD3, TCR-γ/δ, TIA-1, negative for CD4, CD8, TCR-αβ, and perforin	Clonally rearranged *TCR*, isochromosome 7q, trisomy 8
Subcutaneous panniculitis-like T-cell lymphoma	Multiple subcutaneous nodules, may be associated with hemophagocytic syndrome with pancytopenia, fever, and hepatosplenomegaly	Diffuse, lace-like infiltrate in subcutis without sparing septae; epidermis uninvolved; necrosis, karyorrhexis, rimming of fat cells	CD3, CD8, granzyme B, perforin, TIA-1	Clonally rearranged *TCR*
Mycosis fungoides	Long natural history, multiple skin lesions, patch, progressing to plaque, progressing to tumor, frequently on trunk	Epidermotropic infiltrate of tumor cells with "cerebriform" nuclei, Pautrier microabscesses	CD2, CD3, CD5, CD4, TCR-αβ; no expression of CD7	Clonally rearranged *TCR*
Sézary syndrome	Aggressive variant of mycosis fungoides; erythroderma, lymphadenopathy, and circulating Sézary cells	**PB:** Minimum of 1,000 Sézary cells per mm³, "cerebriform" nuclei	Increased CD4/CD8 ratio lacking expression of CD7	Clonally rearranged *TCR*
Angioimmunoblastic T-cell lymphoma	Immunodeficiency secondary to lymphoma, skin rash, edema, pleural effusion, ascites, cytopenia, polyclonal hypergammaglobulinemia, positive rheumatoid factor	Mixture of polymorphous lymphocytes some with clear cytoplasm, plasma cells, eosinophils, and immunoblasts; arborizing HEV; prominence of FDC meshwork outside follicles	CD2, CD3, CD4 with coexpression of CD10, follicular dendritic cells are highlighted by CD21, CD23, CD35, immunoblasts are CD20+ and EBV+	Clonally rearranged *TCR*, trisomy 3, trisomy 5, additional X chromosome

(continued)

TABLE 41.4 Characteristic Features of Different T- and NK-Cell Malignancies (*Continued*)

Disease	Clinical Presentation	Morphology	Immunophenotype	Genetics
Peripheral T-cell lymphoma, unspecified	Predominantly nodal-based lymphomas that cannot be better classified, generalized disease	Broad cytologic spectrum, T-zone variant with preservation of follicles, Lennert variant with many epithelioid clusters	CD2, CD3, mostly CD4, may express CD30	Clonally rearranged *TCR*
Anaplastic large cell lymphoma	10–30% of childhood lymphomas advanced stage (III or IV) with frequent extranodal involvement	Hallmark cells (large cells with abundant cytoplasm and horse-shoe-shaped nuclei)	CD30 (membrane and Golgi), ALK-1 (60–85%), EMA+, CD43, CD2, CD4	Clonally rearranged *TCR*; t(2;5) involving nucleophosmin and ALK

ALK-1 and ALK, anaplastic lymphoma kinase-1; BM, bone marrow; EBV, Epstein–Barr virus; EMA, epithelial membrane antigen; FasL, Fas ligand; FDC, follicular dendritic cells; GI, gastrointestinal; HEV, high endothelial vessels; HLA, human leukocyte antigen; HTLV, human T-lymphotropic virus; LDH, lactate dehydrogenase; LGL, large granular lymphocytes; NK, natural killer; PB, peripheral blood; TCL-1, T-cell leukemia/lymphoma-1; TCR, T-cell receptor; TIA, T-cell intracellular antigen.

TABLE 41.5 Criteria for the Diagnosis of Plasma Cell Myeloma

Panel: Revised International Myeloma Working Group diagnostic criteria

Symptomatic plasma cell myeloma

Clonal bone marrow plasma cells ≥10% or biopsy-proven bony or extramedullary plasmacytoma and any one or more of the following myeloma-defining events:

Evidence of end organ damage that can be attributed to the underlying plasma cell proliferative disorder, specifically: hypercalcemia, renal insufficiency, anemia, bone lesions.

Any one or more of the following biomarkers of malignancy:

Clonal bone marrow plasma cell percentage ≥60%

Involved: uninvolved serum free light chain ratio ≥100

>1 focal lesions on MRI studies

Asymptomatic (smoldering) plasma cell myeloma

Both criteria must be met:

Serum monoclonal protein (IgG or IgA) ≥30 g/L or urinary monoclonal protein ≥500 mg per 24 h and/or clonal bone marrow plasma cells 10–60%

Absence of myeloma-defining events or amyloidosis

TABLE 41.6 Commonly Occurring Cytogenetic Abnormalities in Plasma Cell Myeloma[a]

Abnormality	Occurrence (%)	Prognostic Implications
I. Numerical[b]		Favorable
a. Hyperdiploidy	61–68	Unfavorable
b. Hypodiploidy	10–30	
I. Complex		
Partial or complete deletion of 13 and 11q, del(17q13)	Ranging from 1–25	Unfavorable
t(11;14), t(6;14)[c]	cyclinD1 15–18%, D3 3%	Favorable
t(4;14), t(14;16), t(14;20)[c]	FGFR 15%, MAFB 2%	Unfavorable

[a]Up to 90% of cases show abnormalities using fluorescence in situ hybridization (FISH) techniques; by conventional cytogenetics, 30–50% of patients show an abnormal karyotype.
[b]Most common abnormalities are trisomy 3, 7, 9, and 11; monosomy 13; and, in females, monosomy X.
[c]t(4;14) and t(11;14) are the most common translocations; see text for the oncogenes.

TABLE 41.7 Diagnostic Criteria of Monoclonal Gammopathy of Uncertain Significance (MGUS) and Plasmacytoma (PC)

Type	Marrow Plasmacytosis	Serum M Component	Lytic Lesions	Organ or Tissue Impairment
MGUS	<10%	Less than myeloma levels (IgM/G/A <30 g/dL)	None	None
PC	None	Absent or low	Present	None

Ig, immunoglobulin.

of a monoclonal plasma cell proliferative disorder (serum or urine monoclonal protein, abnormal free light-chain ratio, or clonal plasma cells in the bone marrow).

F. **Immunophenotype.** Neoplastic plasma cells typically express monotypic cytoplasmic immunoglobulin and lack surface immunoglobulin expression. Most cases lack CD19 and CD20 expression, whereas CD79a, CD38, CD138 (syndecan-1), and MUM-1 are found in the majority of cases. CD56 is aberrantly expressed in up to 70% of myelomas. Expression of cyclin D1 is also a feature of plasma cells, specifically in multiple myeloma (see below). Other antigens that are aberrantly expressed and could be helpful in detection of minimal residual disease or targeted therapy include CD20, CD117, CD52, or CD10 (*Blood* 2008; 12:4017; *Am J Clin Pathol* 2004;121:482). CD56-negative myelomas show more extensive marrow infiltration, lower osteolytic potential, frequent plasmablastic morphology, and a tendency toward leukemic transformation (*Br J Haematol* 2002; 117:882).

G. **Plasma Cell Myeloma Genetics.** Plasma cell neoplasms demonstrate clonally rearranged immunoglobulin heavy and light chains by molecular studies; cytogenetic methods to detect chromosomal abnormalities include cytokine-stimulated bone marrow biopsy for conventional karyotyping and FISH. Combined, these modalities increase the frequency of detectable genetic aberrations in myeloma to over 90% (*Cancer Res* 2004; 64:1546). Complex karyotypes with multiple chromosomal gains and losses are the most frequent abnormalities, the most common being gains in chromosomes 3, 5, 7, 9, 11, 15, and 19 and losses in chromosomes 8, 13, 14, and X (*Blood* 1995;85:2490). Monosomy or partial deletion of 13 (13q14) is the most common structural chromosomal abnormality. In about 40% of cases, translocations involving one of five recurrent oncogenes are seen. The most common translocation is t(11;14)(q13;q32) involving the *BCL1* locus on chromosome 11q13 (*CYCLIN D1*) and the immunoglobulin heavy (*IgH*) chain locus on 14q23, which leads to overexpression of cyclin D1 (*J Clin Oncol* 2005;23:6333; *Brit J Hematol* 1998;101:189; *Blood* 2002;99:2185). Other translocation partners for the *IgH* locus include 4p16.3 (*FGFR-3* and *MMSET*), 6p21 (*CCND3*), 16q23 (*C-MAF*), and 20q11 (*MAFB*) (Table 41.6).

VIII. **CASTLEMAN DISEASE.** The Castleman disease is an important consideration in the differential diagnosis of lymphomas due to its clinical presentation. It can occur at any age but has a predilection for young adults, often presenting as a mass most often in the mediastinum, although cervical, abdominal, and axillary nodes may all be sites of origin (*Cancer* 1972;29:670; *Semin Diag Pathol* 1988;5:346; *Mod Pathol* 1992;5:525). In some cases, generalized lymphadenopathy with B-symptoms, anemia, thrombocytopenia, and pemphigus mimic the clinical presentation of lymphoma. Classically, the Castleman disease is divided into two clinical entities.

A. **Hyaline Vascular–Type Castleman Disease** shows capsular thickening and overt nodularity of lymph node architecture. The diagnostic features are generally seen in lymphoid follicles, namely hyperplasia and expanded mantle zones with lymphocytes arranged in concentric layers. The germinal centers appear regressed and vascularized, with some blood vessel that traverse tangentially to impart a lollipop appearance. Multiple germinal centers can be seen per follicle (e-**Figs. 41.30–41.32**). The paracortical areas are also highly vascularized, containing a mix of cells with an increased number of plasmacytoid/monocytoid lymphocytes accompanied in some cases by a variable increase in plasma cells. While immunophenotypic findings do not differentiate lymph node involvement by hyaline vascular Castleman disease from reactive follicles, a CD21 stain is especially helpful for demonstrating expanded concentric meshwork of follicular dendritic cells. However, ancillary studies (including flow cytometry and immunohistochemistry) must be performed must to exclude Hodgkin lymphoma, non-Hodgkin lymphoma, and plasma cell neoplasms. Surgical resection of the node involved is usually curative (*Virchows Arch A Pathol Anat Histopathol* 1993;423:369).

B. **Plasma Cell–Type Castleman Disease** is less common than the hyaline vascular type. It can be unicentric (localized to one site of presentation), although it more commonly presents as multicentric disease (systemic illness with malaise, fevers, night sweats, and cytopenias). Polyclonal plasmacytosis in the bone marrow, hypergammaglobulinemia, and elevated IL-6 levels are important clues to diagnosis; elevated IL-6 levels are more common in the unicentric plasma cell type. Histologically, the paracortical regions show marked polyclonal plasmacytosis (monoclonal lambda-light chains can be seen in up to 30% of cases); the nodal architecture is otherwise well preserved with follicles varying from reactive to regressed. A variety of other disease entities need to be excluded using appropriate ancillary studies including HIV lymphadenopathy, autoimmune/chronic inflammatory conditions, other lymphomas (most importantly HHV-8–associated plasmablastic lymphoma), and even metastatic carcinoma. An association with POEMS syndrome has been noted (see above); HHV-8 plays a pathogenetic role in HIV- and non-HIV–associated settings and can often be documented in lesional tissue by immunohistochemical stains (ORF73/latency-associated nuclear antigen-1) although an HHV-8 association is more commonly seen in cases with monoclonal plasmacytosis (*Human Pathol* 1985;16:162; *Histopathology* 1989;14:11; *AIDS* 1996;10:61). While unicentric plasma cell–type Castleman disease can be cured with surgical excision, systemic therapy may be required in multicentric forms.

IX. **HODGKIN LYMPHOMA.** Hodgkin lymphoma typically presents as a primarily nodal disease characterized by a predominance of reactive cells with a paucity of neoplastic Reed–Sternberg (R-S) cells or variants. Hodgkin lymphoma comprises two distinct entities: classic Hodgkin lymphoma (CHL) and nodular lymphocyte-predominant Hodgkin lymphoma (NLPHL). These two entities differ in their clinical appearance, morphology, immunoglobulin transcription of the neoplastic cells, and immunophenotype.

A. **Classic Hodgkin Lymphoma (CHL)** accounts for ~95% of Hodgkin lymphoma and is subdivided into four categories: nodular sclerosis (~70%), mixed cellularity (~20% to 25%), lymphocyte-rich (~5%), and lymphocyte depleted (<5%). The neoplastic cell is the classical R-S cell or its variants (mononuclear forms, mummified forms, or lacunar cells).

1. Nodular sclerosis CHL commonly presents with a mediastinal mass. Histology reveals scattered R-S cells embedded in a mixed inflammatory background of mostly T-lymphocytes, plasma cells, eosinophils, neutrophils, and histiocytes, compartmentalized into nodules by thick strands of collagen fibrosis (**e-Figs. 41.33–41.35**).

2. Mixed cellularity CHL presents with scattered R-S cells in a diffuse or vaguely nodular mixed inflammatory background without nodular sclerosing fibrosis.

3. In lymphocyte-rich CHL, the nonneoplastic cellular background is composed of predominantly T-lymphocytes. Other inflammatory cells are rare.

4. Lymphocyte-depleted CHL is rare and occurs most commonly in association with HIV infection. Histologically, sheets of R-S cells predominate without a significant lymphocytic or mixed inflammatory infiltrate.

   The main clinical findings of CHL at diagnosis are painless peripheral lymphadenopathy, most commonly involving the cervical region, and constitutional symptoms such as fever, night sweats, weight loss, and infections due to immunosuppression. Many of the pathologic and clinical features reflect an abnormal immune response due to the wide variety of cytokines and chemokines (Table 41.8) produced by the R-S cells (*Blood* 2002;99:4283). The etiology of CHL is largely unknown. Studies based on the month of diagnosis have revealed peaks in February and March, and the lymphoma appears to be more prevalent in adolescents and young adults with higher socioeconomic status (*Hematol Oncol* 2004;22:11). The association between EBV and CHL has been demonstrated in numerous seroepidemiologic studies in which antibody titers to EBV and viral capsid antigens have been consistently found to be higher in cases compared with controls. There also have been reports of clustering of CHL within the same family, especially among siblings of same sex and close age. Certain human leukocyte antigen (HLA) types such as A1, B5, and B18 appear also to be clearly associated with this lymphoma (*Hematol Oncol* 2004;22:11).

B. **Nodular Lymphocyte-Predominant Hodgkin Lymphoma (NLPHL)** is characterized by scattered large neoplastic L&H cells (lymphocytic and/or histiocytic cells, popcorn cells)

TABLE 41.8 Role of Cytokines in Classic Hodgkin Lymphoma

Cytokine	Biologic Activity	Comments
IL-1	Potent proinflammatory cytokine; induction of fever and acute phase proteins	Associated with B-symptoms
IL-5	Eosinophil differentiation, proliferation, and activation	Associated with blood and tissue eosinophilia
IL-6	Plasma cell differentiation, stimulation of IL-1, and TNF-α production	Associated with thrombocytosis and tissue plasmacytosis
IL-8	Neutrophil recruitment factor	Associated with tissue neutrophilia
IL-9	T-cell and mast cell growth factor	May be acting as a growth factor for Reed–Sternberg cells
IL-10	Impaired immune response	Associated with EBV+ cases
IL-13	B-cell proliferation and survival; Ig class switching to IgG4 and IgE	Autocrine growth factor for Reed–Sternberg cells
TGF-β	Inhibition of IL-2R upregulation and IL-2-dependent T- and B-cell proliferation, potent stimulator of fibroblast proliferation, and collagen synthesis	Associated with tissue fibrosis

EBV, Epstein–Barr virus; Ig, immunoglobulin; IL-2R, interleukin 2 receptor; TGF, transforming growth factor; TNF-α, tumor necrosis factor-α.

residing in nodular meshwork of follicular dendritic processes, filled with nonneoplastic lymphocytes mostly of B-cell lineage (e-Figs. 41.36 and 41.37). Clinically, patients present with localized peripheral lymphadenopathy. The disease develops slowly with fairly frequent relapses, but remains responsive to chemotherapy and usually is not fatal. About 3% to 5% of cases evolve into DLBCL.

C. **Pathophysiology.** The cellular origin of neoplastic cells in both CHL and NLPHL was finally determined when clonally rearranged immunoglobulin genes were amplified from purified Hodgkin cells obtained by microdissection (*Proc Natl Acad Sci U S A* 1994;91:10962). In addition, the detection of somatic mutations within the rearranged immunoglobulin genes suggests a germinal center or postgerminal center B-cell to be the precursor of Hodgkin cells. Although tumor cells of both CHL and NLPHL harbor rearranged immunoglobulin genes, these are not expressed in CHL due to lack of immunoglobulin messenger RNA (mRNA). Further studies have shown that the absence of immunoglobulin transcription is caused by inactivation of the immunoglobulin promoter through impaired or absent activation of the octamer-dependent transcription factor OCT2 and/or its coactivator BOB.1. Immunohistochemistry for OCT2 and BOB.1 usually is negative in classic R-S cells, unlike L&H cells in NLPHL that express these two markers (*Blood* 2001;91:496).

Normally, when B-cells are no longer capable of expressing immunoglobulin they rapidly undergo apoptosis. However, even though classical R-S cells do not express immunoglobulin chains due to the absence of immunoglobulin mRNA, they are resistant to apoptosis. One mechanism preventing apoptosis is believed to be persistent activation of the nuclear transcription factor nuclear factor kappa B (NFκB) in classic R-S cells caused by mutations within members of the IκB family (which are natural inhibitors of NFκB) or by aberrant activation of IκB kinase (*Lancet Oncol* 2004;5:11).

D. **Immunophenotype Studies.** Immunohistochemistry markers important in the diagnosis of Hodgkin lymphoma are:

1. CD30 (expressed on classic R-S cells in ~98% of cases)
2. CD15 (expressed on classic R-S cells in ~80% of cases; also in neutrophils, monocytes, and promyelocytes)

3. CD20 (may be expressed in a small subset of classic R-S cells; strongly positive in L&H cells, positive in intermixed nonneoplastic small B-lymphocytes)
4. CD45 (LCA) (negative in classic R-S cells, strongly positive in L&H cells, positive in accompanying nonneoplastic inflammatory cells)
5. CD79a (negative in classic R-S cells, strongly positive in L&H cells, positive in intermixed nonneoplastic small B-lymphocytes)
6. Epithelial membrane antigen (EMA) (negative in classic R-S cells, positive in L&H cells in ~50% of cases)
7. BCL-6 (positive in L&H cells in nearly all cases)
8. CD3 (positive in intermixed T-lymphocytes; L&H cells are ringed by CD3+ T-cells)
9. CD57 (positive in intermixed cytotoxic T-lymphocytes; L&H cells are ringed by CD57+ T-cells)
10. BSAP (product of the *PAX*-5 gene; positive in both classic R-S and L&H cells)
11. EBV (positive in classic R-S cells in ~40% of cases)
12. OCT2 (positive in L&H cells, negative in classic R-S cells)
13. BOB.1 (positive in L&H cells, negative in classic R-S cells)

X. STAGING OF LYMPHOMAS AND PLASMA CELL MYELOMA

A. Hodgkin and Non-Hodgkin Lymphomas. Formal documentation of anatomic extent of disease is required in all patients newly diagnosed with lymphoma prior to therapeutic intervention. Clinical staging takes into account variables such as medical history and physical examination, imaging studies, blood chemistry determination, complete blood count, erythrocyte sedimentation rate (in Hodgkin lymphomas), and bone marrow biopsy. If a patient presents with relapsed disease, determination of anatomic extent of the disease is recommended but a new clinical stage is usually not assigned. The most recent official system adopted by the 2017 Tumor, Node, Metastasis (TNM) American Joint Committee on Cancer (AJCC) (Amin MB, Edge S, Greene F, et al., eds. *AJCC Cancer Staging Manual*, 8th ed. New York: Springer, 2017) for anatomic staging classification for Hodgkin and non-Hodgkin lymphomas is the Lugano classification (see Table 41.9).

TABLE 41.9	Lugano Classification for Hodgkin and Non-Hodgkin Lymphoma[a]
Limited stage	
I	Involvement of a single lymphatic site (i.e., nodal region, Waldeyer ring, thymus, or spleen)
IE	Single extralymphatic site in the absence of nodal involvement
II	Involvement of two or more lymph node regions on the same side of the diaphragm
IIE	Contiguous extralymphatic extension from a nodal site (with or without involvement of other lymph node regions on the same side of the diaphragm)
II bulky	Stage II with disease bulk[b]
Advanced stage	
III	Involvement of lymph node regions on both sides of the diaphragm; nodes above the diaphragm with spleen involvement
IV	Diffuse or disseminated involvement of one or more extralymphatic organs, with or without associated lymph node involvement; or noncontiguous extralymphatic organ involvement in conjunction with nodal stage II disease; or any extralymphatic organ involvement in nodal stage III disease. Stage IV includes any involvement of the CSF, bone marrow, liver, or lungs (other than by direct extension in stage IIE disease)

[a]Adapted from Cheson BD, Fisher RI, Barrington SF, et al. Recommendations for initial evaluation, staging, and response assessment of Hodgin and non-Hodgkin lymphona: the Lugano classification. *J Clin Oncol* 2014;32:3059 and *AJCC Cancer Staging Manual*, 8th ed. New York: Springer, 2017.
[b]The definition of disease bulk varies; in Hodgkin lymphoma it is defined as a mass greater than 1/3 of the thoracic diameter on CT of the chest or a mass >10 cm; for non-Hodgkin lymphoma definitions of bulk vary by lymphoma histology.

TABLE 41.10 Staging Systems for Plasma Cell Myeloma

| | | Durie–Salmon Staging System[a] | | | | RISS Criteria[b] | | | |
| | | Serum | | Serum/Urine M-Immunoglobulins | | | | | |
Stage	Hb	Calcium	Osteolytic Lesion	M-Immunoglobulins	Protein	β2M	Albumin	LDH	Cytogenetics
I	>10 g/dL	≤12 mg/dL	Normal or single lesion	IgG <5 g/dL IgA <3 g/dL	Bence Jones protein <4 g/24 h	<3.5 mg/dL	≥3.5 g/dL	Normal	No high-risk
II	Not stage I or III								
III	<8.5 g/dL	>12 mg/dL	Advanced multiple lytic lesions	>7 g/dL >5 g/dL	>12 g/24 h	>5.5 mg/dL	—	High[c]	High-risk[d]

β2M, β2 microglobulin; Hb, hemoglobin; Ig, immunoglobulin; LDH, lactate dehydrogenase; "—", not required for staging.

[a]Durie–Salmon subclassifications: A. Relatively normal renal function (serum creatinine value <2.0 mg/dL); B. Abnormal renal function (serum creatinine value ≥2.0 mg/dL).

[b]Palumbo A, Avet-Loiseau H, Oliva S, et al. Revised international staging system for multiple myeloma: a report from International Myeloma Working Group. *J Clin Oncol* 2015;33:2863

[c]Per RISS criteria, the presence of >5.5 mg/dL β2M with either elevated LDH or high-risk cytogenetics will result in stage III disease.

[d]High-risk cytogenetics consist of one or more of the following: del(17p), t(4;14), or t(14;16).

Definition of lymph node regions is based on the definitions proposed by the Rye Symposium in 1965 and used by the Lugano system. The currently accepted classification groups of lymph nodes are right cervical (includes cervical, supraclavicular, occipital, and preauricular nodes); left cervical; right axillary; left axillary; right infraclavicular; left infraclavicular; mediastinal; right hilar; left hilar; para-aortic; mesenteric; right pelvic; left pelvic; right inguinofemoral; and left inguinofemoral.

B. Staging of Plasma Cell Myeloma. The AJCC recommends the Durie–Salmon staging system for plasma cell myeloma (Amin MB, Edge S, Greene F, et al., eds. *AJCC Cancer Staging Manual*, 8th ed. New York: Springer, 2017). This system takes into account various complete blood count variables, blood chemistries, M-protein levels, and imaging studies.

A more comprehensive system that incorporates recent cytogenetics advances is the Revised International Staging System (RISS). This system uses three blood parameters, β_2 microglobulin (β_2M), albumin, and lactate dehydrogenase along with high-risk cytogenetics findings for risk stratification. The RISS has been proven to be useful for staging myeloma and is currently recommended by the AJCC for widespread use. A comparison of these two myeloma staging systems is depicted in Table 41.10.

Lymph Node Cytopathology

Cody Weimholt

I. INTRODUCTION. The lymphoid cells (both benign and malignant) from fine needle aspiration (FNA) specimens characteristically are singly distributed with scant cytoplasm, and the background frequently shows lymphoglandular bodies (cytoplasmic fragments of disrupted lymphocytes) and lymphoid tangles (small fragments of lymph tissue with prominent crush artifact). Aspiration of a quiescent benign lymph node shows a monotonous population of small, mature lymphocytes without atypia.

Proper triage of a lymph node FNA at the time of immediate evaluation requires the distinction between a benign lymphadenopathy or lymphadenitis, a lymphomatous process, and a metastasis from a known or unknown primary in order to direct additional passes for appropriate studies. For metastatic malignancy, IHC is imperative to identify the primary site, therefore additional direct passes for cell block are essential. Identifying the etiology of an infectious lymphadenitis requires culture as well as cell block for IHC and special stains. Diagnosis of lymphoma by FNA requires a multifaceted approach that couples cytomorphology with ancillary studies including flow cytometry, IHC, FISH, cytogenetics, and molecular studies. While controversial, FNA alone can successfully subclassify many lymphomas, with a reported accuracy rate of 51% to 95%, although notable limitations exist (*Acta Ctyol* 2016;60:372). Using a combined approach of FNA plus core needle biopsy, diagnosis of NHL has greater than 96% sensitivity and specificity when compared with excisional biopsy (*Am J Clin Pathol* 2011;135:4). A pattern-based approach organized around lymphoid cell size and uniformity is commonly utilized to determine the exact ancillary studies needed to subclassify a lymphoma.

II. BENIGN LYMPHADENOPATHIES

A. Reactive Hyperplasias. This finding is typically nonspecific since an etiology is unknown in most cases. The aspirate is characterized by a polymorphous population of lymphoid cells with variable size and shape that predominantly contains small lymphocytes with smooth nuclear contours and coarse chromatin, intermixed with scattered intermediate cells and large immunoblast-like cells. Scattered plasma cells, histiocytes, and tingible body macrophages are present. Lymphohistiocytic aggregates (follicular center fragments) are also seen, consisting of collections of lymphoid cells and histiocytes held together by dendritic reticular cells (**e-Fig. 41.38**) (*Acta Cytol* 1987;31:8). Care must be exercised as some malignant processes involve a reactive background.

B. **Lymphadenitis.** Etiologies are diverse and can be infectious (e.g., fungal, mycobacterial, viral) or noninfectious (e.g., sarcoidosis, various autoimmune diseases, drugs). Clusters of neutrophils are indicative of suppurative lymphadenopathy. Collections of epithelioid histiocytes are consistent with granulomatous lymphadenitis (e-**Fig. 41.39**) (*Sarcoidosis* 1987;4:38). Fungal hyphae and yeast forms can occasionally be identified as negative images on Diff-Quik–stained smears (e-**Fig. 41.40**).

III. LYMPHOMAS WITH A SMALL CELL PATTERN

A. **Small Lymphocytic Lymphoma.** The aspirate contains a monotonous population of small lymphoid cells with round nuclear contours, characteristic checkerboard-like clumpy chromatin, and indistinct nucleoli (e-**Fig. 41.41**). Scattered large prolymphocytes/paraimmunoblasts with vesicular chromatin, prominent central nucleoli, and pale cytoplasm are present. Richter transformation will appear as a large cell or pleomorphic pattern.

B. **Lymphoplasmacytic Lymphoma.** The smear contains a mixed population of small lymphoid cells, plasmacytoid cells, and plasma cells.

C. **Follicular Lymphoma.** The aspirate is composed predominantly of small centrocytes (that have irregular and grooved nuclear membranes) intermixed with scattered centroblasts (that have a large noncleaved nuclei with multiple small peripheral nucleoli) and immunoblasts (that have single prominent central nucleolus) (e-**Fig. 41.42**). As the grade increases the aspirate becomes more and more polymorphous in appearance which may mimic reactive hyperplasia. Although the cytologic criteria for grading follicular lymphoma are not well established, the percentage of centroblasts on smears has been proposed as a basis for grading by several groups (*Clin Pathol* 2002;117:880; *Am J Clin Pathol* 1997;108:143).

D. **Mantle Cell Lymphoma.** The aspirate is composed of a monotonous population of small to intermediate-sized lymphoid cells with variable nuclear membrane contour irregularity, dispersed chromatin, and inconspicuous nucleoli (e-**Fig. 41.43**) (*Cancer* 1999;87:216). Aspirates with blastoid transformation appear as a monotonous large cell pattern.

E. **Nodal Marginal Zone B-Cell Lymphoma.** The aspirate contains a polymorphous lymphoid population composed predominately of small lymphoid cells with round nuclei and clumpy chromatin, with scattered plasmacytoid cells and immunoblast-like large cells. Some intermediate-sized lymphoid cells that have a monocytoid appearance and exhibit a moderate amount of pale cytoplasm are also present (e-**Fig. 41.44**).

IV. LYMPHOMAS WITH A MONOTONOUS INTERMEDIATE TO LARGE CELL PATTERN

A. **Lymphoblastic Lymphoma.** The aspirate is composed of a monotonous population of intermediate-sized lymphoid cells with fine granular chromatin, irregular nuclear membrane contours, inconspicuous nucleoli, and scant basophilic cytoplasm (e-**Fig. 41.45**). Mitoses are frequently identified.

B. **Burkitt Lymphoma.** The aspirate contains a monotonous population of intermediate-sized lymphoid cells with round nuclei, finely dispersed chromatin, and multiple distinct nucleoli. The cytoplasm is scant, deep blue, and contains small lipid-filled vacuoles (e-**Fig. 41.46**). Tingible body macrophages and mitosis are prominent and are indicative of brisk cell turnover.

C. **Diffuse Large B-Cell Lymphoma/High-Grade B-Cell Lymphoma.** The aspirate shows a monotonous population of large atypical lymphoid cells. The centroblastic variant contains centroblasts with irregular nuclear membrane contours, coarse chromatin, and multiple small nucleoli (e-**Fig. 41.47**). The immunoblastic variant shows immunoblasts with irregular nuclear membrane contours, open chromatin, and single prominent nucleoli. Flow cytometry occasionally results as false negative due to cell fragility. The T-cell/histiocyte-rich B-cell lymphoma (THRBCL) variant is composed predominantly of small mature lymphocytes and rare large immature lymphoid cells with polymorphic nuclei and prominent nucleoli; the cytologic diagnosis of this variant is challenging.

D. **Peripheral T-Cell Lymphoma, Unspecified Type.** The aspirate is polymorphic and contains scattered large atypical lymphocytes with convoluted nuclear membranes. The background shows a reactive pattern and is composed of small mature lymphocytes, plasma cells, neutrophils, eosinophils, and macrophages.

E. **Myeloid Sarcoma** is an extramedullary solid collection of myeloid cells. The disease can present in a lymph node and may be a harbinger of leukemia or evidence of relapsed disease. Aspirates show tumor cells in any stage of myeloid differentiation ranging from blasts to more mature myeloid forms; however, in some cases myeloid differentiation may be entirely absent.

V. LYMPHOMAS WITH A PLEOMORPHIC PATTERN

A. **Anaplastic Large Cell Lymphoma.** The aspirate shows both singly dispersed and poorly cohesive groups of malignant cells with large and pleomorphic nuclei, prominent nucleoli, and a moderate amount of cytoplasm. Horseshoe- and "donut"-shaped nuclei, as well as binucleated and multinucleated R-S–like tumor cells, are also present. Mistaking this entity for carcinoma is a diagnostic pitfall due to the cellular cohesion and pleomorphism.

B. **Hodgkin Lymphoma.** The aspirate of CHL contains rare to scattered R-S cells. The classic binucleated R-S cells have markedly enlarged nuclei, macronucleoli, and a moderate amount basophilic cytoplasm (e-Fig. 41.48). The mononuclear variant has cells with markedly enlarged, irregular, and multilobated nuclei with macronucleoli (e-Fig. 41.49). The characteristic reactive lymphoid background includes mainly mature lymphocytes, scattered eosinophils, neutrophils, plasma cells, and occasional epithelioid histiocytes (e-Fig. 41.49) (*J Clin Pathol* 1986;86:286). Diagnosis can be challenging due to a scarcity of the R-S cells, and flow cytometry is typically not helpful. IHC is a necessity as it yields a positive predictive value over 90% in some studies (*Cytopathology* 1994;5:226; *Acta Cytol* 2001;45:300). The diagnosis of NLPHL from FNA specimens is usually not possible as the distinction from THRBCL is largely based on architecture.

VI. MISCELLANEOUS LESIONS

A. **Thymoma.** FNA of mediastinal lesions designated as "lymph node" must be interpreted with caution. A thymoma shows a pleomorphic pattern consisting of large neoplastic thymic epithelial cells with prominent nucleoli in a background of numerous small lymphocytes. This can be mistaken for T-cell lymphoblastic lymphoma, Hodgkin lymphoma, or primary mediastinal DLBCL.

B. **Plasma Cell Neoplasms** uncommonly involve lymph nodes and are typically a sign of advanced extramedullary spread of a known multiple myeloma. FNA shows numerous well-differentiated plasma cells; however, immature, plasmablastic, or anaplastic variants can prove challenging to identify.

C. **Histiocytic Lesions.** Aspirates in these lesions display characteristic histiocytic cytomorphology (large, elongated nuclei with small nucleoli and moderate to ample amounts of cytoplasm) and variable degrees of atypia, depending on the specific lesion. IHC is required for diagnosis.

VII. METASTATIC MALIGNANCY.
The most common indication for lymph node FNA is metastatic malignancy, for which the reported sensitivity of accurate diagnosis is over 90% with a specificity of over 98% (*Diagn Cytopathol* 2003;28:175; *Cytopathol* 1996;15:382). The aspirate shows a nonlymphoid population of cells with malignant cytologic features, typically seen as cohesive clusters or fragments, but not infrequently as singly dispersed cells in a pattern mimicking a lymphoma. An absence of a background of lymphocytes and nodal elements is important to report if it is uncertain whether the epithelial malignancy represents a nodal metastasis; examples include breast cancers present in the axillary tail which may be mistaken clinically for axillary nodal metastases, and hilar lung masses which may represent central tumors versus metastatic involvement of hilar nodes. In the case of nodal effacement by tumor this distinction is not possible.

ACKNOWLEDGMENT

The authors thank Julie Kunkel for her contribution to the previous edition of this chapter.

SUGGESTED READINGS

Murphy KM, Weaver C. *Janeway's Immunobiology*, 9th ed. New York: W. W. Norton & Company; 2016.

Pambuccian SE, Bardales RH. *Lymph Node Cytopathology*. New York: Springer; 2011.

Swerdlow SH, Campo E, Harris NL, et al., eds. *WHO Classification of Tumours of Haematopoietic and Lymphoid Tissues*. Lyon, France: IARC Press; 2017.

Wieczorek TJ, Wakely PE Jr. Lymph nodes. In: Cibas ES, Sucatman BS, eds. *Cytology: Diagnostic Principles and Clinical Correlates*. 4th ed. Philadelphia, PA: Elsevier Saunders; 2014.

Bone Marrow Pathology

John L. Frater

I. **NORMAL GROSS AND MICROSCOPIC ANATOMY.** The bone marrow is composed of cells derived from a variety of lineages including stromal cells, adipocytes, lymphocytes, and hematopoietic precursors. The most frequently sampled areas are the posterior superior iliac crest and, less frequently, the sternum and long bones. The bone marrow has an orderly microscopic anatomy. The most superficial part consists of a layer of dense cortical bone with an adjacent cover of dense fibrous periosteum. Deep to the cortex are the bony trabeculae, which consist of thin trabecular bone and the marrow cavity itself. The marrow cavity contains islands of maturing hematopoietic cells with intervening areas of fat, the latter of which increases with age.

The cellularity of the bone marrow is defined as the percentage of the marrow cavity composed of hematopoietic cells. In biopsies from the posterior iliac crest, marrow cellularity decreases with age, and is expressed by the following formula:

$$\text{Marrow cellularity} = (100 - \text{patient age})\% \pm 20\%.$$

Thus for example a 50-year-old individual would be expected to have a marrow cellularity of approximately 100% to 50% ± 20%, or 30% to 70%.

Normally, maturing myeloid and erythroid elements occupy different regions of the marrow cavity. Myeloid precursors lie adjacent to the trabecular bone, and erythroid elements form "islands" of cells between trabeculae. The ratio of myeloid to erythroid elements is approximately 2:1. Megakaryocytes are irregularly distributed throughout the bone marrow. Under normal circumstances they are not present in clusters.

It is important to be cognizant of the multidisciplinary nature of hematopathology. Diagnoses in bone marrow pathology are not generally the product of morphologic analysis of the bone marrow core biopsy, peripheral blood, and bone marrow aspirate smears alone. Clinical history may be extremely important in separating morphologically similar diseases and should be provided by the patient's physicians. Also, the pertinent features of the physical examination, such as lymphadenopathy, splenomegaly, or hepatomegaly are important. Other clinical laboratory information, such as complete blood counts and serum and/or urine protein electrophoresis, are often of interest. Radiographic data are of importance, particularly in the evaluation of a patient with a monoclonal protein.

II. **GROSS EXAMINATION AND TISSUE SAMPLING.** The same pathologist should review both the bone marrow aspirate smears and core biopsies whenever possible to avoid ambiguities or outright contradictions. The bone marrow aspirate is generally performed before the biopsy. There are two kinds of aspirate smears: smears prepared directly from the specimen without pretreatment, and smears prepared from concentrated aspirate fluid. Concentrated bone marrow aspirate smears and touch preparations prepared from the bone marrow core biopsy are particularly useful in the evaluation of specimens diluted with peripheral blood. Three to five of the smears are stained using the Wright–Giemsa or similar technique, one is stained for iron using the Prussian blue technique, and additional unstained smears are reserved for ancillary techniques such as fluorescence in situ hybridization (FISH), if necessary. Although examination of bone marrow cells with enzyme cytochemistry is likely to be rendered obsolete in the coming years, its use is still highly recommended by the World Health Organization (WHO) committee for the diagnosis of acute myeloid leukemia, and high-quality aspirate smears should be reserved for this purpose when an acute myelogenous leukemia is suspected. Additional bone marrow aspirates are obtained for flow cytometric, cytogenetic, and/or molecular genetic studies. Aspirate smears are generally reviewed using high power (600× to 1,000×) and are important for evaluating individual cell detail. However, because the process of aspiration disrupts cell cohesion, the relationship of the various cell types and the marrow cellularity cannot be reliably assessed. An adequate bone marrow core biopsy adds this important information.

III. **DIAGNOSTIC FEATURES OF COMMON BENIGN DISEASES.** The number and scope of nonneoplastic bone marrow disorders are vast. Emphasis is given to commonly encountered bone marrow diseases and conditions that may simulate neoplasia.

A. **Megaloblastic Anemia.** It is often not necessary to perform a bone marrow biopsy in patients who present with anemia, because the most common forms of anemia (iron deficiency, megaloblastic, and anemia of chronic disease) may be diagnosed by laboratory analysis of the peripheral blood, clinical history, and response to iron, vitamin B12, and/or folate replacement. Bone marrow biopsy is performed for patients with anemia that is unexplained or therapeutically resistant.

It is important to note that megaloblastic anemia may simulate a neoplastic condition, particularly a myelodysplastic syndrome (MDS). Patients with megaloblastic anemia may present with marked cytopenias and pronounced dyspoiesis (e-**Figs. 42.1** and **42.2**). Clues to discriminate this benign condition from an MDS include normal blast percentage, absence of karyotypic abnormalities, and improvement of cytopenias following administration of vitamin B12/folate in megaloblastic anemia. Also, the degree of dyspoiesis in megaloblastic anemia often exceeds that encountered in most cases of neoplastic myelodysplasia.

B. **Benign Causes of Lymphocytosis.** Numerous benign conditions may cause a transient increase in benign lymphocytes in the peripheral blood and may simulate chronic lymphocytic leukemia/small lymphocytic lymphoma (CLL/SLL), T-cell large granular lymphocytic leukemia, or other lymphoid leukemias. Stress lymphocytosis is a transient increase in morphologically normal peripheral blood lymphocytes encountered in individuals subjected to physiologic stresses, including individuals presenting to hospital emergency departments. An absolute increase in lymphocytes accompanied by "reactive" forms with increased basophilic cytoplasm and inconspicuous nucleoli may be seen in patients infected with the Epstein–Barr virus (EBV; e.g., infectious mononucleosis) or, less commonly, cytomegalovirus or other viral pathogens. Interestingly, in cases of EBV infection the virus particles are present in morphologically normal lymphocytes, and the reactive lymphocytes represent cytotoxic T-cells directed at the infected cells. Correlation with serum viral antibody titers is useful in arriving at the correct diagnosis and in avoiding unnecessary procedures such as bone marrow and lymph node biopsies. Many other infections are associated with lymphocytosis, including pertussis, in which the lymphocytes have characteristic clefted nuclei and thus may simulate peripheral blood involvement by a non-Hodgkin lymphoma. Persistent polyclonal B-cell hyperplasia, as its name implies, is often of longer duration than other benign forms of lymphocytosis. It frequently affects women who smoke, and is associated with the human leukocyte antigen (HLA)-DR7 phenotype (*Hematopathology. Foundations in Diagnostic Pathology.* Philadelphia, PA: Elsevier; 2007;55–66).

C. **The Granulocytic "Left Shift."** Other cases of leukocytosis represent a granulocytic shift to immaturity (colloquially known by the archaic term "left shift," referring to the traditional placement of immature myeloid cell percentages to the left of neutrophils in classical peripheral blood smear reports). Because many of these cases also demonstrate eosinophilia and/or basophilia, it is important to distinguish them from neoplastic conditions, in particular chronic myelogenous leukemia or other myeloproliferative neoplasms. Most commonly, especially in hospitalized populations, a granulocytic shift to immaturity represents an acute response to bacterial or other infections. Transient increases in mature demarginated neutrophils may also follow surgery or other physical trauma. Unusual causes of increased peripheral blood neutrophils with or without immature granulocytes include chronic idiopathic neutrophilia, hereditary neutrophilia, and leukocyte adhesion factor deficiency.

D. **Benign Causes of Erythrocytosis.** Under normal conditions, the circulating red blood cell mass is maintained at a constant level by the actions of the cytokine erythropoietin, which is produced by renal peritubular cells. An absolute increase in circulating red blood cells (polycythemia) may be primary (most commonly due to the myeloproliferative neoplasm polycythemia vera) or secondary (due to increased production of erythropoietin). Thus, in establishing a diagnosis of polycythemia vera, a number of conditions must be excluded that may cause secondary erythrocytosis, including smoking, living at high altitude, and high oxygen-affinity hemoglobins.

E. **Benign Causes of Thrombocytosis.** There are numerous causes of benign thrombocytosis (defined as a peripheral blood platelet count in excess of 450×10^9/L). Common reactive causes of peripheral thrombocytosis include infection, inflammation, malignancy, iron deficiency, hemolytic anemia, postsplenectomy, recovery from thrombocytopenia, and tissue injury due to surgery or burns (Winthobe's Clinical Hematology, 13th ed. Philadelphia, PA: Wolters Kluwer; 2014; 1122–1123).

F. **Aplastic Anemia.** Bone marrow aplasia is usually associated with bi- or pancytopenia rather than isolated anemia, and may be identified in a variety of clinical settings. It may occur secondary to a variety of drugs, most commonly chemotherapeutic agents, benzene, alcohol, and arsenic. It may also occur secondary to exposure to radiation, viral infection (e.g., viral hepatitis, EBV), or tuberculosis. An important cause of infection-mediated isolated anemia is infection with parvovirus B19. Other causes of bone marrow hypocellularity include paroxysmal nocturnal hemoglobinuria, Fanconi anemia, dyskeratosis congenita, and other very rare inherited bone marrow failure syndromes (*Hematology; Am Soc Hematol Educ Program* 2017;2017:79–87).

The common morphologic finding in bone marrow biopsies from patients with aplastic anemia is marked panhypoplasia; a notable exception is parvovirus infection in which there is selective suppression of erythroid precursors. These specimens should be carefully scrutinized for evidence of significant dyspoiesis or increased blasts, because a minority of MDSs and acute myeloid leukemias present with markedly hypocellular bone marrow biopsies. These specimens should also be examined for evidence of infection as evidenced by granuloma formation in the case of tuberculosis, or intranuclear inclusions in the case of viral infection. The inclusions of parvovirus are ill defined and are localized to the nuclei of proerythroblasts and can be illuminated by immunohistochemistry against viral capsid proteins.

G. **Serous Degeneration** (serous atrophy) is a pattern of bone marrow injury most often associated with acquired immunodeficiency syndrome (AIDS) and states of chronic nutritional deficiency such as starvation, chronic alcoholism, and anorexia nervosa (*Histopathology* 2000;37:199). The primary morphologic finding in the bone marrow is stromal edema with associated microvesicular change. The bone marrow is hypocellular in these regions due to loss of normal hematopoietic elements. These findings may be focal, alternating with regions of relatively preserved normal hematopoiesis. It is important to recognize that the subcortical bone marrow is normally hypocellular and occasionally demonstrates edema, possibly related to trauma associated with the biopsy procedure, and thus may mimic serous degeneration.

H. **Granulomas** may be encountered in bone marrow core biopsies and are occasionally noted in aspirate smears. Granulomas may be quite subtle and are usually composed of admixed histiocytes, lymphocytes, and plasma cells. Some granulomas contain foci of necrosis and infiltrating neutrophils. The causes of granuloma formation in the bone marrow are similar to those in other sites: the most common etiologies are infectious, autoimmune, or idiopathic. In addition, granulomas are occasionally encountered in the bone marrow of patients with Hodgkin lymphoma, although their presence is not indicative of marrow involvement by disease. Because it is impossible to predict with certainty the etiology of bone marrow granulomas, their presence usually warrants the use of stains to aid in the identification of acid-fast bacilli and fungi. However, it should be noted that special stains are far less sensitive than microbiologic culture in the detection of most infectious agents in the bone marrow, so microbiologic analysis of fresh bone marrow tissue is recommended when an infectious etiology is considered. An important item in the morphologic differential diagnosis of granulomas is the lipogranuloma, which is generally considered to be nonpathologic and consists of a collection of histiocytes and lymphocytes surrounding an area of fat demonstrating microvesicular change.

I. **Benign Lymphoid Aggregates** are present in the bone marrow of healthy individuals and at increased incidence in elderly individuals. Because they are common, it is important to recognize the attributes of benign aggregates and distinguish them from their malignant counterparts. Benign aggregates are often well circumscribed and are small to medium sized. They are composed of an admixture of cell types including small and mature-appearing lymphocytes (typically CD3+ T-cells), histiocytes, and granulocytes. They frequently contain a central small-caliber vessel. Although they occasionally abut bony trabeculae, they do not demonstrate the paratrabecular pattern of growth seen in follicular lymphoma and other non-Hodgkin lymphomas involving the marrow. In some cases, immunohistochemistry or in situ hybridization for κ and λ immunoglobulin light chains can be used to further evaluate aggregates.

J. **AIDS.** Since the first cases of AIDS were reported in 1981, a number of associated diseases have been identified in the bone marrow. Commonly encountered morphologic changes in the bone marrow of human immunodeficiency virus (HIV)-infected individuals include granulomas, lymphoid aggregates, plasma cell aggregates, and dysplasia in one or more hematopoietic lineages (*Br J Haematol* 2015;171:695). Since the development of combined drug therapy, the incidence of secondary infections has decreased. However, infectious agents are still encountered in the bone marrow of individuals infected with HIV and, because impaired inflammatory responses are a hallmark of HIV infection, it is recommended that all bone marrow biopsies from patients with HIV be examined with special stains for fungi and mycobacteria.

Lymphoid aggregates occur with increased frequency in the bone marrow of HIV-infected individuals, are sometimes large with ill-defined borders, and grow along bony trabeculae; these are all features suggestive of malignancy. They may be extremely difficult to evaluate, especially in view of the increased incidence of non-Hodgkin lymphomas in this population. Ancillary studies may be useful in monoclonal B-cell or phenotypically abnormal/monoclonal T-cell populations.

Dyspoiesis is a common finding in the bone marrow of patients with HIV infection and can be seen in other viral infections such as hepatitis C. The significance of this finding may be difficult if not impossible to interpret because of the increased incidence of neoplastic myelodysplasia and acute leukemias in the HIV+ population. Blasts are not typically increased in HIV-associated dysplasia, and clonal cytogenetic abnormalities are not present.

K. **Hemophagocytic Syndrome** is a potentially deadly condition in which cytokine-stimulated benign histiocytes phagocytose other hematopoietic cells in an uncontrolled fashion. The most common causes of hemophagocytic syndrome are related to activation of benign macrophages by cytokines produced by malignant cells, and unregulated phagocytosis by macrophages following infection. Malignancy-related hemophagocytic syndrome is most commonly associated with peripheral T-cell lymphoma, although other hematopoietic and lymphoid malignancies are also rarely associated with this complication, including acute myeloid leukemias with the translocation t(16;21)(p11;q22). The most common infectious cause of hemophagocytic syndrome is EBV. Regardless of the underlying cause, hemophagocytic syndrome presents with splenomegaly, fever, and wasting. Pancytopenia, elevated liver function tests, and coagulopathy are variably present. Evaluation of the bone marrow aspirate and core biopsy reveals variable numbers of macrophages containing phagocytosed hematopoietic cells (*Blood Reviews* 2016;30:411).

L. **Chédiak–Higashi Syndrome** is an autosomal recessive inherited disorder that is caused by a mutation in the *CHS1/LYST* gene located on chromosome 1q42. The clinical features of this syndrome are related to abnormal lysosomal trafficking and include recurrent infection, oculocutaneous albinism, neurologic disorders, and a bleeding diathesis.

Granulocytes, monocytes, and lymphocytes contain abnormal large granules derived from secondary or cytotoxic granules (e-**Fig. 42.3**) (*Methods Mol Biol* 2014;1124:501).

M. **Mucopolysaccharidoses.** Alder–Reilly anomaly is identified in the granulocytes of patients with a group of uncommon diseases characterized by X-linked or autosomal recessive transmitted defects in the enzymes involved in mucopolysaccharide metabolism (Table 42.1A). Granulocytes in the peripheral blood and bone marrow have coarse azurophilic granules superficially resembling normal primary granules. Classification of cases of mucopolysaccharidosis requires chemical and/or molecular analysis (*Transl Sci Rare Dis* 2017;2:1).

N. **Lipid Storage Disorders.** There are numerous genetically mediated conditions related to defects in enzymes comprising the pathway of lipid metabolism (Table 42.1B). The most commonly encountered are the Gaucher disease and Niemann–Pick disease.

TABLE 42.1	Storage Diseases

A. Mucopolysaccharidoses

Disease	*Enzyme deficiency*
Hurler syndrome (mucopolysaccharidosis type I H)	α-L-iduronidase
Scheie syndrome (mucopolysaccharidosis type I S)	α-L-iduronidase
Hurler–Scheie syndrome (mucopolysaccharidosis type I H-S)	α-L-iduronidase
Hunter syndrome (mucopolysaccharidosis type II)	Iduronate α-sulfatase
Sanfilippo syndrome type A (mucopolysaccharidosis type III A)	Heparin *N*-sulfatase
Sanfilippo syndrome type B (mucopolysaccharidosis type III B)	α-*N*-Acetylglucosaminidase
Sanfilippo syndrome type C (mucopolysaccharidosis type III C)	α-Glucosaminide transferase
Sanfilippo syndrome type D (mucopolysaccharidosis type III D)	*N*-Acetylglucosamine-6-sulfatase
Morquio syndrome type A (mucopolysaccharidosis type IV A)	*N*-Acetylgalactosamine, 6-sulfate sulfatase
Morquio syndrome type B (mucopolysaccharidosis type IV B)	β-Galactosidase
Maroteaux–Lamy syndrome (mucopolysaccharidosis type VI)	*N*-Acetylgalactosamine-4-sulfatase
Sly syndrome (mucopolysaccharidosis type VII)	β-Glucuronidase

B. Lipid storage disorders

Disease	*Enzyme deficiency*	*Substance stored*
Gaucher disease	β-Glucocerebrosidase	Glucocerebroside
Niemann–Pick disease	Sphingomyelinase	Sphingomyelin
Gangliosidosis	β-galactosidase	GM_1 ganglioside
Tay–Sachs disease	Hexosaminidase A	GM_2 ganglioside
Sandhoff disease	Hexosaminidase A	GM_2 ganglioside
Fabry disease	α-Galactosidase	Ceramide trihexalose

1. **Gaucher disease** demonstrates an autosomal recessive pattern of inheritance and is caused by a defect in the enzyme β-glucocerebrosidase. Clinically, patients present with bone pain and splenomegaly related to the proliferation of morphologically abnormal histiocytes at these sites. The cytoplasm of the macrophages has a "wrinkled tissue paper" appearance, which represents the accumulation of glucocerebroside in these cells (e-**Fig. 42.4**). Occasional cases are associated with B-lineage malignancies (including plasma cell dyscrasias) and light chain amyloidosis (*Transl Sci Rare Dis* 2017;2:1).

2. Patients with **Niemann–Pick disease** typically present with organomegaly, neuropathy, and abnormal laboratory findings similar to those identified in the Gaucher disease. The pathophysiology of the Niemann–Pick disease is related to autosomal recessively inherited defects in the enzyme sphingomyelinase, with the presence of sphingomyelin in affected cells. Macrophages in this disorder have been described as "sea-blue" due to the cytoplasmic accumulation of periodic acid–Schiff-positive material representing the sphingomyelin.

3. The remaining lipid storage diseases, which are somewhat less common, have clinical presentations similar to those of Gaucher and Niemann–Pick diseases. Some are associated with additional findings. For example, Hermansky–Pudlak syndrome is associated with platelet storage pool deficiencies and oculocutaneous albinism (*Platelets* 1998;9:21).

IV. DIAGNOSTIC FEATURES OF MALIGNANCIES

A. Myelodysplastic Syndromes

are clonal hematopoietic disorders characterized in most cases by peripheral cytopenias (hemoglobin <10 g/dL, absolute neutrophil count [ANC] $<1.8 \times 10^9$/L, and/or platelets $<100 \times 10^9$/L) and increased bone marrow cellularity (*Am J Hematol* 2016;91:76). The entities comprising this family of diseases are summarized in Table 42.2. Diagnosis is made by assessment of the bone marrow aspirate smear for significant dyspoiesis and correlation with the clinical history, including a failure to respond to iron, vitamin B$_{12}$, and folate replacement. Dyspoiesis is identified in one or more of the hematopoietic lineages. In the myeloid series this most commonly manifests as abnormal nuclear lobation, including cells with pseudo Pelger–Huët (hypolobate) nuclei, and cells with decreased cytoplasmic granules. Erythroid precursors demonstrate nuclear irregularities including budding, with occasional ringed sideroblasts (erythroid precursors with multiple punctate iron granules surrounding the nuclei that reflect iron abnormally trapped in mitochondria). Megakaryocytes contain multiple separate nuclei or are small with decreased nuclear lobation (e-**Figs. 42.5–42.8**). Importantly, these changes must be present in at least 10% of the cells in a given lineage to morphologically establish this diagnosis.

Detection of a cytogenetic abnormality is helpful, although the majority of cases of "low-grade" myelodysplasia (refractory cytopenia with single lineage dysplasia, refractory anemia with ringed sideroblasts, and refractory cytopenia with multilineage dysplasia) have normal karyotypes. Common cytogenetic abnormalities include partial or complete deletions of chromosomes 5 and 7, del(20q), and/or trisomy of chromosome 8. Abnormalities of chromosome 7 or complex karyotypes (>3 cytogenetic abnormalities) carry a poor prognosis. 5q-syndrome is a special type of MDS in which dyspoiesis is most prominent in the megakaryocytic series, accompanied by thrombocytosis. This form of myelodysplasia is associated with long survival.

High-grade myelodysplasia (refractory anemia with excess blasts types 1 and 2) presents with a greater percentage of peripheral blood/bone marrow blasts compared with low-grade cases. In general, refractory anemia with excess blasts is more clinically aggressive than is refractory anemia with or without ringed sideroblasts, and has a variable propensity for progression to acute leukemia or bone marrow failure, both of which are essentially untreatable by any means short of a bone marrow transplant. Outcome in the MDSs may be predicted using the International Prognostic Scoring System (IPSS), which takes into account blast percentage, karyotype, and the presence of cytopenias.

TABLE 42.2 Myelodysplastic Syndromes

Disease	Blood	Bone Marrow	Cytogenetics (Percentage of Cytogenetically Abnormal Cases)	Outcome (Median Survival)
Refractory cytopenia with single lineage dysplasia	Uni- or bicytopenia No/rare blasts	Unilineage dysplasia <5% blasts <15% ringed sideroblasts	<50%	~2% progress to acute leukemia at 5 yrs
Refractory anemia with ringed sideroblasts	Anemia No blasts	≥15% ringed sideroblasts Erythroid dysplasia <5% blasts	<10%	1–2% progress to acute leukemia (6 yrs)
Refractory cytopenia with multilineage dysplasia	Bi/pancytopenia No/rare blasts No Auer rods <1 × 10⁹/L monocytes	Dysplasia in ≥10% of cells in two or more myeloid cell lines <5% blasts No Auer rods <15% ringed sideroblasts	~50%	~11% progress to acute leukemia at 2 yrs
Refractory cytopenia with multilineage dysplasia and ringed sideroblasts	Bi/pancytopenia No/rare blasts No Auer rods <1 × 10⁹/L monocytes	Dysplasia in ≥10% of cells in two or more myeloid cell lines ≥15% ringed sideroblasts <5% blasts No Auer rods	Unknown; probably similar to refractory cytopenia with multilineage dysplasia	Unknown; probably similar to refractory cytopenia with multilineage dysplasia
Refractory anemia with excess blasts-1 (RAEB-1)	Cytopenias <5% blasts No Auer rods <1 × 10⁹/L monocytes	Uni/multilineage dysplasia 5–9% blasts No Auer rods	~30–50%	~25%
Refractory anemia with excess blasts-2 (RAEB-2)	Cytopenias 5–19% blasts ± Auer rods <1 × 10⁹/L monocytes	Uni/multilineage dysplasia 10–19% blasts ± Auer rods	~30–50%	~33%
Myelodysplastic syndrome—unclassifiable	Cytopenias No/rare blasts No Auer rods	Unilineage dysplasia <5% blasts No Auer rods	Unknown	Unknown
Myelodysplastic syndrome associated with isolated del(5q)	Anemia Normal/increased platelet count <5% blasts	Normal/increased megakaryocytes with hypolobate nuclei <5% blasts Isolated del(5q) cytogenetic abnormality No Auer rods	100% (isolated del(5q) cytogenetic abnormality; cases with additional abnormalities should not be classified under this diagnosis)	Unknown median survival—probably many yrs

Notable exceptions: (1) A diagnosis of RAEB-1 can be established if there are 2–4% myeloblasts in the peripheral blood with less than 5% blasts in the bone marrow. (2) Cases with Auer rods and less than 10% bone marrow myeloblasts are designated as RAEB-2.

Adapted from Swerdlow SH, Campo E, Harris NL, et al., eds. *WHO Classification of Tumours. Pathology and Genetics. Tumours of Haematopoietic and Lymphoid Tissues*, 4th ed. Lyon, France: IARC Press; 2017. Used with permission.

B. Myeloproliferative Neoplasms. The myeloproliferative neoplasms are characterized by an expansion of one or more of the hematopoietic lineages as evidenced by increased bone marrow cellularity and increased circulating white blood cells (usually granulocytes), erythrocytes, and/or platelets. Initially, blasts are present in normal to slightly increased numbers in the marrow. Although these are malignant disorders, the affected cell line(s) are usually morphologically normal, and pronounced dyspoiesis is not a characteristic feature of the chronic myeloproliferative disorders. In contrast to myelodysplasia, organomegaly (splenomegaly and/or hepatomegaly) is a common feature of this disease and becomes more pronounced with disease progression as the bone marrow becomes dysfunctional and/or fibrotic.

The current (2017) WHO classification (Swerdlow SH, Campo E, Harris NL, et al., eds. *World Health Organization Classification of Tumours. Pathology and Genetics. Tumours of Haematopoietic and Lymphoid Tissues, 4th ed.* Lyon: IARC Press; 2017) defines the different subclasses of myeloproliferative neoplasm using diagnostic criteria to more confidently distinguish these entities from reactive/nonneoplastic conditions and from other members of this family of diseases.

1. Chronic myelogenous leukemia is a well-characterized clinicopathologic entity because essentially all cases have the characteristic Philadelphia chromosome t(9;22) (q34;q11) and corresponding rearrangement of BCR-ABL (*Br J Haematol* 1991;79 Suppl 1:34). This is a disorder derived from clonal expansion of an abnormal pluripotential hematopoietic stem cell. Affected individuals typically present with nonspecific constitutional symptoms and on physical examination are frequently found to have an enlarged spleen. Patients most often present in the chronic phase, characterized by a peripheral leukocytosis composed of granulocytes (in various stages of maturation) and peripheral and bone marrow basophilia and eosinophilia (e-**Fig. 42.9**). The blast percentage in chronic phase is usually <2% of white blood cells in the peripheral blood and <5% in the bone marrow. Untreated, cases of chronic myelogenous leukemia invariably acquire additional genetic lesions (i.e., additional Ph chromosome, isochromosome 17q, or trisomy 8) resulting in a maturation arrest in the malignant population and terminate in an acute leukemic (blast) phase. The blast phenotype is myeloid in ~80% of cases and lymphoid in most of the remaining cases, and has a biphenotypic or ambiguous phenotype in rare individuals. Chronic myelogenous leukemia in blast phase is essentially untreatable by any means short of a bone marrow transplant. Increasingly, patients presenting with chronic myelogenous leukemia in chronic phase are treated with small molecular inhibitors such as imatinib mesylate, a tyrosine kinase inhibitor with a high degree of specificity for the BCR-ABL–encoded tyrosine kinase. However, an increasing problem is the development of resistance to imatinib mesylate; and second- and third-generation tyrosine kinase inhibitors have been developed.

2. Polycythemia vera is a clonal stem cell disorder in which the majority of disease manifestations are related to expansion of the cells of the erythroid lineage as evidenced by increased hematocrit, blood volume, and blood viscosity (*Am J Hematol* 2015;90:162; *Blood* 2002;100:4272). The clinical features of this disease are directly related to red cell mass expansion: the skin has a plethoric appearance, and there is an increased propensity for vascular thromboses, hemorrhage, and central nervous system phenomena including stroke, tinnitus, headache, and vertigo. The peripheral blood manifestations of disease are also related to expansion of red blood cell mass. There is an increased red blood cell count (approximately 7,000,000 to 10,000,000/mm^3) and hemoglobin (usually >18.5 g/dL in men or >16.5 g/dL in women) without a corresponding increased reticulocyte count. Because polycythemia vera is related to expansion of a pluripotential hematopoietic stem cell, other cell lines are variably affected. Thus, some patients have an associated neutrophilic leukocytosis and/or thrombocytosis. Other clinical laboratory features of disease include an increased leukocyte alkaline phosphatase (LAP) score and increased serum vitamin B12 levels, the latter due to an increase in transcobalamin 1. Bone marrow analysis is performed

TABLE 42.3	WHO Criteria for Polycythemia Vera

Major criteria:

1. Elevated hemoglobin concentration (>16.5 g/dL in men; >16.0 g/dL in women) or elevated hematocrit (>49% in men; >48% in women) or
2. Bone marrow biopsy showing age-adjusted hypercellularity with trilineage growth (panmyelosis), including prominent erythroid, granulocytic, and megakaryocytic proliferation with pleomorphic, mature megakaryocytes (differences in size)
3. The presence of JAK2 V617F or JAK2 exon 12 mutation

Minor criterion:

Subnormal serum erythropoietin level

Diagnosis requires either all three major criteria or the first two major criteria and the minor criterion.
Adapted from Swerdlow SH, Campo E, Harris NL, et al., eds. *WHO Classification of Tumours. Pathology and Genetics. Tumours of Haematopoietic and Lymphoid Tissues*, 4th ed. Lyon, France: IARC Press; 2017. Used with permission.

to exclude other forms of myeloproliferative disorder and to assess baseline fibrosis. Usually, initial bone marrow analysis reveals increased bone marrow cellularity with multilineage expansion of hematopoiesis, and minimal fibrosis.

In establishing a diagnosis of polycythemia vera, nonneoplastic erythrocytosis and erythrocytosis due to cytokine production by nonhematopoietic malignancies must be excluded. Common causes of secondary erythrocytosis include pathologic conditions (such as chronic pulmonary disease and smoking) and physiologic conditions (such as living at high altitude). A *JAK2* mutation (most commonly V617F but mutations in exon 12 have also been identified) is found in the vast majority of cases and thus is now a major criterion for diagnosis. The diagnostic criteria are summarized in Table 42.3.

In most cases, polycythemia vera is a clinically indolent condition. The treatment of choice for most patients is periodic phlebotomy to minimize the risks associated with increased blood viscosity. Less than 10% of patients develop bone marrow failure or acute leukemia.

3. **Essential thrombocythemia** is a clonal neoplasm, derived from a pluripotential hematopoietic stem cell, in which the majority of clinical and pathologic features are related to morphologically and physiologically abnormal megakaryocytes and platelets (*Leuk Lymphoma* 2017;58:2786). There is usually a marked peripheral thrombocytosis, generally in excess of $1,000 \times 10^9$/L, although a sustained count of >450 × 10^9/L is sufficient for diagnosis. The platelets are frequently morphologically abnormal, including forms with decreased granularity. The most prominent characteristic of the bone marrow is marked megakaryocytic hyperplasia. The megakaryocytes are frequently morphologically abnormal, with large overall size and hyperlobate (staghorn) nuclei. A definite diagnosis can be established after other myeloproliferative neoplasms are eliminated from consideration with ancillary studies. JAK2 V617F mutations are found in approximately 50% of cases (both of essential thrombocythemia and primary myelofibrosis). The major pathophysiologic consequences of the thrombocytosis and proliferation of megakaryocytes are episodic bleeding and thrombosis, which are major causes of morbidity and mortality. Less than 1% of cases progress to acute leukemia. The diagnostic criteria are summarized in Table 42.4.

4. **Primary myelofibrosis** (chronic idiopathic myelofibrosis, agnogenic myeloid metaplasia, myelofibrosis with myeloid metaplasia) is another myeloproliferative neoplasm attributed to transformation of a pluripotential hematopoietic stem cell. Classically, there are two phases in the natural history of a disease (*Am J Hematol* 2016;91:1262). The first phase, referred to as the cellular phase, is characterized by a marked expansion of all hematopoietic lineages. Diagnostic criteria are summarized in Table 42.5. The cellular phase is followed by the spent phase, characterized by progressive bone

TABLE 42.4 **WHO Criteria for Essential Thrombocythemia**

Major criteria:

1. Platelet count >450 × 10⁹/L
2. Bone marrow biopsy showing proliferation mainly of megakaryocytic lineage with increased numbers of enlarged, mature megakaryocytes with hyperlobated nuclei; no significant increase or left shift in granulopoiesis or erythropoiesis
3. WHO criteria for CML, polycythemia vera, primary myelofibrosis, or other neoplasms are not met
4. *JAK2*, *CALR*, or *MPL* mutation

Minor criterion:

The presence of a clonal marker or the absence of evidence of reactive thrombocytosis

Diagnosis requires either all four major criteria or the first three major criteria and the minor criterion.
Adapted from Swerdlow SH, Campo E, Harris NL, et al., eds. *WHO Classification of Tumours. Pathology and Genetics. Tumours of Haematopoietic and Lymphoid Tissues*, 4th ed. Lyon, France: IARC Press; 2017. Used with permission.

marrow failure and fibrosis. Criteria for the fibrotic phase are listed in Table 42.6. Because the cellular phase is often clinically silent, the majority of clinical findings are related to increasing bone marrow fibrosis, and include fatigue (due to anemia), bleeding (due to thrombocytopenia), and infection (due to granulocytopenia). Hepatosplenomegaly due to extramedullary hematopoiesis is a common physical finding.

The cellular phase is often characterized by peripheral granulocytic leukocytosis and/or thrombocytosis. The former is sometimes accompanied by eosinophilia or basophilia clinically mimicking chronic myelogenous leukemia. In the cellular phase, the bone marrow is hypercellular due to a panhyperplasia of all hematopoietic lineages. Megakaryocytes cluster in the bone marrow and are characteristically highly atypical including large forms with bulbous/hyperchromatic nuclei. Fibrosis is minimal at this stage of disease. With time, the bone marrow becomes increasingly fibrotic (which is best illustrated by a reticulin stain) and the patient becomes increasingly susceptible to the consequences of decreased peripheral white blood cells, red blood cells, and platelets. Death is most commonly due to infection or hemorrhage. Acute leukemia is an uncommon late sequela, occurring in <10% of individuals.

TABLE 42.5 **WHO Criteria for Primary Myelofibrosis, Prefibrotic/Early Phase**

Major criteria:

1. Megakaryocytic proliferation and atypia without reticulin fibrosis >1, accompanied by increased age-adjusted bone marrow cellularity, granulocytic proliferation, and often decreased erythropoiesis
2. WHO criteria for CML, polycythemia vera, essential thrombocythemia, myelodysplastic syndromes, or other myeloid neoplasms are not met
3. *JAK2*, *CALR*, or *MPL* mutation or the presence of a clonal marker or the absence of reactive bone marrow reticulin fibrosis

Minor criteria:

The presence of at least one of the following, confirmed in two separate determinations

a. Anemia not attributed to a comorbid condition
b. Leukocytosis at least 11 × 10⁹/L
c. Splenomegaly
d. Lactate dehydrogenase level above the upper limit of the institutional reference range

Diagnosis requires that all three major criteria and at least one minor criterion are met.
Adapted from Swerdlow SH, Campo E, Harris NL, et al., eds. *WHO Classification of Tumours. Pathology and Genetics. Tumours of Haematopoietic and Lymphoid Tissues*, 4th ed. Lyon, France: IARC Press; 2017. Used with permission.

TABLE 42.6 WHO Criteria for Primary Myelofibrosis, Overt Fibrotic Phase

Major criteria:

1. Megakaryocytic proliferation and atypia accompanied by reticulin fibrosis grades 2 or 3, accompanied by increased age-adjusted bone marrow cellularity, granulocytic proliferation, and often decreased erythropoiesis
2. WHO criteria for CML, polycythemia vera, essential thrombocythemia, myelodysplastic syndromes, or other myeloid neoplasms are not met
3. JAK2, CALR, or MPL mutation or the presence of a clonal marker or the absence of reactive bone marrow fibrosis

Minor criteria:

The presence of at least one of the following, confirmed in two separate determinations

a. Anemia not attributed to a comorbid condition
b. Leukocytosis at least 11×10^9/L
c. Splenomegaly
d. Lactate dehydrogenase level above the upper limit of the institutional reference range
e. Leukoerythroblastosis

Adapted from Swerdlow SH, Campo E, Harris NL, et al., eds. *WHO Classification of Tumours. Pathology and Genetics. Tumours of Haematopoietic and Lymphoid Tissues*, 4th ed. Lyon, France: IARC Press; 2017. Used with permission.

5. Systemic mastocytosis. Mastocytosis, the abnormal accumulation of mast cells in the skin and other tissues, has a wide range of clinical behavior. A benign form of disease is localized to the skin, occurs predominantly in younger individuals, and is characterized by spontaneous regression. In the systemic form of mastocytosis, mast cells are increased in many organs including the bone marrow (e-**Figs. 42.10–42.12**). The WHO criteria for systemic mastocytosis are summarized in Table 42.7. Systemic mastocytosis represents a clonal disorder in most cases. Mutations in the *kit* proto-oncogene (most commonly D816V) have been identified in many individuals and presumably play a role in the pathophysiology of the disease. In cases with associated eosinophilia, the

TABLE 42.7 WHO Criteria for Systemic Mastocytosis

Major criteria are as follows:

Multifocal infiltrates of mast cells (≥15 mast cells constitute an aggregate) detected in sections of bone marrow and/or other extracutaneous organ(s), and confirmed by tryptase immunohistochemistry or other special stains.

Minor criteria are as follows:

a. In biopsy sections of bone marrow or other extracutaneous organs, >25% of the mast cells in the infiltrate are spindle-shaped or have atypical morphology, or, of all mast cells in the bone marrow aspirate smears, >25% are immature or atypical mast cells.
b. *Kit* point mutation at codon 816 in bone marrow, blood, or other extracutaneous organ(s)
c. Mast cells in bone marrow, blood, or other extracutaneous organs coexpress CD25 with or without CD2.
d. Serum total tryptase persistently >20 mg/mL (unless there is an associated clonal myeloid disorder, in which case this parameter is not valid)

The diagnosis of systemic mastocytosis may be made if one major and one minor criterion are present, or if three minor criteria are fulfilled.

Adapted from Swerdlow SH, Campo E, Harris NL, et al., eds. *WHO Classification of Tumours. Pathology and Genetics. Tumours of Haematopoietic and Lymphoid Tissues*, 4th ed. Lyon, France: IARC Press; 2017. Used with permission.

FIP1L1/PDGFRA fusion gene has been identified. The same fusion gene has been identified in chronic eosinophilic leukemia/hypereosinophilic syndrome.

The clinical course of systemic mastocytosis is highly variable. Cases with cutaneous involvement (urticaria pigmentosa) are more likely to have a benign disease course, whereas individuals with peripheral blood involvement (mast cell leukemia) frequently die within weeks of diagnosis.

C. Neoplasms Characterized by Eosinophilia and Abnormalities of the Platelet-Derived Growth Factor Receptors and Fibroblast Growth Factor 1 Receptor. The WHO 2008 added an additional category of myeloid and lymphoid neoplasms characterized by fusion genes resulting in aberrant signaling of platelet-derived growth factor receptor A (PDGFRA), platelet-derived growth factor receptor B (PDGFRB), and fibroblast growth factor receptor 1 (FGFR1). These cases all present with eosinophilia and thus other causes of eosinophilia should be ruled out, including T-cell non-Hodgkin lymphomas, infection, and drug therapy. See Table 42.8.

D. Acute Leukemia. Compared with myelodysplastic and myeloproliferative neoplasms, acute leukemias frequently present with a greater tumor burden (i.e., with blast percentages of at least 20%) and are broadly categorized as myeloid or lymphoid according to their immunologic and enzyme cytochemical properties, the characteristic features of which are summarized in Table 42.9. There are two important exceptions to the requirement of at least 20% blasts in acute myeloid leukemia. In the current WHO classification, the presence of t(8;21)(q22;q22) [*AML1/ETO*], inv(16)(p13;q22) or t(16;16) (p13;q22) [*CBFβ/MYH11*], and t(15;17)(q22;q12) [*PML/RARα*] are classified as acute myeloid leukemia regardless of the percentage of blasts (e-Figs. 42.13–42.17). The second exception involves acute erythroid leukemia, which is characterized by an expansion of erythroid elements in the bone marrow comprising >80% of bone marrow cells, of which at least 30% of this population consists of proerythroblasts. Immunophenotypic analysis of acute leukemia is discussed in Chapter 41.

Acute leukemias, particularly in children and the elderly, may present with isolated anemia and a lack of circulating blasts. Diagnosis requires detection of at least 20% blasts in the bone marrow and/or the presence of an acute myeloid leukemia–specific cytogenetic abnormality. Although replacement of the bone marrow by fibrosis, carcinoma, sarcoma, or other nonhematopoietic cell may result in anemia, it is generally accompanied by leukopenia and/or thrombocytopenia, reflecting indiscriminate displacement of normal marrow constituents.

B-lymphoblastic leukemia is arbitrarily separated from its tissue analog, lymphoblastic lymphoma, by the presence of a tissue mass and ≤20% bone marrow blasts in the latter (e-Fig. 42.18), and is no longer subdivided on the basis of immunophenotype because genetic features are more predictive of outcome. B-lymphoblastic leukemia is most common in children <6 years old; patients with purely lymphomatous disease are somewhat younger on average. Most cases express HLA-DR, terminal deoxynucleotidyl transferase (TdT), CD10, CD19, CD24, and cytoplasmic CD79a. CD10-negative cases often demonstrate rearrangements of the mixed-lineage leukemia (*MLL*) gene and coexpress one or more myeloid-associated antigens. In the pediatric population, cytogenetic and molecular genetic findings are highly predictive of disease outcome. Predictors of good outcome include the following: age 4 to 10 years at diagnosis, hyperdiploidy (51 to 65 chromosomes) in the blast population, and the presence of the translocation t(12;21)(p13;q22) [*TEL/AML1*]. Predictors of poor outcome include the following: age <4 years or >10 years, hypodiploidy, t(9;22)(q34;q11.2) [*BCR/ABL*], t(4;11)(q21;q23) [*AF4/MLL*], and t(1;19)(q23;q13.3) [*PBX/E2A*]. The prognostic significance of t(1;19) is controversial. Recently, mutations/deletions in the lymphoid transcription factor gene IKZF1 (IKAROS) have been shown to be associated with a high rate of leukemic relapse and a poor outcome; mutations in *PAX5* are also common.

A special category of lymphoblastic leukemia is the leukemic analog of Burkitt lymphoma. Patients with this disease commonly present with an abdominal mass (Western Europe and North America) or jaw lesion (Africa). The bone marrow is commonly

Disease	Common Rearrangement	Clinical	Morphology	Progression to Acute Leukemia	Prognosis (Sensitivity to Imatinib)
Myeloid and lymphoid neoplasms with PDGFRA rearrangement	FIP1L1-PDGFRA (due to cryptic deletion at 4q12 which may require RT-PCR or FISH for detection)	M > F; wide age range; fatigue, splenomegaly and sequelae of high peripheral eosinophil count (>1.5 × 10⁹/L) including pruritus and cardiac failure	Eosinophilia with orderly maturation; mast cells are increased in bone marrow; typically mimics chronic eosinophilic leukemia	Uncommon, may be AML or T-LBL	Likely good if there is no organ damage from high eosinophil count (Yes)
Myeloid and lymphoid neoplasms with PDGFRB rearrangement	ETV6-PDGFRB (t(5;12)(q31; p12)); can be detected by conventional cytogenetics; numerous variants have been reported	M > F, wide age range; splenomegaly and leukocytosis, including monocytes and eosinophils; mimics CMML	Hypercellular bone marrow with granulocytic predominance, including eosinophils, neutrophilic precursors, and monocytes	Rare, typically myeloid	Likely good if there is no organ damage from high eosinophil count (Yes)
Myeloid and lymphoid neoplasms with FGFR1 abnormalities (also known as 8p11 syndrome)	ZNF198-FGFR1 (t(8;13) (p11;q12) most common; numerous variants identified	M > F, median age ~30; variable clinical presentation; extensive extramedullary disease may be present	Varied, ranging from eosinophilia to T-lymphoblastic lymphoma	AML, T-LBL, B-ALL, mixed phenotype acute leukemia have all been reported	Poor (No)

Adapted from Swerdlow SH, Campo E, Harris NL, et al., eds. *WHO Classification of Tumors of Haematopoietic and Lymphoid Tissues*, 4th ed. Lyon, France: IARC Press; 2017, 68–73.

TABLE 42.9 WHO Classification of Acute Myeloid Leukemias

Disease	Clinical	Morphology	Immunophenotype	Prognosis
A. Acute myeloid leukemia with recurrent genetic abnormalities				
Acute myeloid leukemia with t(8;21)(q22;q22); (RUNX1-RUNX1T1)	Often presents with extramedullary disease	Blasts with long slender Auer rods, abnormal granulation	CD13+, CD33+, MPO+, CD19+, CD34+, CD56+	Favorable
Acute myeloid leukemia with abnormal bone marrow eosinophils inv(16)(p13q22) or t(16;16)(p13;q22) (CBFβ/MYH11)	Occasionally presents with extramedullary disease	Abnormal eosinophils with large basophilic granules, decreased lobation	CD13+, CD33+, MPO+; frequently CD4+, CD14+, CD11b+, CD11c+, CD64+, CD36+, lysozyme+	Favorable
Acute promyelocytic leukemia (AML with t(15;17)(q22;q12)); (PML/RARα and variants)	Coagulopathy, normal/low WBC (hypergranular variant); high WBC (hypogranular variant)	Abnormal promyelocytes with multiple Auer rods predominate	CD33+ (heterogeneous), CD33+ (bright); HLA-DR-, CD34-	Favorable
Acute myeloid leukemia with t(9;11)[a]	Frequently occurs in children	Monocytic blasts predominate	Variable CD13 and CD33+, CD4+, CD14+, CD11b+, CD11c+, CD64+, CD36+, lysozyme+	Intermediate survival
Acute myeloid leukemia with t(6;9)(p23;q34); DEK-NUP214[a]	Pancytopenia	Basophilia with multilineage dysplasia	CD13+, CD33+, myeloperoxidase+, HLA-DR+, CD34+, CD117+, TdT +/-	Poor
Acute myeloid leukemia with inv(3)(q21q26.2) or t(3;3)(q21; q26.2); RPN1-EVI1[a]	Normal/elevated platelet count	Multilineage dysplasia including marked dysmegakaryopoiesis	CD13+, CD33+, HLA-DR+, CD34+, CD117+, CD41/CD61 +/-	Poor
Acute myeloid leukemia with t(1;22)(p13;q13); RBM15-MLK1[a]	Infants and young children; hepatosplenomegaly is common	Megakaryoblastic	CD41/CD61+, CD13+, CD33-, CD34-, HLA-DR-	Typically poor

B. Acute myeloid leukemia with multilineage dysplasia

- Following a myelodysplastic syndrome (MDS) or myelodysplastic syndrome/myeloproliferative disorder
- Without antecedent MDS
- **Or** MDS-related cytogenetic abnormality
- **Or** dysplasia in at least 50% of the cells in two cell lineages

C. Acute myeloid leukemia and MDSs, therapy-related

- Alkylating agent-related; typically has a 5–10-yr latency with t-MDS stage
- Topoisomerase type II inhibitor-related (some may be lymphoid); 1–5-yr latency with no t-MDS phase, commonly has balanced translocations including 11q23 abnormalities
- Other types

D. Acute myeloid leukemia not otherwise categorized

Acute myeloid leukemia minimally differentiated	Usually presents in adulthood, cytopenias	<3% of blasts MPO+, <3% of blasts NBE+	Often CD13+, CD33+, CD117+, CD34+, CD38+, HLA-DR+	Unfavorable
Acute myeloid leukemia without maturation	Usually presents in adulthood, cytopenias, occasionally with markedly increased WBC	Blasts comprise ≥90% of nonerythroid cells; ≥3% of blasts MPO+, <3% of blasts NBE+	Often CD13+, CD33+, CD34+, CD117+, MPO+	Unfavorable
Acute myeloid leukemia with maturation	Variable age range and symptomatology	≥3% of blasts MPO+, <3% of blasts NBE+; >10% of maturing granulocytic cells	Usually CD13+, CD33+, CD15+; variable CD117+, CD34+, HLA-DR+	Variable
Acute myelomonocytic leukemia	Anemia, fever, fatigue; WBC usually elevated	>20% blasts (including promonocytes); ≥20% monocytes and precursors; and ≥20% neutrophils and precursors; ≥3% of blasts MPO+, ≥3% of blasts usually NBE+[b]	Usually CD13+, CD33+; often CD4+, CD14+, CD11b+, CD11c+, CD64+, CD36+, lysozyme+	Variable
Acute monoblastic leukemia	Most common in children, often presents with extramedullary disease, bleeding disorders	≥80% monocytic cells, of which ≥80% are monoblasts; <20% neutrophils and precursors; <3% of blasts MPO+, ≥3% of blasts NBE+	Variable CD13+, CD33+, CD117+; often CD14+, CD4+, CD11b+, CD11c+, CD64+, CD68+, CD36+, lysozyme+	Unfavorable

(continued)

TABLE 42.9 WHO Classification of Acute Myeloid Leukemias *(Continued)*

Disease	Clinical	Morphology	Immunophenotype	Prognosis
Acute monocytic leukemia	Most common in adults, often presents with extramedullary disease, bleeding disorders	≥80% monocytic cells, of which the majority are promonocytes; <20% neutrophils and precursors; <3% of blasts MPO+, ≥3% of blasts NBE+	Variable CD13+, CD33+, CD117+; often CD14+, CD4+, CD11b+, CD11c+, CD64+, CD68+, CD36+, lysozyme+	Unfavorable
Acute erythroid leukemia (erythroid/myeloid)	Adults; anemia	≥50% of entire nucleated population is erythroid and ≥20% myeloblasts in nonerythroid population; >3% of blasts may be MPO+	Erythroblasts are glycophorin A+ and hemoglobin A+; myeloblasts are CD13+, CD33+, CD117+, and MPO+	Unfavorable
Pure erythroid leukemia	Extremely rare	>80% of cells are immature erythroid cells; no significant myeloblast component; >30% of erythroid elements are pro-erythroblasts	Blasts are sometimes glycophorin A+ and hemoglobin A+	Unfavorable
Acute megakaryoblastic leukemia	Cytopenias	Dysplastic megakaryocytes, Blasts often have cytoplasmic pseudopods. Abnormal platelets and megakaryocyte fragments in peripheral blood; usually <3% of blasts MPO+ and >3% of blasts NBE+	Usually CD41+, CD61+; occasionally CD13+, CD33+; CD34-, CD45-, HLA-DR-	Poor
Acute basophilic leukemia	Very rare	Blasts are toluidine blue+; usually <3% of blasts MPO+, <3% of blasts NBE+	Usually CD13+, CD33+, CD34, HLA-DR+, CD9+	Difficult to predict due to low number of reported cases, probably poor
Acute panmyelosis with myelofibrosis	Very rare, adults, pancytopenia with no/minimal splenomegaly	Panhyperplasia, dysplastic megakaryocytes; increased reticulin fibrosis	CD13+, CD33+, CD117+, MPO+; some cases express erythroid or megakaryocytic antigens	Poor

E. Common mutations in acute myeloid leukemia

Mutation	Frequency	Clinical	Cytogenetics	Outcome
NPM1 (nucleophosmin)[c]	~30%	Typically de novo disease; high WBC and myelomonocytic morphology common; blasts typically CD34-	Frequently normal	Favorable
CEBPA (CCAAT/enhancer binding protein-alpha)[c]	~8%	High PB blast count; typically AML without/with maturation	Frequently normal	Favorable
FLT3-ITD (FMS-like tyrosine kinase-internal tandem duplication)	~30%	High WBC; varied morphology (including acute promyelocytic leukemia)	Varied	Poor
IDH1/IDH2 (isocitrate dehydrogenase 1 and 2)	~10% (IDH1); ~15% (IDH2)	Typically AML without/with maturation; uncommon in monocytic leukemias	Typically normal (frequently occurs with other mutations with exception TET2)	TBD
DNMT3a (DNA methyltransferase 3a)	~20%	Common in myelomonocytic/ monocytic leukemias	Normal cytogenetics (exclusive of good risk recurrent genetic abnormality AMLs)	Poor
TET2 (Tet oncogene family member 2)	~7%	No distinct clinical presentation	Typically normal (frequently occurs with other mutations with exception IDH mutations)	TBD

Important note: Identification of the translocations t(8;21)(q22;q22); inv(16)(p13q22) or t(16;16)(p13;q22); or t(15;17)(q22;q12) and variants is diagnostic of acute myeloid leukemia, regardless of the blast percentage. For the genetic lesions indicated by (*) it is controversial whether identification of these lesions in a bonemarrow with <20% myeloblasts is diagnostic of acute myeloid leukemia.

"The World Health Organization allows the diagnosis of acute myelomonocytic leukemia in the absence of NBE reactivity if the "cells meet morphologic criteria for monocytes."

[c]Acute myeloid leukemia with mutated NPM1 and CEBPA are provisional entities in WHO 2008.

IDH1, IDH2, DNMT3a, and TET2 mutations have also been identified in other myeloid malignancies.

Other mutations identified in AML include c-KIT, N-RAS, K-RAS, WT1, RUNX1 and partial tandem duplication of MLL. These mutations are not specific for AML and their prognostic significance has yet to be determined in a large cohort of AML patients.

HLA, human leukocyte antigen; MPO, myeloperoxidase; NBE, naphthyl butyrate esterase; TBD, to be determined; WBC, white blood count.

Adapted from Swerdlow SH, Campo E, Harris NL, et al., eds. *Tumours of Haematopoietic and Lymphoid Tissues*, 4th ed. Lyon, France: IARC Press; 2017. Used with permission.

involved, and the blasts have deeply basophilic cytoplasm with many lipid vacuoles that express CD10 and monoclonal surface immunoglobulin light chain, and are generally CD34 and TdT negative (e-Fig. 42.19). Diagnosis requires demonstration of the translocation t(8;14)(q24;q32) [*MYC/IGH*] or, less commonly, the variant translocations t(2;8)(q11;q24) or t(8;22)(q24;q11) involving *MYC* and the κ and λ light chain genes, respectively.

T-lymphoblastic leukemia/lymphoma is less common and involves an older demographic than its B-cell counterpart. Patients typically present with abundant blasts in the peripheral blood and a mediastinal mass. The blasts are generally TdT positive and demonstrate variable expression of other T-lineage antigens, most commonly CD3 and CD7. Genetic aberrations identified in this entity include translocations between the *TCRβ* and *TCRδ* genes and a variety of partners; microdeletions of *TAL1*; activating mutations in *NOTCH*; and del(9q), which results in deletion of the tumor suppressor gene *CDKN2A*. Although T-lymphoblastic malignancies have historically had a poor prognosis, recent innovations in treatment have improved outcome.

E. CLL/SLL and Related Disorders. In patients (particularly elderly individuals) with unexplained lymphocytosis, an absolute increase in lymphocytes may represent peripheral blood involvement by low-grade non-Hodgkin lymphoma or leukemia such as CLL/SLL (Table 42.10). For most non-Hodgkin lymphomas, diagnosis is made following biopsy of an involved lymph node or extramedullary focus of disease, and bone marrow biopsy is performed for staging rather than precise classification. An exception to this is CLL/SLL, in which primary diagnosis is often made following flow cytometric analysis of the peripheral blood and demonstration of the characteristic immunophenotype (CD5+, CD10–, CD19 bright+, CD20 heterogeneously+, CD23+, FMC7–, CD79b–).

The various non-Hodgkin lymphomas have different patterns of marrow involvement. Because B-cell lymphomas are more common than T-cell tumors, the former are better characterized. For example, follicular lymphoma and mantle cell lymphoma have a paratrabecular pattern of marrow involvement, whereas CLL/SLL is never paratrabecular (e-Fig. 42.20). In the case of CLL/SLL, the pattern of involvement of the marrow may be predictive of prognosis: cases with predominantly focal lesions are more indolent, whereas examples with a diffuse pattern of involvement are more aggressive. As in lymph nodes, the bone marrow infiltrate of CLL/SLL may contain proliferation (or growth) centers that represent aggregates of prolymphocytes (paraimmunoblasts) and presumably represent the proliferative component of the tumor mass (e-Figs. 42.21 and 42.22). Marginal zone lymphomas may demonstrate follicular colonization when they occur in bone marrows with lymphoid aggregates. Overall, the likelihood of marrow involvement by non-Hodgkin lymphoma is highly variable depending on the type, ranging from very common (e.g., CLL/SLL) to rare (e.g., extranodal marginal zone lymphoma). Immunohistochemistry is typically not required in non-Hodgkin lymphoma staging biopsies, although it is occasionally helpful in delineating benign from malignant lymphoid aggregates.

F. Hairy Cell Leukemia is a rare form of chronic leukemia. Most commonly the affected individual is a middle-aged man presenting with pancytopenia, including lymphopenia and monocytopenia, and an enlarged spleen. Occasionally, patients present with a leukemic blood picture mimicking CLL. The bone marrow is virtually always involved. Although identified in bone marrow aspirate preparations, hairy cells are more easily identified in the peripheral blood by the presence of cytoplasmic projections (hence the name "hairy cell leukemia"; e-Fig. 42.23). The malignant cells frequently have an interstitial pattern of involvement in the bone marrow and for this reason are occasionally overlooked. Sometimes the pattern of marrow involvement recapitulates the pattern of splenic involvement, with collections of extravasated red blood cells surrounded by ill-defined collections of hairy cells (e-Figs. 42.24 and 42.25). The malignant cells are positive with tartrate-resistant acid phosphatase (TRAP) enzyme cytochemistry. Flow cytometry identifies a characteristic pattern of reactivity: the hairy cells are CD5, CD10,

Disease	Phenotype	Morphology	Cytogenetics (Significance)	Molecular Genetics (Impact on Outcome)
Chronic lymphocytic leukemia/small lymphocytic lymphoma	CD5+, CD10−, CD19+ (bright), CD20+ (dim), CD23+, FMC7−, CD79b−, sIg light chain+ (dim) CD38± (unfavorable if +), Zap70± (unfavorable if +)	Usually small mature-appearing lymphocytes; diffuse, interstitial, or nodular patterns of marrow involvement (never paratrabecular)	13q14 deletions (favorable outcome), +12 (morphologically atypical, unfavorable outcome), 17p (TP53) deletions (unfavorable)	The presence of Ig heavy chain variable region mutation (favorable)
Mantle cell lymphoma	CD5+, CD10−, CD19+, CD20+ (bright), CD23−, FMC7+, CD79b+, sIg light chain+ (usually bright), cyclin D1+	Usually small lymphocytes with clefted/folded nuclei; diffuse, nodular, interstitial, or paratrabecular patterns of marrow involvement	t(11;14) [BCL1/IGH]	—
Follicular lymphoma	CD5−, CD10+, CD19+, CD20+, CD23−, sIg light chain+	Variable cytomorphology; diffuse, nodular, interstitial, or paratrabecular patterns of marrow involvement	t(14;18) [BCL2/IGH]	—
Marginal zone B-cell lymphoma	CD5−, CD10−, CD19+, CD20+, CD23−, sIg light chain+	Small lymphocytes, some with ample cytoplasm	t(11;18)(q21;q21) [API2/MALT1] identified in a subset of extranodal marginal zone lymphoma	—
Lymphoplasmacytic lymphoma/Waldenström macroglobulinemia	CD5−, CD10−, CD19+, CD20+, CD23−, sIg light chain+	Small lymphocytes, some with plasmacytoid features	t(9;14)(q13;q32) [PAX5/IGH] identified in ~50% of cases but is not limited to this type of lymphoma	—

Ig, immunoglobulin; sIg, surface immunoglobulin.

From Swerdlow SH, Campo E, Harris NL, et al., eds. WHO Classification of Tumours. Pathology and Genetics. Tumours of Haematopoietic and Lymphoid Tissues, 4th ed. Lyon, France: IARC Press; 2017. Used with permission.

and CD23 negative, but positive for the pan B-cell antigens CD19 and CD20. In addition, they typically demonstrate bright coexpression of CD11c and CD25, and are also positive for CD103 and FMC7 (*Am J Hematol* 2017;92:1382; *Semin Oncol* 1998;25:6). Identification of this pattern of reactivity in the presence of appropriate cytomorphology essentially excludes other types of B-cell neoplasia such as splenic marginal zone lymphoma and prolymphocytic lymphoma. Although hairy cell leukemia is largely resistant to conventional chemotherapies, it is sensitive to purine analogs (i.e., cladribine) and is associated with a prolonged median survival.

SUGGESTED READINGS

Foucar K. *Bone Marrow Pathology*. Chicago, IL: ASCP Press; 2010.

Orazi A, Weiss LM, Foucar K, Knowles DM, eds. *Knowles Neoplastic Hematopathology*, 2nd ed. Philadelphia, PA: Lippincott Williams & Wilkins; 2013.

Swerdlow SH, Campo E, Harris NL, et al., eds. *World Health Organization Classification of Tumors. Pathology and Genetics of Tumors of Haematopoietic and Lymphoid Tissues*. Lyon: IARC Press; 2017.

43 Spleen

Brooj Abro, Chen Yang, and Anjum Hassan

I. **NORMAL GROSS AND MICROSCOPIC ANATOMY.** The spleen, weighing 50 to 250 g in a normal adult, is the largest lymphatic organ. Anatomically, it is divided into white pulp and red pulp by an ill-defined interface known as the marginal zone (e-**Fig. 43.1A**). For schematic of splenic architecture, see Figure 43.1.

A. **White Pulp.** The white pulp consists of periarteriolar lymphoid sheets (PALS) which contains lymphoid follicles. T-lymphocytes are predominately located in periarteriolar lymphoid nodules and B-lymphocytes are predominately located in the lymphoid follicles. The latter may contain germinal centers that become visible to the naked eye when enlarged, forming splenic nodules (malpighian corpuscles). In routine hematoxylin and eosin stained sections, the white pulp appears basophilic due to the dense heterochromatin in lymphocyte nuclei (e-**Fig. 43.1B**).

B. **Red Pulp.** The red pulp has a red appearance in fresh specimens and in histologic sections because it contains a large number of red blood cells (e-**Fig. 43.1B**). It consists of splenic sinuses separated by splenic cords (the cords of Billroth) which are comprised of a loose network of reticular cells and fibers with a large number of erythrocytes, macrophages, lymphocytes, plasma cells, and granulocytes. Special endothelial cells that express both endothelial and histiocytic markers (known as littoral cells) line the sinuses. The sinusoidal lining epithelium is discontinuous, allowing for transport of blood cells between the splenic cords and sinuses.

II. **GROSS EXAMINATION AND TISSUE SAMPLING**

A. **Biopsy and Fine Needle Aspiration Cytology.** These procedures are rarely attempted because of the risk of hemorrhage and the likelihood of undersampling. However, some studies suggest increased chances of a definitive diagnosis when fine needle biopsy is combined with flow cytometry, with an overall accuracy of 91% and a major complication rate of less than 1% (*Am J Hematol* 2001;67:93).

B. **Splenectomy.** Trauma, staging procedures, and surgical convenience account for greater than 50% of all splenectomies. Therapeutic splenectomy for known diagnoses (idiopathic thrombocytopenic purpura [ITP], chronic myeloproliferative disorders, lymphomas, etc.) accounts for most of the remaining cases (*Cancer* 2001;91:2001). Unexpected pathology is rarely found in splenectomy specimens, but significant splenomegaly (weight greater than 300 g) or localizing lesions warrant careful prosection and ancillary studies.

C. **Processing.** The spleen is weighed, and its outer dimensions are recorded. Hilar fatty tissue is removed and processed for lymph nodes. The capsule should be described, noting the texture and intactness. The spleen should be thinly sliced (every 2 to 3 mm); lesional distribution should be noted, followed by a description of the uninvolved spleen. Sections of any lesions (preferably following overnight formalin fixation of thin sections) and two representative sections of uninvolved spleen should be submitted for microscopic examination.

If clinically indicated, fresh lesional tissue in 1-mm pieces should be placed in RPMI medium and directed immediately to the flow cytometry laboratory with instructions regarding the appropriate protocol. Cytogenetic studies may be useful, especially for the diagnosis of hematologic malignancies; ideally, using sterile technique, lesional material should be procured immediately after removal of the spleen in the operating room and directed to the cytogenetic lab. Samples can also be frozen or fixed for electron microscopy. Freezing preserves many of the antigens for immunohistochemical evaluation in

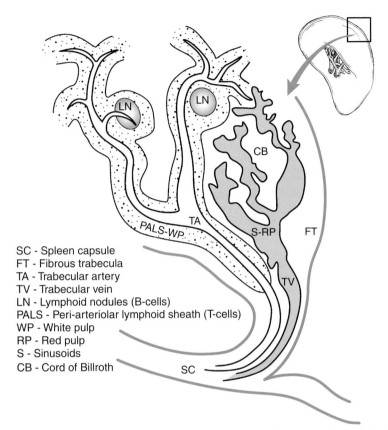

SC - Spleen capsule
FT - Fibrous trabecula
TA - Trabecular artery
TV - Trabecular vein
LN - Lymphoid nodules (B-cells)
PALS - Peri-arteriolar lymphoid sheath (T-cells)
WP - White pulp
RP - Red pulp
S - Sinusoids
CB - Cord of Billroth

Figure 43.1 Diagram of the spleen showing important anatomic landmarks and B- and T-cell distribution.

hematopoietic malignancies and enhances nucleic acid recovery for DNA- and RNA-based molecular diagnostic techniques (although currently most diagnostic molecular tests can be reliably performed on formalin-fixed, paraffin-embedded material).

III. GENERAL CONSIDERATIONS

A. **Splenomegaly.** Often the spleen becomes enlarged due to infectious causes or congestive states. Red pulp congestion is frequently observed and is the most common finding in such cases (Table 43.1).

B. **Hypersplenism.** Hypersplenism refers to destruction of one or more blood cell lines by the spleen (*Eur J Gastroenterol Hepatol* 2001;13:317). It is the most important indication for elective splenectomy. Diagnostic criteria for hypersplenism include cytopenia(s) of one or more blood cell lines, bone marrow hyperplasia, splenomegaly, and correction of cytopenia(s) following splenectomy. Of the many possible etiologies (see Table 43.2), congenital disorders such as hereditary spherocytosis (e-**Fig. 43.2**), infiltrative disorders such as leukemias and lymphomas (e-**Fig. 43.3**), and autoimmune disorders are the most common.

C. **Hyposplenism.** Hyposplenism refers to any deficiency or absence of a functioning spleen and is usually due to splenectomy. Splenic function is usually assessed by

TABLE 43.1 Conditions Associated With Splenomegaly

I. Infection
    A. Infectious endocarditis
    B. Infectious mononucleosis
    C. Tuberculosis
    D. Histoplasmosis
    E. Syphilis
    F. Parasitic infections (e.g., malaria)
    G. Cytomegalovirus
II. Congestive states
    A. Cirrhosis
    B. Splenic vein thrombosis
    C. Heart failure
III. Hematologic malignancy
    A. Non-Hodgkin lymphoma
    B. Hodgkin lymphoma
    C. Myeloproliferative disorders
    D. Multiple myeloma
IV. Immune-related conditions
    A. Rheumatoid arthritis
    B. Systemic lupus erythematous
    C. Storage disorders (e.g., Gaucher disease)

Adapted from Kumar V, Abbas AK, Aster JC. *Robbins & Cotran Pathologic Basis of Disease*, 9th ed. Philadelphia: Elsevier; 2014.

TABLE 43.2 Disorders Associated With Hypersplenism

I. Abnormal sequestration of intrinsically defective blood cells in a normal spleen
    A. Congenital disorders of erythrocytes
        (hereditary spherocytosis, elliptocytosis; hemoglobinopathies, e.g., sickle cell disease, unstable hemoglobins)
    B. Acquired disorders of erythrocytes
        (autoimmune hemolytic anemias, malaria, babesiosis)
    C. Autoimmune thrombocytopenia and/or neutropenia
II. Abnormal spleen causing sequestration of normal blood cells
    A. Disorders of the monocyte/macrophage system
        (chronic congestion, storage diseases, parasitic infections, Langerhans cell histiocytosis, etc.)
    B. Malignant infiltrative disorders
        (leukemias, lymphomas, plasma cell dyscrasias, metastatic carcinoma)
    C. Extramedullary hematopoiesis
        (severe hemolytic states, chronic idiopathic myelofibrosis)
    D. Chronic infections, e.g., tuberculosis, brucellosis
    E. Vascular/stromal abnormalities
        (vascular tumors, peliosis, splenic cysts, hamartomas)
III. Miscellaneous conditions
    A. Hyperthyroidism
    B. Hypogammaglobulinemia
    C. Progressive multifocal leukoencephalopathy

radiologic imaging or morphologic techniques. Peripheral blood smear examination may also be informative; findings suggesting hyposplenism can occur in any blood cell line, including erythrocytes (Howell–Jolly bodies [e-**Fig. 43.4**], poikilocytosis with target cells, acanthocytes, and nucleated red blood cells), platelets (thrombocytosis),

TABLE 43.3 Disorders Associated With Hyposplenism

I. Congenital
  A. Asplenia
  B. Hypoplasia
  C. Immunodeficiency disorders
II. Acquired
  A. Splenectomy
  B. Acquired atrophy and/or infarction
    1. Sickle cell disease
    2. Vascular disorders (vasculitides, thromboembolic conditions)
    3. Essential thrombocythemia
    4. Malabsorption syndromes
    5. Autoimmune diseases
    6. Irradiation
    7. Cytotoxic chemotherapy
    8. Chronic alcoholism
    9. Hypopituitarism
  C. Functional asplenia with normal-sized or enlarged spleen
    1. Infiltration by leukemia, lymphoma, multiple myeloma, mastocytosis
    2. Early (splenomegalic) sickle cell disease
    3. Amyloidosis
    4. Sarcoidosis
    5. Benign and malignant vascular tumors
    6. Malabsorption syndromes
  D. Depressed immune function
    1. AIDS
    2. Status post
      a. Irradiation
      b. Cytotoxic chemotherapy
      c. Immunosuppressive agents, including corticosteroids
    3. Endocrine disorders
      a. Hypothyroidism
      b. Hypopituitarism
      c. Diabetes mellitus
    4. Chronic alcoholism

and leukocytes (lymphocytosis or monocytosis and eosinophilia). Other causes of hyposplenism include congenital hypoplasia (e.g., Fanconi anemia and sickle cell disease [e-**Fig. 43.5**]), infiltrative disorders, old age, and many others (see Table 43.3).

  D. Accessory Spleen. Alternatively termed "spleniculi", these are most commonly located in the splenic hilum, tail of the pancreas, and the gastrohepatic ligament (*N Engl J Med* 1981;304:11). They are found in up to one-third of autopsy cases and share the same histologic and pathologic features as the native spleen (e-**Fig. 43.6**). Accessory spleens are clinically significant in patients requiring splenectomy for hypersplenism.

  E. Splenosis. Splenosis refers to splenic implants or regrowth of splenic tissue after trauma or surgical splenectomy. When associated with trauma, the most common location is in the abdominal cavity, but splenosis has been reported at virtually all anatomic sites, including the brain (*Am J Surg Pathol* 1998;22:894). Usually benign incidental findings, their clinical importance lies in their potential to mimic neoplastic and nonneoplastic splenic lesions.

IV. REACTIVE SPLENIC DISORDERS. These can be divided into diffuse and localized processes. Diffuse disease entities include reactive lymphoid hyperplasia (e-**Fig. 43.7A**), follicular hyperplasia, and disorders such as Castleman disease (see Chapter 41). Localized disease includes granulomatous disorders and infectious processes similar to those in other locations (see Chapter 41).

A. Diffuse Reactive Processes. Reactive lymphoid hyperplasia in the spleen may occur with or without germinal center formation. Because of the reactive nature of the latter and its histologic lack of maturing germinal centers, this entity is variably referred to as "activated A," "early-activated immune reaction," "reactive nonfollicular hyperplasia," and even "immunoblastic hyperplasia." (*Am J Surg Pathol* 1981;5:551) Nongerminal center hyperplasia is often associated with viral infections, especially herpes simplex virus and Epstein–Barr virus (e-**Fig. 43.7B**), which explains the common occurrence of splenomegaly in patients with infectious mononucleosis.

Reactive lymphoid hyperplasia with germinal center formation (e-**Fig. 43.7C**) is commonly referred to as "follicular" hyperplasia. It is the most common pattern of lymphoid hyperplasia in the spleen and is seen in both acute and chronic immune reactions. Follicular hyperplasia is frequently observed in bacterial infection, often as an incidental finding. In fact, splenomegaly is characteristic in subacute bacterial endocarditis, alerting the clinician to this process in the appropriate clinical context is critical to clinical management.

B. Focal Reactive Processes. Localized reactive splenic processes can also present with splenomegaly.

1. Granulomas. The most common form of a focal benign process is granulomatous inflammation, ranging from lipogranulomatous inflammation (of unknown etiology) to caseating or noncaseating granulomatous inflammation. Caseating granulomas are primarily due to infectious disease, including tuberculosis and fungal infection; however, they are also seen in X-linked chronic granulomatous disease. Noncaseating granulomatous disease is most frequently associated with sarcoidosis (e-**Fig. 43.8**). For most granulomas in the spleen, no known etiology can be found (*Arch Pathol Lab Med* 1974;98:261).

2. Infarcts. The spleen is a frequent site of systemic emboli, which commonly arise from cardiac valve lesions or mural thrombi. Infarcts are usually wedge shaped with a hemorrhagic to pale-tan to fibrotic appearance depending on the age of lesion (e-**Fig. 43.9**). Nonwedge-shaped infarcts arise in a variety of intrinsic hematopoietic and nonhematopoietic processes. Essential thrombocythemia and chronic idiopathic myelofibrosis are the hematopoietic disorders most frequently associated with infarcts; less common causes include paroxysmal nocturnal hemoglobinuria, sickle cell disease, and aplastic anemia. Among nonhematopoietic etiologies, vasculitides (polyarteritis nodosa, infections, TTP/ITP associated, etc.) and splenic artery aneurysms are common culprits.

V. NEOPLASTIC DISORDERS OF THE SPLEEN

A. Lymphoid Neoplasms. Lymphoid neoplasms can involve the spleen as a primary disease or as a part of a generalized lymphomatous process. Splenomegaly is a rather nonspecific, but classic component of many hematolymphoid disorders. (Table 43.4)

1. Primary splenic lymphomas. These account for less than 1% of all lymphomas and can be of B- or T-cell origin (see Chapter 41). Not unexpectedly, B-cell lymphomas are more common, and diffuse large B-cell lymphoma (which usually presents as single or multiple circumscribed nodules of varying sizes) accounts for the vast majority of cases (e-**Fig. 43.10**). The diagnostic approach to primary splenic lymphomas is identical to lymphomas presenting elsewhere (see Chapter 41).

2. Secondary splenic lymphomas

a. Hodgkin lymphoma. The spleen is the most common extranodal site of Hodgkin lymphoma, both classic (e-**Fig. 43.11A**) and nodular lymphocyte-predominant Hodgkin lymphoma (NLPHL), although the latter is extremely rare (*Cancer* 1971;27:1277; *Cancer* 1987;59:99). Diagnostic Reed–Sternberg cells or variants (e-**Fig. 43.11B,C**) are a requirement for the diagnosis of classic Hodgkin lymphoma, especially in cases without previously documented history. Immunohistochemical evaluation is often very helpful in the differential diagnosis of classic Hodgkin lymphoma versus NLPHL.

TABLE 43.4	Immunohistochemical Evaluation of Normal and Neoplastic Spleen—Critical Guidelines
GENERAL GUIDELINES TO EVALUATE THE STROMAL COMPARTMENT	Generally speaking, the stromal compartment consists of blood vessels, monocytes/macrophages, and dendritic cells. Together these comprise the "filtration unit" of the spleen and are components of the cords of Billroth.
A. Vascular endothelial cells	CD34, CD31, Factor VIII–related antigen are useful in highlighting both normal and neoplastic lesions.
Littoral cells	Share features of both endothelial cells and monocyte/macrophages; express CD8 uniformly.
B. Monocyte/macrophage	CD68, lysozyme, and antichymotrypsin are useful stains. When evaluation of intracellular material or infectious organisms is desired, PAS, Gram stain, AFB, and GMS stains can be used.
C. Dendritic cells	Two major types: interdigitating (IDC) and follicular (FDC). CD68, S100, CD1a, lysozyme, α_1-antitrypsin may show variable positivity in dendritic cells. FDCs are CD21+ CD35+; IDCs are S100+.
GENERAL GUIDELINES TO EVALUATE THE B- AND T- CELL LYMPHOID COMPARTMENT	In general, most lymphomas involve the white pulp (nodular/follicular low-power appearance), but extensive disease may present as diffuse white pulp expansion.
A. Could this be a metastasis?	CD45 if lesion is not obviously lymphoid.
B. Is it a B- or T- cell process?	B-(CD20, Pax 5, CD79a) and T- (CD3, CD45RO) cell markers are always used in concert to assess number and distribution of cells.
C. Are these malignant B- cells?	Aberrant T-cell markers, CD43, and/or CD5 are often coexpressed in malignant B-cells. By immunohistochemistry (IHC), these must be evaluated with extreme care in B-cell distribution areas (normal T-cells, most marrow-derived (myeloid) cells, and macrophages can all express CD43 by IHC).
D. Are these follicles benign or reactive?	Bcl-2 is particularly helpful in differential diagnosis of follicular lymphoma and reactive follicular hyperplasia. Benign germinal centers retain the capacity to undergo apoptosis and do not express the antiapoptosis protein Bcl-2. About 80% of follicular lymphomas express Bcl-2 in the follicles.
E. How should we subtype the lymphoid malignancies?	Additional B-and T-cell markers must be used to further characterize phenotype of various lymphomas (see also Chapter 41, Tables 41.3 and 41.4)
SOME EXAMPLES OF DISORDERS WITH PREDOMINANTLY RED PULP INVOLVEMENT	In general, disorders with large components of circulating cells have more extensive red pulp involvement.
A. Hairy cell leukemia	DB-44, TRAP, CD25, CD123, and annexin A1–positive
B. Hairy cell leukemia variant	DBA-44+, negative for TRAP, CD25, CD123, and annexin A1
C. Splenic diffuse red pulp small B-cell lymphoma	DBA-44+, negative for CD5, CD10, CD11c, CD25, CD123, and annexin A1
D. Hepatosplenic T-cell lymphoma	CD3+, CD4-, CD8-, often CD56+, markers of cytotoxic molecules (TIA, perforin, granzyme B)+, $\gamma\delta$ rearrangement

TABLE 43.4	Immunohistochemical Evaluation of Normal and Neoplastic Spleen—Critical Guidelines (*Continued*)
E. T-LGL	CD3+, CD8+
F. T-PLL	CD3+, usually CD4+
G. Acute leukemias and myeloproliferative disorders	For granulocytic or monocytic cells: MPO, CD34, CD117, CD68 For erythroid cells: glycophorin, hemoglobin For megakaryocytes: CD41, CD42b, CD61, Factor VIII For precursor lymphoid leukemias: Tdt, CD79a, CD3, CD10

Abbreviations: AFB, acid-fast bacilli; FDC, follicular dendritic cells; GMS, Gomori methanamine silver; IDC, inter-digitating dendritic cells; IHC, immunohistochemistry; MPO, myeloperoxidase; PAS, periodic acid-Schiff; TdT, terminal deoxynucleotidyl transferase; T-LGL, T-large granular lymphocyte lymphoma; TRAP, tartrate-resistant acid phosphatase.

b. Non-Hodgkin lymphomas. More than 50% of cases of low-grade lymphomas show splenic involvement either in the form of splenomegaly or splenic hilar lymph node involvement. Splenic involvement can be categorized as focal or diffuse, the latter mode being more common. Usually there is initial expansion of white pulp in a nodular pattern in cases of low-grade B-cell lymphomas (e.g., small lymphocytic, mantle cell, follicular, or marginal zone) eventually evolving into a diffuse pattern. Both patterns are often observed in appropriately sampled splenectomy specimens. Intermediate and high-grade lymphomas (large cell, Burkitt, lymphoblastic) tend to form single or multiple tumor masses. General histopathologic considerations for the diagnosis of these lymphomas are similar to those occurring in lymph nodes (see Chapter 41).

3. Lymphomas presenting with prominent splenomegaly

a. Splenic B-cell marginal zone lymphoma (SMZL). SMZL is an indolent disease, and splenectomy and/or rituximab therapy is associated with long-term survival (*Leuk lymphoma* 2014;55:1854). SMZL is sometimes accompanied by autoimmune thrombocytopenia or anemia, and circulating villous lymphocytes (with polar projections) are sometimes seen in peripheral blood. The most common genetic aberrations include loss of 7q31-32 with a prevalence of approximately 40%, and somatic mutations effecting *NOTCH2* and *KLF2* genes (*Leukemia* 2014;28:1334; *Leukemia* 2015;29:503). Mutations involving *NOTCH2*, *KLF2*, and *TP53* have been reported to correlate with a worse prognosis (*Clin Cancer Res* 2015;21:4174).

Histologically, expanded PALs are seen, composed of small lymphocytes and monocytoid lymphocytes (e-Fig. 43.12). Flow cytometry should demonstrate a clonal B-cell process (surface light chain restriction), usually lacking coexpression of CD5, CD10, and CD23. Alternatively, immunohistochemistry (IHC) can be performed (to document a B-cell phenotype and coexpression of CD43) coupled with in situ hybridization studies (for kappa and lambda light chains); the latter are usually helpful in highlighting the clonal plasma cell population which forms part of the spectrum of B-cell differentiation in marginal zone B-cell lymphomas.

b. Hepatosplenic T-cell lymphoma (HSTL). This rare lymphoma has a clinically aggressive course and usually afflicts young males. It is characterized by a triad of peripheral cytopenias (anemia and thrombocytopenia), sinusoidal tropism, and hepatosplenomegaly. The disease is somewhat more common in immunosup-pressed settings, such as postsolid organ transplantation, and splenomegaly may exceed 3,000 g. The neoplastic process is based in the red pulp, with conspicuous infiltration of sinuses (e-Fig. 43.13). The differential diagnosis includes other red pulp–based diseases such as hairy cell leukemia (HCL). Immunophenotypic and genetic studies demonstrate a clonal population of T-cells, often double negative for CD4 and CD8, with the majority showing T-cell receptor γδ gene rearrangements. There is strong genetic association with isochromosome 7q10 and trisomy 8 for this entity (*Nat Rev Gastroenterol Hepatol* 2009;6:433).

c. Mantle cell lymphoma (MCL). In MCL, prominent splenomegaly usually represents the leukemic phase or stage III or IV disease. Consequently, the morphologic pattern of involvement can be diffuse, nodular, or both (e-**Fig. 43.14**). Splenic involvement may occur in the absence of significant lymphadenopathy (*Virchows Arch* 2000;437:591). The usual constellation of morphologic, immunophenotypic, and cytogenetic findings is required for diagnosis (see Chapter 41).

d. Hairy cell leukemia (HCL). HCL classically presents with peripheral cytopenias, particularly monocytopenia (*Leuk Lymphoma* 1994;13:307), and splenomegaly in a young male with recurrent opportunistic infections (*Am J Clin Pathol* 1977;67:415). In the spleen, HCL involves and expands the red pulp; the white pulp is usually inconspicuous (e-**Fig. 43.15**). The classic immunophenotype by flow cytometry (CD103+, CD11c+, CD25+) can be easily demonstrated utilizing peripheral blood in the presence of circulating "hairy cells" and is required for diagnosis. This immunophenotype is also helpful in distinguishing HCL from HSTL, T-large granular lymphocyte lymphoma (T-LGL), other T-cell neoplasms, and mast cell disease, all of which can morphologically mimic HCL in the spleen. By IHC, DBA 44, annexin A1, and cyclin D1 stains are helpful (*Lancet* 2004;363:1869; *Hematol Oncol Clin North Am* 2006;20:1051). No common recurrent cytogenetic abnormality is specific; however, numerical abnormalities of chromosomes 5 and 7 have been reported (*Hematol Oncol Clin North Am* 2006;20:1011). The BRAF V600E mutation is specific and detected in approximately 100% of cases of HCL when compared to other B-cell lymphomas (*J Clin Oncol.* 2017;35(9):1002–1010).

e. Splenic B-cell lymphoma/leukemia, unclassifiable. These diseases are, by definition, splenic small B-cell lymphomas that do not fit in any defined category. Two provisional and relatively rare entities include splenic diffuse red pulp small B-cell lymphoma (SDRPL) and hairy cell leukemia variant (HCL-v). These two entities in the spleen are distinct from SMZL based on their pattern of diffuse infiltration by monomorphic lymphocytes in contrast to a nodular pattern of infiltration by biphasic lymphocytes seen in SMZL (*Am J Surg Pathol* 2012;36:1609).

  i. Splenic diffuse red pulp small B-cell lymphoma (SDRPL). Patients present at stage IV disease with involvement of the spleen, bone marrow, and peripheral blood. In the spleen a diffuse pattern of infiltration involving the red pulp is characteristic and an intrasinusoidal infiltrate is evident in the bone marrow. By flow cytometry, SDRPL is typically positive for CD20, DBA-44, and IgG but negative for CD5, CD10, CD11c, CD25, and CD123 (*Discov Med* 2012; 13:253).

  ii. Hairy cell leukemia variant (HCL-v). Even though this is a rare entity, it is important to differentiate HCL-v from HCL and other B-cell lymphomas due to differences in clinical management. It has overlapping features with HCL; however, it shows variant morphologic and clinical findings. Patients present with lymphocytosis and the circulating abnormal cells have an intermediate morphology between prolymphocytes and hairy cells that lack expression of CD25, CD123, TRAP, and annexin A1. (*Am J Hematol* 2017;92:1382).

4. Other B- and T-cell lymphomas. T-prolymphocytic leukemia and T-large granular lymphocytic leukemia commonly involve the spleen (see Chapter 41) as they are usually leukemic at presentation. Likewise B-cell lymphomas, presenting at stage III or IV (see Chapter 41) can also involve spleen. An example of high-stage follicular lymphoma involving the spleen is shown in (e-**Fig. 43.16**).

B. Myeloid Neoplasms

1. Chronic myelogenous leukemia (CML). CML is classically associated with splenomegaly. The spleen is also the most common extranodal site of involvement in the blast phase of CML (e-**Fig. 43.17**). Morphologic findings leading to the diagnosis of CML are best evaluated in touch preparations, although histologic sections are also easy to interpret. Touch preparations are required for optimal enumeration of blasts.

Immunohistochemical stains (CD34, c-kit) and cytochemical stains (Leder, myeloperoxidase) can also be useful in highlighting the blast population. Disease progression (accelerated phase) and transformation in CML is usually obvious both clinically and morphologically.

2. **Acute leukemias.** Acute leukemias present as diffuse involvement of the red pulp (e-**Fig. 43.18**). The spleen is rarely a primary site of myeloid disease, and involvement reflects systemic disease. Histopathologic and immunophenotypic considerations are similar to acute leukemias presenting with peripheral blood and bone marrow involvement (see Chapter 42). Evaluation of spleen specimens for commonly occurring cytogenetic abnormalities, by conventional cytogenetics or FISH, is a standard part of the workup unless there is a prior history of leukemia. Care must be taken to appropriately evaluate for therapy-related morphologic and phenotypic changes, as well as clonal evolution, which may alter the treatment course or effectiveness for targeted therapies.

3. **Mast cell disease and/or systemic mastocytosis.** These myeloproliferative neoplasms frequently involve the spleen. The morphologic patterns of involvement vary from isolated white pulp accentuation with fibrosis, to red pulp involvement with diffuse infiltration, fibrosis, and/or nodular perivascular infiltrates. The presence of eosinophils, plasma cells, and fibrosis are all clues that point to the presence of mast cells. Flow cytometry is often not helpful for mast cell disease primarily because of technical difficulties in gating the desired population, although expression of CD2 and CD25 by flow cytometry is a feature specific to neoplastic mast cells (both benign and neoplastic mast cells are CD45+, CD33+, CD68+, and CD117+). In tissue sections, a Leder stain, CD117, and tryptase are helpful in highlighting mast cells.

C. **Nonhematopoietic Neoplasms and Pseudoneoplasms.** A wide variety of mesenchymal cell types form the complex reticular support network of splenic pulp and consequently a wide variety of mesenchymal tumors can occur as primary splenic neoplasms. These can generally be divided into stromal lesions, vascular lesions, and tumor-like lesions.

1. **Stromal lesions**

   a. **Dendritic cell tumors.** Two different kinds of dendritic cells exist in the normal lymphoid support network: interdigitating dendritic cells (IDCs) which are normally S-100 protein and MHC II positive, and follicular dendritic cells (FDC) which express CD35 and CD21. Splenic involvement can be seen in neoplastic disorders of either IDC and FDC (*Cancer* 1997;79:294; *Am J Surg Path* 2002;26:530). Grossly, involvement is usually nodular, although disseminated systemic disease may present with diffuse splenic involvement. Dendritic cell tumors tend to behave in an aggressive manner despite their bland histologic appearance. In the absence of a preceding history, dendritic cell tumors are diagnoses of exclusion, mandating a thorough immunophenotypic workup to exclude myeloid malignancies, lymphoid B- and T-cell malignancies, and nonhematopoietic malignancies. It is important to note that FDC neoplasia may be associated with the hyaline vascular type of Castleman disease (*Adv Anat Pathol* 2009;16:236).

   b. **Histiocytic lesions.** These lesions range from Langerhans cell histiocytosis (LCH) to histiocytic sarcomas including Langerhans cell sarcoma. Splenic involvement is rare, usually occurring in the setting of disseminated disease and grossly presenting as single or multiple solid nodules.

      Expression of S-100 and CD1a by the neoplastic cells is consistent with a diagnosis of LCH. The sarcomatous forms can be less differentiated and may variably show expression of HLA-DR, CD45, CD68, PLAP, and vimentin (*Am J Surg Pathol* 2004;8:1133).

2. **Vascular lesions.** Vascular tumors are common in the spleen, given its rich vascular framework. Both benign and malignant vascular lesions may present in the spleen. (*Am J Surg Pathol* 1997;21:827).

   a. **Benign lesions**

      i. **Littoral cell angioma** is unique in its presentation in the spleen and grossly is characterized by multiple spongy, cystic nodules. The cystic spaces are lined by cuboidal epithelium with intracytoplasmic eosinophilic globules. The lumina often contain abundant desquamated cells. Vascular markers (CD31, Factor VIII–related antigen) are characteristically expressed; expression of CD68 and CD21 is more variable. CD34, commonly expressed in normal sinusoids, is uniformly negative.

ii. **Peliosis,** characterized by ectatic sinusoids and blood filled cysts, can involve the spleen. The location of the cysts (adjacent to PALS and follicles) is helpful in establishing the diagnosis. The clinical importance of this lesion lies in its propensity to undergo spontaneous rupture.

iii. **Hemangiomas** are a frequent incidental finding at splenectomy (e-Fig. 43.19).

iv. **Sclerosing angiomatoid nodular transformation (SANT)** is a rare nonneo-plastic lesion characterized by angiomatoid nodules surrounded by sclerotic stroma and a lymphoplasmacytic infiltrate (e-Fig. 43.20). It should be dif-ferentiated from vascular neoplasms of the spleen and lymphomas showing lymphoplasmacytic differentiation (*Am J Surg Pathol* 2004;28:1268).

b. **Malignant lesions**

i. **Littoral cell hemangioendothelioma and angiosarcomas** rarely present in the spleen (*Am J Surg Path 2006*;30:1036). They are usually solid, often prompting a differential diagnosis that includes other spindle cell sarcomas. CD31 and Factor VIII–related antigen immunostains establish the vascular nature of these otherwise undifferentiated malignancies; some cases may also show CD34 expression. The translocation t(1;3)(p36.3;q25) that produces a *WWTR1-CAMTA1* gene fusion is a characteristic finding in hemangioendotheliomas (*Sci Transl Med* 2011;3:98ra82; *Genes Chromosomes Cancer* 2011;50:644). Complex cytogenetic abnormalities, none consistent from case to case, have been reported in angiosarcomas (*Cancer Genet Cytogent* 1993;63:171; *Cancer Genet Cytogent* 1998;100:52; *Cancer Genet Cytogent* 2001;129:64).

ii. **Kaposi sarcoma,** in the setting of HIV/AIDS, must be considered in the differential diagnosis of any splenic vascular lesion. Kaposi sarcoma usually shows positive IHC for HHV-8 and a variety of vascular markers.

3. **Pseudoneoplastic lesions.** Examples include splenic hamartoma (well-circum-scribed lesions with an angiomatoid lobular-nodular configuration, resembling red pulp; usually CD8+ and CD68+), splenic cysts (with or without an epithelial cell lining; when an epithelial lining is present it is usually cytokeratin positive [e-Fig. 43.21]), angiomyolipoma (focally HMB-45 positive), and lymphangioma.

Inflammatory pseudotumor is a reactive nodular process that shows a predominance of benign inflammatory cells and stromal cells with sclerosis (e-Fig. 43.22). Inflamma-tory pseudotumor must be distinguished from inflammatory pseudotumor-like FDC tumor (which is usually EBV associated and shows immunohistochemical expression of CD21 and CD35) and lymphomas with lymphoplasmacytic differentiation (mar-ginal zone lymphoma and lymphoplasmacytic lymphoma, see Chapter 41).

4. **Metastatic tumors.** A variety of carcinomas and sarcomas can metastasize to the spleen, although the lack of afferent lymphatics renders the spleen generally less amenable to metastatic disease. Metastases therefore commonly arise in the setting of disseminated disease. The most common metastatic tumors are breast, lung, col-orectal, and ovarian carcinomas and melanoma (*Arch Pathol Lab Med* 2007;131:965). Sarcomas involving the spleen tend to be of dendritic/histiocytic or vascular lineage.

5. **Other neoplasms.** Benign fibromas, osteomas, and chondromas also occur rarely in the spleen.

ACKNOWLEDGMENT

The authors thank Mohammad O. Hussaini for his contribution to the previous edition of this chapter.

SUGGESTED READINGS

Bowdler AJ. *The Complete Spleen*. 2nd ed. Humana Press; 2001.
Neiman RS, Orazi A, eds. *Disorders of Spleen*, 2nd ed. Philadelphia, PA: WB Saunders; 1999.
Rosati S, Frizzera G. Pseudoneoplastic lesions of hematolymphoid system. In: Wick MR, Humphrey PA, Ritter JH, eds. *Pathology of Pseudoneoplastic Lesions*. Lippincott-Raven; 1997, 449.
Swerdlow SH, Campo E, Harris NL, et al. *WHO Classification of Tumors and Haematopoeitic and Lymphoid Tissues*. Lyon: IARC; 2017.

Soft Tissue and Bone

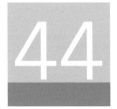

Soft Tissue

John S.A. Chrisinger, John D. Pfeifer, and
Louis P. Dehner

I. TISSUE PROCESSING

A. Biopsy Specimens. The biopsy tissue should be placed immediately into 10% formalin or any other appropriate fixative. The number of biopsy fragments should be recorded, as well as their aggregate dimension, and all the submitted tissue should be processed. Three H&E levels should initially be prepared for microscopic examination. For very small specimens it is strongly recommended that additional unstained slides be cut from the block during initial sectioning in the event additional studies are needed.

B. Resection Specimens. Excisional specimens are often complex and varied, and the macroscopic examination should be guided by tumor location, extent, and type. The margin of all intact specimens should be inked, and the gross distance from the tumor to the closest margin(s) documented. The dimensions of the tumor, the color and consistency of the cut surfaces, and presence and extent of hemorrhage and necrosis should be noted. In general, it is recommended that one section per centimeter of tumor be submitted for microscopic examination. The margins should be evaluated by either shave or radial sections, depending on the nature of the specimen.

Commonly used cytogenetic and molecular analyses can be performed on formalin-fixed paraffin embedded tissue, which plays an ever-increasing role in diagnosis as more types of soft tissue tumors are shown to harbor characteristic genetic aberrations (Table 44.1). A sample of viable tumor can also be snap frozen and stored in the event it is needed for subsequent evaluation.

II. TERMINOLOGY REGARDING THE BIOLOGIC POTENTIAL OF SOFT TISSUE NEOPLASMS

A. Classification. The current WHO Classification of soft tissue tumors (Table 44.2) assigns each neoplasm to one of four categories: benign, intermediate (locally aggressive), intermediate (rarely metastasizing), and malignant. The four categories provide a standard nomenclature to indicate the biologic potential of the various soft tissue tumors.

1. Benign. Most tumors in this category rarely recur. If recurrence does occur, it is typically nondestructive. Complete local excision is curative. The common lipoma is an example of this category.

2. Intermediate (locally aggressive). Tumors in this category have a locally destructive and infiltrative growth pattern, and often locally recur. Wide excision is required for local control, but that is not necessarily an indemnification against a local recurrence. These tumors do not metastasize. Atypical lipomatous tumor is an example of this category.

TABLE 44.1 Recurring Cytogenetic Abnormalities Characteristic of Various Soft Tissue Neoplasms[a]

Tumor Type	Cytogenetic Aberrations	Molecular Alteration
Alveolar rhabdomyosarcoma	t(2;13)(q35;q14) t(1;13)(p36;q14)	PAX3-FOXO1 fusion PAX7-FOXO1 fusion
Alveolar soft part sarcoma	der(17)t(X;17)(p11.2;q25)	ASPSCR1-TFE3 fusion
Anastomosing hemangioma	Limited data, likely simple karyotype	GNAQ mutations
Angiomatoid fibrous histio-cytoma	t(12;22)(q13;q12) t(2;22)(q33;q12) t(12;16)(q13;q11)	EWSR1-ATF1 fusion EWRS1-CREB1 fusion FUS-ATF1 fusion
Atypical lipomatous tumor/well-differentiated liposarcoma	Supernumerary ring and/or marker chromosomes with amplification of 12q14–q15	Amplification of MDM2, CDK4, HMGA2
BCOR-rearranged sarcomas	X chromosome paracentric inversion t(X;22)(p1.4;q13) t(X;4)(p1.4;q31.1)	BCOR-CCNB3 fusion ZC3H7B-BCOR fusion BCOR-MAML3 fusion
Benign deep fibrous histiocytoma	Rearrangements involving 16p12 and 3p21	Fusions involving PRKCB and PRKCD
Calcifying aponeurotic fibroma	ins(2;4)(q35;q25q?) (limited data)	FN1-EGF fusion
Cellular angiofibroma	Deletion of 13q14	Deletion of RB1
Chondroid lipoma	t(11;16)(q13;p12-13)	C11orf95-MKL2 fusion
CIC-rearranged sarcomas	t(4;19)(q35;q13) or t(10;19) (q26;q13) t(X;19)(q13;q13)	CIC-DUX4 fusion CIC-FOXO4 fusion
Clear cell sarcoma of tendons and aponeuroses	t(12;22)(q13;q12) t(2;22)(q32;q12)	EWSR1-ATF1 fusion (majority) EWSR1-CREB1 fusion
Dedifferentiated liposarcoma	Supernumerary ring and/or marker chromosomes with amplification of 12q14-q15	Amplification of MDM2, CDK4, HMGA2
Dermatofibrosarcoma protuberans/giant cell fibroblastoma	t(17;22)(q22;q13) and derivative ring chromosomes	COL1A1-PDGFB fusion
Desmoid fibromatosis	Trisomy 8 or 20; loss of 5q	CTNNB1 or APC mutations
Desmoplastic fibroblastoma	t(2;11)(q31;q12)	Unknown
Desmoplastic small round cell tumor	t(11;22)(p13;q12)	EWSR1-WT1 fusion
Elastofibroma	1q abnormalities	Unknown
Embryonal rhabdomyosarcoma	Gains of 2, 8, and 20, LOH at 11p15	Unknown
Epithelioid hemangioendothelioma	t(1;3)(p36;3q25) t(X;11)(p11;q22)	WWTR1-CAMTA1 fusion YAP1-TFE3 fusion

(*continued*)

Tumor Type	Cytogenetic Aberrations	Molecular Alteration
Epithelioid hemangioma	Rearrangements of 14q24.3 and 19q13.2	*FOS* and *FOSB* fusions
Epithelioid sarcoma	Alterations of 22q11.2	Inactivation of *hSNF5/INI1*
Ewing sarcoma	t(11;22)(q24;q12) t(21;22)(q22;q12)	*EWSR1-FLI1* fusion *EWSR1-ERG* fusion
Extrarenal malignant rhabdoid tumor	Alterations of 22q11.2	Biallelic inactivation of *hSNF5/INI1*
Extraskeletal myxoid chondrosarcoma	t(9;22)(q22;q12) t(9;17)(q22;q11.2) t(9;15)(q22;q21)	*EWSR1-NR4A3* fusion *TAF2N-NR4A3* fusion *TCF12-NR4A3* fusion
Fibroma of tendon sheath (cellular)	Rearrangements of 17p13	*USP6* rearrangement
Fibrous hamartoma of infancy	Translocations involving 2 and 3, and 6, 8, and 12	*EGFR* exon 20 insertion/duplication mutations
Infantile fibrosarcoma	t(12;15)(p13;q25)	*ETV6-NTRK3* fusion
Inflammatory myofibroblastic tumor	Rearrangements of 2p23	*ALK* fusions with a variety of partners
Intimal sarcoma	Amplification of 12q13–14 and 4q12, Gain of 7p12	Amplification of *MDM2*, *KIT* and *PDGFRA*, Gain involving *EGFR*
Intramuscular myxoma	Gains and rearrangements of 8	Activating *GNAS* mutation
Lipoblastoma	Rearrangements of 8q12	Rearrangement of *PLAG1*
Lipoma	Rearrangements of 12q14–q15 and 6p21–22; deletions of 13q12–14	*HMGA2* and *HMGA1* fusions
Low-grade fibromyxoid sarcoma	t(7;16)(q33;p11) t(11;16)(p11;p11) t(11;22)(p11;q12)	*FUS-CREB3L2* fusion *FUS-CREB3L1* fusion *EWSR1-CREB3L1* fusion (rare)
Mammary-type myofibro-blastoma	Deletion of 13q14	Deletion of *RB1*
Melanotic schwannoma	Monosomy of 22q, gains and losses involving 1, 17p, and 21	*PRKAR1A* mutations
Mesenchymal chondrosar-coma	t(8;8)(q13;q21)	*HEY1-NCOA2* fusion
Myoepithelioma/myoepi-thelial carcinoma/mixed tumor	Rearrangements of 22q12, 16q11, or 8q12	*EWSR1* fusions (known partners include: *POU5F1*, *PBX1*, *ZNF444*, and *KLF17*) *FUS* fusions (rare) *PLAG1* rearrangements (mixed tumors)
Myofibroma	Limited data	*PDGFRB* mutations
Myolipoma	t(9;12)(p22;q14)	*HMGA2-C9orf92*

TABLE 44.1 Recurring Cytogenetic Abnormalities Characteristic of Various Soft Tissue Neoplasms[a] (*Continued*)

Tumor Type	Cytogenetic Aberrations	Molecular Alteration
Myxoid liposarcoma	t(12;16)(q13;p11) t(12;22)(q13;q12)	*FUS-DD1T3* fusion *EWSR1-DD1T3* fusion
Myxoinflammatory fibroblastic sarcoma	Amplification of 3p11–12 Alternations involving 7q34	Amplification of *VGLL3* Amplification/rearrangement of *BRAF*
Nodular fasciitis	Rearrangements of 17p13	*USP6* fusions (typically *MYH9-USP6*)
Ossifying fibromyxoid tumor	Rearrangements of 6p21 or Xp11 are most common	*PHF1* or *BCOR* rearrangements in the majority, rarely *CREBBP-BCORL1* or *KDM2A-WWTR1*
Pseudomyogenic hemangioendothelioma	t(7;19)(q22;q13)	*SERPINE1-FOSB*, less commonly *FOSB* rearrangement with an unknown partner
Sclerosing epithelioid fibrosarcoma	t(11;22)(p11;q12) t(11;16)(p11;p11) t(7;16)(p22;p11)	*EWSR1-CREB3L1* fusion *EWSR1-CREB3L2* fusion *FUS-CREB3L2* (rare)
Soft tissue myoepithelioma	Translocations involving 22q12	*EWSR1* fusions with a variety of other genes
Solitary fibrous tumor	Intrachromosomal rearrangements involving 12q	*NAB2-STAT6* fusion
Spindle cell hemangioma	Unknown	*IDH1/2* mutations
Spindle cell/sclerosing rhabdomyosarcoma	Rearrangements of 6q22.1, 8p13.3, and 12q13	*MYOD1* (L122R) mutations *VGLL2* and *NCOA2* rearrangements *TFCP2* rearrangements
Spindle cell/pleomorphic lipoma	Deletion of 13q14	Deletion of *RB1*
Synovial sarcoma	t(X;18)(p11;q11) t(X;20)(p11;q13)	*SSX18-SSX1*, *SSX18-SSX2*, *SSX18-SSX4* fusions *SS18L1-SSX1* fusion (rare)
Tenosynovial giant cell tumor, localized and diffuse types	Translocations involving 1p13, including t(1;2)(p13;q37)	*CSF1* fusions, including *CSF1-COL6A3*

[a]Only select abnormalities are indicated.

3. **Intermediate (rarely metastasizing).** Tumors in this group also have a locally destructive and infiltrative growth pattern. However, they also can metastasize in a small subset of cases (typically less than 2%). The risk of metastasis of an individual tumor cannot typically be predicted on the basis morphologic features. Examples of this category include congenital infantile fibrosarcoma, dermatofibrosarcoma protuberans, and angiomatoid fibrous histiocytoma.

4. **Malignant.** Tumors in this category have a locally destructive growth and metastasize in high percentage of cases; typically low-grade sarcomas have a metastatic rate of 2% to 10%, and high-grade sarcomas metastasize in more than 30% of cases.

TABLE 44.2 | WHO Classification of Soft Tissue Tumors

Adipocytic tumors

Benign
Lipoma
Lipomatosis
Lipomatosis of nerve
Lipoblastoma
Angiolipoma
Myolipoma of soft tissue
Chondroid lipoma
Extrarenal angiomyolipoma
Extra and renal myelolipoma
Spindle cell/pleomorphic lipoma
Hibernoma

Intermediate (locally aggressive)
Atypical lipomatous tumor/well-differentiated liposarcoma

Malignant
Dedifferentiated liposarcoma
Myxoid liposarcoma
Pleomorphic liposarcoma

Fibroblastic/myofibroblastic tumors

Benign
Nodular fasciitis
Proliferative fasciitis and proliferative myositis
Myositis ossificans and fibro-osseous pseudotumor of digits
Ischemic fasciitis
Elastofibroma
Fibrous hamartoma of infancy
Fibromatosis colli
Juvenile hyaline fibromatosis
Inclusion body fibromatosis
Fibroma of tendon sheath
Desmoplastic fibroblastoma
Mammary-type myofibroblastoma
Calcifying aponeurotic fibroma
Angiomyofibroblastoma
Cellular angiofibroma
Nuchal-type fibroma
Gardner fibroma
Calcifying fibrous tumor

Intermediate (locally aggressive)
Palmar/plantar fibromatosis
Desmoid-type fibromatoses
Lipofibromatosis
Giant cell fibroblastoma

Intermediate (rarely metastasizing)
Dermatofibrosarcoma protuberans
Solitary fibrous tumor
Inflammatory myofibroblastic tumor
Low-grade myofibroblastic sarcoma
Myxoinflammatory fibroblastic sarcoma
Infantile fibrosarcoma

TABLE 44.2 WHO Classification of Soft Tissue Tumors (*Continued*)

Malignant
Adult-type fibrosarcoma
Myxofibrosarcoma
Low-grade fibromyxoid sarcoma
Sclerosing epithelioid fibrosarcoma

So-called fibrohistiocytic tumors

Benign
Tenosynovial giant cell tumor, localized-type
Tenosynovial giant cell tumor, diffuse-type
Deep benign fibrous histiocytoma

Intermediate (rarely metastasizing)
Plexiform fibrohistiocytic tumor
Giant cell tumor of soft tissues

Smooth muscle tumors

Benign
Deep leiomyoma

Malignant
Leiomyosarcoma (excluding skin)

Pericytic (perivascular tumors)
Glomus tumor (and variants)
Glomangiomatosis
Malignant glomus tumor
Myopericytoma
Myofibroma
Myofibromatosis
Angioleiomyoma

Skeletal muscle tumors

Benign
Rhabdomyoma (adult, fetal, genital)

Malignant
Embryonal rhabdomyosarcoma (including botryoid, anaplastic)
Alveolar rhabdomyosarcoma (including solid, anaplastic)
Pleomorphic rhabdomyosarcoma
Spindle cell/sclerosing rhabdomyosarcoma

Vascular tumors

Benign
Hemangioma
Synovial hemangioma
Venousl hemangioma
Arteriovenous hemangioma/malformation
Intramuscular hemangioma
Epithelioid hemangioma
Angiomatosis
Lymphangioma

Intermediate (locally aggressive)
Kaposiform hemangioendothelioma

(*continued*)

TABLE 44.2 **WHO Classification of Soft Tissue Tumors (*Continued*)**

Intermediate (rarely metastasizing)
Retiform hemangioendothelioma
Papillary intralymphatic angioendothelioma
Composite hemangioendothelioma
Pseudomyogenic hemangioendothelioma (epithelioid sarcoma-like hemangioendothelioma)
Kaposi sarcoma

Malignant
Epithelioid hemangioendothelioma
Angiosarcoma of soft tissue

Chondro-osseous tumors
Soft tissue chondroma
Extraskeletal mesenchymal chondrosarcoma
Extraskeletal osteosarcoma

Tumors of uncertain differentiation

Benign
Acral fibromyxoma
Intramuscular myxoma (including cellular variant)
Juxta-articular myxoma
Deep ("aggressive") angiomyxoma
Pleomorphic hyalinizing angiectatic tumor
Ectopic hamartomatous thymoma

Intermediate (locally aggressive)
Hemosiderotic fibrolipomatous tumor

Intermediate (rarely metastasizing)
Atypical fibroxanthoma
Angiomatoid fibrous histiocytoma
Ossifying fibromyxoid tumor
Mixed tumor/myoepithelioma/myoepithelial carcinoma
Phosphaturic mesenchymal tumor

Malignant
Synovial sarcoma
Epithelioid sarcoma
Alveolar soft part sarcoma
Clear cell sarcoma of soft tissue
Extraskeletal myxoid chondrosarcoma
Extraskeletal Ewing sarcoma
Desmoplastic small round cell tumor
Extrarenal rhabdoid tumor
Malignant mesenchymoma
PEComa
Intimal sarcoma

Undifferentiated/unclassified sarcomas

Fletcher CDM, Bridge JA, Hogendoorn PCW, Mertens F, eds. *WHO Classification of Tumours of Soft Tissue and Bone.* 4th ed. Lyon, France: IARC Press; 2017. Used with permission.

B. **Histologic Grading of Soft Tissue Sarcoma (STS).** While several grading systems have been proposed over the past 30 to 40 years, including the National Cancer Institute (NCI) system (*Cancer* 1984;53:530), the French Federation Nationale des Centres de Lutte Contre le Cancer (FNCLCC) system (*Int J Cancer* 1984;33:37) (Table 44.3) is the most widely used and has been adopted by the College of American Pathologists and

TABLE 44.3	FNCLCC Grading of Soft Tissue Sarcoma[a]

The FNCLCC grade is determined by three parameters: differentiation (histology specific), mitotic activity, and extent of necrosis. Each parameter is scored: differentiation (1–3), mitotic activity (1–3), and necrosis (0–2). The scores are summed to designate grade.

Grade 1: 2 or 3

Grade 2: 4 or 5

Grade 3: 6–8

Differentiation. Tumor differentiation is histology specific and is generally scored as follows:

Score 1: Sarcomas closely resembling normal, mature mesenchymal tissue

Score 2: Sarcoma of definite histologic type

Score 3: Synovial sarcoma, embryonal sarcoma, undifferentiated sarcomas, and sarcomas of uncertain type

Mitotic count. In the most mitotically active area of the sarcoma, ten successive high-power fields (HPFs) are assessed using a 40× objective.

Score 1: 0–9 mitoses per 10 HPFs

Score 2: 10–19 mitoses per 10 HPFs

Score 3: 20 or more mitoses per 10 HPFs

Tumor necrosis. Evaluated on gross examination and validated with histologic sections.

Score 0: No tumor necrosis

Score 1: Less than or equal to 50% tumor necrosis

Score 2: More than 50% tumor necrosis

[a]Modified from *J Clin Oncol* 1997:15:350; some soft tissue sarcomas in children have their own grading system as outlined in *Cancer* 2010;116:2266. Note: FNCLCC does not apply to all sarcomas.

the American Joint Committee on Cancer (Amin MB et al., eds. *AJCC Cancer Staging Manual.* 8th ed. New York: Springer; 2017). Three histologic features are the basis of this grading system: tumor differentiation, necrosis, and mitotic count. The behavior of some sarcoma types is not well stratified by this system and thus some sarcomas not graded (Table 44.3). Grading systems for select STS in children have also been proposed (*Cancer* 2010;116:2266). It should be noted that it can be difficult to accurately assign a grade to unclassified sarcomas or to tumors distorted by radiation and/or chemotherapy.

III. ADIPOCYTIC TUMORS

A. Benign

1. **Lipoma** is composed of mature adipocytes and is the most common soft tissue neoplasm in adults. Superficial lipomas arise in the subcutis, deep lipomas within the deep soft tissue, parosteal lipomas on the surface of bone, intramuscular lipomas within skeletal muscle, and lipoma arborescens in synovial membranes. Lipomas are well circumscribed and have an oily light yellow cut surface, except in children whose tumors are pale white. Regardless of the anatomic site, the tumor is composed of sheets of mature adipocytes separated into complete and incomplete lobules. Lipomas may have extensive myxoid change (myxoid lipoma), fibrous stroma (fibrolipoma), cartilaginous differentiation (chondrolipoma), osseous differentiation (osteolipoma), or both cartilaginous and osseous differentiation (osteochondrolipoma). Lipomas most commonly show alternations involving 12q13–15 (often resulting in rearrangements of *HMGA2*). Loss of material from 13q and alternations involving 6p21–23 are also observed.

2. **Angiolipoma** typically occurs in the subcutis and consists of mature adipocytes with a variably prominent capillary network with scattered fibrin thrombi. These vessels are typically found at the periphery of the tumor (e-**Fig. 44.1**). These tumors are frequently painful and may be multiple.

3. **Myolipoma** has a female predominance and is usually found in the deep soft tissues of the abdominal cavity, inguinal region, and retroperitoneum. Tumors are well circumscribed and deep tumors are frequently large. Mature adipose tissue is intermixed with fascicles of mature smooth muscle. Atypia, floret-like cells, and thick-walled vessels are absent.

4. **Chondroid lipoma** has a female predominance and mostly occurs in the limb girdle and proximal extremities. Cords and nests of cells displaying different degrees of lipoblastic differentiation (ranging from small bland cells with scant cytoplasm to multivacuolated lipoblasts) are set in a myxoid to chondroid matrix and intermingle with mature adipocytes in the absence of true hyaline cartilage. Surgical excision is curative. Chondroid lipomas have recurrent *C11orf95-MKL2* fusions.

5. **Spindle cell/pleomorphic lipoma** occurs predominantly in middle-aged and elderly men in the posterior neck and upper back, while the majority of tumors in women occur outside the shawl distribution (*Am J Surg Pathol* 2017;41:1267). Patients often present with a mobile dermal or subcutaneous nodule that has been present for many years. Microscopic features are variable: at one end of the spectrum are tumors composed of bland spindle cells set in a myxoid stroma and associated dense ropey collagen bundles and mature adipocytes; at the other end are tumors with small hyperchromatic cells admixed with multinucleated floret cells and mature adipocytes. Tumors are immunopositive for CD34, show loss of Rb, and harbor deletion of *RB1* on 13q14.

6. **Lipomatosis** occurs in several different clinicopathologic settings, all of which are characterized by a diffuse overgrowth of mature adipose tissue. Regardless of the clinical subtype the neoplastic cells are indistinguishable from those found in lipomas, which emphasizes the role of clinical history in arriving at the correct diagnosis.

   a. **Diffuse lipomatosis** preferentially occurs in children less than 2 years old, and involves a substantial part of an extremity as well as the trunk, head and neck, pelvis, abdomen, or intestinal tract. In this setting, the PTEN hamartoma tumor syndrome as expressed in the Proteus syndrome, encephalocraniocutaneous lipomatosis, Bannayan–Ruvalcaba–Riley syndrome, and Cowden disease should be considered (*Genet Med* 2009;11:687).

   b. **Symmetric lipomatosis** occurs predominantly in middle-aged men of Mediterranean ancestry and is characterized by symmetric deposition of fat usually in the upper body.

   c. **Pelvic lipomatosis**, which affects black males over a wide age range, manifests as an overgrowth of fat in perirectal and perivesical areas.

   d. **Steroid lipomatosis** occurs in the setting of adrenocortical hormonal therapy, or with endogenous endocrine abnormalities, and characteristically involves accumulation of fat in the face, sternal region, or middle of the upper back (so-called "buffalo hump").

   e. **HIV-lipodystrophy** affects patients with HIV treated with protease inhibitors and patients receiving other forms of antiviral therapy, and is characterized by the accumulation of visceral fat with fat wasting in the face and limbs.

7. **Lipomatosis of nerve** is most commonly noted in childhood and usually involves the median nerve and its digital branches, followed by the ulnar nerve. Some cases are associated with macrodactyly. Microscopically there is perineurial and epineurial infiltration by a mixture of mature adipose and fibrous tissue which separates individual nerve bundles. Perineural fibrosis is typically seen.

8. **Lipoblastoma** occurs in children (90% of cases occur in children under 3 years old) with a predilection for the extremities and trunk, but tumors can also involve the mediastinum, abdomen, retroperitoneum, head and neck, and viscera (*Am J Surg Pathol* 2009;33:1705). Tumors can have a localized well-circumscribed growth pattern (lipoblastoma) or a diffuse infiltrating growth pattern (diffuse lipoblastoma/lipoblastomatosis). Like other fatty tumors, it has a lobulated architecture and is composed of a mixture of cells showing variable adipocytic differentiation including stellate mesenchymal cells, signet-ring lipoblasts, multinucleated lipoblasts, and mature adipocytes (**e-Fig. 44.2**). Greyish myxoid areas noted grossly have a plexiform

vascular pattern similar to myxoid liposarcoma (MLS), which can be problematic. These tumors are benign and do not metastasize, although approximately 20% to 25% of cases recur. These tumors have the potential for maturation, and some cases have predominantly lipomatous features with residual immature myxoid areas at the periphery of the lobules. Lipoblastomas express S100 protein, desmin (positive cells frequently present at the periphery of lobules), and CD34. Tumors harbor *PLAG1* rearrangements resulting in fusions with a number of different partners.

9. Hibernoma is composed of brown fat admixed with white adipose tissue. It typically occurs in young adults in the neck, axilla, thigh, retroperitoneum, head and neck, trunk, and upper extremities. The cut surface is yellowish to brownish, oily, and spongy; may be lobulated but is well demarcated; and can measure over 20 cm. Microscopically, lobules of finely multivacuolated brown fat cells with round central nuclei and variably pale to eosinophilic granular cytoplasm are admixed with white adipose tissue (e-**Fig. 44.3**).

B. Intermediate (Locally Aggressive)

1. Atypical lipomatous tumor/well-differentiated liposarcoma (ALT/WDLS) usually occurs in adults in the fifth through eighth decade of life in the deep soft tissues of the proximal lower extremity and retroperitoneum; the paratesticular region and mediastinum are less common sites. Tumors arising in the retroperitoneum may attain very large sizes in excess of 50 cm in greatest dimension. Tumors appear well circumscribed and have a lobulated, yellow to white, soft to firm cut surface that varies on the basis of lipomatous, fibrous, inflammatory, and myxoid components. Microscopically, tumors are composed of mature adipocytes with scattered atypical pleomorphic hyperchromatic stromal cells, which are frequently found within vessel walls and fibrous bands with finely fibrillary collagen (e-**Fig. 44.4**). Lymphoid aggregates are common and lipoblasts may be seen. Myxoid areas with branching capillary networks may mimic MLS, and dense inflammatory infiltrates can obscure the underlying tumor. Three histologic subtypes are described: adipocytic (lipoma-like), sclerosing, and inflammatory, but more than one pattern is often present in a single tumor. Fluorescence in situ hybridization testing for *MDM2* amplification characteristic of ALT/WDLS is a sensitive and specific tool for distinguishing ALT/WDLS from histologic mimics. Prognosis is largely determined by anatomic site and size. Smaller, more superficial tumors can be locally resected with negative margins, but those in the retroperitoneum frequently recur. Recurrent tumors may become dedifferentiated (see below).

C. Malignant

1. Dedifferentiated liposarcoma (DDLS) often shows a transition from ALT/WDLS to a pleomorphic and spindle cell sarcoma (e-**Fig. 44.5**), either in the primary tumor (90%) or in a recurrence (10%). DDLS manifests an extremely broad histologic range, including within a single tumor. Many tumors resemble undifferentiated pleomorphic sarcomas (UPS). Myxofibrosarcoma (MFS)-like, meningothelial-like whorls with bone formation, pleomorphic liposarcoma (PLS)-like (homologous dedifferentiation), and heterologous differentiation (leiomyosarcomatous, rhabdomyosarcomatous, osteosarcomatous, chondrosarcomatous, and angiosarcomatous) may be seen, as well as round cell, epithelioid and fibrosarcomatous patterns. Minimum histologic and size criteria for the diagnosis of DDLS have been elusive. Confluent sarcomatous growth and at least 5 mitoses in 10 hpf is a useful cutoff (*Am J Surg Pathol* 2007;31:1); however, it may lead to under-diagnosis in some cases, particularly on biopsy. The transition from ALT/WDLS to DDLS is abrupt or gradual, and ALT/WDLS may not always be identified. Because areas of dedifferentiation may be limited, thorough sampling and careful microscopic examination of all ALT/WDLS is required. *MDM2* amplification is present in the dedifferentiated component.

2. Myxoid liposarcoma (MLS) peaks in incidence at age 30 to 40 years, occurs predominantly in the deep soft tissues of the extremities (more than two-thirds of cases arise in the musculature of the thigh), and is the most common type of liposarcoma in the first two decades of life (*Am J Surg Pathol* 2009;33:645). When the diagnosis of MLS is considered in a retroperitoneal tumor, WD/DDLS with MLS-like features should be excluded; if MLS is confirmed with cytogenetic testing (see below), it likely represents metastatic disease rather than a primary lesion (*Mod Pathol* 2009;22:223). The cut surface of MLS is tan, glistening, and gelatinous; hypercellular areas are associated with a fleshy, white cut surface. Tumors are composed of uniform, round to oval, primitive mesenchymal cells and small lipoblasts embedded in a myxoid stroma with a delicate arborizing ("chicken wire") capillary network (e-**Fig. 44.6**). In contrast, hypercellular (round cell) areas are composed of sheets of primitive round cells, which may obscure the vasculature and stroma. Hypercellular areas are associated with poor outcome and should be reported as an estimated percentage of the tumor volume. *FUS-DDIT3* fusions are present in >95% of tumors, while a small subset harbor *EWSR1-DDIT3* fusions.

3. Pleomorphic liposarcoma (PLS) is a high-grade sarcoma with pleomorphic lipoblasts and a complex genomic profile. This tumor has a predilection for the extremities, often measures in excess of 8 cm, and primarily occurs in individuals over 50 years old. Variable numbers of pleomorphic lipoblasts with enlarged hyperchromatic nuclei that are scalloped by cytoplasmic lipid vacuoles are typically scattered within a pleomorphic and spindle cell sarcoma with storiform growth similar to UPS. Less commonly, pleomorphic lipoblasts are scattered within sheets of atypical epithelioid cells (e-**Fig. 44.7**). MFS-like areas are frequently present. Extreme pleomorphism, brisk mitotic activity including bizarre mitotic figures, and necrosis are common. DDLS can have PLS-like areas (homologous dedifferentiation) (*Am J Surg Pathol* 2010;34:1122; *Am J Surg Pathol* 2010;34:837); however, PLS lacks *MDM2* amplification. PLS carries a poor prognosis with a 30% to 50% metastatic rate.

IV. FIBROBLASTIC/MYOFIBROBLASTIC TUMORS
A. Benign

1. Nodular fasciitis (pseudosarcomatous fasciitis) is a benign, sometimes spontaneously regressing lesion, which occurs in all age groups but has a predilection for young adults. It usually involves the subcutaneous tissue of the head and neck (especially in children), trunk, or upper extremities (e-**Fig. 44.8**). Dermal, fascial, and intramuscular lesions are less common. Tumors may involve small to medium-sized veins (intravascular fasciitis), or the soft tissue of the outer table of the scalp of infants where it displays unusual behavior with bone and meningeal involvement (cranial fasciitis) (e-**Fig. 44.9**). Most lesions are 2 to 3 cm in greatest dimension though some lesions exceed 10 cm. Cystic degeneration is an uncommon gross feature. Microscopically, a variably myxoid to fibrous stroma supports a proliferation of bland myofibroblasts, arranged in storiform and short fascicular patterns, associated with mucoid microcysts, extravasated red blood cells, and inflammatory cells (e-**Figs. 44.8** and **44.9**). The loose growth of tumor cells in a myxoid stroma produces the characteristic "tissue culture" appearance. More collagenized foci can resemble a keloid. Osteoclast-like giant cells may be present. Tumors can be infiltrative and quite mitotically active; however, atypical mitotic figures and atypia are not present. Due to rapid growth, infiltration of the surrounding tissue, high cellularity, and brisk mitotic activity some cases are mistaken for sarcomas, usually leiomyosarcoma (LMS) or MFS. The tumor cells are strongly reactive for SMA and unlike desmoid tumor, are nonreactive for beta-catenin (*Histopathology* 2007;51:509). Nodular fasciitis is characterized by rearrangements of *USP6*, which is most commonly fused with *MYH9* leading to promoter swapping (*Lab Invest* 2011;91:1427; *Mod Pathol* 2017;30:1577).

2. Proliferative fasciitis and proliferative myositis tend to occur in middle-aged and elderly patients. Proliferative fasciitis is most common in the subcutis of the upper extremity (especially the forearm), followed by the lower extremity and trunk. Proliferative myositis is intramuscular and primarily involves the trunk and shoulder girdle. Both lesions are characterized by large ganglion-like cells scattered and clustered within a nodular fasciitis-like proliferation. The ganglion-like cells have basophilic cytoplasm, and one or two eccentric vesicular nuclei with prominent nucleoli. Proliferative myositis infiltrates between skeletal muscle fibers, which produces a checkerboard pattern. Tumors may be mitotically active but atypical mitotic figures are not present. Of note, proliferative fasciitis and proliferative myositis in children manifest with distinct features including hypercellularity, neutrophilic infiltrate, decreased collagen, and necrosis, which can lead to an erroneous diagnosis of sarcoma (*Am J Surg Pathol* 1992;16:364).

3. **Ischemic fasciitis** (atypical decubital fibroplasia) typically occurs over bony prominences in elderly patients, though the tumor has been described in a wide age range of patients. Some cases are associated with prolonged pressure in immobilized individuals. Lesions have a zonal architecture with central areas of degenerative/cystic change with fibrin deposition, and a reactive myofibroblastic and vascular proliferation at the periphery (*Am J Surg Pathol* 1992;16:708; *Am J Surg Pathol* 2008;32:1546).

4. **Myositis ossificans (MO) and fibro-osseous pseudotumor of digits (FOPD)** are histologically similar lesions that occur over a broad age range, though young adults are most frequently affected. MO has a propensity for the extremities, trunk, and head and neck, while FOPD primarily occurs in the subcutis of the proximal phalanx of the digits. Both lesions are thought to be caused by injury; however, this is an area of ongoing investigation. MO has a zonal growth pattern with a cellular (myo)fibroblastic center resembling nodular fasciitis, with surrounding woven bone with osteoblastic rimming which matures to lamellar bone toward the periphery (e-**Fig. 44.10**). FOPD shows similar features; however, a zonal pattern is less consistently present. Biopsies can be quite worrisome as lesions can be quite cellular and mitotically active; however, tumor cells are bland and mitotic figures are not atypical.

5. **Elastofibroma** has a female predominance and is usually found in individuals over 50 years of age between the chest wall and the inferior region of the scapula, deep to the rhomboid major and latissimus dorsi muscles. Rare examples have been described in other locations. The tumor can be unilateral or bilateral and has a gray-white, rubbery to fibrous cut surface with ill-defined margins. Microscopically, mature adipose tissue is admixed with a paucicellular collagenized stroma (e-**Fig. 44.11**), which contains elastic fibers with large, coarse, eosinophilic linear globules arranged in a beads-on-a-string pattern that is highlighted by a VVG or pentachrome stain.

6. **Fibrous hamartoma of infancy (FHI)** is one of the "fibrous tumors of childhood" and is generally seen before 2 years of age. The axillary fold, arm, shoulder, back, thigh, and groin are the preferred sites. The tumor forms an ill-defined mass in the subcutis and has a white fibrocollagenous gross appearance with interspersed fat. Microscopically, intersecting fibrous bands of variable thickness radiate through the subcutis and are associated with discrete nodules of immature mesenchyme (e-**Fig. 44.12**). Without the latter nodules, there is a resemblance to lipofibromatosis. When there is overgrowth of the subcutaneous fat by the fibrous component, the tumor acquires the features similar to fibromatosis. Giant cells within pseudovascular spaces can mimic giant cell fibroblastoma (*Am J Surg Pathol* 2014;38:394). FHI has a low rate of recurrence (10% to 15%). Like most other fibrous tumors in infants and young children, FHI does not express beta-catenin (*Pediatr Dev Pathol* 2009;12:292). *EGFR* exon 20 insertion/duplication mutations have recently been described in these tumors (*Am J Surg Pathol* 2016;40:1713).

7. **Angiomyofibroblastoma** occurs in reproductive age women and commonly involves the subcutis of pelviperineal region (vulva or less commonly vagina), as a painless, well-circumscribed, slow growing mass (*Int J Gynecol Pathol* 2005;24:26). In men, the neoplasm usually involves the paratesticular soft tissue or scrotum. Alternating hyper- and hypocellular zones are composed of epithelioid to spindled cells set in a myxoid/edematous to collagenous stroma. Tumor cells tend to cluster around prominent small, typically thin-walled, vessels (e-**Fig. 44.13**); a subset of cases has a mature fatty component (*Int J Gynecol Pathol* 2005;24:196). Multinucleated cells are

common. Mitotic activity is low to absent. Tumors are immunopositive for desmin, ER, and PR. Some cases have morphologic overlap with cellular angiofibroma.

8. **Cellular angiofibroma** typically involves the superficial soft tissues of the vulva, inguinoscrotal region, or perineum. The tumor is well circumscribed, and has a yellow to tan-brown appearance and soft to rubbery texture. The tumor is evenly cellular and composed of short fascicles of plump bland spindled cells with scant cytoplasm and indistinct borders set in a fibrous to myxoid stroma with delicate collagen fibers. The vascular component is composed of small to medium-sized thick-walled vessels, with or without prominent hyaline. An adipocytic component may be present and rare tumors with sarcomatous features are reported. Tumor cells are immunopositive for ER, PR, and CD34, and show loss of Rb. Like spindle cell lipoma and mammary-type myofibroblastoma, cellular angiofibroma shows loss of 13q14 (the *RB1*) locus.

9. **Nuchal-type fibroma and Gardner fibroma** are both characterized by a haphazard proliferation of dense paucicellular collagenous bundles which involve the dermis, subcutis, and deep soft tissues. However, nuchal-type fibromas have proliferations of nerve twigs (neuroma-like) and older age of presentation compared to Gardner fibromas. Further, Gardner fibromas may be positive for beta-catenin, and rare cases merge with desmoid-type fibromatosis. The possibility of Gardner syndrome should be raised in the presence of Gardner fibroma (*Am J Surg Pathol* 2007;31:410).

10. **Mammary-type myofibroblastoma** occurs most frequently as a subcutaneous mass in the inguinal/groin and vulvovaginal area, followed by the trunk and extremities in adults. Tumors are well circumscribed, unencapsulated, and composed of fascicles of spindle cells with stout nuclei associated with thick hyalinized collagen bundles. A mature adipocytic component is present in the majority of cases. Immunohistochemical studies show that tumor cells are positive for CD34 and SMA (variable) and demonstrate loss of Rb. Mammary-type myofibroblastoma, like spindle cell lipoma and cellular angiofibroma, harbors loss of *RB1*.

11. **Fibromatosis colli** (congenital muscular torticollis; sternocleidomastoid tumor of infancy) afflicts infants (usually less than 6 months old) and presents as a mass in the distal sternocleidomastoid causing torticollis. Microscopically, skeletal muscle fibers are separated by a diffuse bland proliferation of fibroblasts creating a checkerboard pattern. Muscle fibers may show atrophy and degenerative changes, and early lesions are often cellular. Atypia and mitotic activity are absent. The lesion is likely reactive and most cases spontaneously regress.

12. **Juvenile hyaline fibromatosis** is a rare autosome recessive disease usually presenting in infants and children, which is caused by mutations in *ANTXR2* resulting in the growth of tumors in the skin, gums, soft tissue (particularly periarticular), and bones. Tumors are composed of bland round to spindled fibroblasts embedded in abundant amorphous eosinophilic extracellular stroma. Infantile systemic hyalinosis is a more aggressive variant, which presents earlier and in addition to skin, soft tissue, and bone lesions manifests with chronic diarrhea, weight loss, and visceral involvement.

13. **Inclusion body fibromatosis** (infantile digital fibroma/fibromatosis) characteristically presents in infants as a dome-shaped dermal nodule on the dorsal or lateral aspect of the second–fourth digits, with sparing of the first digit. There are rare cases in adults and in nondigital sites. Tumors are composed of bland myofibroblasts with intracytoplasmic eosinophilic inclusions which are frequently perinuclear and may indent the nucleus. Tumor cells are embedded in a collagenous stroma and arranged in whorls and fascicles oriented perpendicular to the epidermis. Entrapment of adnexal structures is typical. Trichrome highlights the intracytoplasmic inclusions. Tumor cells are typically positive for SMA, calponin, and desmin. Beta-catenin may be expressed (*Am J Surg Pathol* 2009;33:1). At least 60% of cases recur, though spontaneous regression is also observed.

14. **Desmoplastic fibroblastoma** (collagenous fibroma) typically presents in middle-aged adults in the deep subcutis of the extremities. Tumors are generally well marginated;

however, infiltration of surrounding adipose tissue or skeletal muscle is not uncommon. Tumors are hypovascular and composed of a paucicellular proliferation of bland spindled, bipolar, and stellate cells in a fibrous to fibromyxoid stroma. Mitotic figures are rare and necrosis is absent. Immunohistochemical studies show variable expression of SMA, while EMA, S100 protein, and CD34 are negative; FOSL1 may be a useful marker of desmoplastic fibroblastoma (*Histopathology* 2016;69:1012). While data are limited, a recurrent t(2;11)(q31;q12) translocation has been observed in these tumors (*Cancer Genet Cytogenet* 2004;149:161).

15. **Calcifying aponeurotic fibroma** is a very rare tumor, which occurs over a broad age range, but is most common in children and adolescents with a male predominance. There is a strong predilection for the distal extremities, particularly the palm and fingers, as well as the plantar foot. The tumor is infiltrative and composed of fascicles of bland fibroblasts with foci of cartilage and fine to course calcification. Osteoclast-like giant cells and epithelioid cells are seen associated with calcifications. The histologic appearance varies with tumor age; early lesions are cellular and lack calcification, while calcification and decreased cellularity are present in late stage lesions. Atypia is absent and mitoses are rare. While only a few cases have been analyzed, recurrent *FN1-EGF* fusions have been identified in these tumors (*J Pathol* 2016;238:502). Recurrences are common in 40% to 50% of cases.

16. **Calcifying fibrous tumor** (calcifying fibrous pseudotumor) has a wide age and anatomic distribution. Tumors involve superficial and deep soft tissue, particularly the extremities, as well as pleura, peritoneum, mesentery, omentum, and viscera. Tumors are well circumscribed, and composed of a paucicellular proliferation of bland spindle cells set in a hyalinized collagenous background with scattered chronic inflammatory cells and dystrophic and/or psammomatous calcifications. Lymphoid follicles are common. Tumor cells are positive for CD34, while negative for ALK1, CD117, and S100 protein. Recently, recurrent molecular alternations have been found in a small number of pleural tumors (*Hum Pathol* 2018;pii: S0046–8177(18)30125–4).

B. Intermediate (Locally Aggressive)

1. **Superficial fibromatoses.** Palmar (Dupuytren contracture) fibromatosis typically develops in adults (with a male to female ratio of 4:1) as a nodule or multinodular mass involving the palmar aponeurosis. Plantar fibromatosis also occurs most frequently in adults; however, a large subset occur in patients below 30 years old. Palmar and plantar have similar microscopic features, which evolve over time. Greater cellularity is present early on, consisting of cellular fascicles of bland uniform spindle cells (e-Fig. 44.14). Older lesions are less cellular and demonstrate greater collagen deposition. These tumors have a high rate of local recurrence. Tumors show variable positivity for beta-catenin, but lack *CTNNB1* and *APC* mutations (*Mod Pathol* 2001;14:695).

2. **Desmoid-type fibromatosis** arises in the mesentery, the abdominal wall (particularly in peripartum women), or in extraabdominal sites, most commonly the limb girdles, chest wall, thigh, and head and neck. Head and neck lesions are overrepresented in children. The tumor may be large (>10 cm) and have a firm white trabeculated cut surface. Microscopically the tumor is infiltrative and composed of long sweeping fascicles of uniform bland myofibroblastic cells with vesicular nuclei and small nucleoli (e-Fig. 44.15). Small elongated blood vessels are characteristic and mitotic figures are often present. The stroma varies from scant in cellular lesions, to myxoid, to sclerotic. Keloid-like fibers may be identified. If skeletal muscle is involved, it is usually infiltrated with remnants of muscle embedded in the fibrous proliferation (e-Fig. 44.16). SMA expression is common, and 70% to 80% of cases show reactivity for beta-catenin. Sporadic tumors have activating mutations in exon 3 of *CTNNB1*, while tumors associated with FAP/Gardner syndrome have germline inactivating mutations in *APC*. *CTNNB1* 45F mutations are associated with increased risk of recurrence (*Am J Pathol* 2008;173:1518).

3. **Lipofibromatosis** (infantile subcutaneous fibromatosis), another fibrous tumor of childhood, is a slowly growing, painless neoplasm most commonly affecting the distal extremities but also occurring in a variety of other sites (*Am J Surg Pathol* 2000;24:1491). Grossly, the tumor is an ill-defined white-tan to yellow mass that usually measures less than 5 cm. Bland uniform spindled fibroblastic cells form bands that surround and separate lobules of fat; the growth pattern resembles FHI but without the nodules of immature mesenchyme. Lipoblast-like cells may be seen at the junction of the adipose and fibrous bands. While high cellularity may be seen, atypia is absent and the mitoses are rare. The tumor expresses CD34, BCL2, S100 protein, actin, and CD99, an unusual phenotypic profile for a fibrous tumor.

4. **Giant cell fibroblastoma** is a variant of DFSP that usually presents in childhood in the subcutis and dermis of the trunk, axilla, and perineum. It is an ill-defined tumor composed of bland wavy spindle cells within a fibrous to myxoid stroma, with scattered multinucleated giant cells lining pseudovascular spaces. Areas of FHI may closely mimic giant cell fibroblastoma. Immunohistochemical studies show that tumor cells are positive for CD34, but negative for S100 protein, desmin, keratin, and SMA. A minority of giant cell fibroblastomas are accompanied by conventional DFSP. Giant cell fibroblastoma recurs in about 50% of cases but metastases have not been described.

C. Intermediate (Rarely Metastasizing)

1. **Solitary fibrous tumor (SFT)** is classically found in the pleura, but can occur in many different locations (including soft tissue, bone, dura, intestinal tract, mesentery, liver, skin, thyroid, lung, and orbit) over a wide age range. In the soft tissue it is usually found in the abdomen, retroperitoneum, limb girdle, and proximal extremities. The tumor is a well-circumscribed, nonencapsulated, firm, white mass measuring 5 to 10 cm on average though much larger tumors can be seen. The tumor is composed of bland plump to spindle cells with a "patternless" architecture associated with gaping branching blood vessels (known as a staghorn or hemangiopericytomatous vascular pattern) (e-**Fig. 44.17**). The stroma is characteristically collagenous, though focal myxoid areas are not uncommon. The cellularity often varies within an individual tumor; some tumors are diffusely cellular and were formerly known as hemangiopericytoma (e-**Fig. 44.18**). Mature adipose tissue is found in the lipomatous variant of SFT and giant cells with or without pseudovascular spaces may be present (giant cell angiofibroma variant). The tumor cells are immunoreactive for STAT6, CD34, and CD99, but a subset of tumors also shows reactivity for SMA, BCL2, EMA, and rare focal positivity for desmin and S100 protein.

As the clinical behavior of an individual tumor is difficult to predict based on histologic features, risk stratification models have been developed and validated to predict behavior based on patient age, tumor size, mitotic rate, and necrosis (*Mod Pathol* 2017;30:1433). A dedifferentiated SFT is characteristically a typical SFT with a transition to a frankly sarcomatous neoplasm. *NAB2-STAT6* fusions are characteristic of all variants of SFT.

As a final note, hemangiopericytoma-like vasculature can be seen in a variety of tumors including synovial sarcoma, malignant peripheral nerve sheath tumor (MPNST), mesenchymal chondrosarcoma, infantile fibrosarcoma, phosphaturic mesenchymal tumor (PMT), thymoma (spindle cell), myopericytoma, deep benign fibrous histiocytoma, and endometrial stromal sarcoma, emphasizing the need for careful clinical correlation, microscopic examination, and immunohistochemical and molecular studies.

2. **Inflammatory myofibroblastic tumor (IMT)** has a predilection for the omentum and mesentery, but can found in a wide range of sites including lung, gastrointestinal tract, bladder, gynecologic tract, head and neck, and central nervous system. The tumor usually presents in children and young adults, however there is a wide age range. Approximately 5% to 10% of IMTs have systemic, constitutional manifestations (fever, anorexia, weight loss, hypochromic microcytic anemia, hypergammaglobulinemia, and thrombocytosis) likely due to IL-6 production by the tumor.

The tumor forms a white to tan, whorled, fleshy to myxoid, circumscribed mass measuring from 1 to 25 cm in diameter which may also show areas of necrosis, hemorrhage, and calcification. Three basic histologic patterns are described: cellular fascicles of spindle cells with a mixed infiltrate of plasma cells, lymphocytes, and eosinophils; foci with a myxoid background resembling nodular fasciitis; and hypocellular, hyalinized foci with chronic inflammatory cells and dystrophic calcifications. An individual tumor may be composed of predominately one pattern or show multiple patterns (e-Fig. 44.19). Mitotic figures are found among the spindle cells, but are not atypical.

Immunohistochemically, approximately 50% to 60% show cytoplasmic staining with ALK (*Am J Surg Pathol* 2001;25:1364). However, virtually all cases are immunoreactive for vimentin; most show reactivity for SMA and variable reactivity for MSA and desmin; 25% to 30% are reactive for cytokeratin. Some IMTs have an IgG4/IgG ratio similar to IgG4-related sclerosing disease; however, this finding does not imply a relationship to the IgG4-related sclerosing disorders (*Mod Pathol* 2011;24:606). *ALK* rearrangements are detected in approximately 50% of cases with a number of different partners; *ALK* rearrangements are less common in adult cases. By immunohistochemistry, ALK-positive tumors may have a more favorable clinical outcome compared ALK-negative tumors (*Am J Surg Pathol* 2007;31:509).

Epithelioid inflammatory myofibroblastic sarcoma is a very aggressive variant of IMT which occurs in the abdomen and is characterized by round to epithelioid morphology, myxoid stroma, neutrophilic infiltrate, nuclear membrane or perinuclear ALK staining, and *RANBP2-ALK* fusion (*Am J Surg Pathol* 2011;35:135).

3. Congenital infantile fibrosarcoma (CIF) are often present at birth or occur within the first year of life. The tumor usually presents in the distal extremities, although trunk and head and neck cases are not uncommon. Of note, the clinical appearance can mimic a vascular lesion.

The tumor, which can be very large especially relative to the patient, ranges from white to tan, fleshy to firm, and may show areas of hemorrhage and necrosis. Careful gross examination usually shows that the tumor has an infiltrative margin. Several histologic patterns are seen, including interlacing, broad fascicles of spindle cells with or without herringbone architecture (e-Fig. 44.20), or the tumor may be composed of more primitive-appearing, round to short spindled cells in a poorly organized pattern; the latter can raise concern for an embryonal rhabdomyosarcoma (ERMS) or an undifferentiated primitive sarcoma. Small foci of palisading necrosis or confluent areas of hemorrhage are helpful diagnostic features in CIF. Mitotic figures are readily identified. Nuclear pleomorphism, atypical mitoses, and a pale background stroma should raise the possibility of ERMS; immunohistochemistry is useful in the exclusion of the latter neoplasm. Demonstration of the t(12;15) (p13;q25) translocation (the same translocation present in cellular mesoblastic nephroma, secretory breast carcinoma, mammary analog secretory carcinoma, a subset of papillary thyroid carcinoma, and a subset of acute myeloid leukemia) may be necessary in problematic cases. Foci resembling CIF may be present in myofibroma and myofibromatosis (*Pediatr Dev Pathol* 2008;11:355). Primitive myxoid mesenchymal tumor of infancy may resemble CIF but lacks the *ETV6-NTRK3* gene fusion and instead harbors *BCOR* internal tandem duplications and shows BCOR expression (*Am J Surg Pathol* 2016;40:1670). Approximately a third of CIF recur; however, metastases are rare.

4. Dermatofibrosarcoma protuberans (DFSP) is a locally aggressive tumor with limited metastatic potential, which occurs over a wide age range. The tumor involves the dermis and subcutis with a predilection for the trunk and proximal extremities. Tumors are composed of monomorphic bland spindle cells with prominent storiform architecture. The tumor entraps adnexal structures and infiltrates the subcutis creating a honeycomb pattern. In addition to giant cell fibroblastoma, other variants include myxoid, pigmented (Bednar tumor), and plaque-like DFSP, as well as DFSP with myoid differentiation. Some tumors have multiple patterns. DFSP may undergo fibrosarcomatous transformation characterized by fascicular, often herringbone, growth with increased atypia and mitotic rate. Rare tumors display pleomorphic sarcoma-like foci. The tumor cells are immunopositive for CD34 (though expression is frequently lost in fibrosarcomatous areas), while negative for S100 protein, desmin, and SMA. Tumors harbor t(17;22)(q22;q13) translocations, which results in the fusion of *COL1A1* with *PDGFB*. The recurrence rate is variable (up to 40%) and appears to be strongly correlated with the completeness of resection. Conventional tumors have extremely limited potential metastasis, while cases with fibrosarcomatous transformation have an approximately 13% metastatic rate.

5. **Myxoinflammatory fibroblastic sarcoma (MIFS)** (acral MIFS; inflammatory myxohyaline tumor of distal extremities with virocyte or Reed–Sternberg-like cells) is typically a low-grade neoplasm arising in the distal extremities of adults, though higher-grade tumors (*Ann Diagn Pathol* 2015;19:157) and involvement of nondistal sites are also seen (*Ann Diagn Pathol* 2002;6:272). Clinically the tumor is a dermal-subcutaneous nodule often measuring 2 to 4 cm. Microscopically, the tumor is infiltrative and multinodular with variable proportions of hyalinized and myxoid stroma, mixed inflammatory infiltrate, spindled to epithelioid cells, ganglion-like cells, Reed–Sternberg-like and virocyte-like cells, multinucleated giant cells, and pseudolipoblasts. Emperipolesis and areas resembling tenosynovial giant cell tumor (TSGT) are frequently observed. The tumor cells are variably immunopositive for CD34 and CD68, while negative for S100 protein, CD15, CD30, desmin, and clusterin. The molecular characterization of MIFS is an area of active investigation. Recurrent *VGLL3* amplifications and *BRAF* alterations have been reported in these tumors whereas *TGFBR3-MGEA5* fusions are rare in pure cases (*Am J Surg Pathol* 2017;41:1456).

6. **Low-grade myofibroblastic sarcoma** (myofibrosarcoma) usually presents in the head and neck or extremities of adults. Tumors are typically infiltrative and comprised of long cellular fascicles or storiform arrays of spindle cells with mild to moderate atypia, indistinct cell borders, prominent collagen deposition, and low mitotic rate. Tumors with greater degrees of atypia may be difficult to distinguish from unclassified sarcomas with myofibroblastic differentiation. Tumors are positive for SMA and/or desmin, while negative for caldesmon, S100 protein, keratin, myogenin, and CD34. Beta-catenin is expressed in a subset of cases. Approximately 30% of cases recur, while metastases are rare.

D. Malignant

1. **Adult-type fibrosarcoma (AFS)** is extremely rare and a diagnosis of exclusion, rendered only after other types of spindle cell neoplasms have been ruled out on the basis of histologic features, immunohistochemical staining profiles, and molecular studies. If these studies are performed, the vast majority of putative AFS can be reclassified into another type of tumor (*Am J Surg Pathol* 2010;34:1504). When strictly defined, AFS is primarily seen in adults, and has a predilection for the deep soft tissues of the head and neck, trunk, and extremities. AFS forms a well-circumscribed or infiltrative firm mass that has a white to tan appearance on cut surface. Sweeping fascicles of compact monotonous spindle cells produce the quintessential herringbone pattern (**e-Fig. 44.21**). The background stroma shows variable collagen content. Immunopositivity is limited to vimentin and, focally, SMA.

2. **Sclerosing epithelioid fibrosarcoma (SEF)** occurs over a wide age range usually in the deep soft tissues of the lower extremities and limb girdles. Rare tumors arise in the abdomen, retroperitoneum, or viscera, as well as bone (*Sarcoma* 2010;2010:431627) where the tumor can closely mimic osteosarcoma. Tumors are well circumscribed and have firm white cut surfaces; cystic and myxoid areas may be present. The rounded or epithelioid cells that compose the mass have minimal eosinophilic to clear cytoplasm; a low mitotic rate; and are arranged in acini, strands, and nests within a very dense collagenous matrix. The appearance can mimic an infiltrating carcinoma or lymphoma. The tumor cells express MUC4 while CD34, S100 protein, SMA,

desmin, HMB-45, SATB2, and CD45 are negative. Occasional cases show focal weak expression of EMA and/or cytokeratin. SEF-like foci can be seen in low-grade fibromyxoid sarcoma (LGFMS). The majority of SEF show *EWSR1* and *CREB3L1* rearrangements and rarely *FUS* and *CREB3L2* rearrangements.

3. **Low-grade fibromyxoid sarcoma (LGFMS)** (including hyalinizing spindle cell tumor with giant rosettes variant) presents over a wide age range (peak in the fourth decade) as a painless deep soft tissue mass in the proximal extremities or trunk that has, in some cases, been present for many years. Other sites include the thoracic cavity, head and neck, abdominal cavity, and retroperitoneum. In younger patients LGFMS is often superficial. Tumors appear well-marginated grossly but are often microscopically infiltrative and composed of bland monotonous spindle cells growing in fascicles and whorls with alternating fibrous and myxoid areas, with increased cellularity and vascularity in the myxoid areas (e-**Fig. 44.22**). Mitotic figures are sparse and necrosis is unusual. Approximately 30% of tumors contain at least focal collagen rosettes composed of a central hyalinized core rimmed by epithelioid cells. Uncommonly, there is increased cellularity and atypia, particularity in recurrent tumors. Tumors are positive for MUC4 and EMA. There is variable expression of keratin, DOG1, SMA, desmin, and CD34, while the tumor is generally negative for S100 protein, CD117, SOX10, and beta-catenin. Approximately 95% of tumors have a demonstrable *FUS-CREB3L2* fusion, while a small subset harbor a *FUS-CREB3L1* fusion. Rare cases show a *EWSR1-CREB3L1* fusion. SEF and LGFMS appear to be distinct though possibility-related neoplasms.

4. **Myxofibrosarcoma (MFS)** occurs over a wide age range, but has a predilection for individuals over 50 years. Most cases occur in the extremities and are superficial; only about one-third occur in the deep soft tissues. WDLS/DDLS should be excluded when MFS-like tumors are encountered in the abdomen/retroperitoneum. A multinodular growth pattern, myxoid stroma, variable cellularity with scattered pleomorphic cells, curvilinear vessels, and incomplete fibrous septa are consistent microscopic features. Pseudolipoblasts are often present. Low-grade tumors are hypocellular with a prominent myxoid matrix that contains only scattered hyperchromatic pleomorphic tumor cells and relatively few mitotic figures. High-grade MFS shows solid growth with marked cellular pleomorphism and a high mitotic rate (e-**Fig. 44.23**). The tumor cells do not have a characteristic immunophenotype, and progression to higher grades can be seen in recurrent MFS. Complex molecular alternations have been identified in MFS, which are similar to these seen in UPS including a subset of tumors with high-level amplifications of genes involved in the hippo signaling pathway (*Cell* 2017;171:950).

V. FIBROHISTIOCYTIC TUMORS
A. Benign
1. **Tenosynovial giant cell tumor (TSGT), localized type** (giant cell tumor of tendon sheath, nodular tenosynovitis) is a well-circumscribed tumor that arises from the synovium of joints, bursae and tendon sheath, or in adjacent tissues. The hand, and less often the wrist, ankle, foot, knee, elbow, and hip are various sites of the tumor, which clinically presents as a painless mass, mainly in adults. Localized tumors form a firm lobulated yellowish-brown to tan circumscribed mass that measures 0.5 to 4 cm; erosion into adjacent bone can be seen in larger lesions. Fibrous septa divide nodules composed of a polymorphous population of histiocytoid to spindled mononuclear cells, larger epithelioid cells, xanthoma cells, siderophages, and osteoclast-like giant cells set in a variably prominent hyalinized stroma (e-**Fig. 44.24)**. Mitotic activity may be brisk. Local recurrence is seen in up to 20% of cases. Translocations involving chromosome 1p13 (specifically the *CSF1* gene) are characteristic.

2. **Tenosynovial giant cell tumor (TSGT), diffuse type** (diffuse-type giant cell tumor, pigmented villonodular synovitis/tenosynovitis) usually presents as an intra-articular or extra-articular proliferation involving the knee or hip joint/periarticular soft tissue. The distal extremities, elbow, shoulder, temporal mandibular joint, and spine are also

rarely involved. Unusual extra-articular tumors have been found in skeletal muscle and the subcutis. Microscopically, diffuse-type TSGT is primarily distinguished from the localized form by the presence of infiltrative growth. In addition, compared to the localized-type, the diffuse-type also tends to have fewer giant cells and more cleft-like spaces; intra-articular diffuse-type tumors form synovial lined villous projections (**e-Fig. 44.25**). Mitotic activity is variable and may be brisk, but atypical mitotic figures are absent. Both localized- and diffuse-type tumors share translocations of chromosome 1p13 involving the *CSF1* gene, which in some cases result in formation of a *COL6A3-CSF1* fusion. Classification of this neoplasm as an intermediate (locally aggressive) tumor is based on the fact that over 45% of intra-articular and up to 60% of extra-articular tumors recur and recurrences may be destructive. Very rare conventional cases metastasize. Malignant diffuse-type TGST are very rare and are defined by clearly sarcomatous proliferations associated with a conventional diffuse-type TSGT or found in a recurrence.

3. Deep benign fibrous histiocytoma is a very rare variant of fibrous histiocytoma/dermatofibroma with a predilection for the subcutis of the extremities and head and neck region, although this tumor is also seen in the retroperitoneum and mediastinum (*Am J Surg Pathol* 2008;32:354). Tumors are well circumscribed, commonly with a fibrous pseudocapsule, and measure less than 4 cm. Histologic features include a storiform or short fascicular proliferation of bland spindle cells with indistinct cytoplasm which may be intermixed with lymphocytes, plasma cells, osteoclast-like giant cells, siderophages, and foamy histiocytes. A hemangiopericytomatous vascular pattern is often present. Necrosis and frequent mitotic figures are unusual. Tumors display variable immunopositivity for CD34 (approximately 50%), SMA, and desmin (rare), while S100 protein, keratin, and EMA are negative. Gene fusions involving *PRKCB* and *PRKCD* have been identified in a minority of cases (*Lab Invest* 2015;95:1071).

B. Intermediate (Rarely Metastasizing)

1. Plexiform fibrohistiocytic tumor (PFHT) primarily occurs in the first three decades of life with a predilection for the extremities (especially the hand and wrist) and less commonly the head and neck (*Ann Diagn Pathol* 2007;11:313). Grossly, it is a firm multinodular poorly circumscribed mass that typically measures less than 3 cm and involves the junction of the dermis and subcutis. Microscopically, nodules and irregular islands of epithelioid to spindled histiocytoid cells with intermixed osteoclast-like giant cells are separated by fascicles of (myo)fibroblastic cells (**e-Fig. 44.26**). Tumors may be predominately fibroblastic, histiocytic, or mixed. The histiocytic variant may resemble giant cell tumor of soft tissue, while the fibroblastic variant with rare histiocytic nodules and few, if any, multinucleated cells mimics fibromatosis. Atypia, necrosis, and brisk mitotic activity are not present. Lymphovascular space invasion may be seen. The spindle cells express SMA; CD68 immunoreactivity is present in the giant cells and mononuclear histiocyte-like cells. MITF may be focally expressed, while immunostains for S100 protein, desmin, and keratin are negative. Approximately 30% to 40% of cases locally recur. Less than 5% metastasize to regional lymph nodes, and metastasis to the lung is even rarer.

2. Giant cell tumor of soft tissue usually involves the subcutis of the extremities in adults, though tumors occur over a wide age and anatomic distribution. Tumors are well circumscribed and nodular with soft, fleshy, gray to red-brown cut surfaces. Microscopically, there are variably sized nodules composed of mononuclear cells with round to ovoid nuclei and osteoclast-like giant cells embedded in a vascular stroma. Nodules are separated by fibrous septa with hemosiderin-laden macrophages and hemosiderin deposition. Mitotic activity can be brisk but atypical mitotic figures, cellular pleomorphism, and atypia are absent. Necrosis is rare. A partial shell of bone is noted in about 50% of cases, and vascular invasion is identified in about 30%. Aneurysmal bone cyst-like changes and foamy macrophages can be seen. The multinucleated giant cells are strongly CD68 immunopositive, whereas the mononuclear cells express SMA and only focal CD68 immunoreactivity. Giant cell tumor of soft tissue does not appear to harbor *H3F3A* mutations as seen in giant cell tumor of bone (*Mod Pathol* 2017;30:728).

VI. SMOOTH MUSCLE TUMORS. Smooth muscle tumors are neoplasms in most cases, but a small subset of lesions are hamartomas that are usually present in children. Neoplasms in this category are ubiquitous in distribution from the skin and soft tissues, to visceral sites including the gastrointestinal and female reproductive tracts. In most cases, the pathologic distinction between benign and malignant is reasonably straightforward, with the exception of leiomyoma of deep soft tissues and some tumors arising in the uterus (*Histopathology* 2006;48:97). Many of the biologic features of this group of tumors can vary with site; for example, superficial, often small LMS of skin may have the same microscopic features as their large deep counterparts even though the former have a more favorable prognosis. Similarly, an entirely benign appearing leiomyoma of the uterus can produce distant metastases, particularly to the lungs.

A. Benign

   1. **Leiomyoma of deep soft tissue** is a rare neoplasm that usually develops in the retroperitoneum and the abdominal cavity, while rarely arising in the extremities. The tumor can measure in excess of 30 cm. It is composed of bland well-differentiated smooth muscle cells with blunt nuclei, eosinophilic fibrillary cytoplasm, and fascicular architecture with perpendicular intersections (e-**Fig. 44.27**). There is no necrosis and a very low mitotic rate (<1/50 hpf in somatic soft tissue tumors and abdominopelvic/retroperitoneal tumors in males, and <5/50 hpf in abdominopelvic/retroperitoneal tumors in females). Fibrosis, myxoid change, hyalinization, and calcification may be seen. Tumors are positive for SMA, desmin, and caldesmon, and may express keratin. The diagnosis of a deep leiomyoma should be approached with caution, particularly in small biopsies. Pilar leiomyoma and uterine smooth muscle tumors are discussed elsewhere (see Chapters 38 and 33, respectively).

B. Malignant

   1. **Leiomyosarcoma (LMS)** typically presents in mid-life and beyond. Tumors are present in multiple clinicopathologic settings: a retroperitoneal mass; a tumor arising from a large blood vessel with a preference for large veins (particular the inferior vena cava); a subcutaneous or intramuscular tumor of the extremities; a dermal-based neoplasm; and a visceral tumor. Uterine and intestinal LMS are not considered in this chapter, although the uterus is the most common primary site overall for LMS.

   Except for cutaneous LMS, these tumors usually measure in excess of 6 cm and have a trabeculated or smooth, glistening, white-gray cut surface. These tumors are composed of spindle cells with eosinophilic fibrillary cytoplasm and elongated nuclei with blunt ends (e-**Fig. 44.28**). Fascicles characteristically intersect at right angles and perinuclear vacuoles are often seen. Tumors range from relatively bland with focal atypia and lower mitotic rates to highly pleomorphic sarcomas with extensive necrosis and brisk mitotic activity, including atypical forms. Generally there is expression of at least two of three smooth muscle markers (SMA, desmin, and h-caldesmon). Focal expression of keratin, EMA, CD34, and S100 may be present. These tumors have complex karyotypes with gains and losses across multiple chromosomes (*Virchows Arch* 2010;456:201).

   2. **Epstein–Barr virus (EBV)–associated smooth muscle tumors** are a distinct clinicopathologic group of smooth muscle neoplasms arising in the immunocompromised setting in all ages in visceral, soft tissue, and cutaneous sites. These tumors are associated with genomic integration of EBV; multifocally is common and results from clonally distinct infections (*Am J Surg Pathol* 2006;30:75). Well-differentiated smooth muscle cells with limited atypia, fascicular architecture, and a predominantly T-lymphocytic infiltrate are typical of these tumors. Rounded primitive-appearing cells are also frequently present. The tumor cells express SMA and about half label with desmin. In situ hybridization testing for EBV-encoded RNA (*EBER*) is helpful to confirm the diagnosis. The prognosis is variable and does not correlate

with histologic features. Mortality in patients with EBV-associated smooth muscle tumors is usually due to other complications of immunosuppression (i.e., infections) rather than to the tumor(s).

VII. PERICYTIC (PERIVASCULAR) TUMORS
A. Benign

1. **Angioleiomyoma** (vascular leiomyoma, angiomyoma) is usually a painful subcutaneous neoplasm occurring in the extremities or less commonly the head and neck. These well-circumscribed tumors, usually measuring less than 2 cm, can be divided into three histologic types: a solid type with fascicles of well-differentiated smooth muscle cells and small slit-like vascular channels; a venous type with thick-walled vessels that merge with bundles of smooth muscle; and a cavernous type with ectatic vessels with variable wall thickness and smooth muscle within the septa. Concentric growth of tumor cells around vessels may be seen. Tumors are immunopositive for SMA, caldesmon, and desmin. Recurrences are quite rare and metastases are not observed.

2. **Glomus tumors** occur over a wide age range and usually manifest in the subungual region of the hand, as well as the wrist and foot, but not to the exclusion of other sites including the bone, lung, and gastrointestinal tract. Tumors are typically small and painful when touched or exposed to cold. Microscopically, these tumors consist of a mixture of glomus cells (small uniform round cells with eosinophilic to amphophilic cytoplasm, a central nucleus, and distinct cell borders), smooth muscle cells, and vascular spaces (e-**Fig. 44.29**). Depending on the relative proportion of these elements, lesions may be divided into three main subtypes: solid type, composed of nests of glomus cells surrounding capillary-sized vessels; glomangioma, composed of small clusters of glomus cells surrounding dilated vessels; and glomangiomyoma, in which there are large vessels and smooth muscle cells in addition to glomus cells. Glomus tumors express SMA and h-caldesmon, but are negative for keratin and S100 protein. Desmin is focally positive in a minority of cases. Type IV collagen highlights pericellular basement material. *NOTCH* rearrangements have been observed in a majority of cases (*Genes Chromosomes Cancer* 2013;52:1075). The recurrence rate is approximately 10%.

   Malignant glomus tumors are rare and manifest with either a spindle cell or round cell sarcoma pattern and are characterized by: (1) marked nuclear atypia with at least 5 mitoses/50 hpf or (2) atypical mitotic figures (*Am J Surg Pathol* 2001;25:1). The diagnosis also requires identification of a benign glomus tumor component or SMA and pericellular type IV collagen labeling.

3. **Myofibroma and myofibromatosis** exhibit variably biphasic growth with immature plump to spindled cells arranged in cellular whorls and fascicles interspersed with relatively paucicellular myoid nodules. A staghorn pattern is often associated with the primitive-appearing spindle cell component. Myoid nodules typically have a basophilic stroma, but can also be hyalinized or calcified, and may be associated with a vessel suggesting an angiocentric origin (e-**Fig. 44.30**). Hypercellular spindle cell foci are present in some cases with a resemblance to CIF, but the tumor cells lack the t(12;15) translocation characteristic of the latter tumor. The tumors are positive for SMA and h-caldesmon, while negative for CD34, keratin, and S100 protein. Myofibromas harbor activating *PDGFRB* mutations (*Am J Surg Pathol* 2017;41:195).

   Three clinicopathologic types of infantile myofibroma/myofibromatosis are recognized: (1) a solitary mass usually in the head and neck of a young child (0 to 3 years old), the most common; (2) multiple tumors involving skin, soft tissue, and bone; and (3) generalized myofibromatosis involving viscera in addition to skin, soft tissue, and bone. Unlike the former types, which are benign, generalized myofibromatosis is frequently fatal (*Pediatr Pathol Lab Med* 1995;15:571). Tumors in adults are typically superficial solitary lesions involving the head and neck or extremities.

4. **Myopericytoma** usually arises as a small superficial tumor in the extremities (*Am J Surg Pathol* 2006;30:104). Tumors are unencapsulated but well circumscribed and

composed of a cellular population of ovoid to spindled cells with eosinophilic to amphophilic cytoplasm, arranged in multilayered concentric profiles around thick- and thin-walled blood vessels. Mitotic figures are inconspicuous. Some tumors show overlapping features with myofibroma, glomangiopericytoma, and angioleiomyoma. There is diffuse immunopositivity for SMA and h-caldesmon. Rare cases of malignant myopericytoma are reported (*Histopathology* 2002;41:450).

Of note, adult and pediatric sarcomas with a prominent myopericytomatous growth pattern and *NTRK1* fusions have been identified (*J Pathol* 2016;238:700). These tumors may respond to targeted therapy.

VIII. SKELETAL MUSCLE

A. Nonneoplastic Disorders.
Histopathologic examination of skeletal muscle biopsies, whether obtained through an open biopsy or through a needle biopsy, continues to have a critical role in the evaluation of patients with suspected myopathy (*Curr Neurol Neurosci Rep* 2004;4:81). One portion of the biopsy should be formalin-fixed and paraffin-embedded according to standard laboratory protocols; another should be frozen for enzyme histochemistry studies; and the remainder should be fixed in glutaraldehyde for electron microscopic studies. While the histopathologic evaluation of skeletal muscle biopsies is a key component in the evaluation of neuromuscular disorders and can be used to diagnose a variety of inherited, inflammatory, and toxic myopathies, it should only be performed in the context of a thorough history and clinical examination that has included appropriate laboratory studies (including measurement of serum creatine kinase) and electromyography. A number of inflammatory, toxic, and axial myopathies have characteristic histopathologic findings, and immunohistochemical studies can be utilized to characterize inflammatory infiltrates when present (*Autoimmunity* 2006;39:161).

1. **Muscular dystrophies and other congenital myopathies** are diagnosed primarily based on clinical and electromyographic features. Increasingly, the histopathologic evaluation of muscle biopsies in these settings has been supplanted by genetic testing as an increasing number of diseases have been characterized at a genetic level (*Pediatr Dev Pathol* 2006;9:427; *Brain Pathol* 2001;11:206).

2. **Mitochondrial myopathies,** which traditionally have been diagnosed based on the demonstration of the so-called ragged-red fibers by Gomori trichrome stain, are increasingly diagnosed based on genetic testing since the genetic abnormalities in mitochondria that underlie these disease have been characterized (*J Submicrosc Cytol Pathol* 2006;38:201; *Biosci Rep* 2007;27:23).

B. Benign Tumors

1. **Rhabdomyomas** include cardiac rhabdomyoma which is usually, but not exclusively, seen in the setting of tuberous sclerosis, or extracardiac rhabdomyoma (fetal, adult, and genital rhabdomyoma).

   a. **Fetal rhabdomyoma** usually involves the head and neck of infants and young children, particularly the periauricular region, but all ages and a wide range of anatomic sites may rarely be affected. Tumors are frequently associated with nevoid basal cell carcinoma syndrome. The tumor usually forms a well-circumscribed small submucosal or subcutaneous nodule. The classic type is composed of bundles of fetal myotubes with interspersed small primitive mesenchymal cells. The intermediate or cellular type (juvenile rhabdomyoma) is characterized by increased cellularity, smooth muscle-like differentiation, and more mature rhabdomyoblastic differentiation. Fetal rhabdomyoma must be differentiated from ERMS, the latter of which has infiltrative growth, atypia, necrosis, and atypical mitotic figures. Tumors express desmin and myogenin.

   b. **Adult rhabdomyoma** usually presents as a well-circumscribed solitary mass in middle-aged to elderly adults and has an overwhelming predilection for the head and neck region (especially the oral cavity, pharynx, and larynx). Microscopically, sheets of large polygonal cells with abundant granular eosinophilic or vacuolated cytoplasm, well-defined cell borders, and round nuclei with prominent nucleoli are supplied by a fine vascular network. Spider cells, cytoplasmic cross-striations, and rod-like inclusions may also be present. Tumors are positive for desmin and myogenin, while negative for keratin, CD68, and chromogranin. Focal S100 protein expression may be seen. More than 40% recur, likely due to incomplete resection (*Hum Pathol* 1993;24:608).

c. Genital rhabdomyoma is very rare and typically presents in the vagina of adult women as a solitary 1- to 3-cm polyp. Tumors in men are also rarely observed. Microscopically, there is a hypocellular haphazard proliferation of differentiated polygonal and spindled rhabdomyoblasts with abundant eosinophilic cytoplasm and cross-striations embedded in a loose stroma. There is little, if any, atypia or mitotic activity; a cambium layer and ulceration are absent. Local excision is curative.

C. Malignant Tumors

1. Embryonal rhabdomyosarcoma (ERMS) is the most common STS of childhood and typically presents before 10 years of age. Older adults and infants are infrequently affected. ERMS has a strong predilection for the head and neck and genitourinary tract. Tumors may arise in the retroperitoneum, abdominopelvic cavity, and viscera. Unlike alveolar rhabdomyosarcoma (ARMS), ERMS rarely presents in peripheral soft tissues. Typically, ERMS is a soft, gelatinous-myxoid infiltrative mass whose shape and size depend on the anatomic site. When the tumor arises in a mucosal site like the nasopharynx, common bile duct, bladder, uterine cervix, or vagina, it has a polypoid configuration with the botryoid pattern of small primitive cells concentrated beneath the surface epithelium (cambium layer). Otherwise, the tumor has a rounded to ovoid configuration without a capsule or pseudocapsule; the cut surface has a faint multilobular appearance in which hemorrhage is more common than necrosis.

It is misleading to characterize ERMS as a "round cell" neoplasm since the morphology of the tumor cells is often quite diverse, ranging from short spindled or round cells, to ovoid cells with or without a delicate cytoplasmic tail, to larger cells with pale vacuolated to eosinophilic cytoplasm (e-**Fig. 44.31**). Tumor giant cells are usually absent. The intercellular space often has a pale mucoid to myxoid appearance. Where there is stroma the tumor cells are larger, more compact, and more likely to have bright eosinophilic cytoplasm. In many tumors, the fact that no two high magnification microscopic fields have identical features reflects the polymorphous character of many ERMS. Diffuse and/or lobular growth patterns are seen either as a dominant or mixed feature.

A difficult assessment is the determination of "viable" tumor in a posttreatment biopsy. By convention, if the biopsy contains tumor cells with features seen in the pretreatment biopsy, residual viable tumor is the appropriate interpretation. Differentiated rhabdomyoblasts with negative Ki-67 (MIB-1) staining are considered nonproliferative and nonviable.

The immunophenotype correlates with the degree of skeletal muscle differentiation. Primitive ERMS may show only vimentin expression. Desmin, myoD1, and/or myogenin nuclear positivity is often present but in a minority of the tumor cells, whereas myogenin tends to display near 100% nuclear positivity in ARMS (*Am J Surg Pathol* 2008;32:1513). Tumors can be risk stratified based on tumor site, stage, patient age, and histologic type.

2. Alveolar rhabdomyosarcoma (ARMS), like Ewing sarcoma (EWS) and hematolymphoid malignancies, is one of the quintessential malignant round cell neoplasms of childhood. Most cases are diagnosed in adolescents and young adults, although ARMS is seen infrequently in infants and older adults. Primary sites most frequently include the extremities, paraspinal and perineal regions, and the head and neck. Microscopically, the tumor has two general patterns: solid sheets of uniform high-grade round cells without extracellular mucin, and the classic alveolar pattern with dyshesive nests of tumor cells separated by incomplete fibrovascular septa (e-**Fig. 44.32**). Both patterns can be seen in metastatic ARMS (the initial encounter with the tumor may be in a lymph node or bone metastasis since ARMS often presents with disseminated disease). Most ARMSs are strongly and diffusely immunopositive for desmin, MyoD1, and myogenin (*Pathol Oncol Res.* 2008;14:233). Expression of keratin, CD99, and neuroendocrine markers may be seen.

Demonstration of a *FOXO1 (FKHR)* gene break apart by FISH is an important adjunct in the diagnosis of ARMS, with a positive result in approximately 75% to 80% of cases (*Am J Pathol* 2009;174:550). The *PAX3-FOXO1* fusion gene (resulting from t(2;13)) is more common (present in 70% to 80% of fusion positive cases) than the *PAX7-FOXO1* fusion gene (resulting from t(1;13)). Fusion negative ARMS have a gene profile and prognosis more like ERMS (*J Clin Oncol* 2010;28:2151). Rare RMS show mixed ARMS- and ERMS-like patterns; these tumors represent a diagnostic dilemma which may be resolved by FISH to determine the fusion status of the tumor.

3. Pleomorphic rhabdomyosarcoma is a highly aggressive sarcoma that presents in the deep soft tissues of adults (*Am J Surg Pathol* 2009;33:1850). Histologically the tumor typically grows as sheets of highly pleomorphic polygonal rhabdomyoblasts with deeply eosinophilic cytoplasm accompanied by a variable spindle cell or round cell component. Brisk mitotic activity (including atypical forms), necrosis, and bizarre multinucleated rhabdomyoblasts are common. Cross-striations are rarely seen and areas of ERMS or ARMS are not present. Desmin, MyoD1, and myogenin are positive; pancytokeratin and CD34 are reactive in a minority of cases. Tumors demonstrate a complex karyotype. The prognosis is poor.

4. Spindle cell/sclerosing rhabdomyosarcoma are rare tumors. They are distinct from embryonal and alveolar RMS (and may include multiple distinct entities). In older children and adults, tumors have a predilection for the head and neck and extremities; tumors in younger children (less than 10 years old) and infants are most common in the paratesticular and head and neck region. Histologically, the tumors are frequently infiltrative and composed of long fascicles of monotonous spindle cells with vesicular nuclei with interspersed rhabdomyoblasts. The mitotic rate is variable and necrosis is infrequent. Dense sclerosis can divide the tumor cells into trabeculae and nests. The tumor cells are positive for desmin, myogenin, and MyoD1. Tumors in young children and infants harbor *VGLL2* and/or *NCOA2* rearrangements and have a favorable prognosis (*Am J Surg Pathol* 2016;40:224), while tumors in older children and adults, which show recurrent L122R mutations in MyoD1, pursue an aggressive course (*Mod Pathol* 2016;29:1532).

Of note, an epithelioid and spindle cell rhabdomyosarcoma with *TFCP2* fusions and ALK expression occurring in bone has also recently been recognized (*J Pathol* 2018;245:29).

IX. VASCULAR TUMORS. Vascular or vasoformative lesions constitute a pathogenetically heterogeneous group of lesions composed of endothelial-lined spaces with a circumscribed or diffuse growth. These lesions are solitary or less often multifocal. The skin and underlying soft tissues are the most common sites of presentation, but there are few, if any, anatomic sites or organs that are excluded from involvement. In terms of pathogenesis, vascular tumors are reactive lesions (etiology known or unknown), malformations, or neoplasms.

A. Inflammatory Lesions. Inflammatory disorders of the vessels are covered in the chapter on the cardiovascular system (see Chapter 9).

B. Benign Vascular Tumors

1. Papillary endothelial hyperplasia (PEH, Masson tumor) is a particular manifestation of thrombus organization. It can be divided into primary (often occurring in a vein in the head and neck or subcutis of the fingers), secondary (arising in a hemangioma, hemorrhoidal vein or thrombohematoma), and extravascular (*Arch Pathol Lab Med* 1993;117:259). Microscopically, there are numerous, small, delicate papillae with fibrin or hyalinized cores that project into vascular lumens (e-**Fig. 44.33**). Often there is a transition between an organizing fibrin clot and PEH. A single layer of plump endothelial cells without appreciable cytologic atypia is characteristic and helps differentiate it from angiosarcoma. With continued organization of the clot, the papillae fuse and form an anastomosing network of vessels with eventual recanalization.

2. **Glomeruloid hemangioma** is an uncommon multifocal primarily intravascular capillary proliferation that is usually associated with POEMS (*p*olyneuropathy, *o*rganomegaly, *e*ndocrinopathy, *M*-protein, and *s*kin changes) syndrome. Glomeruloid capillary proliferations within dilated dermal blood vessels are microscopic features. Glomeruloid capillary tufts have an outer layer of pericytes and are lined by bland endothelial cells with or without cytoplasmic vacuolation and eosinophilic globules.

3. **Lobular capillary hemangioma (LCH, pyogenic granuloma)** is one of the most common vascular lesions and is seen primarily in skin and mucosal sites where satellite lesions may occur, but the anatomic distribution is wide. Microscopically, the lesion is well-circumscribed, frequently pedunculated, and composed of lobular arrays of uniform capillary-sized vessels with a central thick-walled feeder vessel and associated with a collarette of epidermis (**e-Fig. 44.34**). Mitoses may be numerous. Ulceration with inflammation, hemorrhage, and granulation tissue can obscure the underlying pathology (*J Eur Acad Dermatol Venereol* 2001;15:106). Extramedullary hematopoiesis may be seen.

4. **Bacillary angiomatosis** has a close clinical and pathologic resemblance to LCH, but also features an interstitial neutrophilic infiltrate and amorphous deposits of Warthin–Starry positive aggregates of *Bartonella henselae* or *B. quintana*. Virtually all cases of bacillary angiomatosis occur in immunocompromised individuals, usually in the setting of HIV.

5. **Vascular transformation of lymph nodes** (nodal angiomatosis) occurs as a reactive change in lymph nodes often associated with lymphovascular obstruction. Ectatic capillary-sized vessels within the subcapsular space and nodal sinuses are seen, which do not efface the lymph node architecture, unlike Kaposi sarcoma.

6. **Juvenile hemangioma** (infantile hemangioma, hemangioma of infancy) is the most common type of hemangioma in infants (typically found in the first weeks of life). This neoplasm has a female predominance and a predilection for the head and neck. Lesions have rapid proliferative phase followed by prolonged involutional stage; the latter can continue into late childhood. The tumor clinically presents as a purple-reddish macule or nodule centered in the skin or subcutaneous tissue. Cellular lobules of capillaries with compressed vascular lumina and readily identifiable mitotic figures characterize the proliferative phase. With involution, the vascular spaces become well-defined, dilated, and may develop thick hyalinized walls; mitoses are absent, a collagenous stroma becomes prominent, and fatty replacement may be observed. Tumors are diffusely immunopositive for GLUT1, which is in contrast to other histologically similar lesions.

7. **Congenital hemangioma** is present at birth, usually involves the head and neck and extremities, and has two subtypes: rapidly involuting congenital hemangioma (RICH) and noninvoluting congenital hemangioma (NICH) (*J Am Acad Dermatol* 2004;50:875). Early lesions are characterized by lobules of capillaries with dilated centrilobular vessels. Dense fibrous tissue divides the lobules. Unlike infantile hemangioma, these lesions are GLUT1 immunonegative.

8. **Tufted angioma** (angioblastoma of Nakagawa) typically presents in infancy in the dermis of the neck, upper trunk, and shoulders. The tumor is characterized by scattered cellular nodules composed of capillaries with compressed lumina and crescent shaped lumina at the periphery, producing a cannonball-like pattern (*Arch Dermatol* 2010;146:758) (**e-Fig. 44.35**). The mitotic rate is low and atypia is absent. Rare tumors are complicated by Kasabach–Merritt syndrome.

9. **Verrucous hemangioma** is composed of a mixture of cavernous and capillary vessels involving the superficial and deep dermis, associated with overlying epidermal hyperkeratosis, acanthosis, and papillomatosis.

10. **Cherry angioma** occurs in the superficial dermis of the trunk and upper extremities of adults. The tumor is composed of a well-circumscribed proliferation of dilated capillaries with an epidermal collarette.

11. **Cavernous hemangioma** is considered to be a venous malformation and occurs in the same age range and anatomic distribution as infantile hemangioma, but is less common, shows virtually no tendency to regress, and may be locally destructive due to extrinsic pressure on adjacent structures. The microscopic appearance is that of a pattern of grouped, dilated, thin-walled blood vessels with an inconspicuous endothelial lining. The blue rubber bleb nevus syndrome (characterized by cavernous hemangiomas of the skin and gastrointestinal tract) and Maffucci syndrome (cavernous hemangiomas, spindle cell hemangiomas, and enchondromas) are two associated syndromes.

12. **Arteriovenous malformation** is typically found in the head and neck where it is composed of a mixture of arteries, thick-walled veins, capillaries, and arteriovenous shunts.

13. **Venous hemangioma** (venous malformation) is very rare and typically presents during adulthood in the subcutis and deep soft tissue. Lesions are poorly circumscribed and composed to veins of varying caliber and wall thickness. The veins often show thrombosis, PEH, and dystrophic calcification. Arteries are absent, which can be confirmed with an elastic stain.

14. **Spindle cell hemangioma** usually occurs in young adults in the cutis and subcutis of the distal extremities, especially the hand. Multiple lesions are common. The tumor is composed of two components: thin-walled cavernous vessels lined by bland flattened endothelium, and solid areas composed of cellular sheets of spindle cells with compressed vascular channels and round or epithelioid vacuolated cells which may resemble adipocytes. The tumor involves a large preexisting vessel in many cases. Recurrence/growth of multifocal tumors is common (greater than 50% of cases). These tumors frequently harbor mutations in *IDH1/2* (*Am J Pathol* 2013;182:1494).

15. **Synovial hemangioma** arises in intra-articular synovium and bursa, most commonly in the knee of children and young adults. Lesions show cavernous (most common), capillary, or mixed patterns often associated with hyperplastic synovium and hemosiderin deposition.

16. **Intramuscular angioma** (intramuscular hemangioma) most frequently arises in the muscles of the thigh. It is a diffusely infiltrating mass composed of variably sized vessels ranging from large thick-walled veins to cavernous vascular spaces, arteries, lymphatics, and capillaries, and thus has features more in keeping with an arteriovenous malformation than a true neoplasm. Mature adipose tissue is a frequent component of the mass. The local recurrence rate is high.

17. **Epithelioid hemangioma** is slightly more common in females and tends to occur between 20 and 40 years of age as a small, variably colored nodule or plaque on the head and neck, particularly around the ear. Microscopically, it is a well-circumscribed nodule in the dermis or subcutis, or less frequently in the deep soft tissue, that has a vague lobular pattern of capillary-sized vessels around a feeder vessel. The endothelial cells are plump and have abundant eosinophilic, sometimes vacuolated, cytoplasm with impingement upon the vascular lumen (tombstone appearance). The vascular proliferation is frequently accompanied by a mixed inflammatory infiltrate composed largely of lymphocytes, eosinophils, and histiocytes. The neoplasm occurs rarely in the skeletal system and penis (*Am J Surg Pathol* 2004;28:523; *Am J Surg Pathol* 2009;33:270). A subset of cases, particularly those in soft tissue and bone, are characterized by *FOS* rearrangements, while angiolymphoid hyperplasia with eosinophilia is not (*Am J Surg Pathol* 2015;39:1313). *FOSB* rearrangements have been identified in cases with atypical features (*Genes Chromosomes Cancer* 2014;53:951).

18. **Angiomatosis** is a poorly circumscribed, diffuse network of variability sized vascular structures involving multiple tissue planes and/or multiple contiguous muscles. In virtually all cases it presents during childhood or adolescence as diffuse soft tissue swelling. The demonstration that the vessels are GLUT-1 immunonegative

is consistent with the interpretation that angiomatosis is a malformation. There are two histologic patterns: mixed-vessel lesions resembling intramuscular angiomas and capillary-predominant lesions with a lobular pattern. Large thick-walled veins with smaller vessels are often present within the walls, and adipose tissue is frequently admixed. Syndromic associations include Klippel–Trenaunay–Weber, Parkes–Weber, Bannayan–Riley–Ruvalcaba, Maffucci, and Proteus syndromes (*Semin Musculoskel Radiol* 2009;13:255). Local recurrences are very common following resection.

19. **Lymphangioma** is a cavernous and/or cystic lymphatic malformation composed of dilated lymphatic channels that occurs most commonly in the first years of life in the head and neck (e.g., cystic hygroma). Thin-walled dilated irregular lymphatic vessels of varying size are lined by flattened endothelium that is strongly immunopositive with D2-40. Scattered lymphoid aggregates may lie beneath the endothelium (e-**Fig. 44.36**).

20. **Atypical vascular lesion** presents as small papules or areas of erythema several years (average 5 years) after external radiation, usually for mammary carcinoma. These lesions are often composed of relatively well-circumscribed dilated irregular thin-walled vascular channels resembling lymphatics which may show a dissecting pattern of growth. Less commonly, a proliferation capillaries is seen (*Am J Surg Pathol* 2008;32:943). Flat to hobnail endothelial cells line the vascular spaces. Lesions are often confined to the superficial dermis and are wedge shaped. Large size, infiltrative margins, involvement of the subcutis, endothelial multilayering, nuclear atypia, and mitoses should be viewed with concern for angiosarcoma. Clinical correlation is essential, and in difficult cases immunohistochemical studies for MYC (which is positive in radiation-associated angiosarcoma) can be helpful. Rare cases of angiosarcoma arising in atypical vascular lesions have been described.

21. **Epithelioid angiomatous nodule** presents as one or less often multiple nodules involving the dermis. The trunk and extremities are most frequently affected. The lesion is composed of well-circumscribed unilobular sheet-like proliferations of epithelioid cells with vesicular chromatin and prominent nuclei. Focal vascular channels are present and mitoses are frequently identified (*Am J Dermatopathol* 2004;26:14).

22. **Sinusoidal hemangioma** usually presents in adults in the subcutis or deep dermis of the trunk, extremities, and breast. Lesions are typically small and grow as back-to-back dilated thin-walled vascular channels with pseudopapillae. The lesions is generally well circumscribed, but focal infiltrative growth can be seen (*Am J Surg Pathol* 1991;15:1130).

23. **Anastomosing hemangioma** typically occurs in adults and arises in the genitourinary tract, gastrointestinal tract, liver, and soft tissue (particularly paravertebral). The tumor are composed of anastomosing thin-walled capillary-sized vessels with scattered hobnail cells, eosinophilic globules, only mild atypia, and few if any mitoses. Adipocytic metaplasia, fibrin thrombi, and extramedullary hematopoiesis are often seen (*Am J Surg Pathol* 2016;40:1084). While tumors are generally well circumscribed, infiltration of surrounding tissues may be seen. The tumor harbors recurrent *GNAQ* mutations, and given similar histologic and molecular findings, these lesions may be related to hepatic small vessel neoplasm, though hepatic small vessel neoplasm shows more infiltrative growth (*Mod Pathol* 2017;30:722; *Hum Pathol* 2016;54:143).

24. **Hobnail hemangioma** (targetoid hemosiderotic hemangioma) typically occurs in adults in the dermis of the extremities. These lesions show a zonal architecture. Dilated thin-walled vascular channels with papillary projections and hobnail cells are present in the superficial dermis, while the vessels become smaller and compressed in the deeper dermis. Hemosiderin deposition is typical.

C. **Intermediate (Locally Aggressive) Vascular Tumors**

1. **Kaposiform hemangioendothelioma (KHE),** a rare locally aggressive neoplasm, presents most commonly in the first year of life in the extremities, trunk, or retroperitoneum. As the designation KHE implies, individual irregular lobules consist of

a mixture of capillary-sized vessels resembling capillary hemangioma that blend with fascicles of spindle cells with slit-like channels resembling Kaposi sarcoma. Frequent findings include glomeruloid structures, fibrin thrombi, cytoplasmic eosinophilic globules, and stromal and intracytoplasmic hemosiderin deposition. Lymphatic vessels are often present at the periphery of the tumor (*Am J Surg Pathol* 2004;28:559). Significant mitotic activity and atypia are absent. KHE is negative for HHV8, and immunopositive for GLUT1. Approximately 20% of cases are complicated by the Kasabach–Merritt syndrome.

D. Intermediate (Rarely Metastasizing) Vascular Tumors

1. **Retiform hemangioendothelioma,** an uncommon neoplasm, arises in the skin of the distal extremity or trunk in young to middle-aged adults. The tumor is a reddish-purple slowly growing plaque, centered in the reticular dermis, usually measuring less than 2 to 3 cm and often extending into the subcutis. Microscopically, there is an ill-defined proliferation of elongated branching narrow vessels that resemble the rete testis. The endothelial cells are monomorphic with a low mitotic rate, hyperchromatic nuclei, hobnail morphology, and high nuclear to cytoplasmic ratio. A lymphocytic infiltrate is typically present. The recurrence rate is over 50% and multiple recurrences are common. Lymph node metastases are rarely reported.

2. **Papillary intralymphatic angioendothelioma** (Dabska tumor) typically occurs in the skin of children though the tumor affects a wide age range. Ill-defined proliferations of thin-walled cavernous vascular spaces containing intraluminal papillary tufts of hobnail or matchstick-like endothelial cells, with an associated perivascular and intraluminal lymphocytic infiltrate, are typical features. Glomeruloid structures may be seen. Significant mitotic activity and atypia are absent. The tumor cells are immunopositive for D2-40, CD31, and CD34. A subset is associated with vascular malformations.

3. **Kaposi sarcoma** is an endothelial proliferation linked to human herpesvirus 8 (HHV8) infections. The clinicopathologic features of Kaposi sarcoma are discussed in more detail in the chapter on nonmelanocytic tumors of the skin (Chapter 38).

4. **Pseudomyogenic hemangioendothelioma/epithelioid sarcoma-like hemangioendothelioma** typically affects young adults and often arises as multifocal lesions involving multiple tissue planes in the extremities. The tumor is infiltrative and composed of plump spindled and epithelioid cells with relatively uniform round to ovoid vesicular nuclei and prominent eosinophilic cytoplasm. The tumor cells are arranged in sheets, nodules, and fascicles accompanied by a neutrophilic infiltrate (*Am J Surg Pathol* 2003;27:48; *Am J Surg Pathol* 2011;35:190). Rhabdomyoblast-like cells are often seen. While intracytoplasmic lumina may be present, overt vasoformation is absent. The tumor is positive for AE1/AE3, SMA (in a subset of cases, often focal), ERG, CD31 (50% of cases), and FOSB, while negative for CD34, EMA, S100 protein, desmin, and myogenin. INI1 is retained. *FOSB* rearrangements, typically *SERPINE1-FOSB*, are present (*J Pathol* 2014;232:534).

5. **Composite hemangioendothelioma** is likely not a distinct entity and probably includes multiple tumor types. It is defined by a variable admixture of vascular growth patterns; architectural components commonly resemble retiform hemangioendothelioma, epithelioid hemangioendothelioma (EHE), and spindle cell hemangioma. Tumors have a predilection for the distal extremities and usually occur in the cutis and subcutis of adults. A subset with an aggressive clinical course displays a neuroendocrine phenotype (*Mod Pathol* 2017;30:1589). Tumors with areas of angiosarcoma are best regarded as angiosarcomas with multiple growth patterns.

E. Other Intermediate Vascular Tumors With Limited Data

1. **Polymorphous hemangioendothelioma** is a soft tissue or lymph node–based vascular neoplasm in adults with multiple patterns including solid and vasoformative growth without atypia.

2. **Giant cell angioblastoma** is composed of vessels surrounded by ovoid to spindled, histiocytoid, and multinucleated cells.

F. Malignant Vascular Tumors

1. Epithelioid hemangioendothelioma (EHE) is a malignant endothelial neoplasm that occurs in patients of all ages, although it is rare in early childhood. The deep soft tissues, liver, lung, soft tissue, and bone are the most common primary sites. Up to 50% of patients have multifocal involvement at the time of presentation, which has been shown to represent metastatic disease (*Cancer Genet* 2012;205:12). The *WWTR1-CAMTA1* gene fusion is a characteristic feature of the majority of tumors, regardless of anatomic site (*Genes Chromosomes Cancer* 2011;50:44), while *YAP1-TFE3* is found in a small but distinct subset (*Genes Chromosomes Cancer* 2013;52:775). Microscopically, the tumor consists of cords, short strands, solid nests, or individual epithelioid to rounded cells (e-Fig. 44.37). The cells have low-grade nuclear features with a low mitotic rate. Endothelial differentiation is evident by the formation of intracytoplasmic lumina (producing a signet ring-like or blister cell appearance) but distinct endothelial-lined vascular channels are not prominent in conventional cases. Fragments of red blood cells may be seen within intracytoplasmic lumina. The neoplastic cells are embedded within a chondroid-like to myxohyaline stroma. Tumors with *YAP1-TFE3* rearrangements have more abundant eosinophilic cytoplasm, more vasoformative growth, and mild to moderate atypia. While behavior is difficult to predict and histologic features do not correlate well with outcome, increased mitotic rate and larger tumor size may portend a more aggressive course (*Am J Surg Pathol* 2008;32:924). Tumor cells express CD31, CD34, CAMTA1 (in cases with *WWTR1-CAMTA1* fusions), and TFE3 (usually cases with *YAP1-TFE3* fusions). Of note, approximately 30% of tumors show keratin expression.

2. Angiosarcoma is a highly aggressive malignancy that can be divided into several clinicopathologic groups including sporadic cutaneous angiosarcoma (frequently on the scalp of older men), lymphedema-associated cutaneous angiosarcoma (Stewart–Treves syndrome), radiation-associated cutaneous angiosarcoma, angiosarcoma of deep soft tissue, angiosarcoma of breast parenchyma, and tumors involving other viscera (e.g., liver, heart, and spleen). Tumors are poorly circumscribed and hemorrhagic; extensive hemorrhage may cause clinical, and even histologic, confusion with a hematoma. Typical histologic features include infiltrating complex ramifying vascular channels with intraluminal papillae, endothelial multilayering, and enlarged hyperchromatic nuclei. However, angiosarcoma has protean histologic features that vary from hemangioma-like (but with scattered enlarged atypical endothelial cells with occasional mitotic figures and an infiltrating growth pattern) to a poorly differentiated spindle cell sarcoma with a hemorrhagic background (e-Fig. 44.38).

Epithelioid angiosarcoma, a well-recognized variant, typically occurs in deep soft tissues and is predominately composed of sheets or nests of epithelioid cells with abundant eosinophilic or amphophilic cytoplasm, large vesicular nuclei, and prominent nuclei (e-Fig. 44.39). Metastatic lesions without overt vasoformation may give the impression of mesothelioma, melanoma, or carcinoma (*Arch Pathol Lab Med* 2011;135:268).

X. CHONDRO-OSSEOUS TUMORS

A. Benign

1. Chondroma occurs over a broad age range usually in the hands and feet, particularly the fingers, with a juxta-articular and tendinous predilection. Chondromas are typically small, well marginated, and composed of lobules of mature hyaline cartilage often with calcification and ossification. Hypercellularity is common and moderate atypia may be seen; however, the mitotic rate is low and atypical mitoses are not present. The tumor may have myxoid change, fibrosis, or xanthogranulomatous inflammation, which can cause confusion with a TSGT. Tumors with chondroblastoma-like features have been reported. Rearrangements of involving 12q13–15 are seen in a subset of cases.

B. Malignant

1. Extraskeletal osteosarcoma is a highly malignant neoplasm that usually arises in adults in the deep soft tissues of the extremities (most commonly the thigh), trunk, and retroperitoneum. About 10% of patients have history of prior radiation to the site. The tumor is usually composed of highly atypical pleomorphic cells with numerous mitoses, including atypical forms, associated with osteoid deposition. Like osseous osteosarcoma, extraskeletal tumors may be osteoblastic, chondroblastic, fibroblastic, or telangiectatic. Small cell and well-differentiated cases have also been reported. Osteoid deposition is usually most prominent in the center of the tumor while more peripheral regions of the neoplasm tend to be more densely cellular (this zonation is the reverse of the pattern present in MO).

2. **Extraskeletal mesenchymal chondrosarcoma** is an aggressive neoplasm which occurs over a wide age range, but is most common in adolescents and young adults. Tumors usually involve the head and neck (particularly dura and orbit) or proximal lower extremity. Microscopically, small nodules of well-differentiated hyaline cartilage are separated by sheets of undifferentiated small round to spindle cells, with or without hemangiopericytomatous vessels. The tumor cells are immunopositive for vimentin, CD99, NKX2.2, desmin (in a subset of cases), EMA (in a subset of cases), and SOX9, while negative for FLI1 (*Hum Pathol* 2010;41:653; *Appl Immunohistochem Mol Morphol* 2011;19:233). HEY1-NCOA2 fusions are characteristic.

XI. PERIPHERAL NERVE TUMORS. The tumors of presumed peripheral nerve or nerve sheath derivation comprise some of the more common soft tissue neoplasms.

A. Benign

1. **Traumatic neuroma** is a nonneoplastic response to nerve injury, often after a surgical procedure. It is typically a firm, tender nodule measuring less than 5 cm in maximal dimension that consists of a haphazard proliferation of small crowded nerve fascicles and fibrosis (e-**Fig. 44.40**).

2. **Mucosal neuromas** of the lips, mouth, eyelids, and intestines are manifestations of MEN IIB. Microscopically there is a haphazard proliferation of hyperplastic nerve bundles with prominent perineurium.

3. **Neurofibromas** are divided into three types based on growth pattern: localized, diffuse, and plexiform.

   a. **Localized neurofibroma** is usually superficial and solitary, and is not associated with a genetic syndrome. Microscopically, the circumscribed nonencapsulated tumor is composed of a haphazard proliferation of polymorphous spindle cells and strands of collagen (shredded carrot-like). The Schwann cells have wavy/buckled nuclei and indistinct pale eosinophilic cytoplasm, and are admixed with short spindle cells. The background has variable proportions of myxoid and collagenous stroma and scattered mast cells and lymphocytes. The tumor may be intraneural.

   b. **Plexiform neurofibromas** are almost always manifestations of neurofibromatosis 1 (NF1) (*Lancet Neurol* 2007;6:340). These tumors typically develop in early childhood as superficial (more common) or deep masses, and vary in size and extent of local involvement. Extensive intraneural growth can produce a bag-of-worms gross appearance in which the endoneurium of multiple nerve bundles is expanded by tumor, which can also extend into the adjacent soft tissue (e-**Fig. 44.41**). A diffuse pattern may accompany the plexiform component in the surrounding soft tissues. Usually the transformation to MPNST takes the form of an obviously high-grade sarcoma; however, establishing minimum criteria for the diagnosis of malignant transformation is difficult. Foci should be noted that have at least two of the following features: loss of neurofibroma architecture (fascicular growth and/or lack of CD34 positive fibroblasts), increased cellularity, mitotic rate >1/50 hpf but <3/10 hpf, and atypia. A tumor with two of these features may provisionally be diagnosed as atypical neurofibromatous neoplasm of uncertain biologic potential; a tumor with these features in addition to a higher mitotic rate and necrosis represents malignant transformation (*Hum Pathol* 2017;67:1) (e-**Fig. 44.42**). Nuclear reactivity for p53 is an additional finding of concern. It is important to note that nuclear atypia or increased cellularity alone does not justify a diagnosis of MPNST; however, such tumors should be carefully examined for mitoses.

   c. **Diffuse neurofibroma** often presents as a plaque on the trunk or head and neck of young patients. The dermis and subcutis are effaced by an infiltrative loose cellular proliferation within a myxoid and collagenous matrix containing Schwann cells and short spindle cells (e-**Fig. 44.43**). Wagner–Meissner bodies may be seen. The overgrowth of subcutaneous fat is similar to that seen in DFSP and infantile subcutaneous fibromatosis.

Tumors show patchy positivity for S100 protein and CD34; collagen IV is usually expressed whereas EMA is found in a small subset of cases. Diffuse staining for S100 protein is more common in schwannoma. Sporadic and NF1-associated neurofibromas are likely driven by biallelic inactivation of the *NF1* gene.

4. Schwannoma (neurilemoma) most often arises in patients between 20 and 40 years old, but can occur over a wide age range. Schwannoma frequently presents as a solitary mass in the head and neck and on the flexor surfaces of extremities. Bilateral vestibular schwannomas are characteristic of NF2; multiple schwannomas are seen in Gorlin–Koutlas syndrome, NF2, and schwannomatosis (*Annu Rev Pathol* 2007;2:191).

The tumor is usually invested by a true capsule (except for visceral and osseous lesions). Gross features include a white to yellow-white mucoid cut surface with or without cystic degeneration, calcification, and hemorrhage. Most tumors are less than 5 cm, although those that arise in the retroperitoneum can be larger. The characteristic low-power microscopic pattern (e-**Fig. 44.44**) consists of alternating Antoni A areas (organized spindle cells with or without Verocay bodies) (e-**Fig. 44.45**) and Antoni B areas (less cellular regions in which the oval to spindled cells are arranged more haphazardly in a loose myxoid matrix). Thickened hyalinized vessels are prominent in many cases. Degenerative features such as cystic change, ancient change, hyalinization, hemorrhage, hemosiderin deposition, foamy histiocytes, and calcification are frequently present and can be extensive.

There is considerable histologic variability in schwannomas. Despite seemingly atypical findings such as increased mitotic rate and ancient change, these tumors are benign and malignant transformation is exceeding rare. Tumor cells are diffusely immunopositive for S100 protein and SOX10, while negative for EMA, CD34, and claudin-1. GFAP and keratins are expressed in a subset of cases, particularly in tumors in the retroperitoneum, mediastinum, and gastrointestinal tract.

In addition to conventional schwannomas, multiple variants exist including plexiform, cellular, epithelioid, and microcystic/reticular. Plexiform schwannomas tend to occur in younger patients compared with conventional schwannoma, and are typically cellular or conventional schwannomas with extensive intraneural growth creating a plexiform pattern. Cellular schwannomas have a predilection for the retroperitoneum, mediastinum, and pelvis; these tumors generally lack Antoni B areas and Verocay bodies and are composed of cellular fascicles of spindle cells which may have mitotic activity, atypia, and focal necrosis. Epithelioid schwannomas are usually encapsulated superficial tumors composed of epithelioid cells growing in sheets, cords, and clusters with or without areas of conventional schwannoma; these tumors frequently show loss of INI1 (*Am J Surg Pathol* 2017;41:1013). Microcystic/reticular schwannoma is rare, generally occurs in the gastrointestinal tract, and is composed of anastomosing spindle cells creating a reticular and microcystic pattern.

5. Granular cell tumor occurs in virtually all ages, although more frequently in adults. There is a predilection for the skin, base of tongue, and oral cavity. The tumor has irregular borders, and is composed of nests, cords, and confluent sheets of polygonal to slightly spindled cells with small bland nuclei and abundant eosinophilic granular cytoplasm (e-**Fig. 44.46**). Pseudoepitheliomatous hyperplasia may be present in the overlying epidermis or squamous mucosa. Malignant granular cell tumor is rare and is characterized by at least three of the following features: tumor necrosis, spindle cell morphology, vesicular nuclei with prominent nucleoli, increased mitotic activity (>2 mitoses/10 fields at 200× [not 400×] magnification), high nuclear to cytoplasmic ratio, and pleomorphism (*Am J Surg Pathol* 1998;22:779). Immunoreactivity for S100 protein, SOX10, TFE3, NSE, and CD68 is usually present, while there is no expression of HMB-45 and keratins.

6. **Dermal nerve sheath myxoma** is usually found in the dermis of the extremities, particularly the hand and fingers, over a wide age range. Microscopically, lobules composed of epithelioid, spindled, and stellate cells arranged in small nests, reticular arrays, rings, and cords set in abundant myxoid stroma are present, separated by fibrous bands. Atypia is absent and mitoses are rare; the tumor cells are diffusely positive for S100 protein. Cellular neurothekeoma with myxoid stroma may resemble dermal nerve sheath myxoma (e-**Fig. 44.47**).

7. **Perineurioma** is composed of perineural cells and usually involves the extremities or trunk. The tumors is well circumscribed with storiform, whorling, and loose fascicular growth of bland spindle cells with long cytoplasmic processes set in a myxoid to collagenous stroma. Perivascular whorls are characteristic and reticular arrays may be seen. Mitoses are rare and necrosis is absent. The cells of intraneural perineurioma grow concentrically around axons producing onion bulb-like configurations. Sclerosing perineuriomas typically are acral tumors composed to epithelioid to plump spindled cells set in fibrous stroma. Perineuriomas are immunopositive for EMA (may be focal), CD34, and claudin-1, while immunonegative for S100 protein.

8. **Solitary circumscribed neuroma** (palisaded encapsulated neuroma) has a pronounced predilection for the head and neck (particularly the face) of adults, and presents as a solitary dome-shaped dermal nodule (measuring less than 1 cm). The lesion is well circumscribed and partially encapsulated by perineurium. Intersecting short fascicles of bland Schwann cells with interfascicular clefting and lack of zonation are characteristic features. Nuclear palisading is uncommon. Nerve origin and intratumoral axons (highlighted with neurofilament) are frequently seen. The tumor cells are strong and diffusely positive for S100 protein, while the capsule stains with EMA. The tumor is benign and does not recur.

9. **Ectopic meningioma and meningothelial hamartoma** by definition arise completely outside of intracranial or intraspinal areas. Ectopic meningioma occurs over a wide age range and has a strong predilection for the head and neck, while meningothelial hamartoma occurs in neonates and infants typically on the scalp. Ectopic meningioma shows similar histologic features to CNS meningiomas including subtype morphologies and a complete range of tumor grades (WHO I–III), though benign tumors are most common. The meningothelial subtype is most frequently observed and is characterized by uniform ovoid cells with syncytial, lobular, and whorled growth patterns. Nuclear grooves and intranuclear pseudoinclusions are typical.

Meningothelial hamartoma forms pseudovascular and microcystic spaces lined by meningothelial cells; variable nodule formation is also seen.

Infiltrative growth is typical of both ectopic meningioma and meningothelial hamartoma. The tumor cells are positive for EMA and PR, while negative for S100 protein, CD34, CD31, synaptophysin, and chromogranin. While meningothelial hamartoma is wholly benign, the prognosis of an ectopic meningioma depends on the completeness of resection and tumor grade.

10. **Nasal glial heterotopia** (ectopic glial tissue) is largely restricted to neonates and infants and has a strong predilection for the skin on and around the nose, as well as the nasal cavity. The lesion is composed of nests of glial tissue which can be highlighted with a trichrome stain (the nests of glial tissue stain, red), GFAP, and S100 protein. The nests are separated by fibrous bands.

11. **Benign triton tumor** (neuromuscular choristoma) has a strong predilection for large proximal nerves (most commonly the sciatic nerve and brachial plexus) and usually arises in young children, though adults are rarely affected. The tumor causes fusiform expansion of the involved nerve, which correlates with a haphazard endoneurial proliferation of mature skeletal muscle fibers, which may be associated with desmoid fibromatosis in the primary tumor or in a recurrence. *CTNNB1* mutations have been detected in neuromuscular choristoma and associated desmoids (*Am J Surg Pathol* 2016;40:1368).

12. **Hybrid nerve sheath tumors** are a group of lesions composed of more than one conventional peripheral nerve sheath tumor type. The tumors are typically superficial

and have a broad age and anatomic distribution. Schwannoma/perineuroma is the most common combination; it is composed of admixed Schwann and perineurial cells, and typically exhibits perineurioma-like growth with whorls and storiform patterns. Tumors with distinct areas of schwannoma and perineuroma have also been described. Neurofibroma/schwannoma exhibits biphasic morphology with nodules of Antoni A schwannoma embedded in a neurofibroma. Neurofibroma/perineurioma and granular cell tumor/perineurioma are also rarely reported.

B. Malignant

1. **Malignant peripheral nerve sheath tumor (MPNST)** can be difficult to diagnose. A sarcoma can generally be classified as MPNST if it arose in a patient with NF1, arose in a peripheral nerve, arose from a benign nerve sheath tumor (in most cases a neurofibroma), or if it demonstrates histologic, immunophenotypic, and/or ultrastructural features that reflect Schwannian differentiation.

   These tumors are typically large with fleshy mucoid cut surfaces and large areas of hemorrhage and necrosis. Microscopically, they are composed of fascicles of atypical spindle cells that may have wavy or comma-shaped nuclei. The cellular density often varies producing a "marbled" appearance (e-Fig. 44.48). Nuclear palisading and increased cellularity around vessels is present in some tumors. Heterologous differentiation including rhabdomyosarcomatous (malignant triton tumor), chondrosarcomatous, osteosarcomatous, and angiosarcomatous is seen in more than 10% of cases. Glandular differentiation is rare and usually seen in the setting of NF1. Rare epithelioid MPNSTs have extensive epithelioid morphology.

   Lack of specific immunohistochemical markers for MPNST complicates the diagnosis outside of the usual settings. While epithelioid MPNST stain diffusely for S100 protein, less than 50% of conventional tumors show immunoreactivity. Diffuse S100 staining is very unusual in conventional MPNST and if present other diagnoses should be considered, especially spindle cell melanoma. MPNSTs have complex karyotypes.

2. **Ectomesenchymoma** is a rare aggressive neoplasm that typically occurs in children in the peritesticular region, head and neck, and abdomen. It is composed of a rhabdomyosarcomatous component with embryonal, spindle cell, or alveolar features, admixed with a population of cells with a range of neuroectodermal differentiation, including ganglion, Schwannian, and neuroblastic cells. The rhabdomyosarcomatous component expresses desmin and myogenin; S100 protein is positive in the Schwannian cells, and synaptophysin is positive in ganglion and neuroblastic cells. Ectomesenchymoma harbors *HRAS* mutations suggesting a relationship with ERMS (*Am J Surg Pathol* 2016;40:876).

3. **Melanotic schwannoma** usually presents in adults in the posterior spinal nerves roots, though other sites are rarely affected. The tumor is rare in children. Melanotic schwannomas are commonly associated with Carney complex (*Ann Endocrinol (Paris)* 2010;71:486). The tumor is usually composed of sheets and short fascicles of spindled to polygonal cells with pale eosinophilic cytoplasm. Psammoma bodies are seen in approximately half the cases, and melanin pigment is variably prominent. The tumor is positive for S100 protein, HMB-45, MART-1, and tyrosinase. *PRKAR1A* mutations are frequently present. Recurrence (35% of cases), metastasis (15% to 42% of cases), and disease-related mortality are not uncommon (*Am J Surg Pathol* 2014;38:94).

XII. TUMORS OF UNCERTAIN DIFFERENTIATION

A. Benign

1. **Intramuscular myxoma** occurs primarily in adults between 40 and 60 years old as a solitary, painless, slowly growing mass within the muscles of the thigh, buttocks, or limb girdle. Most tumors measure <10 cm and are grossly well circumscribed with a pale gelatinous cut surfaces. Conventional tumors are composed of a hypocellular proliferation of small bland stellate to spindled cells set in an abundant myxoid matrix that contains an inconspicuous vascular network (e-Fig. 44.49). Mitoses are rare. Peripheral infiltrative growth with entrapment of skeletal muscle

is not uncommon. Cellular myxomas are a morphologic variant characterized by increased cellularity and vascularity within a collagenous background (*Am J Surg Pathol* 1998;22:1222; *Histopathology* 2001;39:287). One or more myxomas of the soft tissues associated with fibrous dysplasia characterizes Mazabraud syndrome. The tumor variably expresses CD34 and SMA, but is negative for desmin, S100 protein, and MUC4. Activating mutations in codon 201 of the *GNAS* gene are present in Mazabraud-associated and sporadic tumors.

2. **Juxta-articular myxoma** has a predilection for middle-aged men and usually arises in the vicinity of a large joint (primarily the knee) (*Hum Pathol* 1992;23:639). This tumor has similar histologic and immunohistochemical features as cellular intramuscular myxoma, but has a periarticular location and lacks *GNAS* mutations.

3. **Deep ("aggressive") angiomyxoma** is a slow growing locally infiltrative tumor that usually occurs in the pelvic/perineal soft tissue of reproductive age women, but is also rarely seen in the inguinal and scrotal areas of men. It forms a deep ill-defined mass often measuring more than 10 cm that has a gelatinous cut surface. The tumor is infiltrative and composed of a relatively hypocellular proliferation of small bland stellate to spindled cells set in an edematous/myxoid stroma with fine collagen fibers (e-**Fig. 44.50**). Prominent variably sized thick- and thin-walled vessels are present; spindle cells appear to spin off from intratumoral vessels. The tumor cells express vimentin desmin, ER, and PR. *HMGA2* rearrangements are present in a subset of cases. The tumor has a propensity to recur, particularly if incompletely excised, but does not metastasize.

4. **Pleomorphic hyalinizing angiectatic tumor (PHAT)** is a slow growing poorly circumscribed tumor which usually arises in the subcutis of the distal lower extremity in adults. The neoplasm is characterized by a proliferation of spindled and hyperchromatic pleomorphic cells with nuclear pseudoinclusions and clusters of thin-walled ectatic blood vessels with fibrinoid change or hyalinization. Thrombosis, intracytoplasmic hemosiderin within tumor cells, and a mixed inflammatory infiltrate are typical. The mitotic rate is low. At the tumor periphery areas resembling hemosiderotic fibrolipomatous tumor (HFLT) are frequently present (*Am J Surg Pathol* 2004;28:1417). Tumor cells are often positive for CD34 while negative for S100 protein. Tumors have a recurrence rate of 30% to 50% and rare tumors progress to a myxoid sarcoma. Of note, PHAT is likely related to HFLT based on morphologic features and shared *TGFBR3* and/or *MGEA5* rearrangements, while kinship with MIFS is less convincing (*Adv Anat Pathol* 2017;24:268).

5. **Hemosiderotic fibrolipomatous tumor (HFLT)** usually presents in middle-aged adults in the distal extremities, particularly around the foot and ankle. There is a female predominance. The tumor is ill defined and composed of fascicles of bland spindle cells with intracytoplasmic hemosiderin admixed with mature adipose tissue. The mitotic rate is low and a chronic inflammatory infiltrate may be present; areas with features similar to PHAT may be seen. The tumor cells are positive for CD34 but negative for SMA, desmin, and S100 protein. HFLT and PHAT share rearrangements of *TGFBR3* and/or *MGEA5*. Recurrence occurs in up to 50% of cases, and rare cases progress to a myxoid sarcoma. HFLT and PHAT are likely related (see previous section).

6. **Ectopic hamartomatous thymoma** is found almost exclusively in the lower neck region and generally occurs in adult men. The lesion is composed of a variable admixture of spindle cells, epithelial structures, and mature adipocytes. The bland spindle cells are arranged in fascicles and the epithelial component forms nests with squamous or glandular differentiation. Both the spindle and epithelial components are diffusely positive for keratin.

7. **Atypical fibroxanthoma (AFX)** is a dermal tumor which occurs in sun-damaged skin, usually on the head and neck of the elderly. Tumors are small and composed of highly atypical pleomorphic spindled, epithelioid, and multinucleated cells. Mitotic figures, including atypical forms, are numerous. AFX shows no line of differentiation and is a diagnosis of exclusion; histologic and immunophenotypic evidence of squamous, melanocytic, vascular, and smooth muscle differentiation should be excluded before

the diagnosis of AFX is rendered. AFX follows a benign course without recurrence or metastasis. However, large dermal tumors with similar clinical, histologic, and immunohistochemical features as AFX but which additionally have lymphovascular or perineural invasion, necrosis, or invasion beyond the superficial subcutis are known as pleomorphic dermal sarcomas. These tumors recur (28%) and can metastasize (10%) (*Am J Surg Pathol* 2012;36:1317).

8. Acral fibromyxoma presents over a wide age range but is most common in adults and shows a strong predilection for the nail bed or periungual area. The tumor is composed of monomorphic spindle and stellate cells with loose fascicular, vague storiform, or haphazard growth. The mitotic rate is low and tumor cells are usually bland; however, pleomorphism is rarely observed. Multinucleated cells are frequently present. The stroma is variably myxoid to fibrous. CD34 is frequently immunopositive and there is variable focal positivity for EMA and SMA, but S100 protein, keratin, and desmin are immunonegative.

B. Intermediate (Rarely Metastasizing)

1. Angiomatoid fibrous histiocytoma (AFH) is a slow growing tumor which usually arises in the deep dermis and subcutis of the limbs, trunk, or head and neck of children and young adults. Most cases measure 4 cm or less. The cut surface is multinodular and hemorrhagic; blood-filled cystic spaces are a common feature, but nonhemorrhagic tumors are also seen. The neoplastic population consists of nodules of bland monotonous histiocytoid to spindled cells with indistinct borders, with interspersed pseudo-angiomatoid blood-filled spaces (e-**Fig. 44.51**). The tumor is surrounded by a fibrous pseudocapsule; a dense plasma cell-rich chronic inflammatory cuff is often present at the periphery, which can mimic a lymph node. Atypia and mitotic activity are infrequently present. There is variable expression of EMA, desmin (about 50% of cases), CD99, and CD68; keratin, CD31, CD21, CD23, and S100 protein are generally negative. AFH can harbor *EWSR1-CREB1* (most common), *EWSR1-ATF1* and *FUS-ATF1* (rare) fusions. The recurrence rate is up to 15% and metastases are rare. Of note, AFH, clear cell sarcoma (CCS) of tendons and aponeuroses, CCS-like tumor of the gastrointestinal tract (gastrointestinal neuroectodermal tumor), primary pulmonary myxoid sarcoma, a subset of malignant mesothelioma, and hyalinizing clear cell carcinoma harbor at least one of the same fusions (*Am J Surg Pathol*. 2012;36:e1; *Am J Surg Pathol* 2017;41:980).

2. Ossifying fibromyxoid tumor (OFMT) is usually seen in adults as a long-standing painless mass measuring 3 to 5 cm. The extremities (70% of cases), trunk, head and neck, and retroperitoneum are various primary sites of the tumor (*Am J Surg Pathol* 2008;32:996). Microscopically, lobules of uniform, round to spindled cells are arranged in cords and trabeculae in a fibromyxoid to collagenous matrix; a fibrous pseudocapsule with or without a peripheral incomplete shell of lamellar bone is present. Malignant OFMT are characterized by either high-grade nuclear atypia or high cellularity with mitotic rate >2/50 hpf (*Am J Surg Pathol* 2003;27:421). These tumors express S100 protein while showing variable reactivity for desmin, pankeratin, GFAP, and MUC4. *PHF1* or *BCOR* rearrangements are seen in the majority of cases. Typical tumors have limited potential for recurrence and rarely metastasize, while approximately 60% of malignant OFMT metastasize.

3. Myoepithelioma/myoepithelial carcinoma/mixed tumor comprise a group of neoplasms which display varying proportions of myoepithelial and epithelial elements. These tumors usually present as a painless swelling in the subcutis or deep soft tissues of the extremities. While adults are most commonly affected, a significant proportion of cases occur in children. The tumors are lobulated and composed of epithelioid and spindled cells arranged in cords, nests, sheets, and reticular patterns, set in a chondromyxoid to hyalinized stroma. Mixed tumors additionally show ductal differentiation. Like histologically similar salivary gland tumors, there is a wide range of architectural patterns, divergent differentiation, and a low mitotic rate. These tumors are generally positive for keratins and EMA, and variably positive for S100 protein, SOX10, p63, SMA, calponin, and GFAP; they are negative for desmin and a minority of tumors show loss of INI1. *EWSR1* rearrangements are seen in approximately 50% of myoepithelial tumors, while mixed tumors harbor *PLAG1* rearrangements similar to salivary gland analogues. Histologically aggressive cases are termed myoepithelial carcinomas and are characterized by moderate to severe nuclear atypia; these tumors show increased recurrence and metastatic rates, and are overrepresented in children.

4. **Phosphaturic mesenchymal tumor (PMT; mixed connective tissue variant)** typically arises in soft tissue or bone in adults. The tumor is frequently difficult to locate and patients often have suffered from long durations of oncogenic osteomalacia (usually caused by tumor secretion of FGF23 leading to renal phosphate wasting) before the tumor is identified. Rare cases are not associated with osteomalacia. PMT can mimic a wide range of bone and soft tissue tumors, but is typically characterized by bland spindled to stellate cells embedded in a myxochondroid to hyalinized matrix, with areas of grungy to flocculent calcification (*Am J Surg Pathol* 2004;28:1). The unusual matrix may mimic chondroid or osteoid. Osteoclast-like giant cells, microcystic change, and adipocytes are frequently noted. The tumor is vascular with numerous capillaries and often large vessels which may be ectatic. The tumor cells are positive for SATB2, CD56, SMA (focal), FGFR1, FGF23, ERG, and somatostatin receptor 2A, but negative for desmin, S100 protein, CD34, and STAT6. Rearrangements of *FN1* have been found in about 50% of cases, most commonly fused to *FGFR1* or less frequently *FGF1* (*Am J Surg Pathol* 2017;41:1371). Most tumors are benign, and resection often leads to rapid clinical improvement; rare tumors with overtly sarcomatous histology are malignant.

5. **Perivascular epithelioid cell tumors** (PEComas) are a family of related neoplasms with myomelanocytic differentiation including angiomyolipoma, lymphangiomyomatosis, clear cell "sugar" tumor of the lung, and clear cell myomelanocytic tumor of the falciform ligament/ligamentum teres. PEComas can be found throughout the body including bone, soft tissue, and viscera. Microscopically, PEComas are often composed of trabeculae and nests of large epithelioid cells that have clear to granular eosinophilic cytoplasm and round nuclei. A capillary network surrounds nests and trabeculae. Tumor cells associated with vessel walls may be found. Spindled cells predominate in some tumors. Sclerosing PEComa has extensive sclerotic stroma and trabecular architecture. Increased tumor size, mitotic activity >1/50 HPF, necrosis, marked atypia, and diffuse pleomorphism are associated with aggressive behavior (*Am J Surg Pathol* 2005;29:1558; *Am J Surg Pathol* 2013;37:1769). The tumor cells are immunopositive for HMB-45, MITF, melan-A, SMA, calponin, and less often for caldesmon and desmin; a minority of cells are positive for S100 protein. Loss of *TSC2* is the most common molecular alteration in these tumors, while a subset harbor *TFE3* fusions and express TFE3 (*Am J Surg Pathol* 2010;34:1395).

C. Malignant

1. **Ewing sarcoma (EWS)** most commonly presents in the second decade of life in bone or soft tissue. However, viscera, skin, and other anatomic sites can be affected in patients over a wide age range. Biopsy followed by posttreatment resection is the management sequence in most cases; these biopsies offer many diagnostic challenges because of the frequently associated necrosis and compression artifact. Typically, the tumor is composed of uniform round cells with clear to finely vacuolated cytoplasm and a central nucleus with fine to slightly coarse chromatin. Mitotic figures are present but are not especially numerous in most cases. Architecturally, broad sheets, lobules, nests, and strands are some of the growth patterns (e-**Fig. 44.52**). Homer-Wright rosettes and condensed small cellular nodules within otherwise monotonous sheets of round cells may be seen. Rare findings include larger cells with irregular nuclei and nucleoli (atypical variant), spindle cells, adamantinoma-like morphology, and a pale mucoid background. Clear cytoplasm is usually an indication of abundant diastase digestible glycogen. CD99 characteristically shows strong and diffuse membrane positivity; however, CD99 is expressed in a number of other small round cell tumors including lymphoblastic lymphoma/leukemia, poorly differentiated synovial

sarcoma, CIC-rearranged sarcoma, mesenchymal chondrosarcoma, rhabdomyosar-coma, and desmoplastic small round cell tumor (DSRCT). Punctate cytokeratin reactivity is seen focally in 20% to 25% of cases. NKX2.2 may also be a useful marker particularly when combined with CD99 (*Virchows Arch* 2014;465:599).

Chromosomal translocations that form fusions between the *EWSR1* gene and a member of the *ETS* family of transcription factors (most commonly *FLI1* followed by *ERG*) are characteristic of EWS, though a small minority of cases harbor fusions of *EWSR1* with non-*ETS* genes, or *FUS* rearrangement instead of *EWSR1*. A small fraction of tumors have cryptic fusions that can introduce diagnostic uncertainty (*Cancer Genet Cytogenet* 2010;200:60).

2. Desmoplastic small round cell tumor (DSRCT) characteristically has a marked male predominance and manifests as abdominal masses, frequently with diffuse involve-ment of peritoneal surfaces. Tumors often occur in the second or third decade of life; rare tumors present outside the abdomen and in older adults. The classic histologic features are variably sized nests, sheets, and trabeculae of small round undifferenti-ated cells set in a desmoplastic stroma (**e-Fig. 44.53**); rosette and glandular forma-tions may be seen. Of note, DSRCT can present with a wide range of histologic features, which may complicate diagnosis. Since several other malignant round cell neoplasms also can have desmoplastic stroma, including blastemal predominant Wilms tumor, EWS, and embryonal or alveolar RMS, ancillary testing is extremely helpful. DSRCT is polyphenotypic with expression of keratin, EMA, desmin, and NSE, as well as CD99 and WT1 (antibody to the c-terminus); DSRCT is negative for myogenin and MyoD1. The *EWSR1-WT1* fusion is characteristic of DSRCT.

3. Synovial sarcoma typically presents in patients between the ages of 15 and 40 years old in the periarticular soft tissues, but the tumor can arise in virtually any site. Approximately 8% to 10% of all STS in the first two decades are synovial sarcoma, and the tumor is uncommon in individuals over 50 years of age.

The usual gross appearance is a well-circumscribed mass with a grey-tan surface; cystic and calcified foci are not uncommon. Tumors larger than 5 cm tend to have a worse outcome (*J Clin Oncol* 2000;18:2087). The tumor is composed of a monot-onous population of relatively bland spindle cells with scant cytoplasm growing in cellular fascicles and sheets. The two classic histologic subtypes are the monophasic type (only spindle cell pattern) and the biphasic type (which in addition to the spin-dle cell component contains epithelial glands (**e-Fig. 44.54**) and nests). Masts cell are often present. The mitotic rate is variable and necrosis is uncommon. The tumor can progress to poorly differentiated synovial sarcoma, which is characterized by nuclear atypia and an increased mitotic rate. Poorly differentiated foci can have round cell, spindled, epithelioid, and rhabdoid patterns. The immunophenotype, regardless of subtype, includes the expression of EMA, pankeratin, CK7, CK19, CD99, and TLE1, but no expression of desmin and CD34. S100 protein is focally expressed in approximately a third of cases (*Am J Surg Pathol* 2002;26:1434). The t(X;18) which fuses *SYT* (SS18) with *SSX1*, *SSX2* or rarely *SSX4*, is characteristic of the tumor. Rare cases harbor *SS18L1–SSX1* fusions (*Genes Chromosomes Cancer* 2017;56:296).

4. Clear cell sarcoma (CCS) of tendons and aponeuroses (melanoma of soft parts) typically presents in the distal soft tissues (especially the foot and ankle) of young adults. Tumors are usually deep and associated with a tendon or aponeurosis. Fibrous septa divide nests and fascicles composed of uniform ovoid to spindled cells with pale eosinophilic to clear cytoplasm and vesicular nuclei with prominent nucleoli (**e-Fig. 44.55**). Wreath-like multinucleated tumor cells are a characteristic feature, and melanin pigment can often be found but is typically not prominent. Recurrent and metastatic lesions may show increased pleomorphism, mitotic activity, and an epithelioid morphology. The immunoprofile reflects the melanocytic differentiation of the tumor with S100 protein, SOX10, HMB-45, MITF, and melan-A/MART-1 immunopositivity. The *EWSR1* translocations present in CCS are not seen in mela-noma; greater than 90% of CCS harbor *EWSR1-ATF1* fusions, while a subset shows

EWSR1-CREB1 fusions. Of note, identical fusions are also present in CCS-like tumor of the gastrointestinal tract (gastrointestinal neuroectodermal tumor) and AFH. A prolonged clinical course is often observed, with frequent late recurrence and metastasis including to lymph nodes.

5. **Alveolar soft part sarcoma (ASPS)** is most commonly seen in patients between the ages of 15 and 35 years old and shows a female predominance. The tumor has a predilection for the head and neck (especially the orbit and base of the tongue) in children, while the deep soft tissue of the extremities (especially the buttock and thigh) are the most common sites in adults (*Arch Pathol Lab Med* 2007;131:488). Microscopically, uniform large polygonal cells with abundant eosinophilic granular to clear cytoplasm are arranged in nests with pseudoalveolar growth; delicate fibrous septa and sinusoidal vessels separate nests (e-**Fig. 44.56**). However, the tumor may have a more diffuse, nonalveolar, pattern especially in pediatric cases involving the tongue. Vascular invasion is an almost constant feature. Rare findings include anaplasia, brisk mitotic activity, and necrosis (*J Clin Pathol* 2006;59:1127). Rod-shaped or rhomboid crystalline inclusions, when present, are highlighted by PAS and are diastase resistant. Tumor cells are positive for TFE3 (variable and focal), but negative for HMB-45, keratin, synaptophysin, and chromogranin. The nonreciprocal der(17)t(X;17) translocation is the characteristic cytogenetic feature of this tumor resulting in the *ASPSCR1-TFE3* fusion. Local recurrence is rare, while metastasis (including at presentation and after long intervals) is common.

6. **Extraskeletal myxoid chondrosarcoma (EMC)** typically arises in the deep soft tissues of the proximal extremities, usually presents between 35 and 60 years of age, and has a male predilection. Uncommon other primary sites include the nasopharynx, vulva, heart, and retroperitoneum. Microscopically, fibrous septa divide myxoid nodules populated by small, uniform, bland, round to spindled cells with strikingly eosinophilic cytoplasm that are arranged in interconnecting cords, rings, strands, and reticular networks (e-**Fig. 44.57**). Hemorrhage, necrosis, and hemosiderin deposition are often present. Cellular foci are composed sheets of large epithelioid cells with prominent nucleoli. Rhabdoid features may also be present. The tumor cells are variably positive for S100 protein. Keratin and EMA are rarely expressed, while brachyury is negative. Loss of INI1 may be seen, particularly in tumors with rhabdoid cells; INSM1 may be useful as immunopositivity has been demonstrated in 90% of EMC, with limited expression in histologic mimics (*Am J Clin Pathol* 2015;144:579). The tumor is characterized by *NR4A3* rearrangements, most commonly leading to a *EWSR1–NR4A3* fusion. The clinical course is often protracted with late recurrence and metastasis.

7. **Extrarenal malignant rhabdoid tumor** is an extremely aggressive neoplasm that has a strong predilection for infants and young children, and involves a wide range of anatomic sites including the neck, paraspinal soft tissues, retroperitoneum, abdominopelvic cavity, viscera, and central nervous system (in the latter location it is termed atypical teratoid rhabdoid tumor). This tumor can present in newborns with disseminated disease including placental involvement. Grossly, it is a highly infiltrative neoplasm with a soft, grayish tan, and necrotic cut surface. The tumor is characterized by sheets and trabeculae of rhabdoid cells that have eccentric vesicular nuclei, prominent nucleoli, and a characteristic eosinophilic cytoplasmic inclusion (which is largely composed of cytokeratin) (*Mod Pathol* 2001;14:854). Less commonly, tumors have a small round cell pattern with only rare rhabdoid cells. The tumor cells are positive for vimentin, keratin, and EMA; INI1 expression is absent. Biallelic inactivation of the *SMARCB1* gene is the underlying genetic feature.

8. **Epithelioid sarcoma** can be divided into distal and proximal types. The distal or conventional type of epithelioid sarcoma usually occurs in adolescents and young adults and is found in the fingers, hand, wrist, or the equivalent sites in the distal lower extremity. The more aggressive proximal type typically occurs in middle-aged adults and involves the limb girdle/proximal extremities, pelvis, perineum, and genital tract.

In the distal type, arcades and nodules of uniform relatively bland epithelioid to plump spindled cells with eosinophilic cytoplasm are set in abundant collagen (e-**Fig. 44.58**). The nodules can undergo central necrosis, creating an appearance that resembles a necrobiotic granuloma (*J Cutan Pathol* 1986;13:253). Angiomatoid growth may mimic epithelioid angiosarcoma.

The proximal type is characterized by a multinodular proliferation of large polygonal cells with marked nuclear atypia, vesicular nuclei, and prominent nucleoli, often with prominent rhabdoid morphology (e-**Fig. 44.58**). Necrosis is common, but a granuloma-like pattern is absent.

Both distal and proximal types express EMA, vimentin, cytokeratins, and CD34 (in 40% to 50% of cases), and show loss of INI1 reactivity (approximately 90% of cases) that reflects inactivation of the *SMARCB1* gene (*Am J Surg Pathol* 2009;33:542; *Hum Pathol* 2009;40:349).

9. Intimal sarcoma is a rare, extremely aggressive tumor which by definition involves large vessels (particular the pulmonary trunk and arteries, and abdominal aorta) with predominately intravascular growth. The tumors show a wide range of histologic features, but most appear as a pleomorphic and spindle cell sarcoma often with myxoid stroma. There are amplifications of *MDM2, KIT,* and *PDGFRA*, as well as gains involving *EGFR* (*Am J Surg Pathol* 2014;38:461).

10. Undifferentiated/unclassified sarcomas. Undifferentiated/unclassified sarcoma is a diagnosis of exclusion and is composed of a heterogeneous group of tumors without an identifiable line of differentiation. These include sarcomas with pleomorphic, spindle cell, round cell, epithelioid, and mixed morphologies.

Undifferentiated pleomorphic sarcoma (UPS) are characterized by complex cytogenetic rearrangements that can involve over 30% of the genome (*Virchows Arch* 2010;456:201). The tumor preferentially arises in the extremity in individuals over 40 years of age and presents as a rapidly enlarging mass; about 5% have metastatic disease at diagnosis, usually in the lung. The tumor often measures 15 to 20 cm, if not greater, and has a white to tan-white, fleshy to fibrous cut surface, with areas of necrosis and hemorrhage. The microscopic pattern is often complex (e-**Fig. 44.59**), with field-to-field variation in terms of growth pattern (storiform, fascicular, and sheets), cytomorphology (spindled, polygonal, and rounded to ovoid cells), and background stroma (fibrous to sclerotic, often with focal myxoid foci). An inflammatory infiltrate and multinucleated cells are not uncommon. One consistent microscopic feature is high nuclear grade often with numerous atypical mitotic figures; extensive necrosis with cystic degeneration and hemorrhage are other common findings. In the retroperitoneum, DDLS is a primary differential consideration; sarcomatoid carcinoma should be excluded, particularly in mucosal and visceral sites.

Significant progress has been made in the classification of undifferentiated round cell sarcomas. *CIC*-rearranged sarcomas (*CIC-DUX4* is the most common fusion) are distinct and frequently affect the deep soft tissue of the trunk and extremities of young adults. They are composed of moderately pleomorphic round cells with course chromatin, and foci with spindle cell and epithelioid morphology. Myxoid stroma is a commonly seen. These tumors are frequently immunopositive for WT1, DUX4, and ETV4. These are highly aggressive tumors with a 43% 5-year survival rate, which is significantly worse than EWS (*Am J Surg Pathol* 2017;41:941).

BCOR-rearranged sarcomas are another distinct group. These tumors have a predilection for adolescents, frequently arise in bone, and are composed of monotonous small round cells with focal areas of spindled morphology. The tumor cells are immunopositive for BCOR, CD99 (variable), and CCNB3 (in tumors with *CCNB3* rearrangements). While data are limited, these tumors appear to have a more favorable prognosis compared with EWS. *BCOR* is most frequently fused with *CCNB3*.

XIII. REPORTING. The surgical pathology report for a soft tissue tumor should be tailored to each case. Important elements include the histologic type, tumor grade if applicable (the

FNCLCC system is recommended; see Table 44.3), tumor location, tumor size, resection margin status, and surgical procedure. The extent of tumor necrosis and mitotic rate should be noted if required for grading, or following neoadjuvant treatment. The results of any ancillary studies, including immunohistochemistry, electron microscopy, cytogenetic analysis, and/or molecular testing should also be reported.

SUGGESTED READINGS

Dehner LP. Soft tissue. In: Aliya N Husain, J. Thomas Stocker, Louis P Dehner, eds. *Stocker and Dehner's Pediatric Pathology*, 4th ed. Philadelphia, PA: Lippincott, Williams & Wilkins; 2015.

Fletcher CDM, Bridge JA, Hogendoorn PCW, Mertens F. *WHO Classification of Tumours of Soft Tissue and Bone*. 4th ed. Lyon, France: IARC Press; 2013.

Goldblum JR, Folpe AL, Weiss SW. *Enzinger & Weiss's Soft Tissue Tumors*. 6th ed. Philadelphia, PA: Saunder; 2014.

Hornick JL. *Practical Soft Tissue Pathology: A Diagnostic Approach*. 2nd ed. Philadelphia, PA: Elsevier, Inc; 2018.

Miettinen M, Fetsch JF, Antonescu CR, Folpe AL, Wakely PE. *Tumors of the Soft Tissues. AFIP Atlas of Tumor Pathology, Series 4, Fascicle 20. Amer Registry of Pathology*, Washington, DC; 2015.

Pfeifer JD. *Molecular Genetic Testing in Surgical Pathology*. Philadelphia, PA: Lippincott, Williams & Wilkins; 2006.

Retroperitoneum

Aidas J. Mattis, Louis P. Dehner, John D. Pfeifer, and John S.A. Chrisinger

I. NORMAL ANATOMY. The retroperitoneal space (in some respects a virtual space) is located between the posterior parietal peritoneum and the fascia that covers the muscles of the lumbar region. It extends upward to the diaphragm, downward to the base of the sacrum and iliac crests, and laterally to the external borders of the lumbar muscles and the ascending and descending colon. The retroperitoneum contains loose connective tissue; lymph nodes; the aorta and inferior vena cava with their vascular branches; the adrenal glands; the kidneys and ureters; and portions of the pancreas, duodenum, and large intestine. This chapter will focus on the entities that arise from the tissues of the retroperitoneal space; disorders arising from the organs that are completely or partially retroperitoneal are covered in their respective chapters.

II. NONNEOPLASTIC DISEASES

A. Inflammatory Lesions

1. Sclerosing mesenteritis (mesenteric panniculitis) constitutes a morphologically similar group of idiopathic tumor-forming processes. The usual presentation is a mass in the mesentery; sclerosing changes may extend into the inferior retroperitoneum with similar histologic features as idiopathic retroperitoneal fibrosis (see below). A biopsy reveals a variably intense mixed lymphoplasmacytic infiltrate in a dense, relatively hypocellular collagenous background. Residual adipose tissue may have the features of fat necrosis with dystrophic calcification and panniculitis. The differential diagnosis includes reactive processes (e.g., infection, bowel perforation), a neoplasm, and IgG4-related sclerosing disease. Lesions should be carefully examined for histologic features of IgG4-related sclerosing disease (i.e., obliterative phlebitis and storiform fibrosis), followed by immunohistochemical studies for IgG4 and IgG if the histologic findings warrant further investigation. Of note, metastatic deposits, particularly those originating from neuroendocrine tumors of the small intestine, may be accompanied by a disproportionate fibroinflammatory reaction and thus an inadequate biopsy may show a histologic pattern that mimics sclerosing mesenteritis. Further, counts of IgG4+ plasma cells/hpf and the IgG4/IgG ratio are often elevated in the inflammation accompanying metastatic disease, which can lead to further confusion with IgG4-related sclerosing disease (*Histopathology* 2018; Jun 26. [Epub ahead of print]). Lymphoma should be excluded particularly in the presence of lymphadenopathy. If the biopsy has a prominently spindle cell component, inflammatory pseudotumor, inflammatory myofibroblastic tumor (IMT), and well-differentiated liposarcoma (WDLS) should be considered. Since the histologic findings of sclerosing mesenteritis are nonspecific, even after the other possibilities have been excluded, the diagnostic line in the report may simply read "chronic inflammation and fibrosis."

2. Idiopathic retroperitoneal fibrosis (sclerosing retroperitoneal fibrosis, Ormond disease) is an uncommon inflammatory process which usually affects middle-aged adults (and older) and shows a male predominance. It is characterized by bilateral sclerosing fibrosis of the retroperitoneum that can ultimately cause constriction and obliteration of the ureters. Grossly, there is poorly circumscribed fibrosis, usually at the level of the lower abdominal aorta and its bifurcation. Microscopically, the process is characterized by dense fibrosis/sclerosis associated with predominately lymphocytic inflammation (e-Fig. 45.1). A subset of tumors with features of idiopathic retroperitoneal fibrosis are IgG4-related and show storiform fibrosis, obliterative phlebitis, and a dense lymphoplasmacytic infiltrate with increased IgG4-positive plasma cells (IgG4/IgG ratio >40% and >30 IgG4-positive plasma cells/hpf) (*Mod Pathol* 2012;25:1181). Visceral involvement also suggests IgG4-related sclerosing disease. Fibroinflammatory reactions to radiation, lymphoma, or methysergide and other drugs can be indistinguishable from idiopathic retroperitoneal fibrosis.

3. **Malakoplakia** occasionally affects the retroperitoneal soft tissues in patients over a wide age range. Malignancy and over forms of immunosuppression are predisposing factors. The process is a response to chronic bacterial infection (usually *E. coli*, *Klebsiella*, *Yersinia*, or *Proteus*) and grossly appears as a yellow plaque or mass. Microscopically, it is composed of sheets of granular and vacuolated histiocytes that contain lamellated inclusions known as Michaelis–Gutmann bodies which are von Kossa, iron, and PAS positive (diastase resistant). These distinctive inclusions (e-**Fig. 45.2**) are thought to represent the remnants of bacteria within phagosomes that have been mineralized by calcium and iron.

4. **Retroperitoneal abscesses** are generally secondary to infectious processes of adjacent organs, most commonly of the kidneys. Less frequently, abscesses originate from distant septic foci that propagate via a hematogenous route.

B. **Cystic Lesions.** While most cystic lesions of the retroperitoneum represent a secondary or degenerative change within a benign or malignant neoplasm, several benign primary cystic lesions also occur.

1. **Cystic lymphangioma or cystic lymphatic malformation** of the retroperitoneum accounts for 5% of all retroperitoneal cystic lesions and can occur at any age. Involvement of the mesentery is an associated feature since this malformation is not well circumscribed (*J Surg Oncol* 1996;61:234). Pathologically, multi-or unilocular cysts contain a clear or milky fluid, and are lined with a single layer of flattened endothelium which is D2-40 immunopositive (*J Pediatr Surg* 1999;34:1164).

2. **Multicystic peritoneal inclusion cyst** occurs predominantly in women of reproductive age and, even though rarely seen in the retroperitoneum, is in the differential diagnosis of cystic lesions (especially of multilocular cystic lymphangioma). Prior abdominal surgery is common. Histopathologically, the lesion consists of mesothelial-lined cystic spaces usually containing watery secretions, separated by a delicate fibromuscular stroma. The lining mesothelium is usually immunoreactive for calretinin. As discussed in some detail in Chapter 11, some confusion exists regarding the proper classification of multicystic peritoneal inclusion cyst, as demonstrated by the fact that the lesion has previously been known as multicystic mesothelioma.

3. **Bronchogenic cysts** can rarely occur in a subdiaphragmatic location, including the retroperitoneum, as part of the morphologic spectrum of bronchopulmonary foregut malformations. The related anomaly, extralobar sequestration with features of congenital cystic adenomatoid malformation type 2, presents a solid mass in the same site, usually in infants and young children; its suprarenal location can lead to confusion with neuroblastoma (*J Pediatr Surg* 2007;42:1627). The cysts are lined by respiratory-type, pseudostratified, ciliated columnar epithelium that can focally contain seromucous glands and nodules of hyaline cartilage.

4. **Müllerian cysts** of the retroperitoneum are usually in excess of 10 cm in greatest dimension and are lined by cuboidal to columnar epithelium that often contains ciliated cells; there is no atypia, although stratification and epithelial tufting can be present as in tubal epithelium. Beneath the lining of a Müllerian cyst loose fibrous tissue, dilated vessels, and incomplete smooth muscle bundles can be seen (*Hum Pathol* 2003;34:194). Mucinous cystadenoma with ovarian-type stroma (which is inhibin-immunopositive) occurs rarely as an extrapancreatic cyst in the retroperitoneum.

5. **Enteric duplication cyst** (EDC) is an extremely uncommon congenital lesion and may be detected prenatally (*Pediatr Radiol* 2000;30:671). Although usually intraabdominal and associated with the small intestine, EDC has sporadically been described in the retroperitoneum. The gross appearance is usually a spherical, tubular,

or dumbbell-shaped cyst with a smooth lining and viscous contents. Microscopically, the cyst wall has a variably differentiated enteric mucosa consisting of a simplified cuboidal or cylindrical epithelium, to a more normal appearing mucosa with a muscularis mucosae and a muscularis propria. Focal areas of squamous metaplasia and gastric-type mucosa have also been described in retroperitoneal EDCs (*JOP* 2006;10:492).

C. Additional Nonneoplastic Conditions. Various additional nonneoplastic lesions may be encountered in the retroperitoneum, which in some cases can raise clinical concern for a neoplastic process. Gossypiboma, endometriosis, hemorrhage, bile collection, spillage of gallstones, and extravasation of urine can all be occasionally encountered in the retroperitoneal space.

III. NEOPLASMS. Primary retroperitoneal tumors arise from the extravisceral tissues that comprise the retroperitoneum; the neoplasms for the most part are malignant in adults and originate from lymphoid and various soft tissue elements including fat and neural structures. The histogenesis of some of the high-grade sarcomas is not apparent, and immunohistochemical and molecular studies often provide information that is very helpful for classification. In children and young adults, germ cell neoplasms can present in the retroperitoneum, but the most common neoplasms of the retroperitoneum in children include the neuroblastic tumors (neuroblastoma and its variants) and high-grade lymphomas, in particular Burkitt lymphoma, large cell lymphoma, and Hodgkin lymphoma. The most commonly encountered primary retroperitoneal tumors in adults are sarcomas, followed by lymphomas and germ cell tumors (*Cancer* 2000;88:364). Overall, 70% to 80% of retroperitoneal tumors are malignant and thus the retroperitoneum is the only body site where the frequency of malignant neoplasms exceeds that of benign tumors. The anatomy of the retroperitoneal space makes it possible for primary, as well as metastatic, tumors to attain substantial dimensions before clinical manifestations become evident. Malignant retroperitoneal tumors have a generally poor prognosis since they are often found at an advanced stage of disease, and even apparently resectable tumors often recur.

A. Soft Tissue Tumors. Primary sarcomas arising in the retroperitoneum constitute 10% to 20% of all soft issue sarcomas in adults, most commonly well-differentiated/dedifferentiated liposarcoma (DDLS) and leiomyosarcoma (LMS). Solitary fibrous tumor (SFT), undifferentiated pleomorphic sarcoma (UPS), pleomorphic liposarcoma (PLS), and malignant peripheral nerve sheath tumor (MPNST) are also not uncommon in this site. As a group, retroperitoneal sarcomas are often in excess of 10 cm and weigh more than 500 g. Complete resection is associated with the most favorable outcome, but size and extent of involvement often limits the completeness of the resection; local recurrence is common. Models to predict outcome in retroperitoneal sarcomas accounting for patient age, tumor size, multifocality, extent of resection, FNCLCC grade, and histologic type have been developed and validated (*J Clin Oncol* 2013;31: 1649; *Cancer* 2016;122:1417). As for soft tissue sarcomas arising in other anatomic sites, the FNCLCC system is recommended for grading (if applicable) and the American Joint Committee on Cancer (AJCC) system is utilized for staging of retroperitoneal sarcomas.

1. Adipocytic tumors

    a. Benign

        i. Myolipoma is a rare benign tumor with a predilection for the retroperitoneum. It has a pronounced female predominance. This circumscribed and often at least partially encapsulated lesion has a lobulated fatty appearance with areas of white to grey-white tissue; the large size, usually 10 cm or greater, often raises the question of liposarcoma. Microscopically, the tumor contains an admixture of mature adipocytes and fascicles of smooth muscle (*Am J Surg Pathol* 1991;15:121). Rarely, round cell morphology, degenerative nuclear atypia, and a hypercellular fascicular pattern may be seen; however, there is an absence of mitotic activity and nondegenerative atypia (*Am J Surg Pathol* 2017;41:153). Floret-like cells and thick-walled vessels are also not present. The leiomyomatous component is diffusely and strongly immunopositive for SMA and desmin. While data are limited, *HMGA2* rearrangement has been identified in myolipoma.

ii. **Lipoblastoma,** a benign tumor of early childhood, presents in the retroperitoneum in 5% to 10% of cases. From the retroperitoneum, the tumor may extend into the mesentery and omentum. Lipoblastoma may grow in excess of 6 cm, and grossly has a glistening grey-white mucoid surface with faint lobulation. Microscopically, the lobules contain immature fetal adipocytic cells with progressive differentiation toward mature adipose cells. The lobules are usually separated by connective tissue septa that contain small vessels. Some tumors have a striking resemblance to myxoid liposarcoma (MLS), but lipoblastoma contains desmin-positive cells. Further, lipoblastomas lack *DDIT3* rearrangements, and instead harbor *PLAG1* rearrangements resulting in fusions with a number of different partners.

b. **Intermediate (locally aggressive)**

i. **Well-differentiated liposarcoma (WDLS).** As a group, liposarcomas are the most common primary nonvisceral malignant neoplasms of the retroperitoneum and account for 30% to 50% of retroperitoneal sarcomas; WDLS is the most common subtype of liposarcoma in this site. WDLS is a locally aggressive neoplasm, which, like many retroperitoneal tumors, can grow to enormous sizes before coming to clinical attention. Grossly, a thin external membrane is usually the only structure serving as a "capsule" for an apparently well-circumscribed yellowish-white lipomatous mass. WDLS has a wide morphologic spectrum but is generally composed of variable proportions of mature adipose tissue and fibrous bands with fine collagen, with scattered atypical cells that have enlarged, hyperchromatic, irregular nuclei. Lymphoid aggregates and floret-like cells are common. A dense inflammatory infiltrate that largely obscures the underlying tumor may be present, and may mimic lymphoma or Castleman disease. Lipoblasts may be seen (e-**Fig. 45.3**), but are not necessarily useful for establishing the diagnosis. Fluorescence in situ hybridization testing for *MDM2* amplification can be very helpful in ambiguous cases.

c. **Malignant**

i. **Dedifferentiated liposarcoma** (DDLS) is a malignant neoplasm that often shows an abrupt or gradual transition from WDLS to a pleomorphic and spindle cell sarcoma resembling UPS (e-**Fig. 45.4**). DDLS show a broad range of histologic patterns including within a single tumor. Myxofibrosarcoma-like, meningothelial-like whorls with bone formation, PLS-like (homologous dedifferentiation), epithelioid and round cell morphologies, and heterologous differentiation (leiomyosarcomatous, rhabdomyosarcomatous, osteosarcomatous, chondrosarcomatous, and angiosarcomatous) are patterns that may be seen. While dedifferentiation is obvious in many cases, minimum histologic and size criteria for the diagnosis of DDLS have been elusive. Confluent sarcomatous growth and at least 5 mitoses in 10 hpf is a useful cutoff (*Am J Surg Pathol* 2007;31:1). Both WDLS and DDLS harbor amplification of the *MDM2* and *CDK4* genes.

ii. **Myxoid liposarcoma** (MLS). On the basis of histologic and molecular analysis, it has been shown that most presumed primary retroperitoneal MLS actually represent WDLS/DDLS that have MLS-like morphology (*Mod Pathol* 2009;22:223); however, it is noteworthy that unlike most sarcomas, metastatic MLS has a predilection for soft tissue sites including the retroperitoneum. Therefore, in the absence of a known extraretroperitoneal MLS, suspected MLS of the retroperitoneum should undergo *MDM2* and/or *DDIT3* cytogenetic testing; if a diagnosis of MLS is confirmed, metastasis from another site (usually the thigh) should be excluded. Very few primary retroperitoneal MLS have been identified (*Am J Surg Pathol* 2016;40:1286).

iii. **Pleomorphic liposarcoma** (PLS) is a rare highly aggressive tumor. Microscopically, PLS is characterized by variable numbers of pleomorphic lipoblasts with cytoplasmic lipid vacuoles that scallop enlarged hyperchromatic nuclei. These pleomorphic lipoblasts are typically set within a pleomorphic and spindle cell sarcoma with storiform growth similar to an UPS. Sheets of atypical epithelioid cells (mimicking adrenal cortical carcinoma or other carcinoma), paraganglioma-like areas, or myxofibrosarcoma-like areas may be present. Extreme pleomorphism, brisk mitotic activity including bizarre mitotic figures, and necrosis are common. DDLS should be excluded before a diagnosis of retroperitoneal PLS is rendered as DDLS is much more common, especially in the retroperitoneum, and can have a PLS-like component.

2. **Smooth muscle tumors**

a. **Deep-seated leiomyoma (leiomyoma of deep soft tissue)** is an uncommon benign tumor that primarily occurs in perimenopausal women and is rare in men. Microscopically, the tumor resembles a uterine leiomyoma, exhibiting intersecting fascicles of bland appearing smooth muscle cells. There is no necrosis and a very low mitotic rate (<1/50 hpf in males and <5/50 hpf in females). Fibrosis, myxoid change, hyalinization, and calcification may be seen. The tumor is commonly immunopositive for estrogen and progesterone receptors in women. Deep-seated leiomyoma will occasionally recur after incomplete excision, but metastasis does not occur (*Adv Anat Pathol* 2002;9:351). Explanations for a deep smooth muscle tumor in the abdomen or retroperitoneum of a female include a so-called "parasitized" leiomyoma from the uterus, which has essentially separated from the outer portion of the uterus and gained its principal blood supply from an adjacent structure. Intravenous leiomyomatosis from the uterus also presents as benign appearing smooth muscle tumors in the pelvic soft tissues, often with extension into adjacent lymph nodes; the essential pathologic feature is the identification of circumscribed nodules of benign appearing smooth muscle within vascular or lymphatic spaces.

b. **Leiomyosarcoma** (LMS) accounts for 20% to 30% of all retroperitoneal sarcomas and typically arises in adults middle-aged and older. Like the other retroperitoneal sarcomas, dimensions and weights often exceed 15 cm and 500 g, respectively. Grossly, there is commonly a nodular surface with areas of hemorrhage, necrosis, and cystic degeneration. Histologically, the tumor is composed of atypical spindle cells with elongated, blunt-ended nuclei and eosinophilic fibrillary cytoplasm (**e-Fig. 45.5**). The presence of cytologic atypia, significant mitotic activity, or necrosis in a retroperitoneal smooth muscle neoplasm warrants a diagnosis of LMS. Aggressive metastatic disease and poor prognosis are characteristic of retroperitoneal LMS. It is worth mentioning that some LMS in the retroperitoneum arise from the inferior vena cava or renal vein, or represent a metastasis from a primary LMS of the uterus or paratesticular soft tissues.

3. **Skeletal muscle tumors**

a. Benign skeletal muscle tumors of the retroperitoneum are extremely rare. Only isolated cases of **rhabdomyoma** have been reported, with similar pathologic characteristics as when the tumor occurs elsewhere.

b. **Rhabdomyosarcoma** (RMS) of the embryonal or alveolar subtypes in the retroperitoneum-pelvis is a neoplasm of children between 2 and 10 years of age (**e-Fig. 45.6**). Approximately 10% to 15% of childhood RMS arise in the soft tissues of the pelvis and/or retroperitoneum, and are usually 10 cm or greater in maximal dimension (*Pediatr Blood Cancer* 2004;42:618); the retroperitoneum is an unfavorable site for a childhood RMS (*J Pediatr Hematol Oncol* 2001;23:215). Tumors with features of pleomorphic RMS in the retroperitoneum may represent true pleomorphic RMS, a nongerminal pattern of malignancy in a germ cell tumor, spread of a sarcomatoid carcinoma, or a component of a DDLS (*Am J Surg Pathol* 2007;31:1557).

4. Fibroblastic/myofibroblastic tumors

a. Intermediate (locally aggressive)

  i. **Desmoid-type fibromatosis** usually arises in the mesentery-omentum with extension into the retroperitoneum, but occasionally is limited to the retroperitoneum. Those desmoid tumors arising in the proximal lower extremity can in the course of several local recurrences extend through the sciatic notch into the retroperitoneum as well; the presence of familial adenomatous polyposis in these patients should be addressed. Desmoid fibromatosis is infiltrative and its cut surface shows a firm, trabeculated pattern, which can grossly resemble a smooth muscle tumor. Microscopically, sweeping interlacing bundles of uniform spindle-shaped fibroblasts are present in a collagenous, keloid-like, or myxoid stroma with no evidence of nuclear atypia (e-**Fig. 45.7**). Scattered mitotic figures may be identified and should not be a source of concern unless they are atypical. The tumor is immunopositive for vimentin and smooth muscle actin; nuclear beta-catenin staining is characteristic and seen in 70% to 80% of cases.

b. Intermediate (rarely metastasizing)

  i. **Solitary fibrous tumor** (SFT) is uncommon in the retroperitoneum (*Hum Pathol* 2000;31:1108). The tumor is composed of a variably cellular proliferation of bland plump to spindle cells with a "patternless" architecture associated with gapping branching blood vessels (known as a staghorn or hemangiopericytoma-like vascular pattern). This neoplasm shows a range of clinical behavior that is difficult to predict; however, these tumors can be risk stratified based on patient age, tumor size, necrosis, and mitotic rate (*Mod Pathol* 2017;30:1433). Mature adipose tissue is found in the lipomatous variant of SFT. SFT is positive for CD34 and STAT6; however, even though STAT6 expression is characteristic of SFT, STAT6 positivity is not uncommon in DDLS. Further, SFT is frequently immunopositive for PAX8, which, in the appropriate context, can cause confusion with sarcomatoid renal cell carcinoma. In difficult cases, molecular analysis for the *NAB2–STAT6* fusion characteristic of SFT is helpful.

  ii. **Inflammatory myofibroblastic tumor** (IMT), like desmoid-type fibromatosis, may present in the mesentery-omentum with extension into the retroperitoneum. IMT typically presents in children and young adults. Grossly, it is a firm, grey-white multinodular mass that measures 1 to 25 cm. Microscopically, it is characterized by predominately one or a mixture of three histologic patterns: cellular fascicles of spindle cells with a mixed infiltrate of plasma cells, lymphocytes, and eosinophils; a loose spindle cell proliferation in a myxoid background resembling nodular fasciitis; and a hypocellular hyalinized pattern with chronic inflammatory cells and dystrophic calcifications. The nuclei of the spindle cells have vesicular chromatin and relatively conspicuous nucleoli; mitotic figures are found among the spindle cells but are not atypical. In addition to immunopositivity for vimentin and SMA, approximately 50% of cases are ALK-1 positive (*Am J Surg Pathol* 2007;31:509). Increased IgG4 plasma cells are seen in some cases of IMT (*Mod Pathol* 2011;24:606).

  iii. **Infantile fibrosarcoma** is known to occur in the retroperitoneum (*Fetal Pediatr Pathol* 2011;30:329), but it most commonly presents in the extremities. Cellular mesoblastic nephroma, which arises in the kidney in infancy, has the same morphology and harbors the same t(12;15) translocation.

c. Malignant

  i. **Adult-type fibrosarcoma** is extremely rare and a diagnosis of exclusion. It accounts for less than <1% of all sarcomas. The overwhelming majority of putative adult-type fibrosarcomas actually represent other tumor types

(*Am J Surg Pathol* 2010;34:1504). In the retroperitoneum, DDLS, synovial sarcoma, cellular schwannoma, SFT, LMS, MPNST, and UPS should be considered in the differential diagnosis.

ii. **Other variants of fibrosarcoma,** such as low-grade fibromyxoid sarcoma (*Am J Clin Pathol* 2018;149:128), sclerosing epithelioid fibrosarcoma, and myxofibrosarcoma are rarely encountered in the retroperitoneum. Of note, most retroperitoneal tumors with histologic features of myxofibrosarcoma are DDLS.

5. Neural tumors

a. Benign

i. **Schwannoma** accounts for approximately 1% to 5% of all retroperitoneal tumors, and grossly appears as a large (>10 cm) solitary, encapsulated, firm mass. Histologically it presents with alternating cellular areas with palisading nuclei (Antoni A) and myxoid hypocellular areas (Antoni B). Hyalinized vessels and cystic change are also common features. While AE1/AE3 expression in peripheral schwannomas is rare, retroperitoneal schwannomas frequently show AE1/AE3 expression; staining may be extensive and is thought to result from cross-reactivity with GFAP (*Mod Pathol* 2006;19:115). Cellular schwannomas have a predilection for the retroperitoneum and are characterized by a complete or nearly complete lack of Antoni B areas and Verocay bodies. Necrosis, mitotic activity (generally low), and dense cellularity may be seen in cellular schwannoma.

b. Malignant

i. **Malignant peripheral nerve sheath tumor** (MPNST) represents 5% to 10% of all retroperitoneal sarcomas. Microscopically, the tumor typically features asymmetric spindle-shaped cells arranged in dense fascicles with hyperchromatic nuclei and frequent mitoses (e-**Fig. 45.8**).

c. Tumors of sympathetic nervous tissue

i. **Ganglioneuroma** is composed of a proliferation of Schwann cells with scattered ganglion cells set in a collagenous stroma. Ganglioneuroma can be mistaken for schwannoma in those areas of the tumor with a paucity or absence of ganglion cells.

ii. **Neuroblastoma** may originate from the sympathetic nervous system chain of ganglia, commonly in the retroperitoneum and without involvement of the adrenal gland. In fact, the extra-adrenal retroperitoneum is the site of origin of 30% to 35% of neuroblastomas in the pediatric population.

iii. **Adult neuroblastoma,** though rare, is in the differential diagnosis of malignant round cell tumors of the retroperitoneum of adults. Nonetheless, there is a greater likelihood that a paraspinal malignant round cell neoplasm in a young adult is Ewing sarcoma or lymphoma than a neuroblastoma.

iv. **Paraganglioma** arises from cells in the para-aortic sympathetic chain and at the aortic bifurcation. Similar to adrenal pheochromocytomas and extra-adrenal paragangliomas elsewhere, these retroperitoneal tumors may be functional with associated characteristic signs and symptoms, but most cases are nonfunctional. Grossly, the tumor is rubbery with firm brown to tan cut surfaces, and in large specimens can exhibit a cystic component secondary to central necrosis or hemorrhage. The tumor is composed of well-defined nests of cells surrounded by sustentacular cells; the nests are usually composed of round cells with abundant granular eosinophilic or basophilic cytoplasm (e-**Fig. 45.9**). Nuclear atypia and vascular invasion may also be present. In the retroperitoneum, these tumors tend to have an aggressive course with local invasion and a high incidence of local recurrence, as well as a higher rate of metastasis than adrenal pheochromocytoma (20-42% for the former versus 2% to 10% for the latter) (*Urol Ann* 2010;2:12).

6. Vascular tumors. Vascular tumors, ranging from hemangiomas to angiosarcomas, have been reported as isolated cases in the retroperitoneum.

a. **Kaposiform hemangioendothelioma** (KHE) is a vascular tumor that is particularly common in the retroperitoneum. It is a tumor of childhood that is frequently complicated by the Kasabach–Merritt phenomenon. Though initially described as a distinctive vascular neoplasm of the retroperitoneum, it is now recognized to occur in the skin and soft tissues of the extremities. In the retroperitoneum the tumor tends to be large, poorly circumscribed, and may involve adjacent structures. Microscopically, the tumor is composed of a lobular arrangement of hemangioma-like areas and fascicles of spindle cells; microthrombi, slit-like endothelial-lined vascular channels, and hyaline globules are also present and thus the tumor resembles Kaposi sarcoma. However, KHE lacks nuclear positivity for HHV-8.

7. **Gastrointestinal stromal tumor (GIST).** GIST may rarely apparently present in the retroperitoneum. However, these tumors likely have an origin in the gastrointestinal tract, which may or may not be appreciated clinically or histologically. The unusual site can complicate diagnosis as GIST may mimic DDL, cellular schwannoma, smooth muscle neoplasms and SFT. The prognosis is generally poor (*Am J Surg Pathol* 2017;41:577).

8. **Soft tissue tumors of uncertain lineage and unclassified sarcomas**

   a. **Synovial sarcoma** is typically a firm, gray-pink, circumscribed mass measuring 8 to 10 cm. In contrast to synovial sarcomas elsewhere, retroperitoneal synovial sarcomas tend not to metastasize outside of the abdomen but are difficult to control locally, and thus have an overall poor prognosis (*Histopathology* 2004;45:245; *J BUON* 2008;13:211). A potential diagnostic pitfall may arise due to the fact that retroperitoneal cellular schwannomas may histologically somewhat resemble synovial sarcoma and are often positive for AE1/AE3 cytokeratin expression.

   b. **Undifferentiated pleomorphic sarcoma** (UPS) often has a complex microscopic pattern; however, many tumors are composed of pleomorphic polygonal and spindle cells with high-grade nuclear atypia often arranged in fascicles, loose storiform arrays, or sheets. UPS formerly accounted for up to 30% of sarcomas of the retroperitoneum, but recent studies have shown that the majority of these sarcomas are actually DDLS. Thus, a careful search for areas of WDLS, immunohistochemical studies for MDM2 and CDK4, and/or cytogenetic analysis for *MDM2* amplification (as discussed above in the section on DDLS), should be performed. Other pleomorphic sarcomas should also be excluded (e.g., pleomorphic LMS).

   c. **Malignant small round cell tumors** of virtually every type have been described as primary tumors of the retroperitoneum. **Ewing sarcoma** presents in this location in approximately 5% of cases, usually as a paraspinal mass. **Desmoplastic small round cell tumor** usually arises in the peritoneal cavity, but in some series up to 15% of cases originate in the retroperitoneum.

B. Germ Cell Tumors

1. **Primary retroperitoneal teratomas** typically occur in infancy and childhood, and are rare in adults. About 75% of cases occur in children younger than 5 years of age, and the incidence in females is twice that of males, as is also the case for sacrococcygeal teratomas in children. Grossly, these tumors have a mixed solid and cystic appearance.

   a. **Mature teratomas** in this site, as elsewhere, contain mature tissue from more than one germinal layer, with occasional calcification or ossification. Mature cystic teratomas should be thoroughly sampled (one section per cm) in order to exclude the presence of yolk-sac tumor, especially in a young child. Immature somatic elements such as primitive neural tubules or sheets of neuroblasts with a fibrillary background should not be viewed with concern in an infant or young child.

   b. **Immature teratomas** contain immature or primitive tissue (derived from any or all three germ cell layers) that is usually mixed with areas of mature tissue. The most common immature neural tissues form rosettes, sheets of neuroblasts, or tubules of primitive neural cells. The pathologic grading of retroperitoneal teratomas, specifically in children, on the basis of the extent of immature somatic tissues has no prognostic significance. On the other hand, the presence of yolk sac tumor establishes the malignant nature of the neoplasm.

2. Secondary germ cell neoplasms. A teratoma in an adolescent or young male may be a post-treatment "growing teratoma" which represents residual metastatic disease from a malignant mixed germ cell tumor of the testis. Similarly, the presence of a retroperitoneal tumor in the absence of a known primary testicular germ cell tumor should lead to careful evaluation of the testes since they may harbor a scar (with or without intratubular germ cell neoplasia) as evidence of spontaneous regression of a primary testicular neoplasm. In fact, a retroperitoneal germ cell tumor, in a male, whether seminoma or of another pattern, is metastatic disease from the testis until proven otherwise.

C. Lymphomas and Other Lymphoproliferative Disorders

1. Both non-Hodgkin and Hodgkin lymphoma manifest in retroperitoneum as lymphadenopathy, a localized mass, or retroperitoneal fibrosis. Bulky retroperitoneal lymphadenopathy with or without intestinal or other organ involvement in the first two decades of life usually represents Burkitt lymphoma. In adults, the same presentation usually represents small lymphocytic lymphoma/chronic lymphocytic leukemia or one of the other B-cell lymphomas including follicular lymphoma. Diagnosis can be challenging due to limitations on the adequacy of the specimen, a prominent fibrous reaction, necrosis, and/or a non-representative biopsy.

2. Castleman disease also occasionally presents in the retroperitoneum. The hyaline vascular type, which is most common in the retroperitoneum as elsewhere, is usually localized to a single lymph node and tends to be asymptomatic; the plasma cell type is multifocal and usually presents with a more aggressive course and systemic manifestations. The hyaline vascular type is characterized grossly by homogenous orange-yellowish cut surfaces, and microscopically by giant lymphoid follicles centered on a markedly hyalinized vessel surrounded by lymphocytes concentrically arranged in an onionskin pattern (**e-Fig. 45.10**). The plasma cell type is grossly similar, but on microscopic examination contains more plasma cells with less vascular hyalinization.

D. Tumors of Müllerian Type. Tumors of Müllerian type are occasionally described in the retroperitoneum. As in the ovary, they are usually serous, mucinous, or endometrioid type, and can be benign, borderline, or malignant. In the retroperitoneum, borderline and malignant tumors appear to be more common than their benign counterparts. Tumors are usually large and unilateral, and tend to present with no concomitant ovarian lesions.

E. Metastatic Tumors. Various primary malignant neoplasms arising in retroperitoneal or posterior abdominal wall organs such as the pancreas, kidney, liver, and adrenal gland often present with or are accompanied by direct extravisceral invasion into the retroperitoneum. Retroperitoneal lymph node metastases are also seen in association with many primary tumors of other sites.

ACKNOWLEDGMENT

The authors thank Catalina Amador-Ortiz, author of the previous editions of this chapter.

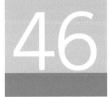

46 Bone Neoplasms and Other Nonmetabolic Disorders

Lingxin Zhang and John S.A. Chrisinger

I. NORMAL MICROSCOPIC ANATOMY. The bones are composed of compact bone, which is derived from intramembranous ossification, and coarse cancellous bone, which is the osseous remnant of endochondral ossification. Compact bone makes up the cortices of long bones and constitutes their diaphyses and the surface portion of their metaphyses, as well as the compacta of the flat and irregular bones. Cancellous bone is present in the medullary cavity and is abundant at the ends of the long bones. In bone, form follows function (Wolff's law). In the shafts of bones, most of the forces act upon the surface. Here, the compact bone, which is 90% solid and only 10% space, bears the compression, tension, shear, and torsional forces. The medulla, shielded from forces, contains less bone. The ends of the bones are supported by the vertical plates and horizontal struts of the cancellous bone, yet cancellous bone is only 25% bone and 75% marrow by volume; here the cortex is very thin.

Bone matrix is classified as woven or lamellar depending on the predominant fiber arrangement of its collagen. In woven bone, the collagen fiber pattern is random. This type of bone is found in the fetal skeleton and in processes in which there is very rapid bone production. In lamellar bone, the bone collagen fibers are arranged in stacks of tightly packed fibers that are parallel in the same stack. In the next layer, the collagen fibers are also parallel to one another, but their direction is different than the collagen in the previous stack so that the bone appears to be layered. Both compact and cancellous bone consists of lamellar bone after the age of 3 years. After this age, woven bone is almost always pathologic, although the etiology is often not discernible without imaging studies (Bullough PG. *Orthopedic Pathology*, 5th ed. St. Louis: CV Mosby; 2010). In compact bone, the lamellae are arranged concentrically around central vascular canals termed Haversian canals; each canal and its associated lamellae are referred to an osteon or Haversian system. Haversian canals are connected to each other by Volkmann canals. In cancellous bone, the lamellae are arranged in linear, parallel plates (**e-Fig. 46.1**). Adjacent osteons are separated from each other and from interstitial lamellae (see the section on circulatory diseases) and circumferential lamellae (which encircle the inner or outer cortex and are remnants of periosteal intramembranous ossification) by basophilic staining cement lines. Cement lines are sliding planes that are richer in calcium than surrounding bone matrix but the exact composition of which is unknown; they are produced by osteoblasts when bone is synthesized following osteoclast resorption (reversal cement lines) or after a period of inactivity (arrest cement lines). In the former type, the lamellae are discontinuous on either side of the cement line and in the latter the lamellae are continuous on either side (**e-Fig. 46.2**).

II. SPECIMEN PROCESSING

A. Gross Handling and Selection of Sections. The approach to specimen handling is largely one of common sense. Small biopsy specimens should be submitted for sectioning in their entirety. If there is any doubt about whether they contain bone, they should be fixed, briefly decalcified, and rinsed. Most bone biopsies performed with needles are sufficiently thin for adequate fixation and decalcification, whereas curettings may sometimes need to be sliced into thinner fragments. The amount of curettings to submit for sectioning depends on their volume and whether the curettings are uniform. When it is feasible, all curettings should be submitted. If the lesion curetted is a hyaline cartilage tumor, as much of the specimen as possible should be reviewed to identify atypical chondrocytes as well as any subtle interface with normal surrounding bone.

Other large specimens such as total joint replacements and bone resections also need to be sliced into thinner fragments. Although this may be accomplished with large band saws or other power-type saws, motorized saws are dangerous and somewhat time consuming to maintain properly, especially in a laboratory that receives a limited number of bone specimens. Vibrating or oscillating saws, which are usually available in autopsy suites, should be avoided if possible, because they do not section uniformly and their oscillating movement creates tension and compression artifacts that often make bone sections impossible to interpret properly.

The handling and disposition of larger resection specimens depends on the reason for the procedure. For malignant tumors in which patients have not received neoadjuvant chemotherapy (after biopsy but prior to resection), grading, staging, and adequacy of resection are the major clinical issues. Amputations from these patients should include sections from the soft tissue and vascular margins as well as those from the tumor itself. Tumor sections should be taken in such a way as to document the pertinent tumor histology, whether the tumor involves the medulla and/or cortex, and how far the tumor extends into soft tissues. The specimen should be cut in such a way as to disclose the greatest extent of tumor; review of the imaging studies can guide the selection process. Careful attention should be paid to taking sections from any areas that are grossly disparate from the appearance of the majority of the tumor. Radical resections for malignant tumors that are not amputations need the same sectioning methods, but any area of the resection constituting a margin must be sectioned and appropriately designated. This includes the bone resection margin, overlying soft tissue dissection margins, and the margins of any skin and soft tissue encompassing a prior biopsy site.

Specimens resected from patients who have received neoadjuvant chemotherapy (currently used in osteosarcoma and in Ewing sarcoma [EWS]) need more extensive sampling to estimate the extent of treatment-associated necrosis. This means that one or more thin slabs should be cut through the entire extent of the bone and tumor, and that the entire slab or slabs should be fixed, decalcified, mapped, and examined not only for tumor stage but for extent of necrosis. The slabs should be photographed so as to produce a section map; if a specimen X-ray machine is available, specimen radiographs can be used both as section maps and as controls for adequate specimen decalcification (e-**Fig. 46.3**). Additional sections may be taken if there are areas not in the slab selected that appear as though they might be viable; the pathologist's task in this enterprise is to find viable tumor if any is present. It is worthwhile to remember that to extrapolate the degree of necrosis in a single slab into necrosis of the tumor as a whole makes the assumption that what is present in that particular slab is representative of the entire lesion.

B. **Decalcification.** The main difference between processing of bone specimens and of softer tissues is the requirement for an extra step of decalcification. Removal of calcium insures that bone collagen is no harder than the paraffin in which it is embedded, and that microtomy of bone tissues will approximate that for other types of specimens. Decalcification may be performed in a number of ways. In acid decalcification, hydrogen ions are in effect substituted for calcium ions. Electrolysis in effect accomplishes the same end, but is performed in an electrolyte solution with a weak electrical current. Ionic exchange is the slowest method but is the most gentle on tissue and results in the fewest artifacts. In practice, most histology laboratories rely on weak acid decalcification because it is the quickest and there is pressure from eager clinicians for rapid turnaround times in diagnosis. With use of acid decalcification methods, a few caveats must be kept in mind. First, the tissue must always be fixed adequately prior to decalcification to prevent artifacts that interfere with adequate staining or that can degrade the tissue after sections are prepared. This means that the tissue must be adequately thin (no more than 3- to 4-mm thick) prior to fixation, and that the tissue has remained in formalin or some other suitable fixative for an interval adequate to coagulate the proteins for routine staining. In addition, if immunohistochemistry needs to be performed, adequate fixation helps to insure that the decalcification process will less alter tissue antigens. Second, when decalcification is performed with acid solutions, specimens must be rinsed in running water to ensure that the residual pH of the tissue is sufficiently neutral for hematoxylin staining. Failure to neutralize the acid not only results in understaining with hematoxylin, but it will cause stained sections to lose their hematoxylin staining in an accelerated manner. If time is insufficient for adequate specimen rinsing, the specimen should be neutralized in a dilute basic solution such as sodium bicarbonate. Third, if sections are left in dilute acid for a much longer period than necessary for calcium removal, tissue hydrolysis will remove the nucleic acids that cause nuclear hematoxylin staining and nuclei will appear acidophilic. This so-called "overdecalcification" artifact is generally not reversible. Overdecalcification may not interfere with many diagnostic interpretations, but it is important not to mistake this artifact for tissue necrosis, particularly in postchemotherapy specimen interpretation.

Adequate decalcification will vary by the tissue being decalcified. For example, woven bone, even though it tends to have higher calcium concentrations than lamellar bone, will often section adequately with incomplete decalcification because the former has less organization and less cutting resistance. The decision regarding whether the tissue is ready for embedding is often subjective and revolves around whether the tissue is pliable, trims easily, or can be penetrated with a needle. Complete decalcification is best judged either by testing the supernatant fluid with a colorimetric indicator or comparing specimen radiographs prior to and after decalcification. These tests are seldom practical in a very busy general surgical pathology practice.

Many cytogenetic and molecular tools have recently emerged to facilitate the diagnosis of bone tumors. Routine acid decalcification methods degrade nucleic acids and thus can interfere with ancillary testing including fluorescence in situ hybridization (FISH) and direct DNA sequence analysis. Therefore, if possible, a section of the tumor should be decalcified in EDTA in case cytogenetic/molecular testing is needed (EDTA chelates calcium ions and has no impact on nucleic acids).

C. **Approach to the Interpretation of Bone Specimens.** Patient complaints related to the musculoskeletal system constitute nearly one-third of physician office visits in the United States, so orthopedic problems are extremely common. While surgical pathologists are often asked to rule out bone tumors as the etiology of a clinical problem, it is useful to keep in mind that fractures alone are about 3,000 to 4,000 times more common than all primary bone tumors combined, and that metastatic tumors to bone are at least 20 times more common than primary bone tumors. The accurate diagnosis of bone diseases requires the correlation of patient demographics along with the clinical history and imaging studies to put the problem in its correct context prior to any histologic examination of the tissue. Symptoms and signs are fairly similar in orthopedic diseases; these consist of pain, loss of function, deformities, and (in the case of tumors) sometimes a mass or a sense of fullness. Pain is the most common symptom, and although it may vary considerably, pain severe enough to wake a patient from sleep is the type suspicious for neoplastic diseases.

D. **Importance of Radiologic Findings.** The surgical pathology of orthopedic diseases most often consists of defining the nature of bone lesions that are space occupying on imaging studies, advising the clinician if an infection may be present, and histologically documenting miscellaneous bone diseases that are not diagnosable by imaging studies alone. Because surgical pathologists usually render biopsy diagnoses with the assumption that a biopsy is representative of the pathologic process, it is natural to assume the same parameters in bone biopsies. This is a potentially dangerous assumption, because most orthopedic diseases are invisible without imaging studies. This means that to assure that a biopsy is representative of a process, the smaller the biopsy specimen, the greater the need to review the imaging studies defining that process. Because bones are deep seated, imaging studies are required to grasp the extent and behavior of bone lesions. For a surgical pathologist, correlating imaging studies with histologic findings depends on knowledge of normal bone and joint anatomy, normal anatomy as represented in radiographic images or other imaging studies, and the rudimentary alterations in imaging studies produced by pathologic processes (not only what a process does to normal bone, but also how normal bone alters the process) (*Adv Anat Pathol* 2005;12:155). The majority of the radiographic image produced by long bones is due to beam attenuation by cortical bone in the shafts and by cancellous bone in the ends (**e-Fig. 46.4**). The attenuation produced by flat bones is primarily due to cortical bone, and that of irregular bones depends on the proportion of bone elements in any given part of the bone.

Space-occupying lesions within bone usually cause bone destruction, bone production, or some combination of the two. Destructive lesions are not seen in a single radiographic view until at least 40% of the bone in the path of the x-ray beam is destroyed. This means that almost an entire thickness of cortex must be destroyed to see the lesion if an intact and a destroyed cortex are superimposed in one view, or that at least 40% of cancellous bone must be destroyed in a bone end. It is partly for this reason that orthogonal views of bones are taken (e.g., posteroanterior and lateral views) so that destructive lesions may be isolated in routine radiographs. Radiodense lesions superimpose on the extant bone, causing more attenuation and easier visibility on a routine radiograph. In contrast, a lesion that is less dense than bone may fill the entire medullary cavity of a bone, but if it does not destroy the cortex it will be invisible regardless of the view because the dominant attenuator of the x-ray beam is the cortex, not the medullary fat or marrow. It is for these reasons that other imaging studies such as computed tomography (CT) scans and magnetic resonance imaging (MRI) are performed. These studies yield information that is complementary to that derived from routine radiographs. While they may be more sensitive in yielding information, a particular type of imaging modality should be used in concert with routine radiographs to answer a particular clinical question not answered by the radiographs.

III. DIAGNOSTIC FEATURES OF BONE LESIONS. There are very few general categories of bone disease (congenital, developmental/acquired, traumatic, circulatory, infectious, iatrogenic, tumor forming, metabolic, and Paget disease), although there are many individual diseases (McCarthy EF, Frassica FJ. *Pathology of Bone and Joint Disorders: With Clinical and Radiographic Correlation*. Cambridge University Press; 2014). Most patients can be separated into general diagnostic categories on the basis of their imaging studies. For example, traumatic diseases, which are among the commonest problems, will demonstrate fractures (with or without bone displacement) or dislocations on routine radiographs. Metabolic bone diseases (discussed in Chapter 47), which characteristically affect the entire skeleton, usually demonstrate generalized radiolucency or osteopenia. Congenital and developmental diseases will usually affect more than one bone, are often symmetrical, and often demonstrate modeling deformities. Infections show a variety of radiographic abnormalities depending on the type of organism present, the localization of the infection, and its chronicity. Avascular necrosis and idiopathic infarction demonstrate radiodensities in end arterial distributions; they are wedge-shaped at the convex ends of long bones and medullary in their diaphyses. Primary tumors of bone are usually localized defects that vary in their radiographic appearance in accordance with their biologic behavior. Metastatic tumors are usually localized defects that affect more than one bone or more than one focus in one bone, but they can be mistaken for primary tumors if they are solitary. Joint diseases change the quality or quantity of the space between the bone ends normally seen in radiographs; they may also produce joint erosions or joint deformities. The salient features of some miscellaneous bone diseases that pathologists sometimes encounter are presented in Table 46.1.

A. Congenital and Developmental Diseases. Very few of these disorders come to the attention of surgical pathologists, since most are diagnosed on the basis of their clinical and imaging appearances. Some of them, such as the histiocytoses and storage disorders, may be confirmed histologically or may be seen incidentally, such as when there is a hip replacement for avascular necrosis associated with Gaucher disease. Many others, such as most of the sclerosing dysplasias exclusive of diseases with specific histologies (e.g., osteopetrosis), demonstrate bone of increased density but are not specific or separable from one another histologically without demonstrating the changes seen in the radiographs (**e-Fig. 46.5**).

Tumor/Lesion	Location	Age (years)	Radiologic Findings	Pathologic Findings	Differential Diagnosis
Congenital/Developmental	Diffuse, sometimes localized; usually symmetrical	<10	Modeling abnormality	Disease-dependent	Very broad
Traumatic	Any part of any bone	Any	Fracture lines; dislocations	Hemorrhage; organization; woven bone and chondroid matrix	Osteosarcoma and chondrosarcoma
Circulatory					
Avascular necrosis	Convex ends of LBs	5–40	Wedge-shaped radio-density; crescent sign; collapse of articular cartilage	Necrotic marrow and bone; subarticular plate fracture	None
Idiopathic infarction	Medulla of LBs	>20	Hazy density sometimes resembling smoke	Necrotic marrow and bone; calcification and ossification of marrow fat	Enchondroma[a]
Paget disease	Any portion of any bone; almost always extending to articular ends	>50	Early: bone resorption in wedge-shaped edge Later: course trabeculation; loss of corticomedullary demarcations	Osteoclastic resorption + increased vascularity and marrow fibrosis; "mosaic" cement lines in middle to late stages	Hyperparathyroidism; myelodysplasia and myelofibrosis; metastatic carcinoma with fibrosis
Infectious					
Hematogenous	Cortex of LBs	2–15	Early: ↑ uptake on bone scan; change of marrow signal on MRI; Later: mixed sclerosis and radiolucency	Marrow fibrosis with osteonecrosis and exudate/mixed inflammatory cell infiltrate	Round cell tumors and Langerhans cell histiocytosis
Direct	Any; open trauma or deep ulcer	Varies	Mixed sclerosis and radiolucency	Marrow fibrosis with osteonecrosis and exudate/mixed inflammatory cell infiltrate	Round cell tumors and Langerhans cell histiocytosis

[a]Radiologic differential diagnosis.

LBs, long bones; MRI, magnetic resonance imaging.

B. Traumatic Disorders. Fractures are numerically the most frequent bone and joint disorders. They do not usually come to the attention of surgical pathologists because most treatment is closed or does not produce tissue for diagnosis. In contrast, open fractures requiring debridement and acute fractures of the femoral neck undergoing joint replacement are sometimes received in pathology laboratories. Acute fractures usually demonstrate some degree of accompanying hemorrhage, reactive changes such as dilated sinusoids in still viable nearby marrow, and fragmented bone trabeculae. Subacute fractures will also demonstrate devitalization of the bone at the fracture site (empty osteocyte lacunae and necrosis of marrow), although histologic evidence of healing is usually not evident for 7 to 10 days. Fractures that do not heal and fractures that are thought to be pathologic are sometimes sampled to rule out the presence of tumor or infection. It is very important to know that there is a history of trauma when reviewing tissue, or there is some danger of misinterpreting microcallus or reactive changes as matrix production by a tumor. Even if the history is not available, imaging studies will reveal if a tumor is present, and it is worthwhile to remember that primary bone tumors that produce bone matrix are rarely the sites of fracture. There are histologic parameters to separate bone and cartilage formation by tumor from that of trauma, although it takes some experience to recognize them. Bone or osteoid production by tumor matrix is often lace-like and becomes sheet-like as more bone is produced. Bone produced as a repair phenomenon may be focally lace-like, but more often it rapidly acquires a microtrabecular architecture and then becomes trabecular as it matures. In reactive bone there is almost always a zonation of maturity that is dependent on both the area in the lesion sampled and the time from trauma. While bone and cartilage are both common findings in both osteosarcoma and in fracture callus, cartilage tends to disappear as callus matures but it persists in osteosarcoma (e-**Fig. 46.6**). In addition, the progression from bone to cartilage back to bone is orderly in reactive processes but is totally random in bone tumors.

C. Circulatory Disturbances

1. Bone necrosis. Osteonecrosis occurs in areas where the bone circulation has an end arterial distribution. The most common sites are near the convex surfaces of joints where epiphyseal arterial branches supply the cancellous bone in the distribution of a cone. When this area of bone is deprived of circulation, avascular or aseptic necrosis of the bone results. The cancellous bone up to the calcified zone of the articular cartilage, deriving its blood supply from nutrient arteries to the epiphysis, undergoes infarction. The overlying articular cartilage, which derives oxygen and nutrients from the synovial fluid, remains viable. These changes are not immediately visible on routine radiographs because there are no changes in density of the necrotic bone. However, radionuclide bone scans do demonstrate early hypervascularity in the zone surrounding the necrotic area, and MRI demonstrates edema and loss of marrow fat because of early adipocyte necrosis. The wedge-shaped area of radiodensity characteristic of late osteonecrosis develops for a variety of reasons, but deposition of calcium salts due to saponification of free fatty acid esters may be of greatest importance (although it is often difficult to recognize calcium salts in decalcified sections because they are dissolved by the decalcification process). Clinical symptoms become severe when the necrosis has extended to the articular cartilage with loss of congruency of the usual convex–concave joint surface and destruction of the subarticular plate. It is not uncommon for the articular cartilage and superficial subarticular plate to detach from the underlying cancellous bone (because dead bone matrix and living bone have the same inherent strength and stiffness, this probably happens because the subarticular bone no longer has the capacity for remodeling in the face of repetitive forces, and accumulated shear stress causes it to detach). When detachment occurs, the radiodense subarticular bone attached to the articular cartilage forms a crescentic shadow that may be seen radiographically (e-**Fig. 46.7**).

2. Bone infarctions. Infarcts are also presumably the result of a disruption in end arterial circulation. In the diaphysis, a bone infarct is largely confined to the medulla.

This portion of the bone derives its blood supply from nutrient arteries that penetrate the cortex to supply the sinusoids of the medullary cavity and the inner cortex. The saponified marrow fat resulting from fat necrosis may appear to contain hazy or smoky radiodensities, and biopsies will reveal fat necrosis and a few scant trabeculae with empty osteocyte lacunae (e-Fig. 46.8).

The outer cortex is supplied mainly by perforating arterioles derived from arteriae comitantes of the periosteum. The cortical portions of this circulation travel longitudinally via Haversian canals and interconnect within the cortex via the Volkmann canals. Because the circulation in the cortex is thereby microscopically collateralized, the cortex of long bones is somewhat more protected against infarction than is the medullary cavity. It is important to remember that within the cortex there are interstitial lamellae derived from the remnants of old Haversian systems, and inner or outer circumferential lamellae that have not fully resorbed but have no active blood supply, and because of this, physiologically there are lamellae that are devoid of osteocytes and are physiologically dead (e-Fig. 46.9); since all cortical bone is compact bone, this means that small foci of empty osteocyte lacunae within the cortex do not necessarily imply that there is avascular necrosis even though the bone is histologically dead. Ordinarily, it is necessary for both nutrient and periosteal blood supplies to be disrupted to cause a true cortical infarction. This happens most often in conjunction with trauma and with infections.

D. **Paget Disease.** This disease has some histologic features in common with high-turnover metabolic bone diseases, but it is not a metabolic disease because it does not diffusely affect the entire skeleton and has no known associated metabolic defect (metabolic bone diseases are covered in Chapter 47). Paget disease is characterized by an imbalance or uncoupling of osteoclastic and osteoblastic activities, with osteoclastic bone resorption predominating early in the disease and osteoblastic activity persisting late in the disease. These histologic manifestations are correlated radiographically with characteristic radiolucency early in the disease, radiodensity in the late stages, and a mixed pattern for most of the interval between (*Skeletal Radiol* 1995;24:173). Because the bone microarchitecture is altered, there is loss of the normal bone contour radiographically, and there is gradual loss of the normal cortical appearance and an increasingly coarse appearance to the bone trabeculations. A biopsy from an early radiolucent lesion demonstrates large bizarre osteoclasts producing large and irregular resorption pits (Howship lacunae) on trabecular surfaces. These are often accompanied by paratrabecular fibrosis and dilated marrow sinusoids. As the resorption pits become filled in by osteoblast activity, irregularly shaped cement lines (sometimes likened to grout lines in a mosaic) mark the demarcation between the old and new bone. The bone on either side of these cement lines demonstrates either lamellar bone, in which the layers are discontinuous on either side, or lamellar bone on one side and woven bone on the other side. As the disease progresses and osteoclast activity slows, the bone becomes thicker and more interconnected than normal but its arrangement and increased irregular cement lines make it more prone to deformities and fractures (e-Fig. 46.10).

E. **Infectious Disorders.** Infections of bone arise either by direct introduction of organisms into the bone due to open trauma or overlying infections of soft tissue, or by secondary hematogenous spread. Most hematogenous osteomyelitis occurs in the first two decades of life. Its usual site in the bone is in the metaphysis adjoining the growth plate of a long bone because the microcirculation is stagnant in this area. Osteomyelitis due to open trauma can occur at any age; osteomyelitis associated with overlying infections is most often associated with peripheral vascular disease and so is seen later in life. Most infections of the bone are bacterial, but infections with fungi and lower virulence organisms may occur in immunocompromised hosts.

The vast majority of hematogenous osteomyelitis is due to coagulase-positive *Staphylococcus aureus*, but many other organisms may infect bones. Histologically, microorganisms are seldom seen in bone biopsies of patients with osteomyelitis because of the very high number of organisms required for high power or oil-immersion microscopy to detect bacteria. Because of this, bacterial cultures should always be taken when infections of bone are suspected clinically, preferably prior to the institution of antibiotic therapy. Bacterial culture is on the order of 10 million times more sensitive than histology, even when special histochemical stains for organisms are used. Infections in bone are often accompanied by necrosis of at least some of the affected bone; the primary reason for this is that edema accompanies inflammation, and edema in the closed confines of the cortex compromises the medullary nutrient arteries and sinusoids due to resulting increased pressure. The innermost cortical circulation may be similarly compromised by increased intramedullary pressure. If the pressurized exudate finds its way into empty Haversian and Volkmann canals, it may push its way through these intracortical spaces and eventually dissect the periosteum, and its perforating arteries, from the cortex. If the cortex is deprived of its dual circulation, then it in turn becomes necrotic; this necrotic bone is called sequestrum. The combination of necrotic bone sequestrum, marrow fibrosis and/or fat necrosis, and mixed inflammatory infiltrates (usually including neutrophils and plasma cells) provides good histologic corroboration of osteomyelitis, but the demonstration of organisms is the gold standard for the diagnosis of infections (**e-Fig. 46.11**).

F. Iatrogenic Disorders. Treatment-related disorders are seldom a major problem in the pathologic diagnosis of orthopedic disease, provided that an accurate clinical history is communicated to the surgical pathologist. For example, the diagnosis of osteosarcoma would be very unusual in a patient of the sixth decade without prior radiation of the site, or without some other underlying premalignant bone lesion. Administration of various therapeutic regimens may lead to secondary alterations in bones; perhaps the most notable of these is the amyloidosis of bones, tendon sheaths, and ligaments that develops from β2-microglobulin accumulation in long-term hemodialysis patients. Substances that have been given parenterally but that are not metabolized may also be deposited in bones or joints; without prior knowledge of therapeutic treatment, it may be difficult to make an accurate diagnosis (**e-Fig. 46.12**).

G. Neoplastic and Tumor-like Lesions. Primary tumors of bone are quite rare, accounting for only 0.2% of all malignancies, or an incidence of 0.8 per 100,000 individuals per year (NCI [2011] SEER Cancer statistics review, 1975–2008.). There is a bimodal age distribution, with one peak in adolescence and a smaller one in patients older than 60 years. Among other characteristics, each bone tumor has its own age predilection, which is very useful from a differential diagnostic standpoint. Primary benign bone tumors are probably less common than primary malignant tumors if the very common nonossifying fibroma, osteochondroma, and enchondromas of the hands are excluded. In addition to benign and malignant bone neoplasms, there are a number of nonneoplastic lesions that can present in a manner similar to neoplastic conditions (Table 46.2); all of these lesions are discussed below, and their main features are presented in Tables 46.3 and 46.4. Pathologic stage should be reported for bone tumors and the American Joint Committee on Cancer (AJCC) staging scheme is recommended for this purpose (Amin MB et al., eds. *AJCC Cancer Staging Manual.* 8th ed. New York: Springer, 2017).

1. Cartilage-forming tumors

a. Osteochondroma is a cartilage-capped bony protrusion (**e-Fig. 46.13**) that arises from the surface of any bone that models or grows by endochondral ossification. On imaging, osteochondromas demonstrate a marrow cavity and a cortex continuous with those of the host bone. Although classified as bone neoplasms, osteochondromas may also result from displacements of the cartilaginous grown plate. This is consistent with their metaphyseal location and the fact that they cease to grow after skeletal maturation. Most osteochondromas are sporadic and solitary; however, multiple lesions are present in hereditary multiple osteochondromas syndrome (HMO), which is an autosomal dominant hereditary condition. Cytogenetic alternations involving 8q22-24.1, the site of the *EXT1* gene are present in 55% to 75% of HMO cases, and approximately 80% of sporadic tumors. *EXT2* alterations are also found HMO. The risk of malignant transformation to

TABLE 46.2 WHO Classification of Bone Tumors

Chondrogenic tumors
Benign
Osteochondroma
Chondroma
   Enchondroma
   Periosteal chondroma
Osteochondromyxoma
Subungual exostosis
Bizarre parosteal osteochondromatous
   proliferation
Synovial chondromatosis
Intermediate (locally aggressive)
Chondromyxoid fibroma
Atypical cartilaginous tumor/Chondrosarcoma
   grade I
Intermediate (rarely metastasizing)
Chondroblastoma
Malignant
Chondrosarcoma grades II and III
Dedifferentiated chondrosarcoma
Mesenchymal chondrosarcoma
Clear cell chondrosarcoma

Osteogenic tumors
Benign
Osteoma
Osteoid osteoma
Intermediate (locally aggressive)
Osteoblastoma
Malignant
Low-grade central osteosarcoma
Conventional osteosarcoma
   Chondroblastic osteosarcoma
   Fibroblastic osteosarcoma
   Osteoblastic osteosarcoma
Telangiectatic osteosarcoma
Small cell osteosarcoma
Secondary osteosarcoma
Parosteal osteosarcoma
Periosteal osteosarcoma
High-grade surface osteosarcoma

Fibrogenic tumors
Intermediate (locally aggressive)
Desmoplastic fibroma
Malignant
Fibrosarcoma of bone

Fibrohistiocytic tumors
Benign fibrous histiocytoma/Non-ossifying
   fibroma

Hematopoietic tumors
Malignant
Plasma cell myeloma
Solitary plasmacytoma
Primary non-Hodgkin lymphoma

Osteoclastic giant cell rich tumors
Benign
Giant cell lesion of the small bones
*Intermediate (locally aggressive, rarely
   metastasizing)*
Giant cell tumor of bone
Malignant
Malignancy in giant cell tumor of bone

Notochordal tumors
Benign
Benign notochordal tumor
Malignant
Chordoma

Vascular tumors
Benign
Hemangioma
*Intermediate (locally aggressive, rarely
   metastasizing)*
Epithelioid hemangioma
Malignant
Epithelioid hemangioendothelioma
Angiosarcoma

Myogenic tumors
Benign
Leiomyoma of bone
Malignant
Leiomyosarcoma of bone

Lipogenic tumors
Benign
Lipoma of bone
Malignant
Liposarcoma of bone

Tumors of undefined neoplastic nature
Benign
Simple cyst
Fibrous dysplasia
Osteofibrous dysplasia
Chondromesenchymal hamartoma
Rosai–Dorfman disease
Intermediate (locally aggressive)
Aneurysmal bone cyst
Langerhans cell histiocytosis
   Monostotic
   Polyostotic
Erdheim–Chester disease

Miscellaneous tumors
Ewing sarcoma
Adamantinoma
Undifferentiated high-grade pleomorphic
   sarcoma

From: Fletcher CDM, Bridge JA, Hogendoorn P, Mertens F, eds. *WHO Classification of Tumours of Soft Tissue and Bone.* Lyon, France: IARC Press; 2017.

TABLE 46.3 Commonest Location(s), Usual Age Distribution, and Salient Pathologic Features of Benign Bone Tumors

Tumor/Lesion	Location	Age (years)	Salient Pathologic Findings
Cartilaginous			
Osteochondroma	Metaphysis of LBs	10–30	Cartilage-capped bony protrusion
Chondroma	Hands/feet; medulla of LBs	Any	Variably cellular hyaline cartilage
Chondroblastoma	Epiphysis/apophysis of LBs	10–20	Chondroid-like matrix; S100-positive cells with grooved nuclei
Chondromyxoid fibroma	Metaphysis of LBs	10–30	Hypocellular chondromyxoid lobules surrounded by more cellular spindle-cell areas
Osseous			
Osteoma	Facial bones	Adults	Mineralized compact bone
Osteoid osteoma	Cortex of LBs	10–30	"Nidus" of immature bone surrounded by sclerotic bone
Osteoblastoma	Vertebrae; cortex of LBs	10–30	Identical to osteoid osteoma but larger; often no sclerosis
Fibrous, fibrohistiocytic, histiocytic, and GCT			
Fibrous dysplasia	Ribs; jaw; LBs-medullary	10–30	Irregular woven bone within fibroblastic stroma
Osteofibrous dysplasia	Tibial cortex	<20	Similar to fibrous dysplasia but with appositional osteoblasts
Desmoplastic fibroma	LBs; jaw; pelvis	20–30	Fibromatosis-like proliferation
Nonossifying fibroma	LBs	5–15	Bland spindle cells in storiform pattern + histiocytes + giant cells
BFH	LBs; pelvis	>20	Identical to nonossifying fibroma but variable
Langerhans cell histiocytosis	Skull; jaw; metaphysis and diaphysis of LBs	5–15	Mixed inflammatory cells and eosinophils; S-100/CD1a-positive cells with grooved/multilobulated nuclei
Erdheim–Chester disease	LBs	>40	Foamy histiocytes and fibrosis
Giant cell tumor	Epiphysis/metaphysis of LBs	20–45	Evenly placed giant cells among mononuclear cells with identical nuclei
Others			
Aneurysmal bone cyst	Vertebrae; flat and LBs	10–20	Blood-filled spaces separated by fibrous septae; giant cells
Simple cyst	Metaphysis of LBs	10–20	Fluid-filled "cysts" lined by connective tissue
Hemangioma	Vertebrae; flat and LBs	20–50	Capillary and/or cavernous sized vessels

BFH, benign fibrous histiocytoma; GCT, giant cell tumor; LBs, long bones.

TABLE 46.4 Commonest Location(s), Usual Age Distribution, and Salient Pathologic Features of Malignant Bone Tumors

Tumor/Lesion	Location	Age (years)	Salient Pathologic Findings
Chondrogenic			
Chondrosarcoma	Flat bones; metaphysis, and epiphysis of LBs		
Conventional (NOS)	Metaphysis	20–80	Variably cellular hyaline cartilage permeating bone
Dedifferentiated	Metaphysis	>30	Conventional chondrosarcoma + high-grade spindle cell sarcoma
Mesenchymal	Metaphysis	20–50	Undifferentiated small cell tumor + hyaline cartilage
Clear cell	Epiphysis	20–70	Conventional tumor with abundant large clear tumor cells
Osseous			
Osteosarcoma	Metaphysis of LBs; jaw	10–20; >40	
Conventional	Medullary		Osteoid formed directly by malignant cells
Low-grade central	Medullary		Mildly atypical fibroblastic proliferation + thick bone trabeculae
Telangiectatic	Medullary		Blood-filled spaces + fibrous septae + highly malignant osteoid
Parosteal	Cortex outside periosteum		Mildly atypical fibroblastic proliferation + thick bone trabeculae
Periosteal	Cortex inside periosteum		Abundant cartilage matrix with variable malignant osteoid
Fibrous/fibrohistiocytic			
Fibrosarcoma	Metaphysis of LBs; may extend to end of bone	20–60	Malignant spindle cells in a fascicular pattern
Undifferentiated high-grade pleomorphic sarcoma	Metaphysis of LBs; may extend to end of bone	20–80	Malignant spindle cells in storiform pattern + histiocytic cells (other patterns may be seen)
Hematolymphoid			
Myeloma	Skull; vertebrae; pelvis; LBs	>40	Variably atypical (monoclonal) plasma cells
Lymphoma	Any	Any	Lymphoid proliferations similar to nonbony lesions
Epithelial			
Adamantinoma	Cortex of tibia and/or fibula	25–35	Epithelial cells + fibroblasts + woven or lamellar bone
Metastatic carcinoma	Any	>40	Malignant epithelial cells; morphology/IHC helps confirm origin
Others			
Ewing sarcoma	Diaphysis of LBs	5–20	Small round blue cells ± rosettes; characteristic IHC; translocation
Chordoma	Base of skull; sacrum	>30	Lobules of vacuolated cells embedded in myxoid matrix
Angiosarcoma		20–60	Anastomosing vascular channels lined by highly atypical cells; characteristic IHC

IHC, immunohistochemistry; LBs, long bones; NOS, not otherwise specified.

peripheral chondrosarcoma is approximately 1% in sporadic cases and 5% to 25% in HMO.

b. **Chondromas** comprise a group of lesions that are composed of variably cellular mature hyaline cartilage (e-**Fig. 46.14**). Enchondromas arise within the medullary cavity and most commonly involve the small bones of the hand and feet or long tubular bones, whereas periosteal chondromas arise on the cortical surface (about half of which involve the humerus). Most chondromas are incidental, but some, especially in long bones, can present with pathologic fractures. Radiographically, chondromas appear as well-demarcated lucent lesions with variable amounts of stippled mineralization (e-**Fig. 46.15**). Ollier disease is characterized by multiple enchondromas, which commonly affects one side of the body more than the other, associated with bone deformities that develop early in life; Maffucci syndrome is characterized by multiple enchondromas with associated extraosseous hemangiomas, typically spindle cell hemangiomas. Both of these developmental disorders are associated with a significantly increased incidence of secondary chondrosarcoma, although the incidence is higher in patients with Maffucci syndrome. Enchondromas in these patients tend to be more cellular and myxoid, so the histologic appearances alone cannot always be used to diagnose malignant transformation. In such cases, clinical (e.g., rapid growth), radiologic (e.g., cortical destruction, soft tissue masses), and/or pathologic (e.g., necrosis, permeation of bone trabeculae) findings must be used in combination to arrive at the correct diagnosis. Somatic *IDH1/2* mutations have been identified in solitary enchondromas, enchondromas in Ollier disease, and enchondromas and spindle cell hemangiomas in Maffucci syndrome.

c. **Chondroblastoma** is a benign neoplasm, which characteristically has a epiphyseal or apophyseal location. It often presents with arthritic pain and/or joint stiffness due to its close proximity to joints. Histologically, the tumor is composed of discrete, round mononuclear cells with ovoid, folded, or grooved nuclei (e-**Fig. 46.16**). A pink extracellular material resembling early cartilage is also present, sometimes with "chicken-wire" calcification, but the lesion very seldom produces true hyaline cartilage. Giant cells are often present; if they are abundant and the matrix is scant, the lesion can be confused with a giant cell tumor (GCT). However, the radiologic identification of a sclerotic rim or a demarcated edge with or without calcification (e-**Fig. 46.17**), as well as the fact that almost all patients with this lesion are young and still have open growth plates, helps distinguish chondroblastoma from GCT. In addition, the neoplastic chondroblasts are positive for S100 protein. The majority of chondroblastomas harbor mutations in the *H3F3B* gene (*Nat Genet* 2013;45:1479).

d. **Chondromyxoid fibroma** presents in the metaphyses of growing individuals. It is characteristically well circumscribed, eccentric, and may demonstrate bone expansion (e-**Fig. 46.18**). Histologically, there are lobular aggregates of spindle-shaped to stellate cells arranged within a chondroid to myxoid matrix. Importantly, these lobules are surrounded by zones of hypercellularity in which mononuclear and multinucleated giant cells are evident (e-**Fig. 46.19**). *GRM1* fusion leading to promoter swapping and *GRM1* upregulation has been identified in chondromyxoid fibroma. The neoplasm is benign.

e. **Osteochondromyxoma** is a rare tumor which occurs in the setting of Carney complex. While the tumor generally has a benign radiographic appearance, aggressive growth including soft tissue extension may be seen. Histologically, hypocellular proliferations of bipolar, stellate, and polygonal cells with bland nuclear features and embedded in myxoid stroma characterize the tumor. Cartilage, osteoid, and bone production may be seen.

f. **Subungual (Dupuytren) exostosis** occurs on the distal phalanx, most commonly on the dorsal aspect of the great toe, and is most common in the second and third decade. The radiographic appearance varies with the age of the lesion, but mature lesions are characterized by a boney mass on the surface of the bone without continuity with the medullary cavity. Microscopically, there is a cellular myofibroblastic proliferation with cartilage undergoing enchondral ossification. The lesion may produce osteochondroma-like architecture.

g. Bizarre parosteal osteochondromatous proliferation (Nora's lesion) occurs on the surface of the bone, most commonly the short tubular bones of the hands and feet; however, long bones are not uncommonly affected. Radiographically, the lesion is well marginated and the underlying cortex is intact. Microscopically, a spindle cell proliferation is associated with cartilage undergoing enchondral ossification; the cartilage is hypercellular and the chondrocytes are enlarged. There is prominent osteoblastic rimming and "blue bone" may be present.

h. Synovial chondromatosis most commonly involves the knee, hip, and elbow joints as well as the tenosynovium of the distal extremities. In this tumor nodules of hyaline cartilage with clusters of chondrocytes grow within the synovium of joints, bursa, and tendon sheaths. The cartilage may undergo enchondral ossification and loose bodies are frequently found. While the lesion is benign, there is a high rate of local recurrence.

i. Chondrosarcoma (not otherwise specified) is one of the few primary malignant tumors that affect adults with fully mature skeletons. It is classified as primary when there is no pre-existing lesion, or secondary when it arises in a pre-existing bone lesion such as osteochondroma or Ollier disease. Chondrosarcoma most commonly involves the flat bones of the trunk and proximal tubular bones of the extremities. Radiographically, it tends to be large and radiolucent, with radiodense stippling, curlicues, and rings due to matrix calcification or ossification. When it is a central (medullary) lesion, there is often cortical destruction and sometimes cortical thickening. When peripheral, the cartilage matrix is usually >3 cm in thickness (e-**Fig. 46.20**).

Histologically, chondrosarcoma is composed of mature appearing hyaline cartilage except that the chondrocytes have varying degrees of increased cellularity, nuclear atypia, and even mitotic activity. Chondrosarcoma can show variable degrees of differentiation, ranging from minimally hypercellular tumors resembling enchondromas with scattered enlarged hyperchromatic tumor cell nuclei that are sometimes binucleate (grade I), to unequivocally malignant tumors with markedly atypical cells and easily identifiable mitotic figures (grade III). Grade II tumors have features intermediate between the two (e-**Fig. 46.21**). Regardless of their grade, chondrosarcomas (when sampled adequately) invariably show permeation of existing marrow spaces between bony trabeculae (e-**Fig. 46.22**); this is a very helpful feature for distinguishing low-grade tumors from enchondromas, especially in the small bones of the hands and feet where enchondromas may show a degree of hypercellularity and/or binucleation quite reminiscent of that seen in low-grade chondrosarcomas of larger, more proximal bones. The presence of tumor cell necrosis can also point to a diagnosis of chondrosarcoma. Nevertheless, there are cartilaginous tumors that remain difficult to accurately categorize, especially when the radiologic features of malignancy are not clearly evident. Occasionally, complementary imaging studies such as CT scans may help to identify true bone destruction in a central cartilage tumor, or MRI will demonstrate the extent of a cartilage cap in a peripheral cartilage tumor, which in turn can help to identify the true biologic nature of the lesion when a small biopsy cannot (e-**Fig. 46.23**). The prognosis of chondrosarcoma is mostly dependent on grade and completeness of resection (as no other modality of treatment is effective), with 5-year survival rates ranging from 90% for low-grade tumors to 53% in higher-grade tumors.

Somatic mutations in the isocitrate dehydrogenase genes *IDH1* and *IDH2* have been identified in over 50% of chondrosarcomas, as well as in both sporadic and syndromic enchondromas. Thus, mutation analysis can be helpful in difficult cases.

j. Dedifferentiated chondrosarcoma. In addition to areas of resembling enchondroma or low-grade conventional chondrosarcoma, this tumor is characterized by the presence of a distinct, second, clearly defined, high-grade noncartilaginous sarcomatous component (e-**Fig. 46.24**). The latter is most frequently represented by a pleomorphic and spindle cell sarcomatous component, but osteosarcoma, fibrosarcoma, and rhabdomyosarcoma have also been reported. The tumor has a very poor prognosis.

k. Mesenchymal chondrosarcoma is a rare tumor also characterized by a dimorphic pattern and is composed of a undifferentiated small round cell component that is often arranged in a hemangiopericytomatous pattern, intermixed with a variable number of islands of hyaline cartilage (e-**Fig. 46.25**). Although it may occur at any age, the peak age incidence of patients with this tumor (second and third decades) is earlier than that seen in patients with other chondrosarcomas. Mesenchymal chondrosarcoma has a high incidence of local recurrence and distant metastasis, although the latter may not occur for 5 to 10 years. Mesenchymal chondrosarcoma harbors a recurrent *HEY1-NCOA2* fusion and lacks *IDH1/2* mutations.

l. Clear cell chondrosarcoma. Another rare type of chondrosarcoma lacking *IDH1/2* mutations, this tumor shows a predilection for the ends of long bones after the growth plates have closed (e-**Fig. 46.26**). It is characterized histologically by the presence of abundant large round clear cells with well-defined cell borders intermixed with areas of conventional low-grade chondrosarcoma (e-**Fig. 46.27**). Prominent woven bone formation within the tumor is typical. The clear cells contain large amounts of intracellular glycogen and stain strongly for S-100 protein. The prognosis is similar to that of low-grade chondrosarcoma. Metastases occur in about 20% of patients and may behave indolently or aggressively. Clear cell chondrosarcoma has a high predilection for metastasis to other bones.

2. Bone-forming tumors

a. Osteoma is a well-circumscribed, radiodense, benign lesion that most frequently arises in the jaws and paranasal sinuses (e-**Fig. 46.28**), but can also be seen in long bones. Some cases are sporadic, whereas others arise in association with familial polyposis coli (see Chapter 14). Histologically, osteomas are composed of mineralized compact bone matrix with a variable admixture of mature and immature bone but no cellular stroma (e-**Fig. 46.28**).

b. Osteoid osteoma. This benign, self-limited tumor usually presents with pain that often wakes patients from sleep but is relieved by aspirin. Although it usually involves the cortices of long bones, osteoid osteoma has been reported in almost every skeletal site. Radiographically, there is a central area of radiolucency surrounded by dense reactive sclerosis (e-**Fig. 46.29**). The quantity of sclerosis varies by location in the bone. If the lesion is cortical, the reactive sclerosis may obscure the lesion such that it can only be seen by thin-cut CT scans. In the medullary cavity, there may be little or no sclerosis.

Histologically, the radiolucent area, termed the "nidus," is composed of vascularized fibroconnective tissue in which immature new bone is being formed. This new bone is usually arranged in microtrabecular arrays lined by plump appositional osteoblasts that lack nuclear pleomorphism (e-**Fig. 46.30**). Simple excision or curettage of the nidus of an osteoid osteoma is curative.

c. Osteoblastoma is virtually identical histologically to osteoid osteoma but, unlike the latter, is not limited in growth potential. When diagnosed, osteoblastomas are usually larger than 2 cm in diameter. Radiographically, they may resemble large osteoid osteomas, they may be expansile like aneurysmal bone cysts (ABCs), or they may even appear as aggressive as malignant tumors. There is also a predilection to involve the axial skeleton, especially the vertebral pedicles and arches. Occasionally, osteoblastomas may be very cellular and their osteoblasts may be several times the size of usual osteoblasts. Tumors having predominant areas of this histologic feature have been termed "aggressive osteoblastoma" or "epithelioid osteoblastoma" (e-**Fig. 46.31**). The prognosis of osteoblastomas is excellent if amenable to excision.

d. **Osteosarcoma** is the most common nonhematopoietic primary malignant neoplasm of bone. The peak incidence of this tumor is late childhood and adolescence; however, there is a second peak in patients older than 40 years, most cases of which develop secondarily in pre-existing bone lesions (e.g., Paget disease) or following irradiation. The metaphyses of long bones (e.g., femur, tibia, humerus) are the most common sites of involvement; isolated diaphyseal involvement is rare, and involvement of the epiphyses of long bones or small bones of the hands and feet is exceptionally rare. Other sites of involvement include the jaws, skull, and axial skeleton. Most cases of osteosarcoma present with pain (often dull and unremitting) with or without a palpable mass. Radiologically, there is almost always evidence of a destructive bony lesion, often with evidence of new bone formation. There may also be an interrupted periosteal reaction and soft tissue involvement (e-**Fig. 46.32**).

The histologic hallmark of osteosarcoma is the presence of osteoid or bone formation directly by tumor cells. Osteoid appears as dense, pink, amorphous material (resembling collagen or amyloid) that has a lace-like or sheet-like appearance (e-**Fig. 46.33**). Intermixed within, and often in direct contact with this osteoid matrix, are the neoplastic tumor cells which can be quite variable in appearance and include polyhedral cells, spindle cells with variable nuclear atypia, small blue cells (resembling EWS, see below), and large markedly atypical cells. The predominant matrix produced by the tumor can be bone or osteoid, cartilaginous, or fibrous. As described below, osteosarcomas are best classified based on radiologic and/or pathologic features that have been shown to have distinct prognostic implications (*Am J Clin Pathol* 2006;125:555). Like other bone forming tumors, osteosarcoma expresses SATB2; however, the utility of immunohistochemistry is limited and the results must be carefully interpreted in the context of the tumor morphology.

i. **Central osteosarcomas** arise within the medullary cavity and include:

(a) **Conventional intramedullary osteosarcoma** is the prototypical osteosarcoma, for which most of the above information refers. Neoplastic tumor cells in conventional osteosarcoma are often polyhedral or spindle-shaped with unequivocally malignant features. Historically, osteosarcomas have been subclassified based on the predominant matrix production (osteoblastic, chondroblastic, or fibroblastic), but this classification has no prognostic importance. Other less common patterns include osteoblastoma-like, chondroblastoma-like, small cell, and giant cell rich. Osteosarcoma with a small cell pattern should be differentiated from other round cell sarcomas including EWS. Given that preoperative chemotherapy for these tumors is the current standard of care (and has significantly improved the 5-year survival rate of this tumor from 20% to over 80%), it is important to carefully map the tumor in the resection specimen (as discussed earlier) to determine the extent of tumor necrosis compared with the volume of viable plus nonviable tumor since a favorable long-term outcome is associated with >90% tumor necrosis. Additional chemotherapy is often offered to patients with less necrosis as a second-line attempt to further improve survival.

(b) **Low-grade central osteosarcoma** is a rare type of osteosarcoma (1% to 2%) composed of a variably cellular spindle cell/fibroblastic proliferation that lacks the degree of cytologic atypia seen in conventional osteosarcoma. In addition, bone production is usually evident as irregular, somewhat thick, anastomosing or branching bony trabeculae. These trabeculae simulate the woven bone of fibrous dysplasia or the longitudinal seams of bone in parosteal osteosarcoma (see below) and are separated by a spindle-cell stroma. Review of the radiologic findings often reveals subtle signs of malignancy that are useful in making the diagnosis (e-**Fig. 46.34**). This tumor has a much more indolent course compared with conventional osteosarcoma; however, there is still a high recurrence rate if the tumor is inadequately excised, often with associated grade progression. The large majority of low-grade central osteosarcoma harbor amplification of 12q13–q15 including *MDM2* and *CDK4*.

(c) **Telangiectatic osteosarcoma** is characterized by large, blood-filled spaces separated by highly cellular fibrous septae that contain markedly pleomorphic cells with a variable amount of osteoid production (e-**Fig. 46.35**). Radiologically, this tumor is radiolucent and expansile, and resembles ABC. Compared with other osteosarcomas, it is more likely to present with a pathologic fracture. Although not necessarily associated with improved survival, this aggressive osteosarcoma is very sensitive to chemotherapy.

ii. **Surface osteosarcomas.** About 1 in 20 osteosarcomas occurs in association with the bone surface rather than in the medullary cavity. The vast majority of these are low-grade tumors showing radiodensity and osseous differentiation. They include:

(a) **Parosteal osteosarcoma** accounts for approximately 4% of osteosarcomas and the majority of surface osteosarcomas. It characteristically involves the posterior distal femur, is associated with the outer fibrous layer of the periosteum, and tends to wrap around the bone. Histologically, it consists of well-formed bony trabeculae, often arranged in parallel streamers separated by a hypocellular spindle stroma as seen in low-grade central osteosarcoma (e-**Fig. 46.36**). Cartilaginous differentiation is also common, often seen as a cartilage cap and sometimes causing confusion with osteochondroma. Radiographically, however, there is no continuity of the interior of parosteal osteosarcoma and the medullary cavity, the adjacent bony cortex is not continuous with the outside of parosteal osteosarcoma (e-**Fig. 46.37**), and the intertrabecular spaces do not contain fatty or hematopoietic marrow. The prognosis of parosteal osteosarcoma is similar to that of low-grade intramedullary osteosarcoma.

If inaccurately diagnosed as benign, or if inadequately excised, these lesions will recur. Recurrences may be low grade, but they may also be high grade; low-grade parosteal sarcoma undergoing high-grade transformation is termed *dedifferentiated parosteal osteosarcoma* and has a prognosis similar to conventional osteosarcoma. *MDM2* amplification is present in the majority of parosteal osteosarcomas.

(b) **Periosteal osteosarcoma** arises between the cortex and overlying periosteum most commonly in the tibial or femoral diaphysis, and is characterized by abundant cartilaginous matrix and a somewhat greater degree of cytologic atypia than is seen in parosteal osteosarcoma.

(c) **High-grade surface osteosarcoma** is histologically identical to conventional intramedullary osteosarcoma except that it arises on the bone surface. The prognosis is similar to that of conventional intramedullary osteosarcoma.

3. Fibrous and fibrohistiocytic tumors

a. **Fibrous dysplasia** usually presents as a solitary lesion, although it may affect multiple bones in a single limb bud distribution, or multiple bones without limb bud distribution. The polyostotic form is one of the manifestations of the McCune–Albright syndrome, which includes pigmented skin lesions and endocrinopathies. Mazabraud syndrome is characterized by fibrous dysplasia and soft tissue myxoma(s).

Fibrous dysplasia may be asymptomatic, but deformities, secondary fractures, and even pain may be the presenting manifestation. Radiographically, the lesion is almost always intramedullary, and it tends to affect those portions of bone formed by endochondral ossification. While secondary cortical atrophy may take place because of intramedullary expansion of the lesion, fibrous dysplasia usually does not involve the cortex; it is often expansile and results in modeling deformities of the host bone. It is well circumscribed and radiolucent, but less radiolucent than the underlying bone that it has replaced; radiologists often refer to its appearance as having a ground glass quality (e-**Fig. 46.38**).

Histologically, fibrous dysplasia consists of various combinations of any tissue present in bone, so fibrous tissue, bone, cartilage, and vascular tissues are produced in various combinations. The usual microscopic pattern, however, consists of loosely arranged, vascularized fibrous tissue in which disconnected curved microtrabeculae of bone are disposed. These trabeculae are not only woven in their collagen fiber pattern, but when a section is examined under polarized light, the fabric of their collagenous background forms a continuum with the fabric of the fibrous tissue (e-**Fig. 46.39**). Cartilage formation is not unusual, and occasionally cartilage is formed in such excess that lesions may be mistaken radiographically and histologically for cartilaginous neoplasms.

Treatment is usually focused on relief of deformities or other morbid symptomatology. The prognosis is usually excellent. Missense mutations in *GNAS* are present in syndromic and non-syndromic fibrous dysplasia, and the same mutations are present in other tumors in McCune-Albright syndrome as well as myxomas in Mazabraud syndrome.

b. Osteofibrous dysplasia is a fibro-osseous lesion and is almost invariably seen in the tibia, fibula, or both. Its peak incidence is in the first two decades of life. Radiographically, the lesion is radiolucent and usually based in the cortex; it may extend to the medullary cavity. The lesion may be unilocular or multilocular; while it tends to be circumscribed, it may also diffusely involve the diaphysis and cause secondary bowing deformities (e-**Fig. 46.40**). Histologically, osteofibrous dysplasia resembles fibrous dysplasia except that the microtrabeculae of bone tend to be rimmed by appositional osteoblasts even at their very earliest synthesis (e-**Fig. 46.41**). The fibrous stroma tends to be more cellular than in fibrous dysplasia, and is less contiguous with the trabeculae under polarized light. The lesional bone also tends to mature at the periphery with the surrounding normal bone. The lesional bone tends to undergo spontaneous involution with time, although sometimes it behaves more aggressively.

c. Nonossifying fibroma (fibrous cortical defect) is the commonest space-occupying lesion of bone, estimated to affect one in four individuals. Even though it is thought to be developmental, in rare cases the lesion behaves as a tumor of limited biologic potential. Unless it is associated with a fracture, patients are generally without symptoms; the lesions are typically discovered incidentally during the course of evaluation for some other condition and the routine radiographs are virtually diagnostic. The lesion is a well-circumscribed radiolucent defect in the metaphyseal cortex with scalloped sclerotic borders, and it is almost always longer in the cephalocaudal than axial direction (e-**Fig. 46.42**). It is most commonly found in the distal femoral or proximal tibia metaphysis.

Histologically, the lesion consists of spindle cells arranged in a distinctly storiform pattern. A fair number of multinucleated giant cells, histiocytic cells with foamy cytoplasm, and histiocytes containing hemosiderin pigment (e-**Fig. 46.43**) may also be present. While bone formation is not observed (hence the name), lesions that have fractures or microscopic infarctions are admixed with reactive bone. Because this lesion may be focally cellular, it is important to review the radiographs to avoid misdiagnosis. Most nonossifying fibromas are self-healing and do not require clinical intervention.

Of note, **benign fibrous histiocytoma** of bone has the same histologic features as nonossifying fibroma (e-**Figs. 46.44**), but differs in clinical and radiographic features including being painful and commonly involving the ilium and ribs, or the diaphysis of long bones. Secondary proliferations in other bone tumors (e.g., GCT) may also produce the same histologic findings as seen in benign fibrous histiocytoma.

d. Desmoplastic fibroma. This rare tumor occurs in adolescents and young adults with the mandible being the most commonly affected site. Radiologically, it often expands the involved bone, is entirely radiolucent, and is usually well circumscribed. Histologically, it is composed of bland fibroblastic or myofibroblastic cells in a background of collagen identical to that found in desmoid-type fibromatosis (e-**Fig**. 46.45). Although it is benign, it behaves similarly to fibromatosis of soft tissue in that there is a high recurrence rate when not completely excised. While desmoplastic fibroma is histologically similar to desmoid tumor, it does not appear to be driven by *APC* or *CTNNB1* mutations.

e. Fibrosarcoma is rare and a diagnosis of exclusion. It is reported to have a relatively uniform age distribution between the second and sixth decades. It usually involves the metaphyses of long bones resulting in pain, swelling, and a destructive radiologic lesion without radiographically detectable matrix. Histologically, fibrosarcomas are usually quite cellular with malignant spindle cells arranged in a fascicular or herringbone pattern (e-**Fig**. 46.46). The differential diagnosis includes other malignant spindle-cell tumors such as fibroblastic osteosarcoma, dedifferentiated chondrosarcoma, leiomyosarcoma, undifferentiated high-grade pleomorphic sarcoma, synovial sarcoma, and desmoplastic fibroma.

4. Osteoclastic giant cell rich tumors

a. Giant cell lesion of the small bones is a provisional term for a benign tumor which occurs in the small bones on the hands and feet of children and adolescents, causing pain and sometimes a pathologic fracture. It appears as an osteolytic and expansile lesion, with cortical thinning without a periosteal reaction on radiograph. The cortex is typically intact but cortical break-through can be seen. Histologically, a bland (myo)fibroblastic proliferation and osteoclast-like giant cells are present, which characteristically cluster around hemorrhage. The giant cells in this lesion are less evenly distributed and have fewer nuclei than seen in GCT. Histologically indistinguishable tumors occur in the setting of hyperparathyroidism (brown tumor) and in the jaw (sporadic giant cell reparative granuloma, or as a manifestation of cherubism). *USP6* rearrangements have been found in giant cell lesion of the small bones providing evidence that these tumors are actually solid ABCs, while gnathic tumors and lesions associated with cherubism and hyperparathyroidism lack this alteration (*Hum Pathol* 2014;45:1147, *Skeletal Radiol* 2008;37:321).

b. Giant cell tumor (GCT) comprises around 4% to 5% of all primary bone tumors and has a peak incidence between 20 and 45 years of age; it is rarely seen in skeletally immature individuals or in patients older than 50 years. It typically affects the ends of long bones and extends to the articular or apophyseal portions of the bone; the pelvis or small bones of the hand or feet are more rarely affected. Given the often juxta-articular location of the tumor, joint swelling and limitation of movement are common presenting symptoms. Radiologically, the tumor is radiolucent and eccentric, may expand the bone, and is well demarcated (e-**Fig**. 46.47). There is almost never a periosteal reaction associated with the tumor.

The histologic hallmark of the tumor is the presence of sheets of round, oval, or elongated mononuclear cells with an open chromatin pattern, evenly intermixed with numerous osteoclast-like giant cells with nuclei similar to those of the mononuclear cells (e-**Fig**. 46.48). The cell borders are often indistinct so that on low power the lesion appears as a syncytium. Mitoses are variable in number; atypical mitoses are occasionally seen and do not necessarily predict malignant behavior. The presence of the characteristic mononuclear cells and the even interposition of the giant cells are essential for the diagnosis since giant cells can be a component of many bone lesions. Other histologic features occasionally seen in GCTs include a focal storiform pattern, which, when abundant foam cells are present, can easily be confused with benign fibrous histiocytoma. There also may be areas of fibrosis, as well as secondary cystic areas resembling ABC (see below). The most important differential diagnosis is the so-called "brown tumor" of hyperparathyroidism (see Chapter 47); the lack of radiologic or biochemical evidence of hyperparathyroidism, as well as the absence of additional bone lesions, can be very helpful in this regard. Another important differential diagnosis is giant-cell reparative granuloma that characteristically involves the mandible and is composed of clusters of giant cells in a fibrovascular stroma, but which lacks the mononuclear cells characteristic of GCT (e-**Fig. 46.49**). Driver mutations in the *H3F3A* gene are present in 70% to 90% of GCTs of bone.

Most cases of GCT behave in a benign fashion; some, however, are associated with local aggressiveness and occasionally with distant metastasis (about 2% of cases), primarily to the lung ("benign metastasizing GCT"). Most of these metastases grow slowly and are rarely lethal.

Denosumab, a monoclonal antibody, can be used in the treatment of GCT, inhibiting receptor activator of NF-κB (RANK) ligand. Denosumab treatment leads to marked histologic alteration of the tumor with giant cell depletion, spindle cell proliferation, and woven bone formation. These changes may mimic benign fibrous histiocytoma, malignant GCT, and low or high-grade de novo osteosarcoma (*Am J Surg Pathol* 2016;40:72).

Malignant GCT is defined as a sarcomatous lesion arising within a GCT, or as a sarcoma that appears in the same area in which a bona fide GCT was treated (e-**Fig. 46.50**). The former instance is sometimes referred to as a primary malignant GCT, the latter as a secondary GCT. The prognosis is related to the histology, size, and grade of the malignant component.

5. Hematopoietic and lymphoid tumors

a. Solitary plasmacytoma and multiple myeloma. These tumors are malignant proliferations of plasma cells that account for the majority of tumors arising primarily in bone. The presentation of myeloma is quite variable (see Chapter 42), but involvement of the skeletal system is usually manifested by bone pain and/or pathologic fractures. Radiologically, plasmacytoma and the lesions of multiple myeloma are lytic, well demarcated, and without a rim of sclerotic bone; however, multiple myeloma may also present with generalized osteoporosis without any detectable foci of discrete bone destruction. Histologically, the tumors are composed of plasma cells and their precursors at various stages of development (e-**Fig. 46.51**). The main differential diagnosis is often other hematolymphoid tumors, although myeloma cells are occasionally quite anaplastic and can resemble carcinoma or high-grade sarcoma. Accordingly, immunohistochemical studies (see Chapter 42) can be useful to confirm the diagnosis.

b. Lymphoma. Most bone lymphomas are secondary to disease elsewhere, but primary bone lymphomas also occur. In general, lymphomas presenting in bone are classified as primary provided no lymph node involvement is present both at the time of presentation and for a long interval afterward (the length of this interval varies according to different authors). Most primary lymphomas of bone represent examples of diffuse large B-cell lymphoma or other high-grade tumor because most lower-grade lymphomas and leukemias present with diffuse marrow involvement rather than as a mass. Primary Hodgkin lymphoma of bone is exceedingly rare. Radiologically, lymphomas usually present as radiolucent lesions, sometimes disproportionately destructive when compared with the patient's clinical symptoms (e-**Fig. 46.52**). In about 20% of cases, the lesions present as radiodensities. The histologic findings recapitulate those seen in extraskeletal sites. The prognosis is dependent on the type of lymphoma and stage.

c. Langerhans cell histiocytosis (LCH) comprises a group of neoplastic Langerhans cell proliferations that can be unifocal (solitary eosinophilic granuloma), multifocal (Hand–Schuller–Christian disease), or disseminated (Letterer–Siwe disease). All can produce bone lesions that tend to present early in multifocal and disseminated forms. LCH most frequently involves the craniofacial bones, but other bones such as the femur, pelvis, and ribs may also be involved. Radiographically, the lesions appear radiolucent and rapidly destructive, sometimes with associated exuberant periosteal new bone formation when they occur in long bones (e-**Fig. 46.53**).

Histologically, there is a mixed inflammatory infiltrate including neutrophils, eosinophils, lymphocytes, and histiocytes (with or without giant cells) in which Langerhans cells are identified. Langerhans cells have eosinophilic to clear cytoplasm and contain oval, grooved, or multilobulated nuclei (e-**Fig. 46.54**); immunohistochemically, they characteristically express S100 protein and CD1a. Because there is a histologic similarity to chronic osteomyelitis, lesions thought to be LCH should be cultured. LCH has a very good prognosis except in the disseminated form, which is associated with a poor outcome (*Pediatr Blood Cancer* 2005;45:37). Recurrent *BRAF* V600E mutations are present in approximately 60% of LCH (*Blood* 2010;116:1919).

d. Erdheim–Chester disease is a rare disorder characterized by the presence of skeletal and extraskeletal foamy histiocytic infiltrates with associated fibrosis (e-**Fig. 46.55**). Most patients are older than 40 years, and there is usually bilateral symmetric or patchy sclerosis of the medullary cavity of the involved bones (most frequently the long bones of the extremity). Given the frequent and progressive infiltration of vital organs (such as the kidney, heart, or lung), most patients succumb within a few years. Recurrent *BRAF* V600E mutations are present in approximately 50% of cases of Erdheim—Chester disease (*Blood* 2012;120:2700).

6. Vascular tumors

a. Hemangioma. Although incidental hemangiomas are relatively common, clinically symptomatic tumors account for <1% of primary bone tumors and tend to present in late adulthood. Hemangioma is most frequently seen in the vertebrae, followed by the craniofacial skeleton and metaphyses of long bones. It appears as a radiolucent often expansive lesion in long bones, but as a vertically striate "corduroy pattern" lesion in intact vertebrae. Histologically, it is composed of capillary sized or cavernous vessels that permeate the marrow and are lined by bland endothelial cells (e-**Fig. 46.56**). The tumor is benign with low rates of recurrence following excision. A *EWSR1-NFATC1* fusion has been reported in one case of hemangioma of bone (*Am J Surg Pathol* 2013;37:613).

b. Epithelioid hemangioma is a locally aggressive neoplasm which occurs over a wide age range but is most common in adults. The tumor is most frequently found in long tubular bones (40%); the small bones of the distal lower extremity and hand, flat bones, and vertebrae are also not uncommonly involved (*Am J Surg Pathol* 2009;33:270). Multifocality is present in approximately 20% of cases. On plain film the lesion is a defined lytic lesion, which many show soft tissue extension. Lobular proliferations of epithelioid endothelial cells, often with intracytoplasmic lumina, form vascular channels and sheets. Myxohyaline chondroid-like matrix is not present. *FOS* rearrangements have been identified in epithelioid hemangioma, while a subset of cases with atypical features harbor *FOSB* fusions (*Genes Chromosomes Cancer* 2014;53:951).

c. Pseudomyogenic hemangioendothelioma/epithelioid sarcoma-like hemangioendothelioma most frequently presents as multiple tumors involving multiple tissue planes in the extremities in young to middle-aged adults. While purely skeletal disease is rare, bone involvement associated with soft tissue tumors is not uncommon. The imaging characteristics of this tumor range from sharply circumscribed to moth-eaten. Microscopically, the tumors are composed of plump spindled and epithelioid cells with relatively uniform round to ovoid vesicular nuclei and prominent eosinophilic cytoplasm. Tumor cells are arranged in sheets, nodules, and fascicles accompanied by a neutrophilic infiltrate (*Am J Surg Pathol* 2003;27:48; *Am J Surg Pathol* 2011;35:190). Rhabdomyoblast-like cells are often seen, while vascular channel formation is absent. Osseous lesions may be accompanied by prominent reactive bone. The tumors are positive for AE1/AE3, SMA (subset of cells, can be a focal finding), ERG, CD31 (50% of cases), and FOSB, while negative for CD34, EMA, S100 protein, desmin, and myogenin. INI1 expression is retained. *FOSB* rearrangements, typically *SERPINE1-FOSB*, are present (*J Pathol* 2014;232:534).

- **d. Epithelioid hemangioendothelioma** (EHE) is a malignant vascular tumor which can involve any skeletal site but is most common in long bones. Approximately 50% of patients have multiple tumors at presentation (e-**Fig. 46.57**), which have been show to represent metastatic disease (*Cancer Genet* 2012;205:12). On imaging, tumors are lytic with well to ill-defined margins. Microscopically, cords, nests, or sheets of plump cells that, in their attempt to form vessels, are often vacuolated; some of the vacuoles may contain erythrocytes. An extracellular myxoid or hyalinized stroma is characteristic, although not always identified. EHE with *YAP1-TFE3* fusions have more abundant eosinophilic cytoplasm, more vasoformative growth, and mild to moderate atypia. Tumor cells express CD31, CD34, ERG, FLI1, CAMTA1 (cases with *WWTR1-CAMTA1* fusions), and TFE3 (usually cases with *YAP1-TFE3* fusions). Of note, tumors may stain with keratin and EMA. The *WWTR1-CAMTA1* gene fusion is a characteristic feature of the majority of EHE, regardless of anatomic site (*Genes Chromosomes Cancer* 2011;50:44), while *YAP1-TFE3* is found in a small but distinct subset (*Genes Chromosomes Cancer* 2013;52:775).

- **e. Angiosarcoma** accounts for less than 1% of bone tumors and presents over a broad age range. Most tumors are radiolucent with poor margination, soft tissue extension, and periosteal reaction. Approximately 30% are multifocal. Angiosarcomas are usually characterized, at least focally, by the presence of irregularly anastomosing vascular channels that are lined by highly atypical endothelial cells, but they may largely consist of solid, patternless aggregates of polyhedral or spindle cells (e-**Fig. 46.58**). Poorly differentiated angiosarcomas may fail to express vascular markers. It should be noted that angiosarcomas express cytokeratins, which is an important consideration when metastatic carcinoma is in the differential diagnosis. Most angiosarcomas are associated with a poor outcome.

7. Epithelial tumors

- **a. Adamantinoma** comprises less than 1% of malignant bone tumors. The tumor occurs over a wide age distribution, with the median age of patients between 25 and 35 years. The tibia is most frequently involved, followed by the fibula, and both sites synchronously. Radiologically, an intracortical radiolucent lesion is evident, which may involve the medullary cavity (e-**Fig. 46.59**).

    Histologically, classic adamantinoma is composed of epithelial cells having a basaloid, tubular, or squamoid appearance; has a predominantly spindle cell pattern; or consists of a mixture of the two patterns (e-**Fig. 46.60**). A storiform fibroblastic proliferation that contains variable amounts of woven or lamellar bone may also be present. Rarely, the tumor is predominantly composed of the latter component, with only rare scattered epithelial cells (single or in small nests, sometimes only detected by immunohistochemistry); such tumors have been termed as having an "osteofibrous dysplasia-like pattern" or as "differentiated adamantinomas," and usually present in patients younger than 20 years. Adamantinomas are invariably immunopositive for various keratins and epithelial membrane antigen, and often also for vimentin. Classic adamantinomas are indolent tumors with a high local recurrence rate but metastasis occurs in about 20% of patients; differentiated adamantinomas almost never metastasize.

- **b. Metastatic carcinoma** is the most common tumor affecting the skeleton, which is the third most common site to be involved by metastatic carcinoma after the lungs and liver. Primary carcinomas of the breast, lung, prostate, kidney, and thyroid gland compose >80% of all bone metastases. Radiologically, metastatic deposits can be radiolucent or radiodense, or can display a mixed pattern (e-**Fig. 46.61**). Given its high incidence, metastatic carcinoma should always be in the differential diagnosis of solitary or multiple bone lesions in patients older than 40 years.

The histology usually resembles that of the primary carcinoma, if it is known. It should be noted that a fibroblastic, osteoblastic, or vascular response to the metastatic tumor may occasionally be quite prominent and overshadow the tumor cells, which may only be focally evident (e-**Fig. 46.62**). Consequently, immuno-histochemistry may reveal isolated subtle tumor cells that are not obvious in small biopsy specimens.

8. Ewing sarcoma and *BCOR*-rearranged sarcomas

a. **Ewing sarcoma (EWS).** In addition to its classic presentation in the diaphyses of long bones, the tumor can involve axial bones such as the pelvis and ribs, as well as soft tissues (see Chapter 44) and other organs. EWS has been described at various ages, but most patients are younger than 20 years. Although patients usually have pain and a mass, they may also present with fever and leukocytosis suggestive of an infectious process. Radiologically, a destructive permeative lesion is usually evident, often with an overlying multilayered but discontinuous "onion-skin" periosteal reaction (e-**Fig. 46.63**). Occasionally, there is a large soft tissue mass with no obvious bone destruction on the routine radiographs, but the intraosseous component becomes evident on a CT scan or MRI.

Histologically, EWS is the prototype for "small round cell tumors" as it is composed of sheets of such cells, often with glycogen-containing clear cytoplasm (e-**Fig. 46.64**). Some tumors show Homer–Wright rosettes which are characterized by groups of tumor cells that surround a central core of eosinophilic extracellular material. Immunohistochemically, EWS shows characteristic strong cell membrane immunoreactivity for CD99, negativity for CD45, and variable reactivity for neural markers such as NSE, synaptophysin, CD57, NF, and S100 protein. Cytokeratins may also be positive.

A characteristic feature of this tumor is the presence of a recurrent balanced reciprocal translocation involving the *EWSR1* gene on chromosome 22 and a member of the *Ets* family of genes, the most common of which (85% of cases) is the *FLI-1* gene on chromosome 11 (*Br J Cancer* 1994;70:908). A small minority of cases harbor fusions of *EWSR1* with non-*Ets* genes, or *FUS* rearrangements instead of *EWSR1*. The prognosis of EWS has greatly improved with multimodality treatment, and 5-year survival rates now approach 70%.

b. ***BCOR*-rearranged sarcomas** have a predilection for adolescents, frequently arise in bone, and are composed of monotonous small round cells with areas of spindled morphology (*Nat Genet* 2012;44:461). The tumor cells are positive for BCOR, CD99 (variable), and CCNB3 (in tumors with *CCNB3* rearrangements). While data are limited, these tumors appear to have a more favorable prognosis compared with EWS. *BCOR* is most frequently fused with *CCNB3*.

9. Notochordal tumors

a. **Benign notochordal cell tumor** (BNCT) is an indolent notochordal cell proliferation which almost always involves the axial skeleton. Unlike chordoma, it usually appears as a sclerotic lesion without extraosseous extension. Histologically, BNCT is composed of sheets of large polygonal cell with distinct cell borders, clear vacuolated to eosinophilic cytoplasm, and minimal nuclear atypia. Tumor cells may resemble adipocytes. Myxoid stroma is not present. The tumor cells are positive for brachyury, keratin, EMA, and S100 protein expression. Tumors with features of BNCT but with minimal soft tissue extension and/or focal myxoid stroma appear to pursue a benign course; however, given the limited available data, such tumors may provisionally be designated atypical notochordal cell tumor (*Am J Surg Pathol* 2017;41:39).

b. Chordomas are malignant tumors with notochordal differentiation and account for approximately 4% of malignant bone tumors. Most tumors present after 30 years of age with a peak incidence between 50 and 60 years of age. The midline of the axial skeleton, particularly the sacrum and the base of the skull, is usually affected. Radiologically, a lucent lesion is seen with scattered calcifications; there is often a large associated soft-tissue component (e-**Fig. 46.65**). Histologically, chordomas are composed of lobules of tumor in which sheets, cords, or nests of vacuolated, eosinophilic to clear cells are embedded in a myxoid matrix (e-**Fig. 46.66**). Areas of hyaline cartilage characterize chondroid chordoma. Chordomas express brachyury, cytokeratins, EMA, and S100 protein. Chordomas are aggressive tumors that are most notable for local recurrence when incompletely excised, but also have metastatic potential. Dedifferentiated chordoma, which has a high-grade sarcomatous component, is associated with a very poor outcome.

10. Cystic/cyst-like lesions

a. Simple bone cyst is an intraosseous space-occupying lesion consisting of an accumulation of fluid. The lesion is usually lined by a thin membrane composed of flattened cells of unknown type that may be involved in the production of the fluid, which usually appears serous. The base of the lesion is usually situated at an active growth plate, and the cyst is more or less maintained by continuous remodeling of the bone around the area of fluid pressure. The lesion is circumscribed and radiolucent, and usually involves the proximal humeral, femoral, or tibial region (e-**Fig. 46.67**). It does not expand the bone or cause deformity unless there has been a fracture with displacement prior to healing, and it tends to be symmetric. While fluid may not be obvious radiographically, the contents are demonstrable by MRI. Histologically, the diagnosis is one of exclusion and depends upon correlation of the imaging, operative findings, and lack of any other diagnostic tissue. Because most simple cysts are treated conservatively by injection of steroids or other sclerosing agents, it is unusual to see the lining of a simple cyst histologically unless there has been repeated fracture.

b. Intraosseous ganglion. This is a subarticular defect in the cancellous bone filled with mucoid fluid. The bone surrounding the defect is remodeled and sometimes sclerotic (e-**Fig. 46.68**). The defect is histologically similar to the subarticular cysts associated with overlying osteoarthritis (geodes), except that the subarticular plate and articular cartilage are radiographically intact in patients with intraosseous ganglia. The lesion is presumed to arise from a microscopic continuity of the subarticular plate with the joint space that either cannot be detected by imaging studies or that has healed; this etiology would allow pressurized synovial fluid to come in contact with the intertrabecular medullary space. There are no diagnostic features histologically as the concentrated fluid is practically acellular and resembles the contents of tenosynovial ganglia.

c. Aneurysmal bone cyst (ABC). This peculiar lesion derives its name from its expansile character. It is not a true cyst, but rather a collection of blood-filled spaces that are separated by fibro-osseous tissue septa containing a varying number of multinucleated giant cells in a varying amount of immature bone. Most ABCs occur prior to 20 years of age. The lesion usually arises as an eccentric radiolucent lesion in metaphyses of long bones (e-**Fig. 46.69**). When it is central and symmetric it can often be distinguished from a simple cyst because it causes the bone to become wider than the growth plate. While its internal edge tends to be well marginated radiographically, ABC sometimes extends across adjacent bones, particularly if it arises in the spine. Complementary imaging studies, particularly MRI, reveal peculiar fluid–fluid levels on T2-weighted axial and sagittal views (e-**Fig. 46.70**); these levels are caused by the signal differences in erythrocytes and plasma, reflect erythrocyte sedimentation, and demonstrate that blood in intact ABC is both unclotted and stagnant or slow moving.

Histologically, the lesion has vascular spaces that progress from very small capillary spaces to very large sinusoids separated by fibrous septae and sometimes by bone (e-**Fig. 46.71**). Within the septae are fibroblasts, scattered multinucleated giant cells, and osteoblasts associated with the bone production. Rarely, the lesion is almost entirely solid, although sometimes the solid variant may demonstrate fluid levels on imaging. In about half of cases there is some other lesion associated with the cyst and admixed with curetted fragments; this has been termed secondary ABC. The associated lesion is usually benign, although malignant tumors have also been described in association with ABC. Primary ABC are neoplasms which harbor rearrangements of the *USP6* gene and/or the *CDH11* gene, while secondary ABC do not have these alternations (*Am J Pathol* 2004;165:1773).

11. **Undifferentiated high-grade pleomorphic sarcoma.** These tumors are similar to their soft tissue counterparts, with most cases developing in patients older than 40 years. It can also complicate Paget disease, or occur after irradiation or infarction. Most cases involve the long bones of the extremities or the pelvis. Histologically, there is a mixed population of spindle cells, histiocytic cells, and giant cells. Pleomorphic tumor cells, abnormal mitotic figures, and the characteristic storiform pattern of growth are also evident (e-**Fig. 46.72**). Almost all of the histologic subtypes described in soft tissue have also been described in bone. The focal identification of osteoid or bone matrix is sometimes the only histologic difference between undifferentiated high-grade pleomorphic sarcoma and osteosarcoma, although most osteosarcomas arising in this age group are secondary to a prior disease or treatment.

12. **Other rare primary bone neoplasms.** There are other benign and malignant soft-tissue neoplasms that can primarily arise in bone, including leiomyoma, leiomyosarcoma, lipoma, liposarcoma, and schwannoma. All of these are histologically similar to their soft-tissue counterparts (see Chapter 44).

ACKNOWLEDGMENT

The authors thank Omar Hameed and Michael J. Klein, authors of the previous editions of this chapter.

47 Metabolic Diseases of Bone

Deborah Veis

I. NORMAL ANATOMY. Because of its accessibility and composition of both cortical and trabecular (cancellous) bone, the iliac crest is the site of choice for evaluation of systemic metabolic bone diseases (MBDs). Cortex forms the external layer of all bones, comprises approximately 80% of bone mass, and supports most of the tissue's mechanical function. Trabecular bone, the meshwork surrounded by marrow or fat, is much more metabolically active than cortex. To support both its mechanical and metabolic functions, bone is dynamically regulated, and the skeleton is replaced completely every 10 years. The process of replacement, known as remodeling or turnover, is accomplished by the coordinated action of bone-forming osteoblasts and bone-resorbing osteoclasts, and is regulated by a variety of systemic factors including calcium, phosphorus, and parathyroid hormone (PTH). The goal of iliac crest biopsy is to assess this process.

In either the cortex or trabeculum, remodeling begins when mononuclear osteoclast precursors (derived from hematopoietic progenitors) arrive at a bone surface, fuse, and differentiate into functional polykaryons (Fig. 47.1). Mature osteoclasts polarize and secrete acid and proteases onto an isolated microenvironment of the bone surface, excavating a pit known as Howship lacuna. This resorption phase ends with the osteoclasts' apoptosis, and a reversal phase follows, characterized by activation of osteoblasts (of mesenchymal origin) to replace the excavated bone; the activity of osteoclasts and osteoblasts is normally tightly coupled, and the amount of bone synthesized matches the amount resorbed. Newly secreted matrix called osteoid becomes mineralized to form mature bone. The remodeling cycle ends when new bone formation is complete, and the osteoblasts are either incorporated into the new bone matrix as osteocytes, or become quiescent surface bone lining cells. The net result of each cycle is the formation of a new osteon, a packet of bone delineated by a "cement line" in which the collagen fibers are aligned. These lamellae of bone are easily seen when decalcified hematoxylin and eosin (H&E)-stained sections are examined under polarized light (e-**Fig. 47.1**). Some osteoblasts become encased in matrix and mature into osteocytes. In normal bone, their long axis is typically parallel to that of their neighbors and the lamellae, but in rapidly formed woven bone, as in repair or high turnover diseases such as Juvenile Paget's Disease, their orientation is random and they have an increased density in the matrix.

Osteoclasts can be identified by their characteristic appearance as multinucleated cells on the bone surface, with discrete nuclei (in contrast to megakaryocytes, which have fused nuclei). The most sensitive method of identifying osteoclasts histologically is expression of tartrate-resistant acid phosphatase (TRAP), which stains osteoclasts bright red (e-**Fig. 47.2**), although this is not usually necessary for diagnosis. Osteoblasts appear as cuboidal cells on the bone surface, often in rows, with abundant cytoplasm and an eccentric nucleus (e-**Fig. 47.3**). The strength of the undecalcified biopsy is in the evaluation of the function of these cells rather than their morphology. Osteoblasts secrete matrix proteins onto the bone surface, but several days are required for mineral deposition. Therefore, the extent of bone surface covered by osteoid (osteoid surface) is one indicator of osteoblast activity. The thickness of the osteoid seams reflects the rate of mineral apposition, because mineralization converts osteoid to bone. Decalcification required for standard paraffin processing removes the distinction between newly synthesized osteoid and mature calcified bone. In contrast, undecalcified plastic sections can be stained in several ways to demonstrate osteoid. The von Kossa stain, a silver-based stain used with a basic fuchsin

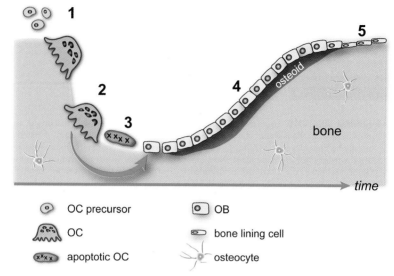

Figure 47.1 The bone remodeling cycle. *1.* Osteoclast (OC) precursors are recruited to the bone surface, where they fuse and differentiate into mature polykaryons. *2.* The osteoclasts resorb both organic and inorganic matrix of bone. *3.* The resorption phase ends with osteoclast apoptosis. *4.* During the reversal phase, osteoblasts (OB) differentiate from mesenchymal precursors under the influence of factors from osteoclasts (*curved arrow*) and secrete new bone matrix known as osteoid. *5.* At the end of the remodeling cycle, some osteoblasts have been incorporated into the bone and become osteocytes, whereas others remain on the surface as synthetically quiescent bone-lining cells.

counterstain, shows calcified bone matrix as dark brown or black, whereas the unmineralized matrix (osteoid) appears pink-red (e-**Fig.** 47.4A). A trichrome stain, either Goldner (e-**Fig.** 47.3) or modified Masson (e-**Fig.** 47.4B), also distinguishes mineralized bone from osteoid. These latter stains allow easier interpretation of cellular morphology than the von Kossa, and also highlight peritrabecular or marrow fibrosis.

A second critical marker of osteoblast function is tetracycline labeling. Tetracycline family antibiotics are calcium-chelating fluorochromes that bind to actively mineralizing bone surfaces, can be taken orally, and are well tolerated. They are given in 2 courses, separated by 2 weeks (see below). If bone formation is active during both intervals, examination of unstained sections by fluorescence microscopy demonstrates two bright bands of labeling (a double label) (e-**Fig.** 47.5). Similarly, active bone formation during only one of the labeling periods yields a single tetracycline label (e-**Fig.** 47.5). Combination of the extent of labeled trabecular bone surface and the distance between labels provides the mineral apposition rate and bone formation rate. In a normal subject, most surfaces with osteoid, as seen on trichrome or von Kossa stains, have single or double labels.

During normal endochondral bone development, cartilage formed at the growth plate is replaced by bone in the primary spongiosa through the action of osteoclasts. Toluidine blue stains cartilage purple, and cartilage may be found within trabeculae near the growth plate in children (e-**Fig.** 47.6). However, a finding of entrapped cartilage in an iliac crest bone biopsy in an adult, or >1 cm from the growth plate in a child, is indicative of osteoclast dysfunction such as in osteopetrosis.

II. INDICATIONS FOR BIOPSY, TISSUE SAMPLING, AND PREPARATION

A. Indications for Biopsy. The most common indications for metabolic bone biopsy are end-stage renal disease (ESRD) and unexplained hypercalcemia or hyperphosphatemia, osteoporosis unresponsive to therapy, or suspected osteomalacia. Patients who have multiple or unexplained fractures (particularly if they are failing to heal), unexplained bone pain, an elevation in serum alkaline phosphatase, or a suspected rare MBD may also be candidates.

B. Biopsy Procedure. A critical component of evaluation of metabolic bone biopsies is in vivo fluorochrome labeling of bone via use of a regimen of tetracycline (250 mg PO qid) orally four times a day or demeclocycline (150 mg qid or 300 mg bid) for 3 days, followed by a 14-day interval, then 3 more days of therapy. Some other tetracycline antibiotics such as doxycycline do not fluoresce well, so care must be taken that pharmacists do not make substitutions. Biopsy is performed 3 to 5 days after the last dose. Biopsy interpretation may therefore be confounded by recent antibiotic use of drugs in the tetracycline family. Similarly, inadequate labeling can be caused by malabsorption syndromes or by taking tetracycline with meals, dairy products, iron-containing medications, antacids, or calcium supplements. For patients on dialysis, biopsy should be one day after, and not the same day.

Biopsy is performed as an outpatient procedure; the most accessible site for biopsy is the anterior iliac crest, typically with a horizontal approach. When obtained, the specimen should be placed directly into 70% ethanol.

C. Sample Preparation. The specimen should be fixed in 70% ethanol for at least 48 hours, and this solution is suitable for shipping and long-term storage at room temperature. Following dehydration with xylene, the specimen is mounted in methyl methacrylate, and the tissue core is sectioned parallel to its long axis at 5 to 7 μm thickness using a tungsten blade. Undecalcified sections are stained with von Kossa, Goldner or modified Masson trichrome, and toluidine blue. Thicker 10-μm sections are coverslipped without staining for examination under fluorescence.

D. Quantitative Versus Qualitative Evaluation. The American Society for Bone and Mineral Research has described a nomenclature for a basic set of structural and kinetic features identified by undecalcified bone biopsy (*J Bone Miner Res* 2013;28:2), and there are two commercially available systems that allow quantitative analysis based on these standards (OsteoMeasure, OsteoMetrics, Inc. and Bioquant Osteo II, BIOQUANT Image Analysis Corporation). Reference values, based on somewhat limited populations, have been published (*J Bone Miner Res* 1988;3:133; *J Bone Miner Res* 2004;19:1628; *Bone* 2000;26:103; *N Engl J Med* 1988;319:1698). Although some laboratories perform quantitative analysis on all specimens, qualitative assessments are often adequate for diagnosis of individual patients. Quantitative analysis is most useful in the setting of research studies.

III. DIAGNOSTIC FEATURES OF METABOLIC BONE DISORDERS

A. Osteoporosis. In the setting of osteoporosis or osteopenia, biopsy establishes the rate of bone remodeling (turnover), degree of mineralization, architectural integrity, and effects of treatment. Iliac crest bone biopsy is a poor indicator of bone mass, as bone volume/tissue volume (BV/TV) is variable within this region. However, trabecular connectivity, which describes the intactness of the trabecular meshwork, correlates with bone mass. In osteoporosis/osteopenia, trabeculae are very small and often appear as isolated islands (low connectivity), rather than as an interconnected grid (good connectivity) (e-**Fig. 47.7**). In high-turnover osteoporosis, osteoid surface is enhanced (e-**Fig. 47.8A**), with normal or increased numbers of osteoclasts and osteoblasts. The extent of double tetracycline-labeled trabecular bone surface is also increased, although the distance between the double labels is usually normal (e-**Fig. 47.8B**). In low-turnover osteoporosis or osteopenia, there is little osteoid, few osteoclasts or osteoblasts, and rare or absent trabecular double tetracycline labels (e-**Fig. 47.9**). Even in low-turnover states, double labeling in the cortex is usually present, and is a good positive control for adequate tetracycline dosing and specimen processing.

Many patients with osteoporosis have been treated with bisphosphonates, often for several years. Although biopsy studies have shown that normal turnover is intact in most patients (*JAMA* 2006;296:2927), some cases of suppressed bone turnover have been reported and are associated with increased fractures (*J Clin Endocrinol Metab* 2005;90:1294; *N Engl J Med* 2006;355:2048; *Clin Cases Miner Bone Metab* 2015;12:273). Bisphosphonates target the osteoclast, decreasing resorption and enhancing apoptosis, producing changes that can readily be seen in tissue sections with osteoclasts appearing either hyperchromatic with pyknotic nuclei (e-**Fig. 47.10A**) or round and unpolarized (e-**Fig. 47.10B**).

B. **Osteomalacia.** In osteomalacia, newly formed organic bone matrix fails to mineralize normally, and the result is wide osteoid seams, often greatly increased in extent along the trabecular bone surface (e-**Fig. 47.11A**). Some osteoid may be completely unlabeled by tetracycline (e-**Fig. 47.11B**), whereas other surfaces may show irregular and diffuse fluorescence (e-**Fig. 47.11C**); double tetracycline labels are infrequent. Florid osteomalacia due to nutritional rickets (vitamin D deficiency) is rare, but milder cases may be found unexpectedly and bone biopsy is the only definitive diagnostic tool. Osteomalacia is also seen in fluorosis, usually caused by excessive fluoride in drinking water (e-**Fig. 47.11D** and E). The degree of osteomalacia in hypophosphatasia, a rare deficiency of alkaline phosphatase activity, can be quite severe (e-**Fig. 47.11F**).

Tumor-induced osteomalacia (TIO, also known as oncogenic osteomalacia) is a rare form of osteomalacia that can occur in both adults and children. Iliac crest bone biopsy in TIO shows the typical features of osteomalacia described above (e-**Fig. 47.12A**). The bone manifestations of TIO are caused by mesenchymal tumors that secrete the phosphatonin FGF-23, leading to hypophosphatemia due to renal phosphate wasting. The tumors are typically small and slow-growing, and can be difficult to detect. If not visible by CT or MRI, sestamibi or octreotide scans may be useful, as well as targeted venous sampling for FGF-23 (*Expert Rev Endocrinol Metab* 2009;4:435). Histologically, the majority of the tumors in cases of TIO are best characterized as **phosphaturic mesenchymal tumor (mixed connective tissue variant)** and have low cellularity, bland spindled cells, distinctive "grungy" calcified matrix, and an incomplete rim of membranous ossification and/or formation of an osteoid-like matrix at least focally (*Am J Surg Pathol* 2004;28:1) (e-**Fig. 47.12B**). They may be locally infiltrative into muscle or fat (e-**Fig. 47.12C**), have prominent vessels reminiscent of hemangiopericytoma, myxoid change, hemorrhage, or osteoclasts. TIO tumors typically stain for FGF23 but not S100, CD34, or smooth muscle actin. Resection of the solitary tumor mass results in complete resolution of hypophosphatemia and clinical symptoms in the majority of cases.

C. **Renal Osteodystrophy.** Chronic kidney disease–metabolic bone disease (CKD–MBD) has been defined as a systemic disorder of bone and mineral metabolism due to CKD manifested by one or more of the following: (1) Abnormalities of calcium, phosphorus, PTH, or vitamin D metabolism; (2) Abnormalities of bone turnover, mineralization, volume, linear growth, or strength; (3) Vascular or other soft tissue calcification (*Kidney Int* 2006;69:1945; *Kidney Int Suppl* 2017;7:1). CKD–MBD is associated with increased morbidity and mortality. Three predominant patterns in bone biopsy have been described: high bone turnover with osteitis fibrosa (hyperparathyroid bone disease), low bone turnover (including low-turnover osteomalacia and adynamic bone disease), and mixed uremic osteodystrophy.

1. The most important role of biopsy is in the setting of **hypercalcemia**, in which a finding of PTH-driven high turnover indicates a need for parathyroidectomy, whereas a finding of low turnover is a contraindication for this surgery. Bone changes can occur relatively early in CKD, and low turnover correlates with increased vascular calcification.

2. **In high turnover renal osteodystrophy,** elevated PTH levels drive bone resorption by many osteoclasts; peritrabecular fibrosis, also known as osteitis fibrosa, may also be present (e-**Fig. 47.13A**). Bone formation is accelerated, often with formation of disorganized woven bone (seen on polarization; e-**Fig. 47.13B**) and increased

tetracycline double labels (e-**Fig. 47.13C**). Trabeculae may be irregular in shape, and the cortex may be porous due to increased resorption.

3. In either form of **low turnover osteodystrophy**, trabecular surfaces appear quiescent, with few osteoblasts or osteoclasts. Trabecular connectivity may also be decreased, and this parameter is more useful than the overall BV/TV (as mentioned above in the discussion of osteoporosis). In the osteomalacic form of renal osteodystrophy, mineralization is delayed and wide osteoid seams identified by von Kossa or trichrome staining (e-**Fig. 47.14A**) are not tetracycline labeled (e-**Fig. 47.14B**). In adynamic bone disease, both osteoid (e-**Fig. 47.14C**) and tetracycline labels (e-**Fig. 47.14D**) are minimal or absent. In the past, aluminum toxicity from dialysis was often the cause of low turnover renal osteodystrophy, but the etiology of the adynamic changes seen more recently is not known.

4. **Mixed uremic osteodystrophy,** as the name implies, shows features of increased PTH and defective mineralization. Additionally, the appearance may vary considerably within the specimen (e-**Fig. 47.15A**), with areas of increased turnover adjacent to more quiescent regions with poor mineralization. Some areas may show abundant osteoid and robust tetracycline double labels (e-**Fig. 47.15B** and **C**) adjacent to broad single labels or unlabeled osteoid (e-**Fig. 47.15D**).

D. **Glucocorticoid-Induced Osteoporosis.** Because long-term glucocorticoid therapy is widely used in chronic inflammatory diseases and in organ transplantation, there is a high prevalence of glucocorticoid-induced bone disease. Early in treatment, glucocorticoids increase bone resorption, but more prolonged therapy eventuates in adynamic bone in which the number of osteoclasts and osteoblasts is decreased, as is tetracycline double labeling.

E. **Primary Hyperparathyroidism.** Diagnosis of most cases of primary hyperparathyroidism is based on elevated serum calcium and PTH levels. However, in normocalcemic patients with variable or borderline PTH levels, bone biopsy can be useful in making the diagnosis because histologic findings represent the net effect of PTH over time. As in secondary hyperparathyroidism, such as in high-turnover renal osteodystrophy, sections typically show increased osteoid surfaces (some with woven bone), increased tetracycline labeling, and elevated numbers of osteoclasts and osteoblasts. Osteitis fibrosa cystica, the formation of cystic bone loss due to elevated osteoclast activity associated with marrow fibrosis, is found only in severe cases and due to routine testing of serum calcium is rarely seen. However, peritrabecular fibrosis may be present. Another effect of PTH is to increase the porosity of the cortex, which may be difficult to distinguish from trabecular bone.

Focal well-demarcated osteolytic lesions known as **brown tumors** are also associated with hyperparathyroidism (e-**Fig 47.16**). Brown tumors consist of clusters of multinucleated giant cells in a fibrotic stroma, and the associated islands of bone are often woven rather than lamellar. Brown tumors can occur in any bone as a single lesion, or be multifocal. They generally resolve when PTH levels are restored to normal.

SUGGESTED READINGS

Carvalho C, Alves CM, Frazao JM. The role of bone biopsy for the diagnosis of renal osteodystrophy: a short overview and future perspectives. *J Nephrol* 2016; 29:617–626.

Dempster DW, Compston JE, Drezner MK, Glorieux FH, Kanis JA, Malluche H, et al. Standardized nomenclature, symbols, and units for bone histomorphometry: a 2012 update of the report of the ASBMR Histomorphometry Nomenclature Committee. *J Bone Miner Res* 2013;28:2–17.

Recker RR, Aguilar Moreira C. In: Bilezikian JP, ed. *Primer on the Metabolic Bone Diseases and Disorders of Mineral Metabolism.* Washington, DC: American Society for Bone and Mineral Research; 2018:310–318.

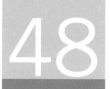

Joints and Synovium

Lingxin Zhang, Peter A. Humphrey, and
John S.A. Chrisinger

I. NORMAL ANATOMY. Joints are composed of the ends of contiguous bones and the associated soft tissue elements, including cartilage, ligaments, tendons, and synovium. The scope of this chapter focuses on diarthrodial (synovial) joint. Grossly, diarthrodial joints are covered by smooth hyaline cartilage. Histologically, this articular cartilage is hypocellular with a glassy extracellular matrix composed mainly of collagen, proteoglycan, and water. Embedded within the matrix are chondrocytes within surrounding spaces (lacunae). There are four zones in the articular cartilage—superficial, mid, deep, and calcified (e-**Fig. 48.1**)—and chondrocytes have a different appearance depending on their location. Those near the surface of the articular cartilage are small and flattened; in the mid and deep zones, the chondrocytes are more rounded and arranged in columns. A thin, basophilic line known as the tidemark, which represents the mineralized front, separates the mid and calcified layers of articular cartilage. The calcified cartilage base interdigitates with the underlying subchondral bone.

Ligaments, which join two adjacent bones, are formed mainly of collagen. Tendons are connective tissue structures connecting the muscle to the bone. Microscopically, there is often an intermediate tissue at the interface between the fibrous tissue and the bone (known as enthesis), which is either a hyaline cartilage or a fibrocartilage. Under polarized light, collagen fibers (Sharpey fibers) pass through this tissue.

The synovium is a glistening white membrane with a flat, single layer of lining cells that lack intercellular junctions and an intact basement membrane (e-**Fig. 48.2**). Biologically, this architecture is believed to allow free exchange of cells and molecules through the synovium. A fibrous or fibroadipose supporting layer lies beneath the synovial cell layer, which is moderately vascular. The synovium also lines tendon sheaths and bursae.

II. GROSS EXAMINATION AND TISSUE SAMPLING. Joint tissue, including bone, cartilage, synovium, enthesis, and meniscus, can be received from orthopedic procedures such as primary and revision arthroplasties, arthroscopic or open excision of intra-articular tumors. If fragments are received, the number, color, shape, and aggregate size of the fragments should be recorded. If chalky white deposits are identified, a fresh wet preparation can be prepared if a polarizing microscope is available. If not, some of the tissue should be placed into absolute (100%) alcohol to preserve the crystals. Bony tissue is sectioned with a bone saw and submitted following decalcification. For both accurate prognostication and quality assurance, tissue sampling for microscopic examination is not only justified but should be mandatory for primary and revision arthroplasties.

A. Revision Arthroplasties. The bone and soft tissue at the implant interface should be examined for the presence or absence of discoloration, loosening, necrosis, a purulent exudate, and wear particles. The explanted prosthesis should be described, including any identification numbers or defects.

B. Soft Tissue Tumors. For excised intra- or extra-articular masses, size, color, consistency, shape, and nodularity (single vs. multiple) should be provided. The outer surface of the specimen should then be inked, and cut sections should be characterized as to the color, presence or absence of hemorrhage and necrosis, and distance of tumor to inked margin. One section per centimeter of tumor is a useful guide for section submission. Demonstration of the tumor in relation to the closest inked margin(s) and to any recognizable normal tissue is important.

C. **Joint Replacement Surgeries.** The hips and knees are the two most commonly replaced large joints. A systemic approach to the macroscopic examination of each joint component is particularly important to discover the underlying pathogenesis. The overall dimensions of the submitted bone and soft tissue, the shape and contour of the articular surfaces, the presence of trauma or dysplasia, should be recorded. When examining the knee joint, an abnormality should be localized to a specific compartment (medial, lateral, or patello-femoral). Articular cartilage color, thickness, and abnormalities such as loss, erosion, cleft or tuft formation, detachment, corrugation, crystalline deposits and bony and cartilaginous overgrowths (osteophytes or exostosis) should be documented. Synovium color, consistency (soft, rubbery), surface proliferation (nodular, villous/papillary), and pannus formation should be described. One or several sections of the synovium should be submitted. Any associated gross bone defects, such as sclerosis, bony necrosis, subchondral fracture, pseudocyst formation, and marrow abnormalities, should be noted. Sections of macroscopically abnormal areas should be submitted for histologic examination as follows: the bone and overlying cartilage should be fixed overnight in formalin, decalcified, and sectioned into 3- to 5-mm slices. One or two sections are usually sufficient to document cartilaginous and associated bone abnormalities; the sections should demonstrate the junction of normal and abnormal cartilage with the underlying bone.

III. **DIAGNOSTIC FEATURES OF COMMON DISEASES OF JOINTS AND SYNOVIUM.** The use of polarizing plates in the histologic examination of joints and synovium is very helpful for analyzing crystals and the nature of connective tissue fibers.

In terms of joint disorders, a two-tier (non-inflammatory, inflammatory) (Klein MJ, Bonar SF, Freemont T, et al. *Atlas of Nontumor Pathology: Non-Neoplastic Diseases of Bones and Joints.* ARP Press, 2011) or three-tier (degenerative, inflammatory, metabolic) (McCarthy EF, Frassica FJ. *Pathology of Bone and Joint Disorders: With Clinical and Radiographic Correlation.* Cambridge University Press, 2014) general classification system applies. Non-inflammatory disorders include the prototypal osteoarthritis, avascular necrosis, subchondral insufficiency fracture, rapidly progressive osteoarthritis, neuropathic arthropathy (Charcot joint), dysplasias, and post-traumatic arthropathy. Rheumatoid arthritis, seronegative spondyloarthropathies and septic/infectious arthritis are the major inflammatory etiologies for joint destruction. Metabolic diseases cause crystal or aberrant chemical component deposition, ultimately increase the risk for degenerative joint diseases. A joint may be affected by more than one disorders. Osteonecrosis can be multifactorial from infection, trauma, or other processes that interrupt blood flow. The convex surfaces of the end of long bones are particularly susceptible. Primary synovial tumors are rare, the four most common are synovial chondromatosis, tenosynovial giant cell tumor (TSGT), lipoma arborescens, and synovial hemangioma, and all typically have a monoarticular distribution.

A. **Osteoarthritis** is a noninflammatory arthropathy which is a common manifestation of a heterogeneous group of disorders. It is the most common disease of the joints; after the age of 65 years the prevalence is about 60% in men and 70% in women. The etiology of osteoarthritis is multifactorial. Major trauma, repetitive joint use, chronic inflammatory arthritis, and congenital malformations are major risk factors. The diagnosis is usually based on clinical and radiographic features.

Grossly, cartilaginous thinning, disruption, and fibrillation can be seen. In areas of complete cartilage loss, the underlying bone is exposed; this bone has a dense polished appearance like marble (known as eburnation). Microscopically, vertical clefts in the cartilage are characteristic (**e-Fig. 48.3**), with reduplication of the tidemark. There may be associated villous hyperplasia and mild chronic inflammation of the synovium (which should not be confused with rheumatoid arthritis). Papillary masses of the metaplastic cartilage, bone, or adipose tissue may form in the synovial membrane; detachment of the masses results in intra-articular loose bodies. In eburnated areas, the bone may show sclerotic thickened bony trabeculae, cysts with fluid and fibromyxoid tissue, and superficial bony necrosis.

Since the 1990s, several entities have been isolated from osteoarthritis due to their distinct clinical, radiologic and histologic features. **Subchondral insufficiency fracture** (*Rev Rhum Engl Ed* 1996;63:859; *Arthritis Rheu* 1999;42:2719) affects elderly patients and has a predilection for women. The fracture occurs beneath the subchondral bony end plate, particularly the hip joint, and incites intense pain that is out of proportion to the subtle radiologic change. **Rapidly progressive osteoarthritis** (*J Bone Joint Surg Am* 2000;82:858; *Ann Rheum Dis* 2008;67:1783) is another recognized entity and a relationship has been suggested between the two. Accelerated joint destruction occurs in the measure of months. Histologically, a large amount of bony and cartilaginous detritus induces dramatic cellular reaction.

B. Neuropathic Joint (Charcot Disease) is a noninflammatory joint disorder affecting weight-bearing joints as a result of denervation. It was originally described in association with tabes dorsalis. Currently, neuropathic damage secondary to diabetes or alcohol is the most common cause. Radiologically, there is severe deformation of the joint. Osteopenia or hyperostosis with osteophyte development may be seen. Histologically, many of the findings overlap with osteoarthritis, such as osteosclerosis, cyst formation, and synovial villous hyperplasia. However, a larger volume of bone and cartilage debris (and a larger size of the individual fragments themselves) with an associated foreign-body–type giant cell reaction within the synovium is more typical of a neuropathic joint.

C. Rheumatoid Arthritis is a chronic multisystem disease of unknown cause. The hallmark of rheumatoid arthritis is a chronic inflammatory synovitis, typically involving multiple joints in the hands and feet in a symmetric distribution. Clinically, the synovial inflammation causes swelling, tenderness, and limitation of motion. Histologically, there is hypertrophy and hyperplasia of the synovium along with a lymphoplasmacytic infiltrate, which together generate a papillary/polypoid chronic synovitis (**e-Fig. 48.4**). Lymphoid follicles and acute fibrinous surface exudate (**e-Fig. 48.5**) can also be seen. Synovial giant cells and bone and cartilage fragments may be present in the synovium. The overall histologic picture is not specific for rheumatoid arthritis, and similar changes may be seen in other arthritides such as systemic lupus erythematosus and psoriasis. Of note, in certain inflammatory arthropathies, subarticular pseudoabscesses can be found and should not be misinterpreted as evidence of infection. These pseudoabscesses have been described in rheumatoid arthritis, but are especially characteristic of psoriatic arthritis.

Destruction of cartilage and joint fusion (ankylosis) can occur due to the formation of pannus (inflamed synovium and granulation tissue) over the surface of the articular cartilage, with invasion into cartilage and even bone and joint capsule.

Extra-articular manifestations of rheumatoid arthritis, which usually occur in patients with high titers of rheumatoid factor, include rheumatoid nodules, vasculitis, pleuropulmonary involvement (such as fibrosis and serositis), and splenomegaly with neutropenia in the Felty syndrome. Rheumatoid nodules develop in about 25% of patients with rheumatoid arthritis. Although common locations include the olecranon bursa, proximal ulna, and Achilles tendon, they can also be found in the heart, lung, pleura, kidney, and meninges. Histologically, there is a central zone of fibrinoid necrosis surrounded by palisading histiocytes (**e-Fig. 48.6**).

D. Synovitis Associated With Loose Large Joint Arthroplasty can be seen when there is failure of a total joint replacement, and can be related to a foreign-body–type inflammatory response or infection. The foreign material can be metal, plastic/polyethylene, and/or methyl methacrylate cement. Microscopically, metallic particles are present as 1- to 3-μm particles within macrophages. Needle-shaped, polarizable fragments of polyethylene plastic usually are found in foreign-body giant cells. Methyl methacrylate cement is lost upon processing, and consequently the cement causes empty spaces within foreign-body–type giant cells in histologic sections after routine processing. These different types of foreign material can also elicit an exuberant fibrohistiocytic response (**e-Fig. 48.7**).

When neutrophils are seen, particularly when they are numerous, the possibility of infection should be considered. Frozen section of the inflamed tissue from a failed joint replacement may be requested, and the number of neutrophils per high-power field

(HPF) should be reported. At least five HPFs on at least two sections should be examined. The presence of ≤5 neutrophils per HPF in tissue (not fibrin) has high specificity (about 95%) for the absence of infection, whereas the presence of >5 neutrophils per HPF has a sensitivity of up to 69% for identification of the presence of infection (*Mod Pathol* 1998;11:427).

E. **Crystal-Induced Synovitis** shows deposition of microcrystals in joints and periarticular tissues results in gout (monosodium urate), pseudogout (also known as chondrocalcinosis, due to calcium pyrophosphate dihydrate crystals), and apatite disease (hydroxyapatite crystals) (*Am J Clin Pathol* 2000;14:773). Gout and pseudogout are definitively diagnosed by polarizing light microscopic detection of crystals in joint fluid.

   1. **Gouty tophi** are formed when urate crystals are deposited in the subcutaneous soft tissue, synovium, bone, or bursae, with a granulomatous response dominated by histiocytes and foreign-body giant cells (e-**Fig. 48.8**). Fixation of the tissue in alcohol is necessary to preserve the crystals. A deGalantha histochemical stain can be used to highlight the crystals. Gout crystals are needle-shaped and negatively birefringent (yellow under polarized light, when aligned parallel to the axis of the interference plate).

   2. **Pseudogout.** The crystals of pseudogout appear rhomboid and purple in nondecalcified H&E-stained slides (e-**Fig. 48.9**); with decalcification, the crystals are lost and what is left are rounded pools of basophilic material surrounding rhomboid areas that mark the prior site of the crystals. These crystal deposits do not typically elicit a histiocytic or foreign-body giant cell reaction (*Semin Diagn Pathol* 2011;28:37). They are positively birefringent (blue under polarized light, when aligned parallel to the axis of the interference plate).

F. **Infectious Arthritis** is often diagnosed by clinical history and joint fluid examination, including Gram stain of a centrifuged cell pellet and microbiologic culture.

G. **Hemosiderotic Synovitis** follows chronic intra-articular hemorrhage which can occur in patients with hemophilia and synovial hemangioma. Microscopically, there are fine villous projections early in the disease course. Hemosiderin is present within synoviocytes and macrophages (e-**Fig. 48.10**). Osteoarthritis usually ensues.

H. **Baker Cyst,** which can be found in osteoarthritis and rheumatoid arthritis, is a synovial-lined cyst in the popliteal space that is formed by herniation. In contrast, ganglia (ganglion cysts) are not synovial lined and do not communicate with the joint.

I. Tissue from a **torn meniscus** from the knee may be submitted as tissue shavings or as a fibrocartilaginous loose body. Histologically, there are few changes in the avascular and collagenized tissue because reparative fibrosis and neovascularization are uncommon.

J. **Intervertebral Disc.** Each intervertebral disc is a type of joint (amphiarthrodial), and tissue fragments from a prolapsed disc may be submitted. Microscopically, fibrous tissue, fibrocartilage, and cartilaginous tissue can be seen. Chondrocyte necrosis and/or groups of proliferating chondrocytes may be found. The presence of neovascularization indicates herniation (*Hum Pathol* 1988;19:406).

K. **Synovial Tumors** are uncommon and can arise from the synovium of the tendon sheaths, bursae, and joint spaces (*Semin Diagn Pathol* 2011;28:37).

   1. **Tenosynovial giant cell tumor (TSGT), localized-type** is the most common benign neoplasm of the tendon sheath and synovium. These giant cell tumors are usually found in adults in the fingers, the knee, and the ankle. Grossly, they are circumscribed nodular masses a few centimeters in diameter, with mottled pink-gray cut surfaces that often show flecks of yellow or brown (representing lipid and hemosiderin, respectively). Fibrous septa divide nodules composed of a polymorphous population of histiocytoid to spindled mononuclear cells, larger epithelioid cells, xanthoma cells, siderophages, and osteoclast-like giant cells set in a variably prominent hyalinized stroma (e-**Fig. 48.11**). Mitotic activity may be brisk. Local recurrence is seen in up to 20% of cases.

   2. **Tenosynovial giant cell tumor (TSGT), diffuse-type** usually presents as an intra-articular or extra-articular proliferation involving the knee or hip joint/periarticular soft

tissue. The distal extremities, elbow, shoulder, temporal mandibular joint, and spine are also rarely involved. Microscopically, diffuse-type TSGT is primarily distinguished from the localized form by the presence of infiltrative growth. In addition, compared with the localized-type, the diffuse type also tends to have fewer giant cells and more cleft-like spaces; intra-articular diffuse-type tumors form synovial-lined villous projections (e-**Fig. 48.12**). Mitotic activity is variable and may be brisk, but atypical mitotic figures are absent. Both localized and diffuse-type tumors share translocations of chromosome 1p13 (CFS1), which in some cases result in formation of a *COL6A3-CSF1* fusion. Classification of this neoplasm as an intermediate (locally aggressive) tumor is based on the fact that over 45% of intra-articular and up to 60% of extra-articular tumors recur and recurrences may be destructive. Very rare conventional cases metastasize. Malignant diffuse-type TGST are very rare and are clearly sarcomatous proliferations; they are associated with a conventional diffuse-type TSGT, or found in a recurrence of TSGT.

3. **Synovial chondromatosis** is a benign nodular cartilaginous proliferation arising in the synovium of joints, bursae, or tendon sheaths. It is usually monoarticular in distribution, involving the knee or hip in adults. Grossly, there are multiple cartilaginous or osteocartilaginous nodules, each measuring <1 mm to several millimeters in diameter, which may be embedded within the synovium and/or mobile as loose bodies. Microscopically, the nodules of hyaline cartilage harbor clusters of chondrocytes that can show nuclear atypia with nuclear enlargement, hyperchromasia, and binucleation (e-**Fig. 48.13**), findings that should not be viewed as evidence of malignancy. Local recurrence after excision occurs in about 15% of cases.

4. **Synovial chondrosarcoma** is extremely rare and is often associated with synovial chondromatosis. Histologic features of malignancy include loss of the "clustering" growth pattern typical of synovial chondromatosis (e-**Fig. 48.14**), with replacement by a sheet-like arrangement of chondrocytes, prominent myxoid change, necrosis, and spindling (*Cancer* 1991;67:155). The prognosis is poor.

5. **Synovial hemangioma** is very rare and usually found in the knee of young adults. Microscopically, most are cavernous hemangiomas; some are capillary or mixed (e-**Fig. 48.15**).

6. **Synovial lipoma** is rare. Grossly, the synovium is yellow, thickened, and exhibits excrescences (lipoma arborescens). Microscopically, the synovium is infiltrated by mature adipose tissue (e-**Fig. 48.16**). Recurrence is rare.

7. A variety of tumors may rarely present as an intra-articular mass including solitary fibrous tumor, synovial sarcoma, epithelioid sarcoma, extraskeletal myxoid chondrosarcoma, undifferentiated pleomorphic sarcoma, nodular fasciitis, and lymphoma.

ACKNOWLEDGMENT

The authors thank Michael J. Klein for his help with this chapter.

Cytopathology

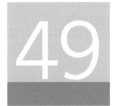

General Principles of Cytopathology

Cory Bernadt

I. **INTRODUCTION.** Cytopathology has developed into a discipline that examines cellular elements from throughout the body collected by a wide variety of methods and procedures. It shares with other anatomic pathology disciplines a morphologic study of cells utilizing patterns and cellular features to identify specific pathologic conditions. Cytopathology provides diagnostic information in a wide variety of clinical settings, and can thus be used to guide patient management both at the time of initial diagnosis and during the course of treatment. In broad terms, there are three main areas of cytopathology, specifically: (1) gynecologic/Pap slides; (2) nongynecologic (Non-Gyn); and (3) fine needle aspiration (FNA).

The utility of cytopathology is underscored by the fact that virtually all ancillary laboratory techniques used in surgical pathology can also be performed on cytology specimens.

A. **Immunocytochemistry.** Special stains are commonly applied to cytologic samples, often to confirm the morphologic diagnosis, to help in determining the possible primary sites of a tumor, or to determine the presence of specific prognostic markers. In general, cell block sections are preferred for immunocytochemical staining because most laboratories have experience processing the formalin-fixed, paraffin-embedded tissue sections that are generated from cell blocks.

B. **Flow Cytometry.** In the presence of a lymphocyte-rich sample, the possibility of a lymphoproliferative process may need to be addressed by flow cytometry. Body fluids, particularly effusions, are amenable to this type of analysis.

C. **Molecular Genetic Methods.** Cytologic preparations, including fluid specimens, brushings, washings, and scrapings, are suitable substrates for molecular analysis. Regardless of the method used to process samples (e.g., whether air dried, ethanol fixed, or used to produce a cell block), it is possible to extract nucleic acids that can be analyzed by a wide variety of genetic assays, including polymerase chain reaction (PCR), DNA sequence analysis (including next-generation sequencing methods), gene expression analysis, and fluorescence in situ hybridization (FISH).

II. **GYNECOLOGIC/PAP SLIDES.** The "Pap test" is the most successful cancer screening test in medicine. After the wide introduction of the Pap smear, the incidence of cervical carcinoma dropped significantly, and the Pap smear remains the mainstay of screening women for cervical carcinoma. Standardized terminology and categorizations for the Pap smear have been developed (*The Bethesda System for Reporting Cervical Cytology.* New York, Springer International Publishing, 2015). The Bethesda Reporting System for Cervical Smears is covered in more detail in the Cytopathology section of Chapter 34.

III. NONGYNECOLOGIC CYTOPATHOLOGY encompasses a wide variety of body sites, organs, and types of specimens. In general, any lesion that can be drained, brushed, washed, or scraped can be a "Non-Gyn" cytopathology specimen.

A. Specimen Types

1. Fluid. These constitute a major category of Non-Gyn specimens and include pleural fluid, ascites/peritoneal fluid, pericardial fluid, and cerebrospinal fluid. Any loculated fluid can be drained and submitted for analysis (neck cyst, hepatic cyst, etc.) including synovial and vitreous fluid. Urine specimens, either voided or catheterized, are also commonly examined.

2. Brush. The endoscope makes it possible to introduce a brush and collect cells and tissue from a wide variety of internal locations. These include the bronchopulmonary tree (bronchial brush), alimentary tract (esophageal brush, gastric brush, and common/pancreatic/hepatic bile duct brushes), peritoneal cavity, and genitourinary tract (urethra brush, ureter brush, and renal pelvic brush).

3. Wash. Lesions sampled by a brush are usually accompanied by a "wash" specimen, which can be collected to sample additional cells. These specimens commonly include lung (bronchial wash, bronchoalveolar lavage), peritoneal cavity (pelvic wash), and urinary bladder (bladder wash, ureter wash, and renal pelvic wash).

4. Scrape. The Tzanck smear of the skin is utilized for the identification of mucocutaneous herpes virus effect.

B. Preparation and Processing

1. Submission. Material can be submitted fresh or fixed. In general, unfixed material should be refrigerated until it can be delivered to the cytopathology laboratory. Even after arrival, it should be refrigerated until processed since unfixed cells in a fluid environment are in a constant state of degeneration, both in situ and after being collected. Specimens delayed in processing that have not been properly handled can be uninterpretable.

2. Fixative and stain. Alcohol is the standard fixative. Alcohol fixation can be utilized at a variety of steps in specimen handling, including at the time of collection (slides prepared from a brush can be placed in 95% ethanol at the patient's bedside, or the brush itself can be placed directly into a liquid fixative container) or after initial processing of the specimen (after preparation of cytospin slides from a fluid sample). Regardless, once cellular material is placed on a slide, it needs to be alcohol fixed as soon as possible. A delay of more than a few seconds can cause air-drying artifact, which renders the cells indistinct and the nuclei "washed out" when subsequently Pap stained. Severe air-drying artifact can render a slide uninterpretable.

a. The **Pap stain** highlights nuclear morphologic details including distinct chromatin and nuclear membrane detail. The cytoplasm tends to have a blue-green coloration with keratinization showing organophilic decoration.

b. A modified **Wright–Giemsa**, commonly referred to as **Diff-Quik**, is the other main cytopathology stain. It is performed on slides which are first air dried. Once completely air dried, slides are placed in a methanol fixative and then stained (total time to complete the stain can be less than a minute). The **Diff-Quik** stain highlights lymphoid elements and a variety of extracellular elements (colloid, matrix, mucin, and so on).

c. The Pap stain and the Diff-Quik stain are complementary and both are frequently utilized in combination on Non-Gyn and FNA specimens.

C. Reporting.
Standardized recommendations for reporting the findings in Non-Gyn cytopathology specimens have recently been developed (*Arch Pathol Lab Med* 2009;133:1743). Uniform reporting enhances patient care and thus implementation of these guidelines in routine practice is strongly recommended.

IV. FINE NEEDLE ASPIRATION. One of the most challenging and dynamic areas of cytopathology is FNA. Virtually any organ or abnormality (either palpable or localized by imaging techniques) can be subjected to FNA. The technique essentially provides a microbiopsy of cellular material (cells and tissue) for microscopic examination and for testing by a wide variety of ancillary methods. FNA permits immediate interpretive evaluation which makes possible real time adjustments of the biopsy procedure, appropriate specimen triage, and directed ancillary testing.

A. Principles. The procedure is minimally invasive and accurate. At its core, FNA involves the use of a thin bore needle with a cutting end moved in a piston motion to obtain cells and tissue. The cellular elements present within the needle are then processed for diagnosis (e-Fig. 49.1).

B. Technique. While simple, proficiency and adequacy require an understanding of the procedure and experience in its use. It is the cutting, beveled end of the needle and capillary action of a repetitive "piston-like" motion movement which provides the cellular elements necessary for diagnosis. The appropriate application of needle movement is critical since insufficient movement will not adequately sample the tissue, and prolonged movement can lead to hemodilution and entrapment of the tissue in a clot. The appropriate number of tissue passes and appropriate negative pressure will vary for each individual case and clinical presentation.

Negative pressure during the procedure (typically applied by an empty 10- or 20-cc plastic syringe attached to the needle) can be useful but is not always necessary. There are many solid cellular lesions/neoplasms that can be adequately sampled without aspiration, including lymph nodes and the thyroid. Vascular organs and neoplasms benefit from a nonaspiration FNA technique since aspiration can lead to bleeding and specimen hemodilution.

Needles utilized can range from 22 to 27 gauge. Larger gauge needles tend to cause more bleeding and, paradoxically tend to be less diagnostic. Needle length can vary significantly (5/8 inch to inches) and will depend on what is required to reach the lesion.

C. Procedure. In broad terms, the needle is directed to the area of interest by either palpation or under image guidance.

  1. Palpable. This method involves any lesion that can be localized or identified by manual palpation. It must be stressed that FNA of every location requires an understanding of the associated local anatomy, especially for areas in the head and neck, thyroid, chest wall, and various soft tissue locations. Superficial FNA of palpable lesions is well tolerated, minimally invasive, and has a very low complication rate.

  2. Image guidance. This method involves utilizing an imaging modality to direct the needle, most commonly ultrasound or CT imaging. The principles of the FNA biopsy itself remain the same. In some cases, a stylet within the needle is helpful; it is used to prevent sampling of organs as the needle moves toward the lesion, and then removed once the needle tip is in the desired location. An immediate assessment of the FNA sample makes it possible for the pathologist to guide the clinician to ensure that a diagnostic sample is collected and that the appropriate ancillary studies are initiated at the time of the procedure.

D. Materials

  1. Palpable. The materials required are simple and readily available. They can be conveniently organized in a small basket or box which can be easily transported from the laboratory (e-Fig 49.2).

  2. Image guidance. The appropriate type of needle and the FNA approach are determined by the clinical setting. On-site presence of the cytopathology team with glass slides, fixative (alcohol), needle rinse tube (normal saline or RPMI), stains (Diff-Quik), and a microscope, will help optimize the likelihood that a diagnostic sample is obtained and that appropriate ancillary studies are initiated.

E. Clinical Application

  1. Immediate evaluation. Immediate evaluation is the standard of care because it provides several advantages. First, it guides the procedure and thus ensures a maximum effort to obtain a diagnosis. By examining the slides during the procedure, immediate evaluation can be used to help decide if more FNAs are necessary; guide the needle position placement by determining if lesion or nonlesional material is present; and if nondiagnostic, support a decision to move to a potential second site. Second, with immediate evaluation, the tradeoff between the length of the procedure and number of biopsies can be managed to balance the requirement for diagnostic tissue without unnecessarily extending the length of the procedure. By assuring a diagnostic procedure, the number of nondiagnostic samples can be minimized and repeat procedures and delays in diagnosis can be avoided. Third, the cytopathologist can identify those cases where tissue for appropriate ancillary studies needs to be collected to enhance diagnostic accuracy. These situations include identifying a lymphoproliferative process where rinse material is sent for flow cytometry analysis, abscess/granulomatous inflammation where microbiologic cultures are indicated, poorly differentiated neoplasms where a cell block can provide material for immunohistochemical evaluation, and lesions where cytogenetics/molecular diagnostics can contribute to the diagnosis.

F. **Specimen Processing**
1. **Direct smears** are stained by the Pap and Diff-Quik methods.
2. **Liquid medium.** FNA samples that are collected in a liquid medium provide a wide variety of options for further analysis. While it is helpful to perform needle washes during the FNA procedure, the best chance for a sufficient cell block involves direct (no slides prepared) dedicated FNA samples placed in the liquid medium (saline or RPMI). Cell block preparation affords a variety of options and advantages; sections of the cell block contribute to the morphologic evaluation of the lesion, and also provide cellular material for immunohistochemical analysis, interphase FISH, and for a wide range of molecular tests.

ACKNOWLEDGMENT

The author thanks Brian Collins, author of the previous edition of this chapter.

SUGGESTED READINGS

Crothers BA, Tench WD, Schwartz MR, et al. Guidelines for the reporting of nongynecologic cytopathology specimens. *Arch Pathol Lab Med* 2009;133:1743–1756.

Gill GW. *Cytopreparation—Principles & Practice*. New York: Springer Science+Business Media; 2013.

Gupta PK. University of Pennsylvania aspiration cart (Penn-A-Cart): an innovative journey in fine needle aspiration service. *Acta Cytol* 2010;54:165–168.

Gupta PK. Progression from on-site to point-of-care fine needle aspiration service: opportunities and challenges. *Cytojournal* 2010;7:6.

Massad LS, Einstein MH, Huh WK, et al. 2012 updated consensus guidelines for the management of abnormal cervical cancer screening tests and cancer precursors. *Obstet Gynecol* 2013;121:829–846.

Ancillary Methods

Frozen Sections and Other Intraoperative Consultations

Peter A. Humphrey and John D. Pfeifer

I. INTRODUCTION. Intraoperative consultations fall into two general categories. Microscopic consultations, usually performed as frozen sections, are undertaken to establish a tissue diagnosis, determine the nature of a lesion that may require ancillary testing, establish that sufficient diagnostic tissue has been obtained, identify the metastatic disease, and assess surgical margins or the extent of disease. Microscopic consultations can also be performed using touch preparations, a practice that has the advantage of preserving valuable tissue. Nonmicroscopic consultations are gross examinations of a specimen that provide the surgeon with real-time information on tissue margins and the anatomic extent of disease processes. They also facilitate the triage of fresh tissue for ancillary diagnostic studies or research protocols.

II. FROZEN SECTIONS. High-quality frozen sections can be produced with remarkable speed if equipment is kept in optimum working condition and if the operator is well versed in the technique. In experienced hands, the entire consultation can often be performed in 10 to 15 minutes from the time of the arrival of the specimen in the frozen section room to the notification of the surgeon of the diagnosis. For larger tissue specimens, proper interpretation requires a thorough gross examination of the tissue prior to sectioning. Good communication with the surgeon regarding operative findings and knowledge of pertinent clinical history are also absolutely essential for optimization of the process.

A. Indications. Frozen sections are indicated to establish a tissue diagnosis (such as the presence of malignancy, which will guide intraoperative patient management and the extent of surgery); for tissue identification (e.g., to confirm the presence of parathyroid tissue in a parathyroidectomy specimen); to determine the nature of a lesion that may require ancillary testing that requires special fixatives or media (e.g., RPMI for flow cytometry or glutaraldehyde for electron microscopy); to establish that sufficient diagnostic tissue has been obtained; to identify metastatic disease; and to assess surgical margins or the extent of disease.

Frozen sections should not be used merely to satisfy a surgeon's curiosity, to compensate for inadequate preoperative evaluation, or as a mechanism to communicate information more quickly to the patient or the patient's family.

B. The Frozen Section Procedure. Frozen sections are performed by freezing the tissue in a block of specialized embedding medium, followed by cutting thin (usually 5 micron) sections from the block using a cryostat (refrigerated microtome). The sections are adhered to glass slides, fixed in ethanol, and stained with hematoxylin and eosin (H&E).

Small specimens may be completely utilized for frozen section slide preparation, but if possible a portion of the tissue should be preserved for routine handling to avoid freezing artifacts that can compromise interpretation of the permanent sections (e.g., in the case of brain biopsies). For larger tissue samples, judgment must be exercised in gross sampling so that the area(s) of highest diagnostic yield is selected for frozen section. Cytologic imprints can be an important adjunct in diagnosis at the time of intraoperative microscopic evaluation by frozen section, especially for hematolymphoid abnormalities, lymph node biopsies, and thyroid lesions.

C. **Interpretation.** The interpretation of frozen sections requires integration of the histologic morphology in the H&E-stained sections; the gross features of the specimen; information from the surgeon regarding the origin of the tissue and the indication for the consultation (including the clinical history, radiologic findings, and intraoperative observations); and the ways in which the frozen section diagnosis will affect the operative strategy. In difficult cases, it may be necessary to request additional tissue for frozen section analysis; if additional tissue cannot be obtained, deferral of a definitive diagnosis pending examination of formalin-fixed paraffin-embedded (FFPE) sections is appropriate. In routine clinical practice, such deferrals are employed in less than 5% of frozen section diagnoses.

D. **Communication of Findings.** Clear communication of a concise diagnosis to the surgeon is the last step of the intraoperative consultation. Usually there is a narrowly defined clinical problem that frozen section is to solve; this should be specifically and unambiguously addressed in the diagnosis. The diagnosis is written and signed, with the date and time, by all interpreting pathologists and made part of the final pathology report. If the written diagnosis is verbally transmitted, the pathologist should first confirm with the recipient of the information the identity of the patient (using two identifiers) and the surgeon. The operating room staff member taking the diagnosis should repeat it back to the pathologist to confirm accurate communication.

Certain phraseologies tend to be resistant to misinterpretation. For instance, "negative for malignancy" or "positive for malignancy" are generally well understood. Since some diagnosis can easily be incompletely heard or misunderstood in a busy operating room, the diagnosis should always be repeated back as a safeguard.

E. **Accuracy of Frozen Sections.** The accuracy of frozen sections will vary from institution to institution based on the types of surgical cases evaluated and the experience of the involved pathologists. Table 50.1 highlights the fact that the accuracy of frozen section diagnosis is dependent on the anatomic site. Regular self audits of the frozen section service help surgeons and pathologists be aware of the performance characteristics of the modality in their own hands. Such audits of single institutions, and pooled data across hundreds of institutions, show that accurate diagnoses are made overall in more than 95% of cases, while discordance with the final diagnosis occurs in 2 to 15% of cases. Deferral of the diagnosis until permanent section diagnosis occurs in 1% to 4% of cases.

F. **Sources of Error in Frozen Sections.** Errors can be divided into errors of interpretation and errors of sampling; both usually result in false-negative diagnoses. False-positive diagnoses are rarer, likely because experienced pathologists tend to appropriately defer to permanent section rather than make an incorrect diagnosis on substandard material.

Discrepancies between a frozen section and the final (permanent section) diagnosis should be documented in the final surgical pathology report, along with the reason for the discrepancy. If the discrepancy is of clinical significance, the pathologist should immediately alert the surgeon to the change in diagnosis.

1. Misinterpretation accounts for about 40% of errors overall (*Arch Pathol Lab Med* 1996;120:804; *Arch Pathol Lab Med* 1996;120:19). Interpretations of frozen sections are more prone to this error than interpretation of permanent sections due to the presence of artifacts that are not encountered in routinely fixed, paraffin-embedded sections. Some tissues are more likely to show significant artifact, especially those with high fat content such as pelvic lymph nodes.

TABLE 50.1 Examples of Frozen Section Evaluation

Tissue	Concordance With Permanent Section Diagnosis	False Negative	Comments on Utility
Breast			Limited (see text)
Cervix	73% for evaluation of dysplasia		Poor for evaluation of dysplasia
Gallbladder	95% when used to evaluate a mural lesion		Useful in the rare instances in which it is required
Liver			Diagnostic dilemmas that generate deferrals: 1. Hamartoma vs. cholangiocarcinoma 2. Regenerative nodule vs. hepatocellular carcinoma 3. Adenoma vs. hepatocellular carcinoma
Lung	99%		Useful; deferral rate of only 3–4%
Axillary sentinel lymph nodes for metastatic breast cancer	90%[a]–96%[b]	15%[a]–37%[b]	Possibly useful (see text)
Lymph nodes for staging	~100%[c]	20–40%[c]	Limited and dependent upon the lymph node location (see text)
Ovary	92%	5%	Useful; errors are disproportionately represented among mucinous tumors
Pancreas	98% when used for diagnosis of primary lesion; almost 100% for margins	1%	Atypical ductal structures, especially in the setting of pancreatitis, may mimic carcinoma; deferral rate of 6–7%
Parathyroid	99% (for parathyroid vs. nonparathyroid tissue)		Useful for distinction of parathyroid vs. nonparathyroid tissue: inadequate for diagnosis of parathyroid carcinoma, or for differentiating adenoma from hyperplasia
Skin, melanoma		Up to 50%	Strongly discouraged (see text)
Skin, nonmelanoma		About 2%, based on recurrence rates following Mohs microsurgery[d]	Useful for the evaluation of margins in the resection of tumors with infiltrating borders and tumors of the face, especially eyes, ears, and nose
Thyroid	98%	10%	Inadequate for follicular lesions, as the sampling required is not practical (see text); better for lesions with papillary architecture; deferral rate is 6%

[a]When nodes with submicrometastases (<0.2 mm) are considered "positive."
[b]When nodes with submicrometastases are considered "negative."
[c]Staging pelvic lymph nodes at prostatectomy.
[d]Data on correlation with permanent sections are sparse, as follow-up permanent sections are not performed.

2. Sampling errors occur in two ways. The first is sectioning error. Diagnostic tissue may be present in the frozen block, but the block may not be faced sufficiently for the lesion to be present on the actual frozen section slides; the diagnostic material may then be found in routine permanent sections of the residual frozen block, a scenario that accounts for 10% to 15% of errors. The second type of sampling error is gross sampling error. This accounts for about 45% of errors overall, and is seen when the diagnostic tissue is not in the portion of the specimen sampled by the frozen section; good gross pathology skills will minimize, but never eliminate, this problem. Furthermore, it is not feasible to completely sample larger lesions by frozen section, and so sampling errors will always exist for large lesions with heterogeneous composition.

G. **Anatomic Sites Deserving Special Mention.** The anatomic sites with the most discrepancies between frozen section and permanent section are skin, breast, lymph nodes for metastatic disease, the female genital tract, and thyroid. While frozen sections have a role in the surgical management of disease in these sites, loss of diagnostic material during the performance of frozen sections is unavoidable, and so each case must be evaluated as to whether frozen section diagnosis will add enough value to warrant this loss.

1. **Skin.** Frozen sections for margin assessment in the excisions of large nonmelanoma skin cancers such as basal cell carcinoma and squamous cell carcinoma are indicated if the lesion has vague infiltrative borders or is in a location in which wide excision is not possible, as in the case of tumors of the eyelid, nose, or ear (*Arch Pathol Lab Med* 2005;129:1536). If the borders of a lesion are well defined by gross examination, frozen sections are not as necessary.

   It is widely agreed that the intraoperative primary diagnosis of pigmented lesions is ill advised. The determination of prognosis and subsequent management of melanoma requires an accurate assessment of Breslow thickness, and frozen artifact may cause so much specimen distortion as to make a depth of invasion assessment meaningless in both permanent and frozen sections. Freezing artifact compounded by actinic damage, frequent in patients with pigmented lesions, also conspires to obscure histology. Subtle changes, such as intraepidermal spread by single melanocytes, are very difficult to appreciate in frozen sections, making the method a poor choice for margin assessment as well. In fact, the false-negative rate for lentiginous spread of melanoma by frozen section evaluation may be as high as 50%.

2. **Breast.** Once commonplace, the initial pathologic diagnosis of breast tumors is now very rarely made intraoperatively by frozen section. Methods for detection of smaller tumors, more sophisticated treatment algorithms (as opposed to mastectomy only), and standardized tissue processing protocols that help ensure the accuracy of subsequent biomarker testing now usually lead to diagnosis based on FFPE needle core biopsy or excision specimens. Margin evaluation is sometimes requested during breast-conserving procedures, but the high fat content of breast tissue makes frozen specimens technically difficult to section and prone to freezing artifact. Evaluation of margins by imprint histology is an alternative to frozen section, but it is insensitive unless the margins are grossly involved, in which case the examination is unnecessary (*Arch Pathol Lab Med* 2005;129:1565).

3. **Lymph nodes for metastatic disease (including axillary sentinel lymph nodes for breast carcinoma)**

   a. **Sentinel lymph nodes.** Although current diagnostic modalities have reduced the need for breast frozen sections, requests for frozen sections of sentinel lymph nodes have increased (**e-Fig. 50.1A,B**). Unfortunately, frozen sections on sentinel nodes consume considerable tissue; if no metastases are identified, further evaluation of the node is significantly hampered (**e-Fig. 50.2**).

   Numerous studies have indicated that the sensitivity of frozen section evaluation of sentinel nodes is about 60%, although the specificity is near 100% (*Mod Path* 2005;18:58). The metastases that are typically missed by frozen section are the so-called "isolated tumor cell clusters" (which by definition are small clusters of cells not larger than 0.2 mm, or single tumor cells, or fewer than 200 cells in a histologic cross section), a class of metastases that is now a component of AJCC reporting and/or staging of malignancies from a variety of sites including breast, uterine corpus, uterine cervix, cutaneous melanoma (Amin MB, Edge S, Greene F, et al., eds. *AJCC Cancer Staging Manual*, 8th ed. New York: Springer, 2017). The low sensitivity of the frozen section approach, combined with the fact that the procedure consumes tissue and thus compromises subsequent evaluation of routinely prepared FFPE sections and immunostains, markedly limits the utility of intraoperative frozen section diagnosis of sentinel lymph nodes. Nonetheless, it is sensible to perform frozen sections when the clinical history and gross examination of the node give a high degree of suspicion for metastasis. Imprint cytology of the fresh lymph node is another possible approach to intraoperative sentinel lymph node evaluation.

  b. **Other lymph node frozen sections.** The intraoperative evaluation of lymph nodes can be performed by frozen section or by imprint cytology, and tissue should be allocated for flow cytometric analysis, routine histology, and molecular diagnostics as indicated by the diagnosis.

4. **Thyroid.** The widespread use of fine needle aspiration (FNA) has altered the approach to frozen section evaluation of the thyroid. Frozen section evaluation of thyroid excision specimens is best performed in conjunction with imprint cytology, the latter of which is more sensitive for the nuclear grooves, inclusions, and chromatin-clearing characteristic of papillary carcinoma. Since the distinction between follicular adenoma and carcinoma by frozen section (e-**Fig 50.3**) would require thorough sampling of the tumor and capsule for invasion and angioinvasion, frozen section is poorly suited to this application (*Can J Surg* 2004;47:29).

5. **Female genital tract.** Of all the neoplastic processes of the female genital tract, ovarian neoplasms are probably the best suited to intraoperative frozen section diagnosis (*Arch Pathol Lab Med* 2005;129:1544; *Int J Gynecol Cancer* 2005;15:192). Even so, borderline mucinous neoplasms of the ovary have a significant rate of discordance between the frozen section and permanent section diagnoses, primarily due to sampling error. The diagnosis of cervical dysplasia is fraught with difficulties due to frozen section artifact and low concordance with permanent section diagnosis.

III. **OTHER INTRAOPERATIVE CONSULTATIONS.** Intraoperative nonmicroscopic consultations are often required even though no frozen section is needed. Indications include gross diagnosis (such as benign simple ovarian cyst or uterine leiomyoma); gross confirmation of the presence of a lesion or mass; identification of a margin or region of interest that requires special sampling for permanent sections; specimen orientation; triage of tissue for ancillary testing modalities that require special processing or fixatives (in which case good judgment is required to ensure a balance between the need for tissue for routine histopathologic evaluation and the need for tissue for specialized testing); and collection of tissue for tumor banking or research studies.

  A. **Opening of a Viscus Organ for Gross Examination and Fixation.** Gastrointestinal specimens commonly require opening in the operating room so that the surgeon can see whether or not lesional tissue has been excised. In partial intestinal excisions for inflammatory disease, in which the risk for malignancy is increased, a careful intraoperative examination may inform the surgeon of a previously undetected tumor which may have implications for additional surgical therapy.

  Similarly, gross examination and opening of the adnexa and/or uterus and can aid in determining the extent of surgery that is required. Such gross examination often leads to frozen sections when ovarian surface papillary excrescences are identified, or when solid or complex architecture features are discovered in an ovarian cyst.

  B. **Tissue Banking.** Tumor for banking must be chosen so that the remaining lesional tissue material will still be suitable for a complete diagnostic evaluation. The banked tissue should not include a surgical margin, or have an important relationship to an anatomic structure that would impact staging or the need for adjuvant therapy. In cases of small specimens, it may be necessary to defer banking for the sake of a thorough diagnostic evaluation.

ACKNOWLEDGMENT

The authors thank Michael E. Hull, an author of the previous edition of this chapter.

SUGGESTED READINGS

Argani P, Cimino-Mathews A. *Intraoperative Frozen Sections: Diagnostic Pitfalls*. New York: Demos Medical; 2013.

Ferreiro JA, Myers JL, Bostwick DG. Accuracy of frozen section diagnosis in surgical pathology: review of a 1-year experience with 24,880 cases at Mayo Clinic Rochester. *Mayo Clin Proc* 1995;70:1137–1141.

Sawady J, Berner JJ, Siegler EE. Accuracy of and reasons for frozen sections: a correlative, retrospective study. *Hum Pathol* 1988;19:1019–1023.

Taxy JB, Husain AN, Montag AG. *Biopsy Interpretation: The Frozen Section*. Riverwoods, IL: Lippincott Williams & Wilkins; 2009.

51 Electron Microscopy

Frances V. White

I. **INTRODUCTION.** Transmission electron microscopy (EM) has been used by surgical pathologists over the past 50 years for the diagnosis of a wide range of diseases in various organ systems (Table 51.1). The method allows for the visualization of subcellular morphology, with appreciation of disease processes and structural abnormalities that cannot be resolved by light microscopy. EM is an essential part of the work-up of medical renal diseases, peripheral nerve diseases, muscle diseases, and primary ciliary dyskinesia (PCD). It is also useful in evaluating metabolic and inherited diseases, providing an initial differential diagnosis, or ruling in or out a specific disease process. The role of EM in the diagnosis of neoplasms has decreased since the advent of immunohistochemical and molecular techniques, but it is still an ancillary tool for the evaluation of atypical tumors or when other techniques yield indeterminate results. Although not usually needed, EM is occasionally used to demonstrate infectious agents or evidence of drug toxicity.

In recent years, EM has been combined with immunohistochemical and in situ hybridization methods, allowing antigen detection and localization at the subcellular level. These combined methods require special fixation and processing protocols. Although immunoelectron microscopy is currently used primarily in research laboratories, the method is now considered to be a promising diagnostic technique in oncologic surgical pathology, in particular for the identification and localization of targets for gene therapy.

II. **METHODOLOGY.** Tissue for EM must be immediately fixed. A thin slice of tissue should be immersed in a cold fixative such as buffered 2% to 4% glutaraldehyde, or buffered glutaraldehyde plus paraformaldehyde, and then diced into 1-mm cubes using a sharp, clean scalpel blade. Specimens are usually postfixed in osmium tetroxide, dehydrated in ethanol, and then embedded in an epoxy resin or plastic. Semi-thin (1-μm-thick) sections are cut from the blocks and stained with toluidine blue or methylene blue, and light microscopic examination of the semi-thin sections is used to select the blocks from which thin sections are cut and placed on grids. The thin sections are usually stained with uranyl acetate and lead citrate; other stains, however, may be selected to enhance electron contrast of specific particles or structures depending on the tissue type and diagnostic question. Tissue processing typically takes a couple of days, but with microwave techniques grids can be ready within 5 hours postfixation.

For some disease processes, if glutaraldehyde-fixed tissue is not available, EM can be performed on formalin-fixed wet tissue or paraffin-embedded tissue. Wet tissue is preferable to paraffin-embedded tissue, but previous prompt fixation in formalin is essential. Autopsy material, whether fixed in glutaraldehyde or formalin, is often unsatisfactory due to the prolonged postmortem interval prior to fixation.

A focused differential diagnosis based on integration of the clinical history and light microscopic findings is essential for the correct interpretation of ultrastructural findings. Except for the most routine specimens, the pathologist should personally review the semithin sections by light microscopy and select the blocks for further processing. In addition, the pathologist should communicate his differential diagnosis to the electron microscopist and specify the cell type and subcellular structures of interest. Obviously, sampling error is minimized and the most information is obtained when the pathologist is directly involved in scanning the tissue grids.

III. **KIDNEY.** EM, in conjunction with routine histology and immunofluorescence, is an essential part of the work-up of medical renal biopsies to diagnose glomerular disease

TABLE 51.1 Examples of Subcellular Features Used for Classification of Disease by Electron Microscopy

Subcellular Feature	Cell/Tissue Type	Diagnostic Setting
Peroxisomes	Liver	Increased number in alcoholic liver disease, chronic passive congestion, oral contraceptive use, various hepatitides
Siderosomes	Mitochondria	Sideroblastic anemia
Genetic diseases		
Cilia	Epithelial cells	Primary ciliary dyskinesia
Lysosomes	Neurons, Skin, Conjunctiva	Identification of lipoidosis and several types of mucopolysaccharidoses
	Hepatocytes	Identification of several types of mucopolysaccharidoses
Peroxisomes	Liver and kidney	Absence in Zellweger syndrome and neonatal adrenoleukodystrophy
Neoplasms		
Intercellular junctions	Epithelial cells; selected mesenchymal nonlymphoid tumors	Distinction between lymphoma and carcinoma
Intracellular or intercellular lumina	Glandular epithelium	Identification of adenocarcinomas
Microvillous core rootlets	Glandular epithelium of alimentary tract	Identification of gastrointestinal origin of metastatic carcinomas
Cytoplasmic tonofibrils	Squamous epithelium	Identification of squamous differentiation in epithelial tumors
Premelanosomes and melanosomes	Melanocytic cells	Identification of melanomas
Neurosecretory granules	Neuroendocrine and neuroectodermal cells	Identification of neuroendocrine and neuroectodermal neoplasms
Birbeck granules	Langerhans cells	Identification of Langerhans proliferations such as Langerhans cell histiocytosis
Other		
Viruses and parasites	Solid tissues, fecal specimens, body fluids	Identification of infectious agent
Electron-dense deposits and/or other basement membrane alterations	Glomeruli	Identification and classification of glomerular diseases
	Adjacent to vascular smooth muscle	CADASIL syndrome

CADASIL, cerebral autosomal dominant arteriopathy with subcortical infarcts and leukoencephalopathy.

(see Chapter 19). It is also performed on renal allograft biopsies when recurrent or de novo glomerular disease is suspected. Because EM makes it possible to visualize the individual components of the glomerular capillary wall, including endothelium, glomerular basement membrane, and visceral epithelial cells, it is used for identification and localization of discrete electron-dense deposits in glomeruli, either of immunoglobulins, amyloid, or amyloid-like proteins. The glomerular basement membrane can also be evaluated for abnormal thickening, thinning, and/or splitting and for the presence of electron lucent, granular, or other deposits. Tubular basement membranes, arterioles, and the interstitium can also be evaluated by EM for pathogenic changes, for example, nonimmune deposits such as amyloid, light chain dense deposits, and cryoglobulins.

IV. **NEOPLASMS.** The role of EM in the diagnosis of neoplasms has decreased since the advent of immunohistochemical and molecular markers. EM, however, is still a useful ancillary method in selected cases and for poorly differentiated tumors for which immunohistochemical and molecular studies are inconclusive. In general, a differential diagnosis is first developed based on light microscopic findings, and EM is then used to look for evidence of cellular differentiation toward the tumors in the differential diagnosis (e-**Fig. 51.1**). For example, desmosomes, tonofilaments, melanosomes, and premelanosomes may be sought in the differential diagnosis of carcinoma versus melanoma. EM does not differentiate reactive, benign, neoplastic, and malignant processes.

V. **INHERITED METABOLIC DISEASES.** Initial studies in the work-up of inherited metabolic diseases often include a biopsy of affected organs (such as liver, skin, conjunctiva, muscle, or peripheral nerve) (*Ultrastruct Pathol* 1992;16:231; *Ultrastruct Pathol* 1997;21:345). For select diseases, EM findings may be pathognomonic. In most cases, however, light microscopy and EM findings are useful in narrowing the differential diagnosis and providing direction for further laboratory studies. Definitive diagnosis typically requires enzyme studies of fibroblast cultures and/or molecular studies.

A. **Prenatal Studies.** EM can be performed on amniotic cells and chorionic villous tissue obtained for prenatal diagnosis (*Arch Gyn Obstetr* 2005;271;3:260). Ultrastructural studies on noncultured amniotic cells can yield a rapid diagnosis or differential for certain metabolic diseases, including type 2 glycogen storage disease, lysosomal storage diseases, and peroxisomal disorders.

B. **Liver.** Inherited metabolic diseases often result in hepatocellular dysfunction, either as part of a **systemic** disorder or as part of disease limited to the liver. In the work-up of hepatitis and cholestatic liver disease in infancy and childhood, a portion of the liver biopsy is routinely placed in glutaraldehyde for possible ultrastructural studies. In cases where obstruction and infection have been ruled out, EM is performed to look for evidence of primary metabolic disease. Certain metabolic diseases have pathognomonic or near-pathognomonic findings, such as types 2 and 4 glycogen storage diseases, alpha-1-antitrypsin disease, and Wilson disease (e-**Fig. 51.2**). Abnormalities in the number and structure of mitochondria and peroxisomes are characteristic of other specific diseases, as are lysosomal inclusions. Ultrastructural findings are always interpreted in conjunction with light microscopic findings, clinical history, biochemical assays, and other laboratory studies.

C. **Lung.** The protocol for lung biopsy in the work-up of interstitial lung disease in infancy includes placing a portion of the specimen in EM fixative so that tissue is **available** for ultrastructural analysis if needed based on the light microscopic findings. Diseases that have characteristic ultrastructural findings (e-**Fig. 51.3**) include pulmonary interstitial glycogenosis and surfactant processing abnormalities (surfactant protein B [SPB] deficiency and adenosine 5′-triphosphate [ATP]-binding cassette transporter A3 [ABCA3] mutations) (*Ultrastruct Pathol* 2005;29:503; *Ultrastruct Pathol* 2013;37:356).

D. **Heart.** Glycogen storage disease type 2 (Pompe disease) can be diagnosed based on ultrastructural findings in cardiac biopsies. Adriamycin toxicity involving the heart results in characteristic cytoplasmic changes that can be seen by light microscopy in semithin sections prepared for EM.

VI. **NEUROPATHOLOGY SPECIMENS.** EM is critical for the evaluation of peripheral nerve biopsies and muscle biopsies, and is also useful in the evaluation of selected neurooncologic specimens (See Chapter 39). EM examination of skin and conjunctival biopsies is used in the diagnosis of neuronal ceroid lipofuscinosis, infantile neuroaxonal dystrophy, and cerebral autosomal dominant arteriopathy with subcortical infarcts and leukoencephalopathy (CADASIL) (e-**Fig. 51.4**).

VII. PRIMARY CILIARY DYSKINESIA. Historically, EM has been considered the gold standard for the diagnosis of PCD using ciliary biopsies and brushings obtained from the nasal mucosa and lower airway. A significant percentage of patients with PCD, however, have normal or nondiagnostic ultrastructural findings, including patients with known mutations affecting ciliary function; in these cases it is important to let the clinicians know that normal ultrastructural findings do not exclude PCD. EM findings should be used in conjunction with other laboratory tests and/or mutational analysis (*Proc Am Thorac Soc* 2011;8:434; *Ultrastruct Pathol* 2017;41:373). The most frequently identified ultrastructural abnormalities in PCD are decreased numbers or absence of outer and/or inner dynein arms (e-**Fig. 51.5**). Ultrastructural abnormalities in other ciliary components have also been reported, but not in a consistent manner. Difficulties in interpretation result from significant overlap of EM findings in chronic inflammatory processes and an inherent difficulty in the visualization of inner dynein arms.

VIII. MICROVILLUS INCLUSION DISEASE. Microvillus inclusion disease presents as intractable secretory diarrhea in the neonate. Characteristic light microscopic findings include villous atrophy and loss of the brush border, but EM is required for diagnosis. Pathognomonic ultrastructural findings include absent or decreased numbers of stubby microvilli on the apical cytoplasmic membrane of enterocytes, along with cytoplasmic membrane–bound inclusions with microvillus projections. Morphologic variants have been reported (*J Pediatr Gastroenterol Nutr* 2004;38:16).

ACKNOWLEDGMENT

The author thanks Ashima Agarwal, an author of the previous edition of this chapter.

SUGGESTED READINGS

D'Agati VD, Jennette JC, Silva FG. *Non-neoplastic Kidney Disease. Atlas of Nontumor Pathology (First series, Fascicle 4).* Washington DC: American Registry of Pathology Press. 2005.

Iancu TC. The ultrastructural spectrum of lysosomal storage diseases. *Ultrastruct Pathol* 1992; 16:231–244.

Sherman PM, Mitchell DJ, Cutz E. Neonatal enteropathies: defining the causes of protracted diarrhea of infancy. *J Pediatr Gastroenterol Nutr* 2004;38:16–26.

Suvarna KS, Layton C, Bancroft J, eds. *Bancroft's Theory and Practice of Histological Techniques E-Book.* 8th ed. Elsevier. 2018.

52

Histology and Histochemical Stains

Kevin D. Selle

I. RECEIPT, ACCESSIONING, AND GROSS DISSECTION. Most, if not all, biopsies and large tissue specimens are routed to the pathology laboratory. Under normal circumstances the specimens are received in 10% neutral buffered formalin (formalin begins the fixation process and prevents autolysis and decomposition). The specimen is first logged into the surgical pathology computer system and given a unique identifying number, referred to as an accession number or case number. Once accessioned, the specimen is taken to the gross dissection room; depending on the practice setting, residents, fellows, Pathologist Assistants, and/or trained technicians are responsible for gross processing of the specimen under the supervision of an attending pathologist. Gross processing entails describing the specimen's size, shape, color, and overall general appearance, followed by placing samples of the tissue in processing cassettes (for biopsies, the entire tissue specimen is placed in a cassette; for larger specimens, regions of tissue are sampled according to established protocols). Each cassette is labeled with the accession number as well as a part designator and number; this numbering scheme is designed to allow the location of a particular section of tissue within the context of the whole specimen.

II. PROCESSING. The loaded cassettes are stored in 10% neutral buffered formalin until automated tissue processing. The normal processing cycle is approximately 8-hours long, although more rapid processing is routinely performed for small tissue specimens. Since, in general, processing is designed to remove the water from the specimen and replace it with paraffin, the individual steps of a processing cycle are often tailored to particular tissue types. Automated, closed-system tissue processors utilize agitation, vacuum, and increased temperature to optimize the process. In general terms, the process is as follows. First, the tissue is subjected to 10% neutral buffered formalin to assure complete fixation. Complete fixation aids in the dehydration steps and prevents tissue shrinkage and other artifacts caused by excessive or rapid dehydration; chemically, the most important result of formalin fixation is the production of methylene crosslinks between nucleic acids and/ or proteins, although formalin also reacts with lipids and carbohydrates. Once the tissue is well fixed, it is subjected to several changes of graduated alcohols in a gradient starting at 70% and ending at 100%, a process that removes water from the tissue at a slow controlled rate designed to prevent excessive shrinkage and disruption of the architecture and cellular components. After complete dehydration of the tissue has been accomplished, a clearing agent is used to remove the alcohol and allow tissue infiltration by paraffin; this clearing agent must therefore be miscible in both alcohol and paraffin. Xylene is most often used for this purpose, although commercial xylene substitutes are available. In the next step of processing, heated paraffin infiltrates into the tissue. Paraffin is solid at room temperature but has a relatively low melting point, and so is a good choice as an infiltration and embedding media. While pure paraffin wax was used in the past, current commercially available paraffins are formulated with various plastic polymers to allow better infiltration and a more rigid crystalline structure, both of which aid subsequent microtomy.

III. EMBEDDING. Properly fixed and processed tissue sections are embedded in molds to prepare them for microtomy. The tissue is removed from the cassette and oriented in the base of a mold that is of a size to allow paraffin to surround the tissue section. During embedding, the tissue is oriented with the understanding that the surface placed down in the mold will become the face of the tissue block, and will thus be the surface cut into first by the microtome blade. Attention must be given to tissues requiring specific orientation such as tubular structures requiring complete cross-sections (e.g., ureteral margins). Orientation is critical to proper tissue representation on the finished slide and leads to proper pathologic diagnosis, and so the importance of proper embedding cannot be overstated. After proper orientation, the mold and tissue are touched to a cold plate to begin to solidify the paraffin so that the tissue is held in place as the mold is filled with paraffin. The empty cassette is placed on top of the mold so that it becomes the back of the tissue block, conveniently retaining the identification of that tissue sample. Finally, the mold is allowed to cool so that the paraffin block containing the oriented tissue can be easily removed.

IV. MICROTOMY. Proper microtomy requires a well-trained and highly skilled microtomist, usually a trained histotechnician or histotechnologist. The microtome instrument is designed to hold the paraffin tissue block firmly in place as it is cyclically presented to a stationary microtome blade. Each turn of the microtome handle (each cycle) advances the tissue block a set distance so microtomes must be kept clean and in good working order. Most tissues are sectioned at 4- to 5-microns thick; however, some tissues are cut thinner at 3 microns (e.g., kidney biopsies and lymph node biopsies), and others thicker at 5 to 6 microns (e.g., bone and brain).

In practice, the paraffin block is first "faced in" to reach a level within the tissue where there is a representative tissue section plane; the block is then cooled on wet ice to further harden the paraffin and aid microtomy. If proper care is taken, individual sections come off of the microtome blade connected to each other, a string of tissue sections called a "ribbon." The tissue ribbon is then floated on a warm water bath at a temperature 6 to 8 degrees below the melting point of the paraffin to make the paraffin very pliable. This aids in mounting the sections on a glass microscope slide labeled with the corresponding accession number and part identifier for that particular block (in addition, the convection currents formed in the water bath help gently stretch the tissue sections, removing any wrinkles).

V. HEMATOXYLIN AND EOSIN STAINING. Slides that have been sectioned are stained to reveal their histologic detail. The primary stain used for pathologic diagnosis is the hematoxylin and eosin stain. Hematoxylin is derived from the logwood tree, and has long been in use in the pathology laboratory. By itself it is not a dye, but once it is oxidized to hematein and combined with a metallic mordant it acquires a strong affinity for nuclear chromatin. Eosin is a dye that at a pH of approximately 4.6 to 5.0 is a strong anion and thus has an affinity for positively charged, cationic, tissue protein groups. At the proper pH, eosin combines at different rates to tissue proteins and thus produces a graduation of distinct shades from light pink to pinkish red.

There are several methods for performing the hematoxylin and eosin stain that can be used to achieve slight variations in the end stain to match the preference of the pathologist. The two general variations of hematoxylin and eosin staining in common use are progressive methods and regressive methods. Progressive methods involve staining slides for a designated period of time, then stopping the reaction as soon as optimal staining has occurred; every tissue stains slightly differently with hematoxylin based on its type, fixation, and prior decalcification, and therefore the length of time in hematoxylin is critical using the progressive method. Regressive methods overstain the tissue sections with hematoxylin then differentiate the hematoxylin using acid alcohol; by overstaining and then differentiating the hematoxylin by the regressive method, a darker, crisper stain can be achieved with the assurance that all hematoxylin positive elements are represented.

The routine regressive staining protocol for the hematoxylin and eosin stain is briefly as follows. The tissue sections are dried completely in an oven since water left on or under the tissue sections can allow the sections to fall off of the slide during the staining process. The slides are then deparaffinized by soaking in xylene, the xylene is removed by alcohol, and the slides are rehydrated by 95% alcohol and then water before staining with hematoxylin. Excess hematoxylin is then removed with a water rinse, the slides are differentiated using acid alcohol, rinsed, and the hematoxylin is "blued" by immersion in a weak ammonia water solution. The slides are rinsed again, placed in 80% alcohol, and stained with eosin. Excess eosin is removed by alcohol rinses, and the slide is prepared for mounting with a coverslip and resinous media by removal of the alcohol using xylene rinses.

VI. OTHER FREQUENTLY USED HISTOCHEMICAL STAINS. Tissue stains range from very simple to complex in methodology, and can be used to demonstrate most major tissue elements relevant to pathologic diagnosis. They are based on the chemistry of various dyes and metals, and most were developed prior to the advent of immunohistochemistry. In general, a histochemical stain consists of the main chemical reaction that demonstrates the specific tissue element of interest, followed by chemical reactions that provide staining of the background uninvolved tissue elements, often including nuclear detail. Histochemical stains are usually grouped by the tissue element they stain.

A. **Carbohydrates.** In humans, carbohydrates exist as various sugars and polymers linked to proteins. Simple sugars cannot be detected by standard histochemical procedures because they are water soluble and thus removed during processing; however, polymers such as glycogen can be detected. Naturally occurring polysaccharides can be classified into four groups based on their histochemical staining differences: neutral polysaccharides (group I), acid mucopolysaccharides (group II), glycoproteins (group III), and glycolipids (group IV). Amyloid must also be included because, even though it is not a carbohydrate, its histochemical staining properties are similar to those of polysaccharides. The histochemical stains most often used to detect carbohydrates and differentiate the various types of carbohydrate are Alcian blue, colloidal iron, mucicarmine, the periodic acid–Schiff (PAS) reaction, Congo red, and Thioflavin T.

1. **Mucicarmine.** The mucicarmine method is used to detect tissue mucins and utilizes the tissue dye carmine. When carmine is reacted with aluminum it forms a compound that has a net positive charge and is attracted to the negative acid groups of epithelial mucins. Metanil yellow and Weigert's hematoxylin are used as counter stains and produce yellow staining of the background tissue elements and blue-black nuclear staining (e-**Fig. 52.1**).

2. **Alcian blue.** Alcian blue, a phthalocyanine basic dye, forms salt bridges with the acid groups in mucopolysaccharides. Staining tissue sections in an Alcian blue solution at pH 1.0 produces staining of only sulfated mucopolysaccharides, while staining at pH 2.5 produces staining of all mucopolysaccharides. These two methods make it possible to differentiate sulfated from carboxylated mucopolysaccharides; further differentiation between mucosubstances of connective tissue origin versus mucosubstances of epithelial origin can be achieved by the addition of hyaluronidase digestion (e-**Fig. 52.2**).

3. **Colloidal iron.** The colloidal iron stain is based on the chemical principle that at low pH colloidal ferric ions can be absorbed by both carboxylated and sulfated mucopolysaccharides, as well as other glycoproteins. The absorbed ferric ions are detected by use of the Prussian blue reaction (see below).

4. **Congo red.** Congo red reacts with cellulose and amyloid. The dye is a linear molecule that attaches to amyloid in a sheet-like fashion resulting in the so-called "apple green" birefringence when subjected to polarized light. This "apple green" birefringence is considered specific for amyloid in Congo red–stained tissue sections (e-**Fig. 52.3**).

5. **Thioflavin T.** Thioflavin T is a fluorescent tissue dye that has an affinity for amyloid. Thioflavin T fluoresces yellow to yellow-green when the tissue section is viewed by fluorescent microscopy, but the dye is not as specific for amyloid as Congo red.

6. **Periodic acid–Schiff (PAS).** The PAS reaction is invaluable in histochemistry because of its versatility. In this reaction, the glycol groups of polysaccharides, mucosubstances, and basement membranes are subjected to oxidation by a solution of periodic acid. The oxidation of the glycols results in the formation of dialdehydes. The dialdehydes are then reacted with the Schiff reagent, a colorless solution created by reducing basic fuchsin in the presence of sulfurous acid. When reacted with the previously oxidized tissue, Schiff reagent is bound to the dialdehyde groups and gains a red color (e-**Fig. 52.4**).

    The differentiation of glycogen from other mucosubstances can be achieved using the PAS stain as follows. Two identical tissue sections are cut. The first section is treated (or digested) with either amylase or diastase to remove any glycogen in the tissue, and then both sections are stained following the PAS procedure. If the substance in question is glycogen it will be present in the undigested section but not in the digested one (e-**Fig. 52.5**).

B. **Connective Tissues.** Connective tissue is made up of three elements in varying amounts, namely cells, a variety of protein fibers, and the so-called ground substance. The commonly used connective tissue stains are used to demonstrate cells and various protein fibers, and include the reticulin stain, trichrome stain, Jones methenamine stain, phosphotungstic acid hematoxylin stain (PTAH), Verhoeff-Van Gieson (VVG) stain, and Oil red O stain. Each of these stains has many different modifications based on the preferences of the laboratory and pathologists involved. Since ground substance is principally composed of mucopolysaccharides, it can be demonstrated by the carbohydrate stains mentioned previously.

1. **Reticulin.** The reticulin stain is similar to the PAS stain in that glycols are first reduced to dialdehydes by the use of an acid. The tissue is next sensitized to accept metallic silver ions with an ammoniacal silver solution, and the silver ions that are attached on and around the dialdehyde groups are then reduced to metallic silver. Finally, the tissue sections are toned from brown to black by replacing the metallic silver with metallic gold; sodium thiosulfate is used to remove any remaining unreacted silver in the tissue to prevent darkening of the slide over time. The end result is that reticulin fibers are stained black against a clear background (e-**Fig. 52.6**).

2. **Jones methenamine silver (JMS).** The JMS stain uses methenamine to form a complex with silver, which is then reacted with dialdehyde groups formed by the reduction of glycol units in the basement membrane in a process similar to that of the reticulin stain (e-**Fig. 52.7**).

3. **Trichrome.** There are a number of variations of the trichrome stain; in general, they all use three dyes with affinities for different connective tissue elements. The first step in the trichrome stain involves mordanting the tissue with a heavy metal fixative such as Bouin fixative. The tissue is then dyed with a nuclear stain, most often an iron hematoxylin. Next, an acidic dye such as acid fuchsin or biebrich scarlet is used to stain the cytoplasm of cells, collagen, and muscle; either phosphotungstic acid or phosphomolybdic acid is then used to remove the acid dye from the collagen (since the cytoplasm of cells is less permeable than collagen, with proper timing the dye can be removed from collagen without complete removal from other tissue elements). Finally, collagen is stained using aniline blue. As the name suggests, the method produces tissue sections that are stained in three colors: black cell nuclei; red cell cytoplasm and muscle; and blue collagen and mucus (e-**Fig. 52.8**).

4. **Verhoeff van Gieson (VVG).** The VVG is another compound stain. The tissue section is first overstained with an iron hematoxylin solution, and then the hematoxylin is differentiated by removal with ferric chloride; since elastic fibers have the greatest affinity for iron hematoxylin, they are the last to decolorize, and so it is possible to halt the differentiation at the point when the elastic fibers are the only tissue elements still stained. The tissue section is then treated with van Gieson's solution which contains the dye acid fuchsin; in a very strong acid solution the dye selectively stains only collagen. Picric acid, used to maintain the proper pH during staining, stains the rest of the tissue elements yellow. The VVG stain demonstrates red stained collagen, black elastic fibers, and a yellow background (e-**Fig. 52.9**).

5. **Phosphotungstic acid hematoxylin (PTAH).** The PTAH stain requires mordanting of the tissue section in Zenker's fixative prior to staining. Because phosphotungstic acid is present in the staining solution in excess over hematoxylin, all of the hematoxylin is bound into a tungsten-hematein lake which selectively binds to cell nuclei, fibrin, and cross-striations in muscle fibers. The excess unreacted phosphotungstic acid stains the remaining tissue elements red to red-brown.

6. **Pentachrome.** The pentachrome stain is a compound stain that essentially combines the elastic fiber staining of a modified VVG stain with a modified trichrome stain. Alcian blue is first used to stain mucosubstances, and then iron hematoxylin is used to

stain elastic fibers. Following the differentiation of the iron hematoxylin, a combined crocein scarlet and acid fuchsin solution is used to stain muscle, cellular cytoplasm, amorphous ground substance, and collagen red. Phosphotungstic acid in solution is then used to decolorize the collagen and amorphous ground substance, which is then subsequently stained yellow using a saturated alcoholic safran solution.

7. **Oil Red O.** This stain is used to demonstrate fat in tissue sections, or lipid droplets in cell cytoplasm. The dye Oil red O is highly soluble in lipids, and when used in solution with isopropanol, is actually more soluble in fat than the alcohol.

This stain requires the use of frozen section tissues because the alcohol and xylene steps in standard paraffin processing remove virtually all lipids from the tissue. The staining itself is fairly straightforward. Frozen tissue sections are cut, fixed with formaldehyde, and then stained in the Oil red O solution. The sections are next rinsed free from any excess stain and then counterstained using hematoxylin. The stain results in blue cell nuclei and bright red staining of fat droplets.

C. **Microorganisms.** There are many different stains that can be performed to demonstrate microorganisms, specifically bacteria and fungi, in tissue sections. The most commonly used stains are the acid fast bacteria or AFB, the Fite modification of the AFB, Gram, Grocott methenamine silver or GMS, Warthin–Starry, and PAS.

1. **Gram stain.** The tissue Gram stain is not much different from the standard Gram stain performed in the microbiology laboratory. In the tissue Gram stain, however, after the use of crystal violet to demonstrate gram-positive bacteria by a blue color, basic fuchsin (a red dye), is used to demonstrate gram-negative organisms as well as cell nuclei. Differentiation of gram-positive and gram-negative bacteria is still a critical step; over-differentiation is a common staining error. The final step in the Brown–Hopps Gram stain involves treating the tissue with a picric acid solution that renders the background yellow. In addition to identification of bacteria, the stains can be used to demonstrate *Actinomyces* infection, *Nocardia* infection, coccidioidomycosis, blastomycosis, cryptococcosis, aspergillosis, rhinosporidiosis, and amebiasis (e-**Fig. 52.10**).

2. **Acid fast bacilli (AFB).** The tissue AFB stain is simply a modification of the standard Ziehl–Neelsen and Kinyoun stains that are based on the fact that carbol-fuchsin, a solution created by reacting basic fuchsin with phenol in alcohol, is soluble in lipids. Tissue sections are first treated with the carbol-fuchsin solution and then differentiated using acid alcohol; bacteria that have waxy, lipid-containing cell walls resist decolorization with acid alcohol and are said to be "acid fast." A methylene blue counterstain is used to highlight other tissue elements and provide a background to highlight the red microorganisms (e-**Fig. 52.11**). A slight modification of this procedure can be used to specifically stain for *Nocardia* species in tissue sections. Another modification of this stain, known as the Fite AFB stain, is used when *Mycobacterium leprae* is suspected (e-**Fig. 52.12**).

3. **Grocott methenamine silver (GMS).** This stain utilizes most of the same chemical reactions and principles as the JMS stain. In the GMS stain, however, a stronger oxidizer, chromic acid, is used instead of the weaker periodic acid. Since the cellular walls of fungi are very thick and contain much more carbohydrate than basement membranes and reticulin fibers of the surrounding tissue, the stronger oxidizer allows for creation of dialdehyde groups from the carbohydrates of the fungi cell walls with overoxidation and subsequent destruction in basement membranes and other carbohydrate structures in the tissue section. The GMS stain utilizes a light-green counterstain, resulting in fungus cell walls that are various shades of black to taupe in a light-green background (e-**Fig. 52.13**).

4. **Warthin–Starry.** The Warthin–Starry method is used primarily for the demonstration of spirochetes, but other bacteria are also stained. The procedure is based on the principle that bacteria in general and spirochetes in particular have the ability to bind silver ions.

The staining procedure therefore involves impregnation of the spirochetes in the tissue with silver ions, with subsequent reduction of these ions to metallic silver using a developer containing hydroquinone. The stain demonstrates black spirochetes against a yellow to pale-brown background. The spiral morphology of this form of bacteria can be fully appreciated by the use of this method (e-**Figs. 52.14** and **52.15**).

5. Periodic acid–Schiff (PAS). This stain is often used for the demonstration of fungi in tissue, but is most helpful when a counterstain of light green is applied. The method used in stains for microorganisms is no different than when used for carbohydrates.

D. Nervous System. Most of the stains used on tissues from the nervous system are for demonstration of either nerve fibers or the myelin sheath. Two commonly used stains for central nervous system tissues are the Bielschowsky and the Luxol Fast Blue.

1. Bielschowsky. The Bielschowsky and all of its modifications are silver stains that follow the principles and general steps of the reticulin stain. In the Bielschowsky technique, the tissue sections are impregnated with a 20% silver nitrate solution and then treated with an ammoniacal silver solution to which formaldehyde has been added. Nerve endings, neurofibrils, neurofibrillary tangles, and neuritic plaques are all stained black.

2. Luxol fast blue. Luxol fast blue, a phthalocyanine dye that is soluble in alcohol, is attracted to bases found in the lipoproteins of the myelin sheath. For this stain, tissue sections are treated with Luxol fast blue over an extended period of time (usually overnight) and then differentiated with a lithium carbonate solution. Since Luxol fast blue has a strong affinity for the lipoproteins of the myelin sheath, it remains bound to these lipoproteins even after removal from other tissue elements. The myelin sheath is stained blue against a colorless background.

E. Pigments and Minerals. Pigments are substances deposited in the interstitium of tissues, or as inclusions or granules in the cytoplasm of cells. Pigments can be derived from minerals such as iron and calcium, or can be endogenous such as melanin. The following staining techniques are used for the demonstration of the most commonly encountered pigments.

1. Iron. The Prussian blue reaction is the most common staining technique for the demonstration of iron in tissue sections. Prussian blue stains only weakly bound iron. Strongly bound iron, such as iron in hemoglobin, will not stain. The principle of this stain is simple: when treated with potassium ferrocyanide in an acidic solution, ferrous ions in tissue react to form an insoluble blue pigment. A nuclear fast red counterstain is usually applied to demonstrate the background tissue morphology (e-**Fig. 52.16**).

2. Urates. A modified GMS stain can be used to demonstrate uric acid crystals. No oxidation of the tissue sections is performed; instead, the sections are reacted in the methenamine solution for an extended period at an elevated temperature. Silver ions deposit on the uric acid crystals which in turn reduce the silver ions to metallic silver, so no toning is necessary. A light-green counterstain is usually applied, and the resulting stained section demonstrates black uric acid crystals in a green background.

This stain requires the use of alcohol fixed tissues because uric acid is soluble in water.

3. Calcium (von Kossa method). The von Kossa method to stain for calcium is very simple. Tissue sections are incubated in a 5% silver nitrate solution under a very strong light source. The silver ions deposit on the calcium and are reduced to metallic silver by the strong light, in much the same process as occurs in a photographic film. The stained section is rinsed free of any unreacted silver ions by a sodium thiosulfate wash, and then counterstained with nuclear fast red to highlight the background tissue morphology (e-**Fig. 52.17**).

4. Copper (rhodanine method). Copper can be demonstrated in tissues using several methods, but the most sensitive method employs rhodanine. Tissue sections are subjected to a saturated solution of 5-(p-dimethylaminobenzylidine) rhodanine in aqueous solution. The rhodanine reacts with proteins that have bound copper rather than directly with the copper itself. The excess stain is rinsed from the sections, and

TABLE 52.1	Common Histochemical Stains	
Stain	Tissue Element Demonstrated	Result
Alcian blue pH 2.5	All acidic mucopolysaccharides	Blue
Alcian blue pH 1.0	Only sulfated acid mucopolysaccharides	Blue
Colloidal iron	Both carboxylated and sulfated muco-polysaccharides and all glycoproteins	Blue
Mucicarmine	Epithelial mucins; *Cryptococcus* capsule	Red
PAS	Neutral mucopolysaccharides, glycogen, basement membranes, and fungi	Rose-red
Congo red	Amyloid	Apple green
Thioflavin T	Amyloid	Yellow
Reticulin	Reticulin fibers	Black
Trichrome	Nuclei, collagen, muscle	Black, blue, red
JMS	Basement membranes	Black
PTAH	Fibrin, muscle striations	Deep purple
Pentachrome	Nuclei, collagen, muscle, elastic fibers Fibrin, muscle, mucin	Black, yellow, red, black Red, red, blue
Oil red O	Fat	Red
VVG	Elastic fibers	Black
AFB	Acid fast bacilli	Red
Fite AFB	*Mycobacterium leprae*	Red
Gram	Differentiating gram-positive from gram-negative bacilli	Gram-positive bacteria: blue; gram-negative bacilli: red
GMS	Fungi	Taupe to black
Warthin–Starry	Spirochetes	Black
Steiner	Bacteria, particularly *Helicobacter pylori*	Black
Dieterle	*Spirochetes* and *Legionella*	Black
Giemsa	Bacteria, primarily *H. pylori*	Blue
Bielschowsky	Nerve endings, neuron fibrils, tangles, and plaques	Black
Luxol fast blue	Myelin	Blue
Iron (Prussian blue)	Iron	Blue
Copper (Rhodanine)	Copper	Red to red-orange
Calcium (von Kossa)	Calcium	Black
Calcium(Alizarin red S)	Calcium	Red
Uric acid (Gömöri)	Urate crystals	Black
(Fontana–Masson)	Argentaffin granules Melanin	Black
Bile pigments (Hall bile)	Bile pigments	Emerald green
Churukian–Schenk	Argyrophil granules	Black
Leder	Cells of myeloid lineage	Red

the sections are counterstained with Mayer's hematoxylin, an aqueous hematoxylin that will not overstain the rhodanine reaction. This tissue stain demonstrates bound copper as a granular red pigment with pale blue cell nuclei (e-**Fig. 52.18**).

5. **Argyrophil staining.** Argyrophil substances within a cell bind silver ions. They are "silver loving" but do not reduce silver to its visible metallic form. There are several different techniques for the demonstration of argyrophil substances, all of which are chemically similar to the Warthin–Starry technique. A solution of silver nitrate is used to impregnate the argyrophilic substances in the tissue, and a reducing solution containing hydroquinone is then used to reduce the bound silver ions to metallic silver. Nuclear fast red is often used as a counterstain. By this approach, argyrophilic substances are stained black.

6. **Argentaffin staining (Fontana–Masson method).** Argentaffin substances not only bind silver ions like argyrophilic substances, but also reduce bound ionic silver to metallic silver without the use of a developer or other reducing agent. This property of argentaffin substances, which include melanin, underlies the Fontana–Masson stain. An ammoniacal silver solution is used to treat tissue sections, and the argentaffin substances within the tissue not only bind the silver ions in the solution, but reduce them to metallic silver. Gold chloride is used as in the reticulin stain to tone the metallic silver from brown to black. Nuclear fast read is the counterstain of choice for this stain (e-**Fig. 52.19**).

7. **Bile pigments.** Bile pigment stains are used on liver sections to distinguish bile pigments from lipofuscin. The use of Fouchet's reagent demonstrates biliverdin, bilirubin, and most other bile pigments. The tissue sections are treated with an aqueous solution of trichloroacetic acid and ferric chloride which renders an emerald-green precipitate, and Van Gieson solution is used as a counterstain (as in the VVG procedure). Stained tissue sections show bile pigments as emerald green, collagen as red, and other tissue elements as yellow.

F. **Enzymes.** Most enzyme stains require the use of frozen section tissues because formalin fixation and paraffin processing tends to inactivate cellular enzymes. The vast majority of enzyme stains are used in the evaluation of diseases that affect the skeletal muscle.

The only enzyme stain performed on routinely processed tissue is the Leder stain, which demonstrates the presence of chloroacetate esterase in cells of myeloid lineage (chloroacetate esterase is an enzyme that can survive the rigors of formalin fixation and paraffin processing but not acid decalcification, so application of the stain to bone marrow specimens requires the use of nonacid decalcification). In the Leder method, tissue is treated with a solution of naphthol-chloroacetate and pararosaniline, and reaction with the cellular chloroacetate esterase forms a red precipitate. Hematoxylin is used as the counterstain to demonstrate nuclear detail (e-**Fig. 52.20**).

G. **Staining Table.** Table 52.1 presents tissue stains listed by their most common name, the tissue element that they demonstrate, and the resulting coloration or specific result.

SUGGESTED READINGS

Carson F, Cappellano CH. *Histotechnology, A Self-Instructional Text.* 4th ed. Chicago, IL: ASCP Press; 2014.

Suvarna KS, Layton C, Bancroft JD. *Bancroft's Theory and Practice of Histological Techniques.* 8th ed. Amsterdam: Elsevier; 2018.

Sheehan DC. *Theory and Practice of Histotechnology.* 2nd ed. Columbus, OH: Battelle Press; 1987.

53 Immunohistochemistry
Marianna Ruzinova and Peter A. Humphrey

I. INTRODUCTION. Immunohistochemistry is one of the most powerful and widely used ancillary methods in surgical pathology. The technique makes it possible to simultaneously visualize cell type and differentiation markers in standard tissue sections by light microscopy, and has revolutionized diagnostic surgical pathology.

Antigens in tissue sections were first detected using antibodies via immunofluorescence performed on frozen sections (*Proc Soc Exp Biol Med* 1941;47:200). Although immunofluorescence is still used in the evaluation of medical kidney biopsies (see Chapter 19) and some skin biopsies (Chapter 38), currently the most common approach for diagnostic detection of antigens uses formalin-fixed paraffin-embedded (FFPE) tissue sections and immunoperoxidase methodology. This enzymatic labeling technique has evolved from simple direct peroxidase conjugation of the primary antibody, to the use of multistep peroxidase–antiperoxidase (PAP), avidin–biotin (and related) conjugate methods, which, along with amplification techniques such as tyramide and polymer-based labeling, allow for much greater sensitivity in antigen detection.

Laboratory utilization of immunohistochemistry (also known as immunohistology and immunostaining) requires appropriate test selection, specimen acquisition and management, methodology, validation, reporting, and interpretation. This chapter provides a concise overview of these elements. Comprehensive guidelines pertaining to these elements have been published by The Clinical and Laboratory Standards Institute (Hewitt SM, Robinowitz M. *I/LA28. Quality Assurance for Design Control and Implementation of Immunohistochemistry Assays.* 2nd ed. Wayne, PA: CLSI; 2011).

II. TEST SELECTION (PREANALYTICAL PHASE). Immunohistochemical stains are usually ordered after examination of hematoxylin and eosin (H&E)-stained sections. Common indications for immunohistochemistry are the diagnosis and characterization of neoplasms, but there are other indications as well such as detection of infectious organisms and evaluation of prognostic and/or predictive factors (Table 53.1). In recent years, mutation-specific antibodies have been introduced as a supplement to or replacement for molecular analysis.

The use of specific immunostains is driven by the clinical and morphologic context of each individual case. Panels of antibodies are often used, which should be devised based on the anticipated value added to the clinical, radiographic, and pathologic differential diagnosis; in other words, the panel of antibodies used in a particular case should be directed toward a specific question. Various approaches have been used to help construct appropriate immunostain panels, including algorithmic approaches and tabular approaches. Web sites with information on the specificity and sensitivity of various immunostains, and on construction of immunostain panels based on differential diagnosis of specific neoplasms, also exist (see below).

III. SPECIMEN TYPE AND TISSUE MANAGEMENT. Immunostains are usually performed on standard histologic tissue sections, although they can also be performed on cytology specimens. Whereas the use of FFPE tissue sections offers obvious logistical advantages, some antigens require the use of fresh tissue or tissue preserved with ethanol-based fixatives. The discussion here focuses on tissues fixed in 10% neutral buffered formalin because this is the tissue type most commonly available for analysis in routine clinical practice.

Immediate fixation in neutral pH formalin for 12 to 48 hours at room temperature is desirable. However, it must be noted that formalin induces cross-links that may mask some epitopes resulting in loss of immunoreactivity. Acid decalcification of bone samples

TABLE 53.1	Examples of Practical Uses of Selected Antigens in Routine Surgical Pathology[a]

Antigen	Predominant Distribution	Common Diagnostic Uses
To identify cellular proteins to help classify a neoplasm		
Cytokeratin	Epithelial cells	Distinction of carcinoma from lymphoma or melanoma
Cytokeratin isoforms	Epithelial cells	Determination of primary site of metastatic carcinoma (pattern of expression of various isoforms is related to the site of origin)
Epithelial membrane antigen	Epithelial cells	Distinction of carcinoma from melanoma
Desmin	Myogenous cells	Identification of smooth muscle or skeletal muscle tumors
Muscle-specific actin	Myogenous cells	Identification of smooth muscle or skeletal muscle tumors
Prostate-specific antigen	Prostatic epithelium	Identification of metastatic prostatic carcinoma
Calcitonin	Parafollicular thyroid epithelium	Distinction of medullary thyroid carcinoma from other thyroid tumors
Alpha-fetoprotein	Neoplastic hepatocytes and selected germ cell tumors	Identification of hepatocellular carcinoma, endodermal sinus tumor, and other germ cell tumors
β-Human chorionic gonadotropin	Placental tissue; trophoblastic and germ cell tumors	Identification of trophoblastic differentiation in germ cell tumors
HMB-45	Melanocytic cells	Identification of melanoma
CD31	Vascular endothelium	Identification of vascular neoplasms
CD34	Vascular endothelium and some soft tissue tumors	Identification of vascular neoplasms, solitary fibrous tumors, dermatofibrosarcoma protuberans
To identify infectious agents to help classify a neoplasm		
Epstein–Barr virus latent membrane protein 1	Lymphocytes	Identification of EBV-associated lymphomas
Human herpesvirus 8	Vascular endothelium	Identification of Kaposi sarcoma
Merkel cell polyomavirus	Neuroendocrine cells	Identification of Merkel cell carcinoma
p16	Epithelium	Surrogate marker for HPV infection
To subclassify a hematolymphoid malignancy[b]		
CD45 (LCA)	Lymphocytes	Distinction of lymphoma from carcinoma or melanoma
CD3, CD4, and CD8	All T cells, helper T cells, cytotoxic T cells (respectively)	Characterization of lymphoid infiltrates

TABLE 53.1	Examples of Practical Uses of Selected Antigens in Routine Surgical Pathology[a] (*Continued*)

Antigen	Predominant Distribution	Common Diagnostic Uses
CD19 and CD20	B cells	Characterization of lymphoid infiltrates
CD34, TdT	Blasts	Detection of acute leukemias
Myeloperoxidase, lysozyme	Myeloid, monocytic cells	Characterization of myeloid neoplasms
CD138, and kappa and lambda cytoplasmic light chains	Plasma cells	Characterization of plasma cell neoplasms
To provide prognostic or predictive information		
Estrogen receptor and progesterone receptor	Mammary epithelium and endometrium	Prediction of clinical response to hormonal therapy
HER2	Epithelium	Level of expression provides prognostic information and predicts clinical response to therapy
PD-L1	Numerous tumor types	Level of expression predicts clinical response to therapy
BRAF V600E mutation	Numerous tumor types	Identification of V600E-activating mutation provides prognostic information and predicts clinical response to therapy in melanoma and thyroid carcinoma
To identify patients likely to have an inherited cancer syndrome		
MLH1, PMS2, MSH2, and MSH6	All cell types	Lack of staining indicates a defect in DNA mismatch repair (MMR), which may suggest the presence of Lynch syndrome
To identify infectious agents		
Helicobacter pylori	Stomach	Identification of organism in gastric biopsies
Treponema pallidum	Numerous organs	Identification of organism in tissue biopsies

[a]This table is not comprehensive and is intended to provide selected examples only. For more detail, see Lester SC, ed. *Manual of Surgical Pathology*. 3rd ed. Philadelphia, PA: Elsevier; 2010:73–106, or the commercial site PATHIQ. Immunoquery at www.immunoquery.com.
[b]See Chapters 41 and 42 for more detail.

can also cause loss of immunoreactivity. "Unmasking" of some epitopes from FFPE tissue (and tissue treated with acid decalcification) can be accomplished by antigen retrieval techniques. Enzyme digestion was used for this purpose in the past, but now simple heat treatment (heat-induced antigen retrieval) is the most commonly used approach to optimize antigen detection.

Unstained tissue sections cut onto charged slides or poly-L-lysine-coated slides (or gelatin- or albumin-coated slides) are typically used for immunohistochemistry. However, it is possible to perform immunostains on sections that have already been stained with H&E (*Am J Clin Pathol* 2005;124:708), but because success with such restaining protocols is variable, unstained tissue sections remain the best resource for immunostains.

Immunostaining should be performed on freshly cut sections from the paraffin block, because unstained sections exposed to air may lose antigen immunoreactivity over the course of days to weeks.

IV. METHODOLOGY

A. The Primary Antibody is an immunoglobulin molecule that binds to the target antigen in the tissue sections. The primary antibody may be either a monoclonal antibody derived via the hybridoma technique, or a polyclonal antibody from an antiserum. In general, polyclonal antibodies tend to be more sensitive but less specific than monoclonal antibodies. Unlike monoclonal antibodies, polyclonal antibodies are not uniform reagents of unlimited supply; different batches of antisera may result in polyclonal antibody heterogeneity.

Each antibody, whether polyclonal or monoclonal in origin, needs to be tested for sensitivity and specificity in target antigen detection, and the reaction conditions for its use need to be optimized. Titration experiments must be performed to achieve a working dilution of the primary antibody that yields the greatest contrast between specific staining and nonspecific staining. If prediluted reagents and kits are used, it is recommended that the manufacturer protocol be followed because validation was performed using those reaction conditions.

B. Background Staining results from nonspecific antibody binding and from endogenous enzymes that nonspecifically interact with the chromogenic substrate. Nonspecific antibody binding is more likely to occur with polyclonal antibodies. Endogenous enzymes that cause background staining are found in normal cells including erythrocytes, neutrophils, eosinophils, hepatocytes, plasma cells, and neoplastic cells; their activity can often be blocked (e.g., endogenous peroxidase can be blocked by incubation with hydrogen peroxide).

C. Detection Systems

1. **Direct conjugate–labeled antibody method.** In this method, the label (e.g., peroxidase or fluorescein) is directly chemically linked to the primary antibody. Disadvantages of this approach include a requirement for a large amount of primary antibody for labeling and a lack of signal amplification.

2. **Indirect or sandwich method.** The primary antibody is unlabeled, and a secondary antibody, reactive against the primary antibody, carries the label.

3. **Unlabeled antibody method.** Also known as the PAP method, this procedure uses an unlabeled primary antibody, an unlabeled bridge antibody, and a complex of an antiperoxidase antibody and the peroxidase molecule itself. The bridge antibody, directed against both the primary antibody and the antiperoxidase antibody, links the primary antibody–tissue antigen reaction to the signal generated by the peroxidase. This approach has largely been replaced by the more sensitive approaches below.

4. **Avidin–biotin or streptavidin–biotin conjugate method.** A biotinylated secondary antibody is used to recognize the primary antibody; avidin or streptavidin complexed with biotinylated peroxidase is then bound to the secondary antibody (both avidin and streptavidin have extremely high affinity for biotin). These reactions deliver several peroxidase molecules to the primary antibody binding site and so boost sensitivity. Streptavidin has several advantages over avidin, including decreased background staining.

5. **Tyramine amplification (catalyzed signal amplification [CSA]) methods.** With these methods, there is increased sensitivity due to greater accumulation of biotin at the antigen–primary antibody reaction site as a result of the catalytic activity of peroxidase on biotinylated tyramine.

6. **Polymer-based labels.** This approach uses dextran chain polymers to localize numerous enzyme molecules to the antigen site by linking multiple antibody and enzyme molecules together along the polymer chain (Fig. 53.1). This method avoids problems due to endogenous biotin.

7. **Alkaline phosphatase** can be used instead of peroxidase when the target antigen is in tissues rich in myeloid cells that contain high levels of endogenous peroxidases, such as bone marrow.

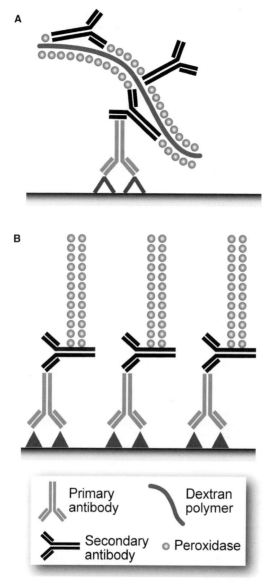

Figure 53.1 Immunohistochemical detection using the polymer method. This technique allows linkage of numerous molecules of enzyme (either peroxidase or alkaline phosphatase) to one (**B**) or more (**A**) molecules of secondary antibody. Delivery of a large number of enzyme molecules to the antigen–primary antibody reaction site yields high sensitivity. (Modified from Taylor CR, Cote RJ, eds. *Immunomicroscopy. A Diagnostic Tool for the Surgical Pathologist.* 3rd ed. Philadelphia: Elsevier; 2006.)

8. **Chromogens** are the color-producing reactants in the detection system. Methods using peroxidase, diaminobenzidine (DAB, produces a brown color), and 3-amino-9-ethyl carbazole (AEC, produces a red color) are commonly used.

9. **Counterstaining** is most often accomplished using the nuclear stain hematoxylin. Care must be taken not to overstain the tissue sections, especially when the target antigen is located in the nucleus.

10. **Antibody cocktails** can be used to detect two or more antigens at the same time. Single-color (*Am J Surg Pathol* 2005;29:579) or two-color (*Am J Clin Pathol* 2005;123:231) approaches can be used.

11. **Automation.** Automated immunostaining devices are in routine use in most laboratories and can improve standardization, throughput, and reproducibility of immunohistochemical procedures.

12. **Quantitative immunohistochemistry.** Immunohistochemical reactions have traditionally been manually scored in a semiquantitative manner by pathologists to estimate staining intensity and percentage of cells stained in the area of interest. Such scoring has been particularly important for a few markers, for example, detection of HER2 immunoreactivity in breast carcinoma to determine the eligibility of breast cancer patients for trastuzumab (Herceptin) therapy (*J Clin Oncol* 2013;31:3997). Because image analysis improves the consistency of quantitative immunohistochemical scoring, it is likely that digital microscopy (see Chapter 61) with image analysis will be increasingly used in this context.

V. **VALIDATION.** Positive and negative controls should be included in every sample run and reviewed along with the test immunohistochemical reaction. A positive tissue or cell control known to express the antigen under investigation should be used, and should be subjected to the same reaction conditions in the same analytical run as the test tissues or cells. Some laboratories place a positive control tissue section on the same slide as the test tissue section; for some immunostains there may be an internal positive control in the test tissue. A negative control can be generated using a tissue known to lack the antigen of interest or by replacing the primary antibody with an irrelevant nonimmune antibody or antiserum; a search should also be made in the test tissues for negative internal controls.

VI. **REPORTING.** Immunohistochemical stain reports should include specific content elements (Table 53.2).

VII. **INTERPRETATION.** The results of the immunostains must be integrated with the interpretation of the clinical, radiographic, gross, and histopathologic findings of the case, as well as the results of any additional ancillary tests (such as molecular genetic tests). After evaluation of positive and negative controls, the test tissue sections should be assessed for presence of the area(s) of interest, localization of immunohistochemical signal (e.g., cytoplasmic,

---

TABLE 53.2	Guidelines for Incorporation of Results of Immunohistochemical Stains in Surgical Pathology Reports[a]

1. All immunostain results should be reported, whether positive, negative, or noncontributory
2. A differential diagnosis justifying immunostain selection should be given
3. The report may also include the following:
   - the nature of the specimen tested: frozen section, paraffin section, cytoprep, etc.
   - the paraffin block number used to obtain sections for immunostaining
   - the antibodies used, including where appropriate, the clone number
   - specific staining details for each antibody, including cellular localization when relevant
4. An interpretation of the findings in the context of the diagnosis, with reference to the associated surgical pathology report if immunohistochemical results are reported separately
5. Exact protocols, antigen retrieval methods, and reaction conditions need not be part of the report but must be available in laboratory manuals and records

[a]Modified from Taylor CR, Cote RJ, eds. *Immunomicroscopy. A Diagnostic Tool for the Surgical Pathologist.* 3rd ed. Philadelphia: Elsevier; 2006:41, Table 1.8.

nuclear, membranous), intensity of signal, and number of immunoreactive cells or foci. In some cases, especially for limited and small tissue samples, the area of interest may not be present in the additional sections used for immunohistochemistry. Specific attention should be directed toward background staining, and artifacts such as localization of signal along tissue edges (edge artifact) or in areas of necrosis.

Immunostain results can profoundly influence a diagnosis or can be noncontributory, so the role of immunostains in arriving at the final diagnosis should be specified in the report. For example, a comment in the report should indicate that immunostains were used to establish, confirm, or support a diagnosis, or that they are noncontributory. For predictive markers such as HER2/*neu* and PD-L1, guidelines for staining and reporting should be followed (*J Clin Oncol* 2013;31:3997; *Appl Immunohistochem Mol Morphol* 2016;24:392).

VIII. SOURCES OF DATA ON ANTIBODIES AND ANTIGENS, INCLUDING CONSTRUCTION OF MARKER PANELS. The chapters in this book provide information on the most useful immunostains for the evaluation of diseases of each organ system and/or tissue type. Other sources for detailed information on useful marker panels include books (Lester SC, ed. *Manual of Surgical Pathology.* 3rd ed. Philadelphia, PA: Elsevier; 2010:73–106) as well as Internet sites (one helpful commercial site is PATHIQ Immunoquery at www.immuno-query.com).

SUGGESTED READINGS

Dabbs DJ, ed. *Diagnostic Immunohistochemistry: Theranostic and Genomic Applications.* 5th ed. Philadelphia, PA: Elsevier; 2014:1–46.

Taylor CR, Cote RJ, eds. *Immunomicroscopy. A Diagnostic Tool for the Surgical Pathologist.* 3rd ed. Philadelphia, PA: Elsevier; 2006.

Immunofluorescence

Aidas J. Mattis and Joseph Gaut

I. **INTRODUCTION.** Immunofluorescence studies are used to support fixed tissue diagnoses and to provide additional diagnostic and prognostic information as it relates to autoimmune diseases, vesiculobullous diseases, transplantation, and glomerular disease. Immunofluorescence requires fresh tissue submitted in a preservative nonfixative transport medium such as Michel medium, or fresh frozen tissue. For fresh tissue, the transport medium should be held at room temperature; temperature extremes should be avoided. A specialized microscope and a room where the majority of ambient light can be extinguished are required for either direct or indirect immunofluorescence examination.

II. **DIRECT IMMUNOFLUORESCENCE**

A. **Skin/Mucosa.** Cutaneous/mucosal biopsies for immunofluorescence are stained with fluorescein-labeled antibodies to immunoglobulin (IgG, IgA, IgM), complement (C3), and collagen IV. The patterns of staining that correlate with specific diseases are discussed in more detail with the corresponding diagnoses in the chapter on inflammatory disorders of the skin (Chapter 38). Patterns of staining include basement membrane (e-**Fig. 54.1**) and intercellular (e-**Fig. 54.2**) positivity.

1. **Bullous pemphigoid.** A biopsy of perilesional tissue to include the edge of a blister is optimal. Some studies have reported a high false-negative rate for tissue from the lower extremity; if possible, tissue for direct immunofluorescence should be obtained from above the knee. Direct immunofluorescence is positive in approximately 85% to 90% of cases of bullous pemphigoid.

2. **Pemphigus vulgaris.** A biopsy of perilesional tissue, without including the edge of a blister, is optimal. Direct immunofluorescence is positive in approximately 90% to 95% of cases of pemphigus vulgaris.

3. **Dermatitis herpetiformis.** A biopsy of perilesional tissue, avoiding excoriated areas, is optimal. Direct immunofluorescence is positive in approximately 80% of cases of dermatitis herpetiformis.

4. **Vasculitis.** A biopsy of lesional tissue is required. Sources vary on recommendations regarding age of the lesion; however, the majority favors a lesion that has been present for <48 hours.

5. **Lupus.** A biopsy of an established lesion that has been present for at least 8 weeks, preferably 12, is required to detect immunofluorescence positivity in discoid lupus. In the past, prognostic information regarding disease activity was associated with immunofluorescence positivity in sun-protected, nonlesional skin in systemic lupus.

B. **Kidney.** Biopsy practices vary, however it is common practice to attempt two or three biopsies to collect sufficient tissue for light microscopy, immunofluorescence, and electron microscopic analysis (*Arch Pathol Lab Med* 2009;133:181). Renal biopsies are usually performed under ultrasound guidance, and the tissue cores are evaluated in the ultrasound suite with a dissecting microscope. Since it is important to avoid air drying of the tissue, the biopsy is placed in a Petri dish with a balanced salt solution while it is examined with the dissecting microscope. Because glomerular diseases are a common indication for renal biopsy, the tissue is distributed in such a way that approximately 2 or more glomeruli are examined by electron microscopy, 2 or more by immunofluorescence, and 10 or more by light microscopy. The tissue assigned to electron microscopy is placed in glutaraldehyde; tissue for immunofluorescence is frozen, and tissue for light microscopy is placed in formalin. When a biopsy needs to be transported to the laboratory from a remote site, it should be placed in a container with transport medium such as Michel medium.

Although FFPE tissue is not routinely used for immunofluorescence evaluation, there are selected circumstances where this may be essential. Immunofluorescence on FFPE tissue may be employed as a salvage technique when frozen specimens are deemed inadequate due to lack of cortical tissue (*Kidney Int* 2006;70:2148). Some renal diagnoses rely on paraffin IF to "unmask" deposits (*Mod Pathol* 2015;28:854). Immunofluorescence on FFPE tissue is performed by deparaffinizing the FFPE tissue and treating the tissue with pronase for antigen retrieval, followed by staining using typical immunofluorescence protocols.

Light microscopic evaluation of the renal biopsy is performed using hematoxylin and eosin, periodic acid–Schiff (PAS), trichrome, and methenamine silver–stained sections. The PAS and silver stains facilitate examination of the basement membranes, and the trichrome stain highlights areas of interstitial fibrosis. Evaluation with fluorescein isothiocyanate (FITC) conjugated antibodies against IgG, IgM, IgA, C3, C1q, fibrinogen, albumin, κ, and λ are performed by direct immunofluorescence.

Transplant kidney biopsies are also stained for C4d using an indirect immunofluorescence technique. C4d is used to assess for humoral rejection, usually seen as immunopositivity of the peritubular capillaries. C4d IHC can be used as a salvage technique when the frozen IF specimen is unsatisfactory. Addition of a 3% Evans Blue counterstain is helpful to decrease the FITC background and to enhance visualization of the tissue (*Am J Transplant* 2009;9:812) (e-**Fig. 54.3**).

C. Lung. In the event of suspected humoral rejection after pulmonary transplantation, biopsy of pulmonary parenchymal tissue acquired via transbronchial biopsy can be submitted in Michel medium for evaluation of complement (C4d) by direct immunofluorescence. It is worth noting that evaluation for the presence of C4d can also be accomplished using an immunoperoxidase method on FFPE.

III. INDIRECT IMMUNOFLUORESCENCE. Blood (5 to 10 mL) drawn into a tube without anticoagulant is required for all indirect immunofluorescence studies. The serum is removed and is applied to an epithelial substrate. The substrate varies with the clinical diagnosis, and the clinical diagnosis should guide the decision to pursue the appropriate indirect immunofluorescence study. For indirect immunofluorescence, serial dilutions (1:10 to 1:1,280) of serum are inoculated onto the tissue substrate together with fluorescein-labeled anti-IgG.

A. Pemphigus Vulgaris. The primary utility for indirect immunofluorescence is for the diagnosis of pemphigus vulgaris and to follow response to therapy. Serial dilutions are performed and the end point of positivity of intercellular IgG is reported (e-**Fig. 54.2**). Commercially prepared slides using guinea pig or monkey esophagus are used. As in other serologic tests, it is possible to get a prozone effect in patients with pemphigus vulgaris, so additional dilutions may be required to avoid a false-negative result.

B. Paraneoplastic Pemphigus. The substrate for evaluation of paraneoplastic pemphigus is murine/rat bladder epithelium. Because this test is not commonly ordered, it is usually only performed at reference laboratories.

C. Bullous and/or Cicatricial Pemphigoid. Circulating antibodies that produce a linear basement membrane zone positivity (e-**Fig. 54.1**) are detected in fewer than half of the patients with documented pemphigoid, making ancillary testing by indirect immunofluorescence minimally useful for this disease process.

D. Dermatitis Herpetiformis. Circulating antibodies are not detectable in the serum of patients with dermatitis herpetiformis; therefore, indirect immunofluorescence is not indicated.

E. Reference Laboratories. Reference laboratories are a useful resource for indirect immunofluorescence testing for rare diseases. Evaluation of epidermolysis bullosa is performed by Beutner Laboratories (Buffalo, NY). Testing for paraneoplastic pemphigus is performed by Mayo Clinical Laboratories (Rochester, MN). Some research laboratories also perform specialized testing for rare vesiculobullous dermatoses, however testing in this setting may not be approved for clinical use.

ACKNOWLEDGMENT

The authors thank Anne C. Lind and Rosa Davila, authors of the previous edition of this chapter.

55 Flow Cytometry

Friederike Kreisel

I. **BASIC PRINCIPLE.** Flow cytometry simultaneously measures and analyzes multiple physical and/or chemical characteristics of single particles, usually cells, as they flow in a fluid stream through a beam of light. With this technique any suspended microparticle, ranging in size from 0.2 to 150 μm can be analyzed.

Many protocols for the preparation of cell suspensions exist. Peripheral blood or bone marrow aspirate specimens already represent a suspension of single cells but they must be prevented from clotting by using collection tubes containing disodium EDTA, sodium citrate, or heparin. Enrichment for leucocytes can be achieved by lysis of accompanying red blood cells with ammonium chloride buffer or utilizing density-gradient separation (*Flow Cytometry in Clinical Diagnosis.* 3rd ed. Chicago, IL: ASCP Press, p31–65, 2001). Solid tissue should be collected in RPMI medium, and the tissue should be minced into small pieces and passed through a fine mesh.

II. **THE FLOW CYTOMETER.** The flow cytometer is composed of three main systems (*Flow Cytometry in Clinical Diagnosis.* 3rd ed. Chicago, IL: ASP, p31–65, 2001) (Figure 55.1):

A. **The Flow System.** The sample is injected into a stream of sheath fluid within the flow chamber. Through the principle of hydrodynamic focusing, the particles are forced into the center of the stream and transported to the laser beam for analysis, where only one particle or cell moves through the laser beam at a given moment. The sample pressure is always greater than the sheath fluid pressure; increasing the sample pressure increases the flow rate of the sample by increasing the width of the sample core, allowing more cells to enter the stream at a given moment. A higher flow rate is generally used for immunophenotyping of cells. A lower flow rate is important in applications where greater resolution is needed, such as DNA analysis.

B. **Optical System.** Lasers illuminate the particles in the sample stream and optical mirrors and filters route the different wavelengths of the generated light scatter and fluorescent signals to the appropriate photodetectors.

1. **Light scatter.** Light scattering occurs when a particle or cell deflects incident laser light. Forward-scattered light (FSC) is in line with the laser light beam and represents a measurement of the cell surface size. Side-scattered light (SSC) is collected perpendicular to the laser light beam and analyses the granularity or internal complexity of a cell. Leukocytes can be separated into different subpopulations utilizing FSC and SSC. For example, lymphocytes will show both a low forward scatter and a low side scatter due to the small size and lack of cytoplasmic granulation. On the other hand, neutrophils are larger in size and show granular cytoplasm as well as a complex nucleus, and therefore will show both a high forward and side scatter (e-**Fig. 55.1**).

2. **Fluorescence**. Another way to identify particular subpopulations is to conjugate fluorescent dyes to monoclonal antibodies directed toward antigens on a particular cell subset. The fluorescent dyes absorb light energy over a range of wavelengths that is characteristic for that fluorophore; with the absorption of light energy an electron in the fluorescent dye is raised to a higher energy level, and subsequently the excited electron returns to its ground state emitting the excess energy as a photon of light. The emitted light, known as fluorescence, is captured by a detector.

The staining procedure can be carried out in a direct or indirect approach staining (*Flow Cytometry, First Principles,* New York: Wiley-Liss, p75–102, 1992). The direct staining procedure involves a single staining incubation, followed by several washes

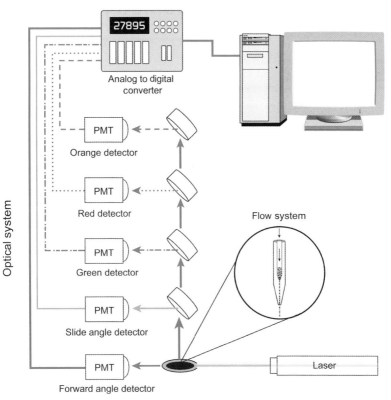

Figure 55.1 The flow cytometer is composed of a flow system, optical system, and electronic system. The flow system transports cells in a stream to the laser beam for analysis. The optical system consists of lasers to illuminate the cells in the sample stream and optical filters to direct the resulting light signals to the appropriate detectors. The electronic system converts light signals into electronic signals that are processed by the computer.

to remove nonspecifically bound antibodies. The indirect staining procedure involves the incubation of cells with a nonfluorescent monoclonal antibody directed toward the specific antigen, that after washing is followed by a second incubation with a fluorescent antibody directed against the monoclonal antibody. Although more time consuming, the indirect staining procedure is less expensive and more sensitive.

Argon ion lasers are the most common lasers used in flow cytometry because the 488-nm light emitted can be absorbed by more than one fluorochrome. Examples of fluorochromes that are conjugated to antibodies are fluorescein isothiocyanate (FITC) and phycoerythrin (PE). FITC absorbs light in the range of 460 to 510 nm and then fluoresces in the range of 510 to 560 nm, with a peak at ~525 nm, giving a green fluorescent color. PE absorbs light in the range of 480 to 565 nm and fluoresces at ~570 nm, creating a red fluorescent color. Although both fluorochromes absorb light in the same range of wavelengths, the difference in the peak emission wavelengths makes it possible to measure them by different detectors, which permits different fluorochromes (FITC, PE, and many others) to be used simultaneously in one sample. Combined with the FSC and SSC data, the staining pattern of each subpopulation will aide in delineating which cells are present in a sample and in what percentage they are present (**e-Fig. 55.2**).

C. Electronic System. Photodetectors convert the generated FSC, SSC, and fluorescent light signals into electrical impulses.

    1. Photodetectors. Generally, two types of photodetectors are used in flow cytometry: photomultiplier tubes (PMTs) and photodiodes. PMTs have voltages applied to them to amplify the electrical current generated from the light signals. These are mostly used to detect weaker signals generated by SSC and fluorescence. Photodiodes are less sensitive to light signals and are used to detect stronger FSC.

    Amplification of a signal detected by a photodetector can also be achieved by increasing the amplification gain, by means of log amplification or linear amplification. Log amplifiers are usually used to separate negative from dim positive signals, and are commonly used to analyze fluorescence signals in cells stained with fluorochrome-labeled antibodies since these cells often exhibit a great range of fluorescence intensities. Linear amplifiers are generally used to analyze forward and side scatter signals.

    2. Conversion to a digital value. The intensity of the electronic impulses derived from the photodetectors is assigned a digital value by means of an analog to digital converter (ADC). The role of the ADC is therefore to convert a continuous distribution of signal intensities into individual channels, where each channel has a defined light intensity range, and then to organize the data into a graphical plot. An electronic threshold is used to limit the number of events to the population of interest (for example, the threshold can be set on FSC to eliminate events that represent debris smaller than the threshold channel number). Once the acquired data are saved, cell populations can be displayed as different data plots. A single parameter, such as FSC or FITC (FL1) can be displayed as a single-parameter histogram, where the horizontal axis represents the signal intensity expressed as the parameter's signal value in channel numbers and the vertical axis represents the number of events per channel (**e-Fig. 55.3**). Signals with identical intensities accumulate in the same channel. Two parameters, such as FITC (FL1) and PE (FL2) can be displayed simultaneously in a dot plot (**e-Fig. 55.4**), in which one parameter is displayed on the x-axis and the other parameter is displayed on the y-axis.

    A subset of data can be defined through a so-called gate. For example, based on the FSC and SSC, a gate can be set on a selected population of interest and analysis restricted to only that subset of the population.

III. USES. Flow cytometry has become a valuable ancillary study methodology for classifying acute leukemias and lymphomas.

A. Cell Markers. Monoclonal antibody technology has provided flow cytometry with a large variety of antibodies specific to nuclear, cytoplasmic, and surface antigens characteristic of particular cell subsets (Table 55.1). These are organized as cluster of differentiation (CD) antigens, which help differentiate hematopoietic and lymphoid cells into different characteristic subpopulations. Selected CD markers that are used in the diagnosis of acute leukemias and lymphomas are discussed in Chapters 41 and 42. Flow cytometric scattergrams of an example of precursor B-lymphoblastic leukemia are shown in **e-Figure 55.5**. Typical flow cytometric findings of chronic lymphocytic leukemia are shown in **e-Figures 55.6** and **55.7**.

B. Multicolor Flow Cytometry with 2 or more lasers and 8 to 10 different antibodies is increasingly used in clinical practice for the diagnosis of hematopoietic malignancies. The larger set of antibodies allows for differentiation of "normal" cell populations from neoplastic populations, and makes it possible to detect minimal residual disease (MRD) at a sensitivity of 1:10,000 to 1:100,000 (i.e., 1 abnormal cell in 10,000 to 100,000 normal cells).

TABLE 55.1 Antibodies Used for Immunophenotyping by Flow Cytometry

CD Designation	Normal Distribution	Use For
CD1a	Immature T-cells	Lymphoblastic lymphoma Langerhans cell histiocytosis
CD2, 3, 4, 5, 7, and 8	T-cells	Lineage of lymphoma/leukemia
CD5	T-cells	SLL/CLL, mantle cell lymphoma
CD10 (CALLA)	Many cell types	Precursor B-ALL, follicular lymphoma
CD11c	Monocytes	Hairy cell leukemia strongly positive; SLL/CLL dim positive
CD13	Monocytes Myeloid cells	Lineage of leukemia Extramedullary myeloid tumor
CD14	Monocytes	AML M5
CD15	Monocytes Myeloid cells	Lineage of leukemia Extramedullary myeloid tumor
CD16	NK, NK-like T-cells	Large, granular lymphocyte leukemia
CD19, 20, 21, 22 and 23	B-cells	Lineage of lymphoma/leukemia
CD23	B-cells	SLL/CLL strongly positive
CD25	Many cell types	Hairy cell leukemia strongly positive
CD33	Monocytes Myeloid cells	Lineage of leukemia Extramedullary myeloid tumor
CD34	Stem cells	Stem cells for transplantation in AML
CD38	Plasma cells, activated T-cells, Myeloid cells	Limited clinical value
CD41, 42	Megakaryocytes	AML M7
CD45 (LCA)	All leukocytes	Lineage of malignancy, used for gating
CD55	GPI-anchored proteins	Paroxysmal nocturnal hemoglobinuria (PNH)
CD56 and 57	NK, NK-like T-cells	Large granular lymphocyte leukemia
CD59	GPI-anchored proteins	PNH
CD61	Megakaryocytes	AML M7
CD64	Monocytes	AML M5
CD71 (Glycophorin A)	Erythroid	True erythroleukemia
CD79a	B-cells (blasts to plasma cells)	Lineage of lymphoma/leukemia
CD103	Subset of intramucosal T-cells	Hairy cell leukemia
CD117 (c-kit)	Hematopoietic progenitor cells	AML
HLA-DR	B-cells Activated T-cells Monocytes	B-cell leukemias/lymphomas AML (except M3) Peripheral T-cell lymphomas
FMC-7	Some B-cells	Prolymphocytic leukemia, hairy cell leukemia, splenic lymphoma
TdT (DNA polymerase)	B- and T-lymphoblasts	B-ALL, T-ALL Lymphoblastic lymphoma AML (M0 or M1)
Myeloperoxidase	Myeloid cells	Lineage of leukemia Extramedullary myeloid tumor
Kappa/lambda	B-cells	Maturity, clonality, SLL/CLL (dim)

An example of MRD testing by flow cytometry is in B-lymphoblastic leukemia, in which MRD testing provides the strongest indicator for event-free survival in the pediatric population. Understanding the normal immunophenotypic maturation pathway of hematogones is crucial in MRD evaluation. Markers most commonly used to distinguish between normal hematogones and neoplastic B-lymphoblasts are CD19, CD20, CD38, CD9, CD45, CD58, CD13/CD33, and CD34. The most common abnormalities in B-ALL include increased expression of CD10, CD19, and CD58, while CD38 and CD45 are often decreased. However, the detection sensitivity of 1:10,000 to 1:100,000 is dependent on the abnormal blast immunophenotype to be sufficiently different from normal in order to distinguish it from regenerating B-cell populations, and the lack of degenerative changes in the sample that could influence interpretation. An example of MRD analysis is shown in e-**Figure 55.8**.

C. **Flow Cytometry Interpretations.** Flow cytometry, in addition to enzyme cytochemistry, is used for basic classification of acute leukemias into a myeloid, lymphoid, or multiple phenotype. The flow is also useful for classification of ALL (B- vs. T-cell) and for classification of non-Hodgkin lymphomas (see below). Most CD markers are on the cell surface (known as "s" markers), but sometimes cells are permealized to allow staining of intracellular/cytoplasmic markers (known as "c" markers).

1. **AML markers**
   Blasts: express CD34, HLA-DR
   Myeloid: express CD13, CD33, CD15, MPO, CD117
   Megakaryoblast: express CD41, CD61
   Monocytic: express CD14, CD64
   Promyelocytes: lack CD34, HLA-DR

2. **ALL markers**
   Precursors: express Tdt (function in B-cell VDJ rearrangement), CD34, HLA-DR, CD45 (dim)
   B-lineage: express CD19 (immunoglobulin), CD20, CD22, cCD79a (immunoglobulin)
   T-lineage: express CD2, CD3, CD5, CD7
   Pre-B-blasts: lack Ig, CD20
   Pre-T-blasts: express CD1, CD4, CD8

3. Indolent non-Hodgkin lymphomas
   Clonality by κ/λ ratio (normal 2:1)
   CD5 neg, CD10 neg: marginal zone lymphoma
   CD5 neg, CD10 pos: follicular lymphoma
   CD5 pos, CD23 pos: SLL/CLL
   CD5 pos, CD23 neg, cyclinD1 pos: mantle cell lymphoma

4. **Hairy cell leukemia**
   Expresses CD 25, CD103, CD11c (newer markers include DBA44 and Annexin A1)
   Negative for CD5, CD10, CD23
   Light chain restriction present

D. **DNA Content.** Besides analyzing surface or cytoplasmic properties of a cell, flow cytometry can also analyze DNA content of a cell (*Flow Cytometry in Clinical Diagnosis,* 3rd ed. Chicago, IL: ASCP Press, p641–662, 2001). Several types of fluorescent stains are available depending on which DNA bases within the helix are targeted; most require the use of laser with significant ultraviolet (UV) output in order to be specific. For example, HOECHST 33342 or DAPI are specific for the adenosine/thymine base pairs, whereas mithramycin and chromomycin A3 preferentially target the guanine/cytosine base pairs. Propidium iodide is not very specific since it stains all double-stranded nucleic acids, but it can be included as a DNA stain in conventional cytometers with low-power argon lasers since it absorbs light at 488 nm.

DNA staining is generally performed to assess the amount of DNA in the nucleus of a cell, or to analyze the rate of cell division. In addition, because most normal cells contain the same amount of DNA (diploid or euploid), measurement of the DNA

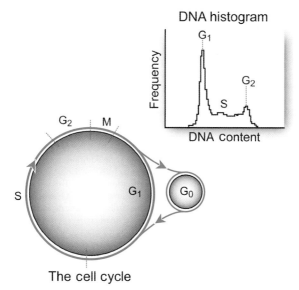

Figure 55.2 Histogram of the DNA distribution in a cycling population of cells that illustrates the distribution of nuclear DNA content present at a particular moment in the population of cells.

content of a cell can also differentiate normal cells from aneuploid malignant cells. The histograms from malignant tumors will show abnormal peaks corresponding to more (hyperdiploid) or less (hypodiploid) DNA than normal cells.

E. **Cell Cycle Analysis.** The cell cycle is composed of four phases. Cells in G0 phase are not cycling. Cells in G1 are recovering from division or are preparing for division. Cells in S phase are in the process of synthesizing new DNA. Cells in G2 phase have finished DNA synthesis and therefore have double the normal amount of DNA (i.e., tetraploid). Cells then undergo mitosis and cytokinesis, producing two daughter cells containing diploid DNA. The cell cycle can be plotted as a histogram with the number of cells per channel on the y-axis and the fluorescence intensity of cells stained for DNA content on the x-axis (Figure 55.2).

SUGGESTED READINGS

Check I. Clinical applications of DNA content analysis. In: Kerren DF, McCoy JP, Carley JL, eds. *Flow Cytometry in Clinical Diagnosis*, 3rd ed. Chicago, IL: ASCP Press; 2001; 641–662.

Longobardi GA. Instrumentation: Beyond the black box. In: Longobardi GA, ed. *Flow Cytometry, First Principles*, New York: Wiley-Liss; 1992; 15–40.

Longobardi GA. Cells from without: Lymphocytes and the strategy of gating. In: Longobardi GA, ed. *Flow Cytometry, First Principles*, New York: Wiley-Liss; 1992; 75–102.

McCoy JP. Basic principles in clinical flow cytometry. In: Kerren DF, McCoy JP, Carley JL, eds. *Flow Cytometry in Clinical Diagnosis*, 3rd ed. Chicago, IL: ASCP Press; 2001; 31–65.

Ormerod MG. Preparing suspensions of single cells. In: Ormerod MG, ed. *Flow Cytometry*, 3rd ed. Oxford: Oxford University Press; 2005; 35–46.

Ormerod MG. Fluorescence and fluorochromes. In: Ormerod MG, ed. *Flow Cytometry*, 3rd ed. Oxford: Oxford University Press; 2005; 23–33.

56 Cytogenetics
Patrick Mann and Julie Neidich

I. **INTRODUCTION.** The first descriptive illustrations of human chromosomes were published by Flemming in 1882 (F. C. W. Vogel, Leipzig). Since then, three significant milestones in the history of clinical cytogenetics are the preparation of chromosome spreads from peripheral blood cultures (*Exp Cell Res* 1960;20:613), the development of hypotonic methods to obtain enhanced chromosome spreads (*Cancer Res* 1960;20:462), and the discovery that fluorescent quinacrine compounds could be used to demonstrate a unique banding pattern for each human chromosome pair (*Hereditas* 1971;67:89). The remarkable advancement of the field of human cytogenetics is emphasized by the fact that it has been only just over 60 years since the correct number of human chromosomes has been established. The various banding methods in current use not only permit identification of each chromosome, but also make it possible to detect specific alterations associated with constitutional and acquired syndromes and neoplasms.

II. **TRADITIONAL CYTOGENETIC ANALYSIS.** While cytogenetic analysis is commonly used in the evaluation of congenital disorders (specifically, to diagnose syndromes associated with abnormalities of chromosomal number or structure, to establish the chromosomal sex in cases of sexual ambiguity, and to screen for karyotypic abnormalities in patients with multiple birth defects) and for prenatal diagnosis, the primary application for karyotype analysis in surgical pathology is in the evaluation of neoplastic disorders. The utility of the technique in surgical pathology rests on the fact that specific cytogenetic abnormalities have been recognized that are closely, and sometimes uniquely, associated with morphologically and clinically distinct subsets of lymphoma and leukemia, and with soft tissue neoplasms. Cancer cytogenetic studies have greatly aided targeted therapy, prognosis, and risk-based stratification of intensity of therapy.

A. **Advantages.** The power of conventional cytogenetics lies in its ability to provide simultaneous analysis of the entire genome without any foreknowledge of the chromosomal regions involved in the disease process. In most cases, the type and location of an identified chromosomal abnormality is either directly diagnostic, or can be used to direct additional testing. Contrary to some predictions, the advent of technologies such as chromosomal microarray analysis has not diminished the importance of traditional cytogenetics; in fact, these novel cytogenomic techniques achieve some of their greatest utility when they are utilized in conjunction with traditional clinical cytogenetics.

B. **Limitations.** The clinical utility of traditional cytogenetic analysis is restricted by two general features of the method. From a technical standpoint, analysis can only be performed on viable tissue specimens that contain proliferating cells (discussed in more detail below). From a sensitivity standpoint, analysis has resolution of only about 3 to 4 Mb at an 850-band level, and only about 7 to 8 Mb at a 400-band level. Traditional cytogenetic analysis is therefore only suited for detection of numerical abnormalities and gross structural rearrangements. The method does not have the sensitivity to detect mutations such as small deletions, duplications, and amplifications, or single base pair substitutions.

C. **Basic Laboratory Procedures.** Chromosomes that can be individually distinguished by light microscopy can only be visualized during cell division; thus the fundamental requirement for traditional cytogenetic analysis is a tissue specimen that contains actively proliferating cells, or cells that can be induced to proliferate in vitro. The general

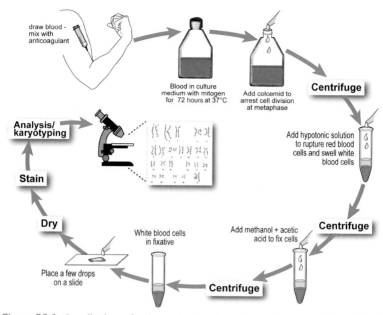

Figure 56.1 Overall scheme for the production of metaphase chromosomes for traditional cytogenetic analysis.

schema for obtaining metaphase chromosomes for cytogenetic analysis is shown in Figure 56.1.

1. **Culture initiation.** Different specimen types have different sample and handing requirements (Table 56.1). Inappropriate handling, as well as delay between specimen collection and culture initiation, can markedly decrease the likelihood that the sample will grow in vitro, so communication and coordination with the cytogenetics laboratory are essential.

   In vitro culture relies on a sterile microenvironment, and so specimens should be collected under sterile conditions. In practice, sterility is most difficult to achieve when sampling solid tissues; in this setting, clean instruments and a clean cutting surface, together with transport of the specimen in medium supplemented with broad spectrum antibiotics, can be used to minimize contamination.

TABLE 56.1	Specimen Requirements
Tissue Type	**Sample Collection**
Peripheral blood	Preservative-free sodium heparin; transport refrigerated or at room temperature
Bone marrow aspirate	Preservative-free sodium heparin; the first several mL of the aspirate usually contains the greatest proportion of cells and so is the optimal sample for cytogenetic analysis; transport at room temperature
Solid tissue	Collect and transport in sterile culture medium containing broad-spectrum antibiotics; carefully select maximally viable tumor for analysis; transport on ice to minimize autolysis and microbial overgrowth

Bone marrow and solid tissue neoplasms consist of cell types that proliferate spontaneously in culture, although often at a low rate. Lymph nodes are composed of cells that have a low intrinsic proliferative rate but that can be induced to divide much more rapidly by the addition of mitogens. Phytohemagglutinin (PHA) stimulates proliferation of T-lymphocytes. Lipopolysaccharide (LPS), protein A, 12-O-tetradecanoly-phorbol-13-acetate (TPA), Epstein–Barr virus, synthetic oligonucleotides, and pokeweed mitogen induce proliferation of B-lymphocytes, and are also required for successful culture of some leukemias and lymphomas of B-cell origin.

2. **Culture maintenance.** The length of in vitro culture depends on cell type. Since bone marrow cultures contain spontaneously proliferating cells, they can be harvested after only a 24- to 48-hour culture interval, as well as directly after specimen collection. Peripheral blood cultures usually require a 72-hour culture interval. The growth rate of solid tissue specimens is difficult to predict; some solid tumors require culture periods of 2 weeks or longer.

3. **Cell harvest.** Colcemid, a synthetic analogue of colchicine (an alkaloid from the bulb of the Mediterranean plant *Colchicum*) prevents separation of sister chromatids and is used to block the proliferating cells in metaphase, thus allowing an accumulation of cells at metaphase stage. A hypotonic solution is then used to swell the cells so that, after fixation, the chromosomes are adequately spread for microscopic analysis.

Since cells in culture do not proceed through the cell cycle in synchrony, chemical synchronization of cell division is often required to obtain an acceptable mitotic index. A common chemical approach involves addition of excess thymidine, which stalls cells at the S-phase of the cell cycle by decreasing the amount of dCTP available for DNA synthesis. When the excess thymidine is removed (or the effect of excess thymidine is eliminated by the addition of deoxycytidine), normal DNA replication resumes, and the collective release of the cells from S-phase produces a transiently high mitotic index. Alternatively, 5-fluorodeoxyuridine (which inhibits the enzyme thymidylate synthetase) can be used to stall cells at the G1/S boundary; in this method, addition of thymidine releases the block.

4. **Banding.** The different techniques that can be used to stain metaphase chromosomes can be divided into two general categories: methods that produce specific alternating light and dark regions (bands) along the length of each chromosome, and methods that stain only a defined region of specific chromosomes (Table 56.2). In general, the

TABLE 56.2	Major Chromosome Staining and Banding Techniques
Method	**Staining Pattern**
Techniques that produce specific alternating bands along each chromosome	
Giemsa banding (G-banding)	Dark bands are AT rich; light bands are CG rich
Quinacrine banding (Q-banding)	Bright regions are AT rich
Reverse banding (R-banding)	AT rich regions stain lightly (have dull fluorescence), CG rich regions staining darkly (have bright fluorescence)
4,6-Diamidino-2-phenylindole staining (DAPI staining)	DAPI binds AT rich regions; produces a pattern similar to Q-Banding
Techniques that stain selective chromosome regions	
Constitutive heterochromatin banding (C-banding)	Stains heterochromatin (α-satellite DNA) around the centromeres; can also be used to demonstrate some inherited polymorphisms
Telomere banding (T-banding)	Technical variation of R-banding used to stain telomeres
Silver staining for nucleolar organizer regions (NOR staining)	Stains the NORs (which contain rRNA genes) on the satellite stalks of acrocentric chromosomes
Fluorescence in situ hybridization (FISH)	Staining pattern is dependent on the probe

dark bands are gene-poor AT-rich regions whereas the light bands comprise gene-rich GC-rich regions. The quality of staining depends on several technical factors, including sufficient separation of the chromosomes in the metaphase spread to allow clear visualization. Most modern cytogenetics labs use a Giemsa dye method (G-banding) as a standard for all karyotype analysis, and add additional stains or fluorescent probes to reveal more detail about individual cases. Although there are no internationally accepted standards for banding resolution, ideograms are used as reference points (e-**Fig. 56.1**). Clinical laboratories aim for resolution at or above the 550 band level for blood chromosome analysis, while analysis of prenatal or neoplasm samples may be closer to 400 to 500 bands. Many countries, including the United States, Canada, United Kingdom, France, Japan, and Australia, have established standards that specify the minimum requirements for the number and quality of cells that must be processed for chromosome analysis depending on sample type, although many cases require even more detailed analysis.

5. Microscopic analysis. The method used to stain the chromosomes dictates whether bright-field microscopy or fluorescence microscopy is used to visualize the chromosomes. Conventional photography was traditionally used to produce high resolution prints of the stained chromosomes, but electronic imaging systems are now a standard.

6. The final step in cytogenetic analysis is the production of a **karyotype**, which consists of the chromosomal complement of the cell displayed in a standard sequence on the basis of size, centromere location, and banding pattern (e-**Fig. 56.2**).

D. Assay Failure. Many of the common causes of failure to obtain a cytogenetic result (Table 56.3) can be avoided by careful selection of viable tissue with prompt specimen transport to the cytogenetics laboratory in the appropriate medium. Nonetheless, several causes of assay failure are inherent to in vitro culture and cannot be eliminated by even the most meticulous laboratory technique.

Cytogenetic analysis of solid tumors highlights a number of these intrinsic technical limitations. First, since benign solid tumors contain few mitotic cells, cultures are susceptible to overgrowth by nonneoplastic cells. Second, even high-grade malignant solid tumors often grow poorly in vitro, especially if grown without the appropriate culture medium and growth factor supplementation. Third, the number of neoplastic cells in a solid tumor sample can be difficult to determine based on gross examination, and the material submitted to the cytogenetics laboratory may consist primarily of stromal cells and inflammatory cells. Fourth, the viability of the neoplastic cells is often uncertain; even tumor samples that are not grossly necrotic may contain predominantly nonviable tumor cells. Fifth, in vitro culture selects for subclones within the neoplastic population that have a growth advantage, and so the karyotype may not be representative of the entire neoplasm. Sixth, contamination is often unavoidable for samples collected in the frozen section area or gross room, or from specimens arising from anatomic sites normally colonized by bacteria, such as the oral cavity, gastrointestinal tract, and skin.

The overall failure rate of conventional cytogenetic analysis is difficult to quantify for many tissue types, neoplasms, and diseases, and so it is difficult to provide

---

TABLE 56.3   **Common Reasons for Failure of Traditional Cytogenetic Analysis**

Culture Failure
No viable cells present in the sample (necrotic tumor sample or improper specimen handling)
Inappropriate sample (peripheral blood without blasts is submitted instead of bone marrow)
Overgrowth by nonneoplastic cells
Overgrowth by a nonrepresentative clone of tumor cells
Microbial overgrowth

Postculture Failure
Technical errors involving cell harvest, slide preparation, or staining
Misdiagnosis (an abnormality is overlooked, or an abnormality is incorrectly interpreted)

objective statements regarding the utility of analysis in routine surgical pathology. In studies that specifically address this issue for hematolymphoid neoplasms, cytogenetic analysis has a success rate for detecting characteristic chromosomal aberrations that varies from 33% to 95% depending on the specific diagnosis, but is about 70% overall (*Am J Clin Pathol* 2004;121:826). For solid tumors, the success rate of analysis is less certain; reports describing cytogenetic abnormalities of many solid tumors often do not provide data on failed analyses or negative cases. Objective measures (including sensitivity, specificity, predictive value of a positive or negative result) of traditional cytogenetic analysis as an ancillary testing methodology in routine clinical practice are therefore often unknown.

III. FLUORESCENCE IN SITU HYBRIDIZATION. Virtually all in situ hybridization analysis is performed using probes that are directly or indirectly labeled with fluorophores. Guidelines for the use of fluorescence in situ hybridization (FISH) in clinical laboratory testing have been developed by the American College of Medical Genetics (https://www.acmg.net/docs/ACMG%20SG%20E9_FISH%20GIM%20July2011%20pdf%20.pdf), and standardized nomenclature for reporting results has been developed (discussed in more detail below).

Metaphase and interphase FISH are essentially modified Southern blots in which the target DNA consists of chromosomes rather than membrane bound DNA. Technically, the method has four steps: the probe and metaphase or interphase target are denatured by a high temperature and formamide, the probe is hybridized to the chromosomal target, unbound probe is removed by post-hybridization washes, and finally, the bound probe is detected by fluorescence microscopy. A fluorochrome-based counterstain is virtually always used to help detect the chromosomes or nuclei during microscopic examination; the use of DAPI as a counterstain makes it possible to localize the position of the bound probe to specific chromosomal bands.

A. Probes. A variety of fluorophores can be incorporated into FISH probes either directly or indirectly. The choice of labels is largely governed by practical issues, such as the excitation and emission filters on the microscope that will be used to view the chromosome spreads.

Several probe kits have been cleared by the United States Food and Drug Administration (FDA) for in vitro diagnostic testing, although many probes for FISH are classified as analyte-specific reagents (ASRs) and so are exempt from FDA approval. Standards and guidelines for clinical use of ASRs have been established by the American College of Medical Genetics, as have recommendations for interpretation of a metaphase or interphase FISH result (see https://www.acmg.net/docs/ACMG%20SG%20E9_FISH%20GIM%20July2011%20pdf%20.pdf).

1. Repetitive sequence probes. The most widely used repetitive sequence probes bind to α-satellite sequences of centromeres; these probes produce strong signals since α-satellite sequences are present in hundreds of thousands of copies. Chromosome-specific centromere-specific probes have been developed for most human chromosomes based on differences in α-satellite sequences, and are particularly useful for demonstrating aneuploidy. These FISH probes can be used on both metaphase and interphase preparations, and simultaneous analysis of more than one locus is possible when a cocktail of differentially labeled probes is used in the same hybridization. Other repetitive sequence probes include probes that recognize β-satellite sequences (located on the short arms of acrocentric chromosomes), and probes that recognize the telomeric repeat sequence TTAGGG.

2. Unique sequence probes. Probes of this type are used to detect sequences that are present only once in the genome. They are usually derived from genomic clones, but can also be produced from cDNA or by PCR. Different cloning vectors are used to produce unique sequence probes of different length, including plasmids for probes 1 to 10 kb long, bacteriophage λ for probes up to 25 kb long, bacterial artificial chromosomes (BACs) for probes up to about 300 kb long, and yeast artificial chromosomes (YACs) for probes from 100 kb to 2 Mb long. The availability of mapped BAC libraries, originally developed as part of the Human Genome Project, has greatly

simplified the production of probes for any locus (http://genome.ucsc.edu/cgi-bin/hgGateway and https://bacpacresources.org/).

Unique sequence probes (also known as locus-specific identifier probes, or LSI probes) are used primarily to detect changes in the copy number of a specific locus, to confirm the presence of rearrangements involving a specific locus, or to detect so-called cryptic rearrangements that cannot be identified by examination of chromosomes stained by routine banding methods (e-Fig. 56.3). The advantages and disadvantages of metaphase FISH analysis using unique sequence probes directly parallel those of interphase FISH (as discussed in Chapter 58).

3. Whole chromosome probes (WCPs). WCPs, also known as chromosome painting probes or chromosome libraries, consist of thousands of overlapping probes that recognize unique and moderately repetitive sequences along the entire length of individual chromosomes. They are isolated through flow sorting of specific chromosomes, microdissection of specific chromosomes accompanied by PCR amplification, or via production of somatic cell hybrids. WCPs are used to identify rearrangements that are not evident by routine banding methods, to confirm the interpretation of aberrations identified by routine banding methods, or to establish the chromosomal origin of rearrangements that are difficult to evaluate by other approaches. These probes are designed for use with metaphase chromosome preparations because hybridization to the decondensed chromatin in interphase nuclei gives a splotchy, undefined hybridization pattern. WCPs for each human chromosome are commercially available.

IV. MULTIPLEX METAPHASE FISH. Multiplex FISH (also known as multicolor FISH) and spectral karyotyping (SKY) are related techniques in which metaphase chromosome spreads are hybridized with a combination of probes labeled with different fluorophores. Since N different fluorophores can produce (2^N-1) different color combinations, five different fluorophores yield sufficient different color combinations to uniquely label WCPs so that all 24 different human chromosomes can be identified in one hybridization.

For both multiplex FISH and SKY, a cocktail consisting of labeled probes for each of the 24 chromosomes is hybridized to metaphase chromosome spreads, and the fluorescent emissions are measured by computerized imaging systems. Specialized software is used to determine the combination of fluorophores present along the length of each chromosome, which makes it possible to assemble a karyotype.

A. Advantages. Multiplex FISH and SKY are used to detect aneuploidy, detect interchromosomal rearrangements, and identify marker chromosomes (chromosomal material of unknown origin). In many cases, multiplex FISH or SKY make it possible to establish the chromosomal origin of rearrangements that cannot be defined based on routine cytogenetic analysis.

B. Disadvantages. The lower limit of the size of individual DNA chromosomal fragments that can be visualized by either technique is in the range of 1 to 2 Mb, although neither technique provides direct information on the involved chromosomal bands. Similarly, multiplex FISH and SKY will only reveal intrachromosomal deletions and duplications that are large enough to result in a change in size of the affected chromosome; neither technique is designed to detect intrachromosomal rearrangements such as inversions, and neither is informative in regions with repetitive DNA. Due to the expense of the probe sets, hardware, and software, many clinical labs do not perform SKY or multiplex FISH assays.

C. Modifications of Multiplex FISH and SKY. Mixtures of so-called partial chromosome paints, each of which hybridizes to only a band or sub-band of an individual chromosome, can be used to produce a pseudocolor banded karyotype at a resolution of about 550 bands (*Cytogenet Cell Genet* 1999;84:156). The use of partial chromosome paints makes it possible to employ multiplex FISH and SKY methodology to identify translocation breakpoints and to detect interchromosomal rearrangements. While these techniques may reveal more detail about any aberration, they are not usually available as clinical assays, but are instead research tools.

V. COMPARATIVE GENOMIC HYBRIDIZATION. While comparative genomic hybridization (CGH) often has a higher sensitivity than conventional cytogenetic analysis, of even greater significance is the fact that CGH can be performed using DNA extracted from fixed as well as fresh tumor samples. The technique therefore makes it possible to perform a genome-wide scan for structural alterations even on those cases for which conventional cytogenetic analysis is not feasible or is unsuccessful. CGH essentially opens the entire formalin-fixed tissue archive to at least limited cytogenetic analysis.

For a typical CGH test, genomic DNA from a tumor sample is labeled with a red fluorophore, and genomic DNA from a paired normal tissue sample is labeled with a green fluorophore. The green and red probes are mixed and used in a single hybridization.

A. Metaphase CGH. This technique is basically a variation of metaphase FISH used to survey the entire genome for chromosomal deletions and amplifications (*Science* 1992;258:818; *Trends Genet* 1997;13:405). At this point, most laboratories do not perform metaphase CGH, and have incorporated array CGH (see below) or other microarray methods to detect losses and gains of chromosomal material using DNA extracted from the sample. The patient's labeled probe mixture is used in a hybridization to metaphase chromosomes prepared from normal cells, and the ratio of the green to red fluorescent signals is measured along the length of each chromosome. Areas where the ratio deviates significantly from the expected one-to-one relationship indicate a change in DNA copy number in the tumor; areas where the red to green ratio is significantly greater than 1 are areas of chromosomal gain (usually amplifications), and areas where the red to green ratio is significantly lower than 1 are areas of chromosomal loss (deletions). The smallest chromosomal alterations that can be reproducibly detected are about 3 Mb long.

B. Array CGH (aCGH). This approach utilizes a microarray consisting of an ordered arrangement of DNA molecules (features) linked to a solid matrix support. The labeled probe mixture is hybridized to the microarray, and the ratio of the green to red fluorescent signals is measured for each feature (Fig. 56.2). Because each DNA feature has been mapped to a specific region of the genome, the ratio of the green to red fluorescent signal for each feature provides information on the gain or loss of the corresponding chromosomal region. The resolution of aCGH is in theory limited only by the number of features in the array; commercially available arrays currently provide a resolution of under 10 Kb. Genomic microarrays (aCGH and related microarray based methods) are currently clinically applied to detect genomic copy number changes as well as copy neutral changes (uniparental disomy [UPD]/loss of heterozygosity [LOH]).

VI. MICROARRAY ANALYSIS. Since the advent of the use of genomic microarrays the clinical laboratory, the technology has rapidly become the standard of care to evaluate patients for genomic imbalance, especially in diagnostic testing for patients with congenital anomalies, developmental delay, and intellectual disabilities. However, adaptation of genomic microarrays in cancer diagnostics, especially in solid tumors, is not currently widespread.

A. Advantages. Microarray testing offers several advantages over traditional cytogenetic techniques. With a markedly increased resolution over conventional chromosome analysis, genomic imbalances less than 50 to 100 kb are routinely detectable using array based copy number methodology. In addition, there is no requirement for cell viability since DNA serves as the starting material. Testing can therefore be performed on a variety of specimen types including peripheral blood lymphocytes, bone marrow, lymph nodes, formalin-fixed paraffin-embedded tumor tissue, amniocytes, products of conception, fresh tissue samples, and buccal cells, among others.

Although BAC arrays utilizing cloned DNA targets of approximately 160 kb served as the first generation of aCGH diagnostics in the clinical lab, oligonucleotide arrays (utilizing probes that are 25 to 75 bp long) are easier to design and manufacture, and provide markedly increased probe coverage across the genome. Consequently, oligonucleotide arrays have replaced BAC arrays in clinical laboratories; their use employs two general strategies, namely aCGH and single nucleotide polymorphism (SNP) analysis. Although the aim of both techniques is the detection of genomic gain or loss, the method for doing so differs between each assay.

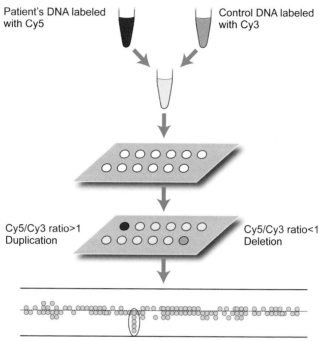

Patient's DNA labeled with Cy5

Control DNA labeled with Cy3

Cy5/Cy3 ratio>1 Duplication

Cy5/Cy3 ratio<1 Deletion

Figure 56.2 Array CGH methodology. **Top:** Method. A patient's DNA is labeled with a red dye and a control genomic DNA preparation is labeled with green dye. The DNA preparations are mixed and cohybridized to an array of BACs or oligonucleotides on a glass slide. The DNA bound to each spot (known as a feature) of the array is quantified using a laser scanner. In the patient's DNA, normal regions will be indicated by a yellow balanced color; regions of duplication will be identified as red, and regions of deletion will be identified as green. **Bottom:** Data presentation. The data from each feature of the array (represented by *circles*) are plotted in relation to the features' positions along the chromosome and a balanced copy number (*horizontal line*). In this illustration, a cluster of adjacent features that falls significantly below a balanced copy number result (*oval*) indicates the presence of a deletion. The resolution of array CGH is in theory limited only by the number of features in the array; commercially available arrays currently provide a resolution of less than 10 Kb. (Figure adapted from Beaudet AL, Belmont JW. Array-based DNA diagnostics: let the revolution begin. *Annu Rev Med* 2008;59:113–129.)

As discussed above, aCGH detects copy number imbalances through the comparison of a normal control sample against a patient sample. In contrast, SNPs are evaluated by comparing signal intensities from the assay substrate (derived from the DNA of the patient sample) to that of an in silico reference model in order to determine relative gains and losses. The ability to probe for SNPs is advantageous for several reasons. First, the approach makes it possible to perform simultaneous copy number quantification and SNP detection. Second, the use of SNP arrays allows for detection of regions with a copy neutral LOH which may be used to identify genetic alterations in tumor samples, heterodisomy, the parental chromosome of origin for a de novo deletion or duplication, and more generally, consanguinity and uniparental disomy. Ultimately, SNP detection helps maximize the potential for detecting disease-associated abnormalities and also offers mechanistic evidence for the molecular basis of the disease. A comparison of SNP and oligo arrays is shown in Table 56.4.

TABLE 56.4 Comparison Between SNP and Oligo Arrays

Array Attributes	Single Nucleotide Polymorphism Arrays	Oligonucleotide Arrays
Number of markers	Greater than 1,000,000 markers	Less than 200,000 markers
DNA input requirement	200–500 ng	1–5 µg
Probe types	SNP and oligo probes	Oligo probes
Limits of resolution	Less than 10–20 kb	As low as 10–20 kb
Threshold for detection of mosaicism	May be as low as 5%	20–30%
Ability to detect copy neutral LOH	Yes	No
Ability to detect uniparental disomy	Yes	No
Ability to detect consanguinity	Yes	No
Method of assessment of copy number imbalance	Probe signal intensities (derived from the patient sample) compared to an in silico reference model	Patient sample directly hybridized against control DNA to detect relative gains and losses
Detection of balanced chromosomal rearrangements	No	No

The technique of allelic discrimination by SNP analysis differs between commercially available platforms, but nonetheless involves hybridization of fragmented single-stranded DNA (derived from the patient sample) to arrays that contain unique nucleotide probe sequences (2 million or more). One widespread commercial approach is based on allele-specific hybridization to probes representing the possible alleles; signal intensities that correspond to the level of binding (Fig. 56.3) are measured by scanning technology. The other widespread commercial approach utilizes a single base extension technique with differentially labeled nucleotide terminators to distinguish the SNP alleles; the signal intensity generated from this reaction is used to make a base call at that SNP (Fig. 56.3).

Finally, exon level arrays have been designed to allow for the identification of very small losses and gains. These arrays concentrate probes over exons within expressed genes, usually genes of clinical interest, in order to assay for deletions and duplications as small as one exon in a gene of interest. Since deletions and duplications have been identified as pathogenic variants in numerous genes, this type of assay has proven a useful diagnostic tool when used in conjunction with next-generation sequencing panels, whole exome analysis, and whole genome analysis.

B. Limitations. While copy number changes are often readily discernable, balanced chromosomal rearrangements cannot be detected with this technology, including balanced translocations, inversions, and insertions. In addition, regions containing segmental duplications, those with a complex genomic structure, and those containing other repetitive sequences will have limited detection. Low level mosaicism may not be detectable, and LOH is demonstrable only using SNP-based platforms.

VI. HUMAN CHROMOSOME NOMENCLATURE. Technical advancements, together with an ever more complete understanding of human chromosomal structure, necessitate periodic revision of nomenclature guidelines. The document in current use is the *International System for Human Cytogenetic Nomenclature* from 2016, abbreviated ISCN 2016, which includes ideograms for all of the chromosomes that serve as useful reference points because of their universal acceptance and availability.

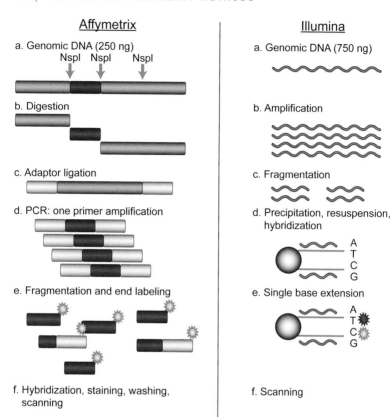

Figure 56.3 SNP array procedures. In the Affymetrix platform (ThermoFisher Scientific; Waltham, MA), genomic DNA is digested with the NspI restriction enzyme and the resulted DNA fragments are ligated to adaptors and subsequently amplified; the amplification products are fragmented, end-labeled, and hybridized to the array. In the Illumina platform (Illumina, Inc., San Diego, CA), the entire genome is amplified and then hybridized to a bead array; allelic discrimination is achieved by a single base extension reaction. In both platforms, the signal intensity is measured for each probe and compared with an *in silico* reference to evaluate DNA copy number. (Figure adapted from Schoumans J, Ruivenkamp C. Laboratory methods for the detection of chromosomal abnormalities. *Methods Mol Biol* 2010;628:53–73.)

A. Chromosome Region and Band Designations. The centromere divides each chromosome into a short or p arm, and a long or q arm. Each chromosome arm ends in a terminus, designated pter and qter for the short and long arms, respectively. A list of the more frequent symbols and abbreviations used to describe human karyotypes is shown in Table 56.5.

Chromosome arms are divided into regions based on landmarks, defined as consistent and distinct morphologic areas that aid in the identification of that chromosome. The regions adjacent to the centromere of the short arm and long arm are designated as p1 and q1, respectively, the next distal as p2 and q2, and so on. Chromosome regions are divided into bands, and the bands are divided into subbands, both of which are

TABLE 56.5	Common Symbols and Abbreviations Used in Karyotype Designations
Abbreviation or Symbol	Description
add	Additional material of unknown origin
square brackets []	Number of cells in each clone
cen	Centromere
single colon (:)	Break
double colon (::)	Break and reunion
comma (,)	Separates chromosome number, sex chromosomes, and abnormalities
del	Deletion
der	Derivative chromosome
dmin	Double minute(s)
dup	Duplication
i	Isochromosome
idem	Identical abnormalities as in prior clone
inv	Inversion
ins	Insertion
mar	Marker chromosome
minus sign (−)	Loss
multiplication sign (×)	Multiple copies, also designates copy number with ISH
plus sign (+)	Gain
question mark (?)	Uncertainty of chromosome identification or abnormality
r	Ring chromosome
rcp	Reciprocal
slash (/)	Separates cell lines or clones
semicolon (;)	Separates chromosomes and breakpoints in rearrangements involving more than one chromosome
t	Translocation

numbered sequentially. The terminal band on the long arm of chromosome 11 is therefore written as 11q25, indicating chromosome 11, long arm, region 2, band 5, and is referred to as "eleven q two-five."

B. **Description of Karyotypes.** ISCN nomenclature provides rules for karyotype designations. The first item of the designation is the total number of chromosomes (including the sex chromosomes) followed by the sex chromosomes. Chromosomal abnormalities follow the sex chromosome designations using established symbols and abbreviations. The sex chromosomes are described first, followed by abnormalities in the autosomal chromosomes in numerical order. For each chromosome described, numerical changes are listed before structural aberrations. Table 56.6 provides examples of the karyotypic designation of numerical and structural abnormalities detected by traditional cytogenetic analysis. The rules for designating the karyotype of constitutional abnormalities are also used for designating the abnormalities associated with neoplasms, although the biology of tumors requires additional definitions and guidelines.

C. **Description of FISH and Microarray Results.** ISCN 2016 also includes rules for designating cytogenetic findings derived from various in situ hybridization techniques (a summary of the more common symbols and abbreviations is shown in Table 56.5)

TABLE 56.6	Examples of Human Chromosome Nomenclature
Designation	**Description**
Description of karyotypes	
Constitutional sex chromosome aneuploidies	
45,X	Turner syndrome
47,XXY	Klinefelter syndrome
Autosomal chromosome aneuploidies	
47,XY,+21	Male with trisomy 21 (Down syndrome)
48,XY,+21c,+21[20]	Male with trisomy 21, with gain of an additional chromosome 21 in his tumor cells. The number in brackets designates the number of cells that were analyzed and contain the additional chromosome 21.
Abnormalities in Neoplasms	
47,XX,+10,t(11;22) (q24;q12)[5/20]	Female whose tumor cells have two cytogenetic abnormalities: an additional chromosome 10, and a reciprocal translocation between the long arm (q) of chromosome 11 at region 2, band 4, and the long arm (q) of chromosome 22 at region 1, band 2. The first number in brackets designates the number of cells with the observed abnormalities and the last number designates the total number of cells that were analyzed.
Description of metaphase FISH results	
47,XY,+mar.ish der(3) (wcp3+)	In this tumor, traditional cytogenetic analysis shows a marker chromosome; metaphase FISH using a whole chromosome paint for chromosome 3 shows that the marker is derived from chromosome 3

as well as microarrays. For metaphase chromosome in situ hybridization, the results of conventional cytogenetic analysis (if performed) are listed first, followed by the results of in situ hybridization analysis, and finally the nomenclature for the microarray findings. Ideally, loci are designated according to the HUGO Gene Nomenclature Committee (http://www.genenames.org/); when HUGO designations are unavailable, probe names are used.

ACKNOWLEDGMENT

The authors thank Shashikant Kulkarni, Hussam Al-Kateb, and Catherine Cottrell, authors of the previous edition of this chapter.

SUGGESTED READINGS

Beaudet AL, Belmont JW. Array-based DNA diagnostics: let the revolution begin. *Annu Rev Med* 2008;59:113–129.

Gersen SL, Keagle MB, eds. *The Principles of Clinical Cytogenetics*. 2nd ed. Totowa: Humana Press; 2005.

Kallioniemi OP, Kallioniemi A, Sudar D, et al. Comparative genomic hybridization: a rapid new method for detecting and mapping DNA amplification in tumors. *Semin Cancer Biol* 1993;4:41–46.

LaFramboise T. Single nucleotide polymorphism arrays: a decade of biological, computational and technological advances. *Nucleic Acids Res* 2009;37:4181–4193.

McGowan-Jordan J, Simons A, Schmid M, eds. *ISCN 2016: An International System for Human Cytogenetic Nomenclature*. Basel: S Karger; 2016.

Miller DT, Adam MP, Aradhya S, et al. Consensus statement: chromosomal microarray is a first-tier clinical diagnostic test for individuals with developmental disabilities or congenital anomalies. *Am J Hum Genet* 2010;86:749–764.

Rooney DE, ed. *Human Cytogenetics: Constitutional Analysis: A practical approach*. 3rd ed. Oxford: Oxford University Press; 2001.

Schoumans J, Ruivenkamp C. Laboratory methods for the detection of chromosomal abnormalities. *Methods Mol Biol* 2010;628:53–73.

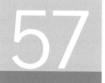

57 Fluorescence in Situ Hybridization (FISH)

Jennifer K. Sehn, Lily Zhang, Yi-Shan Lee, and Anjum Hassan

I. **INTRODUCTION.** Fluorescence in situ hybridization (FISH) is a molecular technique for the evaluation of specific DNA sequences in a cellular context. Fluorescently labeled probes are hybridized to DNA regions of interest based on the Watson–Crick base pairing. Given the size of FISH probes (usually in the range of 100 to 200 kb), FISH is most commonly utilized for the evaluation of structural or numeric chromosomal abnormalities, including translocations, gene deletion/amplification, and aneusomy (e-**Figs. 57.1–57.4**). FISH is not useful for the evaluation of alterations less than around 20 kb in size (such as single-nucleotide variants, small structural rearrangements, or smaller insertions/deletions).

For surgical pathologists, one of the most useful features of FISH is that it is performed directly on cells, allowing for the evaluation of molecular aberrations in the context of intact tissue morphology. Most surgical pathology FISH tests are performed on nondividing (interphase) cells from formalin-fixed, alcohol-fixed, or air-dried specimens, including sections from routine surgical pathology tissue blocks, cytology smears, and blood or bone marrow smears (Table 57.1). Importantly, while EDTA decalcification is suitable for specimens in which FISH will be performed, acid decalcification is not compatible with FISH or other DNA-based analyses.

In surgical pathology, FISH is used primarily to detect somatic cancer-associated mutations (particularly aneusomy, gene deletion/amplification, and translocations) with known diagnostic, prognostic, or therapeutic implications (Tables 57.2 and 57.3). A marked H&E-stained guide slide is usually used to specify which areas are best for interpretation, designating the regions with high tumor cellularity (mostly tumor cells, with little background inflammation, stroma, vessels, etc.) and viability (avoiding areas of necrosis). In addition, sex chromosome (XY) FISH can be useful in evaluating engraftment in patients with sex-mismatched bone marrow or organ transplants (e-**Fig. 57.5**). FISH also can be performed on dividing (metaphase) cells from cell cultures, as is typically done for samples of multiple myeloma or products of conception (chorionic villi).

II. **FISH APPLICATIONS AND PROBE TYPES**

A. **Aneusomy and Gene Copy Number Changes: Centromere Enumeration Probe (CEP).**
CEP are highly robust probes that target repetitive DNA sequences that are specific to the centromere of each chromosome (e.g., CEP7 hybridizes to the centromere of chromosome 7). They are most useful clinically in the detection of aneusomies (including polysomy or monosomy of entire chromosomes) or as a reference for chromosome copy number in gene amplifications/deletions (distinguishing when there are more or fewer signals from a gene-targeted probe versus the total number of copies of that chromosome in each cell); in deletion/amplification analysis, CEP probes are used in combination with locus-specific identifier (LSI, also known as gene specific) probes to evaluate the copy number of the locus of interest compared with the number of chromosomes present in the cell (e-**Figs. 57.6 and 57.7**). A normal cell shows two signals for each CEP probe (representing the maternally and paternally inherited copies of each chromosome). Examples of common applications for CEP probes in surgical pathology are listed in Table 57.3.

Chromosomal polysomy/monosomy and gene amplification/deletion are amongst the most common alterations detected in neoplasms by FISH (Table 57.3). It can be difficult to distinguish specific tumor-associated polysomies and monosomies from

TABLE 57.1	Examples of Specimen Types Suitable for FISH Analysis

Fresh/frozen tissue

Cytology specimens
  Body fluids (e.g., urine)
  Intraoperative smears
  Cell culture preparations

Formalin-fixed paraffin-embedded tissue
  Thin sections (4–6 microns)
  Disaggregated nuclei
  Archived unstained sections

Previously stained sections (e.g., negative immunohistochemistry controls)

nonspecific gains and losses that are secondary changes due to tumor genomic instability (e-**Fig.57.8**). The use of CEP reference probes helps to distinguish polysomy/monosomy (gain or loss of the entire chromosome) from true gene amplification/deletion.

B. **Structural Variants: Break-Apart and Fusion LSI Probe Sets.** Multiple types of FISH probes are available for the detection of structural variants (particularly translocations) in surgical pathology specimens, including break-apart (FISH-BA), fusion (FISH-F), and extra-signal (ES-FISH). Which type of probe is employed depends on whether or not the fusion partner gene is relevant. It is important to remember that usually only one of the two cellular copies of a gene is involved in a structural aberration such as a translocation or inversion, such that tumor cells harboring a translocation also still harbor one normal copy of each gene. Examples of common applications in surgical pathology for these types of probes are listed in Table 57.3.

1. **Dual-color fusion probes.** Dual-color fusion probes employ two locus-specific probes with different fluorophores which target two different partners in a translocation (e.g., *BCR* on 22q and *ABL* on 9q). Translocation-negative cells yield separated or "split" signals (e.g., two green, two red signals; e-**Fig. 57.4A**). Translocation-positive cells yield "fusion" yellow or red-green signals as the loci of interest are brought together by the translocation (e.g., one fusion, one green, one red signal; e-**Fig. 57.4B**). Cells must be scored carefully to avoid overinterpretation of small populations of cells where green and red signals overlap purely by chance. Based on signal proximities in normal controls, typical conservative cutoffs for a positive FISH-F test result require the presence of fused signals in >30% cells (*Mod Pathol* 2006;19:1).

TABLE 57.2	Examples of Diagnostic Tests Performed by FISH

Prenatal testing
  Trisomy 13, 18, 21
  XY aneusomies

Microdeletion syndromes
  Cri-du-Chat syndrome (5p)
  Prader–Willi/Angelman syndrome (15q)
  DiGeorge syndrome (22q)

Transplant pathology
  XY FISH on sex-mismatched organ transplant
  Disease relapse using known genetic alterations in primary tumor

Oncology (diagnostic, prognostic, and/or predictive markers)
  Chromosomal aneusomies
  Gene/locus deletions
  Gene amplifications
  Translocations

TABLE 57.3	Cancer-Associated Alterations Commonly Detected by FISH		
Type	**Tumor Type (References)**	**Alterations/Probes**	**Association**
Aneusomies/ deletions	Oligodendroglioma	1p- with 19q-	Diagnostic, prognostic, predictive
	Urothelial carcinoma	+3, 7, or 17; 9p-	Diagnostic
	Lung carcinoma	+7p, 8q, 5p, or 6	Diagnostic
	CLL	13q-, 11q-, 17q-	Diagnostic, prognostic
	GBM	+7, -10	Diagnostic
	Prostatic carcinoma	8p-, 8q+	Prognostic
	Medulloblastoma	17p-, 17q+; (i17q)	Diagnostic
	Leukemias/MDS	+8, +12; -5, -7	Diagnostic, prognostic
	MRT, AT/RT	*INI1/hSNF5* (22q-)	Diagnostic
	Meningioma	*NF2* (22q-)	Diagnostic
	Multiple myeloma	*RB1* (13q-), *TP53* (17p-)	Prognostic
	MPNST	*NF1* (17q-)	Diagnostic
Amplifications	Breast carcinoma	*HER-2/neu*	Prognostic, predictive
	Neuroblastoma	*N-myc*	Diagnostic, prognostic
	GBM	*EGFR*	Diagnostic
	Medulloblastoma	*MYCN, c-myc*	Diagnostic, prognostic
	Gastric carcinoma	*HER-2/neu*	Prognostic, predictive
Translocations	EWS/PNET	*EWS-FLI1*, EWS-BA	Diagnostic
	Synovial sarcoma	*SYT-SSX*, SYT-BA	Diagnostic
	Alveolar RMS	*PAX3-FKHR*, FKHR-BA	Diagnostic
	DSRCT	*EWS-WT1*, EWS-BA	Diagnostic
	M/RC liposarcoma	CHOP-BA	Diagnostic
	Clear cell sarcoma	*EWS-ATF1*, EWS-BA	Diagnostic
	IMT	*ALK-TPM3, ALK-TPM4, ALK-CARS*, ALK-BA	Diagnostic, prognostic
	Burkitt lymphoma	*MYC-IGH*, MYC-BA	Diagnostic
	MALT lymphoma	*API2-MALT1, IGH-MALT1,* MALT1-BA	Diagnostic
	Follicular lymphoma	*IGH-BCL2*	Diagnostic
	ALCL	ALK-BA	Diagnostic, prognostic, predictive
	Mantle cell lymphoma	*IGH-CCND1*	Diagnostic
	Multiple myeloma	*IGH-CCND1, IGH-FGFR3,* IGH-BA	Prognostic
	CML	*BCR-ABL*	Diagnostic, MRD, predictive
	AML	*AML1-ETO,* CBFB-BA, *PML-RARA,* RARA-BA, MLL-BA, *BCR-ABL*	Diagnostic, prognostic, predictive
	ALL	*TEL-AML1, BCR-ABL,* MLL-BA	Diagnostic, prognostic, predictive
	BCL, unclassifiable with features intermediate between DLBCL and Burkitt lymphoma	*IGH-BCL2; MYC-IGH,* MYC-BA	Diagnostic, prognostic
	Myeloid and lymphoid neoplasms with eosinophilia	*PDGFRA, PGDFRB, FGFR1; FIP1L1-PDGFRA*	Diagnostic, prognostic, predictive

ALCL, anaplastic large cell lymphoma; ALL, acute lymphoblastic leukemia; AML, acute myelogenous leukemia; AT/RT, atypical teratoid/rhabdoid tumor; BA, break-apart probe set; BCL, B-cell lymphoma; CLL, chronic lymphocytic leukemia; CML, chronic myelogenous leukemia; DLBCL, diffuse large B-cell lymphoma; DSRCT, desmoplastic small round cell tumor; EWS, Ewing sarcoma; GBM, glioblastoma; IMT, inflammatory myofibroblastic tumor; M/RC, myxoid/round cell; MDS, myelodysplastic syndrome; MPNST, malignant peripheral nerve sheath tumor; MRD, minimal residual disease assessment; MRT, malignant rhabdoid tumor; PNET, primitive neuroectodermal tumor, RMS, rhabdomyosarcoma.

2. Break-apart probes. Break-apart probes comprise two probes localizing just prox-imal and distal to a breakpoint of interest. In translocation-negative cells, the two probes are in proximity to one another, resulting in fusion signals. Translocation-positive cells will result in at least one pair of split signals (e.g., one fusion, one green, one red signal). Compared with dual-color fusion probes, break-apart probes offer several advantages. False-positive results are rare, as split signals should not occur purely by chance. Also, commercial break-apart probes are often more than 500 kb in size, yielding large, easily interpretable signals. Most importantly, this strategy identifies translocations that involve multiple partner genes, although the resulting disadvantage of break-apart probes is that they provide no information regarding the identity of the fusion partner.

For example, *EWSR1* is known to have multiple possible fusion partners, within the same tumor type (e.g., the many known *EWSR1* rearrangements characteristic of the Ewing sarcoma) or in different tumor types (e.g., *EWSR1-FLI1* fusions in the Ewing sarcoma vs. *EWSR1-WT1* in desmoplastic small round cell tumor vs. *EWSR1-ATF1* in clear cell sarcoma of soft parts). In many cases, it is complicated and unnecessary to identify the partner gene in a translocation; merely identifying that the target gene (e.g., *EWSR1*) is rearranged is sufficient to answer the clinical question. In normal cells, the probes are located close enough to result in one over-lapping signal (which appears yellow); each normal cell will have two yellow signals (one for each copy of the chromosome) (e-**Fig. 57.4C**). In cells with a rearrangement of the target gene, the probes are split (broken apart) and seen as two signals—one red and one green; positive cells have one red, one green, and one yellow signal (split signals for the rearranged copy of the gene, and a fused signal for the other copy of the gene) (e-**Fig. 57.4D**). Typical conservative cutoffs for a positive FISH-BA test results require the presence of split signals in >15% of cells (*Mod Pathol* 2006;19:1).

3. Other approaches. ES-FISH (extra signal) is a strategy that has been used to increase the sensitivity and decrease the false-positivity rate of FISH-F. One of the probes in ES-FISH is particularly large and spans the breakpoint region. In the presence of a translocation, the large probe is split, leading to an extra signal that is smaller than the nonsplit, nonfused signals (e.g., one fusion, one normal green, one normal red, and one ES red signal). Since it is unlikely that individual cells will contain both a fusion signal and an extra signal, the probability of scoring cells with chance overlap of red and green signals as translocation positive is close to zero.

III. FISH NOMENCLATURE. FISH results are reported using standardized nomenclature, according to the *International System for Human Cytogenomic Nomenclature* (ISCN), which was most recently revised in 2016 (McGowan-Jordan J, Simons A, Schmid A, eds. *ISCN 2016: An International System for Human Cytogenomic Nomenclature.* Basel, Switzerland: Karger, 2016.). A summary of the more common symbols and abbreviations is shown in Table 57.4.

If interphase in situ hybridization is performed, results are presented in the following order: the abbreviation nuc ish is listed first, followed by the chromosome band to which the probe maps, followed by the locus designation, a multiplication sign, and the number of signals present (Table 57.5). If both conventional cytogenetic analysis and metaphase in situ hybridization are performed, the result of the conventional cytogenetic analysis is listed first, followed by a period, followed by the abbreviation ish, followed by the in situ hybridization results presented in the same order described above. If conventional cytoge-netic analysis is performed in conjunction with interphase in situ hybridization, the results are described on separate lines of nomenclature. Ideally, loci are designated according to Genome Data Base (GDB) nomenclature (http://gdbwww.gdb.org). When GDB designa-tions are unavailable, probe names are used. If two or more probes for the same or different loci are used, they are separated by commas.

By ISCN guidelines, aneusomy or amplification/deletion is reported as the number of signals present for the probes of interest, as described above. A positive result for structural variants (rearrangements, translocations) is reported as con (for "connected," in cells in

TABLE 57.4	Examples of Symbols and Abbreviations Used in Interphase FISH Nomenclature
Abbreviation or Symbol	Description
plus sign (+)	Present on a specific chromosome
minus sign (−)	Absent on a specific chromosome
++	Duplication on a specific chromosome
X	Precedes numbers of signals seen
;	Separates probes on different derivative chromosomes
period (.)	Separates cytogenetic results from ish results
amp	Amplified signal
con	Connected or adjacent signals
ish	When used by itself, refers to hybridization to chromosomes
nuc ish	Nuclear or interphase in situ hybridization
pcp	Partial chromosome paint
sep	Separated signals (which are usually adjacent in normal cells)
subtel	Subtelomeric
wcp	Whole chromosome paint

TABLE 57.5	Examples of Nomenclature Used for Neoplasms Evaluated by Interphase FISH
Designation	Description
nuc ish 11p13(WT1x2),22q12(EWSR1x2), (WT1 con EWSR1x1)	Interphase FISH of a tumor cell using single-fusion probes. A probe for WT1 at 11p13 shows two signals, as does a probe for EWSR1 at 22q12. However, one WT1 and one EWSR1 signal are juxtaposed (or connected), consistent with a t(11;22)(p13;q12) translocation.
nuc ish 22q12(EWSR1x2)(5′EWSR1sep 3′EWSR1x1)	Interphase FISH of a tumor cell using a break-apart probe set for the EWSR1 locus at 22q12. Two sets of EWSR1 signals are present, but on one copy of chromosome 22 the probes are separated (most likely as a result of a rearrangement of the EWSR1 locus).
nuc ish 22q12(5′EWSR1,3′EWSR1 con 5′EWSR1,3′EWSR1)x2	Interphase FISH using the same break-apart probe set as in the above example. However, in this tumor, the two probes remain juxtaposed on both copies of chromosome 22 (which provides no evidence of a rearrangement of the EWS locus).
nuc ish 8q24(MYCx2)(5′MYC sep 3′MYCx1)[119/200]	Interphase FISH using a break-apart probe set. In this tumor, a split of red and green signals was detected. This is consistent with a c-myc-containing chromosomal rearrangement in 119 of 200 nuclei evaluated.
nuc ish 8q24(5′MYC,3′MYC con 5′MYC,3′MYC)x2[174/200]	Interphase FISH was performed utilizing a commercial c-myc (8q24) break-apart probe set. In this particular case, a split of red and green signals was not detected in 174 of 200 nuclei evaluated.

which fusion probes are normally present on separate chromosomes but are juxtaposed on the same chromosome in cells harboring the target rearrangement) or sep (for "separated," in cells in which break-apart probes normally flank the gene of interest but are separated due to rearrangement). Examples of FISH results are described in Table 57.5.

IV. **LIMITATIONS.** The basic steps for surgical pathology FISH protocols are similar to those of immunohistochemistry and include deparaffinization, pretreatment/target retrieval, probe and target DNA denaturation, hybridization (a few hours to overnight), posthybridization washes, detection, and microscopic interpretation/imaging. FISH is therefore typically a 2-day assay, although same day assays are possible if the probes are particularly robust.

Several factors can complicate interpretation of FISH results, including artifacts in probe hybridization secondary to fixation and processing techniques; truncation artifact (underestimation of copy number due to transection of individual nuclei in FFPE tissue sections); autofluorescence (background fluorescence signal from the tissue itself, separate from true probe signals and frequently present at multiple wavelengths of light); and partial hybridization failure (most problematic when combining a highly robust probe with a comparatively weak probe, such as a CEP with a small locus-specific probe). In addition, fluorescent signals fade over time and with exposure to light. In some cases, chromogenic in situ hybridization (CISH) can be used instead of FISH to allow for more permanent signals (e.g., CISH for HER2 gene amplification or human papilloma virus DNA detection).

V. **USE OF FISH VERSUS OTHER MOLECULAR TECHNIQUES.** When compared with metaphase cytogenetics (see Chapter 56), interphase FISH has several clear advantages. One advantage is the lack of a requirement for mitotically active cells via cell culture, which removes potential artifacts due to in vitro growth selection biases such as overgrowth of nonneoplastic stromal elements. On the other hand, FISH is not a genomic screening tool; it provides a targeted approach for alterations that have been initially identified by more global molecular techniques, such as classic cytogenetics, loss of heterozygosity (LOH) screening, comparative genomic hybridization (CGH), array CGH (aCGH), array single-nucleotide polymorphism (SNP) analysis, and gene expression profiling.

In terms of resolution, FISH is more sensitive than conventional karyotypic analysis and CGH (both of which are limited to alterations of several Mb in size) but less sensitive than PCR-based assays for detecting small alterations (which can be designed to detect even single base pair changes). Since FISH probes are typically at least 20-kb long, and most average 100- to 200-kb long, alterations need to be fairly large for reliable detection by FISH, and consequently FISH cannot detect small intragenic mutations, deletions, or insertions.

Minimal residual disease or early recurrences are better detected by PCR of blood or fresh tissue specimens rather than FISH. Minimal residual disease detection usually involves detection of as few as one abnormal per million normal cells, a level of sensitivity that cannot be attained by FISH techniques to date. In contrast, FISH is very sensitive for identifying gene deletions or amplifications from samples of mixed cellularity, such as neoplasms with clonal heterogeneity or contaminating nonneoplastic elements. This setting, in which morphologic analysis can be used to guide evaluation of only the cell population of interest, FISH can typically detect gains, translocations, or amplifications in as few as 5% and deletions in 15% to 30% of the cells within a sample.

ACKNOWLEDGMENT

The authors thank Arie Perry, Tu-Dung Nguyen, and Diane Robirds, authors of the previous edition of this chapter.

SUGGESTED READING

Perry A. Fluorescence in situ hybridization. In: Pfeifer JD. *Molecular Genetic Testing in Surgical Pathology*. Philadelphia, PA: Lippincott Williams & Wilkins; 2006.

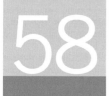

58 Direct and Indirect Methods for DNA and RNA Sequence Analysis

John D. Pfeifer

I. INTRODUCTION. Clinical molecular diagnostic methods have been integrated into many laboratory disciplines, and guidelines and recommendations from both professional societies and regulatory agencies have been developed to assist in the development and performance of clinical molecular pathology testing (Table 58.1). Most molecular tests performed in surgical pathology focus on somatic or acquired DNA variations in the cells of the disease process that provide information that aids in diagnosis, identifies prognostic indicators, stratifies patients into effective treatment options, helps monitor treatment response, and/or identifies patients at increased risk of disease. Polymerase chain reaction (PCR)-based approaches and so-called next generation sequencing (NGS)-based approaches have become the central technologies for much of clinical sequence analysis.

II. SPECIMEN REQUIREMENTS, HANDLING, AND PROCESSING. Nucleic acid sequencing in the setting of surgical pathology requires the same attention to detail regarding efficient specimen collection, identification, preparation, and routing as any other pathology test.

A. Specimens. Specimen requirements are dictated by the disease process, including the type of tissue, amount of tissue, type of sample (fresh or frozen tissue, formalin-fixed paraffin-embedded tissue, cytology specimen, and so on), and the extent of the disease in the sample. The amount of tissue required for PCR-based testing or NGS-based analysis is relatively small which contributes to the clinical utility of the technique.

Regardless of specimen type, two general features of the tissue sample influence molecular assays. First, there must be a sufficient quantity of the specific target cell (and therefore target DNA or RNA) in the sample. Second, the size or integrity of the nucleic acid molecules after isolation from the tissue can dramatically affect the sensitivity of the detection of specific alterations, thus nucleic acid degradation (whether due to fixation, or enzymatic, heat, pH, or mechanical forces) can reduce the sensitivity of testing.

1. Tissue type. Fresh peripheral blood, bone marrow, solid tissue biopsies, cytology specimens, enriched cell populations (e.g., from flow cytometry), and formalin-fixed paraffin-embedded tissue sections are all sources of nucleic acids for molecular analysis. For fresh tissue, specimens should be collected and transported to the molecular pathology laboratory using aseptic techniques, if possible. Transport on ice reduces cell lysis, minimizes nuclease activity, and reduces nucleic acid degradation.

2. Tissue quality

a. Fresh tissue and cell suspensions are the optimal templates for sequence analysis. The preferred method of preservation of fresh tissue prior to isolation of nucleic acids is ultra-low temperature frozen storage at −70°C, which permits indefinite preservation with virtually no effect on the quality of the extracted nucleic acids. Low temperature frozen storage around −20°C can adequately preserve DNA and RNA for several months.

Cell suspensions (including hematologic specimens such as peripheral blood and bone marrow) should be collected in the presence of an anticoagulant, preferably EDTA or ACD; heparin should be avoided because heparin carry-over after nucleic acid isolation may inhibit subsequent PCR steps. Freezing of hematologic specimens presents distinct obstacles to the preparation of good quality nucleic acid and should generally be avoided.

b. Nucleic acids extracted from fixed tissue can also be used for sequence analysis, although the type of fixative and length of fixation both have a profound effect

TABLE 58.1	Selected Resources for Clinical Molecular Pathology Laboratory Operational Guidelines	
Entity	Site	Tool(s)
Clinical Laboratory Improvement Amendments '88	http://www.cms.hhs.gov/clia/	Clinical Laboratory Accreditation requirements and compliance lists
College of American Pathologists (CAP)	http://www.cap.org	Laboratory Accreditation (LAP) Molecular Pathology Laboratory Inspection Checklist Proficiency Surveys • Molecular Oncology (MO) • Medical Genetics (MGL) • Pharmacogenetics (PGX) • Monitoring Engraftment (ME) • Molecular Microbiology (HIV, HCV, ID) • Microsatellite Instability (MSI) • Sarcoma Translocation (SARC) • Nucleic Acid Testing (viral; NAT)
Clinical and Laboratory Standards Institute (CLSI; *formerly National Committee for Clinical Laboratory Standards, NCCLS*)	http://www.nccls.org	Molecular Methods Guidelines • Genetic diseases • IGH and TCR Gene rearrangements • Nucleic Acid Amplification • Nucleic Acid Sequencing • Collection and Handling of Specimens • Proficiency Testing
American College of Medical Genetics (ACMG)	http://www.acmg.net	Standards and Guidelines for Clinical Genetics Laboratories Policy Statements for Molecular Testing of Genetic Diseases
US Food and Drug Administration (FDA)	Http://www.fda.gov	Medical Devices 21CFR809.30 In Vitro Diagnostic Products for Human Use • Analyte Specific Reagents (ASRs)
Association for Molecular Pathology (AMP)	http://www.amp.org	Molecular Pathology professional organization Test Directories • Solid Tumors • Hematopathology • Infectious Disease

on their recovery. Non cross-linking fixatives such as ethanol provide the most consistent preservation of amplifiable nucleic acids, with more variability from tissues fixed with formalin, Zamboni's and Clark's fixatives, paraformaldehyde, and formalin-alcohol-acetic acid. Tissues processed in Carnoy's, Zenker's, Bouin's, and B-5 fixatives are poor substrates for sequence analysis since little amplifiable DNA or RNA can be recovered from them.

The effects of formalin fixation have been evaluated in some detail, not surprising given that most surgical specimens are fixed in formalin. Formaldehyde reacts with nucleic acids and proteins to form a mixture of end products that are covalently linked by methylene bridges, engenders oxidation and deamination reactions, and leads to the formation of cyclic base derivatives. Thus, the quality of DNA and RNA isolated from formalin-fixed tissue is critically dependent on the length of fixation, with a deterioration of nucleic acids with increasing fixation time. In general, tissue fixed in neutral buffered formalin for less than 8 hours contains DNA and RNA from which PCR products greater than 600 bp in length can be reliably amplified, but fixation extended for greater than 8 to 12 hours decreases the length of PCR products that can consistently be amplified.

3. Tissue quantity. Minimum sample requirements are determined by the assay methodology and extent of target cell involvement in the tissue. A typical sequencing based assay requires only 10 to 200 ng of DNA (about 10^3 to 10^4 cells).

B. Histopathologic Review. Prior to nucleic acid extraction from the tumor specimen, formal review of the pathologic specimen by an anatomic pathologist is required to ensure the presence of malignant tissue, and to assess the quality and quantity of the material submitted for testing. The pathologic assessment is an important quality control step since it permits evaluation of possible analytic confounders including the percentage of nonneoplastic tissue, necrosis, cautery artifact, and so on, and thus helps ensure that the specimen is adequate for the validated assay. Obtaining an approximate value of the percentage of tumor involvement in a given sample may also be useful during interpretation of the sequencing data. Unfortunately, although pathologist review of cancer samples is required to select the regions of tumor with high cellularity and viability, the estimates are unreliable (*Mod Pathol* 2014;27:168; *Arch Pathol Lab Med* 2013;137:1545).

It is important to recognize that **tissue heterogeneity** is different from **intratumoral heterogeneity**. Tissue heterogeneity refers to the fact that no tumor specimen is composed of 100% neoplastic cells. Instead, cancer samples contain a varying proportion of nonneoplastic cells including stromal cells (benign parenchymal cells and fibroblasts), inflammatory cells (primarily neutrophils, lymphocytes, and macrophages), and endothelial cells (of blood vessels and lymphatics). Intratumoral heterogeneity is a term used to refer to the fact that malignant neoplasms usually demonstrate clonal heterogeneity. Consequently, even with a relatively pure tumor sample identified by histopathologic review, the number, type, and frequency of sequence variants detected in that sample may or may not be an accurate reflection of the range and frequency of the variants elsewhere in the tumor.

III. GENERAL FEATURES OF NUCLEIC ACID SEQUENCING TESTS

A. Factors That Affect Testing on a Diagnostic Level. The intrinsic biologic variability of disease has the greatest impact on the diagnostic sensitivity and specificity of molecular testing. Since only a subset of patients with a specific disease may harbor a characteristic mutation, more than one genetic variant may characterize a specific disease, the same mutation may be characteristic of more than one disease, a mutation characteristic of disease may be present in healthy individuals (reduced penetrance), and so on, even a molecular genetic method with perfect analytic performance will have a lower sensitivity and specificity when used for diagnostic testing of patient samples.

Another diagnostic limitation of the use of PCR in routine clinical testing is a result of the fact that the technique is so sensitive that it amplifies target DNA and RNA sequences from cellular debris as well as viable cells (*Cancer* 1997;80:1393). Consequently, in the absence of histologic confirmation of the presence of live tumor cells, the significance of PCR-based detection of tumor derived nucleic acids in lymph nodes or even peripheral blood is uncertain.

B. Factors That Affect Testing on an Operational Level. Purely operational factors can introduce uncertainty into the interpretation of results when testing is performed prospectively in routine clinical practice. If the probability that a case is subjected to additional analysis depends on the initial test result itself, clinical variables, or both, selection bias (also called verification bias, posttest referral bias, and work-up bias) is introduced into the test. Discrepant analysis (also known as discordant analysis) can also introduce uncertainty in the interpretation of test results. Finally, even mundane factors such as differences in disease prevalence can have a marked effect on the predictive value of positive and negative test results.

C. Implications for Clinical Testing. Taken together, the analytic/technical features of molecular genetic assays, biologic variability, variation in assay design, and differences in distribution of disease in the patient populations have many implications for testing applied in routine clinical practice.

1. **Characteristics of tests with clinical utility.** The criteria used to evaluate the clinical utility of other hospital laboratory tests should also be applied when considering the role of a sequencing test in patient care (Table 58.2).

   a. The relative merit of the testing should focus on the ability of the test findings to improve patient care. For clinical utility, the sequencing test must provide an improvement in the standard of patient care by providing new or refined information with the potential for clinical stratification of disease subtypes, prognostic categories, treatment regimens, gene-targeted therapies, survival statistics, or disease progression. The test results should complement the findings of established tests, such as cytogenetics, immunohistochemistry, and cell surface marker analysis. In the context of surgical pathology, the test results must be correlated with the histopathologic features of the case.

   b. Routine clinical use of sequencing tests must consider practical aspects of clinical prevalence (the disease should represent a significant health problem or diagnostic dilemma), test run frequency, clinically relevant turnaround time, sensitivity, and specificity. Testing for diseases which are common in many populations (e.g., cancer, microbial infections, genetic predispositions) and have well-defined molecular markers will be performed in many laboratories. Molecular genetic testing for rare disorders will be routinely available only at selected laboratories with specific clinical programs or areas of institutional focus and expertise.

   c. Testing must include steps to validate the result, and will include positive and negative assay controls, definition of the details and limits of interpretation of test results, and provisions for proficiency testing of the analytic method, competency of the technologists, and interpretive expertise of the laboratory director.

   d. Results must be reported in a context that explains the data and integrates the findings with other pathology results to avoid seemingly contradictory reports in comparison with other laboratory tests that possess different levels of resolution or detection.

   e. Biosafety, legal, ethical, and privacy issues must consistently be observed.

TABLE 58.2 Characteristics of Sequencing Tests With Clinical Utility

Criterion	Utility
The disorder must be a significant health problem.	Disease prevalence and adverse effect on affected individuals are measurable and serious.
Treatment alternatives are available to alter disease course.	The genotype does affect the patient's clinical outcome.
A reliable molecular test is available to distinguish true positive and false positive results.	Focus on molecular changes known to be associated with disease pathology.
Pretest and Posttest counseling resources are available.	Interpretation of molecular findings with the data from the clinical presentation and other pathology tests.
The test is cost-effective and/or cost-beneficial.	More costly or invasive disease monitoring methods are unnecessary. Specific treatment options and/or prognostic outcomes are indicated by the molecular results.
Referring clinicians accept the test as worthwhile to aid their decision-making.	Diagnosis, treatment, and/or clinical outcome are enhanced by the addition of the molecular pathology results to other medical tests.

2. Discordant cases. Cases will arise in which there is a lack of concordance between the diagnosis suggested by the molecular test results and the morphologic diagnosis. The debate over the best approach to resolve the ambiguity presented by these cases reflects the fundamental impact of molecular genetics on the classification of disease as well as the status of morphology as the historical standard of diagnosis by which new methods are measured. Rather than arbitrarily assuming that genetic testing or morphology is superior in all cases, the most reasonable way to handle discordant cases is to acknowledge the presence of the discrepancy, and then reappraise the clinical data, pathologic findings, and therapeutic implications of all the test results.

For those cases in which the diagnosis suggested by morphology and genetic testing are different, prospective clinical trials are required to assess whether stage, prognosis, and response to treatment are more accurately predicted by the molecular test results than by the morphologic findings on which most staging and treatment protocols are based. Epidemiologically, there is a distinction between diagnostic testing and prognostic testing, with different study designs required to assess the performance of tests in these different settings (*J Clin Epidemiol* 2002;55:1178; *Ann Intern Med* 2003;139:950).

IV. BASIC PCR METHODOLOGY

A. Amplification. Selective amplification of the target sequence is achieved through the use of oligonucleotide primers that hybridize to the 5' and 3' ends of the DNA target sequence (Fig. 58.1). In addition to the two primers and input (template) DNA, the reaction mixture also includes the four deoxynucleotide triphosphates (dATP, dCTP, dGTP, dTTP) and a heat-stable (thermostable) DNA polymerase. The first step of the PCR itself involves heating the mixture to a high temperature to denature the target DNA; in the second step, the reaction is cooled to allow the primers to anneal to their complementary sequence in the target DNA; in the third step, the reaction is heated to the temperature at which the heat-stable DNA polymerase has optimal activity. As a result of this three-step denaturation, annealing, and polymerization cycle, the two primers will initiate synthesis of new DNA molecules from opposite strands of the input DNA heteroduplex. With each repetition of the three step cycle, the newly synthesized DNA strands will also act as templates for further DNA synthesis, and so DNA duplexes in which both strands have the fixed-length of the target sequence (so-called amplicons) accumulate exponentially.

PCR makes it possible to selectively amplify a specific DNA target sequence within a background of heterogeneous DNA sequences such as total genomic DNA or cDNA derived from unfractionated cellular RNA. The sensitivity of PCR for detection of a few target molecules in a large background of unaltered DNA molecules (1 in 10^5 or lower) is one of the principle strengths of the methodology. However, each of the components in a PCR, including the input DNA, the oligonucleotide primers, the thermostable polymerase, the buffer, and the cycle parameters, has an effect on the sensitivity, specificity, and fidelity of the reaction.

B. Factors That Affect PCR Testing on an Analytic/Technical Level

1. Advantages of PCR

a. PCR is simple, quick, and inexpensive. A single PCR cycle of melting, annealing, and extension is usually completed within several minutes, and consequently an entire PCR amplification of 25 to 35 cycles can be performed in only a few hours. Because of the high level of amplification achieved by PCR, the product DNA can be visualized after simple gel electrophoresis, avoiding the hazards and expense of radiolabeling methods.

b. PCR has high sensitivity and specificity. When optimized, PCR can detect one abnormal cell in a background of 10^5 normal cells, and can even be used to analyze single copy genes from individual cells (*Methods Enzymol* 2002;356:295; *Methods Enzymol* 2002;356:334). PCR can also be used to detect a broad range of genetic abnormalities ranging from gross structural alterations such as translocations to single base pair changes.

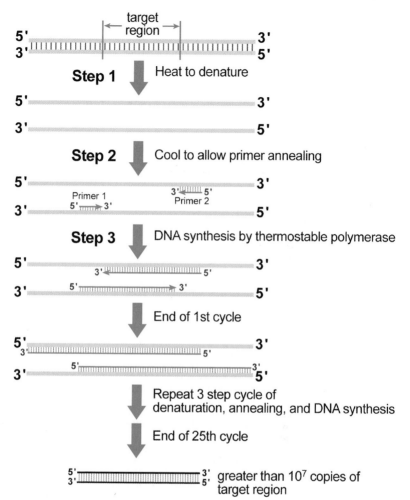

Figure 58.1 Schematic diagram of PCR. Each cycle consists of three steps: the reaction mix is heated to denature the double-stranded DNA template, the reaction mix is cooled to permit annealing of oligonucleotide primers to sequences that flank the target region, and then the reaction mix is warmed to permit the heat-stable polymerase to synthesize new DNA strands. Each newly synthesized DNA strand then acts as a template in subsequent three step cycles of denaturation, annealing, and DNA synthesis, producing exponential amplification of the target region.

    c. PCR products are easily labeled for detection. For primer mediated labeling, a labeled chemical group (usually a fluorophore) is attached to the 5' end of either or both oligonucleotide primers. Alternatively, the PCR product can be directly labeled by including one or more labeled nucleotide precursors into the PCR reaction mix.

    d. Phenotype–genotype correlations are possible. When performed on tissue sections, PCR provides only an indirect correlation of morphology with underlying genetic abnormalities. Microdissection, in which the region of interest is carved out of the formalin-fixed paraffin-embedded tissue block, scraped from tissue sections or cytology slides, or collected more precisely with a micromanipulator apparatus, provides some enrichment for morphologic-genetic correlations. More precise phenotypic–genotypic analysis is achieved by collecting individual cells by laser capture microdissection, by flow cytometry, or even immunomagnetic methods. In situ PCR performed on histologic tissue sections themselves is perhaps the ultimate method for providing morphologic-genotypic correlation; however, the technique is so technically demanding that it has limited use in clinical laboratories.

2. Limitations of PCR

   a. PCR only analyzes the target region. Testing only provides information on the target segment amplified by the specific primer set employed.

   b. PCR only amplifies intact target regions. Mutations that damage a primer binding site (including insertions, deletions, and even point mutations) preclude amplification of the target region by PCR and can easily lead to errors in test interpretation. Similarly, mutations that alter the structure of the target region in ways not accounted for during primer set design (e.g., large insertions, deletions, inversions, or translocations) may preclude amplification.

   c. Amplification bias. PCR bias refers to the fact that some DNA templates are preferentially amplified versus other templates within the same reaction. PCR bias can be caused by differences in template length, random variations in template number (especially with very low target abundance, producing an artifact known as allele dropout), and random variations in PCR efficiency with each cycle. Amplification bias can even result from differences in the target sequence itself as small as a single base substitution. PCR bias can cause over tenfold differences in amplification efficiency in some settings, a difference that can influence quantitative PCR test results and loss of heterozygosity analysis. PCR bias can be a particularly troublesome problem in multiplex PCR.

   d. Technical factors. There are several technical factors that can lower the sensitivity and specificity of PCR in routine clinical practice below that obtained in optimized research settings. Nonspecific inhibitors of PCR are sometimes present in patient samples, including heparin and uncharacterized components of CSF, urine, and sputum. Given the extreme sensitivity of PCR, strict attention to the physical organization and methodologies of the laboratory are required to avoid cross-contamination of specimens.

   However, the most important technical limitations are introduced when fixed rather than fresh tissue specimens are used for testing due to the degradation of DNA and mRNA that occurs prior to and during fixation, as noted above. Test sensitivity and specificity are compromised by degradation since it makes it necessary to amplify shorter target sequences or employ a nested PCR approach, both of which increase the risk of amplification of nonspecific sequences and cross-contamination (*Am J Surg Pathol* 2002;26:965).

V. VARIATIONS OF PCR

   A. Nested PCR. In this technique, two consecutive PCR reactions are performed on the same DNA sample; an initial amplification of a longer target sequence followed by a second amplification of a shorter sequence contained within the first. The second PCR may involve two internal primers (fully nested) or one internal primer and one of the original primers (semi nested). Nested PCR provides a marked increase in sensitivity compared with traditional PCR, and is desirable when the target sequence is present at an extremely low copy number (such as when the mutation is present in only a small subset of the cell population under study), when the nucleic acids have been degraded as a result of tissue fixation, or, for reverse transcriptase-PCR as discussed below, when the target mRNA is expressed at an extremely low level. Since the increased sensitivity carries an increased risk of cross contamination, reproducible nested PCR results require strict attention to laboratory technique, rigorous use of controls, and confirmation of product identity.

B. **Reverse Transcriptase PCR (RT-PCR).** RT-PCR makes it possible to amplify RNA extracted from a tissue sample; a complementary DNA (cDNA) strand is synthesized from the RNA template using the enzyme reverse transcriptase, and the cDNA is then amplified by conventional PCR. Fresh (or fresh frozen) tissue is the preferred source of RNA for RT-PCR. RNA from fixed tissue is an acceptable substrate for testing (e-Fig. 58.1), even though it always suffers some degree of degradation depending on the prefixation interval, the type of fixative, the length of fixation, and the method used to isolate the RNA.

1. **Advantages of RT-PCR.** RT-PCR permits direct amplification of multi-exon sequences by eliminating the intervening introns, and thus greatly simplifies mutation scanning methods. Similarly, RT-PCR makes it much simpler to demonstrate the presence of translocations that create fusion genes by making it possible to directly detect the fusion transcripts encoded by the translocations (e-Fig. 58.2). RT-PCR can also be used to detect changes in mRNA structure that result from alternative splicing, to demonstrate aberrant splicing due to mutations, and to evaluate the level of gene expression through the quantitative methods discussed below.

2. **Limitations of RT-PCR.** RNA is a more technically demanding substrate with less stability than DNA. Tissue samples must be processed rapidly (ideally, within 20 minutes) to avoid mRNA degradation, especially since many mutations render transcripts more susceptible to cellular mechanisms that clear abnormal transcripts from the cell. A nested PCR approach is often necessary when the target RNA is present at very low levels, and in this setting RT-PCR carries an increased risk of contamination and amplification of nonspecific sequences because the transfer of the first PCR product to a separate tube for the nested PCR entails transmission of a highly amplified DNA preparation.

C. **Quantitative PCR.** An ideal PCR would generate a perfect 2-fold increase in the number of copies of the amplicon in each cycle of the reaction. In reality, inhibitors of the reaction, accumulation of pyrophosphate molecules, decreasing polymerase activity, and reagent consumption all contribute to a plateau phase in the later stages of the reaction during which the amplicon is no longer accumulating at an exponential rate (*Clin Chem Lab Med* 2000;38:833). Reliable quantitation of PCR therefore involves more than simple measurement of the amount of product DNA present at the end of 30 to 40 cycles of the reaction. Real-time PCR, also referred to as quantitative-PCR (Q-PCR), employs real-time measurements of DNA accumulation (usually via fluorescence-based approaches) during the early exponential phases of PCR progress to provide precise estimates of the initial concentration of the target sequence(s).

A wide variety of different chemistries for Q-PCR are in routine use, including the so-called *Taq* Man (also known as 5' exonuclease or hydrolysis real time-PCR), molecular beacon (which can be designed to distinguish targets differing by only a single nucleotide), scorpion (also known as self-probing amplicons), hybridization probe, and intercalating dye methods. Regardless of the chemistry, changes in fluorescence that result from target amplification are measured by a detector for each cycle of the reaction, and used by a computer to construct an amplification plot of fluorescence versus the cycle number to quantify the concentration of the input target DNA sequence.

1. **Advantages of Q-PCR.** The method can be applied to fresh as well as formalin-fixed paraffin-embedded tissue, and phenotype-genotype correlations are possible through analysis of specific cell populations collected via microdissection, laser capture microdissection, and so on. Q-RT-PCR is also a robust analytic approach (e-Fig. 58.3).

2. **Disadvantages of Q-PCR.** Even for optimized assays, testing can be complicated by amplification bias, which in the context of Q-PCR has two major sources; PCR drift due to random fluctuations in amplification efficiency in the early cycles of the reaction when the templates are present at very low concentration, and PCR selection due to mechanisms that systematically favor amplification of some particular target(s).

For Q-RT-PCR, the reverse transcription reaction can introduce additional variables into the analysis.

3. Use of Q-PCR in nonquantitative settings. Since the probes used in Q-PCR (and Q-RT-PCR) have specificity for the target amplicon, the amplification plot not only confirms the presence of the DNA product, but also confirms its identity. Intercalating dyes can also provide confirmation of both the presence and identity of the DNA product when coupled with subsequent melting curve analysis. Because Q-PCR eliminates the need for gel electrophoresis to demonstrate successful amplification while simultaneously confirming product identity, Q-PCR is often used as a "one-step" alternative to conventional PCR or RT-PCR even when quantitation is not required.

D. Multiplex PCR. Multiplex PCR is the simultaneous amplification of multiple target sequences in a single reaction through the simultaneous use of multiple primer pairs. The technique saves time and money, is ideal for conserving templates that are in short supply, and has been successfully applied to many amplification approaches including nested PCR and Q-PCR. However, even in optimized reactions, multiplex PCR may be complicated by amplification bias due to PCR drift and PCR selection. Rigorous optimization of primer design and careful titration of the relative primer concentration among separate primer pairs are essential for robust, reproducible multiplex PCR.

E. Methylation-Specific PCR. Methylation of CpG sites in human DNA has been associated with transcriptional inactivation of imprinted genes, is important for X chromosome inactivation, and is an important mechanism for developmentally regulated and tissue specific gene regulation. An altered pattern of methylation is also characteristic of many human diseases (e-**Figs. 58.4** and **58.5**). Changes in the CpG methylation pattern in some malignancies have been associated with differences in response to specific chemotherapeutic agents and overall survival.

Recently developed methylation-specific PCR techniques exploit the sequence differences produced when methylated CpG (abbreviated as meCpG) and unmethylated CpG are treated with sodium bisulfite (*Proc Natl Acad Sci USA* 1996;93:9821). This chemical modification will not alter methyl cytosine but will depurinate cytosine to produce a transversion, which results in replacement by thymidine in subsequent DNA synthesis during PCR. Since the two strands of genomic DNA are no longer complimentary after sodium bisulfite treatment, PCR with specifically designed primers for meC and T substituted sequences makes it possible to infer the methylation status of the original untreated DNA (e-**Fig. 58.6**). Methylation-specific PCR can be applied to DNA extracted from fresh tissue, FFPE tissue, and even archival cytology specimens.

VI. SEQUENCE ANALYSIS BY SANGER SEQUENCING. The **dye terminator cycle sequencing method** for direct DNA sequencing, a derivative of so-called Sanger sequencing, is currently used for virtually all routine DNA sequence analyses. This technique (e-**Fig. 58.7**) utilizes synthetic oligonucleotide primers complimentary to a known sequence of the template strand to be analyzed, and is greatly simplified by the use of fluorescently labeled, chain-terminating dideoxynucleotide triphosphates. As initially described, enzymatic extension of the primer was performed only once per sequencing reaction, but the utility of the method is greatly increased by the modification known as cycle sequencing (or linear amplification sequencing). Cycle sequencing is similar to conventional PCR in that it employs a thermostable DNA polymerase and a temperature cycling format for DNA denaturation, annealing, and enzymatic DNA synthesis, but only one primer (the sequencing primer) is added to the reaction mixture.

VII. SEQUENCE ANALYSIS BY NEXT GENERATION SEQUENCING. The high throughput of massively parallel sequencing methods (also known as next generation sequencing methods, or simply NGS), coupled with their low cost and high accuracy, makes them ideally suited for the analysis of cancer specimens in clinical settings where diagnosis or choice of therapy requires the information about the presence of mutations in several different areas of the same gene, and/or in several different genes. Enthusiasm for the use of NGS is due to the fact that NGS can be used to comprehensively evaluate multiple genetic loci when only a limited quantity of DNA is available for testing, which is important given the increasing number of targeted chemotherapy drugs (which requires analysis of an ever increasing number of genes) while ever smaller tissue specimens are available for testing (a result of current trends to shift from large excisional biopsies to needle or aspiration biopsies for diagnosis).

The genetic complexity of cancer specimens underscores the importance of NGS's capability to evaluate the full spectrum of sequence variations in dozens to thousands of genes in a single assay. The genomes of all cancer cells carry somatic (often referred to as acquired) alterations which fall into four general classes, single nucleotide variants (SNVs), small insertions and deletions (indels, which are generally less than a few dozen bases long), copy number variants (CNVs), and structural variants (SVs, such as translocations). Some of the mutations are so-called "driver mutations" because they confer selective clonal growth advantage or evasion from apoptosis and are casually involved in oncogenesis, others of which are so-called "passenger mutations" since they do not contribute to development of cancer but are secondary changes with little diagnostic or therapeutic importance.

Identifying somatic driver mutations in cancer has several direct clinical applications. First, the pattern of mutations itself can be diagnostic in cases in which traditional histopathologic examination is not definitive (*Am J Surg Pathol* 2014;38:534). Second, somatic mutations can be used to predict how a patient may respond to a drug with respect to toxicity or efficacy. For example, alterations in exon 19 of *EGFR* in patients with nonsmall cell lung cancer (NSCLC) are responsive to treatment with gefitinib. Similarly, the majority of patients with NSCLC whose tumor carries an inversion in *ALK* or a translocation in *ROS1* respond to treatment with crizotinib. Other somatic mutations predict resistance to therapy with tyrosine kinase inhibitors (TKIs), such as *KRAS* mutations in lung cancer. Third, somatic mutations can provide prognostic information on the risk of disease progression or relapse. For example, an internal tandem duplication in the *FLT3* gene is associated with poor prognosis in acute myeloid leukemia (AML) while mutations in nucleophosmin (*NPM1*) are associated with a favorable prognosis.

Amplification-based as well as hybrid capture-based NGS assays can be used for the analysis of cancer specimens. Similarly, assays that target a panel of genes (from several genes, to several hundred genes), the exome, or the entire genome have been developed. However, as with all lab tests, the utility of the various assays is extremely dependent on the clinical setting. In general, since clinical utility has been defined for only a few thousand different mutations in a few hundred genes, sequence analysis of the exome or entire genome in a clinical setting is currently unjustified, and so currently the most common assays focus on panels of genes with well documented roles in diagnosis, prognosis, or prediction of response to therapy.

A. Amplification-Based Methods. Amplification-based NGS methods rely on exponential amplification of the target region utilizing sequence-specific primers. When compared with hybrid capture-based methods, amplification methods have a simpler workflow, with reduced hands-on time and more rapid turnaround time, and so have popularity in clinical settings. Highly multiplexed microfluidic and microdroplet methods (e.g., RainDance Technologies, Fluidigm) have substantial upfront hardware costs but can increase cost efficiency via sample pooling. Several amplification enrichment systems have been optimized for compatibility with benchtop sequencing instruments (e.g., Ion Torrent, Illumina MiSeq), which makes amplification-based technology accessible to any size laboratory for clinical use. However, amplification-based approaches have several limitations. First, there are significant limits on the size of the target region that can be sequenced because of practical issues with the number of PCR reactions that can be multiplexed in a single amplification. Second, only a subset of variant types can be detected; in general SNVs and small indels can be identified, while detection of CNVs and SVs is challenging unless specific assay designs are employed. Third, as with any amplification-based test, there is the potential for amplification bias, polymerase sequencing errors, contamination, and primer binding artifacts. Fourth, amplification-based NGS requires prior knowledge of the sequences and the nature of the mutations to be targeted; the assay lacks the potential for identifying novel disease-associated mutations outside the targeted regions.

While many clinical NGS labs have internally developed amplification-based tests, commercially available assays are the most popular. They require as little as 10 ng of input DNA (or less) and work well with different types of tumor samples including archived FFPE samples. The turnaround time (TAT) from receiving samples to reporting can be as short as 3 to 5 days.

B. Hybrid Capture-Based Methods. NGS by targeted hybridization capture is a sensitive and specific method to detect somatic alterations in tumor samples. With appropriate assay design, the approach enables detection of all four classes of genomic alterations in cancer specimens, with very high analytic sensitivity and specificity, a very low limit of detection, and very high reproducibility. Given the genetic heterogeneity that is such a fundamental characteristic of cancer, particularly in solid tumors, the efficient and cost-effective targeting of multiple classes of mutations in a large number of genes in a single assay maximizes the usefulness of the approach. Hybrid capture methodologies have the flexibility for use with a range of target region sizes, from one gene to the entire exome.

However, hybrid capture-based tests have several disadvantages. DNA library preparation generally takes 3 to 5 days (compared with one day for amplicon-based enrichment library preparation), with a large proportion of this time allocated to probe hybridization (typically 24 to 48 hours incubation time for the hybridization step itself) and, therefore, clinical hybrid capture tests have a longer TAT. Although automation can be used to decrease TAT, it requires specialized equipment and is thus associated with an initial capital investment. Hybridization-based NGS clinical tests also frequently suffer from design restrictions, including problems with high GC content, repetitive regions, and gene family members that share sequence homology (pseudogenes). The bioinformatics and interpretive component of hybrid capture-based testing has emerged as particularly problematic, since the ease with which massive amounts of sequence can be generated on the current generation of platforms can easily overwhelm a laboratory's ability to analyze the data.

C. Assay Scope

1. Targeted gene panels. Panels for acquired mutations in cancer specimens focus on genes that are considered clinically actionable in that there is well-established literature providing evidence for their diagnostic, predictive, and/or prognostic value. The panels may be quite narrow (e.g., only a few dozen genes) based on the specific cancer being evaluated such as colon adenocarcinoma, lung adenocarcinoma, or gastrointestinal stromal tumor (*J Mol Diagn* 2012;14:357; *J Mol Diagn* 2014;16:89), or much broader (e.g., hundreds of genes) based on recurrently mutated genes across multiple cancer types (http://foundationone.com/learn.php-2).

Smaller and larger panels each have distinct advantages and disadvantages. For clinical testing, limiting the number of targeted genes avoids an excessive number of distracting VUSs, decreases incidental findings, and can provide a more rapid TAT. Assays with a smaller target region also usually have better coverage and are easier to multiplex, providing for greater sequencing depth and therefore increased analytical sensitivity for detecting mutations with low variant allele frequencies (VAFs), increased efficiency, and a lower cost. Another important advantage of small panels that target only loci with well-established relevance is higher rates of reimbursement, a difference that is critical in the clinical setting where testing is paid for by health insurance carriers rather than by research grants or philanthropy. In contrast, large panels are more likely to include genes relevant to clinical trials or drug development, and so have much more utility in investigational settings. In the end, panel design is determined by examining factors such as clinical need, expected sample volume, practicality of running multiple small disease-directed panels versus a single more general cancer-based panel, and sources of revenue.

2. Exomes and whole genomes. Exome and genome sequencing are often applied to the study of cancer as a discovery tool in the investigative setting. Exome or genome sequencing is helpful for detection of CNVs and is especially well-suited to detection of SVs which often involve noncoding DNA breakpoints.

However, there are several limitations to the use of exome and whole genome in routine clinical practice. First, because of the high depth of coverage (about 1,000×) required for sensitive and specific identification of somatic variants in cancer samples due to the admixture of benign and malignant cells within the tumor, clonal heterogeneity of the tumor cells, and variation in coverage across different regions of DNA, the cost is often prohibitive in clinical practice. Second, the utility of sequencing genes without established clinical significance is an issue. Beyond the genes evaluated by focused panels, there are relatively few loci for which sufficient clinical-grade evidence exists to support interpretation of functional or therapeutic consequences for the variants identified; thus, most variants identified are VUSs and do not meaningfully contribute to patient management. Third, intensive bioinformatic analysis is required to manage the vast amounts of data provided by such large scale sequencing.

D. Library Complexity. The number of independent DNA template molecules (sometimes referred to as genome equivalents) sequenced in an NGS assay has a profound impact on the sensitivity and specificity of variant detection. While it is possible to perform NGS analysis of even picogram quantities of DNA (*Cancer Res* 2013;73:2965; *Nature Methods* 2014;11: doi:10.1038/nmeth.2771), this technical feat is accomplished by increasing the number of amplification cycles during library preparation. However, the information in 1,000 sequence reads derived from one genome is clearly quite different than the information present in 1,000 sequence reads from 1,000 different genomes. Thus, library complexity and sequence depth (see below) are independent parameters in NGS assay design.

E. Depth of Coverage. Coverage is defined as the number of aligned reads that contain a given nucleotide position, and sufficient depth of coverage is critical in clinical NGS assays for identification of sequence variants with the required level of sensitivity and specificity. There are many factors that influence the required level of coverage. The first variable is the sequence complexity of the target region. Target regions with homology to multiple regions of the genome, a higher number of repetitive sequence elements, pseudogenes, and increased GC content generally have decreased coverage. Second, the method used for targeted enrichment can impact coverage depth; amplification-based approaches often provide higher depth (although the complexity of the sequence data may be uncertain, as discussed above). Third, in a multiplexed clinical assay where multiple samples are sequenced simultaneously, the size of the target region (e.g., 400 kb for a typical panel of genes, versus 30 to 75 Mb for an exome, versus over 3 Gb for a genome) will impact the depth of coverage that can be reasonably achieved for each sample.

The relationship between depth of coverage and the reproducibility of variant detection from a given sample is straightforward: a higher number of high-quality sequence reads lends confidence to the base called at a particular location, whether the base call from the sequenced sample is the same as the reference base (no variant identified) or is a nonreference base (variant identified), and thus increases assay sensitivity and specificity. However, the depth of coverage required to make accurate variant calls is also dependent upon the type of variant being evaluated, and whether the variant is germline or somatically acquired. In general, a lower depth of coverage is acceptable for constitutional testing where germline alterations are more easily identified since they are in either a heterozygous or homozygous state; a minimum of 30x coverage with balanced reads (forward and reverse reads equally represented) is usually sufficient for this purpose. However, much higher read depths are necessary to confidently identify somatic variants in tumor specimens due to tissue and tumoral heterogeneity (see below); an overall coverage on the order of 1,000× is often required (*Cancer Genet* 2013;206;420). For NGS of mitochondrial DNA, an average coverage of greater than 20,000 is required to reliably detect heteroplasmic variants present at 1.5% (*Genet Med* 2013;15:388).

The need for high read depths reflects the complexity involved in somatic variant detection. As discussed below in more detail, tumor biopsy specimens represent a heterogeneous mixture of tissue encompassing malignant cells, as well as supporting stromal cells, inflammatory cells, and uninvolved tissue; malignant cells harboring somatic variation can become diluted out in this admixture. Of additional consideration, intramural heterogeneity creates tumor subclones so that only a small proportion of the total tumor cell population may harbor a given mutation, and so the read depth of the assay should be sufficiently high to compensate for this variation.

F. Analytic Issues. NGS tests are somewhat unique in that the analytic portion of the test itself consists of three individual components, specifically the sequence platform itself; the so-called wet bench procedures that are involved in the extraction of nucleic acids and DNA library preparation; and the bioinformatics associated with base calling, reference genome alignment, variant identification, variant annotation, and variant interpretation. The general features of all three of these components as they apply to NGS analysis of cancer specimens are similar to those for constitutional testing. However, there are some additional issues that must be considered in the analysis of tumor samples, specifically in the bioinformatic analysis.

As with all NGS testing, after the sequencing reads are generated from the DNA extracted from a tumor specimen, bioinformatics tools are used to align the reads against a reference genome and identify differences between the tumor's sequence and the reference. Given the intrinsic genomic instability of malignancies, and their often complicated intratumoral heterogeneity due to the presence of various tumor subclones, maximum clinical utility of cancer specimens can only be achieved using a bioinformatic pipeline designed to detect all four classes of genomic variants (SNVs, indels, CNVs, and SVs) at allele frequencies that are physiologically relevant. The four main classes of variants each require different computational approaches for sensitive and specific identification (assuming the assay is designed to permit their detection); various informatics pipelines are known to have different levels of accuracy for the various classes of variants, and even for specific variants, and so optimization of the pipeline used for a clinical NGS test is imperative.

G. Orthogonal Validation. As with any laboratory test, clinical NGS assays used to detect sequence variants in cancer specimens require confirmation of test results by orthogonal methods during assay development, as well as to confirm unexpected or puzzling results that arise in routine clinical use. Test validation in general includes three steps, namely establishment of the analytic sensitivity and specificity of the test, definition of the range of detectable mutations and the limits of detection of the assay, and demonstration of the capability of the NGS test to detect mutations in undiagnosed patients. Given that the bioinformatics associated with base calling, reference genome alignment, and variant identification, annotation, and interpretation are such a key component of an NGS test, the bioinformatic pipeline itself must be separately evaluated.

While each orthogonal validation approach has its own advantages and disadvantages, several issues are common to all in the setting of NGS tests of tumor specimens. First, although the lower limit of sensitivity of optimized conventional approaches is similar to that of routine NGS tests for SNVs, enhanced NGS bioinformatic pipelines enable detection of variants present at a frequency of less than 1%, a level of sensitivity significantly better than can be achieved by conventional techniques. Second, some of the discrepancies between SNVs detected by NGS assays and an orthogonal validation method may actually represent tissue heterogeneity and/or intratumoral heterogeneity rather than technical errors. Third, orthogonal validation used as confirmatory testing of positive results but not of negative results can raise the issue of discrepant analysis (also known as discordant analysis or review bias) that may poorly estimate test performance (*Clin Chem* 1998;44:108; *J Clin Microbiol* 200;38:4301; *J Clin Epidemiol* 1998;51:219). This last issue is especially problematic since some current guidelines recommend the use of confirmatory testing for positive results without associated testing of negative results (i.e., wild type results).

Conventional orthogonal validation approaches that have been used to confirm SNVs in NGS test results include Sanger sequencing, restriction fragment length polymorphism (RFLP) analysis, allele-specific PCR, and SNP arrays. Similar approaches are well suited to confirm the presence of indels identified by NGS. Common technologies used for orthogonal CNV validation are quantitative real-time PCR (qPCR), interphase FISH, and array CGH; the optimal choice depends on the size and scope of CNVs being validated. Classical cytogenetics, metaphase FISH, and interphase FISH are the approaches that are commonly used to confirm the presence of SVs identified by NGS.

H. Annotation. Use of NGS for clinical testing of cancer specimens is a paradigm shift that has profound implications for variant annotation. Unlike focused testing for genes with well-established clinical correlations, NGS involves analysis of numerous genes for which the spectrum of variation has not been well characterized and for which there is often only limited evidence for a disease association. Essentially, many of the evidence-gathering and analysis activities traditionally performed for diagnosis, prognosis, or prediction of response to therapy have migrated from their classical position prior to the test (in the clinic), to a position where they follow the test (interpretation of test results). This poses challenges to interpretation of whether the variant has a plausible contribution to the cancer phenotype (whether that is the tumor type itself, its prognosis, or its response to a specific therapy). The annotation of the clinical significance of an identified sequence variant is therefore often a difficult and time-consuming process to gather the relevant scientific and medical evidence. The major factors that complicate annotation of sequence variants include the lack of clinical standards for interpreting primary NGS results, inconsistencies in reporting clinical variants in commonly used file formats, and a lack of systematized communication among clinical (and research) laboratories and the scientific literature.

Fortunately, an increasing number of resources is being created to support the task. First, common variants not known to be disease-related must be filtered. Large-scale efforts such as HapMap and the 1000 Genomes Project that characterize genetic variation in diverse population groups support assessments of the frequency of human variation (Table 58.3); ClinVar, dbSNP, and Variation Viewer support searching and filtering functions related to allele frequencies; and dbSNP provides files of common variants not known to be disease related. Then, the disease associations of the variant must be considered. Many centralized reference databases (Table 58.4), such as those at NCBI, are designed for representing relationships between variants and phenotypes; for example, dbGaP is a catalogue of variation-disease associations and MedGen harmonizes phenotype terminologies and supports computational access to phenotype data.

1. Variants of unknown significance (VUSs). The issues associated with annotation of variants are so important because, even with gene panels, exome, or whole genome

---

TABLE 58.3   Selected Reference Databases and Datasets for Human Variation

Name/URL	Overview
International HapMap Project http://hapmap.ncbi.nlm.nih.gov/	International collaboration to assess common variation in multiple populations and identify haplotype blocks.
1000 Genomes Project http://www.1000genomes.org/	International collaboration to assess common variation in multiple populations using NGS approaches.
NHLBI GO Exome Sequencing Project (ESP) https://esp.gs.washington.edu/drupal/	Multicenter collaboration using NGS approaches to identify variation in exomes; includes rich phenotypic data.
dbSNP Database of Short Genetic Variations http://www.ncbi.nlm.nih.gov/snp	Archive of short (<50 bp) sequence variants; includes both common and rare variants, both germline and somatic.
dbVar http://www.ncbi.nlm.nih.gov/dbvar	Archive of longer (>50 bp) sequence variants; includes copy number changes and complex rearrangements.

TABLE 58.4	Selected Databases and Datasets for Variants in the Context of Phenotype
Resource	**Content**
OMIM http://omim.org/	Subset of variants in genes reported in human phenotypes and genes. Curated from the published literature.
dbGaP http://www.ncbi.nlm.nih.gov/gap	Archive of studies and datasets of genotype and phenotype. Provides both unrestricted and controlled forms of access.
ClinVar http://ncbi.nlm.nih.gov/clinvar/	Archive of submitted interpretations of medically related variants.
HGMD http://www.hgmd.org/	Collation of published genetic germline variation in nuclear genes underlying or associated with human inherited disease. Public and professional versions.
HGVS Locus Specific Mutation Databases http://www.hgvs.org/dblist/glsdb.html	Aggregation of gene-specific databases of observed variation.
COSMIC – Catalogue of somatic mutations in cancer http://cancer.sanger.ac.uk/cancergenome/projects/cosmic/	Curated catalogue of genes that undergo somatic mutation in human cancers, supported by the Wellcome Trust Sanger Institute. Contains information on neoplasms and other related samples, with somatic mutation frequencies. Data are extracted and curated from the primary literature.
The Cancer Genome Atlas (TCGA) http://cancergenome.nih.gov/abouttcga/overview	Comprehensive effort to accelerate the understanding of the molecular basis of cancer through the application of genome analysis technologies.
GeneReviews http://www.ncbi.nlm.nih.gov/books/NBK1116/	Expert-authored, peer-reviewed disease descriptions presented in a standardized format; focused on clinically relevant and medically actionable information for the diagnosis, management, and genetic counseling of specific inherited conditions.
PharmGKB http://www.pharmgkb.org/	Collects, curates, and disseminates information about the impact of human genetic variation on drug responses.
GTEx (The Genotype-Tissue Expression (GTEx) project) browser http://www.ncbi.nlm.nih.gov/gtex/test/GTEX2/gtex.cgi/	Resource database and associated tissue bank for study of the relationship between genetic variation and gene expression in human tissues.

tests optimized for clinically relevant sensitivity and specificity, the majority of variants identified currently fall into the category of VUSs. By definition, for a VUS there is insufficient existing evidence to support a definitive annotation regarding the effect of the variant on protein function, cell function, tumor behavior, and/or response to treatment. VUSs are particularly abundant in the sequence of tumor specimens due to the intrinsic genetic instability of most malignancies.

There are two general categories of VUSs. The first is a sequence change affecting the coding region of a well-established gene in a particular tumor type, but not following the pattern of somatic mutation typical for that gene; the second is previously undescribed variants occurring in DNA sequences that do not encode amino acids, including splice sites and regulatory regions (promoters, enhancers, UTRs, or even more broadly acting regulatory elements like microRNAs or long noncoding RNAs).

I. **Postanalytic/Reporting.** For ease of interpretation, most clinical laboratories classify variants identified in constitutional testing into five categories, as follows: (1) Pathogenic, (2) Likely pathogenic, (3) Uncertain significance, (4) Likely benign, and (5) Benign. This five-level classification scheme has recently been proposed as the standard for interpretation of variants in inherited disorders through a joint recommendation of the American College of Medical Genetics and Genomics (ACMG), the Association of Molecular Pathology (AMP), and the College of American Pathologists (CAP) (*Genet Med* 2015;17:405).

Similarly, consensus guidelines have been published for classification of somatic (acquired) variants with regard to the disease and in relation to the actionability of the given variant with respect to prognosis, diagnosis, or therapeutic decision making using four categories (*J Mol Diagn* 2017:19:4). Since predicted responsiveness to targeted therapy is often the primary reason for NGS testing, variants expected to be sensitive or resistant to a given therapy should be documented; driver and passenger variants should also be reported even in the absence of a direct role in choice of therapy. When a variant is identified that is known to be associated with a familial cancer predisposition syndrome (and when paired tumor-normal analysis is not performed), follow-up formal genetic counseling and germline analysis should be suggested in the report since it can be difficult to ascertain the etiology of a given variant as germline or somatic based on the VAF from NGS analysis of a tumor sample alone.

J. **Solid Tumor Versus Cell-Free Analytes.** In the setting of oncology, NGS methodologies have traditionally been used to sequence solid tumor specimens, and a wide range of NGS assays has been validated for use with fresh tissue, FFPE tissue, or both. When tissue samples are the analyte, the requirements for high tumor cellularity, high tumor viability, and so on (as discussed above) are important to obtain results that have utility for diagnosis or prediction of response to therapy.

Given the high sensitivity and throughput of NGS, it is not surprising that the technique has also been applied to the analysis of cell free DNA (cfDNA) present in plasma. In patients with cancer, a subset of cfDNA molecules is derived from the neoplasm, and this subset is known as circulating tumor DNA (ctDNA). NGS of cfDNA has several practical advantages in that it is a noninvasive test (cfDNA can easily be obtained from plasma from routine blood draws) and can be used in appropriately designed tests to detect all four classes of mutations (*Ther Clinical Risk Manag* 2017;13:1363). However, questions persist regarding the clinical validity and utility of the majority of cfDNA NGS tests performed in early stage cancer treatment monitoring or residual disease detection. In addition, numerous studies have demonstrated discordance between the results of NGS performed on cfDNA versus solid tumor specimens, although it is unclear whether the discordance is due to technical artifacts, assay design issues, or the intrinsic biologic heterogeneity of most malignancies (*Arch Path Lab Med* 2018;142:1242).

VIII. **INDIRECT DNA SEQUENCE ANALYSIS.** Indirect identification of normal and mutant alleles at a specific locus which correlate with the presence of disease can be of clinical utility and substitute for direct determination of specific nucleotide sequences. Virtually all of the indirect methods are based on PCR and can be applied to a broad range of clinical specimens. Examples of indirect methods include the following.

A. **Allelic Discrimination by Size.** Alleles that vary by small insertions or deletions can be distinguished based on the size of the PCR product after gel electrophoresis, perhaps the most straightforward method for indirect DNA sequence analysis (e-**Figs. 58.7** to **58.9**).

B. **Allelic Discrimination Based on Susceptibility to a Restriction Enzyme.** Using the technique known as RFLP analysis, mutations that either create or destroy a restriction endonuclease site can easily be distinguished by a two-step process that involves DNA digestion with the restriction endonuclease followed by gel electrophoresis to size fractionate the digested DNA. Virtually all RFLP analysis is performed on PCR product DNA (e-**Figs. 58.9** to **58.11**).

C. **Allele-Specific PCR.** Allele-specific PCR (also known as the amplification refractory mutation system, or ARMS) employs oligonucleotide primers designed to discriminate between normal and mutant target DNA sequences that may differ by a single base (*J Mol Diagn* 2007:9:272). Simultaneous analysis of multiple loci via a multiplex PCR format is possible if the amplicons from the different loci are of different sizes. PCR conditions must be optimized with sufficient stringency so that amplification only occurs when complete DNA sequence complementarity exists between primer and target molecules.

IX. **CLONALITY ASSAYS.** Demonstration that the cells in a lesion share a common genetic alteration can be used to support classification as a neoplasm rather than as a polyclonal reactive process, although it is important to emphasize that clonal neoplasms are not necessarily malignant.

A. **Assays Based on Immunoglobulin and T-cell Receptor Genes.** Most PCR clonality assays performed clinically are used to assess lymphoid infiltrates based on evaluation of immunoglobulin gene or T-cell receptor gene rearrangements. PCR primer design is an important component of these assays. Since generation of immunoglobulin and T-cell receptors involves deletions, template-independent nucleotide additions, and single base-pair changes, consensus primers are designed to bind to conserved sequence regions, and multiple sets of primers are used in order to insure that a broad range of rearrangements can be detected. Demonstration of a monoclonal or oligoclonal population of cells within an infiltrate is very often indicative of malignancy, but not always, since oligoclonal or monoclonal gene rearrangements may characterize reactive lymphoid proliferations.

B. **Clonality Assays Based on Specific Gene Mutations.** This class of assays focuses on detection of specific mutations in individual genes, including single base pair changes and larger scale structural changes (such as deletions, or insertions of viral genomes). This type of analysis can be useful when attempting to show that two neoplasms represent independent synchronous tumors rather than one tumor with metastases.

X. **MICROSATELLITE INSTABILITY ASSAYS.** Defects in the DNA mismatch repair system produce a characteristic pattern of mutations known as microsatellite instability (MSI). Direct analysis of the genes responsible for mismatch repair is not usually performed in routine clinical practice because it requires complete DNA sequencing of (at least) four causative genes, there are no specific mutation "hot spots," and the genes may be inactive as a result of epigenetic silencing rather than mutation. PCR-based analysis offers a more efficient, though indirect, method to identify defects in the DNA mismatch repair system via detection of the short increases or decreases in the length of the short tandem repeat (STR, or microsatellite) sequences that are the characteristic feature of MSI. Mutations in the genes which normally monitor the fidelity of DNA replication of these repeated sequences results in generation of variable lengths of the repeats in the tumor cells.

Laboratory testing regimens for MSI have only been formally addressed in the context of colorectal cancer (*Cancer Res* 1998:58;5248). For all other tumor types, MSI testing is not yet standardized in terms of the number and identity of microsatellite loci that must be analyzed, or in terms of the number of loci that need to show length alterations to be considered indicative of MSI.

DNA derived from either fresh tissue or FFPE tissue can be analyzed in the MSI assay. Comparison of the size of the PCR products from the target STR loci in the neoplasm versus normal tissue is used to detect changes in the length of the microsatellite sequences indicative of MSI. In most cases the profile of PCR-amplified sequences permits straightforward classification as indicative of MSI or not; however, there are no uniform criteria for interpretation of marginal test results, although standards have been proposed (*Mutat Res* 2001:461;249). Sources of variation in MSI analysis include the presence of contaminating nonneoplastic tissue (which can limit test reliability because demonstration of MSI in even the most sensitive testing regimens requires that neoplastic cells comprise at least 10% of the total population), the identity of the microsatellite markers used in the analysis (the susceptibility of a given microsatellite to instability is highly dependent both on the number of repeats and the length of the repeat units), and the potential for biased amplification of some alleles.

XI. INFECTIOUS DISEASE TESTING. PCR-based molecular genetic approaches frequently have higher sensitivity than standard special stains, and can often provide information not typically available from special stains such as species-specific identification and drug sensitivity. Molecular methods are also a useful way to detect organisms that cannot be cultured (e.g., human papilloma virus [HPV]) or that are notorious for their slow growth in culture (e.g., *Mycobacterium tuberculosis*).

A. Bacteria

1. **Mycobacteria.** In most assays, PCR targets the highly conserved gene that encodes the 65 kDa heat shock protein, but other target loci include the genes encoding 16S rRNA or the repetitive insertion element IS6110. PCR testing has been successfully applied to FFPE tissue from a wide variety of sites, including the respiratory tract, GI tract, GU tract, skin, bone, liver, and lymph nodes, and also to cytology specimens. Alternative isothermal amplification approaches originally developed for use in the clinical microbiology laboratory have also been adapted for use with processed tissue specimens (*Expert Rev Mol Diagn* 2004;4:251).

2. **Helicobacter pylori.** Although the genome of *H. pylori* is remarkable for the polymorphism between different clinical isolates, PCR-based methods have nonetheless been developed that permit successful detection of virtually all reported forms of *H. pylori* by PCR from either fresh or FFPE tissue, including the nonculturable coccoid form (*MethodsX* 2015;2:1) The most common target loci in PCR assays include the 16S rRNA gene, urease gene, or arbitrary regions chosen empirically based on their utility. Recently developed real time quantitative PCR methods that target the 23S rRNA gene permit simultaneous detection of *H. pylori* and antibiotic resistant testing.

3. **Other bacterial pathogens.** PCR has been used to detect *Bacillus anthracis* organisms in formalin fixed tissue specimens associated with bioterrorism or accidental environmental release from bioweapons facilities (*J Clin Microbiol* 2002;40:4360).

B. Fungi. Most PCR assays target sequences within the fungal rRNA genes. PCR can be performed using universal primers that bind to highly conserved sequences in the region, followed by direct or indirect DNA sequence analysis of the PCR product to identify the specific fungal pathogen. Alternatively, sequence differences in the 18S rRNA gene can be used to design primers that are specific for individual fungal pathogens. Sequence polymorphisms of the mitochondrial large subunit rRNA gene have also been used as a target in PCR tests to identify fungal pathogens in tissue specimens, and quantitative PCR methods (Q-PCR) have also been developed for detection of fungal pathogens in tissue specimens.

C. Viruses

1. **HPV.** Most PCR protocols for HPV testing make use of consensus primers targeted to the viral L1 gene that are potentially capable of detecting all HPV types that affect the anogenital region. Following amplification using consensus primers, the HPV type can be determined by either DNA sequence analysis or membrane hybridization with type-specific probes. However, both approaches are labor intensive and difficult to automate, which makes them poorly suited for screening a large volume of patient specimens. For this reason, HPV testing of cytology specimens is usually performed using liquid-based methodologies.

2. **Hepatitis C virus (HCV).** RT-PCR methods used to detect HCV in liver biopsy specimens focus on the 5' noncoding region of the virus that is highly conserved between the (at least) six genotypes and more than 90 subtypes of HCV that have been described worldwide. Maximal RT-PCR test sensitivity can only be achieved via a nested RT-PCR approach, or when the PCR products are evaluated by Southern blot hybridization.

3. **Epstein–Barr virus.** A quantitative PCR methodology has been described that targets five highly conserved segments of the EBV genome (*J Mol Diagn* 2004;6:378). The method can be applied to FFPE tissue, but maximum test sensitivity is only obtained when analysis involves all five marker loci.

4. **Respiratory viruses.** PCR assays for use with FFPE specimens have been developed for many individual respiratory viruses, for example influenza types A and B (*J Mol*

Diagn 2011;13:123) and adenovirus (*J Infect* 1993;27:43). A nested RT-PCR assay has been described for detection of the coronavirus responsible for severe acute respiratory syndrome (SARS) (*Am J Clin Pathol* 2004;121:574); the method can be applied to FFPE tissue from both open lung biopsies as well as necropsy specimens, a feature of the assay that is important given the virulence of the pathogen. The rapidity and simplicity of the approach make it ideally suited for diagnosis given the epidemiology of SARS outbreaks.

D. Protozoans

1. Toxoplasmosis. Several different PCR-based assays (for use with either fresh or FFPE tissue) have been developed for detection of *Toxoplasma gondii*, the etiologic agent of toxoplasmosis. The assays have clinical utility because serologic diagnosis of active infection is unreliable since IgM levels do not correlate with recent infection, and since reactivation of disease is not always accompanied by changes in antibody levels.

2. Leishmaniasis. A number of different loci serve as targets in PCR-based tests for leishmaniasis, including repetitive nuclear DNA sequences, genes encoding rRNA, and kinetoplast DNA. In fact, PCR utilizing primers that amplify a 120-bp fragment of kinetoplast DNA has a higher sensitivity than all other diagnostic methods that have been evaluated, including serologic testing, microbiologic culture, routine histopathologic evaluation, and immunohistochemical staining. Methods for use with FFPE tissue have recently been developed (*Mol Cell Probes* 2015;29:507).

3. Intestinal parasites. A number of molecular approaches for diagnosis of microsporidia have been described that can be used with FFPE for species-specific detection (*Emerg Infect Dis* 1996;2:183). Since different pathogenic microsporidia can have different sensitivities to antimicrobial agents, testing provides an opportunity to establish the diagnosis as well as direct therapy.

XII. IDENTITY DETERMINATION. Although the advantages of DNA-based identification analysis have been most widely publicized in forensics and parentage studies, this testing also has a role in the routine practice of surgical pathology including resolution of specimen identity issues (*Am J Clin Pathol* 2011;135:132), evaluation of tumors in transplant recipients, evaluation of bone marrow engraftment, diagnosis of hydatidiform moles (e-**Fig. 58.12**), and demonstration of natural chimerism.

PCR-based approaches for DNA typing have greatly expanded the range of testing because they require such small amounts of DNA and can be performed on fresh, fixed, or even partially degraded specimens. Virtually all DNA typing is currently performed based on a core set of STR loci chosen by the Federal Bureau of Investigation (FBI) of the United States for use in a national database of convicted felons known as the Combined DNA Index System (CODIS). Commercial kits for either monoplex or multiplex PCR amplification of CODIS loci have greatly simplified STR typing and made the method accessible to most molecular genetic laboratories.

ACKNOWLEDGMENT

The author thanks TuDong Nguyen and Barbara Zehnbauer, authors of the previous editions of this chapter.

SUGGESTED READINGS

Kulkarni S, Pfeifer J. *Clinical Genomics*. London: Academic Press; 2015.
Leonard DGB. *Molecular Pathology in Clinical Practice*. 2nd ed. New York: Springer; 2016.
Pfeifer JD. *Molecular Genetic Testing in Surgical Pathology*. Philadelphia, PA: Lippincott Williams & Wilkins; 2006.
Strachan T, Read AP. *Human Molecular Genetics*. 4th ed. London: Garland Science; 2010.

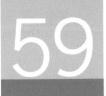

59 Gene Expression Profiling

Mark A. Watson

I. INTRODUCTION. In principle, gene expression profiling involves the simultaneous (multiplexed), quantitative measurement of numerous gene transcripts (RNA) from a cellular biospecimen. The premise of this analytical approach is that the composite and often synergistic measurement of multiple gene products can provide additional molecular information about a biosample that cannot be completely inferred from the measurement of any single gene product. Gene expression profiling has been used for almost two decades in research laboratories, and several applications are used in clinical testing. Historically, gene expression profiling has been performed using nucleic acid microarray technology, but over the past few years, this technology has been significantly supplanted by several other technologies (Fig. 59.1). This chapter reviews the biosample requirements, technology platforms, and data analysis approaches associated with gene expression profiling assays.

II. ASSAY DESIGN

A. Approach. Gene expression profiling studies are often expensive, high complexity assays that generate large amounts of data. Therefore, assay design should be considered carefully to generate meaningful results. Most gene expression studies are designed as biomarker discovery experiments, with the aim of defining a panel of multiple biomarkers that can then be transitioned into a more directed, conventional clinical assay. Experimental paradigms fall into several categories.

1. Class discovery. In such studies, experimental specimens are classified based solely upon their gene expression patterns, and the results of the classification are reviewed to identify new, previously unappreciated clinical or pathologic classifications. Perhaps the most elegant and clinically translatable illustration of this approach has been the reclassification of breast adenocarcinoma based upon microarray-generated gene expression profiles (*Cancer Treat Rev* 2018;62:74).

2. Class distinction. This type of study is designed to identify novel predictive, patterns of gene expression that demonstrate a correlation to an already known parameter such as clinical outcome or treatment response (*Ann Oncol* 2017;28:733).

3. Single sample classification. Ultimately, to achieve clinical utility, it is necessary to create a robust molecular signature that can be prospectively applied to individual patient specimens to accurately predict a clinical phenotype. Typically, a specific subset of gene expression values is examined and a weighted discriminate index is calculated. The resulting index provides a probability measure that a given specimen falls into a specific, predefined diagnostic category. Studies that independently validate a previously identified signature are still relatively rare but are obviously a critical step in transitioning any assay into routine clinical use (*BMC Med* 2016;4:67).

B. Target Molecules. Most gene expression profiling studies involve the analysis of protein-coding mRNAs. However, an increasing appreciation for the significant biologic role of micro RNAs (miRNAs), long noncoding RNAs (lncRNAs), and other RNA species in human pathology have made these attractive analytes for biomarker assessment (*BMC Med Genomics* 2018;11:48; *PLoS One* 2017;12:e0186795). Because of their smaller, uniform size, miRNAs may require specialized isolation or preparation protocols, particularly if analysis is performed from cell-free or acellular (exosome) biospecimens. For assay platforms that involve capture or sequence-specific amplification, specific miRNA probe design may be challenging given their short, relatively homologous sequence composition. Finally, continuous refinements to human genome annotation, particularly for

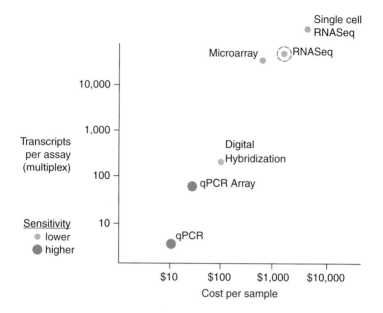

Figure 59.1 Technology platforms for gene expression profiling. Assay platforms described in this chapter are shown, relative to their cost, throughput, sensitivity, and level of RNA transcript multiplexing.

less well-characterized miRNA and lncRNA species, creates additional challenges for data interpretation and validation using orthogonal technology platforms.

C. **Statistical Considerations.** In principle, gene expression profiling is no different than evaluating whether a single biomarker demonstrates a statistically significant difference between defined sample classes using traditional statistics. By definition, a traditional significance threshold of p = 0.05 allows for a 5% false-positive (false discovery) rate. Therefore, when analyzing 35,000 independent gene transcript measurements, as many as 1,750 values will appear to be "significant" by chance alone. To contend with this problem of "multiple testing," several methods have been applied to calculate a true significance threshold when analyzing thousands of variables in relatively few numbers of samples. Although these approaches minimize false-positive results for a given sample set, they can in no way substitute for more robust data validation using multiple, independent sets of samples across different technology platforms and laboratories.

D. **Specimen Requirements.** Because of the inherent complexity of gene expression profiling, specimen quality assurance is essential.

1. **Specimen collection.** Careful consideration must be given to controlled and documented biospecimen collection. Global changes in gene expression can occur in tissue biospecimens as a result of tissue warm ischemia time (*PLoS One* 2013;8:e79826), creating artificial differences in gene expression patterns seen between specimens based on collection procedures rather than important clinical differences. For peripheral blood, bone marrow, and other cellular biospecimens, the method in which a specimen is collected and processed can also influence gene expression signatures (*Proc Natl Acad Sci USA* 2014;111:16802). Finally, most tissue specimens are inherently heterogeneous collections of many cell types. Variable cellular composition between tissue specimens may lead to differences in transcriptional profiles. For example, two tumor samples,

one of which contains 5% neoplastic cellularity and a second which contains 70% neoplastic cellularity, may demonstrate two different gene expression signatures based simply on the content of neoplastic cells present in the tissue. Techniques such as laser microdissection, spatial expression profiling (*Science* 2015;348:6090), or single cell RNA sequencing (*Science* 2017;358:58) can circumvent some complexities in gene expression profiles associated with cellular heterogeneity.

2. **Specimen processing.** Generally, diagnostic surgical pathology tissue specimens are subjected to formalin fixation and paraffin embedding (FFPE), a process that results in chemical cross-linking. Until recently, RNA extracted from FFPE was deemed unsuitable for gene expression profiling analyses. However, newer methods and technologies have rendered RNA isolated from these samples amenable to PCR-, hybridization-, and sequence-based assays. Main determinants of RNA sample quality derived from FFPE tissue include (*JCO Precis Oncol,* 2018):

   a. **Oxidation.** Fixed tissue exposed to ambient atmosphere further degrades (oxidizes) RNA species. Tissue sections stored on glass slides or tissue cut from the exposed surface of a tissue block often yield material unsuitable for even the most robust assay platforms.

   b. **Fixation.** Although most larger pathology departments utilize 10% neutral buffered formalin (NBF) fixation techniques, tissues processed in alternate fixatives or specialized tissue processing, such as decalcification, may render extracted RNA unsuitable for analysis. Prolonged fixation, even in NBF, may result in severely degraded RNA. Since some institutions may not mandate, or may not accurately document specific fixation times, RNA quality may be highly variable between FFPE tissues.

   c. **Cellularity.** Obviously, RNA yield, quality, and patterns of RNA expression may differ considerably based upon the total percentage of transcriptionally active cells in the sample.

   d. **Age.** Although there is some correlation between tissue block age and resulting RNA quality, surprisingly, many studies have anecdotally shown that even 10- to 15-year old, archived FFPE blocks can yield suitable quality material for expression studies.

   Despite these advances, freshly procured, snap frozen or otherwise molecularly preserved biospecimens remain the gold standard for gene expression profile analyses and are absolutely required for some assays, such as single cell RNA sequencing. Since many clinical centers may not have access to resources needed for the processing and storage of frozen samples, a number of commercial solutions have been developed to preserve tissue and cell specimens for gene expression assays, without the need for immediate snap freezing and cryostorage (*PLoS One* 2016;11:e0151383).

E. **Sample Preparation.** Protocols for sample preparation will depend upon the intended analyte (mRNA, miRNA), the source specimen (fixed tissue, fresh tissue, biofluid), and the downstream assay (PCR, microarray, RNA sequencing) used for expression profiling. Many protocols are platform specific, but general considerations include:

1. **RNA isolation.** Most downstream assays require high purity RNA that is free of contaminating genomic DNA. Methods for RNA isolation include organic extraction, column- or bead-based purification, or direct cell lysis. Column- or bead-based purification often yields the highest quality RNA and can be automated, but may exclude some species such as miRNA, unless special measures are used. For limited cell numbers or single cell profiling, direct cell lysis is the method of choice. Isolation of cell free miRNA or exosomal miRNA from biofluids usually requires column- and/or bead-based protocols to handle large sample volumes.

2. **Preamplification.** In cases where quantities of RNA are limiting, such as the case in performing gene expression profiling from tissue needle core biopsies or subsets of limited cell numbers, protocols may involve various forms of molecular preamplification (*BMC Mol Biol* 2015;16:5). Methods may implement limited cycles of polymerase chain reaction (PCR), isothermal amplification, or linear transcript

amplification. Since expression profiling data are meant to be quantitative, it is important that any preamplification protocol used maintain relative copy number of all target transcripts and avoid biased amplification based on transcript size, initial abundance, or sequence content.

3. Enrichment. When gene expression profiling studies are focused on gene-encoding messenger RNAs (mRNAs), various approaches for enrichment can eliminate interference and contamination of other RNA species (ribosomal RNA, transfer RNA, unprocessed mRNA, miRNA, lncRNA) which typically constitute over 95% of total cellular RNA. When high quality RNA is isolated from fresh or snap-frozen tissue, mature mRNA may be isolated by bead- or column-based poly-A capture. While this method enriches for polyadenylated mRNA species, the method requires a relatively large quantity of input RNA (3 to 10 μg) to isolate nanogram quantities of RNA required for downstream analyses. Conversely, ribosomal RNA (rRNA, which constitutes nearly 80% of cellular RNA) can be removed from RNA preparations by a similar bead-based affinity capture method. This approach is particularly useful to remove rRNA from fragmented RNA samples derived from FFPE or other degraded samples. In addition, when RNA is used for sequence library preparation and RNA sequencing (see below), libraries may be selectively enriched for exon coding regions using affinity capture, similar to other methods used for exome and targeted next generation sequencing of DNA. This method maximizes the amount of quantitative sequence data generated from targeted, mRNA coding sequences and eliminates undesired data from other cellular RNA species (*J Mol Diagn* 2014;16:440).

III. TECHNOLOGIES

A. PCR. RNA may be converted into complementary DNA (cDNA), which can then be used as a template for "real-time" or quantitative PCR (qPCR) assays. In its linear phase, the accumulation of fluorescent PCR product can be computationally related to the original amount of input RNA, creating a method for quantifying absolute or relative RNA abundance. Although it is a sensitive method with a large dynamic range for measuring individual gene expression, PCR is generally not used for expression profiling studies because of its limited ability to measure multiple RNA species in a single reaction (multiplexing). However, microfluid microarray platforms can allow the conduct of over 9,200 (i.e., 96 × 96 array) individual, nanoliter-scale qPCR reactions on a single chip assay device (*Lab Invest* 2015;95:113). Such platforms provide extensive multiplexing capabilities for gene expression profiling using conventional qPCR methodology.

B. Microarrays. Nucleic acid microarrays are an ordered arrangement of DNA molecules (probes) on a solid surface. For gene expression profiling, RNA derived from cells or tissue is hybridized to the array to quantify the level of nucleic acid corresponding to each probe. By hybridizing cellular RNA to microarrays with probes directed to mRNA, microRNA (miRNA), or other RNA targets, it is possible to perform qualitative (i.e., detection of alternative splicing) and quantitative gene expression analysis simultaneously on 30,000 to 50,000 genes from a single RNA sample. Nucleic acids microarrays may be fabricated using several different technologies and probe types:

1. cDNA microarrays. Some of the earliest microarray designs utilized cDNA probes. Messenger RNA (mRNA) from a defined tissue or cell source is converted into a double stranded cDNA clone library. Plasmid DNA from each clone is then spotted onto the microarray surface. Genome sequence information is not necessarily required for microarray design, a particular advantage for studying the few remaining experimental organisms where genome sequence information is not available. However, because cDNA probes correspond to relatively long stretches of transcribed mRNA, cross-hybridization and lack of specificity can often limit the accuracy of cDNA microarray results. The effort and infrastructure necessary to store, grow, purify, monitor quality control, and track individual cDNA clones is considerable and not easily standardized. This last constraint limits the use of cDNA microarrays as clinical diagnostic tools.

2. Oligonucleotide microarrays. The availability of the completely sequenced and annotated human genome, coupled with improved synthesis chemistries, has rapidly shifted the fabrication of nucleic acid microarrays toward the use of synthetic oligonucleotide probes, usually 60 to 75 nucleotides in length. Probe sequences may be customized for specific genes, gene transcripts, or gene transcript segments using defined nucleic acid sequences. Sophisticated bioinformatics programs can select optimized oligonucleotide sequences for any gene or transcript of interest to minimize cross reactivity with other sequences, while at the same time standardizing hybridization properties such as melting temperature and G/C sequence content. This customization provides a level of standardization and flexibility to the design of sequence content on nucleic acid microarrays that is aptly suited for clinical diagnostic assays.

3. In situ synthesized microarrays. Another strategy for microarray design involves simultaneously synthesizing specific oligonucleotide probes in situ using combinatorial photochemistry. Affymetrix GeneChip microarrays use a series of micron-scale "masks" to direct light to specific locations on the microarray surface. Photoreactive nucleotides (A,C,G,T) are sequentially passed over the array surface in the presence of each mask. Depending upon the mask pattern, a specific nucleotide is added to the growing chain of oligonucleotides at a specific position. In this combinatorial method, the use of 25 different masks sets (A, C, G, T) in 100 sequential nucleotide addition steps can result in 4^{25} (1×10^{15}) different sequences that are simultaneously created on the array surface.

4. Bead arrays. An alternate approach to traditional microarray design involves the use of a beaded microarray. In this approach, micron-sized beads, each containing a unique oligonucleotide gene sequence in tandem with a unique nucleotide address sequence, are allowed to randomly assemble onto a solid surface. By repeated interrogation of each bead address sequence, the identity of each bead at each position is deduced. The "decoded" array can then be used for its intended hybridization assay.

C. Digital Hybridization. A method commercialized by Nanostring technologies, this approach involves hybridization of probes to target RNA in solution. Each probe for a specific RNA target contains a unique sequential combination of fluorophores, or "barcodes." After hybridization in solution, RNA-probe complexes are captured, passed through a nanoscale fluidics system, and individually counted by instrument optics. The fluorescent barcode identifies the RNA species and the count relates to the absolute number of target RNA molecules in the sample. A large number of possible barcodes that can be assigned to each specific probe means that hundreds of assays (gene transcripts) can be multiplexed in a single reaction. Like microarray technology, detection is hybridization based rather than amplification based. However, unlike conventional microarrays, the assay result is digital (counts of transcripts) rather than analog (hybridization signal intensity), which can provide greater sensitivity and precision for multiplexed gene expression measurements (*Cancer Res* 2015;75:2587). Although the technology platform is complex and more expensive than other methods, it has become a popular approach for both research and limited diagnostic use (*Breast Cancer Res* 2018;20:79).

D. RNA Sequencing. New nucleic acid chemistries and decreasing prices of next generation sequencing technologies have made RNA sequencing a powerful and cost-effective alternative to microarrays for comprehensive gene expression profiling (*Cancer Inform* 2015;14(Suppl 1):57). RNA is converted to cDNA and the cDNA template is used for library generation and sequencing, similar to DNA-based approaches. Digital counts of sequencing reads that map to specific transcriptional units in the genome provide an absolute measure of RNA abundance (gene expression) in the biologic sample. Because the library selection and sequencing process are completely unbiased, the entire representation of cellular RNAs (mRNA, miRNA, lncRNA, and others) is sequenced, mapped, and counted. On the other hand, by selecting or excluding specific populations of cellular RNA (see above), the approach can be applied to enrich for specific RNA sequences, such as mRNA, miRNA, or even mRNA from targeted protein-encoding gene sets (*J Mol Diagn* 2014;16:440). Like other technology platforms, RNA sequencing can be performed on total cellular RNA (after depletion of the prominent rRNA fraction), poly-A selected mRNA, or highly degraded RNA purified from formalin fixed, paraffin embedded tissue sections (*JCO Precis Oncol,* 2018).

E. Single Cell Sequencing. Because of the extensive transcriptional heterogeneity in complex tissues and cell populations, single-cell RNA sequencing has rapidly become an important tool for understanding biologic complexity in human development and disease. In this method, cells are captured based on cell surface markers and individual viable cells are either sorted into individual chambers or packaged into lipid vesicles. RNA isolation, cDNA synthesis, and library construction for individual cells are performed *in situ*. Each cell library is coded with a unique molecular barcode. Libraries from each cell are pooled and sequenced. As in "bulk" RNA sequencing methods, sequencing, mapping, and counting of sequencing reads provides a digital readout of transcript abundance, while the barcode sequence of each individual read assigns the transcript to a specific cell of origin. Depending upon the total number of molecules sequenced in a given experiment, it is possible to sequence (count) hundreds of thousands of individual transcripts from a population of tens of thousands of individual cells (*Cell* 2015;163:799). Obviously, analysis of such enormous data sets is complex. The cost of such experiments is still very expensive given the amount of data generated, but the decreasing cost of next generation sequencing itself is rapidly making even this type of analysis more affordable.

F. In Silico Analysis. For investigators solely interested in the computational aspects of gene expression profiling, and for others who may not have the financial or sample resources to conduct their own studies, a very large number of publicly accessible gene expression data sets (conducted on a wide variety of technology platforms) are available. The Gene Expression Omnibus (GEO – https://www.ncbi.nlm.nih.gov/geo/) is an NIH-sponsored repository of gene expression data. Similar repositories such as The Cancer Genome Atlas (TCGA – https://cancergenome.nih.gov) can provide disease-specific data sets. The EMBL Expression Atlas (https://www.ebi.ac.uk/gxa/home) is a similar resource developed by the European genomics community. Although all of these data sets can be obtained at no cost, it is important to remember that the quality and the clinical and biologic annotation of the data may be highly variable and suboptimal, depending upon the intended analysis. Moreover, as each data set may be generated using a different technology platform (e.g., array type) and under different experimental protocols, a meta-analysis of multiple data sets can be challenging.

IV. DATA ANALYSIS. Data analysis is by far the most complicated and critical aspect of gene expression profiling. Proper analysis and valid conclusions drawn from any gene expression profiling assay require supervision by an experienced genome informaticist and biostatistician. Principal steps in data analysis involve the following (e-**Fig. 59.1**):

A. Primary Data Analysis. Depending upon the technology platform, raw data are converted into transcript-level information using different approaches. Software and algorithms to transform data are either commercially developed and proprietary, or widely available and fairly standardized. For example, analog signal intensity data from microarray hybridization experiments is converted into averaged intensity values and this, in turn, is converted into gene- or transcript-level expression values using algorithms such as Robust Multi-Array Averaging (RMA) which are integrated into commercial software products or available in open-source software packages such as Bioconductor (http://bioconductor.org). Expression data generated from RNA sequence reads are created by mapping and annotating reads to a standard genome build, again either using commercial software packages or open-source software suites such as STAR (*Curr Protoc Bioinformatics* 2015;51:1). When multiple samples are compared in an analysis, or when differential gene expression analysis between samples is required, data processing also involves normalizing signals to account for sample-to-sample variability, and statistical modeling to identify transcripts whose abundance (expression level) is significantly different between samples or sample groups (*PLoS One* 2017;12:e0190152). Although many investigators are only interested in gene-level transcript expression data, it is important to remember that platforms like RNA sequencing and even some specialized microarray assays are capable of assessing qualitative differences in RNA splicing patterns and expression of noncoding RNAs. Moreover, as multiple genes may encode multiple, overlapping, alternatively spliced RNA transcriptional units, deconvolution of complex patterns of transcript splicing can be challenging and often requires specialized software or analytical approaches. The remainder of this section describes the more straightforward, quantitative, gene-level analysis of gene expression profile data.

B. **Data Reduction and Visualization.** Given the size of most gene expression profile data sets (e.g., 35,000 gene expression values × 50 samples = 1.75 million data points), methods for data reduction and visualization to recognize biologically relevant gene expression patterns are required (e-**Fig. 59.2**). There are a number of relatively standard methods in which voluminous and multidimensional gene expression data can be visualized.

1. **Hierarchical clustering.** Samples are organized based upon their similarity in gene expression values, and genes are organized based upon their similarity across samples. Several different measures of similarity can be used, and several different algorithms can be applied to perform the clustering. While hierarchical clustering is a useful tool to provide a manageable view of immense data sets, it does not necessarily impart any underlying "truth" to the data.

2. **Heat maps.** A colorimetric representation of numerical data, usually presented in combination with hierarchical clustering. This visualization scheme provides a convenient method to identify patterns or blocks of similarity between genes and/or samples.

3. **k-Means clustering and principal components analysis (PCA).** These data reduction methods are particularly useful for reducing the level of gene expression data complexity. A large number of variables (i.e., gene expression values) are placed into a finite number of bins based upon their similarity of values across a much smaller number of observations (i.e., samples). The number of bins created (the "k" in k-means) can be adjusted to create a much smaller set of similar, collective values (sometimes referred to as meta-genes) that can then be used as the basis for further analysis. In PCA, samples are plotted in "gene expression space" where the distance between samples in this space is related to their similarity based upon gene expression values. However, for 35,000 independent gene expression values, gene expression space is represented in 35,000 different dimensions. Therefore, the goal of PCA is to reduce 35,000 dimensions into two to three principle components. Then, relatedness between samples can be plotted and visualized.

C. **Annotation and Biologic Classification.** A final significant challenge in data analysis is to determine how patterns of gene expression can be related to biologically meaningful results. As annotation and understanding of the human genome continue to improve, investigators have been able to classify a large number of human genes into ontologies based on function, cellular location, and structural determinants. Several commercial and open-source software programs are available that can map lists of genes to these ontologies and determine whether they constitute a statistically significant over-representation of the ontology, which often results in a clearer view of altered biologic processes associated with differential gene expression. Gene Set Enrichment Analysis (GSEA – http://software.broadinstitute.org/gsea/index.jsp) is one example of an open-source package. For single-cell and simple multicellular organisms, this approach has led to sophisticated models of cell signaling and transcriptional regulatory networks, whereas for complex multicellular human tissues this type of analysis is still evolving.

D. **Validation.** Like any other method, the results of a gene expression profiling analysis should be validated through independent sample testing. Validation of expression profiling data is particularly problematic for many reasons. First, most assays involving comprehensive gene expression analysis (i.e. RNA sequencing, microarrays) are relatively expensive (in the range of $200 to $800 per sample), which creates financial constraints on the number of samples that can be analyzed. Second, the number of independent, adequate samples with a given clinical or biologic phenotype (i.e., rare tumor tissues or other disease pathologies) may be limiting. Finally, as discussed above, the large number of variables associated with a gene expression data set requires that a relatively large number of observations (e.g., samples) must be analyzed to create a degree of statistical confidence. Investigators have devised a number of approaches to perform data validation under these limitations.

1. **Cross validation.** One of the most popular approaches for data validation is sequential sampling or "leave-one-out" cross validation analysis in a single sample set. In an analysis of N study samples, $N-1$ samples are used for the initial statistical analysis to identify groups of "signature genes." The ability of these genes to correctly classify the Nth sample is then calculated and the gene list modified, discarding biomarkers that perform poorly and solidifying those with the best performance. This process is repeated, removing all N samples, one at a time, until a list of genes with the best class prediction score is created. The advantage of this method is that no additional data or experimentation is needed for validation. However, because the cross-validation is still applied to a single set of samples (i.e., the "test" and "validation" sets are one in the same), the ability to generalize conclusions to independent or larger sample sets may still be limited (*Clin Cancer Res* 2008;14:5977).

2. **Sample set splitting.** If an initial sample set is large enough, it is also possible to divide the experiment into independent sets of test data and validation data. In this scheme, patterns of "significant" gene expression are identified using the first set of samples, and patterns are validated in a second set of samples. Although this approach utilizes two truly independent data sets, it necessarily limits the number of independent samples available for the discovery phase and validation phase. The desire to split a limited number of samples into test and validation sets raises the question of sample size requirement for performing expression profiling studies with sufficient statistical power (*Cancer Inform* 2014;13(Suppl 6):1). While multiple methods have been proposed to calculate required sample sizes, the number of samples required will ultimately depend upon the expected biologic result. For example, relatively few study samples may be necessary to identify fundamental genomic differences between squamous cell carcinomas and adenocarcinomas of pulmonary origin, as these tumor cell types are biologically very distinct. On the other hand, a considerably larger study set may be required to identify reliable differences in molecular signatures associated with clinical outcome among stage I lung adenocarcinoma patients if the intrinsic biologic basis for patient outcome is more subtle (*J Natl Cancer Inst* 2010;102:464).

3. **Meta-analyses.** Gene expression profiling results can be validated using multiple independent study data sets. As an ever-increasing number of gene expression studies are published and corresponding data sets are made publicly available in data repositories (see above), it has become increasingly possible to validate patterns of gene expression identified in one experiment using other microarray experiments in the published literature, although caveats regarding appropriate selection and normalization of multiple data sets must be considered (*Nucleic Acids Res* 2012;40:3785).

4. **Orthogonal validation.** If a putative gene signature panel is sufficiently small (5 to 100 genes), a number of lower-multiplexed gene expression analysis platforms may be used to validate findings in an independent sample set. Multiplexed-qPCR, targeted (cDNA capture) RNA sequencing, and digital hybridization can all be performed for $10 to $50 per sample, which makes large sample validation studies possible, if such independent sample sets are available.

V. CLINICAL APPLICATIONS. Gene expression profiling is a powerful approach for understanding basic biologic processes at the genomic and molecular level, but is also used extensively in translational research to discover and validate patterns of gene expression that have relevance to human disease. Although many translational studies have focused on oncology and tumor pathology, gene expression profiling is used in other fields of pathology and clinical medicine such as neuropathology (Alzheimer Disease, Parkinson Disease, epilepsy, schizophrenia), immunopathology (systemic lupus, multiple sclerosis), organ transplantation, reproductive endocrinology, trauma and sepsis, and cardiovascular disease. An obvious requisite to performing gene expression profiling studies is the availability of the appropriate target cell population for study which may be elusive, multifactorial, or difficult to obtain for some diseases. In addition, known and unknown variability within a disease processes and between individual patients with the same disease creates challenges for establishing definitive associations between patterns of gene expression and a disease phenotype.

A. **Gene Expression Profiling as an Ancillary Diagnostic Tool for the Pathologist.** Perhaps one of the earliest, practical applications of gene expression profiling has been its use to more accurately diagnosis histologically ambiguous tumor specimens. Gene expression profiles have been used to molecularly define the cell lineage of metastases of unknown origin (particularly adenocarcinoma) with 80% to 90% accuracy based upon thorough retrospective analysis of clinical data (*J Clin Oncol* 2013;31:217). Gene expression data have also been used to discriminate histologic "look-alikes" with distinct cell origins, such as small round blue cell tumors (*J Mol Diagn* 2007;9:80). Most of these studies have not reached clinical translation, as these often expensive and complex assays have been supplanted by the use of equally effective 1 or 2 immunohistochemical biomarkers.

More importantly, gene expression profiling can subclassify histologically indistinguishable tumors into biologically relevant subtypes. For example, gene expression profiling can segregate diffuse large B-cell lymphoma into aggressive and indolent molecular profiles that also have significance for patient survival (*Clin Cancer Res* 2015;21:2367). Gene expression profiles of invasive ductal breast carcinoma can also clearly define "basal-cell" and "luminal cell" tumor types (among others) that have unique biologic characteristics and therapeutic response profiles (*Cancer Treat Rev* 2018;62:74). There is also on-going interest in using gene expression profiling to completely reclassify tumors and some types of autoimmune disease based not on anatomic site or histopathologic features, but by patterns or modules of gene expression (*CA Cancer J Clin* 2016;66:75). Given that the phenotypic behavior of cells and their response to therapy may be more dependent upon molecular profiles than organ site, this approach has the potential to significantly alter the role of diagnostic pathology and the practice of personalized medicine.

B. **Predicting Disease Behavior.** Gene expression profiles of primary tumor samples have been used to develop predictive signatures of local and distance metastasis, both for specific tumor types and more globally. Further clinical validation of such signatures could, for example, define a new diagnostic category of "metastasis potential positive" tumors which might play an important role for staging cancer patients and therapeutic decision making. Similar approaches have been used to predict clinical quiescence or rapid progression in autoimmune and neurologic degenerative diseases.

C. **Predicting Patient Survival.** Several large clinical studies have identified gene expression signatures that predict patient survival in breast cancer, lung cancer, leukemia, lymphoma, and many other tumor types. While results from these studies are usually validated using statistical methodology or through independent training and test patient populations, an increasingly worrisome finding is that clinically predictive gene expression signatures are not reproducible across multiple studies of the same tumor type. Proposed explanations for these discordant findings include the use of differing and nonstandardized assay platforms, the examination of patient cohorts that are not exactly matched for clinical and treatment parameters, and the relatively complex phenotype of survival which is dependent upon many variables in addition to molecular signatures.

D. **Predicting Therapeutic Response.** Particularly in the context of neoadjuvant cancer chemotherapy trials, gene expression profiling of pretreatment tumor biopsy specimens has been used to develop predictive signatures of treatment response. Although there have been few, large prospective studies published to date, the ability to use gene expression data to prospectively manage patient treatment, avoid adverse toxicities, and optimize therapeutic efficacy is an important but elusive goal in translating these assays to the clinical laboratory.

VI. **GENE EXPRESSION PROFILING IN THE CLINICAL LABORATORY.** Despite a 20-year history of gene expression profile studies that have been published in the peer-reviewed scientific literature, only a handful of "signatures" have achieved a level of validation and adoption so as to be used as a standard-of-care clinical diagnostic. Several factors and considerations may further promote (or limit) full clinical adoption in the future.

A. **Reproducibility.** A well-known limitation of gene expression profiling studies is an inability to validate results across platforms, samples, and laboratories. The FDA has established the Microarray Quality Control (MAQC) Consortium and, more recently, the Sequencing Quality Control (SEQC) Consortium, to systematically evaluate sources of variability that can potentially contribute to irreproducibility of gene expression profiling results (*AAPS J* 2016;18:814). Potential sources of variability include:

1. **Technology platforms.** Different assay platforms (microarrays, qPCR, RNA sequencing) may interrogate an RNA target using different probe sequences or annotation algorithms. Therefore, the specific transcript or transcript variant that is measured could differ between studies using different assay formats.

2. **Sample populations.** Expression profile results that are not equally diagnostic across studies may be related to the fact that study populations are either knowingly or unknowingly disparate. The diagnostic power of a gene expression profile may be closely associated with a specific pathology or clinical phenotype that either is not or cannot be replicated across different studies.

3. **Preanalytical variability.** Unlike DNA sequence and sequence variants, quantitative levels of RNA are dynamic and may be altered by preanalytical variables such as sampling bias, warm ischemia time, and clinical processing method. Unless these variables are identified and controlled, gene expression profiles may not be reproducible across studies and sample sets.

4. **Analytical algorithms.** Although some steps in assay data preprocessing are standardized (**e-Fig. 59.1**), other algorithms and software used to develop and validate a specific gene expression signature that correlates with a phenotype can be highly variable between studies and study groups. Given the same exact data set, strikingly different predictive gene expression signatures may be defined that appear equally accurate.

5. **Statistical errors.** Given the complexity of gene expression profile data, lack of appropriate statistical and genome informatics expertise can lead to erroneous conclusions (i.e., gene expression signatures) that are not reproducible across laboratories, even using the same data set.

6. **Controlled phenotypes.** The reproducibility of a gene expression profile is closely related to the extent of its biologic underpinnings. For example, a signature that can classify one tissue histology from another is far more likely to be reproducible across laboratories than a signature that can predict survival or disease progression, as these phenotypes are multifactorial and potentially unrelated to the intrinsic molecular profile of the cells or tissue under study.

B. **Automation and Standardization.** Most early gene expression profiling studies were performed using robotically spotted DNA microarrays. Advances in nanotechnology, microfluidics, and nucleic acid chemistry have generated a new generation of assay platforms that are highly automated, standardized, faster, and miniaturized. Despite the remaining complexity and interpretative challenges of the assays themselves, this has removed many of the previous technical (i.e., instrumentation) barriers from implementing gene expression profiling assays in clinical laboratories.

C. **Clinical Relevance.** Although gene expression profiling is a significant research tool, there are only a few clinical examples where the measurement of multiple gene expression (RNA) biomarkers provides added diagnostic information as compared with the use of more traditional methods in diagnostic pathology such as immunohistochemical stains or multimarker flow cytometry. In oncology, notable examples include the Onco-Type DX and Prosigna assays used for breast cancer patient management, which are only available at commercial or a subset of academic laboratories. However, as knowledge leads to the potential reclassification of cancer and other human pathologies based upon specific molecular and genomic attributes, in addition to histologic or cellular features, gene expression profiling may find increasing utility in the clinical laboratory as a standard of care diagnostic.

Biospecimen Banking

Brian Goetz, Heidi Miers, and Mark A. Watson

I. SIGNIFICANCE TO PATHOLOGY AND TRANSLATIONAL RESEARCH. The advent of personalized medicine and new technologies for the genomic and molecular analysis of human disease have fundamentally changed the operations and requirements of modern biorepositories over the past decade. Significant developments and their impact on biobanking include:

A. Personalized Medicine. Biomarkers and the biospecimens needed for their assessment are playing an increasing role in the therapeutic management of patients with cancer and other diseases. The progression of science from translational research study, to accredited biomarker validation, to routine clinical utilization is becoming more rapid and integrated. This may create a competition for limited tissue resources (i.e., a tissue needle core biopsy) between clinical diagnostics and research use. Modern biorepositories must often function in both the translational research and clinical diagnostic roles, necessitating a level of regulatory compliance and oversight not normally required of a traditional research laboratory.

B. "Next Generation" Analytes. Discovery of novel disease biomarkers based on extracellular vesicles (*Int J Mol Sci* 2016;17:13), cell-free nucleic acid (*Ann Lab Med* 2018;38:1), rare circulating cells (*Adv Clin Chem* 2016;75:1), and protein phosphorylation states has required new methods for the collection, processing, and storage of biospecimens. These may include the use of novel blood collection tubes (*PLoS One* 2016;11:e0166354), "molecular-friendly" tissue fixatives (*PLoS One* 2016;11: e0151383), and specialized isolation and preservation protocols.

C. Immunobiology. An increased understanding of the role and complexity of the immune system in human diseases (e.g., autoimmunity, cancer, infectious disease) has generated research questions that require the collection (often multiple collections over disease progression), specific subfractionation, and preservation of diverse and often rare cell populations. This, in turn, has required biorepositories to develop advanced protocols for cell processing and separation, and/or to more closely align their operations with clinical immunology laboratories.

D. The Human Microbiome. Similarly, an increased appreciation for the role of the microbiome in human disease has generated interest in collections of swabs, sputum, aspirates, feces, and other "nontraditional" biospecimens from body sites populated with microorganisms. The development of new methods to isolate nucleic acid and other biomolecules from microbial populations found within human biospecimens is also often required.

E. New Era of Biomedicine. Several important principles embody the necessity and rationale for biospecimen bank operations in this new era of biomedicine.

1. Required access to large biospecimen cohorts. A large number of biospecimens may be required to generate statistically meaningful results in a clinical correlative biomarker study. For rare disease presentation, collection of a sufficient cohort may require months or years of accrual. Depending upon the research question, multiple collections from a single participant over time may also be necessary. If additional time is required to reach a desired clinical correlative endpoint (i.e., disease progression or survival), the time interval between first biospecimen collection and assay performance may be years. Biorepositories (as opposed to individual research laboratory freezers) provide a stable, sustainable approach for long-term biospecimen collection and storage.

2. **Biospecimen quality assurance.** Preanalytical variability with regard to biospecimen handling and processing can seriously compromise or confound translational research studies (*Clin Biochem* 2014;47:258). Accurate, robust, and unambiguous schemas for sample labeling and maintenance of "chain-of-identity" to link biospecimens to required correlative data sets are critical. Particularly for tissue biospecimens, diagnostic mislabeling can seriously impede supervised learning approaches to identify new biomarkers. In addition to issues of diagnostic accuracy, knowledge of the precise cellular make-up of biospecimens (particularly for heterogeneous tissues) is often important to properly interpret molecular and genomic data. An added level of complexity in longitudinal studies is that multiple biospecimens collected from the same patient must be accurately coded and tracked to ensure that the correct biospecimen (e.g., initial presentation vs. relapse) is used for downstream analyses.

3. **Availability of biospecimens with high molecular integrity.** Although genomic DNA is relatively stable and unaffected by variables in clinical biospecimen processing and storage, the same is not true for cellular RNA, protein, phosphoproteins, and cell-free nucleic acid. Cellular RNA and proteins may be degraded in cells ex vivo if clinical biospecimens are not rapidly and properly processed and stored. More insidiously, the mRNA and protein complement of cells may rapidly change as a function of processing time and methodology.

4. **Specialized processing and preservation.** An increasing number of translational research studies require use of specialized analytes such as rare circulating cells, extracellular vesicles, cell-free nucleic acid isolated from peripheral blood and plasma, and disaggregated and cryopreserved cell suspensions isolated from patient and animal model solid tissues. A centralized facility with validated protocols for performing these high-complexity tasks is often needed.

5. **Maximal utilization of diverse but limited biospecimens.** Because of the number and diversity of potential biomarkers that can be evaluated from banked biospecimens, repositories can process and preserve a variety of biospecimens in a format that can be distributed to many different study investigators (Fig. 60.1). For example, preoperative serum from cancer patients may be useful for identifying tumor-associated serum markers for early detection, while nucleated cell fractions from bone marrow, peripheral blood, or cavity washings from the same patient may be used to evaluate markers for tumor metastasis. Serial collections of stabilized plasma for isolation of cell-free circulating nucleic acids may prove useful in the detection and/or surveillance for recurrent disease. Collected biospecimens may be rare or small in size, so strategies to efficiently consolidate biospecimen resources (such as tissue microarrays [TMAs]) or to molecularly amplify limiting amounts of genomic material from needle biopsies, tissue touch preps, or washings are critical to providing a useful biospecimen resource.

6. **Biospecimen annotation.** Given the cost and effort often associated with molecular and genomic analyses of clinical biospecimens, molecular data associated with human biospecimens is arguably more valuable than the biospecimen itself. A data system that can accurately track individual samples within large clinical biospecimen sets and that allows for accurate integration and correlation of genomic, molecular, biomarker, and clinical data is obviously crucial (*J Biomed Inform* 2015;57:456). A large and viable biospecimen resource is only useful if it is linked to complete and accurate clinical data that can be used to substantiate or refute clinical hypotheses. At the same time, increasing concerns for medical record privacy and in particular, genetic data privacy require proper measures to protect patient confidentiality (*BMC Med Ethics* 2015;16:32).

7. **Biospecimen custodianship.** There have been increasing concerns regarding ownership of tissue biospecimens and the intellectual property that is generated from their use. There is also a continuing need to appropriately honor the intent and privacy of patient donors. This requires the establishment of an unbiased agent (the "honest broker") who can judiciously administrate and regulate the collection and distribution of biospecimens.

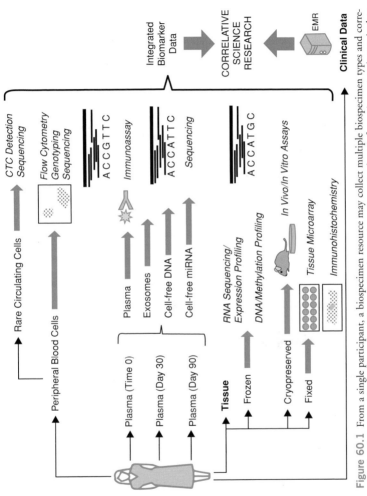

Figure 60.1 From a single participant, a biospecimen resource may collect multiple biospecimen types and corresponding data to enable a wide variety of translational research projects. A robust informatics system is required to track and maintain these data.

8. Guidelines. Because biospecimen banks are an integral part of medical research, and are rapidly becoming an integral part of clinical medicine, several national and international agencies, such as the National Cancer Institute (NCI), the International Society of Biological and Environmental Repositories (ISBER), and the College of American Pathologists (CAP) have created dedicated offices and guidelines for biorepository operations (*Biopreserv Biobank* 2018;16:16). The principles of biospecimen banking obviously relate to the general practice of pathology and therefore it is usually the pathologist and the pathology department that have sufficient expertise to govern these activities. However, an equal understanding of the principles for clinical trial development, drug discovery and development, pharmacologic modeling, biomarker discovery, and downstream correlative science strategies are also relevant expertise not necessarily associated with traditional pathology service. The development and maintenance of a biospecimen resource involves many policies and processes which are outlined in Figure 60.2 and summarized in this chapter.

II. BIOSPECIMEN COLLECTION. The types of biospecimens collected and the methods used to process and store them depends greatly on their projected use, although for many biospecimens the intended use is unknown. Since the comprehensive cost associated with biospecimen procurement, processing, annotation, and storage is not insignificant ($100 to $1,000 per biospecimen, which is highly dependent upon biospecimen type), careful consideration should be given to the scope and focus of the biorepository's operation.

A. Defining the Scope of Operation. The type and number of participants from whom biospecimens are collected depends upon the stated mission and available resources of the biorepository. In some cases, small biorepositories may collect only defined biospecimens from participants enrolled in specific clinical trials. In other cases, the biorepository may be disease-based and seek to universally collect all available biospecimens for a given disease type. When resources or institutional barriers do not permit the creation of a large centralized facility, several small facilities may elect to create a federated system where each bank operates independently, but is linked by a common informatics network. A biorepository may need not be a "bank" at all, but may simply serve to collect, process, de-identify, and immediately distribute biospecimens; the Cooperative Human Tissue Network (CHTN) and the National Disease Research Interchange (NDRI) generally operate as such tissue brokers. A biorepository may also simply exist as a research-based portal for controlled access of diagnostic paraffin block tissue biospecimens, already available in the pathology department.

B. Regulatory Requirements. Many aspects of a biorepository are considered an organized human subjects research activity, and therefore must conform to regulatory requirements that are different than those applicable to a clinical laboratory. Policies have evolved significantly at the national level over the past five years, including recent proposed changes to the "Common Rule" (45 CFR part 46), and also vary greatly between states and institutions. Generally, the following points should be considered with regard to biospecimen-based human subjects' research.

1. Institutional review board (IRB) review. The intended purpose, scope, and policies of the biorepository must be reviewed by the IRB. In some cases, a Certificate of Confidentiality, a document that asserts the right of the biorepository director (or honest broker) to protect the confidentiality of biospecimen data even under court order, may be required.

2. Participant consent. In most cases of prospective biospecimen collection, some form of informed participant consent is required. Explicit informed consent for the retrospective use of existing biospecimens may be waived if it is impossible or impractical to obtain, and the risk to the participant is minimal. Rarely, some institutions have ruled that generic language present in a hospital admissions document or surgical consent form provides sufficient consent for biospecimen collection, assuming that the biospecimens are distributed and utilized in a de-identified ("coded") or anonymized (without any link to PHI) manner. Generally, however, explicit written consent for biospecimen banking should be obtained from the participant. Many

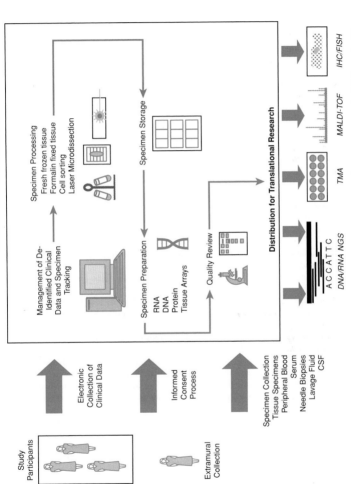

Figure 60.2 Flow diagram of the many processes and resources required to operate a typical full service bio-specimen resource.

generic templates for the language used in such a document are available. Since the main risk to an individual participating in a biospecimen banking program is loss of confidentiality, measures used to protect confidentiality and the risks associated with its loss are the main risks to convey to the participant. However, when human biospecimens are being used for genomic and disease-predisposition studies, and when research results generate patentable biomarker inventions, properly documented, more specific informed participant consent may be critical.

3. Investigator agreements. In addition to IRB requirements that must be satisfied by the biorepository for the initial collection, coding, and storage of biospecimens, investigators seeking to utilize biospecimens from the biorepository may need to meet additional regulatory requirements, which usually require approval of an independent IRB protocol. In addition, investigators may be expected to sign a Data Use Agreement or other investigator agreement that establishes what will or will not be done with distributed biospecimens. If biospecimens are to be distributed to an investigator outside of the biorepository's institution, a material transfer agreement (MTA) may also be necessary.

C. Biospecimen Types

1. Tissues. Collected tissues may be snap-frozen, fixed in a variety of cross-linking or precipitating fixatives, or cryoprotected and frozen to maintain cell viability. Snap-frozen tissue provides the highest quality protein and nucleic acid derivatives, and is often required for genomic or proteomic studies. Tissue that is cryoprotected and frozen is increasing desirable for transport, long-term storage, later thawing for cell dissociation procedures (single cell sequencing and flow cytometric analyses), and development of human-in-mouse xenograft models. However, the logistics of frozen tissue collection and transport are difficult, and proper storage (optimally in liquid nitrogen [LN_2] vapor) is relatively expensive. Formalin-fixed, paraffin-embedded (FFPE) tissue blocks are easy to obtain, easy to store, and very familiar to any pathology service. The quality of molecular derivatives from such tissues is vastly inferior, although several recent technical advances allow FFPE tissue to be used for the generation of DNA sequence and RNA expression data. Fixation of tissue in precipitating fixatives such as ethanol, acetone, and other commercial fixatives designed for molecular diagnostics, followed by embedding in low temperature polymers, provides tissue with excellent histologic detail and molecular material that is superior to that of traditional FFPE tissue (e-**Fig. 60.1**). However, RNA and protein quality still do not match that of material derived from frozen tissue.

2. Blood components. Peripheral blood serum and plasma (often collected at multiple time points throughout a patient's clinical course) are often banked, given the minimally invasive and relatively inexpensive approach to collection. They are the preferred biospecimens for proteomic analysis and conventional biomarker studies. More recently, there is considerable scientific interest in plasma collected in specialized stabilization tubes which can provide a unique source of cell-free extracellular vesicles and circulating, cell-free nucleic acid. However, when properly aliquoted from multiple patients and multiple time points, this material can rapidly occupy a large amount of frozen storage space. Peripheral blood leukocytes (PBL) are the ideal source for germline DNA, and can be stored or processed without the need for additional cell separation protocols such as mononuclear cell isolation. In translational cancer research, isolation and characterization of circulating tumor cells (CTC), which are present in very low numbers in the peripheral blood of advanced stage cancer patients, can be accomplished using immunoaffinity capture reagents or size-based microfluidic instruments; generally, these highly specialized isolation procedures are performed in individual research laboratories. Bone marrow may also be banked, particularly for analyses involving hematologic malignancies, bone marrow dyscrasias, immunologic disorders, or occult tumor cell detection.

3. Other body fluids. Urine, sputum, cavity lavages, and effusions serve as useful analytes. However, large fluid volume biospecimens (such as urine) may be difficult and expensive to process and store for long periods of time, particularly for a future unknown use. Furthermore, analysis of such biospecimens may require only a small amount of material per assay, which then necessitates that collections be excessively aliquoted to prevent multiple freeze/thaw cycles of the same biospecimen. As an alternative, the cellular component of these fluids may be isolated by centrifugation and stored as cell pellets.

D. **Collection Methods.** Depending upon the biospecimen type and its intended application, there are a number of important considerations involved in collecting biospecimens for a biospecimen bank.

1. **Biospecimen acquisition.** For most general tissue bank activities, tissue biospecimens are collected in the course of routine treatment, such as a surgical resection of a solid tumor, a therapeutic needle aspiration to remove joint or body cavity fluid, or a diagnostic bone marrow biopsy. In these cases, it is important that biospecimen collection for research purposes not compromise the diagnostic utility of the biospecimen. In many cases, such as the resection of a breast tumor or colon tumor, it is important that biospecimen procurement occur under the direct guidance of a pathologist who can supervise and assure that diagnostic integrity (e.g., an intact tumor margin) is not compromised. In cases where the diagnostic tissue biospecimen is limiting, properly supervised *ex vivo* sampling by core needle biopsy instrument or skin punch may be used to acquire sufficient material for research without compromising the diagnostic biospecimen. Other protocols may allow for redundant tissue sampling at the time of a diagnostic procedure; for example, for a patient with a suspicious liver mass, standard of care may dictate that two biospecimens from a CT-guided needle biopsy be submitted for diagnostic evaluation, while two additional needle cores may be taken for the research biorepository. In certain cases, the research biorepository may receive tissue samples that harbor clinically relevant diagnostic findings that are not present in the routinely processed tissue samples; for this reason, the pathology department should develop policies regarding clinical versus research biospecimen collection, which may include holding all research biospecimens in escrow until a final clinical diagnosis is rendered. Finally, an IRB-approved study protocol may dictate the collection of "research use only" biospecimens above and beyond what is needed for routine standard of care. This may include something as routine as a peripheral blood draw or may involve image-guided tissue biopsies at multiple time points during the course of a therapy. In these cases (which are usually clinical trial activities), the cost for biospecimen collection is usually supported by the investigator and their study budget.

2. **Biospecimen preservation.** For molecular and genomic analyses, proper tissue preservation is critical. A biospecimen's molecular profile (i.e., gene expression, protein phosphorylation) can rapidly change from the time it is first collected until the time when it is ultimately preserved by freezing or fixation due to "warm ischemia time." Although few evidence-based guidelines exist, warm ischemia time should be limited and at least documented so as not to introduce additional preanalytical variability. Although snap-frozen tissue is the preferred substrate for many studies, several commercial and "home-brew" tissue preservatives are available that provide acceptable biospecimen preservation for molecular studies. Delays in blood processing can affect proteomic biomarker profiles; unlike tissue, whole blood cannot be immediately snap frozen but must be centrifuged to remove the specific plasma or serum component that then, in turn, must be aliquoted and rapidly frozen. As with tissue, a number of commercial products are available to preserve blood cell components at ambient temperature without freezing, although these products are relatively expensive and require specialized downstream isolation procedures.

3. **Remote site collection.** For multi-institutional research protocols, it may be necessary to collect biospecimens from remote sites, often from health centers or medical offices that have little experience in supporting intricate biospecimen collection requirements such as snap-frozen tissue. Proper and efficient collection of

biospecimens from such sites may require preassembled biospecimen procurement kits (e-**Fig. 60.2**) and personnel training to ensure the uniform collection of biospecimens.

4. **Biospecimen quantity.** Modern molecular amplification protocols for DNA (sequence) and RNA (gene expression) analyses often allow investigators to use nanogram quantities of input DNA and RNA. Instrumentation for proteomic analysis has also become considerably more advanced and, although it is not possible to amplify protein analytes from biospecimens, tissue requirements have been minimized even for these technologies. Therefore, even limited size biospecimens such as needle aspirates, tissue touch preps, and core biopsies are valuable and frequently amenable to molecular analyses. Obviously, such biospecimens must be judiciously distributed to maximize their research potential. Conversely, the collection of large tissue biospecimens is not necessarily desirable; they may not be properly preserved when fixed or frozen in their entirety. For such cases, tissue biospecimens should be divided into samples no greater than 1 cm³ for fixation and/or freezing.

5. **Associated data collection.** Clinical and pathologic data corresponding to the patient and biospecimen (for clinical applications), and the participant and biospecimen (for research applications), are as important as the biospecimen itself. Without these associated data, the utility of the biospecimens for clinical or correlative studies is lost. The scope of the data that are collected and stored with the biospecimen will depend upon the mission of the biorepository. It is usually impractical to gather detailed clinical information represented as written notes in a clinical chart or report; instead, it may be more efficient to rely on electronic sources of data. Although data are usually represented in text format, surgical pathology reports provide an accurate and detailed source of pathology information for tissue biospecimens that are collected and diagnosed as part of routine clinical care. In some centers, the electronic medical record (EMR) may provide access to basic patient demographics and clinical diagnostic data (*BMC Genomics* 2016;17:434). For cancer patients and their biospecimens, the hospital tumor registry is often a reasonably detailed and standardized source for cancer-related clinical and pathology data. Except for specific studies, it is generally advisable to collect a limited but standardized data set corresponding to each collected case rather than an exhaustive (and inevitably incomplete) data set for every biospecimen.

E. Biospecimen Data Management. As depicted in Figure 60.1, biospecimen banks may house a complex array of biospecimens and associated data. It is critical that biospecimens be accurately tracked and annotated if they are to be useful. While smaller banks may rely on written logbooks and electronic spreadsheets to track biospecimen information, these methods become rapidly constraining as the bank becomes larger and more diversified. Basic data types that may be required in a biorepository information system include the following.

1. **Receipt, study association, and consent tracking.** An accurate record must be maintained of when and from where biospecimens were received, and whether they are intended for clinical or research use. For research biospecimens, the corresponding research protocol must also be identified, as well as the record of consent under which the biospecimens were collected, since consent regulates how the biospecimens may be used.

2. **Inventory and storage.** It is important to accurately maintain the available quantity and storage location of every biospecimen so that it can be rapidly retrieved on demand.

3. **Quality assurance.** Quality assurance measures such as tissue histology review, warm ischemia time, details of biospecimen processing, and nucleic acid quality should be maintained for each biospecimen.

4. **Clinical annotation.** As discussed above, a minimal set of clinical and pathology annotation data should be associated with each biospecimen.

5. **Distribution and utilization.** The efficacy of a biorepository is judged almost entirely upon its distribution of biospecimens for clinical testing or productive translational

research. Therefore, detailed data concerning biospecimen distribution is essential in justifying the activity and operation of the facility.

Several commercial software packages are available to assist in the management of biospecimen banks. Some of these are stand-alone applications while others are "modules" of more complex clinical trial management systems. Frequently, individual biorepositories, particularly nascent facilities, develop their own data systems, often creating rather arbitrary and custom data schemes and data definitions. While such applications may serve the immediate needs of the bank, they present a significant obstacle to collaboration among different biospecimen resource centers when data standardization and semantic interoperability are required. A number of "open-source" (aka "no cost") alternatives exist in the form of community supported biorepository software applications. Although no informatics system is truly "no cost," these applications provide a balance of data standardization and robustness found in more expensive commercial packages with the relatively lower cost of the software application itself.

III. **BIOSPECIMEN PROCESSING.** The same principles of biospecimen processing used in the clinical laboratory apply to biospecimens banked for clinical and/or research purposes. However, since biospecimens collected for research purposes may be used for experimental studies that are not a part of traditional diagnostic histopathology, special biospecimen processing needs must be considered.

A. **Frozen Tissue.** Although the histologic quality of frozen tissue is inferior to that of FFPE tissue, many molecular studies require high-grade DNA, RNA, and protein extracts for optimal data generation, which can only be obtained from frozen biospecimens. Tissue may be frozen in LN_2, an isopentane cryobath (such as is available in most pathology frozen section rooms), or a make-shift dry ice ethanol bath. Tissue biospecimens should be no larger than 1 cm^3 to ensure rapid and consistent freezing throughout the biospecimen. If the biospecimen is to be used for histologic sectioning for quality review or laser microdissection (LM), it may first be embedded in freezing media such as Optimal Cutting Temperature (OCT) compound. Since OCT material does not interfere with nucleic acid isolation, but may have an effect on proteomic studies, it may be advisable to freeze both embedded and nonembedded tissue to ensure the widest range of downstream uses. Once frozen, tissue may be stored in cassettes in −80-degree ultralow freezers or LN_2 vapor inventory systems. While the latter is more expensive and less efficient with regard to space management and inventory consolidation, biospecimens stored in LN_2 are immune to the power failures and mechanical breakdowns that can occur with electric freezers. Any frozen storage system should be equipped with a temperature recording device to document appropriate storage conditions and a remote alarm system that can contact laboratory personnel in the event of machine failure or power loss prior to breaching storage temperature limits that would put biospecimen quality in jeopardy.

B. **Fixed Tissue.** FFPE tissue biospecimens are not as well suited for molecular and genomic analyses as frozen tissue. However, the quality of fixed tissue biospecimens can be improved using several quality control measures.

1. **Control and documentation of fixation and processing times.** By minimizing or optimizing the time for which tissues are fixed, overfixation (which leads to excessive crosslinking and molecular degradation) can be avoided. When possible, documentation of processing times for each biospecimen can assist in troubleshooting sources of preanalytical variability in tissue biospecimens collected over different time periods or from different locations.

2. **Use of "molecularly friendly" fixatives.** Several commercially available and "home brew" precipitating fixatives preserve tissue and tissue histology while minimizing the damaging effects to protein antigens and nucleic acids caused by crosslinking fixatives such as formalin.

3. **Tissue oxidation.** Whenever possible, fixed tissues should be stored as tissue blocks in a cool, temperature- and humidity-controlled environment. Once fixed tissue

sections are cut to slides, they should be utilized quickly and not stored for long periods of time. Tissue sections cut to slides oxidize quickly, compromising both antigenic targets used for immunohistochemical studies as well as isolated nucleic acid. When institutional surgical pathology departments are unwilling to distribute diagnostic blocks for research biobanking, collection of tissue "scrolls" or 1 to 2 mm tissue punches, stored in a sealed vial, may serve as an adequate substitute for moderate term storage.

C. **Blood Components.** For isolation and storage of serum and plasma, whole blood must be immediately spun and the appropriate liquid component removed from cellular material, aliquoted, and frozen. Processing must be performed rapidly before cell lysis and protein degradation occurs. Consortia of proteomics investigators have published recommendations on blood processing for proteomic studies and while some of these guidelines are evidenced based, robust guidelines have not been firmly established. More recently, clinicians and researchers collect peripheral blood plasma for the isolation and sequencing of exosomal or cell-free nucleic acid. To avoid contamination by cellular nucleic acid from white blood cells and platelets, specialized blood cell stabilization tubes (available from several commercial sources) are utilized, and high-speed centrifugation is performed to create platelet-free plasma for subsequent nucleic acid extraction. Many institutions freeze whole blood at the site of collection as a convenient way to store blood for future genomic DNA isolation; however, freezing blood in glass vacutainer tubes presents a safety hazard, requires considerably more freezer space to store, and inevitably causes cell lysis which results in DNA that is frequently lower in yield, degraded, and contaminated with heme products that can effect downstream assays. Although more labor intensive, immediate spinning of whole blood followed by selective removal, washing, aliquoting, and freezing of the "buffy coat" creates a high-quality biospecimen that is easy to store and results in higher DNA yield and quality. In some cases it may be desirable to isolate the mononuclear cell fraction (PBMC) from peripheral blood and preserve these cells; this approach has the advantage of removing peripheral blood granulocytes and preserving the monocyte fraction which can be manipulated for future uses such as flow cytometry and cell immortalization. However, viable preservation of PBMCs is expensive, requires additional expertise, and is seldom necessary for simple DNA isolation. When PBMC isolation is not a consideration, whole blood may be stored at 4 degrees for as long as 72 hours with little loss in PBMC viability.

D. **Laser Microdissection (LM).** For some types of molecular and genomic analyses, it may be desirable to have material derived from homogeneous or enriched cell populations. LM is a method that uses a laser to either "capture" or cut desired cells away from surrounding tissue under direct microscopic visualization (e-**Fig. 60.3**). The isolated cells may be used for DNA, RNA, or protein isolation for molecular analyses (*Am J Cancer Res* 2014;4:1). Although LM instrumentation is expensive, and the technique is time consuming and requires expertise, its use for translational pathology research studies is routine in many biospecimen banks.

E. **Tissue Dissociation.** An alternative to LM for the dissection of histologically complex tissue biospecimens involves dissociation and epitope-based enrichment of specific cell populations for downstream analyses. This is accomplished using fresh tissue (and sometimes properly cryopreserved and thawed tissue biospecimens) which are subjected to enzymatic digestion, gentle mechanical dissociation, and either cell sorting or immunomagnetic bead capture to isolate specific cell subpopulations. To date, this is largely a tedious processes relegated to research laboratories. However, as methods such as single cell RNA sequencing and CyTOF become more routine platforms for biomarker assessment, it is likely that methods for tissue dissociation and cell capture will also become more robust and automated.

F. **Tissue Microarrays (TMAs).** TMAs provide another format to maximize utilization of limiting tissue biospecimens. TMAs are constructed by sampling one to three 0.8 mm (up to as large as 3 mm) tissue cores from a donor paraffin tissue block, and assembling them into an array of as many as 300 cores in a recipient block (**e-Fig. 60.4**). The resulting recipient block can then be sectioned as a traditional tissue block, making it possible to perform simultaneous immunohistochemistry or fluorescence in situ hybridization on each of the 300 cores, on a single slide. TMAs allow researchers to easily validate patterns of biomarker expression in a large sample series using relatively inexpensive technology. Few special reagents are required and basic TMA instrumentation is relatively inexpensive, but expert review and informatics tracking of the individual case cores on each slide is still required. Another recognized disadvantage of the TMA format is that it is prone to sampling error, as only a small sample from each tissue block is incorporated into the array for analysis.

G. **Nucleic Acid.** An increasing number of genomic-based biomarker studies (DNA sequencing, RNA expression profiling, SNP genotyping) have made the isolation of DNA and RNA from tissue and fluid biospecimens a nearly standard service in most larger biorepositories. Nucleic acid can be effectively isolated from frozen and fixed tissue using several standard protocols, although the quality from the latter is often inferior, as discussed above. Microbial nucleic acid can be isolated from human stool, urine, saliva, body swabs, and other sources, but often requires specialized protocols that differ from those used to isolate eukaryotic cellular nucleic acid, particularly to obtain the comprehensive complement of material from gram-positive organisms. In some cases, it may be desirable to isolate nucleic acid directly from collected biospecimens, such as DNA from peripheral blood or saliva (for genotyping studies) or cell-free DNA from blood plasma samples (for cancer sequencing or other biomarker assays). Nucleic acids are more stable once purified, and can be more conveniently stored as compared with the parent tissue or fluid. However, the initial cost and effort to isolate DNA and/or RNA from every collected biospecimen as it is received can be prohibitive, so prospective preparation of nucleic acids should only be considered when material will be of immediate use.

IV. **QUALITY ASSURANCE.** A biospecimen resource should only provide material that is subjected to rigorous quality control. In fact, the rationale for a pathologist-supervised biospecimen resource is that it is often pathologists who best understand the approach to, and importance of, clinical biospecimen quality control.

A. **Biospecimen Identification.** Just as in any clinical laboratory, proper biospecimen labeling and identification are critical; because a biorepository may store biospecimens for prolonged periods of time, maintenance of proper biospecimen identification is important. As biorepositories become subject to regulatory review similar to that of clinical laboratories, they will need to implement standard clinical laboratory practices to prevent sample mislabeling, including use of preprinted barcode labels, double data entry, and routine data auditing.

B. **Representative Tissue Sampling.** In most cases, biospecimens that are submitted for clinical diagnosis and those that are submitted to a research biorepository are not identical. They may be collected at slightly different times or locations, or may involve sampling bias. For example, in a heterogeneous prostate tumor, a tissue biopsy collected for research may contain no neoplastic cells, although the routinely processed tissue for diagnosis contains high grade adenocarcinoma. Distribution of the banked biospecimen, under the false assumption that it truly reflects the diagnostic material, may result in a compromised research study. Consequently, it is important that individual biospecimens (particularly heterogeneous tissue samples) received by the biorepository are histologically reviewed either prospectively or prior to distribution. Such a review of tissue or cellular samples may involve confirmation of a histopathologic diagnosis as well as notation of general cellular features such as histologic preservation, tissue cellularity, and necrosis. A special circumstance arises when a novel finding or diagnosis is observed in a banked research biospecimen that was not reported from the material used for pathologic diagnosis; resolution of such a problematic circumstance will depend upon the policies of both the IRB and pathology service, and should be documented as part of the biorepository's standard operating procedures.

C. Tissue Preservation and Molecular Integrity. When the biorepository will be responsible for generating and distributing nucleic acids (DNA and RNA), it is important that their molecular integrity is verified. As discussed above, the quality of nucleic acid is directly related to the manner in which the biospecimen was collected and preserved. Fixation and delays in biospecimen processing (warm ischemia time) can compromise nucleic acid quality, as can repeated freeze/thaw cycles (e-**Fig. 60.5**). Inherent necrosis and tissue cellularity in the biospecimen can also affect the quality of nucleic acids. Documentation of molecular biospecimen quality can be accomplished by readily available (albeit often expensive) instrumentation designed for quality review of small amounts of nucleic acid, including fiberoptic spectrophotometers and capillary microelectrophoresis systems. Metrics have been developed which relate quantitative results from these instruments to expected performance in downstream applications and assays (*Sci Rep* 2018;8:6351).

V. BIOSPECIMEN UTILIZATION. The success of any biorepository is measured by the utilization of collected biospecimens. Distribution of biospecimens for patient care or funded research projects is also an important revenue source to support the larger biospecimen banking effort. It is important to note that there is often a 3- to 5-year "lag phase" while the biorepository is developing and maturing its collection before a newly established biospecimen resource is routinely utilized for translational research.

A. Publication of Available Resources. This is best accomplished through a web-based catalog of available resources. Examples of such web-based directories of cancer-related biospecimens on a national level include the NCTN Biospecimen Navigator (https://navigator.ctsu.org) and the NCI Specimen Resource Locator (https://specimens.cancer.gov).

B. Streamlined Administrative Processes. Often, clinicians and researchers are unfamiliar with procedures for requesting biospecimens, obtaining appropriate IRB approval, and creating necessary MTAs. Having a standardized and facilitated process for completing the regulatory steps necessary for biospecimen banking and subsequent distribution will greatly enhance utilization of a biospecimen resource.

C. High-Quality Annotated Biospecimens. Clinical testing and translational research can only be accelerated when the biospecimens distributed are properly quality controlled and "assay ready." Minimal but sufficient clinical and/or pathology data should be supplied with each biospecimen in order to easily enable correlative analyses.

D. Facilitated and Judicious Distribution. The process of case selection, biospecimen retrieval and processing, biospecimen annotation, and distribution can be time consuming and expensive. As a biorepository matures, increasing requests may overwhelm its available personnel resources and can result in significant delays in providing biospecimens. Competing interests for limited biospecimens may also become problematic as utilization increases. Therefore, a biorepository should establish a utilization review committee so that its finite effort and physical resources can be fairly allocated. The utilization committee should be an unbiased representation of pathologists and scientists, with allocation decisions based on clinical necessity, scientific merit of proposed projects, investigator track record with previous requests, funding status, and likelihood that distributed biospecimens will meaningfully contribute to patient care, grant funding, and scientific publication.

VI. SUPPORT. The cost to develop and sustain a fully functional biorepository is substantial, and any plans to develop such a resource should include an approach to long-term financial sustainability (*Biopreserv Biobank* 2017;15:31). Frequent sources of support include the following.

A. Clinical Activities. Although generally viewed as a research activity, some biospecimen banking may directly or indirectly support patient care (i.e., for diagnosis and to direct therapy). These activities should be compensated in a way consistent with their value. Costs may be subsidized by the hospital or medical institution, since clinical biobanking can be considered a component of the general hospital infrastructure required to support best patient care. Clinical biobanking, as might be required for new approaches to personalized medicine, can also be compensated by establishing specific billing codes that reflect the technical components (specimen handling, quality assurance, informatics, and storage) and professional components (selection of appropriate tissue, microscopic review of banked biospecimens) of biospecimen banking. Currently, however, no such clinical billing codes exist.

B. Research Activities

1. **Institutional support.** Academic institutions or departments often support the initial development and operation of a biorepository, which is not surprising considering the central importance of the resource in the mission of translational research. The institution may expect a return on its investment in terms of the number of biospecimen-based projects, publications, and research grants that can be garnered through such a resource.

2. **Extramural funding.** Unlike traditional, hypothesis-based research grants, there are few extramural (noninstitutional) funding mechanisms to specifically support biorepositories. A tissue procurement shared resource facility may, however, be a key funded component of larger initiatives such as NIH program project grants, center grants, or disease-focused programs (e.g., Specialized Programs of Research Excellence, or SPOREs).

3. **Investigator fees.** A viable biospecimen resource must develop investigator fees for the services it provides, including biospecimen collection, storage, processing, and distribution. These fees should be calculated realistically and account for all operations and resources that are required, from the initial collection of a biospecimen to its final distribution to an investigator. Such fees should be structured to also allow for resource growth and further development. At the same time, fees should not be so burdensome as to deter the conduct of sound research, particularly for pilot translational studies where investigator funding may be limited, or where a unique opportunity exists to collect biospecimens (perhaps in the context of a clinical trial), store them, and utilize them at a later date once additional research funding is obtained. Obviously, the greater a biorepository's participation in funded research, the easier it will be to maintain long-term support for the operation, and the more likely that the resource will contribute significantly to impactful, translational biomedical research.

SUGGESTED READINGS

Boeckhout M, Douglas CMW. Governing the research-care divide in clinical biobanking: Dutch perspectives. *Life Sci Soc Policy* 2015;11:7. doi:10.1186/s40504-015-0025-z.

De Souza YG, Greenspan JS. Biobanking past, present and future: responsibilities and benefits. *AIDS* 2013;27(3):303–312. doi:10.1097/QAD.0b013e32835c1244.

Felmeister AS, Masino AJ, Rivera TJ, Resnick AC, Pennington JW. The biorepository portal toolkit: an honest brokered, modular service oriented software tool set for biospecimen-driven translational research. *BMC Genomics* 2016;17(Suppl 4):434. doi:10.1186/s12864-016-2797-9.

Goldenberg AJ, Maschke KJ, Joffe S, et al. IRB practices and policies regarding the secondary research use of biospecimens. *BMC Medical Ethics* 2015;16:32. doi:10.1186/s12910-015-0020-1.

Henderson GE, Edwards TP, Cadigan RJ, et al. Stewardship practices of U.S. biobanks. *Sci Transl Med* 2013;5(215):215cm7. doi:10.1126/scitranslmed.3007362.

Kelly SM, Wiehagen LT, Schumacher PE, Dhir R. Methods to improve sustainability of a large academic biorepository. *Biopreserv Biobank* 2017;15(1):31–36. doi:10.1089/bio.2016.0076.

Legres LG, Janin A, Masselon C, Bertheau P. Beyond laser microdissection technology: follow the yellow brick road for cancer research. *Am J Cancer Res* 2014;4(1):1–28.

Loibner M, Buzina W, Viertler C, et al. Pathogen inactivating properties and increased sensitivity in molecular diagnostics by PAX gene, a novel non-crosslinking tissue fixative. *PLoS ONE* 2016;11(3):e0151383. doi:10.1371/journal.pone.0151383.

McIntosh LD, Sharma MK, Mulvihill D, et al. caTissue Suite to OpenSpecimen: developing an extensible, open source, web-based biobanking management system. *J Biomed Inform* 2015;57:456–464. doi:10.1016/j.jbi.2015.08.020.

Medina Diaz I, Nocon A, Mehnert DH, Fredebohm J, Diehl F, Holtrup F. Performance of streck cfDNA blood collection tubes for liquid biopsy testing. *PLoS ONE* 2016;11(11):e0166354. doi:10.1371/journal.pone.0166354.

Mora EM, Álvarez-Cubela S, Oltra E. Biobanking of exosomes in the era of precision medicine: are we there yet? *Int J Mol Sci* 2016;17(1):13. doi:10.3390/ijms17010013.

Qiu X, De Jesus J, Pennell M, Troiani M, Haun JB. Microfluidic device for mechanical dissociation of cancer cell aggregates into single cells. *Lab Chip* 2015;15(1):339–350. doi:10.1039/c4lc01126k.

Shabihkhani M, Lucey GM, Wei B, et al. The procurement, storage, and quality assurance of frozen blood and tissue biospecimens in pathology, biorepository, and biobank settings. *Clin Biochem* 2014;47(4-5):258–266. doi:10.1016/j.clinbiochem.2014.01.002.

Ulrich BC, Paweletz CP. Cell-free DNA in oncology: Gearing up for clinic. *Ann Lab Med.* 2018;38(1):1–8. doi:10.3343/alm.2018.38.1.1.

Vaught J, Lockhart N. The evolution of biobanking best practices. *Clin Chim Acta* 2012;413(19–20):1569–1575. doi:10.1016/j.cca.2012.04.030.

Wimmer I, Tröscher AR, Brunner F, et al. Systematic evaluation of RNA quality, microarray data reliability and pathway analysis in fresh, fresh frozen and formalin-fixed paraffin-embedded tissue samples. *Scientific Reports* 2018;8(1):6351. doi:10.1038/s41598-018-24781-6.

Zhang J, Chen K, Fan ZH. Circulating tumor cell isolation and analysis. *Adv Clin Chem* 2016;75:1–31. doi:10.1016/bs.acc.2016.03.003.

ADDITIONAL RESOURCES

Biobanking and Biopreservation Journal. https://home.liebertpub.com/publications/biopreservation-and-biobanking/110/overview

Hansel DE, Jewell SD. Developing and Organizing an Institutional Biospecimen Repository. CAP Publication #PUB314. https://www.cap.org

International Society for Biological and Environmental Repositories. http://www.isber.org/

NCI Office of Biorepositories and Biospecimen Research. http://biospecimens.cancer.gov

OpenSpecimen Open Source Biobanking Software. https://www.openspecimen.org

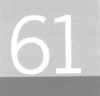

Imaging Technologies in Surgical Pathology: Virtual Microscopy and Telepathology

Mike Isaacs and John D. Pfeifer

I. **CONVENTIONAL LIGHT MICROSCOPY** remains the core tool in diagnostic surgical pathology. Increasingly, electronic modes of image presentation are being used in routine practice in addition to conventional light microscopy, since digitized images of glass slides increase the clinically useful information that can be obtained from a pathologic specimen, including electronic consultations, archiving, and digital image analysis.

II. **VIRTUAL MICROSCOPY** is the technique whereby entire glass slides or selected areas of slides are scanned and converted to digital data files (also known as virtual slides), which can then be viewed on a computer screen. The characteristics of the displayed image, in terms of resolution and range of magnification, are primarily determined by the optical features of the scanning system and are overall comparable with those of glass slide microscopy. However, in contrast to conventional light microscopy where the magnification, focus, and condenser setting can be adjusted at any time, for digital scanning the so-called "scanning depth" must be determined prior to image acquisition. The "scanning depth" includes the region of interest, the scanning power, and the number of horizontal levels to be obtained in the plane of the tissue section (scanning power includes the physical magnification [e.g., 20×] and resolution [e.g., 2,048 × 4,800 pixels], while the number of horizontal levels [so-called z-stacking] is dependent on the section thickness and the need to be able to focus up and down through the tissue and cells in the final virtual image). Depth of focus is a requirement for interpretation of specimens that rely on a 3-dimensional assessment of cellular morphology, for example cytology specimens (*Cancer Cytopathol* 2007;111:203).

A. **Whole Slide Imaging (WSI).** WSI refers to the scanning of glass slides to produce electronic images. Currently there are about a dozen major vendors that market platforms for WSI. The average time to digitize a 15 × 15 region of tissue on glass slide at 40 × for most WSI platforms of a single horizontal level of a slide (non-z-stacked) ranges from 2 to 4 minutes and generates a data file that is enormous (ranging from about 200 MB to 2.5 GB). Although a universal file format known as Dicom has been developed (ftp://medical.nema.org/medical/dicom/DICOMWSI/index.html), it has not been broadly adopted and so scanning platforms are currently built in a closed environment with a proprietary file format. Until the Dicom standard is widely adopted, conversion tools must therefore be used to translate image files between the different virtual slide file formats.

Each virtual file consists of multiple parts, called file segments, which include an identification tag, a barcode (generated by the laboratory Information system [LIS]), a low-power overview, and the images at the selected power. While image acquisition methods vary (linear, meander, array), currently all available systems produce tiled images, that is, small images that are retrieved and stitched together to form the final image on the computer screen at the selected power. Most interfaces allow electronic zooming (i.e., additional magnification) beyond the original scanned magnification.

Resolution and functionality of virtual slides have achieved levels that are comparable with conventional light microscopes. Scanning time has improved over time, but is still time consuming since scanning time is mainly dependent on computational speed and optical physics, the latter of which is determined by the magnification of the scanning objective. The actual image acquisition step occurs via a charged coupled device (CCD) which consists of several hundred thousand individual picture elements (pixels) that transform the optical image into a virtual image; whole slide images are therefore acquired via an optical lens that moves over the slide. Some platforms shorten scanning time by using a meander rather than a linear scanning pattern to acquire images, but both the meander and linear methods have inherent physical limitations that become most apparent when acquiring multiple images within each plane of section (i.e., when z-stacking). The technology known as "lens array microscopy" uses arrays of detectors (miniaturized lenses) to simultaneously capture information from larger areas of the tissue section and can shorten scanning times but still meet the high standards of diagnostic pathology (*Hum Pathol* 2004;35:1303).

B. Image Stitching is the technology by which a larger image is produced via combining several smaller images that have overlapping areas. As a technology, image stitching is already in extremely widespread use in as much as it is the computational process employed by smartphones to produce panoramic photographs from a single lens moved slowly across a field of view. However, recognition of the utility of image stitching as a rapid, automated process that can be used with microscope images captured by a digital camera has been recognized only recently (*Micron* 2013;48:17).

In practice, image stitching for virtual microscopy is a simple process that offers several advantages over conventional WSI. Several commercial vendors market high quality digital cameras (that can be mounted on most major brands of light microscopes) with associated stitching software, at a price that is often 10- to 100-fold lower than a WSI platform. In addition, a small light microscope with an image stitching camera, together with a tablet or laptop computer connected to the internet, can function as a mobile slide scanning and telepathology instrument. Manual operation makes it possible for the pathologist to scan regions of interest during case sign-outs in 1 to 2 minutes, streamlining the workflow to obtain a virtual slide. The utility of panoramic digital images obtained via image stitching has been demonstrated for both cytopathology and surgical pathology (*J Am Soc Cytopathol* 2015;4:S66; *J Pathol Inform* 2016;7:26).

C. Implementation of Virtual Microscopy in the cytopathology or surgical pathology laboratory requires an electronic and organizational infrastructure as well as a slide scanning instrument. The infrastructure requires an efficient interaction between information technology (IT) and LIS personnel. Dedicated and trained technical personnel (e.g., image technologists) are required to load and maintain the scanning instrument, perform initial screening (and rescanning if necessary), monitor scan quality, and distribute the virtual files in a manner that can be conveniently viewed by the pathologist (*J Pathol Inform* 2011;2:36; *Arch Pathol Lab Med* 2017;141:944). A file server with the necessary storage capability (upgradeable tera- to petabyte range or beyond), databases for the virtual files (linked and updated to the LIS), and the necessary maintenance and updates must be managed by a knowledgeable IT person (*Human Pathol* 2003;34:968). For optimal use in routine patient care, high-quality LCD monitors of sufficient size (at least 53 cm diagonal) for peripheral vision are required (*Hum Pathol* 2006;37:1543), with extended desktop computer functionality to be able to simultaneously view the LIS, the gross description and gross images of the specimen, and the virtual slide viewer.

D. Diagnostic and Clinical Applications of virtual microscopy include diagnostic consultations, archiving, primary diagnosis, and quality assurance (QA).

1. The use of virtual microscopy for **diagnostic consultation** (so-called e-consultation) is one of the most useful applications of virtual slide microscopy. In addition to convenience (no packing or mailing of slides is required), there are several advantages to e-consultations. Electronic distribution is virtually instantaneous and allows consulting pathologists to review the scanned slides at any time and location. Online, real-time conferencing and simultaneous viewing by two or more pathologists is easily achieved. In addition, there are no risks of losing the primary data (i.e., tissue blocks or glass slides).

2. Scanning of selected cases for archiving. Virtual slide creation of selected slides sent in consultation makes it possible for the consulting institution to have a permanent record of the diagnostic slides (the medicolegal climate in the United States dictates return of all diagnostic materials to the referring institution). Such an archive enhances patient care by providing an immediately-available permanent record of the slides to guide frozen section diagnosis, or final diagnosis at the time of definitive excision. In addition, the virtual slides are available for subsequent clinicopathologic conferences (*Hum Pathol* 2010;41;751).

3. Primary diagnosis based on review of virtual slides has been shown in many studies to have the same accuracy as primary diagnosis based on routine light microscopy (*Arch Path Lab Med* 2011;135;372; *Arch Pathol Lab Med* 2017;141:944), although the use of virtual slides for primary diagnosis requires an extensive validation procedure. The use of virtual slides for primary diagnosis achieved a major milestone in 2017 when the USA Food and Drug Administration (FDA) cleared a digital pathology system to perform primary diagnosis. This regulatory clearance is expected to not only drive most commercial vendors of digital pathology systems to pursue clearance of their devices, but also markedly increase interest in the routine clinical use of digital pathology.

The utility of virtual slides has clear applications for improved pathology services to underserved areas, as has been known for some time (*Natl Med J India* 2002;15:363; *Ethiop Med J* 2005;43:51). Integration of digital pathology into routine clinical workflows to support routine clinical diagnosis has also been described, but requires significant changes to work flows (*J Digit Imaging* 2017;30:555). However, there is little evidence that digitizing all slides in routine practice results in a cost or time savings (*J Path Inform* 2011;2:39; *Anal Cell Pathol* 2012;35:57).

4. QA programs may be enhanced by review of virtual slides from cases with diagnostic discrepancies. Files can be flagged for subsequent review, and trends in diagnostic errors easily identified (*Dis Markers* 2007;23:459).

E. Education. Virtual microscopy is already an indispensable tool for medical education in pathology, including medical student teaching, teaching of pathology residents and fellows, and continuing medical education for practicing pathologists. Many national pathology conferences and slide seminars now post virtual slides on websites before the meeting itself, and some organizations have built collections of teaching cases (e.g., The United States and Canadian Academy of Pathology [USCAP] at http://uscapknowledgehub.org/index.htm?vsbindex.htm, and the Digital Pathology Association at https://digitalpathologyassociation.org/whole-slide-imaging-repository). Other examples of educational activities based on virtual slides include teaching of histology to medical students (*Anat Rec* 2006;289B:128), a tutorial on Gleason grading of prostatic adenocarcinoma (*Hum Pathol* 2005;36:381), and didactic presentations using a combination of text and virtual microscopy (*Ann Diagn Pathol* 2003;7:67).

Education and experience with interpretation of virtual slides is critical for pathology residents and fellows; at the very least, it prepares trainees for the American Board of Pathology examination (www.abpath.org/VMInstr.htm).

F. Research Applications for virtual microscopy in surgical pathology include consensus review of slides, quantitative image analysis, and imaging of tissue microarrays used to study patterns of gene and protein expression. Virtual images can also provide documentation of specimens or tissue microarrays retained in tissue banks (*Eur J Cancer* 2006;42:3110), or for patients enrolled in clinical trials. As for diagnostic pathology, virtual slides make it possible to easily share specimens among investigators at different sites, anytime. Virtual slides also allow for the electronic publication of whole slides rather than selected fields of slides, which facilitates the transfer of new information to practicing pathologists.

G. Image Analysis can be performed on any of the virtual slide file formats produced by the current generation of slide scanners, and widely accepted freeware and a variety of sub-programs are available to support clinical applications. One versatile solution for image processing and analysis is the NIH freeware named ImageJ (*Biophot Int* 2004;11:36, available at http://rsb.info.nih.gov/ij/). The versatility of this program derives from its open architecture that allows users to implement small and typically customized sub-programs (called "plug-ins"). Over the years, many plug-ins (mostly research-derived) have been developed; for example, "Image J for microscopy" (https://imagej.net/mbf/) includes numerous tools such as intensity and time analysis, particle analysis, colocalization analysis, intensity processing, color processing, stack-slice manipulation, z-functions, t-functions, deconvolution, and annotation.

There has been recent success in the development of more advanced algorithms for so-called artificial intelligence (AI), also generally known as machine learning or cognitive computing. The use of convolutional neural nets (CNNs), coupled with increases in available computing power and dataset sizes, has led to increased interest in the use of computerized image analysis for computer-assisted diagnosis (CAD).

Recent studies of breast malignancies have emphasized the potential of AI methodologies to not only recognize but also classify tumors (*PLoS One* 2017;12:e0177544; *Sci Rep* 2017;7:4172). Other reports have demonstrated the utility of deep learning approaches for evaluation of tissue components at the time of frozen section to increase diagnostic accuracy (*IEEE Trans Med Imaging* 2018; doi: 10.1109/TMI.2018.2851150). While these reports have generated a great deal of interest in the popular press with suggestions that AI will soon replace the role of pathologists in histopathologic diagnosis, this outcome is unlikely in the foreseeable future in as much as, thus far, the published studies have used model systems composed of highly preselected slides, from a very limited set of diagnoses, classified into diagnostic categories of little (if any) clinical utility. In addition, questions regarding the appropriate gold standard for validation of AI approaches remain unresolved (*Arch Pathol Lab Med* 2017;141:1267).

III. TELEPATHOLOGY is the practice whereby pathologists render diagnoses from a distance by viewing electronically transmitted images rather than by examination of the glass slides themselves by light microscopy. Electronic images can be transmitted by ordinary telephone lines, high-speed digital lines, or satellites, but increasingly the images are transmitted via the Internet. With some overlap, three systems are currently available: dynamic, static, and virtual.

A. Dynamic Telepathology Systems. In these systems, pathologists view images in real time by electronic control of a distant robotic microscope that has motorized optics and a motorized stage. Dynamic-robotic telepathology has been primarily used to provide intraoperative frozen section diagnoses to hospitals without on-site pathologists (*Hum Pathol* 2007;38:1330). Typically, in less than a minute a digital overview of the slide is created; virtual controls enable the pathologist to remotely control the movement of the slide on the microscope. Reported diagnostic accuracy is comparable to that of conventional light microscopy.

A variation of the dynamic method is the submission of a live ("streaming") image from the remotely located microscope either with or without robotic control; in the latter paradigm, manipulation of the slide and magnification are simply controlled via instructions to the person using the microscope.

One important disadvantage of either dynamic telepathology method is the extra time needed to review the virtual slides compared with standard slides. In one study (*J Neuropathol Exp Neurol* 2007;66:750) the lack of an on-site presence affected every stage of intraoperative consultation including the gathering of patient information, gross specimen examination and handling, frozen section and smear preparation, communication between various parties involved, and documentation of the consultation process. Thus, implementation of telepathology requires substantial planning, communication, and training of both pathologists and support personnel.

B. Static Telepathology Systems use static images (e.g., .jpeg or .tiff files) that have been selected, stored, and forwarded to the pathologist. Static systems are mainly used to obtain second opinions on difficult cases. Overall, the diagnostic accuracy approaches conventional glass slide optical microscopy. Problems leading to discordance include field selection and poor image quality (*Hum Pathol* 2003;34:1228). For large or complex specimens, the handicaps of preselected images are more pronounced.

C. **Virtual Slide Telepathology.** The use of virtual microscopy in telepathology has been shown to have clinical utility, even in time-sensitive settings such as intraoperative frozen section diagnosis (*J Pathol Inform* 2011;2:36). However, for WSI platforms, the scanning time to produce a whole slide image, the required infrastructure, and the large file sizes may limit the usefulness of virtual slide telepathology in many practice settings. As noted above, the image stitching approach addresses some of these issues.

IV. **OBSTACLES.** Significant issues must be addressed to allow the routine implementation of virtual microscopy and telepathology in diagnostic surgical pathology. First, there are unresolved licensure and reimbursement issues concerning diagnostic surgical pathology practice from a distance. Second, integration with LISs, and validation and incorporation of digital pathology images into the electronic medical record remain haphazard and are not standardized (*J. Biomed Opt* 2007;12:051801). Third, although regulatory issues surrounding scanning platforms have begun to be addressed, the regulatory environment governing the algorithms for image analysis of the various AI paradigms remain undefined. Despite these uncertainties, there is little question that recent advances in imaging technologies provide unique opportunities to improve the accuracy of diagnosis and slide-based biomarker evaluation.

ACKNOWLEDGMENT

The authors thank Jochen K. M. Lennerz and Erika Crouch, authors of the previous edition of this chapter.

Index

Note: Page numbers followed by f and t indicate figures and tables, respectively.